THE PILL BOOK, 13th REVISED EDITION:
THE ILLUSTRATED GUIDE TO THE MOST PRESCRIBED DRUGS IN THE UNITED STATES
Illustrated with 32 pages of actual-size color photographs

With more than 17 million copies in print, THE PILL BOOK is the bestselling consumer drug reference ever, offering the most up-to-date, comprehensive information in a newly redesigned format that is even easier to use.

This new 13th edition of *The Pill Book* contains more profiles of commonly prescribed drugs than any other consumer reference. Compiled by a team of eminent pharmacologists, it is based on official, FDA-approved information usually available only to doctors and pharmacists, plus the latest information gathered from computer databases and online resources. It synthesizes the most important facts about each drug in a concise, readable, easy-to-understand entry.

Here are complete profiles on more than 1800 of the most commonly prescribed drugs, including:

- Generic and brand names
- What the drug is for and how it works
- Usual dosages, and what to do if a dose is skipped
- Side effects and possible adverse reactions, highlighted for quick reference
- Interactions with other drugs and foods
- Alcohol-free and sugar-free medications
- The most popular self-injected medications and their safe handling
- Information for seniors, pregnant and breast-feeding women, and others with special needs

This completely revised and updated 13th edition contains dozens of new brand names and more than 20 important new drugs recently approved by the FDA now on sale for the first time.

THE
PILL BOOK
13th EDITION

Editor-in-Chief
HAROLD M. SILVERMAN, Pharm. D.

Production
ButterWorks Limited
High Text Graphics, Inc.
mouse+tiger
The Stonesong Press, LLC

Consultants
**DRUG INFORMATION SERVICE
ROBERT WOOD JOHNSON UNIVERSITY HOSPITAL
AND RUTGERS COLLEGE OF PHARMACY**

**JUDITH I. BROWN
JENNIFER KITCHIN, MD**

Digital Photography and Color Separations
**CORAL GRAPHICS
STUDIO 365**

Photography
BENN MITCHELL

**Original Creators of THE PILL BOOK
LAWRENCE D. CHILNICK
HAROLD M. SILVERMAN, Pharm. D.
GILBERT I. SIMON, Sc.D.
BERT STERN**

BANTAM BOOKS
NEW YORK · TORONTO · LONDON · SYDNEY · AUCKLAND

In Canada *Aspirin* is a registered trademark owned by Sterling Winthrop Inc.

THE PILL BOOK

A Bantam Book

PUBLISHING HISTORY

Bantam edition published June 1979
Bantam revised edition / October 1982
Bantam 3rd revised edition / March 1986
Bantam 4th revised edition / February 1990
Bantam 5th revised edition / May 1992
Bantam 6th revised edition / June 1994
Bantam 7th revised edition / June 1996
Bantam 8th revised edition / May 1998
Bantam 9th revised edition / May 2000
Bantam 10th revised edition / May 2002
Bantam 11th revised edition / May 2004
Bantam 12th revised edition / May 2006
Bantam 13th revised edition / May 2008
This revised edition was published simultaneously in
trade paperback and mass market paperback.

Published by
Bantam Dell
A Division of Random House, Inc.
New York, New York

ISBN: 978-0-553-58893-4

Manufactured in the United States of America
Published simultaneously in Canada

OPM   10 9 8 7 6

Contents

How to Use This Book   **vii**

In an Emergency!   **xi**

The Most Commonly Prescribed Drugs in the United States, Generic and Brand Names, with Complete Descriptions of Drugs and Their Effects   **1**

Twenty Questions to Ask Your Doctor and Pharmacist About Your Prescription   **1239**

Safe Drug Use   **1241**

Safety Tips for Self-Injectibles   **1242**

Medicine and Money   **1245**

The Top 200 Prescription Drugs in the United States   **1246**

Index
   Generic and Brand-Name Drugs   **1249**

Color Plates
   Pill Identification Charts

The purpose of this book is to provide educational information to the public concerning the majority of various types of prescription drugs that are presently used by physicians. It is not intended to be complete or exhaustive or in any respect a substitute for personal medical care. *Only a physician may prescribe these drugs and their exact dosages.*

While every effort has been made to reproduce products on the cover and insert of this book in an exact fashion, certain variations of size or color may be expected as a result of the printing process. Furthermore, pictures identified as brand-name drugs should not be confused with their generic counterparts. In any event, the reader should not rely solely upon the photographic image to identify any pills depicted herein, but should rely upon the physician's prescription as dispensed by the pharmacist.

How to Use This Book

How to Find Your Medication in *The Pill Book*

- *The Pill Book* lists most medications in alphabetic order by generic name because a medication may have many brand names but has only 1 generic name. Most generic medications produce the same therapeutic effects as their brand-name equivalents but are much less expensive. Drugs that are available generically are indicated by the **G** symbol.

- When a medication has 2 or more active ingredients, it is listed by the most widely known brand name. In some cases, pill profiles are listed by drug type (e.g., Sulfonylurea Antidiabetes Drugs).

- *The Pill Book* includes the names of the top 100 brand-name drugs (cross-referenced to their generic name) in alphabetic order with the pill profiles.

- Most over-the-counter (OTC) medications are not included in *The Pill Book*. For complete information on OTC medications, refer to *The Pill Book Guide to Over-the-Counter Medications*.

- All brand and generic names are listed in the Index. Brand names are indicated by boldface.

- Sugar-free and alcohol-free brand-name drugs are indicated by the **S** and **A** symbols in the beginning of each pill profile.

The Pill Book, like pills themselves, should be used with caution. Viewed properly, this book may save you money and, perhaps, your life. It contains life-size pictures of the most prescribed brand-name drugs in the U.S. *The Pill Book*'s product identification system is designed to help you check that the medication you are about to take is the one your doctor prescribed. Although many dosage forms are included, not all available forms and strengths of every medication have been shown. While every effort has been made to create accurate photographic reproductions of the products, some variations in size or color may be expected as a result of the printing process. Do not rely solely on the photographic images to identify your pills; check with your pharmacist if you have any product identification questions.

Each pill profile in *The Pill Book* contains the following information:

Generic and Brand Name: The generic name is the common name of the drug approved by the Food and Drug Administration (FDA). It is listed along with the current brand names available for each generic drug. Medications that are available in a generic form are indicated by the G symbol.

Most prescription drugs are sold in more than one dosage strength. Also, some drugs, such as oral contraceptives, come in packages containing different numbers of pills. A few manufacturers indicate these variations by adding letters or numbers to the basic drug name; for example, Loestrin 21 1.5/30 and Loestrin 21 1/20. (The numbers here refer to the number of tablets in each monthly packet, 21, and the amount of medication found in the tablets.) Other drugs come in different strengths: This is often indicated by a notation such as "DS" (double strength) or "Forte" (stronger).

The Pill Book lists generic and brand names together only where there are no differences in basic ingredients (e.g., Loestrin). However, the amount of the ingredient may vary from product to product. In most cases, the brand names and generic versions listed for each medication are interchangeable; you can use any version of the drug and expect that it will work for you. *The Pill Book* identifies within the profile those medications for which generic versions are not considered equivalent and which should not be interchanged with a brand-name product or another generic version of the same drug.

Type of Drug: Describes the general pharmacologic class of each drug: "antidepressant," "sedative," "decongestant," "expectorant," and so on.

Prescribed For: All drugs are approved for some symptoms or conditions by federal authorities, but doctors also commonly prescribe drugs for other, as yet unapproved, reasons; in some cases, these are also listed in *The Pill Book*. Check with your doctor if you are not sure why you have been given a certain pill.

General Information: Information on how the drug works, how long it takes for you to feel its effects, or a description of how this drug is similar to or different from other drugs.

Cautions and Warnings: This information alerts you to important and more dangerous reactions. Physical conditions, such as heart disease, that can have serious consequences if the medication is prescribed for you, are in bold type.

Possible Side Effects: Side effects are generally divided into 4 categories—those that are most common, common, less common, and rare—to help you better understand what to expect from your pills. If you are not sure whether you are experiencing a drug side effect, ask your doctor.

Drug Interactions: Describes what happens when you combine your medication with other drugs and lists which drugs should not be taken at the same time as your medication. Some interactions may be deadly. At every visit, be sure to inform your doctor of any medication you are already taking.

Food Interactions: Provides information on foods to avoid while taking your medication, whether to take your medication with meals or on an empty stomach, and other important facts.

Usual Dose: Tells you the largest and smallest doses usually prescribed and gives dosage instructions for children and seniors, when applicable. You may be given different dosage instructions by your doctor. Do not change the dosage of ANY medication you take without first calling your doctor.

Overdosage: Describes overdose symptoms and what to do if you take too much medication.

Special Information: Includes symptoms to watch for, when to call your doctor, what to do if you forget a dose of your medication, and any special instructions.

Special Populations: *Pregnancy/Breast-feeding:* For women who are or might be pregnant, and what to do if you must take a medication during the time you are nursing your baby. *Seniors:* This section presents the special facts an older adult needs to know about every drug and explains how reactions may differ from those of a younger person.

In an Emergency!

Each year over 1 million people experience drug-related poisoning in the U.S., and about 10% of those cases result in death. In fact, drug overdose is a leading cause of fatal poisoning in the U.S.

Although each of the pill profiles in *The Pill Book* has specific information on drug overdose, there are a few general rules to remember if you are faced with an accidental poisoning:

1. Make sure the victim is breathing, and call for medical help immediately.
2. Learn the phone number of your local poison control center and post it near the phone. Call the center in an emergency. When you call, be prepared to explain

   - What drug was taken and how much
   - Status of the victim (e.g., conscious, sleeping, vomiting, or having convulsions)
   - The approximate age and weight of the victim
   - Any chronic medical problems of the victim (e.g., diabetes, epilepsy, or high blood pressure), if you know them
   - What medications, if any, the victim takes regularly

3. Remove anything that might interfere with breathing. A person who is not getting enough oxygen will turn blue (the tongue or the skin under the fingernails changes color first). If this happens, lay the victim on his or her back, open the collar, place one hand under the neck, and lift, pull, or push the victim's jaw so that it juts outward. This will open the airway between the mouth and lungs as wide as possible. Begin mouth-to-mouth resuscitation ONLY if the victim is not breathing.
4. If the victim is unconscious or having convulsions, call for medical help immediately. While waiting for the ambulance, lay the victim on his or her stomach and turn the head to one side. Should the victim throw up, this will prevent inhalation of vomit. DO NOT give an unconscious victim anything by mouth. Keep the victim warm.

5. If the victim is conscious, call for medical help and give the victim an 8-oz. glass of water to drink. This will dilute the poison.

Only a small number of poisoning victims require hospitalization. Most may be treated with simple actions or need no treatment at all.

The poison control center may tell you to make the person vomit. The best way to do this is to use ipecac syrup, which is available over-the-counter at any pharmacy. Specific instructions on how much to give infants, children, or adults are printed on the label and will also be given by your poison control center. Remember, DO NOT make the victim vomit unless you have been instructed to do so. Never make the victim vomit if the victim is unconscious, is having a convulsion, or is experiencing a painful, burning feeling in the mouth or throat.

Be Prepared

The best way to deal with a poisoning is to be prepared for it. Do the following now:

1. Write the telephone number of your local poison control center next to your other emergency phone numbers.
2. Decide which hospital you will go to, if necessary, and how you will get there.
3. Buy 1 oz. of ipecac syrup from your pharmacy. The pharmacist will tell you how to use it. Remember, this is a potent drug to be used only if directed and stored out of reach of children.
4. Learn to give mouth-to-mouth resuscitation.

Reduce the Risk of Drug-Related Poisoning

1. Keep all medications in a locked place out of the reach of young children.
2. Do not store medications in containers that previously held food.
3. Do not remove the labels from bottles so that the contents are unknown.
4. To avoid taking the wrong medication, do not take your medicine in the dark or in a dimly lit room.
5. Discard all medications when you no longer need them by flushing them down the toilet.

The Most Commonly Prescribed Drugs in the United States, Generic and Brand Names, with Complete Descriptions of Drugs and Their Effects

Abilify   *see Aripiprazole, page 107*

see Aripiprazole, page 107

Generic Name

Acamprosate (ah-CAM-pro-sate)

Brand Name
Campral

Type of Drug
Synthetic neurochemical similar to the amino acid homotaurine.

Prescribed For
Alcoholism.

General Information
Acamprosate is used to help alcoholic patients stay alcohol-free after they have stopped drinking. Unlike other drugs used to help people stay away from alcohol, it does not cause people to have a physical reaction to alcohol. Acamprosate restores the balance between two chemical systems in the brain, glutamate and GABA, that are known to become unbalanced in alcoholics, but its exact action is not known. It may reduce alcohol craving. Acamprosate should be part of a program that includes counseling and support, and it should be started as soon as possible after alcohol withdrawal and continued even if the patient starts drinking again. This medication has not been proven to help patients if they are still drinking when they start treatment. Acamprosate has not been studied in patients who abuse other substances together with alcohol. Tolerance or addiction has not developed with acamprosate. It passes out of the body through the kidneys.

Cautions and Warnings
Do not take acamprosate if you are **allergic** or **sensitive** to any of its ingredients or if you have **severe kidney disease.** People with moderate kidney disease require a lower dosage of acamprosate.

Acamprosate does not eliminate or ease alcohol withdrawal symptoms.

People taking acamprosate may become depressed or have suicidal thoughts.

Acamprosate can affect your judgment, thinking, or coordination. Do not drive or operate dangerous machinery if you are taking this medicine.

Possible Side Effects

Almost 2 of every 3 people who take this medicine will experience a drug side effect.
▼ Most common: diarrhea.
▼ Common: headache, weakness, anxiety, depression, and sleep problems.
▼ Less common: pain, accidental injuries, nausea, stomach gas, dizziness, dry mouth, tingling in the hands or feet, itching, sweating, chest pain, loss of appetite, weight gain or loss, impotence, abnormal vision, rash, vomiting, and constipation.
▼ Rare: heart or kidney failure, psoriasis, hypothyroidism, rheumatoid arthritis, and urinary tract infections. Rare side effects can occur in almost any part of the body. Contact your doctor if you experience any side effect not listed above.

Drug Interactions
● Mixing acamprosate with naltrexone can increase the levels of both drugs in the blood, but no dose adjustments are needed.

Food Interactions
Acamprosate may be taken without regard to food or meals.

Usual Dose
Adult: two 333-mg tablets 3 times a day.
Child: not recommended.

Overdosage
The only symptom associated with acamprosate overdose has been diarrhea. Overdose victims should be taken to a hospital emergency room for observation and treatment. ALWAYS bring the prescription bottle or container.

Special Information
Call your doctor if you are breast-feeding, pregnant, or thinking about becoming pregnant while taking this medicine.

Take care while driving a car or performing complex tasks.

If you forget to take a dose, take it as soon as possible. If you do not remember until it is almost time for your next dose, skip the dose you forgot and continue with your regular schedule. Call your doctor if you forget to take 2 or more doses in a row. Do not take a double dose.

Acamprosate must be part of an ongoing treatment program. Do not stop taking it on your own, even if you start drinking again.

Special Populations

Pregnancy/Breast-feeding: Acamprosate can damage animal fetuses in doses that are approximately equal to those taken by people on this medicine. Women of childbearing age should use an effective contraceptive while taking this drug. The potential benefits of acamprosate must be weighed against its risks if your doctor considers it a crucial treatment during your pregnancy.

Acamprosate passes into breast milk. Nursing mothers who must take this drug should use infant formula.

Seniors: Dosage reduction may be needed in seniors because of a general decline in kidney function due to age.

Generic Name

Acebutolol (ah-seh-BUTE-uh-lol) G

Brand Name
Sectral

Type of Drug
Beta-adrenergic blocking agent.

Prescribed For
High blood pressure and abnormal heart rhythms.

General Information
Acebutolol hydrochloride is one of many beta-adrenergic blocking drugs, or beta blockers. These drugs interfere with the action of adrenaline and other chemicals in the body that affect many body functions. Individual beta blockers have different characteristics that can make them more suitable for certain conditions or people.

Cautions and Warnings

Do not take acebutolol if you are **allergic** or **sensitive** to any of its ingredients or to beta blockers.

You should be cautious about taking acebutolol if you have **asthma, severe heart failure,** a **very slow heart rate,** or **heart block** (disruption of the electrical impulses that control heart rate) because the drug may worsen these conditions.

People with **angina** taking acebutolol for high blood pressure risk aggravating their angina if they suddenly stop taking the drug. These patients should have their acebutolol dosage reduced gradually over 1–2 weeks.

Acebutolol should be used with caution if you have **liver or kidney disease** because your ability to eliminate this drug from your body may be impaired.

Acebutolol reduces the amount of blood pumped by the heart with each beat. This reduction in blood flow may aggravate the condition of people with **poor circulation** or **circulatory disease.**

If you are undergoing **major surgery,** your doctor may want you to stop taking acebutolol at least 2 days before surgery.

People with a history of **severe anaphylactic reaction** to allergens may be unresponsive to usual doses of epinephrine while taking beta blockers.

Possible Side Effects

Side effects are relatively uncommon and usually mild; normally they develop early in the course of treatment and are rarely a reason to stop taking acebutolol.

▼ Most common: fatigue.

▼ Common: dizziness and headache.

▼ Less common: chest pain, swelling in the legs or arms, depression, sleeplessness, abnormal dreams, rashes, constipation, diarrhea, upset stomach, stomach gas, nausea, frequent urination, back pain, joint and muscle pain, difficulty breathing, stuffy nose, and vision changes.

▼ Rare: cough, low blood pressure, slow heart beat, anxiety, impotence, changes in response to touch stimulation, itching, vomiting, abdominal pain, painful urination, nighttime urination, liver changes, sore throat, wheezing, eye irritation, pain or dry eye, and lupus erythematosus (extremely rare). Contact your doctor if you experience any side effect not listed above.

Drug Interactions

- Acebutolol may interact with surgical anesthetics to increase the risk of heart problems during surgery. Some anesthesiologists recommend gradually stopping the drug by 2 days before surgery.
- Acebutolol may interfere with the normal signs of low blood sugar and with the action of oral antidiabetes drugs.
- Acebutolol increases the blood-pressure-lowering effects of other blood-pressure-reducing agents, including clonidine, guanabenz, and reserpine, and calcium channel blockers such as nifedipine.
- Aspirin-containing drugs, nonsteroidal anti-inflammatory drugs (NSAIDS), and sulfinpyrazone may interfere with the blood-pressure-lowering effect of acebutolol.
- Cocaine may reduce the effectiveness of all beta blockers.
- Acebutolol may worsen the problem of cold hands and feet associated with ergot alkaloids, used to treat migraine. Gangrene is a possibility in people taking both an ergot and acebutolol.
- Acebutolol will counteract thyroid hormone replacements.
- Calcium channel blockers, flecainide, hydralazine, contraceptive drugs, cimetidine, propafenone, haloperidol, phenothiazine sedatives (molindone and others), quinolone antibacterials, and quinidine may increase the amount of acebutolol in the bloodstream and lead to increased acebutolol effects.
- Acebutolol should not be taken within 2 weeks of taking a monoamine oxidase inhibitor (MAOI) antidepressant.
- Acebutolol may interfere with the effects of some antiasthma drugs, including theophylline and aminophylline.
- Combining acebutolol with digitalis drugs may result in excessive slowing of the heart, possibly causing heart block.
- If you stop smoking while taking acebutolol, your dose may have to be reduced because your liver will break down the drug more slowly afterward.
- Aluminum salts, barbiturates, calcium salts, cholestyramine, colestipol, ampicillin, and rifampin may reduce the effectiveness of acebutolol.
- Beta blockers may block the effects of epinephrine.

Food Interactions

None known.

Usual Dose

High Blood Pressure

Adult: starting dose—100 mg a day, taken all at once or in 2 divided doses. The daily dose may be gradually increased. Maintenance dose—400–800 mg a day.

Senior: Older adults may respond to lower doses and should be treated more cautiously, beginning with 100 mg a day, increasing gradually to a maximum of 400 mg a day.

Child: not recommended.

Abnormal Heart Rhythms

Adult: starting dose—200 mg a day. Maintenance dose—200–600 mg a day in 2 divided doses.

Senior: Older adults may respond to lower doses and should be treated more cautiously, beginning with 100 mg a day, increasing gradually to a maximum of 400 mg a day.

Child: not recommended.

Overdosage

Symptoms of overdose include extremely slow or irregular heartbeat, very low blood pressure, breathing difficulties, and seizures. The victim should be taken to a hospital emergency room. ALWAYS bring the prescription bottle or container.

Special Information

Acebutolol is meant to be taken continuously. When ending acebutolol treatment, dosage should be reduced gradually over a period of about 2 weeks. Do not stop taking this drug unless directed to do so by your doctor.

Do not take other medications, including over-the-counter medications, without consulting with your doctor. The use of some nasal decongestants with acebutolol may result in severely high blood pressure.

Acebutolol may cause drowsiness or dizziness. Be careful when driving or performing complex tasks.

It is best to take acebutolol at the same time each day. If you forget a dose, take it as soon as you remember. If you take acebutolol once a day and it is within 8 hours of your next dose, skip the dose you forgot and continue with your regular schedule. If you take acebutolol twice a day and it is within 4 hours of your next dose, skip the missed dose and continue with your regular schedule. Never take a double dose.

Special Populations

Pregnancy/Breast-feeding: Acebutolol crosses into the placenta. Infants born to women who took a beta blocker while pregnant had lower birth weights, low blood pressure, and slow heart rates. Acebutolol should be taken during pregnancy only if the potential benefit outweighs the risk.

Large amounts of acebutolol pass into breast milk. Nursing mothers taking acebutolol should use infant formula.

Seniors: Seniors taking acebutolol may need a reduced dosage.

Generic Name

Acetaminophen (uh-SEE-tuh-MIN-uh-fen) Ⓖ

Brand Names

Acephen	Mapap*
Aceta	Mapap Children's
Acetaminophen Uniserts	Mapap Extra Strength
Apacet	Mapap Infant Drops
Aspirin Free Anacin Maximum Strength	Maranox
	Neopap
Aspirin Free Pain Relief	Oraphen-PD
Dynafed, Children's JR	Panadol*
Dynafed EX	Redutemp
Dynafed Extra Strength	Silapap
Feverall	Silapap Children's
Feverall, Infants	Silapap Infants
Genapap*	Tapanol
Genebs	Tempra*
Liquiprin	Tylenol*

*Some products in this brand-name group are alcohol- or sugar-free. Consult your pharmacist.

Type of Drug

Antipyretic and analgesic.

Prescribed For

Relief of pain and fever for people who cannot or do not want to take aspirin or a nonsteroidal anti-inflammatory drug (NSAID). Acetaminophen may be given to children about to receive a

DTP vaccination to reduce the fever and pain that commonly follow the vaccination.

General Information

Acetaminophen is generally used to relieve pain and fever associated with the common cold, flu, viral infections, or other disorders where pain or fever may occur. It is also used to relieve pain in people who are allergic to aspirin, or those who cannot take aspirin because of potential interactions with other drugs such as oral anticoagulants. It can be used to relieve pain from a variety of sources, including arthritis, headache, muscle ache, menstrual cramping, and tooth and periodontic pain, although it does not reduce inflammation.

Cautions and Warnings

Do not take acetaminophen if you are **allergic** or **sensitive** to any of its ingredients. Do not take acetaminophen for more than 10 days in a row (5 days for children) unless directed by your doctor. Do not take more than is prescribed or recommended on the package.

Use this drug with extreme caution if you have **kidney or liver disease** or **viral infections of the liver**. Large amounts of alcohol increase the liver toxicity of large doses or overdoses of acetaminophen. **Avoid alcohol** if you regularly take acetaminophen. Some people are more sensitive to this effect than others.

Possible Side Effects

This drug is relatively free from side effects when taken in recommended doses. For this reason it has become extremely popular, especially among those who cannot take aspirin.

▼ Rare: large doses or long-term use may cause liver damage, rash, itching, fever, lowered blood sugar, stimulation, yellowing of the skin or whites of the eyes, and/or a change in the composition of your blood. Contact your doctor if you experience any side effect not listed above.

Drug Interactions

- Large doses of barbiturate drugs, carbamazepine, phenytoin and similar drugs, izoniazid, rifampin, and sulfinpyrazone may increase the chances of liver toxicity if taken with acetaminophen.

- Alcoholic beverages increase the chances for liver toxicity and possible liver failure associated with acetaminophen.

Food Interactions

None known.

Usual Dose

Adult and Child (age 12 and over): 325–650 mg 4–6 times a day, or 1000 mg 3–4 times a day. Avoid taking more than 4 g (twelve 325-mg tablets) a day for long periods of time.

Child (age 11): 480 mg 4–5 times a day.

Child (age 9–10): 400 mg 4–5 times a day.

Child (age 6–8): 320 mg 4–5 times a day.

Child (age 4–5): 240 mg 4–5 times a day.

Child (age 3): 160 mg 4–5 times a day.

Child (age 1–2): 120 mg 4–5 times a day.

Child (age 4–11 months): 80 mg 4–5 times a day.

Child (under age 4 months): 40 mg 4–5 times a day.

Overdosage

Acetaminophen is a commonly used ingredient in many over-the-counter (OTC) medications. Always check the list of ingredients when using more than one OTC medication to ensure that the combined dosage is within guidelines and to avoid accidental overdose.

Acute acetaminophen overdose may cause nausea, vomiting, sweating, appetite loss, drowsiness, confusion, abdominal tenderness, low blood pressure, abnormal heart rhythms, yellowing of the skin and whites of the eyes, and liver and kidney failure. Liver damage has occurred with 12 extra-strength tablets or 18 regular-strength tablets, but most people need larger doses—20 extra-strength or 30 regular-strength tablets—to damage their livers. Regular use of large doses for long periods—3000–4000 mg a day for a year—can also cause liver damage, especially if alcohol is involved. In case of overdose, induce vomiting as soon as possible with ipecac syrup—available at any pharmacy—and take the victim to a hospital emergency room. ALWAYS bring the acetaminophen bottle or container.

Special Information

Unless abused, acetaminophen is a beneficial, effective, and relatively nontoxic drug. Follow package directions and call your doctor if acetaminophen does not relieve pain in 10 days for adults or

5 days for children. Call your doctor if fever gets worse or persists longer than 3 days.

Alcoholic beverages will worsen the liver damage that acetaminophen can cause. People who take this drug on a regular basis should limit their alcohol intake.

If you forget to take a dose, take it as soon as you remember. If it is within an hour of your next dose, skip the dose you forgot and continue with your regular schedule. Do not take a double dose.

Special Populations

Pregnancy/Breast-feeding: Acetaminophen is considered safe during pregnancy when taken in usual doses. Taking continuous high doses of the drug may cause birth defects or interfere with fetal development. Three cases of congenital hip dislocation appear to have been associated with acetaminophen. Check with your doctor before taking this drug if you are or might be pregnant.

Small amounts of acetaminophen may pass into breast milk, but the drug is considered harmless to nursing infants.

Seniors: Seniors may take acetaminophen as directed by a doctor.

Generic Name

Acetazolamide (uh-sete-uh-ZOLE-uh-mide) Ⓖ

Type of Drug

Carbonic-anhydrase inhibitor.

Prescribed For

Glaucoma and prevention or treatment of mountain sickness; also prescribed for epilepsy and treatment of drug-induced swelling or swelling due to congestive heart failure.

General Information

By blocking an enzyme in the body called carbonic anhydrase, acetazolamide produces a weak diuretic effect that helps to treat glaucoma by reducing pressure inside the eye. Acetazolamide's antiseizure properties are also produced by its effect on carbonic anhydrase, though exactly how acetazolamide prevents seizure is not well understood.

Cautions and Warnings

Do not take acetazolamide if you are **allergic** or **sensitive** to any of its ingredients or to sulfa drugs.

Do not take acetazolamide if you have **low blood sodium or potassium, diabetes,** or serious **kidney, liver, or Addison's disease**.

Possible Side Effects

Side effects of short-term therapy are usually minimal.
▼ Most common: nausea or vomiting; tingling feeling in the arms, legs, lips, mouth, or anus; appetite and weight loss; a metallic taste; increased frequency in urination; diarrhea; not feeling well; occasional drowsiness; and weakness. You may also experience rash, drug crystals in the urine, painful urination, low back pain, urinary difficulty, and low urine volume.
▼ Rare: Rare side effects can affect the liver, mental state, blood sugar, muscles, and senses. Contact your doctor if you experience any side effect not listed above.

Drug Interactions

- Avoid over-the-counter drug products that contain stimulants or anticholinergics, which tend to aggravate glaucoma and cardiac disease.
- Acetazolamide may increase blood concentrations of cyclosporine (used to prevent the rejection of transplanted organs).
- Acetazolamide may block or delay the absorption of primidone (prescribed for seizure).
- Avoid aspirin because it may enhance acetazolamide side effects.
- Combining diflunisal and acetazolamide can result in an excessive lowering of eye pressure.

Food Interactions

Acetazolamide may be taken with food if it upsets your stomach. Because acetazolamide can increase potassium loss, take this drug with potassium-rich foods such as bananas, citrus fruits, melons, and tomatoes.

Usual Dose

Glaucoma
    Adult: 250–1000 mg a day.
    Child: 4.5–6.75 mg per lb. a day in divided doses.

Diuresis in congestive heart failure or drug-induced swelling
    Adult: 250–375 mg a day.
    Child: 2.25 mg per lb., once daily in the morning.

Epilepsy: 375–1000 mg a day in divided doses.

Mountain Sickness: 500–1000 mg a day. If possible begin medication 24–48 hours before ascent.

Overdosage

Symptoms of overdose include drowsiness, loss of appetite, nausea, vomiting, dizziness, tingling in the hands or feet, weakness, tremors, or ringing or buzzing in the ears. In case of overdose, induce vomiting as soon as possible with ipecac syrup—available at any pharmacy—and take the victim to a hospital emergency room. ALWAYS bring the prescription bottle or container.

Special Information

Acetazolamide may cause minor drowsiness and confusion, particularly during the first 2 weeks of therapy. Be careful when driving or doing any task that requires concentration.

Call your doctor if you develop sore throat, fever, unusual bleeding or bruises, tingling in the hands or feet, rash, or unusual pains.

Acetazolamide can increase sensitivity to the sun. Avoid prolonged sun exposure and protect your eyes while taking this drug.

Be sure to drink plenty of water or fluids while taking acetazolamide.

If you forget a dose, take it as soon as you remember. If it is almost time for your next dose, skip the dose you forgot and continue with your regular schedule. Do not take a double dose.

Special Populations

Pregnancy/Breast-feeding: High doses of this drug may cause birth defects or interfere with fetal development. When this drug is considered crucial by your doctor, its potential benefits must be carefully weighed against its risks.

Small amounts of acetazolamide may pass into breast milk. Nursing mothers who must take this drug should use infant formula.

Seniors: Seniors are more sensitive to this drug's side effects.

Aciphex   see **Proton-Pump Inhibitors**, page 939

Generic Name

Acitretin   (ah-sih-TREH-tin)

Brand Name
Soriatane

Type of Drug
Antipsoriatic.

Prescribed For
Severe psoriasis; also prescribed for a variety of other skin conditions.

General Information
Acitretin is related to vitamin A and prescription drugs such as etretinate and isotretinoin. Acitretin is produced when etretinate is broken down in the body and its effects are very similar to etretinate. The way that acitretin works is not known. Its full benefit is not likely to be seen until you have taken it for 2 or 3 months. Your doctor is urged to use this medication only in cases of severe psoriasis that have not responded to other treatments because of the risks associated with acitretin.

Cautions and Warnings
Do not take acitretin if you are **allergic** or **sensitive** to any of its ingredients. **Women** who take acitretin must not be **pregnant** during treatment or for 3 years after the completion of treatment. It is not known if acitretin taken by men before conception is also a risk to the fetus.

A small number of people taking this drug have developed liver damage including jaundice (symptoms include yellowing of the skin and whites of the eyes). Acitretin has also been associated with hepatitis. People with kidney failure have much less acitretin in their blood than people with normal kidneys. Caution is advised for people with **liver or kidney damage**.

Cholesterol levels rise in 25–50% of people taking acitretin. Very large increases in triglycerides may be responsible for the few cases of pancreatitis (pancreas inflammation) that have been reported. Your doctor should measure your blood fat levels before you start taking acitretin and monitor them weekly or biweekly until your response to the medication has been determined. People with **diabetes,** who are **obese,** or who have a **history of these conditions** are at increased risk for high cholesterol levels as are people who **drink alcohol excessively.**

Drugs similar to acitretin have been associated with pseudo-tumor cerebri (increased pressure in the brain). Symptoms of pseudotumor cerebri include visual disturbances, headache, nausea, and vomiting. Report these or any unusual symptoms to your doctor at once.

People taking acitretin who had **spine or bone—including knee or ankle—problems** before starting the drug may find that their problems worsen while on the drug.

People with **diabetes** may find it more difficult to control their blood sugar while on acitretin.

Possible Side Effects

▼ Most common: hair loss or change in texture, peeling skin, and inflammation of the lips.

▼ Common: dry eyes, chills or stiffness, dry skin, fingernail problems, itching, rash, tingling in the hands or feet, increased sensory awareness, loss of some sections of skin, sticky skin, and runny nose.

▼ Less common: drying and thickening of eye tissue; eye irritation; eyebrow or eye lash loss; changes in appetite; swelling; fatigue; hot flashes; flushing; sinus irritation; headache; pain; earache; insomnia; depression; Bell's palsy; crusting of the eyelids; blurred vision; conjunctivitis (pink-eye); double vision; itchy eyes or eyelids; cataracts; swelling inside the eye; unusual sensitivity to bright light; dry mouth; nausea; stomach pain; diarrhea; bleeding gums; joint; back; and muscle pain; and worsening of existing spinal problems.

▼ Rare: Rare side effects can occur in almost any part of the body. Contact your doctor if you experience any side effect not listed above.

Drug Interactions

• People combining acitretin and glyburide (an antidiabetic) may have unusually low blood-sugar levels. Your doctor may have to adjust your diabetic treatment program while you are taking acitretin.

- Combining acitretin with methotrexate increases the risk of liver damage.
- Acitretin reduces the effectiveness of low-progestin oral contraceptives (the "mini-pill"). If you are taking one of these contraceptives, switch to another type of birth control and use at least one other contraceptive method for at least 3 years after treatment is completed.
- Combining alcohol with acitretin produces acitretin's parent compound, etretinate. Etretinate stays in the body much longer than acitretin and may therefore affect the fetus for an even longer period of time than might acitretin. Avoid alcoholic beverages.
- Do not take a vitamin A supplement that has more than the standard minimum daily requirement (1000 mcg). Excess vitamin A plus acitretin exposes you to possible vitamin A toxicity.
- Combining acitretin with tetracyclines may increase the risk of severe pressure on the brain.
- Notify your doctor if you are taking etretinate, isotretinoin, oral or topical tretinoin, or cyclosporine.

Food Interactions

Acitretin is best absorbed when taken with food or meals.

Usual Dose

Adult: 25–50 mg a day with your main meal. Dosage may increase after 4 weeks to 25–75 mg a day. Dosage must be individualized to your specific needs.

Child: not recommended.

Overdosage

Symptoms of acitretin overdose include vomiting, headache, and vertigo. Call your local hospital emergency room or local poison control center for more information. ALWAYS bring the prescription bottle or container.

Special Information

Contact your doctor at once if you become pregnant while taking acitretin or in the 3 years following treatment. The risk of birth defects persists as long as the drug is in your body. In one case, small amounts of etretinate were found in blood plasma and fatty tissue more than 5 years after treatment.

Some people have experienced decreased night vision while taking acitretin. Be careful when driving at night.

Report visual disturbances, headache, nausea, vomiting, or anything unusual to your doctor at once.

Do not drink any alcoholic beverages during acitretin treatment and for at least 2 months after treatment has been completed.

Avoid excess vitamin A (see "Drug Interactions").

Some birth control methods, including low-dose progestin contraceptives and tubal ligation may fail while taking this drug. Use at least one additional form of contraception while taking acitretin to avoid pregnancy.

You may have problems tolerating contact lenses while you are taking acitretin.

Do not donate blood while taking acitretin or for 3 years afterwards because your blood might be given to a pregnant woman.

Avoid exposure to excessive sunlight or to sunlamps because of unusual sensitivity caused by acitretin.

If you forget to take a dose of acitretin, take it with food as soon as you remember. If it is almost time for your next dose, skip the one you forgot and continue with your regular schedule. Do not take a double dose.

A worsening of psoriasis may initially occur with treatment, and the full benefit of acitretin may not be seen for 2–3 months.

Special Populations

Pregnancy/Breast-feeding: Acitretin causes birth defects and may damage the fetus. Women who take acitretin must be sure they are not pregnant before starting therapy by using reliable contraception for at least 1 month before starting the drug and taking a pregnancy test within 1 week of starting treatment. Women must use 2 reliable contraceptive methods during treatment and for 3 years following the completion of treatment.

Acitretin may pass into breast milk. Nursing mothers who must take this drug should use infant formula.

Seniors: Seniors have twice as much acitretin in their blood as do younger adults but may take acitretin without special precaution.

Actonel   *see **Bisphosphonates**, page 164*

Actos *see Glitazone Antidiabetes Drugs, page 528*

Generic Name

Acyclovir (ae-SYE-kloe-vir) Ⓖ

Brand Name
Zovirax

Type of Drug
Antiviral.

Prescribed For
Initial treatment and maintenance of genital herpes outbreaks; treatment of herpes zoster (shingles); and treatment of varicella (chickenpox).

General Information
Acyclovir is the only oral drug that reduces growth rates of the herpes virus and the related viruses, Epstein-Barr, varicella, and cytomegalovirus (CMV); both oral acyclovir and oral ganciclovir work against CMV. Intravenous drugs, including acyclovir injection, may also be used for these viral infections; however, intravenous antiviral drugs are usually reserved for patients with HIV, cancer, or otherwise compromised immune systems.

Acyclovir is selectively absorbed into cells that are infected with the herpes simplex virus, where it is converted into its active form. Acyclovir works by interfering with the reproduction of viral DNA, slowing the growth of existing viruses. It has little effect on recurrent infections. To treat both local and systemic (whole-body) symptoms acyclovir must be given by intravenous injection or taken by mouth. Local symptoms may be treated with the ointment alone. Oral acyclovir may be taken every day to reduce the number and severity of herpes attacks in people who suffer 10 or more attacks a year; it may also be used to treat intermittent attacks as they occur, but treatment must be started as soon as possible to have the greatest effect.

Cautions and Warnings
Do not use acyclovir if you are **allergic** or **sensitive** to any of its ingredients. Do not use acyclovir ointment if you have had an

allergic reaction to it or to the major component of the ointment base, polyethylene glycol. Do not apply acyclovir ointment inside the vagina because the polyethylene glycol base may cause irritation and swelling of sensitive vaginal tissue. Acyclovir ointment is not intended for use in the eye and should not be used to treat a herpes infection of the eye.

Renal failure has occurred in patients using oral acyclovir, in some cases resulting in death. People with **kidney impairment** should have dosages adjusted accordingly.

Maintain adequate hydration while taking oral acyclovir.

Animal testing indicates that acyclovir may affect fertility in men. These effects may be reversible.

Possible Side Effects

Capsules, Suspension, and Tablets

▼ Most common: feeling unwell, headache, diarrhea, nausea, and vomiting.

▼ Less common: appetite loss, stomach gas, constipation, fatigue, rash, leg pains, sore throat, a bad taste in the mouth, sleeplessness, and fever.

▼ Rare: aching joints, weakness, and tingling in the hands or feet. Contact your doctor if you experience any side effect not listed above.

Ointment

▼ Most common: mild burning, irritation, rash, and itching. These effects are more likely to occur when treating an initial herpes attack than a recurrent attack. Women are 4 times more likely to experience burning than men.

Drug Interactions

- Do not apply acyclovir together with any other ointment or topical medication.
- Oral probenecid may decrease elimination of acyclovir from the body, which increases blood levels of oral or injected acyclovir, increasing the risk of side effects.
- Combining acyclovir and zidovudine (an HIV drug—also known as AZT) may lead to severe drowsiness and lethargy.

Food Interactions

Acyclovir may be taken with food if it upsets your stomach.

Usual Dose

Capsules, Suspension, and Tablets

Adult: genital herpes attack—200 mg every 4 hours, 5 times a day for 10 days. Recurrent infections—400 mg 3 times a day or 200 mg 5 times a day for 5 days. Suppressive therapy for chronic herpes—800 mg a day, every day for up to a year. Herpes zoster—800 mg 5 times a day for 7–10 days.

Child (age 2 and over): Acyclovir has been given to children in daily doses as high as 36 mg per lb. of body weight without any unusual side effects.

Child (under age 2): not recommended.

If you have kidney disease, your doctor should adjust your dose according to the degree of functional loss.

Ointment: Apply every 3 hours, 6 times a day for 7 days. Apply enough medication to cover all visible skin lesions. About ½ in. of ointment should cover about 4 sq. in. of lesions. Your doctor may prescribe a longer course of treatment to prevent the delayed formation of new lesions over the duration of an attack. Begin using ointment at the first sign of an attack.

Overdosage

Overdose of oral acyclovir may lead to kidney damage due to deposits of acyclovir crystals in the kidneys. Other side effects include agitation, seizures, lethargy, and coma. The risk of experiencing toxic side effects from swallowing acyclovir ointment is quite small. In the case of overdose or accidental ingestion, call your poison control center. ALWAYS bring the prescription bottle or container.

Special Information

Use a finger cot or rubber glove when applying acyclovir ointment to protect against inadvertently spreading the virus. Be sure to apply the medication exactly as directed and to completely cover all lesions. Keep affected areas clean and dry. Loose-fitting clothing will reduce possible irritation of a healing lesion. If you skip several doses, or a day or more of treatment, the drug will not exert its maximum effect.

Acyclovir is not a cure for genital herpes. Herpes may be transmitted even if you do not have symptoms of active disease. To avoid giving the condition to a sexual partner, do not have intercourse while visible herpes lesions are present. A condom offers some protection against transmission of the herpes virus, but spermicidal products and diaphragms do not. Acyclovir alone will not prevent herpes transmission.

Initiate therapy at the first sign of symptoms.

Women with genital herpes have an increased risk of cervical cancer. Speak with your doctor about the need for an annual Pap smear.

Call your doctor if acyclovir does not relieve your symptoms, if side effects become severe or intolerable, or if you become pregnant or want to begin breast-feeding. Check with your dentist if you notice swelling or tenderness of the gums.

Avoid exposure to excessive sunlight or sunlamps because of unusual sensitivity caused by oral acyclovir.

Special Populations

Pregnancy/Breast-feeding: Acyclovir crosses into the circulation of the fetus. Animal studies have shown that large doses—up to 125 times the human dose—cause damage to both mother and fetus. While there is no information to indicate that acyclovir affects a human fetus, do not use it during pregnancy unless it is specifically prescribed by your doctor and the possible benefit outweighs the risk.

Acyclovir passes into breast milk in concentrations up to 4 times the concentration in blood, and it has been found in the urine of a nursing infant. Although no side effects have been found in nursing babies, mothers who must take acyclovir should use infant formula.

Seniors: Shingles attacks in people over age 50 tend to be more severe and respond best to acyclovir treatment if the drug is started within 48–72 hours of the appearance of the first rash. Seniors with reduced kidney function should be given a lower dose of oral acyclovir than younger adults.

Generic Name

Adapalene (uh-DAP-uh-lene)

Brand Name
Differin

Type of Drug
Anti-acne.

Prescribed For

Acne.

General Information

Adapalene is similar to a retinoid. Retinoids are compounds related to vitamin A and are used in acne treatment. When adapalene is applied to an acne lesion, it modifies several of the processes involved in skin cell function. It reduces inflammation in the acne lesion and slows the formation of the material that fills the lesion. Very little adapalene is absorbed through the skin.

Cautions and Warnings

Do not use adapalene if you are **allergic** or **sensitive** to any of its ingredients. If you are **sunburned,** wait until your sunburn clears before applying adapalene to your skin. **Avoid sun or sunlamp exposure** while using adapalene. If you must be in the sun, be sure to apply sunscreen or wear protective clothing over areas where you have applied adapalene. Extreme wind or cold can also be irritating to skin where adapalene has been applied.

Adapalene can irritate the skin if used in combination with products such as medicated or abrasive soaps or cleansers, astringents, or soaps and cosmetics with a strong drying effect. Avoid products containing sulfur, resorcinol, or salicylic acid.

Adapalene can be highly irritating if it gets into your eyes or if it is applied to your lips, the angles of your nose, mucous membranes, cuts, abrasions, or sunburned or damaged skin. Avoid using depilatories or waxing while using adapalene.

Possible Side Effects

▼ Most common: redness, irritation, dryness, scaling, itching, and burning are common after applying adapalene to your skin. These effects usually occur during the first 2–4 weeks of adapalene use and subside as treatment continues. Symptoms may be severe enough to cause you to stop using adapalene; call your doctor if this happens to you.

▼ Rare: skin irritation, stinging sunburn, and worsening acne. Contact your doctor if you experience any side effect not listed above.

Drug Interactions

None known.

Usual Dose

Adult and Child (age 12 and over): Wash affected areas with a mild or soapless cleanser and apply a thin layer of adapalene at bedtime.

Child (under age 12): not recommended.

Overdosage

Chronic ingestion of adapalene can cause liver toxicity and other side effects associated with swallowing large amounts of vitamin A. Swallowing adapalene gel is extremely dangerous for pregnant women, who should not take more vitamin A than is contained in their prenatal vitamins. Infants who swallow adapalene should be taken to a hospital emergency room for treatment.

Special Information

Stop using adapalene and call your doctor if you develop a severe skin reaction or any sign of drug allergy or reaction (symptoms include rash, hives, itching, changes in complexion, and breathing difficulties or irregularities).

Adapalene may exacerbate your acne at first, but you should see improvement within 2 weeks.

If you must be in the sun, be sure to apply sunscreen or wear protective clothing over areas to which you have applied adapalene.

Using more than a thin film of adapalene does not produce better results and may be more irritating to the skin.

If you forget to apply a dose of adapalene, apply it as soon as you remember. If it is almost time for your next application of adapalene, skip the dose you forgot and continue with your regular schedule.

Special Populations

Pregnancy/Breast-feeding: Animal studies of adapalene have shown no effects on the fetus. Since the effect of adapalene on pregnant women is not known, the drug should be used only when the possible benefits outweigh the risks.

It is not known if adapalene passes into breast milk. Nursing mothers should use infant formula.

Seniors: Seniors may use this drug without special precautions.

Brand Name

Adderall

Generic Ingredients

Dextroamphetamine Sulfate + Dextroamphetamine Saccharate + Amphetamine Aspartate + Amphetamine Sulfate

Other Brand Names
Adderall XR

The information in this profile also applies to the following drugs:

Generic Ingredient: Dextroamphetamine Sulfate Ⓖ
Dexedrine   Dextrostat

Generic Ingredient: Lisdexamfetamine Dimesylate
Vyvanse

Type of Drug
Central-nervous-system (CNS) stimulant.

Prescribed For
Attention-deficit hyperactivity disorder (ADHD) and narcolepsy (uncontrollable desire to sleep).

General Information
Amphetamines are stimulants that work on the brain's feeding center. Adderall, which is a mixture of two forms of amphetamine, may be used as a short-term aid in weight reduction. It should not be taken for longer than a few months for this purpose.

Amphetamines may also be prescribed for childhood ADHD, a condition characterized by distractibility, short attention span, hyperactive behavior, emotional instability, and difficulty controlling impulses. They should be used only after a complete evaluation of the child has been done. Frequency and severity of symptoms and their appropriateness for the age of the child determine whether drug therapy is required. Many experts believe that amphetamines offer only a temporary solution because they do not permanently change behavioral patterns. Psychological, educational, and social measures must also be taken to ensure successful treatment in the long term.

Cautions and Warnings

Do not take Adderall if you are **allergic** or **sensitive** to any amphetamine or have **heart disease, a heart defect, high blood pressure, hardening of the arteries, liver or kidney disease, tics or Tourette's syndrome, seizures or abnormal brain wave tests, thyroid disease, glaucoma,** or a **history of drug abuse**.

Amphetamines should be used with extreme caution because they are highly addictive and easily abused.

New or worsening thought patterns, bipolar illness, aggressive or hostile behavior, psychotic behavior, and new manic symptoms can develop during treatment with amphetamines.

Stimulants like amphetamines are not effective and may be dangerous for **children** whose symptoms are related to environmental factors or primary **psychiatric conditions**, including psychosis.

Stimulants can cause weight loss and stunted growth in **children under age 10**. Blurred vision and difficulty focusing can occur.

Possible Side Effects

▼ Common: heart palpitations, restlessness, overstimulation, dizziness, sleeplessness, increased blood pressure, rapid heartbeat, upper abdominal pain, and weight loss.

▼ Less common: euphoria (feeling "high"), hallucinations, muscle spasms and tremors, headache, dry mouth, unpleasant taste in the mouth, diarrhea, constipation, upset stomach, nausea, vomiting, rash, itching, changes in sex drive, and impotence.

▼ Rare: psychotic drug reactions. Contact your doctor if you experience any side effect not listed above.

Drug Interactions

- Combining an amphetamine and a monoamine oxidase inhibitor (MAOI) antidepressant may cause a severe increase in blood pressure as well as bleeding inside the skull. Wait at least 2 weeks after stopping an MAOI before taking an amphetamine.
- Amphetamines may reduce the effectiveness of high blood pressure medicines.
- Gastrointestinal and urinary acidifying agents such as methenamine reduce the effectiveness of amphetamines.

- Gastroinstestinal alkalizing agents, such as sodium bi-carbonate, and urinary alkalizing agents (acetazolamide, some thiazides) may increase and prolong the effects of amphetamines.
- Antipsychotic medications such as chlorpromazine, haloperidol, and lithium carbonate inhibit the stimulatory effects of amphetamines and can cause amphetamine poisoning.
- Amphetamines may enhance the effects of tricyclic antidepressants, norepinephrine, phenobarbital, phenytoin, and meperidine.
- Amphetamines may decrease the effectiveness of beta blockers.
- Amphetamines may counteract the sedative effect of antihistamines.
- Amphetamines can delay the absorption of ethosuximide into the bloodstream.
- Propoxyphene increases the CNS-stimulating effect of amphetamines. Fatal convulsions have occurred in propoxyphene overdose with amphetamines.

Food Interactions

These drugs may be taken without regard to food or meals.

Usual Dose

Dextroamphetamine and Adderall

ADHD

Child (age 6 and older): 5–40 mg once or twice a day.

Child (age 3–5): 2–5 mg a day. Dose may be increased weekly until maximum response is achieved.

Narcolepsy: 5–60 mg a day.

Weight Control: 5–30 mg a day in divided doses 30–60 minutes before meals; alternately, a single, long-acting dose may be taken in the morning.

Adderall XR

Adults: 20 mg a day.

Child (age 13–17): 10–20 mg every morning.

Child (age 6–12): 10–30 mg every morning.

Child (under age 6): not recommended.

Lisdexamfetamine

Child (age 6–12): 30 mg every morning. Daily dose may be increased up to 70 mg.

Child (under age 6): not recommended.

Overdosage

Symptoms include tremors, muscle spasms, restlessness, exaggerated reflexes, rapid breathing, dry mouth, constipation, hallucinations, confusion, panic, and overaggressive behavior. These may be followed by depression, exhaustion, abnormal heart rhythms, blood pressure changes, nausea, vomiting, diarrhea, convulsions, and coma. Take the victim to a hospital emergency room immediately. ALWAYS bring the prescription bottle or container.

Special Information

Amphetamines should be used very cautiously and only when considered absolutely necessary.

When taken for weight control, this drug should be used only when other methods have failed, and will gradually lose its effectiveness as the body starts breaking it down faster. Do NOT increase your dosage when this occurs. The drug must be discontinued.

Amphetamines are addictive and commonly abused. If you feel you have developed a tolerance or dependence to Adderall, contact your doctor. Do not increase your dosage without your doctor's approval.

Amphetamines may impair your ability to drive or operate heavy machinery. Use with caution. To prevent this drug from interfering with sleep, take it at least 6–8 hours before bedtime.

Do not crush or chew the sustained-release form.

If you forget your once-daily dose, skip it and go back to your regular schedule the next day. If you take the drug 2–3 times a day and miss a dose, take it as soon as you remember. If it is within 3 hours of your next dose, skip the one you forgot and continue with your regular schedule. Never take a double dose.

Special Populations

Pregnancy/Breast-feeding: Use of amphetamines during the early stages of pregnancy may cause birth defects. Amphetamines also increase the risk of premature delivery and low-birth-weight infants and may cause drug withdrawal symptoms in newborns. When this drug is considered crucial by your doctor, its potential benefits must be carefully weighed against its risks.

Amphetamines pass into breast milk. Nursing mothers who must take them should use infant formula.

Seniors: Seniors are more sensitive to this drug's effects.

Generic Name

Adefovir (ah-deh-FOE-veer)

Brand Name

Hepsera

Type of Drug

Antiviral.

Prescribed For

Chronic active hepatitis B in adults.

General Information

Hepatitis B is one of several different types of hepatitis, a viral infection of the liver. Adefovir is an antiviral drug that can reduce the amount of hepatitis B virus in the bloodstream and slow its spread to healthy liver tissue, however, it cannot cure chronic hepatitis B. People with chronic hepatitis B may develop liver cirrhosis or liver cancer and it is not known if adefovir can prevent these conditions from occurring. Like other viruses and bacteria, the hepatitis B virus can become resistant to the effects of adefovir.

Adefovir works against the hepatitis C virus in a way similar to that of certain human immunodeficiency virus (HIV) drugs. It interferes with an enzyme called *reverse transcriptase,* which is an essential component of the viral reproduction process. Almost half of each dose is eliminated via the urine within 24 hours of taking it.

Cautions and Warnings

Do not take adefovir if you are **allergic** or **sensitive** to any of its ingredients.

Adefovir can be toxic to the kidneys, especially in people who already have some **kidney problems**. Since it is eliminated from the body through the kidneys, people with **kidney disease** are often given lower doses of adefovir.

In some cases, hepatitis can become severely aggravated upon discontinuation of adefovir. Your doctor should check your liver for 12 weeks after the drug is stopped. It is possible that antiviral therapy may have to be re-started.

Adefovir has some activity against the **human immunodeficiency virus (HIV)**. An HIV blood test is recommended before starting adefovir treatment. If you are HIV positive, adefovir could make the HIV virus resistant to future antiviral drugs.

People taking adefovir can develop liver disease, liver enlargement, fat degeneration, and lactic acidosis (potentially fatal metabolic imbalance). This may be a reason for your doctor to stop your adefovir treatment. This occurs most frequently in **obese women**.

Possible Side Effects

In studies, side effects reported in the treated group were similar in frequency to placebo.

▼ Most common: weakness, headache, stomach pain, and nausea.

▼ Less common: intestinal gas, diarrhea, and upset stomach.

Drug Interactions

This drug was studied extensively in an attempt to predict possible drug interactions. No major interaction problems have been revealed.

- Taking drugs that can be toxic to the kidneys (such as aminoglycosides, cyclosporine, nonsteroidal anti-inflammatory drugs (NSAIDs), tacrolimus, and vancomycin) together with adefovir can lead to the more rapid appearance of kidney damage.
- Ibuprofen, when taken in dosages of 800 mg 3 times a day, will increase adefovir blood levels by about 20%, however the importance of this finding is unknown.

Food Interactions

Adefovir may be taken without regard to food or meals.

Usual Dose

Adults: 10 mg once a day. People with kidney disease requiring dialysis may take only 10 mg a week. The exact dosage is based on the severity of kidney disease.

Child: not recommended.

Overdosage

Gastrointestinal symptoms are the most likely outcome of an adefovir overdose. Take the victim to a hospital emergency room. ALWAYS bring the prescription bottle or container.

Special Information

Practice safe sex and safe needle use. People taking adefovir may still spread hepatitis B through sexual contact or by sharing needles. Practice safe sex using condoms and dental dams.

Do not share personal items that can have blood or body fluids on them, such as toothbrushes or razor blades.

Try to take adefovir at the same time every day.

Adefovir must be taken continuously to maintain its effectiveness. Be sure to keep enough adefovir on hand so that you do not run out of medicine.

If you take adefovir on a regular schedule and forget a dose, take it as soon as you remember. If it is almost time for your next dose, skip the forgotten dose and continue with your regular schedule. Do not take a double dose of this medicine. Call your doctor if you forget 2 or more doses in a row. Skipping or forgetting too many doses can make the hepatitis C virus resistant to adefovir.

Call your doctor at once if you feel very weak or tired, cold (especially in your arms and legs), dizzy or lightheaded, have unusual muscle pain, trouble breathing, stomach pain with nausea and vomiting, or have a fast or irregular heartbeat. These could be signs of lactic acidosis.

Call your doctor if you experience jaundice (symptoms include yellowing of the skin or whites of the eyes), appetite loss for a few days or more, lower stomach pain, nausea, dark urine, or bowel movements that are light in color. These could be signs of liver toxicity.

Special Populations

Pregnancy/Breast-feeding: Animal studies with adefovir have revealed a tendency for some birth defects when the dosage administered was more than 20 times the average human dose. There is no information on the effect of adefovir during pregnancy. The company that produces adefovir has established a registry to collect information on pregnant women who take this drug. When this drug is considered crucial by your doctor, its potential benefits may be carefully weighed against its risks.

It is not known if adefovir passes into breast milk. Nursing mothers who must take it should use infant formula.

Seniors: Seniors may be more sensitive to adefovir's side effects because of the natural loss of kidney function that occurs with advancing age.

Advair Diskus   see **Salmeterol**, page 1013

Brand Name

Aggrenox

Generic Ingredients

Dipyridamole + Aspirin

Type of Drug

Antiplatelet.

Prescribed For

Prevention of recurrent stroke or transient ischemic attack (TIA)— "mini-stroke."

General Information

Stroke is often the result of a clot blocking flow in a blood vessel supplying the brain. Aggrenox helps prevent blood clot formation by reducing the "stickiness" of platelets, blood cells that stick together to form the beginnings of all clots. In one study, Aggrenox reduced the risk of stroke by over 30% compared to placebo in people who had recently had a stroke or TIA.

Cautions and Warnings

Do not use this drug if you are **allergic** or **sensitive** to any of its ingredients or any nonsteroidal anti-inflammatory drug (NSAID). People who have **asthma, nasal polyps,** or **chronic runny nose,** are likely to be sensitive to aspirin.

The aspirin in Aggrenox can cause Reye's syndrome, a severe reaction (vomiting, lethargy, and belligerence, and possibly worsening to coma) in **children under age 16**.

People with a history of **stomach ulcers or stomach problems** should avoid Aggrenox.

People who have **angina** or have had a recent **heart attack** should be very cautious about taking this drug. It may worsen chest pain.

People with **low blood pressure, liver disease, or kidney failure** should be cautious about taking this drug.

People taking Aggrenox may bleed for longer amounts of time. Those with **bleeding disorders** should avoid Aggrenox.

Possible Side Effects

▼ Most common: headache, upset stomach, abdominal pain, nausea, and diarrhea.

▼ Common: pain, tiredness, and vomiting.

▼ Less common: convulsions, rectal bleeding, blood in the stool, hemorrhoids, back pain, accidental injuries, stomach bleeding, feeling unwell, weakness, fainting, memory loss, arthritis, joint or muscle pain, coughing, and respiratory infection.

▼ Rare: Rare side effects can occur in almost any part of the body. Contact your doctor if you experience any side effect not listed above.

Drug Interactions

- Avoid alcohol. People who take 3 or more drinks a day while using any aspirin-containing product are more likely to develop stomach ulcers or bleeding.
- Aspirin may reduce the blood-pressure-lowering effects of angiotensin-converting enzyme (ACE) inhibitor drugs, beta blockers, and diuretics.
- Combining aspirin and acetazolamide or an NSAID can cause kidney problems.
- Aspirin can increase the blood-thinning effects of anticoagulant (blood-thinning) drugs such as warfarin. Avoid this combination.
- Aspirin can increase the effects of oral antidiabetes drugs, possibly leading to low blood sugar.
- Aspirin counteracts the uric-acid-eliminating effects of probenecid and sulfinpyrazone.
- Aspirin can increase the toxic effects of anticonvulsant drugs and methotrexate.
- Dipyridamole increases the level of adenosine in the blood and may increase cardiovascular-related side effects. The adenosine dosage may need to be adjusted when these two drugs are combined.
- Dipyridamole may interfere with cholinesterase inhibitors used to treat myasthenia gravis.

Food Interactions

Aggrenox is best taken on an empty stomach but may be taken with food if it upsets your stomach.

Usual Dose

Adult: 1 capsule (200 mg of sustained-release dipyridamole and 25 mg of aspirin) morning and evening.

Child: not recommended.

Overdosage

Symptoms include a sensation of warmth, flushing, sweating, restlessness, weakness, dizziness, low blood pressure, and rapid heartbeat. Take the victim to a hospital emergency room. ALWAYS bring the prescription bottle or container.

Special Information

Call your doctor if you experience blood in your stool, persistent diarrhea, or abdominal or stomach pain.

Avoid alcohol while taking this drug.

In people taking Aggrenox, minor cuts may take longer than normal to stop bleeding.

If you forget a dose, take it as soon as you remember. If it is almost time for your next dose, skip the one you forgot and continue with your regular schedule.

Swallow Aggrenox tablets whole; do not crush or chew them.

Special Populations

Pregnancy/Breast-feeding: Pregnant women should avoid Aggrenox because of its aspirin content. Aspirin can cause bleeding problems in mother and fetus and result in a low-birth-weight infant. When this drug is considered crucial by your doctor, its potential benefits must be carefully weighed against its risks.

Both ingredients in Aggrenox pass into breast milk. Nursing mothers who must take this drug should use infant formula.

Seniors: Seniors may need a reduced dose of Aggrenox.

Generic Name

Albuterol (al-BUE-tuh-rawl) Ⓖ

Brand Names

AccuNeb	Proventil HFA
ProAir HFA	Ventolin HFA
Proventil*	Vospire ER

Combination Products

Generic Ingredients: Albuterol + Ipratropium Bromide

Combivent	DuoNeb

The information in this profile also applies to the following drugs:

Generic Ingredient: Levalbuterol
Xopenex

Generic Ingredient: Pirbuterol
Maxair

Some products in this brand-name group are alcohol- or sugar-free. Consult your pharmacist.

Type of Drug
Bronchodilator.

Prescribed for
Bronchospasm associated with asthma or other obstructive pulmonary diseases, or induced by exercise.

General Information
Albuterol is similar to other bronchodilator drugs, such as metaproterenol and isoetharine, but it has a weaker effect on nerve receptors in the heart and blood vessels; therefore, it is somewhat safer for people with heart conditions. Levalbuterol is a special form of albuterol that carries a lower risk of side effects.

Cautions and Warnings
Do not use Albuterol if you are **allergic** or **sensitive** to any of its ingredients. Albuterol should be used with caution by people with a history of **angina pectoris** (a condition characterized by brief attacks of chest pain), **heart disease, irregularities in heart beat, high blood pressure, stroke** or **seizure, diabetes, thyroid disease, prostate disease,** or **glaucoma**. Excessive use of albuterol inhalants may worsen **asthma** or other respiratory conditions, and may increase breathing difficulties rather than relieve them. In the most extreme cases, people have had heart attacks after using excessive amounts of inhalant.

Possible Side Effects

▼ Most common: worsening of asthma, ear infection, upper respiratory infection, stuffy nose, dizziness, headache, nausea, vomiting, and muscle cramps.

▼ Less common: angina, abnormal heart rhythms, rapid heartbeat and heart palpitations, allergic reaction, fever, and tremors.

Drug Interactions

- Albuterol's effects on the cardiovascular system may be increased by monoamine oxidase inhibitor (MAOI) and tricyclic antidepressants. These drugs should not be administered together or within 2 weeks of discontinuation of MAOIs or tricyclic antidepressants.
- Beta-blocking drugs such as propranolol not only block the effects of albuterol but may cause severe bronchospasm in people with asthma.
- Albuterol may reduce the amount of digoxin in the blood of people taking both drugs. Digoxin dose adjustment may be required.
- Albuterol may exacerbate certain effects of non-potassium sparing diuretics (loop or thiazide diuretics).

Food Interactions

Albuterol tablets are more effective when taken on an empty stomach—1 hour before or 2 hours after meals—but can be taken with food if they upset your stomach.

Usual Dose

Albuterol and Pirbuterol Inhalation

Adult and Child (age 4 and over): 1–2 puffs every 4–6 hours. Asthma triggered by exercise may be prevented by taking 2 puffs 15 minutes before exercising.

Albuterol Inhalation Solution

Child (age 2–12): starting dose—0.63 mg or 1.25 mg 3 or 4 times a day. Deliver over 5–15 minutes by nebulizer.

Levalbuterol Inhalation Solution

Adult and Child (age 12 and over): 0.63 mg 3 times a day every 6–8 hours. Some people may benefit from 1.25 mg at each dose. Deliver over 5–15 minutes by nebulizer.

Child (age 6–11): 0.31 mg 3 times a day every 6–8 hours, by nebulizer.

Albuterol Inhalation Aerosol

Adult and Child (age 4 and over): 2 inhalations every 4–6 hours. Adults and children age 4 and over may prevent asthma brought on by exercise by inhaling twice 15 minutes before exercising.

Albuterol Sustained-Release Tablets

Adult and Child (age 12 and over): 4–8 mg every 12 hours. Dosage may be cautiously increased to a maximum of 32 mg a day. People being switched from regular to sustained-release tablets generally take the same dosage per day, in fewer tablets—for example, a 4-mg tablet every 12 hours (1 dose) instead of a 2-mg tablet every 6 hours (2 doses).

Child (age 6–12): 4 mg every 12 hours.

Overdosage

Overdose of albuterol inhalation usually results in exaggerated side effects, including chest pain and high blood pressure. People who inhale too much albuterol should see a doctor. Overdose of albuterol tablets may lead to changes in heart rate, palpitations, unusual heart rhythm, chest pain, high blood pressure, fever, chills, cold sweats, nausea, vomiting, and dilation of the pupils. Convulsions, sleeplessness, anxiety, and tremors may also develop, and the victim may collapse. If the albuterol overdose was taken within the past ½ hour, give the victim syrup of ipecac to induce vomiting. Do not give ipecac if the victim is unconscious or convulsing. If symptoms have already begun to develop, the victim may need to be taken to a hospital emergency room. Call for instructions, and ALWAYS bring the prescription bottle or container.

Special Information

If you are inhaling albuterol, be sure to follow the inhalation instructions that come with the product. The drug should be inhaled during the second half of your inward breath, since this will allow it to reach deeper into your lungs. Wait about 1–2 minutes between inhalations. Do not inhale albuterol if you have food or anything else in your mouth.

Do not take more albuterol than your doctor prescribes. Taking more than you need can worsen your symptoms. If your condition worsens after taking your medicine, call your doctor at once and stop taking it.

Call your doctor immediately if you develop chest pain, palpitations, rapid heartbeat, muscle tremors, dizziness, headache, facial flushing, or urinary difficulty, or if you continue having breathing difficulties after taking the medicine.

Do not crush or chew the extended-release tablets.

If you forget a dose of albuterol, take it as soon as you remember. If it is almost time for your next dose, skip the one you forgot. Do not take a double dose.

Special Populations

Pregnancy/Breast-feeding: When used during childbirth, albuterol can slow or delay natural labor. It can cause rapid heartbeat and high blood sugar in the mother and rapid heartbeat and low blood sugar in the baby. Albuterol also causes birth defects in animal studies. When your doctor considers this drug crucial, its benefits must be cautiously weighed against its risks.

It is not known if albuterol passes into breast milk. Nursing mothers who must take it should use infant formula.

Seniors: Seniors with cardiovascular disease should use albuterol with caution.

Type of Drug

Aldosterone Blockers (al-DOH-stir-own)

Brand Names

Generic Ingredient: Eplerenone
Inspra

Generic Ingredient: Spironolactone G
Aldactone

Combination Product
Generic Ingredients: Hydrochlorothiazide + Spironolactone
Aldactazide

Prescribed For

High blood pressure, cirrhosis, and congestive heart failure (CHF); also used for people with low blood potassium who require a diuretic.

General Information

Aldosterone blockers limit the access of aldosterone—a hormone that helps to regulate several different body functions—from its receptor. Too much aldosterone results in high sodium levels, which can lead to water retention and potassium loss; it can also affect the size, shape, and function of the heart. Aldosterone blockers are generally combined with other medicines in the management of disease. These drugs are useful in removing excess body fluids in conditions associated with high aldosterone levels.

One in every ten people with high blood pressure has excess aldosterone in their systems. In people with congestive heart failure (CHF), aldosterone levels can be 20 times higher than normal, which can worsen their condition, making the use of aldosterone blockers an important part of their treatment. Aldosterone blockers also help the heart return to normal size, shape, and function in people with heart failure. Eplerenone is broken down in the liver, primarily by an enzyme system known as CYP3A4.

Cautions and Warnings

Do not take aldosterone blockers if you are **allergic** or **sensitive** to any of their ingredients.

Do not use aldosterone blockers if you have **kidney failure** or **high blood potassium**.

People with **liver disease** should be cautious about using aldosterone blockers.

People taking an aldosterone blocker should have their potassium levels checked periodically.

People with **diabetes** who have albumin in their urine should not take aldosterone blockers.

Possible Side Effects

Eplerenone
▼ Less common: dizziness, diarrhea, fatigue, flu-like symptoms, coughing, abdominal pain, elevation of blood cholesterol and/or triglyceride levels, elevation of blood potassium levels, and albumin in the urine.
▼ Rare: enlargement of the breasts in males, irregular menstrual cycles in women, and painful breasts. Contact your doctor if you experience any side effect not listed above.

Spironolactone
▼ Less common: drowsiness, lethargy, headache, gastrointestinal upset, cramps and diarrhea, rash, mental confusion, fever, feeling unwell, enlargement of the breasts in males, impotence, and irregular menstrual cycles or deepening of the voice in women.

Drug Interactions

- Do not combine eplerenone with itraconazole or ketoconazole. These drugs can cause the amount of eplerenone in the blood to increase by up to 500% and may cause fatal increases in blood potassium.
- Mixing eplerenone with erythromycin, fluconazole, saquinavir, or verapamil increases the amount of eplerenone in the blood. People taking this combination must watch for signs of high

blood potassium (see "Special Information") and have their blood potassium levels checked regularly.

- Combining a potassium supplement and an aldosterone blocker can lead to dangerously high blood levels of potassium. Do not use a salt-substitute or take any extra potassium unless prescribed by your doctor.
- Combining an aldosterone blocker with an ACE inhibitor or an angiotensin II receptor blocker (ARB) may significantly raise blood potassium. Be sure your doctor monitors your potassium levels if you combine these drugs.
- Spironolactone may interfere with anticoagulant (blood-thinning) drugs and mitotane (an anticancer drug).
- Aspirin can interfere with the diuretic effect of spironolactone but does not alter its effect on high blood pressure or CHF.
- Combining spironolactone with alcohol, barbiturates, or narcotics can lead to dizziness or fainting when rising suddenly from a sitting or lying position.
- Combining spironolactone and a corticosteroid can lead to very low blood potassium.
- Spironolactone may alter your response to drugs used during general anesthesia.
- Lithium generally should not be combined with any diuretic.
- Combining nonsteroidal anti-inflammatory drugs (NSAIDs) with aldosterone blockers can lead to severe elevations of blood potassium and reduce the blood-pressure-lowering effect of the diuretic.
- Spironolactone may raise digoxin blood levels and increase the risk of severe digoxin side effects. Your doctor may have to adjust your digoxin dosage.
- St. John's wort (a CYP3A4 inducer) may decrease eplerenone levels by about 30%.

Food Interactions

Food appears to increase the amount of spironolactone absorbed into the blood. Take this drug with food at the same time every day. Eplerenone may be taken without regard to food or meals. Taking this drug with grapefruit juice increases the amount of drug absorbed into your body.

Usual Dose

Eplerenone
   Adult: 50–100 mg a day.
   Child: not recommended.

Spironolactone

Adult: Starting dosage is 50–100 mg a day in divided doses for high blood pressure; 25–200 mg a day in divided doses for high fluid levels related to other diseases; and 25–100 mg a day for low potassium levels related to diuretic use.

Child: 1–2 mg per lb. of body weight a day.

Spironolactone + Hydrochlorothiazide

Adult: 1–4 tablets daily.

Overdosage

Eplerenone overdose may lead to low blood pressure and high blood potassium. Spironolactone overdose may lead to drowsiness, confusion, rash, nausea, vomiting, dizziness, and diarrhea. Rarely, coma may occur in people with severe liver disease. High blood potassium may also occur, especially in people with kidney disease. Call your local poison control center or a hospital emergency room for more information. If you seek treatment, ALWAYS bring the prescription bottle or container.

Special Information

Take aldosterone blockers exactly as they are prescribed.

High blood levels of potassium associated with aldosterone blockers may cause weakness, lethargy, drowsiness, muscle pain or cramps, and muscular fatigue. Use caution while doing anything that requires intense concentration, like driving or operating machinery.

Do not use a salt substitute or take anything else that is a source of extra potassium, including many multivitamin or supplement products.

People with high blood pressure should not self-medicate with over-the-counter cough, cold, or allergy remedies containing stimulants. These drugs can raise blood pressure effectiveness and have an adverse effect on the heart.

If you forget a dose, take it as soon as you remember. If it is almost time for your next dose, skip the one you forgot and continue with your regular schedule. Do not take a double dose.

Special Populations

Pregnancy/Breast-feeding: Animal studies with eplerenone showed no effects on a developing fetus. Spironolactone crosses into the fetal circulation. When your doctor considers either of these drugs crucial, their potential benefits must be carefully weighed against their risks.

Aldosterone blockers pass into breast milk. Nursing mothers who must take aldosterone blockers should use infant formula.

Seniors: Seniors may be more sensitive to the effects of these drugs, especially high blood-potassium levels.

Generic Name

Aliskiren (ah-LISS-kih-ren)

Brand Name
Tekturna

Combination Product
Generic Ingredients: Aliskiren + Hydrochlorothiazide
Tekturna HCT

Type of Drug
Direct renin inhibitor.

Prescribed For
High blood pressure.

General Information
Renin is produced by the kidney in response to a reduction in blood volume and the amount of blood passing through the kidney. Once in the blood, renin reacts with other hormones to form a very powerful blood vessel constrictor called angiotensin II that directly raises blood pressure. Renin also works with a hormone called aldosterone to raise blood pressure and it prevents sodium from being eliminated from the body. This increases the amount of water in the system, raising blood volume and increasing blood pressure. Aliskiren inhibits renin and all of its actions, thereby lowering blood pressure. The blood pressure lowering is usually seen with 2 weeks of starting on treatment. When aliskiren treatment is stopped, blood pressure gradually rises to pre-treatment levels. Only about 2½% of any dose is absorbed into the blood and it takes about a week to reach a steady level in the blood. Most of the drug that is absorbed is broken down in the liver. The rest passes out of the body unchanged in the urine. Aliskiren may be used alone or with other hypertensives, however its use with maximum doses of an ACE inhibitor has not been adequately studied.

Cautions and Warnings

Do not take aliskiren if you are **allergic** or **sensitive** to any of its ingredients.

Angioedema swelling of the face, hands or feet, tongue, or throat can occur at any time during aliskiren treatment. If this happens, stop taking the medicine and go to your doctor's office or a hospital emergency room for treatment. This reaction can interfere with your breathing.

The safety of aliskiren in people with moderate to severe **kidney disease** is not known.

The combination of aliskiren and an **ACE inhibitor** can lead to high blood levels of potassium.

Aliskiren may be less effective in some **black patients** with high blood pressure, especially when dietary salt intake is high. Nevertheless, it should still be considered a useful blood pressure treatment.

Possible Side Effects

▼ Common: nausea, dizziness, and sleeplessness.
▼ Less common: diarrhea, abdominal pain, upset stomach, GERD, cough, rash high blood uric acid levels, gout, kidney stones, headache, nose and throat irritation, fatigue, upper respiratory infection, and back pain.
▼ Rare: difficulty breathing; swelling of the hands, face, eyes, or whole body; and seizures. Contact your doctor if you experience any side effect not listed above.

Drug Interactions

- Mixing aliskiren with irbesartan can reduce the amount of aliskiren into the blood by 50%. This may reduce the effectiveness of aliskiren.
- Aliskiren has been studied together with both hydrochlorothiazide and valsartan and can be combined with them in blood pressure management. It has been used with amlodipine but may not be better than high dose amlodipine alone.
- Aliskiren's interaction with ACE inhibitors is not yet fully known.
- Atorvastatin and ketoconazole slow the breakdown of aliskiren, resulting in an increase of aliskiren blood levels by 50% or more. Dosage adjustment may be necessary.

- Aliskiren can reduce blood levels of the diuretic furosemide, reducing the diuretic's effect.

Food Interactions

Aliskiren can be taken without regard to food or meals. Avoid taking it with high fat meals because they can drastically reduce the amount of aliskiren absorbed into the blood.

Usual Dose

Adult (age 18 and over)
  Tekturna: 50–300 mg at the same time every day.
  Tekturna HCT: 1 tablet a day.

Child: not recommended.

Overdosage

The most likely symptom of overdose is low blood pressure (symptoms include dizziness and fainting). If you think you have taken an overdose, call your doctor or go to a hospital emergency room. ALWAYS bring the prescription bottle or container.

Special Information

Call your doctor at once if you develop swelling of the face, eyes, lips, tongue, or throat; difficulty swallowing or breathing; hoarseness; or other signs of a drug reaction or allergy.

If you forget a dose, take it as soon as you remember. If you do not remember until it is almost time for your next dose, skip the dose you forgot and continue with your regular schedule. Do not take a double dose.

Special Populations

Pregnancy/Breast-feeding: Aliskiren can injure or kill a developing fetus. Pregnant women should not take aliskiren. Women who suspect they are pregnant must call their doctor at once and stop taking aliskiren when pregnancy is confirmed. In those rare cases where aliskiren is considered life-saving for the mother and there is no substitute for aliskiren, your doctor may advise that you continue on the medicine and then check your baby's development with periodic ultrasound examinations.

It is not known if this drug passes into breast milk. Nursing mothers should use infant formula.

Seniors: Seniors may have higher blood levels of aliskiren and be more susceptible to drug side effects, but starting dose adjustment is not required.

Generic Name

Alitretinoin (al-ih-TRET-in-oin)

Brand Name
Panretin

Type of Drug
Retinoid.

Prescribed For
Skin lesions of Kaposi's sarcoma (KS).

General Information
Alitretinoin binds to and activates retinoid receptors in human cells. Once activated, these receptors help stimulate the body's natural mechanisms for limiting tissue growth—in this case, the growth of KS cells. KS lesions, which are primarily associated with human immunodeficiency virus (HIV), can respond to alitretinoin in as little as 2 weeks, but most people do not start to see results for 4–8 weeks or, in some cases, 14 weeks or more.

Cautions and Warnings
Do not use alitretinoin if you are **allergic** or **sensitive** to retinoids or to any of its ingredients.

Alitretinoin is applied to individual KS lesions. It does not treat systemic KS or prevent new KS lesions from forming.

People requiring **systemic KS treatment** (those who have developed more than 10 new KS lesions within a month) should not use alitretinoin.

People with **swollen lymph glands, KS that affects the lungs** or **other major organ involvement** should not use alitretinoin.

Possible Side Effects

▼ Most common: rash and burning pain at application site.
▼ Common: itchy, flaking, peeling, cracking, oozing, swelling, and inflammation at application site.

Drug Interactions
- Do not use insect repellant products that contain DEET, a widely used chemical repellant. Alitretinoin increases DEET toxicity.

Usual Dose

Adult: Apply 2–4 times a day to KS skin lesions. Seniors should use this drug with caution.

Child: not recommended.

Overdosage

Little is known about the effects of accidental ingestion. Call your local poison control center or a hospital emergency room for information. If you seek treatment, ALWAYS bring the prescription bottle or container.

Special Information

Apply enough alitretinoin gel to cover the entire skin lesion. Allow the gel to dry for 3–5 minutes before covering the area with clothing. Avoid showering, bathing, or swimming for at least 3 hours.

If you use a bandage or dressing, be sure it is not tight and that air can circulate freely over the area.

Avoid applying alitretinoin to unaffected skin because it may be irritated by the drug. Avoid applying near the nose, eyes, or mouth.

Alitretinoin contains alcohol. Always keep it away from any open flame.

Retinoids can cause unusual sensitivity to the sun. While this has not been seen with alitretinoin, you should avoid prolonged exposure to the sun or use sunscreen while taking this drug.

If you forget a dose, apply it as soon as you remember. If it is almost time for your next dose, apply the forgotten dose and then space the rest of your doses throughout the day. Continue with your regular schedule the next day.

Special Populations

Pregnancy/Breast-feeding: Alitretinoin can harm the fetus when sufficient levels of the drug are present in the mother's bloodstream, but it is not known if these levels are achieved during routine use of alitretinoin. Women who are or might be pregnant should only use this drug after discussing its potential benefits and risks with their doctors.

It is not known if alitretinoin passes into breast milk. Nursing mothers who must use alitretinoin should use infant formula.

Seniors: There is no information on use of alitretinoin by seniors. Seniors should use it with caution.

Allegra-D *see Antihistamine-Decongestant Combination Products, page 95*

Generic Name

Allopurinol (al-oe-PURE-in-nol) Ⓖ

Brand Name
Zyloprim

Type of Drug
Antigout medication.

Prescribed For
Gout or gouty arthritis; also prescribed to counter the effects of certain therapies for cancer, ulcers, abnormal heart rhythms in heart bypass patients, seizures, and other conditions that may be associated with too much uric acid in the body.

General Information
Unlike other antigout drugs, which affect the elimination of uric acid from the body, allopurinol acts on the system that manufactures uric acid in your body. A high level of uric acid can indicate that you have gout, psoriasis, cancer, or any of a number of other diseases. High levels of uric acid can also be caused by taking certain drugs.

In mouthwash form, allopurinol helps to prevent mouth, stomach, and intestinal ulcers caused by fluorouracil, an antineoplastic drug. Allopurinol may be given before heart bypass surgery to reduce abnormal rhythms and other surgical complications. It can be used to reduce the relapse rates of duodenal ulcers associated with *Helicobacter pylori* infection and to reduce the vomiting of blood from stomach irritation caused by nonsteroidal anti-inflammatory drugs (NSAIDs). Allopurinol has also been used to control seizures in people for whom standard treatments are not effective.

Cautions and Warnings
Do not take allopurinol if you are **allergic** or **sensitive** to any of its ingredients, or if you have ever developed a **severe reaction** to it. Stop taking the medication immediately and contact your doctor if you develop a rash or any other adverse effects while taking

allopurinol. Do not start taking allopurinol again if you stopped it because of a severe reaction.

Allopurinol should be used by **children** only if they have high uric acid levels due to **neoplastic disease** or to **rare metabolic conditions**.

A few cases of liver toxicity have been associated with allopurinol; they improved when the drug was stopped. People taking allopurinol should periodically be tested for liver and kidney function. People with severely **compromised kidney function** should take a reduced dose of allopurinol.

Possible Side Effects

▼ Most common: rash associated with severe, allergic, or sensitivity reaction to allopurinol. If you develop an unusual rash or other sign of drug toxicity, stop taking this medication and contact your doctor.

▼ Less common: nausea, vomiting, diarrhea, intermittent stomach pain, gas, upset stomach, headache, insomnia, tingling or numbness in the hands and feet, muscle or joint pain, and drowsiness or lack of ability to concentrate.

▼ Rare: Rare side effects can occur in almost any part of the body. Contact your doctor if you experience any side effect not listed above.

Drug Interactions

- Large doses of drugs that make your urine more acidic, like megadoses of vitamin C, may increase the risk of kidney stone formation.
- Alcohol, diazoxide, mecamylamine, or pyrazinamide can increase the amount of uric acid in your blood; an increase in your allopurinol dose may be required.
- Allopurinol may increase the action of azathioprine, mercaptopurine, or cyclophosphamide and other anticancer drugs, leading to possible toxicity, bleeding, or infection.
- Allopurinol may prolong the effects of chloropropamide, and can lead to hypoglycemic reactions in patients with kidney disease.
- Taking allopurinol with probenecid or sulfinpyrazone may cause excessive reduction of uric acid.
- Allopurinol may interact with some anticoagulant (blood-thinning) medications, reducing the rate at which the anti-

coagulant is broken down in the body. Dosage reduction may be necessary.

- People who are susceptible to ampicillin, amoxicillin, bacampicillin, or hetacillin rash are more likely to develop such a reaction while also taking allopurinol.
- Combining a thiazide diuretic or an ACE inhibitor (for high blood pressure or heart failure) with allopurinol increases the risk of a drug-sensitivity reaction.
- Combining vidarabine with allopurinol may increase the risk of neurotoxic effects and anemia, nausea, pain, and itching.
- Large doses of allopurinol—more than 600 mg a day—may increase the effects of and risk of toxic reactions to theophylline by interfering with its clearance from the body.

Food Interactions

Take each dose with food or a full glass of water. Drink 10–12 glasses of water, juices, soda, or another liquid each day to avoid the formation of crystals in your urine or kidneys.

Usual Dose

Adult and Child (age 11 and over): 100–800 mg a day, depending on disease and response.

Child (age 6–10): 300 mg a day.

Child (under age 6): 150 mg a day.

The dose should be reviewed periodically by your doctor to be sure that it is producing the desired therapeutic effect.

Overdosage

The expected symptoms of overdose are exaggerated side effects. Allergic skin reactions to allopurinol can be severe and at times fatal. Allopurinol overdose victims should be taken to a hospital. ALWAYS bring the prescription bottle or container.

Special Information

Allopurinol can make you drowsy or make it difficult to concentrate: Take care while driving a car or operating hazardous equipment.

Gout attacks may actually increase during the first few months of taking allopurinol. These attacks should subside.

Call your doctor at once if you develop rash, hives, itching, chills, fever, nausea, muscle aches, unusual tiredness, fever, yellowing of the whites of the eyes or skin, painful urination, blood in the urine, irritation of the eyes, or swelling of the lips or mouth.

Avoid large doses of vitamin C, which can cause the formation of kidney stones during allopurinol treatment. Be sure to drink 10–12 8-oz. glasses of water a day while taking this medication.

If you forget to take a dose of allopurinol, take it as soon as possible. If it is almost time for your next regular dose, double this dose. For example, if your regular dose is 100 mg and you miss a dose, take 200 mg at the next usual dose time.

Special Populations

Pregnancy/Breast-feeding: Allopurinol may cause birth defects or interfere with fetal development. Check with your doctor before taking it if you are or might be pregnant.

Allopurinol passes into breast milk. Nursing mothers who must take allopurinol should use infant formula.

Seniors: No special precautions are required. Follow your doctor's directions and report any side effects at once.

Type of Drug

Alpha Blockers

Brand Names

Generic Ingredient: Alfuzosin
Uroxatral

Generic Ingredient: Terazosin Hydrochloride Ⓖ
Hytrin

Prescribed For

High blood pressure (terazosin) and benign prostatic hyperplasia (BPH) (alfuzosin and terazosin).

General Information

Alpha blockers block nerve endings known as alpha$_1$ receptors. They reduce blood pressure by dilating (widening) and reducing pressure within the blood vessels. The maximum blood-pressure-lowering effect of terazosin is seen between 2 and 6 hours after taking a single dose. Terazosin's effect lasts for 24 hours.

In BPH, alpha blockers work by relaxing smooth muscles in the prostate and neck of the bladder. This effect is produced by blockage of alpha$_1$ receptors in the affected muscles. Despite the fact that terazosin alleviates the urinary symptoms of BPH, the drug's long-term effect on complications of BPH or the need for urinary surgery is not known. Alpha blockers are broken down in the liver.

Cautions and Warnings

Do not take alpha blockers if you are **allergic** or **sensitive** to any of their ingredients.

Alpha blockers may cause dizziness and fainting, especially after the first few doses. This is known as the "first-dose effect" and may be minimized by limiting the first dose to 1 mg at bedtime. The first-dose effect occurs in about 1% of people and may recur if the drug is stopped for a few days and then restarted.

Do not take alfuzosin if you have moderate to severe **liver disease** since this can drastically increase blood concentrations of the drug.

Alpha blockers should be taken with caution if you have **kidney disease**, since blood concentrations may be increased by 50%.

Do not take these medicines if you are already taking an alpha-blocker for either high blood pressure or prostate problems.

Terazosin may slightly reduce cholesterol levels and improve the high-density lipoprotein (HDL) to low-density lipoprotein (LDL) ratio, a positive step for people with blood-cholesterol problems.

Terazosin may reduce the counts of red and white blood cells.

People taking terazosin may experience a weight gain of about 2 lbs.

Possible Side Effects

Alfuzosin

▼ Most common: dizziness, fatigue, upper respiratory infection, and headache.

▼ Less common: pain, abdominal pain, upset stomach, constipation, nausea, impotence, bronchitis, sinusitis, sore throat, low blood pressure, dizziness, and fainting.

▼ Rare: rash, rapid heartbeat, chest pain, and painful and persistent erection. Contact your doctor if you experience any side effect not listed above.

Terazosin

▼ Most common: dizziness, weakness, and headache.

▼ Rare: depression, reduced sex drive or abnormal sexual function (including painful and persistent erection), fluid retention, and weight gain. Contact your doctor if you experience any side effect not listed above.

Drug Interactions

- When taken with other blood-pressure-lowering drugs, terazosin severely reduces blood pressure.
- Verapamil may increase blood levels of terazosin.
- Antifungal drugs such as itraconazole and ketoconazole and protease inhibitors interfere with the breakdown of alfuzosin in the liver, raising the amount of drug in the blood.
- Alfuzosin moderately increases the amount of diltiazem in the blood.
- Alpha blockers should not be taken with ritonavir.

Food Interactions

Alfuzosin should be taken with food.

Usual Dose

Alfuzosin: one 10-mg tablet taken after the same meal every day. Do not crush or chew the tablets.

Terazosin: starting dosage—1 mg at bedtime. Dosage may be increased in increments of 1–5 mg to a total of 20 mg a day. Dosages of 10 mg a day are generally needed to control the symptoms of BPH.

Overdosage

Symptoms may include drowsiness, poor reflexes, and very low blood pressure. Take the victim to a hospital emergency room. ALWAYS bring the prescription bottle or container.

Special Information

Take alpha blockers exactly as they are prescribed and do not stop taking it unless directed to do so by your doctor. Avoid over-the-counter drugs that contain stimulants because they may increase your blood pressure.

Alpha blockers may cause dizziness, headache, and drowsiness, especially 2–6 hours after taking your first dose, though these effects may persist after the first few doses. Wait 12–24 hours after taking the first dose before driving, operating machinery, or performing any other task that requires intense concentration. You may take alpha blockers at bedtime to minimize this problem.

Some people undergoing eye surgery who take alpha blockers can experience an unusual effect called "floppy iris syndrome." Make sure to tell your eye surgeon if you are taking or have ever been treated with an alpha blocker. There is no benefit to stopping alpha-blocker treatment before cataract surgery.

Prostate cancer and BPH may have similar symptoms. Talk to your doctor about ruling out prostate cancer before beginning treatment for BPH.

Call your doctor if you develop severe dizziness, heart palpitations, or any bothersome or persistent side effect.

If you forget a dose, take it as soon as you remember. If it is almost time for your next dose, skip the forgotten dose and continue with your regular schedule. Do not take a double dose.

Special Populations

Pregnancy/Breast-feeding: Alfuzosin is not indicated for use in women. Large dosages of terazosin damage the fetus in animal studies. When alpha blockers are considered crucial by your doctor, their potential benefits must be carefully weighed against their risks.

It is not known if terazosin passes into breast milk. Nursing mothers who must take this drug should use infant formula.

Seniors: Seniors may be more sensitive to the effects of terazosin.

Generic Name

Alprazolam (al-PRAY-zoe-lam) Ⓖ

Brand Names

Niravam   Xanax   Xanax XR

Type of Drug

Benzodiazepine sedative.

Prescribed For

Generalized anxiety disorder and anxiety associated with depression; panic disorder with or without agoraphobia.

General Information

Alprazolam is a member of a group of drugs known as benzodiazepines. Benzodiazepines directly affect the brain. They can relax you and make you more tranquil or sleepier, or they can slow nervous system transmissions in such a way as to act as an anticonvulsant. Many doctors prefer benzodiazepines to other drugs that can be used to similar effect because they tend to be safer, have fewer side effects, and are usually as effective, if not more so.

Cautions and Warnings

Do not take alprazolam if you know you are **allergic** or **sensitive** to it or to another benzodiazepine drug, including clonazepam.

Alprazolam can aggravate **narrow-angle glaucoma,** but you may take it if you have open-angle glaucoma and are receiving therapy for it.

Other conditions where alprazolam should be avoided are: severe **lung disease**, **sleep apnea** (intermittent cessation of breathing during sleep), **liver disease**, **drunkenness**, and **kidney disease**. In each of these conditions, the depressive effects of alprazolam may be enhanced or could be detrimental to your overall condition.

Alprazolam should not be taken by **psychotic patients** because it is not effective for them and can trigger unusual excitement, stimulation, and rage.

Alprazolam is meant to be used for no more than 3–4 months in a row. Your condition should be reassessed before continuing your medicine beyond that time.

Alprazolam may be addictive. When used to treat panic disorder, alprazolam is frequently prescribed in doses exceeding 4 mg a day. Studies show that these higher doses may cause physical and emotional dependence, making it very difficult to stop taking the drug. Drug withdrawal may develop if you stop taking it after only 4 weeks of regular use but is more likely after longer use and at higher doses. It may start with anxiety and progress to tingling in the hands or feet, sensitivity to bright light, sleep disturbances, cramps, tremors, muscle tension or twitching, poor concentration, flu-like symptoms, fatigue, appetite loss, sweating, and changes in mental state. Severe withdrawal symptoms may include seizures.

Your dosage should be reduced gradually (0.5 mg decrease every 3 days) to prevent drug withdrawal symptoms.

Possible Side Effects

▼ Most common: mild drowsiness during the first few days of therapy. Weakness and confusion may occur, especially in seniors and in those who are sickly. If these effects persist, contact your doctor.

▼ Less common: depression, lethargy, disorientation, headache, inactivity, slurred speech, stupor, dizziness, tremors, constipation, dry mouth, nausea, inability to control urination,

---

Possible Side Effects *(continued)*

sexual difficulties, irregular menstrual cycle, changes in heart rhythm, low blood pressure, fluid retention, blurred or double vision, itching, rash, hiccups, nervousness, inability to fall asleep, and occasional liver dysfunction. If you experience any of these symptoms, stop taking the medicine and contact your doctor immediately.

▼ Rare: withdrawal seizures. Rare side effects can occur in almost any part of the body. Contact your doctor if you experience any side effect not listed above.

Drug Interactions

- Alprazolam is a central-nervous-system depressant. Avoid alcohol, other sedatives, narcotics, barbiturates, monoamine oxidase inhibitor (MAOI) antidepressants, antihistamines, and antidepressants. Taking alprazolam with these drugs may result in excessive depression, tiredness, sleepiness, breathing difficulties, or related symptoms.
- Smoking may reduce the amount of alprazolam in your blood by 50%. Smokers may need larger doses.
- The effects of alprazolam may be prolonged when taken together with cimetidine, contraceptive drugs, disulfiram, fluoxetine, isoniazid, itraconazole, ketoconazole, metoprolol, probenecid, propoxyphene, propranolol, and valproic acid.
- The effects of some benzodiazepines may be decreased by rifampin.
- Theophyllines may reduce alprazolam's sedative effects.
- If you take antacids, separate them from your alprazolam dose by at least 1 hour to prevent them from interfering with the absorption of alprazolam into the bloodstream.
- Alprazolam may raise digoxin blood levels and the chances of digoxin toxicity.
- The effect of levodopa + carbidopa may be decreased if it is taken together with alprazolam.
- Combining alprazolam with phenytoin may increase phenytoin blood concentrations and the chances of phenytoin toxicity.

Food Interactions

Alprazolam is best taken on an empty stomach but may be taken with food if it upsets your stomach.

Usual Dose

Anxiety Disorder
Adult: 0.25–0.5 mg 3 times a day. Dosage must be tailored to your individual needs with a maximum dose of 4 mg a day.
Child (under age 18): not recommended.

Panic Disorder
Adult: 1–10 mg a day.
Child (under age 18): not recommended.

Overdosage

Symptoms of overdose are confusion, sleepiness, poor coordination, lack of response to pain such as a pinprick, loss of reflexes, shallow breathing, low blood pressure, and coma. The victim should be taken to a hospital emergency room. ALWAYS bring the prescription bottle or container.

Special Information

Alprazolam can cause tiredness, drowsiness, inability to concentrate, or related symptoms. Be careful if you are driving, operating machinery, or performing other activities that require concentration.

Anyone taking alprazolam for more than 3 or 4 months at a time may have a drug withdrawal reaction if the medicine is stopped suddenly (see "Cautions and Warnings"). Do not stop taking alprazolam, or increase or decrease the dosage, without first consulting your doctor.

If you forget a dose of alprazolam, take it as soon as you remember. If it is almost time for your next dose, skip the dose you forgot and return to your regular schedule. Do not take a double dose. If you take Xanax XR, take your full daily dose once a day in the morning. Do not chew or crush Xanax XR tablets.

Special Populations

Pregnancy/Breast-feeding: Alprazolam may cause birth defects if taken during the first 3 months of pregnancy. You should avoid alprazolam while pregnant.

Alprazolam may pass into breast milk. Nursing mothers who must take alprazolam should use infant formula.

Seniors: Seniors, especially those with liver or kidney disease, are more sensitive to the effects of alprazolam and generally require smaller doses to achieve the same effect.

Generic Name

Alprostadil (al-PROS-tuh-dil) Ⓖ

Brand Names

| Caverject | Edex | Muse |

Type of Drug

Erectile dysfunction agent.

Prescribed For

Erectile dysfunction; also prescribed for atherosclerosis (hardening of the arteries), gangrene, and pain due to blood vessel disease.

General Information

A male erection happens when blood flows into blood vessels and holding areas inside the penis. Problems occur when blood cannot move into the penis as it normally should. Alprostadil (prostaglandin E1 or PGE1) helps men get and keep an erection by dilating blood vessels that supply the penis and by relaxing muscles to help expand holding areas. Alprostadil also dilates other vessels and reduces platelet stickiness—which slows blood-clotting rates—and relaxes some muscle groups. Alprostadil must be injected into the tissue of the penis or inserted into the urethra.

Cautions and Warnings

Do not take alprostadil if you are **allergic** or **sensitive** to any of its ingredients or to other prostaglandin drugs. Alprostadil can cause **priapism** (painful erection lasting more than 6 hours). People with diseases where priapism is a possibility—**sickle cell anemia or trait, multiple myeloma, leukemia**—those with **penile deformities,** or **penile implants, women, children,** or **those for whom sexual activity could be dangerous** should not use alprostadil.

Penile pain is common after using either form of alprostadil, although it is usually mild or moderate.

Possible Side Effects

Injection
▼ Most common: penile pain.
▼ Less common: prolonged erection; penile fibrosis (deformity); blood blister or black-and-blue marks at the injection site, usually caused by poor injection technique;

Possible Side Effects (continued)

penis disorders, including yeast infection, numbness, irritation, sensitivity, itching, redness, and torn skin; penile rash or swelling; headache; dizziness; fainting; respiratory infection; flu-like symptoms; sinus inflammation; runny or stuffed nose; cough; blood pressure changes; local pain; prostate problems; back pain; and general pain.

▼ Rare: Rare side effects can affect the penis, kidney and urinary tract, heart and blood, skin, and eyes. Contact your doctor if you experience any side effect not listed above.

Pellets

▼ Most common: penile pain.

▼ Common: urethral pain, burning or bleeding, and testicular pain.

▼ Less common: headache, dizziness, respiratory infection, flu-like symptoms, runny nose, sinus inflammation, low blood pressure, back pain, pelvic pain, and general pain.

▼ Rare: Rare side effects can affect the kidney and urinary tract, heart and blood, skin, and eyes. Contact your doctor if you experience any side effect not listed above.

Drug Interactions

- Alprostadil can increase the effect of anticoagulant (blood-thinning) drugs. Your doctor may have to adjust the dose of your anticoagulant.
- Alprostadil may decrease the amount of cyclosporine in your blood.
- The safety of combining alprostadil with other drugs that affect blood vessels is not known. These combinations should be used with caution.

Food Interactions

None known.

Usual Dose

Dosage must be individualized to your need and response.

Overdosage

Alprostadil overdose can lead to an extended and painful erection, as well as other side effects. If this occurs, call your doctor or go to the nearest emergency room. Overdose victims should seek medical attention. ALWAYS bring the prescription container.

Special Information

Patient information leaflets are included with each alprostadil prescription. Read this information before you use your prescription.

You must be trained in proper injection technique by your doctor. Self-injection should be permitted only after your doctor has made sure you know how to do it properly. For more information on how to properly administer this drug, see page 1242.

Alprostadil begins working within 5–10 minutes after taking it. Dosage should be set so that your erection lasts for about 30–60 minutes. Use the lowest dose that works.

You should generally not use alprostadil more than 3 times a week, and wait at least 24 hours between uses.

Do not increase the dosage without consulting your doctor.

Contact your doctor or seek medical assistance if your erection lasts longer than 4 hours.

Special Populations

Pregnancy/Breast-feeding: This product should not be used by women. Men using alprostadil must use a condom if they have intercourse with a pregnant woman. Alprostadil passes into semen and will affect the development of a fetal heart if a condom is not worn.

Seniors: Seniors may use alprostadil without special precaution.

Altace   *see **Quinapril**, page 947*

Ambien   *see **Zolpidem**, page 1232*

Generic Name

Aminolevulinic Acid   (ah-MEE-noe-lev-ue-LIH-nic)

Brand Name

Levulan Kerastick

Type of Drug

Photodynamic therapy (PDT) sensitizer.

Prescribed For

Actinic keratoses.

General Information

Actinic keratoses are skin lesions that develop on sun-exposed areas of the face or hands in older adults with fair skin. Dermatologists consider them precancerous. Aminolevulinic acid solution is applied to the lesions in the doctor's office in preparation for PDT. By enhancing light sensitivity in treated skin, aminolevulinic acid increases the effectiveness of PDT, a form of light therapy that slows the growth of skin cells. PDT is administered 1 day after application of this drug.

Cautions and Warnings

Do not use this drug if you are **allergic** or **sensitive** to any of its ingredients or to porphyrins, or have **porphyria**. Aminolevulinic acid should not be applied around the eyes or inside the nose or mouth.

This drug causes increased sensitivity to the sun and bright indoor lighting. Skin reactions that may occur as a result of this sensitivity cannot be prevented by using sunscreen (see "Special Information").

Possible Side Effects

▼ Most common: scaling, crusting, itching, and changes in skin color. During PDT, which lasts for about 17 minutes, you will experience tingling, stinging, and a prickling or burning sensation in the treated lesions. These effects should begin to go away at the conclusion of PDT, though the lesions and surrounding skin will appear red. Swelling and scaling may also occur. These effects are temporary and should completely resolve within 4 weeks.

▼ Common: skin erosion and welts.

▼ Less common: pain, tenderness, swelling, skin ulcers, small blisters, oozing, loss of sensation in the area of application, scabs, and scratch marks.

Drug Interactions

- Other drugs that enhance your sensitivity to light may increase the effects of aminolevulinic acid. These drugs include griseofulvin, thiazide diuretics, sulfonylureas, phenothiazines, sulfonamides, and tetracycline medications.

Usual Dose

Aminolevulinic acid is applied to lesions in the doctor's office 14–18 hours prior to PDT.

Overdosage

Little is known about the effects of accidental ingestion, which is unlikely to occur because this drug is administered in a doctor's office.

Special Information

Only qualified medical personnel should administer this drug.

After application of the drug, avoid exposing the lesions to sunlight or bright indoor lighting for at least 40 hours. Wear a wide-brimmed hat and protective clothing during this period; sunscreen is not effective. Do not wash treated lesions until PDT has been administered.

If you experience a stinging or burning sensation, you may be able to alleviate these effects by shielding the lesions from light.

Special Populations

Pregnancy/Breast-feeding: The safety of using aminolevulinic acid during pregnancy is not known. When this drug is considered crucial by your doctor, its potential benefits must be carefully weighed against its risks.

It is not known if aminolevulinic acid passes into breast milk. Nursing mothers who must use it should use infant formula.

Seniors: Seniors may use this drug without special precaution.

Generic Name

Amiodarone (ah-mee-OE-duh-rone) Ⓖ

Brand Names

Cordarone   Pacerone

Type of Drug

Antiarrhythmic.

Prescribed For

Abnormal heart rhythms.

General Information

Amiodarone should be prescribed only in situations where the abnormal rhythm is so severe as to be life-threatening and does not respond to other drug treatments. Amiodarone works by decreasing the sensitivity of heart tissue to nervous impulses within the heart. It has not been proven that people taking this drug will live longer than those with similar conditions who do not take it. Amiodarone may exert its effects 2–5 days after you start taking it, but often takes 1–3 weeks to affect your heart. Amiodarone's antiarrhythmic effects can last for weeks or months after you stop taking it.

Cautions and Warnings

Do not take amiodarone if you are **allergic** or **sensitive** to any of its ingredients or if you have **heart block** or a very **slow heart rate**. Amiodarone can also cause heart block, a drastic slowing of electrical impulse movement between major areas of the heart, or extreme slowing of the heart rate. Amiodarone heart block occurs about as often as heart block caused by some other antiarrhythmic drugs, but its effects may last longer than those of the other drugs. Amiodarone can also **worsen existing abnormal heart rhythms** in 2–5% of people who take the drug. These effects can be fatal.

Amiodarone can cause potentially fatal drug side effects. At high doses, 10% or more of people taking this drug can develop potentially fatal lung and respiratory effects, beginning with cough and progressive breathing difficulties. Liver damage caused by amiodarone is usually mild. In rare cases, amiodarone has been associated with liver failure that resulted in death.

People taking amiodarone may develop optic nerve irritation, leading to partial or complete loss of vision. Most adults who take amiodarone for 6 months or more develop tiny deposits in the corneas of their eyes. These deposits may cause blurred vision or halos in up to 10% of people taking amiodarone. Some people develop dry eyes and sensitivity to bright light.

One in ten people taking amiodarone can experience unusual sensitivity to the effects of the sun. Use an appropriate sunscreen product and reapply it frequently.

Amiodarone can cause thyroid abnormalities. It may worsen an already sluggish thyroid gland in 2–10% of people taking the drug, and increase thyroid activity in 2% of people taking it. Amiodarone has also been associated with an increase in risk of thyroid tumors.

Antiarrhythmic drugs are less effective and cause abnormal rhythms if **blood potassium** is low.

Possible Side Effects

About 75% of people taking 400 mg or more of amiodarone a day develop some drug side effects. As many as 18% have to stop taking the drug because of a side effect.

▼ Common: fatigue, not feeling well, tremors, unusual involuntary movements, loss of coordination, an unusual walk, muscle weakness, low blood pressure, dizziness, tingling in the hands or feet, reduced sex drive, sleeplessness, headache, nervous-system problems, nausea, vomiting, constipation, appetite loss, abdominal pain, dry eyes, unusual sensitivity to bright light, and seeing halos around bright lights. Unusual sun sensitivity is the most common skin reaction to amiodarone, but people taking this drug can develop a blue skin discoloration that may not go away completely when the drug is stopped. Other skin reactions are sun rashes, hair loss, and black-and-blue spots.

▼ Rare: inflammation of the lung or fibrous deposits in the lungs, changes in thyroid function, changes in taste or smell, bloating, unusual salivation, and changes in blood clotting. Amiodarone can cause heart failure, reduced heart rate, and abnormal rhythms. Up to 9% of people taking amiodarone develop abnormalities in liver function. Contact your doctor if you experience any side effect not listed above.

Drug Interactions

● Amiodarone increases the effects of metoprolol and other beta blockers, calcium channel blockers such as verapamil and diltiazem, cyclosporine, dextromethorphan, digoxin, disopyramide, flecainide, fentanyl, lidocaine, methotrexate, procainamide, quinidine, theophylline, and warfarin and other anticoagulants. These interactions can take from 2 or 3 days to several weeks to develop. Some can be life threatening, and for others, drug dosage adjustments may be enough to avoid a serious problem.

- Fluoroquinolones, azole antifungals, and macrolide antibiotics increase the effects of amiodarone, which can cause life-threatening abnormal heart rhythms.
- When amiodarone and phenytoin are taken together, both drugs can be affected. Amiodarone can be antagonized by phenytoin and other hydantoin anticonvulsants, and the effect of phenytoin can be increased by amiodarone.
- Cholestyramine interferes with the absorption of amiodarone into the bloodstream.
- Cimetidine and ritonavir interfere with the breakdown of amiodarone, leading to high drug blood levels and the increased possibility of side effects.
- Azithromycin can interfere with the effectiveness of amiodarone. This interaction may lead to dizziness and cardiac instability.

Food Interactions

Amiodarone should be taken on an empty stomach, as food delays its absorption into your bloodstream. If amiodarone upsets your stomach, however, you may take it with food but then always take it with food to be consistent. Do not drink grapefruit juice during treatment with amiodarone because grapefruit juice affects how amiodarone is absorbed in the stomach.

Usual Dose

Starting dose—800–1600 mg a day, taken in 1 or 2 doses, usually for 1–3 weeks. Then, 600–800 mg a day for approximately a month. Maintenance dose—400 mg a day. You should take the lowest effective dose in order to minimize side effects.

Overdosage

The effects of amiodarone overdose include low blood pressure, shock, slow heartbeat, and liver toxicity. Overdose victims should be taken to a hospital emergency room for treatment. ALWAYS bring the prescription bottle or container.

Special Information

Side effects are very common with amiodarone; 75% of people taking the drug will experience some drug-related problem. Amiodarone stays in the body for months, so side effects may remain even after the drug is stopped.

Call your doctor if you develop chest pain, breathing difficulties, spitting up blood, nausea, vomiting, abnormal heartbeat, bloating in your feet or legs, tremors, fever, chills, sore throat, unusual bleeding or bruising, changes in skin color, unusual sunburn, or any other unusual side effect. See your doctor for an eye exam if your vision changes at all while taking amiodarone.

Amiodarone can make you dizzy or lightheaded. Take care while driving a car or performing complex tasks.

If you take amiodarone once a day and forget to take a dose, but remember within 12 hours, take it as soon as possible. If you do not remember until later, skip the dose you forgot and continue with your regular schedule. If you take amiodarone twice a day and remember within 6 hours of your regular dose, take it as soon as you remember. Call your doctor if you forget to take 2 or more doses in a row. Do not take a double dose.

Special Populations

Pregnancy/Breast-feeding: In high doses, amiodarone has been found to be toxic to animal fetuses. Women of childbearing age should use an effective contraceptive while taking amiodarone. If you are or might be pregnant and this drug is considered crucial by your doctor, its potential benefits must be weighed against its risks.

Amiodarone passes into breast milk. Nursing mothers who must take this drug should use infant formula.

Seniors: Dosage reduction may be needed in seniors with poor liver function.

Generic Name

Amlexanox (am-LEX-an-ox) [G]

Brand Name

Aphthasol

Type of Drug

Skin-ulcer treatment.

Prescribed For

Canker sores in people with normal immune systems.

General Information

Amlexanox slows the production or release of factors involved in the body's inflammatory response. It aids in the healing of mouth ulcers, but the exact way that it accelerates the healing process is not known.

Cautions and Warnings

Do not use amlexanox if you are **allergic** or **sensitive** to it or to any ingredient in the paste. Stop using this drug if you develop a persistent rash or irritation.

Possible Side Effects

▼ Less common: transient local pain, stinging, or burning after application.
▼ Rare: mouth irritation, diarrhea, and nausea. Contact your doctor if you experience any side effect not listed above.

Drug Interactions

None known.

Food Interactions

Do not apply amlexanox while you have any food in your mouth.

Usual Dose

Adult: Apply a small amount (¼ in.) to each mouth ulcer 4 times a day, preferably after breakfast, lunch, and dinner, and at bedtime.
Child: not recommended.

Overdosage

Swallowing even a whole tube of amlexanox would probably cause only upset stomach, nausea, diarrhea, and vomiting. Call your local poison control center or hospital emergency room for more information. If you seek treatment, ALWAYS bring the prescription container.

Special Information

Begin using amlexanox as soon as possible after noticing a mouth ulcer and use it until your ulcers heal. Call your doctor if the pain does not get better or the sores do not heal after 10 days of using amlexanox.

Make sure your teeth and mouth are clean before applying amlexanox paste. Squeeze ¼ in. of the paste onto your finger and apply it to each mouth ulcer using gentle pressure.

Wash your hands immediately after using amlexanox. If you get the paste into your eyes, wash it out at once using cool water.

If you forget a dose of amlexanox, use it as soon as you remember. If it is almost time for your next dose, skip the dose you forgot and continue with your regular schedule. Do not apply more than the recommended amount at any time.

Special Populations

Pregnancy/Breast-feeding: The effect of amlexanox on pregnancy is not known; use it only after discussing the possible risks and benefits with your doctor.

Amlexanox passes into the milk of nursing animals, but its effect in humans is not known. Nursing mothers should use this drug with caution.

Seniors: Seniors may use amlexanox without special precaution.

Generic Name

Amlodipine (am-LOE-dih-pene) Ⓖ

Brand Name

Norvasc

Combination Products

Generic Ingredients: Amlodipine + Atorvastatin
Caduet

Generic Ingredients: Amlodipine + Benazepril Ⓖ
Lotrel

Generic Ingredients: Amlodipine + Valsartan
Exforge

Type of Drug

Calcium channel blocker.

Prescribed For

Angina pectoris, Prinzmetal's angina, and high blood pressure; has also been studied for heart failure and Raynaud's phenomenon.

General Information

Amlodipine is one of many calcium channel blockers available in the United States. These drugs block the passage of calcium, an essential factor in muscle contraction, into the heart and smooth muscles. Such blockage interferes with the contraction of these muscles, which in turn dilates (widens) the veins and vessels that supply blood to them. This dilating effect reduces blood pressure, the amount of oxygen used by the heart muscles, and the risk of blood-vessel spasm. Amlodipine is therefore useful in treating not only high blood pressure but also angina pectoris (brief attacks of chest pain), a condition related to poor oxygen supply to the heart muscles.

Amlodipine affects the movement of calcium only into muscle cells; it has no effect on calcium in the blood.

The brand-name products Caduet, Lotrel, and Exforge contain combinations of amlodipine and other antihypertensives. For more information for Caduet, see Statin Cholesterol-Lowering Agents, page 1052; for Lotrel, see Benazepril, page 145; for Exforge, see Angiotensin II Blockers, page 80.

Cautions and Warnings

Do not take amlodipine if you are **allergic** or **sensitive** to any of its ingredients.

Amlodipine may, in rare instances, cause low blood pressure in some people taking it for reasons other than hypertension. This is more of a problem with other calcium channel blockers.

Amlodipine may worsen **heart failure** in some people and should be used with caution if heart failure is present. This drug does not protect against the side effects of suddenly stopping **beta-blocking drugs**.

Calcium channel blockers, alone and with aspirin, have caused bruises, black-and-blue marks, and bleeding due to an anticoagulant effect. This is mostly a problem with nifedipine but should be considered for all members of the group.

Amlodipine may cause angina when treatment is first started, when the dosage is increased, or if the drug is rapidly withdrawn. This can be avoided by gradually reducing the dosage.

Studies have shown that people taking calcium channel blockers—usually those taken several times a day, not those taken only once daily—have a greater chance of having a heart attack than people taking beta blockers or another medicine for the same purposes. Discuss this with your doctor to be sure you are receiving the best possible treatment.

People with severe **liver disease** may require reduced dosage. People taking the combination product Caduet may be more likely to develop liver problems because of the addition of atorvastatin, a drug that has been associated with liver disease.

Possible Side Effects

▼ Most common: headache, dizziness or lightheadedness (especially with Caduet), anxiety, nausea, swelling in the arms or legs, heart palpitations, and flushing.

▼ Less common: sleepiness, muscle weakness, cramps or abdominal discomfort, itching, rash, sexual difficulties, wheezing or shortness of breath, muscle cramps, pain, and inflammation.

▼ Rare: Rare side effects can occur in almost any part of the body. Contact your doctor if you experience any side effect not listed above.

Drug Interactions

• Amlodipine may interact with beta-blocking drugs to cause heart failure, very low blood pressure, or an increased incidence of angina.

• Amlodipine may cause unexpected blood-pressure reduction when combined with other antihypertensive drugs and with erectile dysfunction drugs; however, this interaction is more likely with other calcium channel blockers.

• The combination of quinidine (prescribed for abnormal heart rhythms) and amlodipine must be used with caution because it can produce low blood pressure, very slow heart rate, abnormal heart rhythms, and swelling in the arms or legs.

• Amlodipine can increase the effects of theophylline—prescribed for asthma and other respiratory problems—and related drugs.

• Patients taking amlodipine who are given fentanyl as a short-term surgical anesthetic may experience very low blood pressure.

• Calcium channel blockers may cause bleeding when taken alone or combined with aspirin.

Food Interactions

Grapefruit juice may increase the effects of amlodipine.

Usual Dose

Adults: 5–10 mg once a day. Do not stop taking amlodipine abruptly. The dosage should be gradually reduced over a period of time.

Child (age 6–17 years): 2.5–5 mg once a day for high blood pressure. Doses larger than 5 mg have not been studied in children.

Overdosage

Overdose of amlodipine can cause nausea, weakness, dizziness, confusion, and slurred speech. Take overdose victims to a hospital emergency room, or call your local poison control center for directions. You may be asked to make the patient vomit to remove the medication from the stomach. If you go to the emergency room, ALWAYS bring the prescription bottle or container.

Special Information

Call your doctor if you develop constipation, nausea, weakness or dizziness, swelling in the hands or feet, breathing difficulties, or increased heart pains, or if other side effects are bothersome or persistent.

The combination of amlodipine and atorvastatin may cause dizziness, especially when rising from a sitting or lying position. Rise slowly to prevent dizziness and a possible fall. Also, use caution when driving or performing hazardous activities until you know how the medication affects you.

Make sure the doctor who prescribed the combination product Caduet for you knows if you have liver disease.

If you are taking amlodipine for high blood pressure, be sure to continue taking your medication even if you feel well, and follow any instructions for diet restriction or other treatments.

It is important to maintain good dental hygiene while taking amlodipine and to use extra care when using your toothbrush or dental floss because of the chance that the drug will make you more susceptible to certain infections.

If you forget a dose of amlodipine, take it as soon as you remember. If it is almost time for your next dose, skip the dose you forgot and continue with your regular schedule. Do not take a double dose.

Special Populations

Pregnancy/Breast-feeding: Animal studies of amlodipine show that it may damage a fetus. Other calcium channel blockers can be used to treat severe high blood pressure associated with pregnancy, so there is no reason for women who are or might become pregnant to take amlodipine. When this drug is considered crucial by your doctor, its potential benefits must be carefully weighed against its risks.

It is not known if amlodipine passes into breast milk. Nursing mothers who take amlodipine should use infant formula.

Seniors: Seniors, especially those with liver disease, are more sensitive to the effects of this drug and may require reduced dosage. When this drug is considered crucial by your doctor, its potential benefits must be carefully weighed against its risks.

Generic Name

Amprenavir (am-PREN-ah-vere)

Brand Name
Agenerase

The information in this profile also applies to the following drug:

Generic Ingredient: Fosamprenavir
Lexiva

Type of Drug
Protease inhibitor.

Prescribed For
Human immunodeficiency virus (HIV) infection.

General Information
Protease inhibitors revolutionized the fight against acquired immunodeficiency syndrome (AIDS) because, when combined with other drugs, they reduce the amount of HIV virus in the bloodstream to levels that are often undetectable by current methods, such as CD_4 cell immune system counts and viral load measurements (amount of virus in the blood). Amprenavir is taken together with other anti-HIV medications in "drug cocktails" to take advantage of different avenues of attack against the HIV virus. Fosamprenavir is rapidly and almost completely converted to amprenavir by the body and then exerts its protease inhibitor effects. It has no anti-HIV effect on its own. Triple-drug cocktails were responsible for the reduction in the AIDS death rate that began in 1996. Protease inhibitors are always taken together with 1 or 2 nucleoside antiviral drugs, such as efavirenz, emtricitabine, lamivudine, tenofovir, or zidovudine (AZT). Multiple-drug therapy has changed the current view of HIV from a fatal disease to a manageable chronic illness.

Protease inhibitors work in a unique way, but they are not a cure for HIV infection or AIDS. When the HIV virus attacks a cell, it must be converted into viral DNA. Other drugs, known as reverse transcriptase inhibitors, interfere with this step, but they need help in fighting HIV. Protease inhibitors work at the end of the HIV reproduction process, when proteins are "cut" by a protease enzyme into strands of exactly the right size to duplicate HIV. Protease inhibitors prevent the mature HIV virus from being formed by interfering with this cutting process. Proteins that are cut incorrectly or that remain uncut are inactive.

People taking a protease inhibitor may still develop secondary infections or conditions associated with HIV disease. Because of this, it is very important for you to remain under the care of a doctor or other health care provider. The long-term effects of amprenavir are not known. You may be able to pass the HIV virus to others even if you are on triple-drug therapy.

Cautions and Warnings

Do not take amprenavir if you are **allergic** or **sensitive** to any of its ingredients. People allergic to **sulfa drugs** may also be allergic to amprenavir.

Do not use amprenavir oral solution in **children under age 4** due to the risk of toxicity.

People with **liver disease** may require reduced dosage.

Severe and life-threatening skin reactions can develop in people taking amprenavir. Call your doctor right away if this happens.

Amprenavir may raise your blood sugar, worsen **diabetes**, or bring out latent diabetes. Treatment with insulin or an oral diabetes drug may be required in such cases.

The risk of bleeding may be increased in people with **hemophilia** who take protease inhibitors.

Protease inhibitors can cause the redistribution of body fat, leading to buffalo hump, breast enlargement, abnormal thinness, or a round, moon-shaped face. The long-term effects of this are unknown.

Possible Side Effects

Amprenavir is always taken with other drugs, so the side effects listed here are associated with multiple-drug therapy rather than amprenavir taken alone. Amprenavir has been

Possible Side Effects (continued)

studied in children age 4–12 and side effects are the same as in adults.

▼ Most common: nausea, vomiting, diarrhea, mild rash, itching, high blood sugar, and high blood-triglyceride levels.

▼ Common: changes in sense of taste and tingling in or around the mouth or in the hands or feet.

▼ Less common: depression and high blood-cholesterol levels.

▼ Rare: life-threatening rash, diabetes, and buffalo hump. Contact your doctor immediately if you notice signs of a worsening rash, especially if it is accompanied by fever, flu-like symptoms, swelling, blisters, red eyes, or if you experience any side effect not listed above.

Drug Interactions

Amprenavir can interact with many drugs. Be sure to tell your doctor about all the medications you are taking.

- Astemizole, bepridil, dihydroergotamine, ergotamine, lidocaine injection, midazolam, triazolam, ergot derivatives, tricyclic antidepressants, and quinidine should never be combined with amprenavir because of the risk of severe, life-threatening reactions.
- St. John's wort should not be used with amprenavir because it can cause amprenavir resistance.
- You may require dosage adjustments of amiodarone, lidocaine injection, and warfarin when you start taking amprenavir.
- Do not combine rifampin with amprenavir because it reduces drug levels by 90%. Rifabutin reduces the amount of amprenavir in the blood by 15%.
- Combining amprenavir and sildenafil or vardenafil drastically increases the risk of their side effects including low blood pressure, visual changes, and a persistent and painful erection.
- Amprenavir can reduce the effectiveness of birth control pills. Use another means of contraception while taking amprenavir.
- Amprenavir must be taken at least 1 hour before or after antacids.
- Combining amprenavir with statin cholesterol-lowering drugs increases the risk of drug toxicity.

- Carbamazepine, phenytoin, and phenobarbital reduce the effectiveness of amprenavir.
- Other drugs that could interact with amprenavir and should be used with caution are erythromycin, itraconazole, alprazolam, clorazepate, diazepam, flurazepam, calcium channel blockers, delavirdine, efavirenz, nevirapine, estrogens, progestogens, corticosteroids, clozapine, loratidine, and pimozide.
- Ritonavir must be added to the combination of fosamprenavir and nevirapine, an NNRI-type antiviral; they are prescribed together to obtain maximum benefit.
- Fosamprenavir should be used with caution with anti-arrhythmic drugs, bepridil, trazodone, anticonvulsant drugs, ketoconazole, itraconazole, rifabutin, diltiazem, felodipine, nifedipine, nicardipine, nimodipine, verapamil, dexamethasone, drugs for excess stomach acidity, statins, immune suppressants, methadone, contraceptive drugs, and erectile dysfunction drugs because of the increased risk of drug side effects.
- Amprenavir capsules contain large amounts of vitamin E. Do not take a vitamin E supplement while taking this drug.

Food Interactions

This drug can be taken without regard to food or meals, but high-fat foods may reduce the effectiveness of amprenavir.

Usual Dose

Amprenavir Capsules

Adult and Child (age 13–16): 1200 mg (8 capsules) twice a day with other anti-HIV drugs. Adults with moderate to severe liver disease should take 300–450 mg twice a day.

Child (age 4–12): 9 mg per lb. twice day or 6.8 mg per lb. 3 times a day with other anti-HIV drugs, up to 2400 mg a day. This dosage also applies to older children who weigh less than 110 lbs.

Child (under age 4): not recommended.

Amprenavir Oral Solution

Child (age 4–12): 10.2 mg per lb. twice a day or 7.7 mg per lb. 3 times a day with other anti-HIV drugs, up to 2800 mg a day. This dosage also applies to older children who weigh less than 110 lbs.

Child (under age 4): not recommended.

Fosamprenavir

Adult: first-time treatment—1400 mg twice daily (without ritonavir); or 1400 mg once daily with 200 mg ritonavir once daily; or 700 mg twice daily with 100 mg ritonavir twice daily. Previous treatment with another protease inhibitor—700 mg twice daily plus ritonavir 100 mg twice daily.

Child: not recommended.

Overdosage

Overdose symptoms are likely to be exaggerated side effects. Overdose victims should be taken to a hospital emergency room. ALWAYS bring the prescription bottle or container.

Special Information

Amprenavir is not a cure for HIV. It will not prevent you from transmitting the HIV virus to another person; you must still practice safe sex. You may still develop opportunistic infections or other complications associated with advanced HIV disease.

Amprenavir oral solution is absorbed less efficiently than the capsules. They cannot be interchanged for each other on a milligram for milligram basis. Avoid alcohol while taking amprenavir oral solution.

Tell your doctor about all other prescription and over-the-counter drugs you are taking because of the risk of drug interactions.

It is very important to take amprenavir exactly as prescribed. If you forget a dose of amprenavir, take it as soon as you remember. If you miss a dose by more than 4 hours, skip the forgotten dose and continue with your regular schedule. Never take a double dose.

Contact your doctor if you have a rash, nausea, diarrhea, or vomiting, or any intolerable drug side effect.

Special Populations

Pregnancy/Breast-feeding: Amprenavir caused abortions and birth defects in pregnant animals. Its effect on pregnant women is not known and the drug should be taken only after risks and possible benefits have been discussed with your doctor.

Nursing mothers who must take amprenavir should use infant formula.

Seniors: Amprenavir was not studied in seniors. Seniors taking this drug must use caution.

Generic Name

Anagrelide (ah-NAG-rel-ide)

Brand Name

Agrylin

Type of Drug

Antiplatelet.

Prescribed For

Essential thrombocythemia (ET), to reduce blood-platelet count and the risk of excess blood clotting associated with high blood-platelet levels.

General Information

Blood platelets play an important role in the body. They help to form blood clots that "seal off" minor cuts and wounds and prevent excessive bleeding. When platelet counts are too high, as in ET, unwanted clots may form almost anywhere in the body. These clots may obstruct blood vessels, leading to leg cramps, heart attack, stroke, or other medical problems. Exactly how anagrelide reduces blood-platelet count is not known, but it may interfere with the formation of new platelets. Anagrelide is not approved for general use by children under age 16, but it has been used without apparent harm by 8 children between the ages of 8 and 17, who took it in doses up to 4 mg a day.

Cautions and Warnings

Do not take anagrelide if you are **allergic** or **sensitive** to any of its ingredients. This drug should be used with caution by people who have **heart disease**. Use of anagrelide may cause heart palpitations, rapid heart rate, and congestive heart failure.

Unusually low blood-platelet counts can develop in people treated with anagrelide. Platelet counts should be periodically checked while you are taking this drug; they usually rise soon after the drug is stopped.

People with **liver or kidney disease** should use this drug with caution. Anagrelide can cause liver or kidney toxicity and worsen diseases of those organs.

Possible Side Effects

▼ Most common: heart palpitations, diarrhea, abdominal pain, nausea, gas, headache, weakness, swelling, pain, dizziness, and difficulty breathing.

▼ Common: chest pain, rapid heartbeat, vomiting, upset stomach, appetite loss, rash or itching, tingling in the hands or feet, back pain, and not feeling well.

▼ Less common: fever, flu-like symptoms, chills, neck pain, sensitivity to bright light, abnormal heart rhythms, bleeding, heart disease, stroke, angina pain, heart failure, dizziness when rising from a sitting or lying position, flushing, migraine, fainting, depression, confusion, tiredness, high blood pressure, nervousness, memory loss, itching, skin disease, hair loss, stomach bleeding, blood in the stool, stomach irritation, vomiting, anemia, thrombocytopenia (low blood-platelet count), black-and-blue marks, swollen lymph glands, painful urination, blood in the urine, muscle and joint ache, leg cramps, runny nose, nosebleeds, lung disease, sinus inflammation, pneumonia, bronchitis, asthma, double vision, other visual difficulties, ringing or buzzing in the ears, liver inflammation, and dehydration.

Drug Interactions

- Sucralfate may interfere with the absorption of anagrelide. Do not combine these drugs.

Food Interactions

Anagrelide may be taken without regard to food or meals.

Usual Dose

Adult: 0.5 mg 4 times a day or 1 mg twice a day, to start. After at least a week, the lowest effective dose should be sought.

Child (age 17 and under): Limited information is available for the use of anagrelide in children. Children ranging in age from 7–17 have been given starting dosages similar to adults with similar side effects.

Overdosage

Little is known about the effects of anagrelide overdose, but symptoms are likely to include a sudden drop in blood-platelet count and heart or central-nervous-system side effects which could result in abnormal bleeding. Overdose victims should be taken to a hospital emergency room at once. ALWAYS bring the prescription bottle or container.

Special Information

Blood-platelet counts should be checked every two days when beginning anagrelide for 1 week. Until a maintenance dose has been established, platelet counts should then be taken once a week.

Women who might become pregnant should use a reliable form of birth control while taking anagrelide.

If you forget a dose, take it as soon as possible. If it is almost time for your next dose, skip the dose you forgot and continue with your regular schedule. Call your doctor if you forget 2 or more doses in a row. Do not take a double dose.

Special Populations

Pregnancy/Breast-feeding: At high doses, anagrelide caused birth defects in animal studies. When this drug is considered crucial by your doctor, its potential benefits must be carefully weighed against its risks.

It is not known if this drug passes into breast milk. Nursing mothers who must take anagrelide should use infant formula.

Seniors: Seniors may take anagrelide without special precaution.

Generic Name

Anakinra (an-ah-KIN-rah)

Brand Name

Kineret

Type of Drug

Immune system modulator.

Prescribed For

Moderate to severe rheumatoid arthritis in adults.

General Information

Anakinra blocks the biological activity of a substance called interleukin-1, which is produced in response to inflammation. Anakinra may be prescribed together with methotrexate, azathioprine, leflunomide, sulfasalazine, or other drugs for the treatment of rheumatoid arthritis. It must be injected under the skin every day.

Cautions and Warnings

Do not use this drug if you are **allergic** or **sensitive** to any of its ingredients.

Serious infections and malignancies are possible in people using anakinra because of its ability to suppress the immune response. This may be more common in people with other conditions that predispose them to infections such as **asthma** or advanced or uncontrolled **diabetes**.

The safety and effectiveness of anakinra in people whose **immune systems** are suppressed has not been established.

Levels of some white blood cells may be reduced in rare cases, leading to persistent fever or pale skin color. Contact your doctor if any of these symptoms develop.

Anakinra is cleared through the kidneys. People with **severe kidney disease** may accumulate anakinra in their blood.

People taking anakinra should not receive any **live vaccines,** because the body may not be able to respond as expected to the vaccine.

Possible Side Effects

▼ Most common: infections and injection-site reactions.
▼ Common: reduced white-blood-cell counts, headache, nausea, and diarrhea.
▼ Less common: sinusitis, flu-like symptoms, and abdominal pain.

Drug Interactions

- Do not mix anakinra in the same syringe as another drug.
- Anakinra should not be used in combination with etanercept or any other TNF-blocking agent because of the increased risk of infection.

Food Interactions

None known.

Usual Dose

Adult (age 18 and over): 100 mg a day, at the same time each day, injected under the skin via pre-filled syringe. Inject the entire contents of the syringe.

Child: not recommended.

Overdosage

In animal studies, doses up to 35 times the maximum human dose have been used with no evidence of serious toxicities. Call your doctor or local poison center for more information. If you do go to a hospital emergency room, ALWAYS bring the prescription bottle or container.

Special Information

Do not use a syringe of anakinra if the contents are discolored or contain particles. Keep anakinra dosages refrigerated.

Reactions may develop at the site where anakinra is injected. Injection sites should be rotated among the thigh, abdomen, and upper arm to avoid excessive bruising or other skin damage.

If you forget a dose of anakinra, take it as soon as you remember. If it is almost time for your next dose, skip the dose you forgot and continue with your regular schedule.

For more information on how to properly administer this drug, see page 1242.

Special Populations

Pregnancy/Breast-feeding: Animal studies at doses 100 times the human dose indicate no harm to the fetus. However, there is no information on the use of anakinra by pregnant women. When this drug is considered crucial by your doctor, its potential benefits must be weighed against its risks.

It is not known if anakinra passes into breast milk. Nursing mothers who must use anakinra should use infant formula.

Seniors: The risk of anakinra side effects is greater in seniors because of the natural decline in kidney function.

Generic Name

Anastrozole (ah-NAS-troe-zole)

Brand Name

Arimidex

The information in this profile also applies to the following drug:

Generic Ingredient: Letrozole
Femara

Type of Drug

Aromatase inhibitor.

Prescribed For

Breast cancer in postmenopausal women.

General Information

Anastrozole is used for breast cancer that has advanced or spread despite treatment with tamoxifen, as an initial treatment for estrogen-receptor-positive breast cancer or for breast cancer in which the hormone receptor status is unknown. Anastrozole reduces the amount of estradiol, an estrogenic hormone, in the blood. It does this by interfering with the action of the aromatase enzyme, an element involved in the manufacture of estradiol. Most of anastrozole is broken down in the liver.

Cautions and Warnings

Do not take anastrozole if you are **allergic** or **sensitive** to any of its ingredients. Anastrozole increases blood-cholesterol levels.

Women with **estrogen-receptor negative disease** and those who did not respond at all to tamoxifen are not likely to respond to anastrozole.

Deterioration of bone density may occur in women taking anastrozole or letrozole.

People with severe **liver disease** may need reduced dosages of letrozole.

Possible Side Effects

▼ Most common: weakness, nausea, headache, flushing, pain, and back pain.

▼ Less common: muscle and joint pain; cough; diarrhea; constipation; abdominal pain; appetite loss; bone pain; sore throat; dizziness; rash; dry mouth; swelling in the arms, legs, or feet; pelvic pain; unexpected vaginal bleeding; depression; chest pain; and tingling in the hands or feet.

▼ Rare: Rare side effects can occur in almost any part of the body. Contact your doctor if you experience any side effect not listed above.

Drug Interactions

• Usual doses of anastrozole do not affect other medications; however, high doses of anastrozole can reduce the ability of the liver to break down certain drugs.

- Tamoxifen reduces blood levels of anastrozole without increasing treatment benefit. These drugs should not be taken together.
- Estrogen-containing therapies should not be used with anastrozole.

Food Interactions

Anastrozole may be taken with or without food.

Usual Dose

Anastrozole
   Adult: 1 mg once a day.

Letrozole
   Adult: 2.5 mg once a day.

Overdosage

Symptoms of overdose can be exaggerated side effects. Overdose victims should be taken to a hospital emergency room. ALWAYS bring the prescription bottle or container.

Special Information

Call your doctor if your side effects become severe or intolerable.

Use a condom, diaphragm, or other non-hormonal contraceptive while taking anastrozole.

If you forget a dose of anastrozole, take it as soon as you remember if it is within 12 hours of the missed dose. If it is over 12 hours, skip the missed dose and continue with your regular schedule. Call your doctor if you forget more than 2 doses in a row.

Special Populations

Pregnancy/Breast-feeding: Anastrozole is intended only for postmenopausal women. Animal studies have shown that exposure to anastrozole can harm the fetus. Women who think they may become pregnant while taking this drug should use a condom, diaphragm, or other non-hormonal contraceptive.

Seniors: Seniors may take this drug without special precaution.

Type of Drug

Angiotensin II Blockers (AN-jee-oe-TEN-sin)

Brand Names

Generic Ingredient: Candesartan Cilexetil
Atacand

Generic Ingredients: Candesartan Cilexetil + Hydrochlorothiazide
Atacand HCT

Generic Ingredient: Eprosartan Mesylate
Teveten

Generic Ingredients: Eprosartan Mesylate + Hydrochlorothiazide
Teveten HCT

Generic Ingredient: Irbesartan
Avapro

Generic Ingredients: Irbesartan + Hydrochlorothiazide
Avalide

Generic Ingredient: Losartan Potassium
Cozaar

Generic Ingredients: Losartan Potassium + Hydrochlorothiazide
Hyzaar

Generic Ingredient: Olmesartan Medoxomil
Benicar

Generic Ingredients: Olmesartan Medoxomil + Hydrochlorothiazide
Benicar HCT

Generic Ingredient: Telmisartan
Micardis

Generic Ingredients: Telmisartan + Hydrochlorothiazide
Micardis HCT

Generic Ingredient: Valsartan
Diovan

Generic Ingredients: Valsartan + Hydrochlorothiazide
Diovan HCT

Generic Ingredients: Valsartan + Amlodipine
Exforge

Prescribed For

High blood pressure; nephropathy in type 2 diabetes (losartan and irbesartan); heart failure (candesartan and valsartan; and treatment following heart attack (valsartan).

General Information

These drugs work by blocking the effects of angiotensin II, a hormone found in blood vessels and other tissue. Angiotensin II plays an important role in regulating blood pressure. Unlike angiotensin-converting enzyme (ACE) inhibitors—another group of blood-pressure-lowering medication—angiotensin II (AII) blockers do not cause chronic cough. AII blockers can be used alone or with a thiazide diuretic such as hydrochlorothiazide, as in Hyzaar, Avalide, and Diovan HCT, for example. While these are single tablets, your doctor may prescribe an AII blocker and a diuretic as separate pills. Combining an AII blocker and a diuretic may reduce blood pressure twice as much as an AII blocker alone.

AII blockers may be useful in treating heart failure and may slow the progression of kidney disease in people with diabetes and high blood pressure.

Many AII blockers contain combinations of antihypertensives. For more information see Amlodipine, page 65, and Hydrochlorothiazide, page 1113.

Cautions and Warnings

Do not take an AII blocker if you are **allergic** or **sensitive** to any of its ingredients. You may be sensitive to one AII blocker and tolerant of another.

Do not take AII blockers if you are or think you might be **pregnant**.

Patients with **heart failure** given an AII blocker generally experience a drop in blood pressure. If this happens, a temporary dosage reduction may be needed. People being treated with diuretics may also experience a sudden drop in blood pressure (symptoms include dizziness and fainting). Once your body has adjusted to a diuretic-AII blocker combination, this problem should subside.

Telmisartan is noticeably less effective in **black patients.** Irbesartan, candesartan, and losartan are also somewhat less effective in black patients although the addition of a diuretic such as hydrochlorothiazide is usually beneficial.

People with serious **liver disease** or **cirrhosis** should receive a lower starting dosage of losartan. Telmisartan should be used with caution by people with liver disease and related problems; alternate drug therapy should be considered. People with liver disease or cirrhosis should be cautious about taking valsartan, although no dosage adjustment is required.

Some people who take an AII blocker develop kidney function changes similar to those associated with ACE inhibitor drugs. Valsartan and telmisartan dosages may have to be modified in the presence of severe **kidney disease.** No adjustment is required for other AII blockers.

Losartan can be used in **children** age 6 and over. Other AII blockers have not been studied in children under age 18.

Possible Side Effects

AII blockers are generally very well tolerated. In clinical studies, the risk of side effects was about the same for an AII blocker as for a placebo (sugar pill).

Candesartan
▼ Common: respiratory infection.
▼ Less common: dizziness, headache, fatigue, diarrhea, nausea and vomiting, abdominal and other pain, joint pain, sinus problems, sore throat, runny nose, bronchitis, chest pain, and swollen arms or legs.
▼ Rare: Rare side effects can occur in almost any part of the body. Contact your doctor if you experience any side effect not listed above.

Eprosartan
▼ Common: respiratory infection.
▼ Less common: changes in urinary frequency or painful urination, dizziness, headache, sleeplessness, diarrhea, upset stomach, muscle pain or cramps, cough, sore throat, runny nose, and swelling.
▼ Rare: Rare side effects can occur in almost any part of the body. Contact your doctor if you experience any side effect not listed above.

Irbesartan
▼ Less common: dizziness, headache, fatigue, anxiety, nervousness, diarrhea, upset stomach, heartburn, nausea and vomiting, abdominal and other pain, cough, sinus problems, sore throat, runny nose, flu-like symptoms, swelling, chest pain, rash, rapid heartbeat, and urinary infection.
▼ Rare: Rare side effects can occur in almost any part of the body. Contact your doctor if you experience any side effect not listed above.

Possible Side Effects *(continued)*

Losartan
▼ Common: respiratory infection.
▼ Less common: dizziness, sleeplessness, diarrhea, upset stomach, heartburn, pain, muscle cramps, muscle aches, cough, stuffy nose, rash, rapid heartbeat, and sinus problems.
▼ Rare: Rare side effects can occur in almost any part of the body. Contact your doctor if you experience any side effect not listed above.

Olmesartan
▼ Common: dizziness and respiratory infection.
▼ Less common: swelling of the arms and legs, weakness, rash, headache, diarrhea, upset stomach, kidney damage, heartburn, pain, muscle cramps, muscle aches, cough, stuffy nose, sinus problems, and vomiting.
▼ Rare: Rare side effects can occur in almost any part of the body. Contact your doctor if you experience any side effect not listed above.

Telmisartan
▼ Common: respiratory infection.
▼ Less common: dizziness, headache, fatigue, anxiety or nervousness, diarrhea, upset stomach, heartburn, nausea and vomiting, abdominal pain, back pain, muscle aches, cough, sinus irritation, sore throat, influenza, chest pain, urinary infection, rash, swelling in the arms or legs, and high blood pressure.
▼ Rare: Rare side effects can occur in almost any part of the body. Contact your doctor if you experience any side effect not listed above.

Valsartan
▼ Less common: dizziness, sleeplessness, headache, fatigue, diarrhea, upset stomach, heartburn, abdominal pain, joint pain, respiratory infection, cough, sore throat, sinus problems, runny nose, virus infection, and swelling.
▼ Rare: Rare side effects can occur in almost any part of the body. Contact your doctor if you experience any side effect not listed above.

Drug Interactions

- Alcohol and narcotic and barbiturate drugs may increase the blood-pressure-lowering effects, such as dizziness or fainting, of AII blockers.
- Telmisartan may slightly reduce warfarin blood levels, but not enough to require a change in warfarin dosage.
- Combining telmisartan and digoxin can increase digoxin blood levels by up to 50%, leading to possible drug side effects. This combination should be used with caution.
- Rifampin may reduce the effectiveness of losartan.
- Fluconazole may increase the effects of losartan.
- Combining an AII blocker and another blood-pressure-lowering drug, especially a diuretic, reduces blood pressure more efficiently than either drug used alone. People taking a diuretic who start an AII blocker may initially experience a rapid blood pressure drop and should start with a lower AII blocker dosage.
- Combining losartan with the diuretic hydrochlorothiazide can increase the risk of developing low blood potassium (hypokalemia). Your doctor should check your blood electrolytes periodically if you are taking this combination.

Food Interactions

For optimal effectiveness, take valsartan at least 1 hour before or 2 hours after meals. Other AII blockers can be taken with or without food.

Usual Dose

Candesartan
Adult: 8–32 mg once a day. Usual starting dosage is 16 mg a day.

Child: not recommended.

Eprosartan
Adult: 400–800 mg a day in one or two doses. Usual starting dosage is 600 mg.

Child: not recommended.

Irbesartan
Adult: 150 mg once a day to start, increasing to 300 mg once a day if necessary. A lower dosage (75 mg) may be prescribed for people who are dehydrated or salt-depleted.

Child: not recommended.

Losartan

Adult: 25–50 mg once a day to start, increasing gradually up to 100 mg in 1 or 2 doses a day.

Child (age 6 and over): 3 mg per lb. of body weight a day to start and then adjusted as necessary. Dosage not to exceed 100 mg per day.

Child (under age 6): not recommended.

Olmesartan

Adult: 20–40 mg a day. Usual starting dose is 20 mg a day.
Child: not recommended.

Telmisartan

Adult: 20–80 mg a day. Usual starting dosage is 40 mg a day.
Child: not recommended.

Valsartan

Adult: 40–320 mg a day. Usual starting dosage is 80–160 mg a day.

Child: not recommended.

Overdosage

Little is known about AII blocker overdose, although it could be fatal. The most likely overdose symptoms are very low blood pressure, dizziness, and rapid heartbeat. Overdose victims should be taken to a hospital emergency room. ALWAYS bring the prescription bottle or container.

Special Information

Avoid strenuous exercise and very hot weather because heavy sweating or dehydration can cause a rapid blood pressure drop.

People on dialysis who take telmisartan may become dizzy or faint when rising quickly from a sitting or lying position at the beginning of treatment.

Avoid over-the-counter diet pills, decongestants, and stimulants because they may contain ingredients that can raise blood pressure. People taking losartan should avoid using potassium supplements.

Call your doctor if you develop any of the following symptoms: dry mouth, thirst, weakness, tiredness, drowsiness, restlessness, confusion, seizures, muscle pains or cramps, muscular fatigue, dizziness or fainting, drastically reduced urine output, rapid heartbeat, and nausea or vomiting.

If you take an AII blocker once a day and forget a dose, take it as soon as you remember. If it is within 8 hours of your next dose, skip the one you forgot and continue with your regular schedule. If you take an AII blocker twice a day and forget a dose, take it as soon as you remember. If it is within 4 hours of your next dose, take 1 dose right away and another in 5 or 6 hours, then go back to your regular schedule. Never take a double dose.

Special Populations

Pregnancy/Breast-feeding: AII blockers should not be taken during the last 6 months of pregnancy because they can cause fetal injury or death. If necessary, you should take another drug for high blood pressure if you are or might be pregnant.

It is not known if AII blockers pass into breast milk, although they do in animal studies. Nursing mothers who must take an AII blocker should use infant formula.

Seniors: Seniors may take AII blockers without special precautions.

Brand Name

Anthelios SX Cream (an-THEL-e-ose)

Generic Ingredients

Avobenzone + Ecamsule + Octocrylene

Type of Drug

Sunscreen.

Prescribed For

Sunburn prevention.

General Information

Anthelios SX is an over-the-counter moisturizer used to help prevent sunburn and to help provide protection from UVA (short- and long-wave) and UVB rays.

Cautions and Warnings

Do not use this product if you are **allergic** or **sensitive** to any of its ingredients.

Do not apply this product to **broken or burned skin**.

Do not swallow this cream or apply it directly to your eye or to the inside of the mouth, nose or vagina.

Possible Side Effects

▼ Rare: Skin irritation or rash.

Drug Interactions

None known.

Food Interactions

None known.

Usual Dose

   Adult and Child (age 6 months and over): Apply evenly before sun exposure. Reapply as needed or after towel drying, swimming, or perspiring.

Overdosage

Call your local poison control center or hospital emergency room for more information. If you seek treatment, ALWAYS bring the bottle or container with you.

Special Information

One of the ingredients in this product, ecamsule, was approved for use in the US in June, 2007, though it has been available in Europe since 1993.

   Do not forget to reapply this product periodically.

Special Populations

Pregnancy/Breast-feeding: No information available.

Seniors: Seniors may use this product without special precaution.

Type of Drug

Antiemetics (5HT$_3$ Type)

Brand Names

Generic Ingredient: Alosetron
Lotronex

Generic Ingredient: Dolasetron
Anzemet

Generic Ingredient: Granisetron G
Kytril

Generic Ingredient: Ondansetron Ⓖ
Zofran   Zofran ODT

Prescribed For

Nausea and vomiting caused by chemotherapy and other cancer treatments and general anesthesia. Alosetron is prescribed only for women with severe irritable bowel syndrome (IBS) whose main symptom is diarrhea. Ondansetron is also prescribed for psychosis due to levadopa + carbidopa, bulimia, social anxiety disorder, and itching due to morphine treatment.

General Information

These drugs prevent nausea and vomiting by interfering with a form of the neurohormone serotonin (5HT) known as $5HT_3$. They block its effects in the part of the brain that controls vomiting and in the vagus nerve in the stomach and intestines. These drugs are very effective and often work in cases in which older antiemetics have failed. Aloestrin works against IBS by blocking the action of serotonin in the intestines. This reduces the cramping, abdominal discomfort, urgency, and diarrhea caused by IBS. Blood concentrations of alosetron are 30–50% higher in women than in men.

Cautions and Warnings

Do not use antiemetics if you are **allergic** or **sensitive** to any of their ingredients.

Serious and possibly fatal colitis and serious complications of constipation leading to hospitalization, blood transfusions, and surgery have developed in people taking alosetron. People with a history of **gastrointestinal difficulties** including chronic or severe constipation, colitis, intestinal obstruction, or diverticulitis should not take this drug.

People with **heart rhythm problems,** especially those taking diuretics and antiarrhythmic drugs, should be cautious about taking dolasetron.

People with **liver problems** need lower doses of alosetron and may consider using other drugs in this group.

These drugs should only be used when the risk of nausea and vomiting is relatively high.

Possible Side Effects

Alosetron

▼ Most common: constipation.

Possible Side Effects *(continued)*

▼ Common: nausea and abdominal or GI discomfort or pain.
▼ Rare: Rare side effects can occur in any part of the body. Contact your doctor if you experience any side effect not listed above.

Dolasetron

▼ Common: headache, low blood pressure, slowed heart rate, and dizziness.
▼ Less common: high blood pressure, abdominal pain, diarrhea, rapid heartbeat, fever or chills, and tiredness.
▼ Rare: blood in the urine; chest pain; kidney problems; painful or difficult urination; pain; severe stomach pain with nausea or vomiting; rash; hives; itching; swollen face, feet, or lower legs; and breathing difficulties. Contact your doctor if you experience any side effect not listed above.

Granisetron

▼ Most common: headache, constipation, weakness, and low white-blood-cell count.
▼ Common: abdominal pain, diarrhea, nausea, vomiting, appetite loss, chills, and anemia.
▼ Less common: dizziness, fever, anxiety, sleeplessness, hair loss, and low blood-platelet count.
▼ Rare: drug sensitivity reactions, chest pain, and fainting. Contact your doctor if you experience any side effect not listed above.

Ondansetron

▼ Most common: headache, feeling unwell, and constipation.
▼ Less common: anxiety, agitation, dizziness, fever, light-headedness, diarrhea, gynecological problems, itching, abnormal heart rhythms, and low blood pressure.

Drug Interactions

● Alosetron may reduce the amount of hydralazine, isoniazid, and procainamide in the blood.
● Fluvoxamine and alosetron should not be taken together.
● Ketoconazole may increase blood concentrations of alosetron by 30%.
● Combining rifampin and dolasetron may reduce the level of antiemetic in the blood.

- Blood levels of dolasetron may be increased when combined with cimetidine or atenolol.

Food Interactions

These drugs may be taken with or without food.

Usual Dose

Alosetron

Adult: 0.5 mg twice a day to start. Dosage may be increased to 1 mg twice a day if the lower dose is not working. Alosetron should be discontinued if adequate results are not seen after 4 weeks at 1 mg twice a day.

Dolasetron

Adult and Child (age 17 and over): a single dose of 100 mg.
Child (age 2–16): 0.8 mg per lb. of body weight, up to 100 mg.

Granisetron

Adult and Child (age 17 and over): 1 mg twice a day.
Child (age 2–16): not recommended.

Ondansetron

Adult and Child (age 12 and over): 8 mg twice a day. People with liver failure should take no more than 8 mg a day. A single 24-mg dose 30 minutes before starting chemotherapy may be recommended.
Child (age 4–11): 4 mg 3 times a day.
Child (age 3 and under): not recommended.

Overdosage

Symptoms may include severe constipation, temporary blindness, high blood pressure, fainting, and mild headache. Call your local poison control center or a hospital emergency room for more information. If you go for treatment, ALWAYS bring the prescription bottle or container.

Special Information

Call your doctor if you develop chest tightness, wheezing, breathing difficulties, chest pain, or any bothersome or persistent side effect.

Call your doctor at once and immediately stop taking alosetron if you develop constipation or symptoms of ischemic colitis including abdominal pain, cramps, nausea, vomiting, and bloody diarrhea.

Maintain good dental hygiene while taking these drugs. Chronic dry mouth can increase the risk of tooth decay and gum disease.

If you forget a dose, take it as soon as you remember. If it is almost time for your next dose, skip the dose you forgot and continue with your regular schedule. Missing more than 1 dose may increase the risk of vomiting.

To use Ondansetron ODT, make sure your hands are dry. Peel back the foil on a blister and gently remove the tablet. Do not push the tablet through the foil. Immediately place the tablet on top of the tongue, where it will dissolve in seconds, then swallow with saliva.

Special Populations

Pregnancy/Breast-feeding: There are no adequate studies of the effects of these drugs in pregnant women. When your doctor considers any of these drugs crucial, its potential benefits must be carefully weighed against its risks.

These drugs may pass into breast milk. Nursing mothers who must take any of these drugs should consider using infant formula.

Seniors: Seniors may take these drugs without special precaution, although elderly women taking alosetron may be at increased risk of serious constipation.

Type of Drug

Antihistamine Eyedrops

Brand Names

Generic Ingredient: Azelastine
Optivar

Generic Ingredient: Emedastine
Emadine

Generic Ingredient: Epinastine
Elestat

Generic Ingredient: Olopatadine [G]
Patanol

Generic Ingredient: Levocabastine
Livostin

Prescribed For

Eye itching due to allergy.

General Information

Azelastine, emedastine, and epinastine clear conjunctivitis (pink-eye) by preventing the release of chemicals from mast cells in the eye that cause allergic symptoms. They also work to minimize the response of nerve endings to any of these allergy-causing chemicals that might be present. Livostin only affects nerve endings to minimize the allergic response.

Cautions and Warnings

Do not use antihistamine eyedrops if you are **allergic** or **sensitive** to any of their ingredients.

Do not use these drugs to treat redness caused by contact lens irritation.

Possible Side Effects

Side effects are generally mild and subside as your body gets used to the medicine.

Azelastine
▼ Most common: burning or stinging sensation in the eyes, headache, and bitter taste in the mouth.
▼ Less common: asthma, conjunctivitis (pinkeye), difficulty breathing, eye pain, fatigue, flu-like symptoms, sore throat, itching, runny nose, and temporary blurring.

Emedastine
▼ Common: headache.
▼ Less common: mild burning or stinging of the eye, eye fatigue, itching of the eye, weakness, abnormal dreams, bad taste in the mouth, blurred vision, staining of the cornea, dry eyes, red eye, eye discomfort, sensation that something is in your eye, inflammation of the cornea, sinus irritation, rash, runny nose, and tearing.

Epinastine
▼ Most common: burning sensation in the eye and itching.
▼ Less common: headache, runny nose, sinus irritation, cough, and sore throat.

Possible Side Effects (continued)

Levocabastine
▼ Most common: mild stinging or burning in the eyes.
▼ Common: headache.
▼ Less common: dry mouth, visual disturbances, red eyes, tearing or discharge from the eyes, eye pain or dryness, swollen eyelids, fatigue, sore throat, cough, nausea, skin rash or redness, and breathing difficulty.

Food and Drug Interactions
None known.

Usual Dose
Azelastine
   Adult and Child (age 3 and over): 1 drop twice a day in the affected eye.

Emedastine
   Adult and Child (age 3 and over): 1 drop in the affected eye up to 4 times a day.

Epinastine
   Adult and Child (age 3 and over): 1 drop twice a day in the affected eye.

Levocabastine
   Adult and Child (age 12 and over): 1 drop 4 times a day.

Overdosage
Little is known about overdose of antihistamine eyedrops, but it is unlikely to lead to drug side effects. Accidental ingestion of either of these drugs is not likely to be severe because each bottle contains small amounts of active drug. Call your local poison center or hospital emergency room for more information. If you seek treatment, ALWAYS bring the prescription bottle or container.

Special Information
If you wear soft contact lenses and your eye is not red, you may wear your lenses during treatment. Wait at least 15 minutes after using these medicines before putting in your lenses.

   To avoid infection, do not touch the dropper tip to your finger, eyelid, or any other surface. Wait at least 5 minutes before using another eyedrop or eye ointment.

If you forget a dose, administer it as soon as you remember. If it is almost time for your next dose, skip the one you forgot and continue with your regular schedule. Do not take a double dose.

Special Populations

Pregnancy/Breast-feeding: These drugs can cause birth defects at extremely high oral doses in laboratory animals but there is no information on their effect in women. When these drugs are considered crucial by your doctor, their potential benefits must be carefully weighed against their risks.

Emedastine and levocabastine may pass into breast milk. It is not known if azelastine or epinastine pass into breast milk. Nursing mothers who must use antihistamine eyedrops should use infant formula.

Seniors: Seniors may use these drugs without special precaution.

Type of Drug

Antihistamine-Decongestant Combination Products

Brand Names

Generic Ingredients: Acrivastine + Pseudoephedrine
Semprex-D

Generic Ingredients: Azatadine + Pseudoephedrine
Trinalin Repetabs

Generic Ingredients: Brompheniramine + Pseudoephedrine Ⓖ

Allent	Brovex SR
Andehist NR Syrup *	Dimaphen Elixir *
BidHist-D	Dimetapp Cold & Allergy Elixir *
Brofed	Endafed
Bromadrine	Histex SR
Bromadrine PD	Iofed
Bromanate Elixir *	Iofed PD
Bromfed	J-Tan D PD *
Bromfed-PD	Lodrane *
Bromfenex	Lodrane 12 D
Bromfenex PD	Lodrane 24 D
Bromhist NR *	Lodrane D
Bromhist PD *	Lodrane LD

Lo-Hist 12
Lo-Hist LQ *
LoHist-PD
Q-Tapp *
Respahist

Rondec Drops*
Touro Allergy
ULTRAbrom
ULTRAbrom PD
Uni-Tex 120/10 ER

Generic Ingredients: Brompheniramine + Phenylephrine

Alacol *
Alenaze-D *
BroveX-D *
Dimetapp Cold & Allergy
   Chewable Tablets

J-Tan D *
Rhinabid
Rhinabid PD
VaZol-D *

Generic Ingredients: Carbinoxamine + Phenylephrine

Histamax D   Norel LA   XiraHist PD *

Generic Ingredients: Carbinoxamine + Pseudoephedrine Ⓖ

Andec
Andehist NR Drops
Carbaxefed *
Carbaxefed RF *
Carbic-D
Carbic-DS *
Carbiset
Carbiset TR
Carbodec
Carbodec TR
Carboxine-PSE
Cardec

Cardec-S
Coldec-D
Cordron-D *
Cydec
Hydro-Tussin CBX
Maldec
Palgic-D
Palgic-DC
Palgic-DS
Pediatex-D *
Sildec

Generic Ingredients: Cetirizine + Pseudoephedrine

Zyrtec-D 12-Hour

Generic Ingredients: Chlorpheniramine Maleate + Phenylephrine Hydrochloride

Actifed Cold and Allergy
Allerest PE
Cardec *
Ceron *
CP DEC *
Dallergy Drops
Dallergy JR *
Ed A-Hist

Histatab
NoHist
PD Hist D *
Phenabid *
Rescon JR
Rondec *
Rondex *
Sudafed PE

Generic Ingredients: Chlorpheniramine Maleate +
Pseudoephedrine 🅖

AccuHist
Aller-Chlor
Biohist-LA
Clorfed
Clorfed II
Colfed-A
Deconamine *
Deconamine SR
Deconomed SR
Hayfebrol
Histade
Histalet

Histex
Kronofed-A
Kronofed-A Jr.
ND Clear
Pediox Chewable
PSE CPM
QDall
RE2 + 30 *
Rescon-Ed
Sudafed Sinus & Allergy
Tibamine LA
Time-Hist

Generic Ingredients: Chlorpheniramine Maleate +
Phenyltoloxamine + Phenylephrine Hydrochloride

Chlorex A
Nalex-A *

NoHist A *
Rhinacon A

Generic Ingredients: Chlorpheniramine Polistirex +
Pseudoephedrine Polistirex

Sudal-12 *

Generic Ingredients: Chlorpheniramine Tannate + Pyrilamine
Tannate + Phenylephrine Tannate 🅖

AllerTan
AlleRx
Atrohist Pediatric
Chlorex-A12
Nalex-A12 *
Rhinatate
Rhinatate Pediatric
Rynatan

Rynatan-S Pediatric
Triotann
Triotann Pediatric
Triotann S
Triotann S Pediatric
Tri-Tannate Pediatric
Tritan

Generic Ingredients: Chlorpheniramine Tannate + Phenylephrine
Tannate

Dallergy JR Suspension *
Ed Chlor-PED
NuHist
PediaPhyl D *
PediaTan D *

P-Tann D *
Rhinatate-NF Pediatric
R-Tanna
Rynatan Pediatric

Generic Ingredients: Desloratadine + Pseudoephedrine
Clarinex-D 12-Hour   Clarinex-D 24-Hour

Generic Ingredients: Dexbrompheniramine + Pseudoephedrine
Dexaphen-SA   Drixoral Cold & Allergy
Drixomed

Generic Ingredients: Dexchlorpheniramine Maleate + Pseudoephedrine Hydrochloride
Hexafed

Generic Ingredients: Diphenhydramine Hydrochloride + Phenylephrine Hydrochloride
Benadryl-D Allergy & Sinus *
Children's Benadryl-D Allergy & Sinus *

Generic Ingredients: Diphenhydramine Tannate + Phenylephrine Tannate
DiphenMax D   Dytan-D   D-Tann

Generic Ingredients: Fexofenadine + Pseudoephedrine
Allegra-D 12-Hour   Allegra-D 24-Hour

Generic Ingredients: Loratadine + Pseudoephedrine
Alavert Allergy & Sinus D-12   Claritin-D 24-Hour
Claritin-D 12-Hour   Clear-Atadine D

Generic Ingredients: Promethazine + Phenylephrine Hydrochloride Ⓖ
Phenergan VC   Prometh VC Plain

Generic Ingredients: Pyrilamine Tannate + Phenylephrine Tannate
AllenVan-S   Ryna-12 S
Duonate-12   RY-T-12
K-Tan   Tanavan
K-Tan 4   V-Tann
R-Tanna 12   Viravan-T
Ryna-12

Generic Ingredients: Pyrilamine + Pseudoephedrine + Phenyltoloxamine + Pheniramine
Quadra-Hist D Pediatric

*Generic Ingredients: Triprolidine Hydrochloride +
Pseudoephedrine Hydrochloride*

Actifed	Genac
Allerfrim	SilaFed
Aprodine	Sudafed Sinus Nighttime

*Some products in this brand-name group are alcohol- or sugar-
free. Consult your pharmacist.*

Prescribed For

Sneezing, watery eyes, runny nose, itchy or scratchy throat, nasal
congestion, and other symptoms of the common cold, allergies,
and upper respiratory conditions.

General Information

The basic formula for each of these antihistamine-decongestant
combinations is the same: An antihistamine is used to relieve allergy symptoms and a decongestant to treat the symptoms of either a cold or allergy.

Most of these products are taken several times a day, while others are long-acting and are taken once or twice a day. Since nothing can cure a cold or allergy, the best you can hope to achieve
from a cold and allergy remedy is relief from symptoms.

Cautions and Warnings

Do not use antihistamines if you are **allergic** or **sensitive** to any
of their ingredients.

Antihistamines in these products may cause drowsiness. Decongestants may cause anxiety and nervousness and may interfere with sleep.

People with **narrow-angle glaucoma, prostate disease,** certain **stomach ulcers, bladder obstruction,** and those having
asthma attacks should not use these products.

A recent FDA panel recommended that pediatric use of antihistamines and decongestants should be banned for **children
under age 6**.

Possible Side Effects

▼ Most common: restlessness, nervousness, sleeplessness,
drowsiness, sedation, excitation, dizziness, poor coordination, and upset stomach.

Possible Side Effects *(continued)*

▼ Less common: low blood pressure, heart palpitations, rapid heartbeat and abnormal heart rhythms, chest pain, anemia, fatigue, confusion, tremors, headache, irritability, euphoria (feeling "high"), tingling or heaviness in the hands, tingling in the feet or legs, blurred or double vision, convulsions, hysterical reaction, ringing or buzzing in the ears, fainting, increase or decrease in appetite, nausea, vomiting, diarrhea or constipation, frequent urination, difficulty urinating, early menstrual periods, loss of sex drive, breathing difficulties, wheezing with chest tightness, stuffed nose, itching, rash, unusual sensitivity to the sun, chills, excessive perspiration, and dry mouth, nose, or throat.

Drug Interactions

- Combining these products with alcoholic beverages, anti-anxiety drugs, sedatives, or narcotic pain relievers may lead to excessive drowsiness or difficulty concentrating.
- Avoid these products if you are taking a monoamine oxidase inhibitor (MAOI) antidepressant or if you have stopped taking an MAOI in the past 14 days. The MAOI may cause a very rapid rise in blood pressure or increase side effects such as dry mouth and nose, blurred vision, and abnormal heart rhythms.
- The decongestant component of these products may interfere with the normal effects of blood-pressure-lowering medications and can aggravate diabetes, heart disease, hyperthyroid disease, high blood pressure, prostate disease, stomach ulcer, and urinary blockage.
- If your doctor has prescribed one of these products, do not self-medicate with an additional over-the-counter drug for the relief of cold symptoms. This combination may aggravate high blood pressure, heart disease, diabetes, or thyroid disease.

Food Interactions

These drugs are best taken on an empty stomach but may be taken with food if they upset your stomach.

Usual Dose

Dosages vary. Generally, these products are taken every 4–12 hours.

Overdosage

Symptoms of overdose are drowsiness, chills, dry mouth, fever, nausea, nervousness, irritability, rapid or irregular heartbeat, chest pain, and urinary difficulties. Most cases should be treated by inducing vomiting as soon as possible with ipecac syrup—available at any pharmacy. Then call your local poison control center for more information or take the victim to a hospital emergency room. ALWAYS bring the prescription bottle or container.

Special Information

Use extra caution while doing anything that requires concentration, such as driving a car or operating hazardous machinery.

Call your doctor if your side effects are severe or become intolerable.

If you forget to take a dose of your medication, take it as soon as you remember. If it is almost time for your next dose, skip the dose you forgot and continue with your regular schedule. Do not take a double dose.

Special Populations

Pregnancy/Breast-feeding: Animal studies suggest that some older antihistamines cause birth defects but the antihistamines in these products have not been proven harmful. If you are or might be pregnant, do not take any of these products without your doctor's knowledge.

Small amounts of antihistamine or decongestant pass into breast milk. Nursing mothers who must use these products should use infant formula.

Seniors: Seniors are more sensitive to the side effects of these medications.

Generic Name

Apraclonidine (ah-prah-KLON-ih-dene)

Brand Name

Iopidine

Type of Drug

Sympathomimetic.

Prescribed For

Post-surgical increases in eye pressure; also prescribed as additional short-term treatment in people who are using other glaucoma medicines.

General Information

Apraclonidine hydrochloride reduces both elevated and normal fluid pressure inside the eye and selectively blocks certain nerve endings without acting as a local anesthetic. The exact way it works is not known, but apraclonidine, like other drugs that reduce eye pressure, may work by decreasing the production of eye fluid. The drug starts to work within 1 hour after it is put into the eye and reaches its maximum effect in 3–5 hours.

Cautions and Warnings

Do not use apraclonidine if you are **allergic** or **sensitive** to any of its ingredients or to clonidine. This drug can cause an allergic-like reaction, including red eye, swelling of the lid and white of the eye, itching, burning, and the feeling of something in your eye. If this happens, stop using the drug and call your doctor.

Taking this drug with a **monoamine oxidase inhibitor (MAOI) antidepressant** may result in severe side effects—do not combine them.

Using this medicine with other eye-pressure-lowering drugs may not provide additional benefit: Other drugs work in the same way and a further effect may not be possible.

The ability of apraclonidine to lower eye pressure decreases over time. Most people continuously benefit for less than 1 month.

People with **kidney, heart, or vascular disease** should be monitored by their doctors while taking this medicine.

Apraclonidine has been associated with depression. People with **depression** or a history of depression should be monitored by their doctors while taking this medication.

Possible Side Effects

▼ Most common: eye redness, dry eye, discharge from the eye, tearing, eye discomfort, lid swelling, feeling of something in your eye, itching, dry nose, changes in taste, dizziness, drowsiness, dry mouth, headache, and weakness.

Possible Side Effects *(continued)*

▼ Less common: blanching of the eye; lid crusting; abnormal vision; eye pain; runny nose; sore throat; worsening asthma; constipation and nausea; abnormal heart rhythms; chest pain; difficulty sleeping; depression; body pain; nervousness; distorted sense of smell; decreased coordination; pain, numbness, or tingling in the hands or feet; and rash.

Drug Interactions

- Apraclonidine can reduce pulse and blood pressure. If you are also taking drugs to treat high blood pressure or other cardiovascular drugs, check your pulse and blood pressure.
- MAOI antidepressants can slow the breakdown of apraclonidine and increase the risk of drug side effects. This combination should be avoided. You should also wait 14 days after stopping an MAOI before starting apraclonidine.

Usual Dose

Adult: 1–2 drops in the affected eye 3 times a day.

Overdosage

Exaggerated side effects, especially those that affect the nervous system, are symptoms of overdose. Call your local poison control center for more information. ALWAYS take the prescription bottle or container with you if you go to the emergency room.

Special Information

Apraclonidine can cause dizziness and tiredness. Be careful doing anything that requires concentration, coordination, or alertness while taking this medication.

To prevent infection, do not touch the dropper tip to your finger or eyelid. Wait 5 minutes before using any other eyedrop or ointment.

Remove contact lenses before applying apraclonidine and wait 15 minutes before reinserting them.

If you forget a dose of apraclonidine, take it as soon as you remember. If it is almost time for your next dose, take one dose as soon as you remember and then go back to your regular schedule. Do not take a double dose.

Special Populations

Pregnancy/Breast-feeding: In animal studies, apraclonidine was toxic to embryos when given by mouth. It should be used with caution during pregnancy.

It is not known if this drug passes into breast milk. Nursing mothers who must take this medication should use infant formula.

Seniors: Seniors may use this medicine without special precautions.

Generic Name

Aprepitant (ah-PRE-pih-tant)

Brand Name

Emend

Type of Drug

Antinauseant and antiemetic (an agent that prevents or relieves nausea and vomiting).

Prescribed For

Acute and delayed nausea and vomiting associated with chemotherapy, and prevention of nausea and vomiting following anesthesia.

General Information

Aprepitant works against nausea and vomiting by selectively inhibiting the substance P/neurokinin 1 (NK 1) receptor. This is a unique approach to nausea therapy and it complements other nausea therapies, such as corticosteroids and 5-HT receptor antagonists that should be used together with aprepitant. Aprepitant is broken down in the liver.

Cautions and Warnings

Do not take aprepitant if you are **allergic** or **sensitive** to any of its ingredients.

Aprepitant should be used with caution if you have **severe liver disease.** People with mild to moderate liver disease can tolerate the drug.

Aprepitant is not intended for normal nausea and vomiting in those not undergoing chemotherapy treatment or for chronic continuous therapy. It should not be used for the chronic management of nausea and vomiting.

Possible Side Effects

▼ Most common: fatigue, nausea, appetite loss, hiccups, and constipation or diarrhea.
▼ Common: dizziness, dehydration, heartburn, headache, and vomiting.
▼ Less common: abdominal pain, fever, upset stomach, stomach pains, ringing or buzzing in the ears, mucous membrane swelling, and sleeplessness.
▼ Rare: Rare side effects can occur in almost any part of the body. Contact your doctor if you experience any side effect not listed above.

Drug Interactions

- Aprepitant is often given with cancer chemotherapy drugs that are broken down by the same enzymes. This combination might be expected to raise the amount of chemotherapeutic in the blood, but this was not a problem in clinical studies of the drug. Drugs that may have this effect, and should be used with caution, include docetaxel, paclitaxel, etoposide, irinotecan, ifosfamide, imatinib, vinorelbine, vinblastine, and vincristine.
- Aprepitant may slow the breakdown of astemizole, cisapride, pimozide, or terfenadine, leading to serious drug side effects. Do not combine these medicines with aprepitant.
- Aprepitant increases blood levels of midazolam, increasing the chances for drug side effects. Levels of other benzodiazepine sedatives (such as alprazolam and triazolam) may rise as well.
- Clarithromycin, diltiazem, itraconazole, ketoconazole, nefazodone, nelfinavir, ritonavir, and troleandomycin may raise blood levels of aprepitant, increasing the chances for drug side effects and toxicity. These drugs should be combined with caution.
- Amiodarone, carbamazepine, nevirapine, phenobarbital, phenytoin, rifampin, and St. John's wort may reduce the effectiveness of aprepitant.
- Aprepitant can increase the amount of corticosteroid drug that is absorbed into your blood. Oral dexamethasone and methylprednisolone doses should be decreased by half when combined with aprepitant.

- Aprepitant may decrease blood levels of tolbutamide and phenytoin when given concurrently, reducing their effectiveness.
- Blood levels of the hormones ethinyl estradiol and norethindrone—used in many hormonal contraceptive products—can be reduced, compromising the effectiveness of these products. Use a non-hormonal contraceptive method while taking aprepitant.
- Blood levels of aprepitant and paroxetine are both reduced by about 25% when they are combined.
- The breakdown of warfarin may be increased by aprepitant, reducing the blood thinner's effectiveness. If you take warfarin and have to use aprepitant, your doctor should closely monitor your warfarin in the 2-week period (especially days 7–10) after the beginning of each aprepitant cycle.

Food Interactions

This drug may be taken without regard to food or meals.

Usual Dose

Adult: 125 mg 1 hour before starting chemotherapy, followed by 80 mg on the 2 days following chemotherapy. Aprepitant should be used in combination with a corticosteroid (such as dexamethasone) and a 5-HT_3 receptor antagonist (such as ondansetron).

Child: not recommended.

Overdosage

There is limited information about aprepitant overdose, but drowsiness and headache may occur. Overdose victims should be taken to a hospital emergency room. ALWAYS bring the prescription bottle or container.

Special Information

Aprepitant is given in a 3-day cycle. Take the first dose 1 hour before chemotherapy. Take the next 2 doses on the morning of the 2 days following your chemotherapy treatment.

Special Populations

Pregnancy/Breast-feeding: While animal studies of aprepitant revealed no adverse effects on a developing fetus, there is no information on how this drug will affect pregnant women and it should be used only if it is clearly needed. This drug should only be used during pregnancy after carefully weighing its potential benefits against its risks.

Aprepitant passes into milk in animal studies. Nursing mothers who must take it should consider using infant formula.

Seniors: Seniors may be more sensitive to the effects of aprepitant, but dosage adjustments are not needed.

Aricept see Cholinesterase Inhibitors, page 237

Generic Name

Aripiprazole (ah-rih-PIP-rah-zole)

Brand Names

Abilify   Abilify Discmelt

Type of Drug

Antipsychotic.

Prescribed For

Schizophrenia, bipolar disorder, and major depression.

General Information

Aripiprazole is a new type of antipsychotic that works on serotonin and dopamine receptors in the brain. Unlike other newer antipsychotics that only decrease dopamine, it may both increase and decrease dopamine, targeting specific areas of the brain where the neurotransmitter is too plentiful or too reduced. However, the exact way it works is not known.

The effectiveness of aripiprazole was established by studying hospitalized schizophrenics for 4–6 weeks, and later studies also proved its effectiveness for 6 months or beyond.

Cautions and Warnings

Do not take aripiprazole if you are **allergic** or **sensitive** to any of its ingredients.

Aripiprazole has been associated with increased mortality in seniors with **dementia** or **Alzheimer's disease**. The specific causes of death related to atypical antipsychotic drugs were either due to a heart-related event or infection, mostly pneumonia.

People taking this medicine have developed high blood sugar and diabetes. People with a diagnosis of **high blood sugar levels** or **diabetes** should have their blood sugar levels checked regularly while taking aripiprazole. People with a family history of diabetes or other diabetes risk factors should be tested periodically during treatment. Others should be monitored for symptoms of diabetes (increased thirst, increased food consumption, increased urination, and fatigue).

People with **liver or kidney disease** may have higher blood levels of aripiprazole than healthy people, but this is not a reason to adjust the drug dose.

A serious set of side effects known as neuroleptic malignant syndrome (NMS) may occur while taking aripiprazole. Symptoms include high fever, convulsions, difficult or fast breathing, rapid heartbeat, rapid or irregular pulse or blood pressure, increased sweating, muscle rigidity, and mental changes. NMS can be fatal and requires immediate medical attention. This condition has been associated with most antipsychotic medicines.

Tardive dyskinesia (a group of severe side effects associated with antipsychotic and other drugs) may occur while taking aripiprazole and is often considered a reason to stop taking this drug. Symptoms include lip smacking or puckering, puffing of the cheeks, rapid or worm-like movements of the tongue, uncontrolled chewing motions, and uncontrolled arm or leg movements. Symptoms can increase with the length and dosage of antipsychotic drug therapy and may become permanent. Report any of these side effects to your doctor.

Aripiprazole can cause dizziness or fainting when rising from a sitting or lying position, especially when people start taking the drug.

Seizures occur in a small number of people taking aripiprazole. It should be taken with care if you have had or are at increased risk of seizures.

Avoid exposure to **extreme heat**. Antipsychotics can upset your body's temperature-regulating mechanism, making you more prone to heatstroke.

Swallowing problems and inhaling food can be a problem with all antipsychotics, including aripiprazole.

Suicide is a danger with all antipsychotics. To reduce the possibility of possible overdose, people taking this drug should have no more than a 30-day supply of medication at any one time.

Possible Side Effects

In studies of aripiprazole, reported side effects were similar in people taking aripiprazole and those taking an inactive placebo (sugar pill) medicine.

▼ Most common: headache, nausea, vomiting, constipation, anxiety, lightheadedness, tiredness, sleeplessness, and an uncontrollable feeling of restlessness.

▼ Common: weakness and rash.

▼ Less common: fever, tremors, runny nose, cough, blurred vision, abnormal heart rhythms, and weight gain.

▼ Rare: Rare side effects can occur in almost any part of the body. Contact your doctor if you experience any side effect not listed above.

Drug Interactions

- Carbamazepine reduces blood levels of aripiprazole. If carbamazepine is added to aripiprazole treatment, the dose of aripiprazole should be doubled. Aripiprazole dosage should be reduced to normal levels when carbamazepine is stopped.
- Aripiprazole has the potential to increase the effects of certain drugs used to treat high blood pressure.
- Fluoxetine, ketoconazole, paroxetine, and quinidine increase blood levels of aripiprazole. If any of these drugs are combined with aripiprazole, the dosage of aripiprazole should be reduced in half until the other drug is stopped.
- Other drugs often associated with drug interactions (such as dextromethorphan, famotidine, lithium, omeprazole, valproate, and warfarin) are not a problem with aripiprazole.

Food Interactions

This drug may be taken without regard to food or meals.

Usual Dose

Adult: 10–15 mg once a day.
Child: not recommended.

Overdosage

Symptoms include tiredness and vomiting. Take the victim to a hospital emergency room. ALWAYS bring the prescription bottle or container.

Special Information

Aripiprazole may cause drowsiness. Use caution when doing anything that requires intense concentration, like driving or operating machinery.

Avoid alcoholic beverages while taking aripiprazole.

If you get dizzy while taking aripiprazole, avoid sudden changes in posture and avoid climbing stairs.

Do not open the blister pack until you are ready to take aripiprazole. Do not push the tablet through the foil but instead peel the foil back. Handle the tablet with clean, dry hands.

If you forget to take a dose of aripiprazole, take it as soon as you remember and continue with your regular dose on the next day. Tell your doctor or pharmacist if you forget more than one dose of aripiprazole. Do not take a double dose of this medication unless advised to do so by your doctor.

Be sure to tell your doctor about any other medicines you are taking, including over-the-counter remedies.

Special Populations

Pregnancy/Breast-feeding: This medication caused birth defects in animal studies. When this drug is considered crucial by your doctor, its potential benefits must be carefully weighed against its risks. Women who are or might be pregnant should talk with their doctor before taking aripiprazole.

Aripiprazole passes into breast milk. Nursing mothers who must take it should use infant formula.

Seniors: Seniors eliminate 20% less aripiprazole than younger adults, but there is no need for dosage adjustments.

Generic Names

Aspirin, Buffered Aspirin (AS-prin) Ⓖ

Brand Names

There are many brand-name aspirin products, most of which are available over the counter. Check with your pharmacist about which specific brands are available buffered or with antacids.

Type of Drug

Analgesic and anti-inflammatory agent.

Prescribed For

Mild to moderate pain, fever, arthritis, and inflammation of bones, joints, or other body tissues. People who have had a stroke or transient ischemic attack (TIA)—oxygen shortage to the brain—may have aspirin prescribed to reduce the risk of having another such attack. Aspirin may also be prescribed as an anticoagulant (blood-thinning) drug in people with unstable angina and to protect against heart attack. Aspirin has a definite beneficial effect if it is taken as soon as possible after having a heart attack.

General Information

Aspirin may be the closest thing we have to a wonder drug. It has been used for more than a century for pain and fever relief and is now used for its effect on the blood as well.

Aspirin is the standard against which all other drugs are compared for relieving pain and for reducing inflammation. Chemically, aspirin is a member of the group of drugs called salicylates. Other salicylates include sodium salicylate, sodium thiosalicylate, choline salicylate, and magnesium salicylate (trilisate). These drugs are no more effective than regular aspirin, although two of them—choline salicylate and magnesium salicylate—may be a little less irritating to the stomach. They are all more expensive than aspirin.

Aspirin reduces fever by causing the blood vessels in the skin to open, allowing heat to leave the body more rapidly. Its effects on pain and inflammation are thought to be related to its ability to prevent the manufacture of complex body hormones called prostaglandins. Of all the salicylates, aspirin has the greatest effect on prostaglandin production.

Many people find that they can take buffered aspirin but not regular aspirin. The addition of antacids to aspirin can be important to people who must take large doses of aspirin for chronic arthritis or other conditions. In many cases, aspirin is the only effective drug and can be tolerated only with the antacids present.

Cautions and Warnings

Do not take aspirin if you are **allergic** or **sensitive** to any of its ingredients, or to nonsteroidal anti-inflammatory drugs (NSAIDs) such as indomethacin, sulindac, ibuprofen, fenoprofen, naproxen, tolmetin, and meclofenamate sodium or to products containing tartrazine (a commonly used orange dye and food coloring). People with **asthma, a history of hives,** or **nasal polyps** are more likely to be allergic to aspirin.

Reye's syndrome is a life-threatening condition characterized by vomiting and stupor or dullness and may develop in children with influenza (flu) or chickenpox that is treated with aspirin or other salicylates. Up to 30% of people who develop Reye's syndrome can die, and permanent brain damage is possible in those who survive. Because of this, authorities advise against giving **children under age 16** aspirin or another salicylate, especially those with **chickenpox** or **flu**; acetaminophen should be given instead.

People with **liver damage** should avoid aspirin.

Alcoholic beverages may worsen the stomach irritation caused by aspirin. Alcohol increases the risk of aspirin-related ulcers.

Stop taking aspirin if you develop dizziness, hearing loss, or ringing or buzzing in your ears.

Aspirin interferes with normal blood clotting and should therefore be avoided for 1 week **before surgery**. Ask for your surgeon or dentist's recommendation before taking aspirin for pain after surgery.

Aspirin should not be taken by people with **hemophilia** or **bleeding ulcers**, or those who are in a state of **bleeding**.

Possible Side Effects

▼ Most common: nausea, upset stomach, heartburn, loss of appetite, and small amounts of blood in the stool.

▼ Less common: hives, rashes, liver damage, fever, thirst, and visual difficulties. Aspirin may contribute to the formation of stomach ulcers and bleeding. People who are allergic to aspirin and those with a history of nasal polyps, asthma, or rhinitis may experience breathing difficulty and a stuffed nose.

Drug Interactions

- People taking anticoagulant (blood-thinning) drugs should avoid aspirin because it increases the effect of the anticoagulant.
- Aspirin may increase the possibility of stomach ulcer when taken together with alcoholic beverages.
- Aspirin will counteract the uric-acid-eliminating effect of probenecid and sulfinpyrazone. Aspirin may counteract the blood-pressure-lowering effect of ACE inhibitor and beta-blocking drugs. Aspirin may also counteract the effects of some diuretics in people with liver or kidney disease.

- Aspirin may increase blood levels of methotrexate and of valproic acid when taken with either of these drugs, leading to increased chances of drug toxicity. Mixing aspirin and nitroglycerin tablets may lead to an unexpected drop in blood pressure.
- Do not take aspirin with an NSAID. There is no benefit to the combination, and the chance of side effects—especially stomach irritation—is vastly increased.
- Coadministration of aspirin and corticosteroids decreases blood levels of aspirin.
- Urinary acidifiers such as ammonium chloride, ascorbic acid, and methionine may increase the effects of aspirin.
- Large aspirin doses (2000 mg a day or more) can lower blood sugar. This can be a problem in people with diabetes who take insulin or oral antidiabetes drugs to control their condition.

Food Interactions

Because aspirin can cause upset stomach and bleeding, take each dose with food, milk, or a glass of water.

Usual Dose

Adult

Aches, pains, and fever: 325–500 mg every 4 hours; 650 mg every 4–6 hours; or 1000 mg every 6 hours.

Arthritis and rheumatic conditions: up to 5400 mg a day in divided doses. Rheumatic fever, up to 7800 mg a day in divided doses.

Heart attack prevention, stroke, or TIA: 80–325 mg a day or 325 mg every 2 days. Some people may need as much as 1000 mg a day.

Child (under age 16): not recommended because of the risk of Reye's syndrome (see "Cautions and Warnings").

Overdosage

Aspirin may be lethal for adults in overdoses of 30 regular-strength tablets—325 mg each—or 20 maximum-strength tablets—500 mg. Aspirin may be lethal for children in overdoses of 12 regular-strength tablets or 8 maximum-strength tablets.

Aspirin is a commonly used ingredient in many over-the-counter (OTC) medications. Always check the list of ingredients when using more than one OTC medication to ensure that the combined dosage is within guidelines and to avoid accidental overdose.

Symptoms of mild overdose are rapid and deep breathing, nausea, vomiting, dizziness, ringing or buzzing in the ears, flushing, sweating, thirst, headache, drowsiness, diarrhea, and rapid heartbeat.

Severe overdose may cause fever, excitement, confusion, convulsions, liver or kidney failure, coma, and bleeding.

The initial treatment of aspirin overdose involves inducing vomiting to remove any drug remaining in the stomach. Further treatment depends on how the situation develops and what must be done to maintain the patient. Do not induce vomiting until you have spoken with your doctor or poison control center. If in doubt, go to a hospital emergency room. ALWAYS bring the aspirin bottle or container.

Special Information

Contact your doctor if you develop continuous stomach pain or ringing or buzzing in the ears.

Do not use an aspirin product if it has a strong odor of vinegar. This is an indication that the product has started to break down in the bottle.

Do not crush or chew a sustained-release preparation of aspirin.

Check with your doctor if pain lasts more than 10 days, if pain worsens, or redness or swelling develop. Also, report a fever that persists for longer than 3 days.

If you are taking aspirin regularly report to your doctor if you notice a ringing or buzzing in your ear or experience severe or continuing headache.

If you forget to take a dose of aspirin, take it as soon as you remember. If it is almost time for your next dose, skip the dose you forgot and continue with your regular schedule. Do not take a double dose.

Special Populations

Pregnancy/Breast-feeding: Check with your doctor before taking any aspirin-containing product during pregnancy. Aspirin may cause bleeding problems in the fetus during the last 2 weeks of pregnancy. Taking aspirin during the last 3 months of pregnancy may extend the length of pregnancy, prolong labor, and lead to a low-birth-weight infant. It can also cause bleeding in the mother before, during, or after delivery. Anemia may also result from taking aspirin during pregnancy.

Aspirin passes into breast milk, but has not caused any problems in nursing babies. Nursing mothers should speak to their doctors before using aspirin.

Seniors: Aspirin, especially in larger doses that a senior may take for arthritis and rheumatic conditions, may be irritating to the stomach. Seniors with liver disease should not use aspirin.

Generic Name

Atazanavir (at-ah-ZAN-ah-veer)

Brand Name
Reyataz

Type of Drug
Protease inhibitor.

Prescribed For
Advanced human immunodeficiency virus (HIV) infection.

General Information
Atazanavir is a member of the group of anti-HIV drugs called protease inhibitors, which is an important part of the multidrug "cocktail" responsible for gains in the fight against acquired immunodeficiency syndrome (AIDS). These drugs work at the end of the HIV reproduction process, when an enzyme known as protease "cuts" proteins into strands of exactly the correct size to duplicate HIV. Protease inhibitors prevent the mature HIV virus from being formed by inhibiting this cutting process. Proteins cut to the wrong length or those that remain uncut are inactive.

Protease inhibitors are always taken with 1 or 2 nucleoside antiviral drugs such as efavirenz, emtricitabine, lamivudine, tenofovir, or zidovudine (AZT). Protease inhibitors have revolutionized HIV management because, when taken with other antivirals, they reduce the amount of HIV virus in the bloodstream to levels that are often undetectable by current methods such as CD4 cell (immune system cell) counts and viral load (amount of virus in the blood) measurements. Multiple-drug therapy has changed the view of HIV from a fatal disease to a manageable chronic illness.

This drug is broken down in the liver. People with mild to moderate liver disease may have more atazanavir in their bloodstream and require a lower dose of this medicine.

Cautions and Warnings

Do not take this drug if you are **allergic** or **sensitive** to it.

If a serious toxic reaction occurs while taking atazanavir, you should stop taking it until your doctor can determine the cause or until the reaction resolves itself. Then treatment can be resumed.

This drug can cause jaundice (yellow discoloration of the skin or whites of the eyes). Use caution if you have moderate **liver disease**. People with severe liver disease should not take atazanavir.

Atazanavir may raise blood sugar levels, worsen **diabetes**, or trigger latent diabetes. People with diabetes who take atazanavir may need to adjust the dosage of their antidiabetes medication.

HIV virus may become resistant to atazanavir or other protease inhibitors. For this reason it is essential that you take atazanavir exactly according to your doctor's directions.

People with **hemophilia** have experienced bleeding while taking this drug.

Atazanavir causes changes in heart conduction, as shown on an electrocardiogram. People with **AV heart block**, a condition affecting the heart's conduction system, should use this drug with caution.

Atazanavir may cause the redistribution or accumulation of body fat, leading to buffalo hump, breast enlargement, abnormal thinness, or a round, moon-shaped face. The long-term effects of this are not known.

Possible Side Effects

Most side effects are mild. Other side effects become more prominent when atazanavir is taken together with antiretroviral drugs; these include weakness, muscle pain, and mouth ulcers.

▼ Most common: nausea and headache.

▼ Common: vomiting, diarrhea, abdominal pain, rash, infection, drowsiness, insomnia, and jaundice (yellow discoloration of the skin or whites of the eyes).

▼ Less common: fever, fat accumulation, joint pain, depression, dizziness, and tingling or other unusual sensation in the arms, hands, legs, or feet.

Possible Side Effects *(continued)*

▼ Rare: Rare side effects can occur in almost any part of the body. Contact your doctor if you develop any side effect not listed above.

Drug Interactions

- Rifampin, proton pump inhibitors, and St. John's wort substantially reduce atazanavir blood levels. Do not combine these drugs.
- Nevirapine may reduce the effects of atazanavir; they should not be taken together.
- Cimetidine, famotidine, and ranitidine can also reduce atazanavir blood levels. Separate these drugs from atazanavir by at least 12 hours.
- Both atazanavir and indinavir cause elevated levels of bilirubin in the blood. Do not combine these medicines.
- Atazanavir increases levels of cisapride, ergot drugs, irinotecan (an anticancer drug), midazolam, pimozide, and triazolam leading to potentially serious drug toxicities. These drugs should not be combined with atazanavir.
- Combining atazanavir with the antibiotic clarithromycin may lead to an increased chance of clarithromycin-related cardiac toxicity. Clarithromycin dose should be halved.
- Atazanavir may increase side effects of the statin-type blood cholesterol drugs. Do not take this drug with atorvastatin, lovastatin, or simvastatin. Other statins may not be as affected because of how they are broken down in the body.
- If you also take other buffered medications or use antacids, take atazanavir with food, 1 hour before or 2 hours after you take the other medications.
- If you must take efavirenz and atazanavir, your doctor should also be prescribing ritonavir to increase the effectiveness of atazanavir.
- Atazanavir can increase blood levels of the hormones in contraceptive drugs. Your doctor should prescribe the lowest effective dose to avoid undesirable hormone side effects.
- Atazanavir may raise blood levels of amiodarone, calcium channel blockers, cyclosporine, lidocaine, quinidine, rifabutin, sirolimus, tacrolimus, tricyclic-type antidepressants, and warfarin. It may be necessary for your doctor to reduce drug

dosage by as much as half to avoid drug side effects if you start taking atazanavir.

- Protease inhibitors, including atazanavir, may drastically increase sildenafil, vardenafil, and taldenafil blood levels, increasing the risk of side effects including low blood pressure, visual changes, and persistent, painful erection. A lower dose may be required.
- Atazanavir should be used with caution in people taking atenolol. Serious cardiac adverse events may occur.
- Prolonged or increased sedation or breathing difficulties may occur if atazanavir is coadministered with benzodiazepines.

Food Interactions

Take atazanavir with a full meal. The amount of atazanavir absorbed into the blood is vastly reduced when it is taken on an empty stomach, thus negating its antiviral effects.

Usual Dose

Adult: 300–400 mg daily, taken with food. Patients with moderate liver disease should take only 300 mg a day.

Child (under age 16): consult your doctor.

Overdosage

A drug overdose may cause cardiac problems. Possible overdose symptoms may include yellowing of the skin or whites of the eyes. Take the victim to a hospital emergency room for evaluation and treatment. ALWAYS bring the prescription bottle or container.

Special Information

Atazanavir does not cure HIV infection or AIDS. It will not prevent you from transmitting the HIV virus to another person; you must still practice safe sex. You may still develop opportunistic infections or other illnesses associated with advanced HIV disease. The long-term effects of this drug are not known.

Call your doctor if you become dizzy or lightheaded. This could be a sign that the drug is affecting your heart.

Take this medication exactly according to your doctor's instructions. Skipping doses of atazanavir increases the risk that you will become resistant to the drug. It should be taken after meals with your nucleoside antiviral drug. If you forget a dose of atazanavir, take it as soon as you remember and continue with your regular schedule. Do not take a double dose.

Special Populations

Pregnancy/Breast-feeding: While animal studies of atazanavir reveal minor damage to the fetus at double the human dosage, this drug should only be used during pregnancy after carefully weighing its potential benefits against its risks. The company making atazanavir has established a registry to gather information on pregnant women who take this drug.

It is not known if atazanavir passes into breast milk. Nursing mothers with HIV should always use infant formula, regardless of whether they take this drug, to avoid transmitting the virus to their child.

Seniors: Seniors can take this drug without special precaution.

Generic Name

Atenolol (ah-TEN-uh-lol) Ⓖ

Brand Name
Tenormin

Combination Products
Generic Ingredients: Atenolol + Chlorthalidone Ⓖ
Tenoretic

The information in this profile also applies to the following drug:

Generic Ingredient: Nebivolol
Bystolic

Type of Drug
Beta-adrenergic blocking agent.

Prescribed For
Atenolol alone or in combination is prescribed for high blood pressure, abnormal heart rhythms, angina pectoris, and prevention of second heart attack and migraine. It is also used to treat alcohol withdrawal, stage fright, and other anxieties. Nebivolol is currently approved only to treat high blood pressure. Both are used together with other blood-pressure-lowering medications.

General Information
Atenolol is one of many beta-adrenergic blocking drugs, or beta blockers and primarily blocks the beta$_1$ receptor. Nebivolol blocks

both the beta₁ and beta₂ receptors when taken at high doses by people whose liver breaks down the drug more slowly than average. These drugs interfere with the action of adrenaline and other chemicals in the body that affect many body functions. Individual beta blockers have different characteristics that can make them more suitable for certain conditions or people.

When used to treat high blood pressure, atenolol may be used either alone or concurrently with other antihypertensive drugs, particularly with a thiazide-type diuretic.

Cautions and Warnings

Do not take these drugs if you are **allergic** or **sensitive** to any of their ingredients or to other beta blockers. People with a severe allergy to any substance may be more sensitive to that allergen while taking a beta blocker.

People with **angina** who take these medicines for high blood pressure risk aggravating their angina if they suddenly stop taking the drug. These people should have their drug dosage reduced gradually over 1–2 weeks.

Atenolol should not be used by those with **slow heartbeat**, moderate to severe **heart block** (a condition affecting the heart's conduction system), **congestive heart failure** unless it is due to a quickened heart rate that can be treated with atenolol, or **acute heart failure**.

Atenolol and nebivolol should be used with caution if you have **liver or kidney disease**, because your ability to eliminate these drugs from your body may be impaired. Dose adjustments may be needed.

These drugs reduce the amount of blood the heart pumps. This reduction in blood flow may aggravate the condition of people with **poor circulation** or **circulatory disease**.

If you are undergoing **major surgery**, your doctor may want you to stop taking these drugs at least 2 days before surgery.

If you have **pheochromocytoma** (adrenal gland tumor), use atenolol with caution.

Atenolol should be used with caution in those with **chronic bronchitis**, **emphysema**, or other nonallergic bronchospastic diseases.

People with a history of **severe anaphylactic reaction** to allergens may be unresponsive to usual doses of epinephrine while taking beta blockers.

Possible Side Effects

Atenolol

Side effects are relatively uncommon and usually mild; they usually develop early in the course of treatment and are rarely a reason to stop taking atenolol.

▼ Most common: impotence.

▼ Less common: unusual tiredness or weakness, slow heartbeat, heart failure (symptoms include swelling of the legs, ankles, or feet), dizziness, breathing difficulties, bronchospasm, depression, confusion, anxiety, nervousness, sleeplessness, disorientation, short-term memory loss, emotional instability, cold hands and feet, constipation, diarrhea, nausea, vomiting, upset stomach, increased sweating, urinary difficulties, cramps, blurred vision, rash, hair loss, stuffy nose, facial swelling, itching, chest pain, back or joint pain, colitis, drug allergy (symptoms include fever and sore throat), and liver toxicity.

▼ Rare: lupus erythematosus (chronic condition affecting the body's connective tissue). Contact your doctor if you experience any side effect not listed above.

Nebivolol

Side effects increase with rising dosage and are generally mild.

▼ Common: headache.

▼ Less common: fatigue, dizziness, diarrhea, nausea, sleeplessness, chest pain, slow heart beat, breathing difficulty, rash, swelling in the legs and arms.

▼ Rare: weakness, abdominal pain, high blood cholesterol and uric acid levels, and tingling in the hands or feet. Contact your doctor if you experience any side effect not listed above.

Drug Interactions

- Atenolol may interact with surgical anesthetics to increase the risk of heart problems during surgery. Some anesthesiologists recommend gradually stopping the drug by 2 days before surgery.
- Atenolol may interfere with the normal signs of low blood sugar and with oral antidiabetic drugs.

- Atenolol increases the blood-pressure-lowering effects of other blood-pressure-reducing agents, including clonidine, guanabenz, and reserpine; and calcium channel blockers, such as nifedipine.
- Aspirin-containing drugs, indomethacin, and sulfinpyrazone may interfere with the blood-pressure-lowering effect of atenolol.
- Cocaine may reduce the effectiveness of all beta blockers.
- Atenolol may worsen the problem of cold hands and feet associated with taking ergot alkaloids, used to treat migraine. Gangrene is a possibility in people taking both an ergot and atenolol.
- Atenolol will counteract thyroid hormone replacements.
- Calcium channel blockers, diphenhydramine, flecainide, hydralazine, contraceptive drugs, propafenone, haloperidol, phenothiazine sedatives—molindone and others—quinolone antibacterials, and quinidine may increase the amount of atenolol in the bloodstream and lead to increased atenolol effects.
- Atenolol should not be taken within 2 weeks of taking a monoamine oxidase inhibitor (MAOI) antidepressant.
- Cimetidine increases the amount of atenolol absorbed into the bloodstream from oral tablets.
- Atenolol may interfere with the effectiveness of some anti-asthma drugs, including theophylline and aminophylline, and especially ephedrine and isoproterenol.
- Combining atenolol with phenytoin or digitalis drugs may result in excessive slowing of the heart, possibly causing heart block (disruption of the electrical impulses that control heart rate).
- If you stop smoking while taking atenolol, your dose may have to be reduced because your liver will break down the drug more slowly.
- Aluminum salts, barbiturates, calcium salts, cholestyramine, colestipol, ampicillin, and rifampin may reduce the effectiveness of atenolol.
- Beta blockers may increase the effects of gabapentin, lidocaine, or prazosin, leading to undesirable reactions or toxicity.
- Beta blockers may block the effects of epinephrine.
- Fluoxetine, paroxetine, bupropion, propafenone, quinidine, duloxetine, and terbinafine can substantially increase the

amount of nebivolol in the blood by interfering with its breakdown by liver enzymes. Amiodarone, cimetidine, and sertraline also have this interaction but the effect is smaller. Avoid these combinations.

- Other drugs that can increase nebivolol levels but to a much smaller extent are antihistamines, celecoxib, chlorpheniramine, chlorpromazine, citalopram, clemastine, clomipramine, diphenhydramine, doxepin, doxorubicin, escitalopram, halofantrine, histamine, hydroxyzine, levomepromazine, methadone, metoclopramide, mibefradil, midodrine, moclobemide, perphenazine, ranitidine, haloperidol, ritonavir, ticlopidine, and tripelennamine.

- Dexamethasone, rifampin, and sildenafil reduce blood levels of nebivolol but the combined effect on blood pressure is moderate.

Food Interactions

These drugs may be taken without regard to food or meals.

Usual Dose

Atenolol

Adult: 50 mg a day. Some people may require doses of 100–200 mg a day. Dosages over 100 mg a day are not likely to produce additional benefit to those being treated for hypertension. People with kidney disease may need only 50 mg every other day. Older adults should be treated more cautiously and may need a lower dose.

Child: not recommended.

Nebivolol

Adult: 5 mg a day to start, increasing gradually to 40 mg a day as needed.

Child: not recommended.

Overdosage

Symptoms of overdose include changes in heartbeat—unusually slow, unusually fast, or irregular—severe dizziness or fainting, breathing difficulties, bluish-colored fingernails or palms, and seizures. Heart failure and shock may also result from a beta blocker overdose. The victim should be taken to a hospital emergency room. ALWAYS bring the prescription bottle or container.

Special Information

These drugs are meant to be taken continuously. When ending treatment, dosage should be reduced gradually over a period of about 2 weeks. Do not stop taking these drugs unless directed to do so by your doctor. Abrupt withdrawal may cause chest pain, breathing difficulties, increased sweating, and unusually fast or irregular heartbeat.

Call your doctor at once if you develop back or joint pain, breathing difficulties, cold hands or feet, depression, rash, or changes in heartbeat. Atenolol may produce an undesirable lowering of blood pressure, leading to dizziness or fainting; call your doctor if this happens. Call your doctor if you experience persistent or bothersome anxiety, diarrhea, constipation, impotence, headache, itching, nausea or vomiting, nightmares or vivid dreams, upset stomach, insomnia, stuffy nose, frequent urination, unusual tiredness, or weakness.

Atenolol may cause drowsiness, lightheadedness, dizziness, or blurred vision. Be careful when driving or performing complex tasks.

It is best to take beta blockers at the same time each day. If you forget a dose, take it as soon as you remember. If you take nebivolol and do not remember until your next dose, continue with your regular schedule. If you take atenolol once a day and it is within 8 hours of your next dose, skip the dose you forgot and continue with your regular schedule. If you take atenolol twice a day and it is within 4 hours of your next dose, skip the one you forgot and continue with your regular schedule. Never take a double dose of atenolol or nebivolol.

Special Populations

Pregnancy/Breast-feeding: Infants born to women who took a beta blocker while pregnant had lower birth weights, low blood pressure, and reduced heart rates. These drugs should be avoided by pregnant women and women who might become pregnant while taking them.

Atenolol and nebivolol pass into breast milk. Nursing mothers should use infant formula.

Seniors: Seniors taking atenolol should use the lowest effective dose as this group is more likely to have decreased heart, kidney, and liver function, and to be taking additional medications. Dosage adjustment of nebivolol is not necessary in seniors.

Generic Name

Atomoxetine (ah-tom-OX-eh-teen)

Brand Name
Strattera

Type of Drug
Selective norepinephrine reuptake inhibitor.

Prescribed For
Attention-deficit hyperactivity disorder (ADHD).

General Information
Atomoxetine is used for attention deficit hyperactivity disorder (ADHD). This drug may be used by children, teenagers, and adults. Unlike most other medicines used for ADHD, it is not a stimulant.

Cautions and Warnings
Do not take atomoxetine if you are **allergic** or **sensitive** to any of its ingredients.

Suicidal thoughts and actions have occurred in **children** and **teens** taking atomoxetine. Warning signs to look for include agitation, irritability, and unusual behavior changes, especially during the first few months of drug therapy or when drug dosage is increased or decreased.

Separate atomoxetine from any **monoamine oxidase inhibitor (MAOI) antidepressant** by at least 2 weeks. Serious, sometimes fatal, symptoms including body temperature elevations, rigidity, muscle stiffness, or rapid changes of vital signs or mental status (including extreme agitation, progressing to delirium and coma) may occur.

Atomoxetine is not recommended for people with **narrow-angle glaucoma**.

In rare cases, atomoxetine may cause severe liver injury. Atomoxetine should be discontinued in patients with jaundice or evidence of liver dysfunction.

Atomoxetine can increase blood pressure and heart rate. People with **high blood pressure, rapid heartbeat,** or **cardiovascular or cerebrovascular disease** should use it with caution.

People with **liver disease** may require a lower dosage of atomoxetine.

People taking atomoxetine may feel dizzy or faint when rising quickly from a sitting or lying position.

Children taking atomoxetine grow more slowly and gain less weight than other children their age for the first 9–12 months they are taking the medicine. After that, they start growing more quickly and generally catch up with their peers after 3 years.

People with **bipolar disorder** who take atomoxetine may be at risk for experiencing a manic reaction and should be carefully monitored.

Atomoxetine may cause an increase in aggression or hostility, which should be reported to a doctor immediately.

Possible Side Effects

Children
In clinical studies, drug side effects were similar to those reported by people taking an inactive placebo (sugar pill).
▼ Most common: headache, upper abdominal pain, vomiting, and coughing.
▼ Common: dizziness, tiredness, and irritability.
▼ Less common: constipation, upset stomach, runny nose, appetite loss, weight loss, crying, mood swings, and skin rash.

Adults
▼ Most common: dry mouth, headache, nausea, and sleeplessness.
▼ Common: urinary hesitation or difficulty urinating, constipation, upset stomach, tiredness or fatigue, sinus infection, appetite loss, dizziness, sleeping problems, painful menstruation, erectile dysfunction, and reduced sex drive or other sexual concerns.
▼ Less common: heart palpitation, abdominal gas, fever and chills, weight loss, abnormal dreams, sinus headache, tingling in the hands or feet, muscle ache, impotence, delayed onset of menstruation, irregular or other menstrual issues, prostate irritation, skin rash, increased sweating, and hot flushes.
▼ Rare: chest pain and heart palpitations. Contact your doctor if you experience any side effect not listed above.

Drug Interactions

- Atomoxetine should not be used 2 weeks before or after taking an MAOI antidepressant (see "Cautions and Warnings").
- Atomoxetine increases the effects of albuterol, causing high blood pressure and rapid heartbeat. Dosage adjustments may be required.
- Fluoxetine, paroxetine, and quinidine substantially increase the amount of atomoxetine in the blood. Atomoxetine dosages adjustments may be necessary.
- Atomoxetine raises blood pressure and should be given with caution to people who are already taking medicines that raise blood pressure. It may counter the effects of some drugs used to treat high blood pressure.

Food Interactions

Atomoxetine may be taken without regard to food or meals.

Usual Dose

Adult and Child (155 lbs. and over): 40–80 mg a day in a single or divided dose. Maximum dose is 100 mg a day. Divided doses should be taken in the morning and late afternoon or early evening.

Child (age 6 and over and less than 155 lbs.): starting dose— 0.23 mg per lb. of body weight. Dose can be gradually increased up to 0.55 mg per lb. as a single dose in the morning or 2 doses, one in the morning and the second in the late afternoon or early evening. The maximum daily dose is 100 mg.

People with moderate liver disease should take half of the regular dose and those with severe liver disease should take one-quarter of the regular dose.

Overdosage

Little is known about the effects of atomoxetine overdose. Call your local poison control center or a hospital emergency room for information. If you seek treatment, ALWAYS bring the prescription bottle or container.

Special Information

If you forget a dose of atomoxetine, take it as soon as you remember. If it is almost time for your next dose, skip the one you forgot and continue with your regular schedule. Do not take a double dose.

Use caution while driving or operating machinery when you start taking atomoxetine until you can determine how it will affect your abilities.

Special Populations

Pregnancy/Breast-feeding: Animal studies show that atomoxetine may affect a developing fetus. When this drug is considered crucial by your doctor, its potential benefits must be carefully weighed against its risks.

Atomoxetine may pass into breast milk. Nursing mothers who must take this drug should use infant formula.

Seniors: Atomoxetine has not been studied in older adults.

Generic Name

Atovaquone (ah-TOE-vuh-quone)

Brand Name

Mepron [$]

Type of Drug

Anti-infective.

Prescribed For

Prevention and treatment of mild to moderate *Pneumocystis carinii* pneumonia (PCP).

General Information

Atovaquone is an anti-infective with specific activity against PCP, an infection commonly associated with HIV. It is used in people who cannot take the combination of trimethoprim and sulfamethoxazole. In studies comparing atovaquone with trimethoprim-sulfamethoxazole (TMP-SMX), approximately 60% of people with PCP improved on each drug. However, more people died of PCP and other infections while being treated with atovaquone. Of those who died, most had less atovaquone in their bloodstream than those who lived. In studies comparing oral atovaquone with intravenous pentamidine for treating PCP in people with HIV, both drugs were equally effective, at 14%. Again, there was a direct correlation between the amount of atovaquone in the blood and survival.

The drug stays in the body for several days and is eliminated through the liver.

Cautions and Warnings

Do not take atovaquone if you are **allergic** or **sensitive** to any of its ingredients.

This drug has not been studied for severe PCP or in those who are failing on TMP-SMZ.

Atovaquone only works against PCP. People with PCP who have **bacterial, viral, fungal, or other infections of the lung** may continue to worsen despite atovaquone therapy. If this happens, it may be a sign that another kind of infecting organism is the cause. Additional medicine will be necessary.

Atovaquone absorption is strongly influenced by food. People with **gastrointestinal disorders** or those who are unable to take atovaquone with food may not be able to absorb enough medicine for it to be effective. Intravenous treatments of other PCP anti-infectives may be necessary.

Possible Side Effects

Because atovaquone was evaluated in people with advanced HIV, it is difficult to discern side effects of the drug use from those caused by the disease. Overall, only 4–7% of people studied stopped taking the drug because of side effects, a much smaller percentage than occurs with other PCP treatments.

▼ Most common: rash, nausea, diarrhea, headache, vomiting, fever, sleeplessness, weakness, itching, oral fungal infections, abdominal pain, upset stomach, appetite loss, constipation, cough, dizziness, pain, increased sweating, anxiety, sinus inflammation, and runny nose.

▼ Less common: changes in sense of taste, low blood sugar, and low blood pressure.

Drug Interactions

- Atovaquone may increase blood levels of warfarin, oral anti-diabetes drugs, digoxin, and other drugs that bind strongly to blood proteins.
- Rifampin and rifabutin may reduce blood levels of atovaquone, possibly diminishing its effectiveness.

- Taking atovaquone with TMP-SMZ has resulted in reduced blood levels of TMP-SMZ. This should not reduce TMP-SMZ's effectiveness.
- Taking atovaquone with zidovudine (AZT) drastically reduces the rate at which zidovudine is eliminated from the body. For most people, this is not a problem.

Food Interactions

Take atovaquone with food or meals to improve drug absorption. A high-fat meal can increase the amount absorbed by 300%.

Usual Dose

Prevention: 1500 mg daily with food.
Treatment: 750 mg twice a day for 3 weeks, taken with food.

Overdosage

Little is known about the effects of atovaquone overdose; symptoms are likely to be exaggerated drug side effects. Call your local poison control center or hospital emergency room for more information. If you go to the hospital, ALWAYS bring the prescription bottle or container.

Special Information

Taking atovaquone regularly and with food is essential to the drug's effectiveness. If you cannot eat 2 meals a day, your doctor may have to prescribe another PCP treatment.

Call your doctor if you develop any persistent or bothersome side effects.

If you forget a dose, take it as soon as you remember. If it is almost time for your next dose, space your remaining doses equally throughout the rest of the day so that you can still take a total daily dose of 1500 mg, or 2 tsp.

Special Populations

Pregnancy/Breast-feeding: In animal studies, atovaquone has affected fetal development. This drug should only be used during pregnancy after carefully weighing its potential benefits against its risks.

Atovaquone is likely to pass into breast milk because of its affinity for body fat. Nursing mothers should use infant formula.

Seniors: This drug has not been tested systematically in people over age 65. Seniors, especially those with kidney, heart, or liver disease, may be more sensitive to atovaquone side effects.

Avalide   *see Angiotensin II Blockers, page 80*

Avandia   *see Glitazone Antidiabetes Drugs, page 528*

Avapro   *see Angiotensin II Blockers, page 80*

Avelox   *see Fluoroquinolone Anti-Infectives, page 495*

Aviane   *see Contraceptives, page 287*

Generic Name

Azithromycin (uh-ZIH-throe-MYE-sin) Ⓖ

Brand Names

Zithromax   Zmax

Type of Drug

Macrolide antibiotic.

Prescribed For

Upper and lower respiratory tract infections, skin infections, sexually transmitted diseases (STDs), middle ear infections, tonsillitis, pharyngitis, and bacterial sinusitis.

General Information

Azithromycin is an azalide antibiotic, a subgroup of the macrolides. Macrolide drugs are either bactericidal (bacteria-killing) or bacteriostatic (inhibiting bacterial growth) depending on the organism in question and amount of antibiotic present.

Cautions and Warnings

Do not take azithromycin if you are **allergic** or **sensitive** to any of its ingredients or any macrolide antibiotic.

Azithromycin is excreted primarily through the liver. People with **liver disease or damage** should consult their doctors. Those on long-term therapy with this drug should have periodic blood tests.

Colitis (bowel inflammation), ranging from mild to life-threatening, has been associated with all antibiotics (see "Possible Side Effects").

Azithromycin is considered appropriate only for the treatment of more mild forms of **pneumonia** in non-hospitalized patients. People with other underlying conditions, those who are **immune-compromised,** and those who contract pneumonia in a hospital or other institutional setting probably should be treated with other antibiotics.

Possible Side Effects

Most side effects are mild and go away once you stop taking azithromycin.

▼ Most common: nausea, vomiting, abdominal pain, and diarrhea. Colitis (symptoms include severe abdominal cramps and severe, persistent, and possibly bloody diarrhea) may develop.

▼ Less common: heart palpitations; chest pain; vaginal irritation; stomach upset; gas; dizziness; headache; tiredness; unusual sun sensitivity; rash; itching; swelling; fungal infection of the mouth or vagina; dark, tarry stools; kidney inflammation; and vertigo.

Drug Interactions

- Pimozide should not be taken by anyone also taking a macrolide antibiotic. Two people died while taking this combination.
- Antacid products containing aluminum magnesium may delay the absorption of azithromycin into the blood. Separate your antacid dose from azithromycin by at least 1 hour.
- All macrolide antibiotics increase blood levels of cyclosporine and may cause kidney damage.
- Combining azithromycin and a statin cholesterol-lowering drug increases the risk of developing a painful and potentially fatal condition involving severe muscle degeneration.

- Combining azithromycin and nelfinavir may increase azithromycin side effects.

Food Interactions

It is important to take azithromycin liquid on an empty stomach, 1 hour before or 2 hours after meals. Tablets may be taken with or without food.

Usual Dose

Respiratory Tract Infections, Skin Infections, STDs, and Bacterial Sinusitis

Adult (age 16 and over): 500 mg as a single dose for 3 days, or 500 mg as a single dose on day 1, then 250 mg once a day on days 2–5 of treatment. STDs are treated with a single dose of 1000–2000 mg.

Middle Ear Infections and Bacterial Sinusitis* (Child)

1-Day Regimen: 13.6 mg per lb. of body weight a day for 1 day.
3-Day Regimen: 4.5 mg per lb. of body weight a day for 3 days.
5-Day Regimen: 4.5 mg per lb. of body weight a day for day 1, and 2.25 mg per lb. a day for days 2–5.

3-day regimen for bacterial sinusitis preferred.

Tonsillitis and Sore Throat

Child (age 2 and over): 5.5 mg per lb. of body weight a day for 5 days.

Overdosage

Overdose may cause severe side effects, especially nausea, vomiting, stomach cramps, and diarrhea. Call your local poison control center or hospital emergency room for more information. If you seek treatment, ALWAYS bring the prescription bottle or container.

Special Information

Call your doctor if you develop nausea, vomiting, diarrhea, stomach cramps, or severe abdominal pain. Stop taking this drug and immediately call your doctor if you experience breathing difficulties, chest pain, hives, rash, itching, mouth sores, or unusual sensitivity to light.

It is crucial that you follow your doctor's directions on how to take the drug and how many days to take it—even if you feel well sooner. This drug's effectiveness may be severely reduced otherwise. Taking azithromycin at the same time each day may help you remember your medication.

If you forget a dose of azithromycin, take it as soon as you remember. If it is almost time for your next dose, skip the dose you forgot and go back to your regular schedule.

Special Populations

Pregnancy/Breast-feeding: It is not known if azithromycin taken during pregnancy will harm a fetus. This medication should be taken by pregnant women only if it is clearly needed.

It is not known if azithromycin passes into breast milk, but other macrolide antibiotics do. Nursing mothers who must take this drug should use infant formula.

Seniors: Seniors with liver disease should use caution. Seniors who have pneumonia or are especially sickly or debilitated probably should be treated with other medications.

Type of Drug

Azole Antifungals

Brand Names

Generic Ingredient: Fluconazole Ⓖ
Diflucan

Generic Ingredient: Itraconazole Ⓖ
Sporanox

Generic Ingredient: Ketoconazole Ⓖ

Extina	Nizoral
Ketozole	Xolegel

Generic Ingredient: Posaconazole
Noxafil

Generic Ingredient: Voriconazole
Vfend

Prescribed For

Fungal infections of the blood, mouth, throat, vagina, or central nervous system.

Fluconazole, posaconazole, and itraconazole can be used to treat opportunistic fungal infections that inflict many people with HIV or cancer whose immune systems have been compromised.

General Information

Azole antifungals are used to treat a variety of fungal organisms, including Candida, aspergillus, cryptococcus, blastomycosis, fusarium, histoplasmosis, and Scedosporium. They work by inhibiting important enzyme systems in the organisms they attack. These drugs are broken down in the liver.

Cautions and Warnings

Do not take azole antifungals if you are **allergic** or **sensitive** to any of their ingredients. People who are allergic to similar antifungals may also be allergic to these drugs, but cross-reactions are not common and serious allergic reaction is rare.

Azole antifungals can affect heart rhythm and should be used with caution if you have a history of **abnormal heart rhythms.**

Rarely, azole antifungals can cause liver damage. The drugs should be used with caution in people with **liver disease.** At least one in every 10,000 people who take ketoconazole develop liver inflammation. The inflammation generally subsides when the drug is discontinued.

Voriconazole tablets contain lactose. They should not be taken by patients with rare hereditary problems of **galactose intolerance, Lapp-lactase deficiency,** or **glucose-galactose malabsorption.**

Rash may be an important sign of drug toxicity, especially in people with HIV or others with compromised immune function. Report any rashes, especially ones that do not heal readily, to your doctor.

These drugs can have very serious effects if combined with other medicines. See "Drug Interactions" for specific information.

Possible Side Effects

Side effects are generally more common among people with HIV.

Fluconazole

▼ Most common: nausea, headache, rash, vomiting, abdominal pain, and diarrhea.

▼ Less common: liver toxicity, as measured by increases in specific lab tests. These changes in lab values are more common in people with HIV or cancer, who are more likely to be taking several drugs.

Possible Side Effects *(continued)*

▼ Rare: seizures and exfoliative skin disorders. People with HIV or cancer who take fluconazole for fungal infections may develop severe liver or skin problems. Contact your doctor if you experience any side effect not listed above.

Itraconazole

▼ Most common: nausea, vomiting, and rash.
▼ Less common: diarrhea, abdominal pain, appetite loss, swelling in the legs or feet, fatigue, fever, feeling unwell, itching, headache, dizziness, reduced sex drive, tiredness, high blood pressure, liver or kidney function abnormalities, low blood potassium, and impotence.
▼ Rare: gas, sleeplessness, depression, ringing or buzzing in the ears, bronchitis, chest pain, coughing, and swollen or painful breasts in men or women. Contact your doctor if you experience any side effect not listed above.

Ketoconazole

▼ Common: nausea, vomiting, upset stomach, abdominal pain or discomfort, itching, and swollen breasts in men. Most of these side effects are mild and only a small number of people—1.5%—have to stop taking the drug because of severe side effects.

Posaconazole

▼ Most common: fever, headache, chills, swelling in the legs, appetite loss, dizziness, fluid accumulation, weakness, blood pressure changes, anemia, low white-blood-cell counts with or without fever, vaginal bleeding, diarrhea, nausea, vomiting, abdominal pain, constipation, upset stomach, mucous membrane irritation, rapid heart beat, bacteria in the blood, herpes infection, CMV infection, infection, sore throat, low blood potassium, low blood magnesium, high blood sugar, muscle and joint pain, back pain, low blood-platelet levels, black-and-blue marks, sleeplessness, cough, difficulty breathing, nosebleeds, and rash and itching.
▼ Common: upper respiratory infection, low blood calcium, and anxiety.
▼ Less common: tiredness, weakness, blurred vision, taste changes, and heart rhythm changes.

Possible Side Effects *(continued)*

Voriconazole

▼ Most common: visual disturbances.

▼ Common: fever, rash, nausea, blood infections, swelling in the arms or legs, and respiratory disorder.

Drug Interactions

- Do not mix astemizole, cisapride, halofantrine, pimozide, quinidine, or terfenadine with itraconazole, ketoconazole, or posaconazole. Severe cardiac side effects may occur. Similarly, combining fluconazole with cisapride may cause cardiac events. Do not mix these medicines.

- Antacids interfere with the absorption of ketoconazole and itraconazole. Take antacids more than 2 hours after taking these drugs.

- Fluconazole and ketoconazole may increase the amount of the sulfonylurea-type antidiabetes drugs (eg. tolbutamide, glyburide, and glipizide) in the blood, causing low blood sugar. Cyclosporine, phenytoin, theophylline, warfarin, and zidovudine (an HIV drug—also known as AZT) are similarly affected. Dosage adjustments of these drugs and monitoring may be required.

- Ketoconazole may also increase blood levels of HIV drugs including protease inhibitors and didanosine (ddI).

- Use caution when combining fluconazole with rifabutin, rifampin, tacromilus, and terfenadine. Dose adjustments may be necessary.

- Fluconazole and ketoconazole may interfere with contraceptive drugs. Consider using an alternative form of birth control.

- Hydrochlorothiazide may increase blood levels of fluconazole up to 40%.

- Do not mix ketoconazole with triazolam.

- Ketoconazole increases the effects of benzodiazepine sedatives, buspirone, carbamazepine, corticosteroids, digoxin, donepezil, felodipine, nisoldipine, tacrolimus, tricyclic antidepressants, vinca-type alkaloids, and zolpidem. Dosage adjustments may be required.

- Do not mix itraconazole with dofetilide, ergot alkaloids, midazolam, or triazolam.

- Use caution when combining itraconazole with alfentanil, aripiprazole, buspirone, calcium channel blockers, carbamazepine, cilostazol, clarithromycin, corticosteroids, digoxin, erythromycin, halofantrine, haloperidol, sirolimus, tacrolimus, verapamil, vinca-type alkaloids, warfarin, and zolpidem. Dose adjustments may be necessary.

- Rarely, people who combine itraconazole or posaconazole with a statin-type blood-fat lowering drug experience muscle pain and destruction. The statin drug dose should be reduced. Some people who have experienced this interaction were also taking cyclosporine. Cyclosporine dosages should be lowered when combined with itraconazole and a statin drug. Do not combine itraconazole with lovastatin or simvastin.

- Cimetidine, didanosine, famotidine, isoniazid, nizatidine, phenytoin, protease inhibitors, ranitidine, rifabutin, rifampin, and rifapentine may interfere with the effectiveness of itraconazole and posaconazole.

- Voriconazole should not be combined with astemizole, barbiturates, carbamazepine, cisapride, efavirenz, ergot drugs for migraines, pimozide, quinidine, rifabutin, rifampin, sirolimus, and terfenadine.

- Serious increases in levels of cyclosporine and tacrolimus have been reported when mixed with posaconazole. Dosage adjustments are required.

- Posaconazole and an ergot drug should not be mixed.

- Voriconazole and posaconazole should be used with caution with benzodiazepine sedatives, calcium channel blockers, cyclosporine, methadone, statin-type drugs, sulfonylurea-type antidiabetes drugs, tacrolimus, vinca-type anti-cancer drugs, and warfarin. Dosage adjustments of these drugs may be needed to avoid side effects.

- Combining voriconazole and contraceptive drugs, omeprazole, phenytoin, or a protease inhibitor (excluding indinavir) may require dose adjustments and frequent monitoring for drug toxicity.

- Combining voriconazole with an NNRTI for HIV can either increase or decrease blood levels of voriconazole and increase blood levels of the NNRTI. Drug side effects may occur.

Food Interactions

Take voriconazole at least 1 hour before or 2 hours after a meal. Take ketoconazole and itraconazole with food or meals. Posaconazole must be taken with food or a nutritional supplement. Another treatment should be considered if this requirement cannot be met.

Usual Dose

Fluconazole
Adult and Child (age 14 and over): 100–400 mg once a day.
Child: 1.3–5.5 mg per lb. of body weight once a day; no more than 400 mg a day.

Itraconazole
Adult: 200–600 mg once a day.
Child (age 3–16): 100 mg a day has been prescribed, but the long-term effects of itraconazole in children are not known.

Ketoconazole
Oral
Adult: 200–400 mg once a day. Treatment may continue for several months, depending on the type of infection being treated.
Child (age 2 and over): 1.5–3 mg per lb. of body weight once a day.
Child (under age 2): not recommended.

Topical: Apply to affected and immediately surrounding areas 1–2 times a day for 2–6 weeks, depending on the type of infection being treated.

Posaconazole
Adult and Child (age 13 and over): 200 mg (5 ml) 3 times a day. This product includes a measuring spoon.
Child (under age 13): not recommended.

Voriconazole
Adult: 100–300 mg every 12 hours.
Child: not recommended.

Overdosage

Overdose is likely to result in exaggerated drug side effects. Doses of posaconazole up to 1600 mg a day have been taken without any adverse reactions. Take the victim to a hospital emergency room. ALWAYS bring the prescription bottle or container.

Special Information

When taking fluconazole, regular doctor visits are necessary to monitor liver function and general progress. Call your doctor if you develop severe diarrhea; vomiting; reddening, loosening, blistering, or peeling of the skin; darkening of the urine; jaundice (yellowing of the skin or whites of the eyes); loss of appetite; or abdominal pain, especially on the right side. Report other symptoms that are bothersome or persistent.

Itraconazole must be taken for at least 3 months to determine its effectiveness; otherwise, the infection may return.

If you forget a dose of one of these medicines, take it as soon as you remember. If it is almost time for your next dose, skip the one you forgot and continue with your regular schedule. Do not take a double dose.

Special Populations

Pregnancy/Breast-feeding: Animal studies with these medicines show effects on the fetus that have not been seen in humans. Pregnant women should not use azole antifungals unless the possible benefits outweigh the risks.

These drugs pass into breast milk. Nursing mothers who must these drugs should use infant formula.

Seniors: Seniors may require a reduced dosage of fluconazole due to age-related loss of kidney function. No dosage adjustments are necessary with other azole antifungals.

Generic Name

Baclofen (BAK-loe-fen) Ⓖ

Brand Name

Kemstro

Type of Drug

Skeletal muscle relaxant.

Prescribed For

Muscle spasms associated with multiple sclerosis (MS), spinal cord injury or disease, or other nervous system conditions; may also be used to treat trigeminal neuralgia (tic douloureux), hiccups, acid reflux, and as migraine prevention.

General Information

Baclofen may work by interfering with nervous system reflexes at the spinal cord, although it may also have some effect outside the spinal cord. Baclofen is chemically similar to a natural nerve transmitter known as GABA; baclofen's effect on muscle spasm may be related to its effect on GABA nerve receptors.

Cautions and Warnings

Do not take baclofen if you are **allergic** or **sensitive** to any of its ingredients. It should not be taken for muscle spasm resulting from **rheumatic disease, stroke, cerebral palsy,** or **Parkinson's disease** because its benefit in these situations has not been proven. The condition of people with **epilepsy** or **psychotic disorders** may worsen while taking baclofen.

About 4% of **women with MS** who take baclofen for less than 1 year develop ovarian cysts that usually disappear on their own. This is within the normal range for all women—1–5%—for developing ovarian cysts.

Baclofen is excreted primarily through the kidneys, so patients with **kidney disease** or **impaired kidney function** should use baclofen with caution.

Abruptly stopping baclofen can lead to hallucinations and seizure. Dosage should always be gradually reduced, except in cases of severe side effects.

Possible Side Effects

Baclofen may affect lab tests for liver function and can raise blood sugar levels.

▼ Most common: drowsiness, low blood pressure, weakness, dizziness, lightheadedness, nausea and vomiting, headache, and sleeplessness.

▼ Less common: frequent urination, fatigue or lethargy, confusion, euphoria, excitement, depression, hallucinations, tingling in the hands or feet, muscle pain, ringing or buzzing in the ears, coordination difficulties, tremors, rigidity, weakness, loss of muscle tone, unusual eye movement and other muscle-control problems, double vision, pinpoint or wide-open pupils, breathing difficulties, heart palpitations, dry mouth, appetite loss, changes in sense of taste, abdominal pain, diarrhea, bedwetting, difficulty urinating, painful urination, impotence, rash, itching, swelling of the ankle, excessive sweating, weight gain, and stuffy nose.

▼ Rare: slurred speech, blurred vision, seizure, fainting, chest pain, blood in the urine, and testing positive for blood in the stool. Contact your doctor if you experience any side effect not listed above.

Drug Interactions

- Avoid alcoholic beverages and other nervous system depressants such as antihistamines, sedatives, or narcotic pain relievers while taking baclofen.
- Combining a monoamine oxidase inhibitor (MAOI) antidepressant with baclofen may cause drowsiness, nervous system depression, and low blood pressure.
- Combining a tricyclic antidepressant with baclofen may lead to severe muscle weakness.
- Baclofen may increase blood sugar. Diabetics may need to increase their dosage of antidiabetic drugs to account for this effect.
- Combining blood-pressure-lowering drugs with baclofen may lead to dizziness or fainting due to severe lowering of blood pressure.

Food Interactions

This drug may be taken without regard to food or meals.

Usual Dose

Adult and Child: 5 mg 3 times a day for 3 days, gradually increased every 3 days until the desired effect is achieved, usually at 40–80 mg a day. People with kidney disease require lower doses.

Overdosage

Symptoms of baclofen overdose include vomiting, loss of muscle tone, twitching, convulsions, pinpoint or wide-open pupils, drowsiness, blurred or double vision, breathing difficulties, seizure, and coma. Overdose victims should be taken to a hospital emergency room for treatment. ALWAYS bring the prescription bottle or container.

Special Information

Baclofen is a nervous system depressant. Take care when driving or doing anything that requires concentration and physical coordination.

Call your doctor if you develop persistent symptoms such as a frequent urge to urinate, painful urination, constipation, nausea, headache, sleeplessness, or confusion.

Do not stop taking baclofen on your own. Abruptly stopping this drug may lead to hallucinations or seizure.

Your pharmacist may prepare a baclofen liquid. This mixture should be kept in the refrigerator and must be thrown away after 1 month.

If you forget a dose of baclofen and remember within 1 hour of your scheduled time, take it immediately. If you do not remember until more than 1 hour later or if you forget it completely, skip the dose you forgot and continue with your regular schedule. Do not take a double dose.

Special Populations

Pregnancy/Breast-feeding: Baclofen increases the chances of certain birth defects in lab animals. Pregnant women should only take baclofen after carefully weighing its possible benefits against its risks.

Baclofen taken by mouth passes into breast milk. Nursing mothers who must take this drug should use infant formula or receive the drug by injection directly into the spinal cord, because baclofen administered by injection does not pass into breast milk.

Seniors: Seniors may be more sensitive to nervous system side effects including hallucinations, depression, drowsiness, and confusion.

Generic Name

Becaplermin (beh-CAP-ler-min)

Brand Name

Regranex

Type of Drug

Human growth factor.

Prescribed For

Diabetic foot and leg wounds.

General Information

Becaplermin is a type of human growth factor produced in a laboratory. While it is not a substitute for good wound care, becaplermin can stimulate wound tissue to heal faster. Studies of the drug have produced mixed results. In some studies, people using becaplermin were 1½–2 times more likely to have complete healing of their wounds. In another study, the results with becaplermin were the same as those with good wound care alone.

Cautions and Warnings

Do not use becaplermin if you are **allergic** or **sensitive** to any of its ingredients.

Becaplermin should not be used to speed the healing of wounds that are healing by themselves.

Becaplermin should not be applied to **skin cancer** or **tumors** or exposed bones, joints, tendons, or ligaments because its effect on these body structures is not known.

Becaplermin should not be used for wounds that do not extend to subcutaneous tissue or are caused by poor circulation.

Possible Side Effects

People treated with becaplermin plus wound care had a slightly larger risk of developing a rash than those who received wound care alone.

Drug and Food Interactions
None known.

Usual Dose
Adult and Child (age 16 and over): Apply a thin layer to the wound and leave in place for 12 hours. Then, remove the becaplermin bandage, rinse the wound, and cover it with a plain saline-soaked bandage for the rest of the day. Continue this process until the wound has healed completely.

Child (under age 16): not recommended.

Overdosage
Little is known about the effects of accidental ingestion. Call your local poison control center or a hospital emergency room for information. If you seek treatment, ALWAYS bring the prescription container.

Special Information
Call your doctor if your wound worsens or is irritated by becaplermin.

Wash your hands before applying becaplermin.

Do not allow the tip of the becaplermin tube to touch any surface, including the wound being treated.

Your doctor should reassess your treatment if the wound is not 30% smaller in 10 weeks and completely healed in 20 weeks.

Applying more becaplermin than recommended will not make your wound heal better or faster.

If you forget a dose, apply it as soon as you remember. If it is almost time for your next dose, skip the missed dose and continue with your regular schedule.

Special Populations

Pregnancy/Breast-feeding
The safety of using becaplermin during pregnancy is not known. The drug should only be used during pregnancy if it is absolutely necessary.

It is not known if becaplermin passes into breast milk. Nursing mothers who must take this drug should use infant formula.

Seniors
Seniors may take this drug without special precaution.

Generic Name

Benazepril (ben-AY-zuh-pril) Ⓖ

Brand Name
Lotensin

Combination Product
Generic Ingredients: Benazepril + Hydrochlorothiazide Ⓖ
Lotensin HCT

Type of Drug
Angiotensin-converting enzyme (ACE) inhibitor.

Prescribed For
High blood pressure. Also prescribed for renal failure, kidney hypertension, heart failure, post–heart attack management, the management of people with a high risk of heart disease, diabetes, chronic kidney disease, prevention of a second stroke, and non-diabetic neuropathy.

General Information
Benazepril hydrochloride and other ACE inhibitors prevent the conversion of a hormone called angiotensin I to another hormone called angiotensin II, a potent blood-vessel constrictor. Preventing this conversion relaxes blood vessels, thus reducing blood pressure and relieving symptoms of heart failure. Benazepril also affects the production of other hormones and enzymes that

participate in the regulation of blood-vessel dilation. Benazepril starts working in 1 hour and continues to work for about 24 hours.

Cautions and Warnings

Do not take benazepril if you are **allergic** or **sensitive** to any of its ingredients.

Swelling of the face, extremities, or throat has been known to occur with benazepril, which can be dangerous (see "Special Information").

Benazepril occasionally causes very low blood pressure.

Benazepril may affect **kidney function.** Your doctor should check your urine for protein content during the first few months of treatment. Dosage adjustment is necessary if you have reduced kidney function.

Benazepril can affect white-blood-cell counts, possibly increasing your susceptibility to infection. Your doctor should monitor your blood counts periodically.

Benazepril can cause serious injury or death to the fetus if taken during **pregnancy**. Pregnant women should not take benazepril.

ACE inhibitors may be less effective in some **black patients** with high blood pressure, especially when dietary salt intake is high. Nevertheless, they should still be considered useful blood pressure treatments. Swelling beneath the skin to form welts is more common among black patients.

Possible Side Effects

▼ Most common: dizziness, tiredness, headache, nausea, and chronic cough. The cough usually goes away a few days after you stop taking the medication.

▼ Rare: Rare side effects can occur in almost any part of the body. Contact your doctor if you develop any side effect not listed above.

Drug Interactions

- Combining 325 mg a day or more of aspirin with benazepril carries a higher risk of death than taking lower doses (less than 160 mg a day). People taking aspirin to prevent a heart attack should use the lower dose.
- Mixing any ACE inhibitor with an NSAID pain reliever can increase the chance of kidney failure.

- Benazepril may increase the effect of lithium; this combination should be used with caution.
- Severe sensitivity reactions with an ACE inhibitor can occur in hemodialysis patients, in patients undergoing venom immunization, or in those taking allopurinol.
- The blood-pressure-lowering effect of benazepril is additive with diuretics and beta blockers. Any other drug that causes a rapid drop in blood pressure should be used with caution if you are taking benazepril.
- Benazepril may increase blood-potassium levels, especially if taken with dyazide or other potassium-sparing diuretics. Left untreated, this can be fatal.
- Antacids and benazepril should be taken at least 2 hours apart.
- Capsaicin may trigger or aggravate the cough associated with benazepril therapy.
- Indomethacin may reduce the blood-pressure-lowering effects of benazepril.
- Phenothiazine sedatives and antivomiting drugs may increase the effects of benazepril.
- Combining allopurinol and benazepril increases the risk of side effects.
- Benazepril increases blood levels of digoxin, which may increase the chance of digoxin-related side effects.

Food Interactions

You may take benazepril with food if it upsets your stomach.

Usual Dose

Adult: maintenance dose—20–40 mg a day as a single dose or in 2 equally divided doses. People with poor kidney function may need less medication.

Child (age 6 and over): 0.045–0.27 mg per lb. of body weight once a day.

Child (under age 6): not recommended.

Overdosage

The principal effect of benazepril overdose is a rapid drop in blood pressure, as evidenced by dizziness or fainting. Take the overdose victim to a hospital emergency room immediately. ALWAYS bring the prescription bottle or container.

Special Information

Benazepril can cause swelling of the face, lips, hands, and feet. This swelling can also affect the larynx (throat) and tongue and interfere with breathing. If this happens, go to a hospital at once. Call your doctor if you develop a sore throat, mouth sores, abnormal heartbeat, sudden difficulty breathing, chest pain, persistent rash, or loss of taste perception.

Some people who start taking benazepril after they are already on a diuretic (agent that increases urination) experience a rapid drop in blood pressure after their first dose or when their dosage is increased. To prevent this from happening, your doctor may tell you to stop taking your diuretic 2 or 3 days before starting benazepril or to increase your salt intake during that time. The diuretic may then be restarted gradually.

You may get dizzy if you rise to your feet too quickly from a sitting or lying position when taking benazepril.

Avoid strenuous exercise or very hot weather because heavy sweating or dehydration can cause a rapid drop in blood pressure.

While taking benazepril, avoid over-the-counter diet pills, decongestants, and other stimulants that can raise blood pressure. Also, do not use potassium supplements or salt substitutes containing potassium without consulting your doctor.

If you take benazepril once a day and forget a dose, take it as soon as you remember. If it is within 8 hours of your next dose, skip the dose you forgot and continue with your regular schedule. If you take benazepril twice a day and miss a dose, take the missed dose right away. If it is within 4 hours of your next dose, take 1 dose immediately and another in 5 or 6 hours, and then go back to your regular schedule. Never take a double dose.

Special Populations

Pregnancy/Breast-feeding: ACE inhibitors can cause fetal injury or death. Women who are or might become pregnant should not take ACE inhibitors. If you become pregnant, stop taking the medication and call your doctor immediately.

Small amounts of benazepril pass into breast milk. Nursing mothers who must take this drug should consider using infant formula.

Seniors: Seniors may be more sensitive to the effects of this drug due to age-related losses in kidney or liver function.

Benicar   *see Angiotensin II Blockers, page 80*

Generic Name

Betaine (BEE-tane)

Brand Name
Cystadane

Type of Drug
Homocysteine antagonist.

Prescribed For
Homocysteinuria.

General Information
Homocysteinuria is a group of 3 disorders of the metabolism characterized by too much homocysteine in the blood and urine. People with this problem tend to have skeletal problems, problems with the lens of the eye, and blood-clotting problems that can cause chest pain or heart attack. Virtually all people treated with betaine experience a decrease of homocysteine in their blood. When used together with other homocysteinuria treatments, including folate and vitamins B_{12} and B_6, betaine's effect has been additive to those treatments. Betaine starts working in several days and has been used for several years with no loss of effect. Most patients treated with betaine have been children. The effects of homocysteinuria can be devastating in children and include developmental problems, lethargy, seizures, and eye problems.

Cautions and Warnings
None known.

Possible Side Effects

Side effects, which are uncommon, include nausea, upset stomach, diarrhea, choking if the powder is inhaled, and bad odors. Reported psychological changes from betaine are questionable.

Drug Interactions

None known. Betaine has been used successfully together with folate and vitamins B_{12} and B_6.

Food Interactions

Betaine should be taken with food.

Usual Dose

Adult and Child: 3 g twice a day. Dosage for children under age 3 may be started at about 45 mg per lb. a day and then increased in weekly 45-mg steps. Dosage should be increased in all patients until homocysteine is either undetectable in the blood or present in small amounts; doses up to 20 g a day have been required. Carefully measure all doses with the scoop provided. Each level scoopful is equal to 1 g of betaine.

Overdosage

Little is known about the effects of betaine overdose. People have been safely and successfully treated at doses up to 20 g a day. Call your poison control center or a hospital emergency room for more information. If you go to a hospital emergency room, ALWAYS bring the prescription bottle or container.

Special Information

Shake the bottle lightly before removing the cap to loosen the powder. Protect the powder from moisture.

Mix each dose with 4–6 oz. of water until it dissolves completely, then drink it at once.

Do not use the product if the final solution is either not clear or colored, or if the powder does not completely dissolve.

If you forget a dose, take it as soon as you remember. If it is almost time for your next dose, skip the dose you forgot and continue with your regular schedule. Tell your doctor about any missed doses.

Special Populations

Pregnancy/Breast-feeding: The safety of using betaine during pregnancy is unknown. This drug should only be used during pregnancy if it is absolutely necessary.

It is not known if betaine passes into breast milk. Nursing mothers who must take this drug should use infant formula.

Seniors: Seniors may use this drug without special precaution.

Generic Name

Betaxolol (bay-TAX-uh-lol) [G]

Brand Names

Betoptic   Kerlone
Betoptic S

The information in this profile also applies to the following drugs:

Generic Ingredient: Carteolol [G]
Ocupress

Generic Ingredient: Levobunolol [G]
AK Beta   Betagan

Generic Ingredient: Metipranolol [G]
Optipranolol

Type of Drug

Beta-adrenergic blocking agent.

Prescribed For

High blood pressure and glaucoma.

General Information

Betaxolol hydrochloride is one of many beta-adrenergic blocking drugs, or beta blockers, which interfere with the action of a specific part of the nervous system. Beta receptors are found all over the body and affect many body functions. Each beta blocker has particular characteristics that make it more suitable for certain conditions or people. Beta-blocker eyedrops reduce ocular pressure (pressure inside the eye) by slowing the production of eye fluids and by slightly increasing the rate at which these fluids flow through and leave the eye. Small amounts of these drugs are absorbed into the general blood circulation after they are instilled in the eye and may affect areas of the body other than the eye.

Cautions and Warnings

Do not take betaxolol if you are **allergic** or **sensitive** to any of its ingredients. You should be cautious about taking betaxolol if you have **asthma, chronic bronchitis, emphysema, severe heart failure,** a **very slow heart rate,** or **heart block** (disruption of the electrical impulses that control heart rate) because the drug may aggravate these conditions.

People with **angina** risk aggravating their angina if they suddenly stop taking the drug. These people should have their beta-blocker eyedrops dosage reduced gradually over 1–2 weeks.

Liver or kidney problems may reduce your ability to eliminate beta-blocker eyedrops from your body.

Beta-blocker eyedrops may mask the physical signs of **hypoglycemia (low blood sugar)**. People with **diabetes** who must take insulin or oral medications to lower blood sugar and those subject to **hypoglycemia** should use beta-blocker eyedrops with caution.

Beta-blocker eyedrops may reduce the amount of blood your heart pumps with each beat. This reduction in blood flow may aggravate the condition of people with **poor circulation** or **circulatory disease**.

If you are undergoing **major surgery,** your doctor may want you to stop using beta-blocker eyedrops at least 2 days before surgery.

Betaxolol eyedrops should be avoided by people who cannot take oral beta-blocking drugs such as propranolol.

People with a history of **severe anaphylactic reaction** to allergens may be unresponsive to usual doses of epinephrine while taking beta blockers.

Possible Side Effects

Side effects are relatively uncommon and usually mild.

▼ Common: discomfort in the eye.

▼ Less common: blurred vision, inflammation of the cornea, sensation of having something in the eye, sensitivity to light, tearing, itching, dry eye, redness, inflammation, discharge, eye pain, cloudy vision, and crusting of the lashes.

▼ Rare: unusual tiredness or weakness, slow heartbeat, heart failure, dizziness, breathing difficulties, bronchospasm, depression, rash, and hair loss. Contact your doctor if you experience any side effect not listed above.

Drug Interactions

- Beta-blocker eyedrops may interact with surgical anesthetics to increase the risk of heart problems during surgery. Some anesthesiologists recommend gradually stopping the drug by 2 days before surgery.

- Combining beta-blocker eyedrops and oral beta blockers will increase the effects of each drug. These drugs should be combined cautiously.
- Cocaine may reduce the effectiveness of all beta-blocker eyedrops.
- Betaxolol will counteract thyroid hormone replacements.
- Calcium channel blockers, reserpine, phenothiazine compounds, and quinidine may increase the amount of beta-blocker eyedrops in the bloodstream and lead to low blood pressure and heart rate disturbances.
- Betaxolol should not be taken within 2 weeks of taking a monoamine oxidase inhibitor (MAOI) antidepressant.
- Combining betaxolol with digitalis drugs can result in excessive slowing of the heart, possibly causing heart block.
- If you use other glaucoma eye medications, separate your doses to avoid physically combining them.
- Small amounts of beta-blocker eyedrops are absorbed into the bloodstream and may interact with other drugs in the same way as oral beta blockers, although this is unlikely.
- Beta blockers may block the effects of epinephrine.
- If you stop smoking while taking betaxolol, your dose may have to be reduced because your liver will break down the drug more slowly afterward.

Food Interactions

None known.

Usual Dose

Adult

Glaucoma: 1–2 drops in the affected eye twice a day.

Hypertension: 10 mg tablet a day. May increase to 20 mg a day after 7–14 days. For seniors or people with severe kidney impairment, starting dose is 5 mg.

Child: not recommended.

Overdosage

If overdose occurs in the eye, flush it with water or saline. If accidentally ingested, symptoms of overdose of beta-blockers taken orally may occur. These include changes in heartbeat—unusually slow, unusually fast, or irregular—severe dizziness or fainting, breathing difficulties, bluish-colored fingernails or palms, low blood pressure, heart failure, shock, and seizures. If these symptoms occur, the victim should be taken to a hospital emergency room. ALWAYS bring the prescription bottle or container with you.

Special Information

Call your doctor at once if you develop back or joint pain, breathing difficulties, cold hands or feet, depression, rash, or changes in heartbeat. Beta-blocker eyedrops may produce an undesirable lowering of blood pressure, leading to dizziness or fainting; call your doctor if this happens to you. Also call your doctor if you experience persistent or bothersome anxiety, diarrhea, constipation, impotence, headache, itching, nausea or vomiting, nightmares or vivid dreams, upset stomach, trouble sleeping, stuffy nose, frequent urination, unusual tiredness, or weakness.

Do not use with your contact lenses in your eye. Do not touch the dropper to any surface.

If you forget a dose of beta-blocker eyedrops, administer it as soon as you remember. If it is almost time for your next dose, skip the dose you forgot and continue with your regular schedule. Do not take a double dose.

Special Populations

Pregnancy/Breast-feeding: In animal studies, betaxolol given orally at doses much higher than is absorbed through administration in the eye was associated with miscarriage. There is little information about the effects of betaxolol in pregnant women. Betaxolol should be used during pregnancy only if the benefit outweighs the risk.

Some beta blockers pass into breast milk. Nursing mothers taking beta-blocker eyedrops should use infant formula.

Seniors: Seniors may take betaxolol without special precautions.

Generic Name

Bicalutamide (bye-kal-UTE-uh-mide)

Brand Name

Casodex

The information in this profile also applies to the following drug:

Generic Ingredient: Nilutamide
Nilandron

Type of Drug
Antiandrogen.

Prescribed For
Prostate cancer.

General Information
Antiandrogens are prescribed together with another hormone product for prostate cancer. Bicalutamide competes with testosterone and other natural androgens (male hormones) by binding to the same places in body tissue where androgens normally bind. Prostate cancer is androgen sensitive and responds to treatments that counteract the effects of androgen or remove the sources of androgen.

Cautions and Warnings
Do not take this drug if you are **allergic** or **sensitive** to it or any of its ingredients.

People taking this medication may develop severe liver injury. People with **liver disease** may be at greater risk for serious side effects.

Almost 40% of men taking bicalutamide as single therapy for **prostate cancer** develop breast pain and enlargement. Bicalutamide may also reduce sperm count.

Two of every 100 people taking nilutamide develop interstitial pneumonitis (symptoms include cough, chest pain, fever, and breathing difficulties). People with **lung disease** and **Asians** may be at greater risk. Report any breathing difficulty or worsening of pre-existing breathing difficulty to your doctor immediately.

Isolated cases of aplastic anemia (a potentially fatal blood disorder) have been reported in people taking nilutamide, but the relationship between the drug and the disease is not established.

Possible Side Effects
▼ Most common: hot flashes, hot flushes, general pain, headache, weakness, back pain, nausea, constipation, sleeplessness, breathing difficulties, and swollen breasts. Nilutamide—difficulty seeing in the dark and loss of testicle function.

▼ Common: diarrhea and pelvic pain.

Possible Side Effects *(continued)*

▼ Less common: vomiting, abdominal pains, chest pain, flu-like symptoms, high blood pressure, swelling in the ankles or lower legs, high blood sugar, weight loss, dizziness, tingling in the hands or feet, sweating, rash, nighttime urination, blood in the urine, urinary or other infection, loss of libido, impotence, breast pain, painful urination, anemia, and bone pain.

▼ Rare: Rare side effects can occur in almost any part of the body. Contact your doctor if you experience any side effect not listed above.

Drug Interactions

- Bicalutamide and nilutamide increase the effect of oral anti-coagulant (blood-thinning) drugs such as warfarin. Dosage adjustment may be necessary.
- Nilutamide may increase the risk of the potentially serious side effects of phenytoin, theophylline, or vitamin K antagonists.

Food Interactions

None known.

Usual Dose

Bicalutamide
 Adult: 50 mg once a day, morning or night.

Nilutamide
 Adult: 300 mg a day, reduced to 150 mg a day after 30 days.

Overdosage

Symptoms of overdose may include nausea, vomiting, tiredness, headache and dizziness. Overdose victims should be taken to a hospital emergency room. ALWAYS bring the prescription bottle or container.

Special Information

Report anything unusual to your doctor, especially pain or tenderness in the upper right abdomen, yellowing of skin or whites of eyes, severe itching, dark urine, persistent appetite loss, and unexplained flu-like symptoms. These may be signs of severe liver toxicity. Also report any breathing difficulties, cough, chest pain, or fever.

Up to half of people taking nilutamide can take from a few seconds to a few minutes to adapt to darkness. This can be a problem especially when driving at night or through tunnels. Wearing tinted glasses will minimize this effect.

Up to 5% of people taking nilutamide may experience intolerance to alcohol. Symptoms include flushing, tiredness, and lightheadedness. If you experience this reaction, you should avoid alcohol.

Bicalutamide should be taken at the same time each day for best results. If you forget a dose of bicalutamide, take it as soon as you remember. If it is almost time for your next dose, skip the dose you forgot and continue with your regular schedule. Call your doctor if you forget to take more than 1 dose.

Special Populations

Pregnancy/Breast-feeding: Antiandrogens are not intended for use by women.

Seniors: Seniors may take this drug without special precaution.

Brand Name

BiDil

Generic Ingredients

Isosorbide Dinitrate + Hydralazine Hydrochloride

Type of Drug

Vasodilator combination.

Prescribed For

Heart failure in black patients, in combination with other heart-failure treatments.

General Information

BiDil is a combination of two drugs that dilate (open) both arteries and veins. It is the first drug product to be specifically approved for people in a single racial group for any indication. The 2 ingredients in BiDil have been available generically for years and are prescribed for a variety of uses. Isosorbide dinitrate is prescribed for angina, heart failure, and spasms of the esophagus. Hydralazine hydrochloride is prescribed to treat high blood pressure and heart failure. When people with heart failure take this drug combination, it makes it easier for the heart to pump blood throughout the body by widening arteries and veins.

Cautions and Warnings

Do not take BiDil if you are **allergic** or **sensitive** to any of its ingredients.

Do not use erectile dysfunction drugs with BiDil.

This drug may be inappropriate for you if you have had a recent **heart attack** or have **cardiomyopathy** (loss of blood-pumping ability due to damaged heart muscle) or **low blood pressure,** especially postural low blood pressure (symptoms include dizziness or fainting when rising from a sitting or lying position).

Long-term administration of more than 200 mg a day of hydralazine may produce symptoms of lupus erythematosus (a chronic condition affecting the body's connective tissue), including muscle and joint pain, skin reactions, fever, kidney inflammation, and anemia, although they usually disappear when the drug is discontinued. Report any fever, chest pain, feelings of ill health, or other unexplained symptoms to your doctor. The risk of developing lupus increases with higher dosages; approximately 5 out of 100 and 10% of people taking 200 mg a day of hydralazine develop lupus. The daily dosage of hydralazine when you take BiDil can be as high as 225 mg.

Hydralazine may cause a very rapid heartbeat, potentially leading to angina pain or a heart attack.

Taking pyridoxine (vitamin B_6) may relieve tingling or numbness in the hands or feet caused by hydralazine.

Possible Side Effects

▼ Most common: headache and flushing—which should disappear after your body adjusts to the drug—nausea, dizziness, weakness, and chest pain.

▼ Common: low blood pressure.

▼ Less common: blurred vision and dry mouth; sinus irritation, rapid heartbeat, heart palpitations, high blood sugar, runny nose, numbness or tingling in the hands or feet, vomiting, and high blood-fat levels.

Possible Side Effects *(continued)*

▼ Rare: flushing, tearing, itching, or redness of the eyes, tremors, muscle cramps, depression, disorientation, anxiety, itching, rash, fever, chills, occasional hepatitis (symptoms include yellowing of the skin or whites of the eyes), constipation, urinary difficulties, and adverse effects on normal blood composition. Other side effects may affect any organ or organ system. Contact your doctor if you experience any side effect not listed above.

Drug Interactions

- Do not take sildenafil, vardenafil, or taldenafil with Bidil. The combination can result in a rapid and potentially fatal drop in blood pressure.
- Taking this drug with a monoamine oxidase inhibitor antidepressant may increase the blood-pressure-lowering effect of the hydralazine component of BiDil. This combination should be used with caution.
- Do not self-medicate with over-the-counter appetite suppressants and cough, cold, and allergy remedies, since many contain ingredients that may aggravate heart disease.
- Taking this drug with large amounts of alcohol may rapidly lower blood pressure, resulting in weakness, dizziness, and fainting.

Food Interactions

Take this drug on an empty stomach. It is unknown how food affects BiDil.

Usual Dose

Adult: 1 or 2 tablets 3 times a day, 1 hour before or 2 hours after eating.

Overdosage

There have been no reports of BiDil overdose. Symptoms of BiDil overdose would be related to the specific effects of each active ingredient and can include reduced oxygen supply to heart muscle, leading to a heart attack, abnormal heart rhythms, and profound shock. Fainting, coma, and death may follow unless the victim is treated. Overdose victims must be taken to a hospital emergency room at once. ALWAYS bring the prescription bottle or container.

Special Information

Avoid alcohol.

Call your doctor if you develop a persistent headache, dizziness, facial flushing, blurred vision, or dry mouth.

It is important to make sure you drink plenty of fluids every day and pay attention to hot weather and exercise situations in which you might lose unusual amounts of fluids and salts. Fluid loss may lead to low blood pressure, dizziness, and possibly fainting.

If you forget to take a dose of BiDil, take it as soon as you remember. If it is almost time for your next dose, skip the dose you forgot and continue with your regular schedule. Never take a double dose.

Special Populations

Pregnancy/Breast-feeding: Isosorbide dinitrate crosses into the fetal circulation, and hydralazine can cause low blood pressure in pregnant women and their babies. The potential benefits of BiDil must be carefully weighed against its risks when your doctor considers this drug crucial.

It is not known if BiDil passes into breast milk. Nursing mothers who must take it should consider using infant formula.

Seniors: Specifics about how seniors react to this drug are not known. The lowest effective dose of BiDil should always be used, especially in people with reduced kidney and/or liver function.

Generic Name

Bisoprolol (bye-SOPE-roe-lol) Ⓖ

Brand Name

Zebeta

Combination Product

Generic Ingredients: Bisoprolol + Hydrochlorothiazide Ⓖ
Ziac

Type of Drug

Beta-adrenergic blocking agent.

Prescribed For

High blood pressure; may also be used for angina pectoris, and stable congestive heart failure.

General Information

Bisoprolol fumarate is one of many beta-adrenergic blocking drugs, or beta blockers, which interfere with the action of a specific part of the nervous system. Beta receptors are found all over the body and affect many body functions. Each beta blocker has particular characteristics that make it more suitable for certain conditions or people. Hydrochlorothiazide is a diuretic that lowers blood pressure.

Cautions and Warnings

Do not use bisoprolol if you are **allergic** or **sensitive** to it or other beta blockers.

Beta blockers should not be used by people with a **slow heart rate**, a condition called **heart block** (a disorder of the heart's conduction system), or those in **cardiac shock** or overt **heart failure**.

People with **angina** who take bisoprolol for high blood pressure risk aggravating their angina if they suddenly stop taking the drug. These people should have their dosage reduced gradually over 1–2 weeks.

Bisoprolol should be used with caution if you have **liver or kidney disease,** because your ability to eliminate the drug from your body may be impaired.

People with **chronic bronchitis** or **emphysema** should use bisoprolol with caution.

Bisoprolol reduces the amount of blood pumped by the heart with each beat. This blood flow reduction may aggravate the condition of people with **poor circulation** or **circulatory disease**.

If you are undergoing **major surgery,** your doctor may want you to stop taking bisoprolol at least 2 days before surgery.

People with a history of **severe anaphylactic reaction** to allergens may be unresponsive to usual doses of epinephrine while taking beta blockers.

Possible Side Effects

Side effects are relatively uncommon and usually mild.

▼ Most common: impotence.

▼ Less common: unusual tiredness or weakness, slow heartbeat, heart failure, dizziness, breathing difficulties, bronchospasm, depression, confusion, anxiety, nervousness, sleeplessness, disorientation, short-term memory loss,

---

Possible Side Effects (continued)

emotional instability, cold hands and feet, constipation, diarrhea, nausea, vomiting, upset stomach, increased sweating, urinary difficulties, cramps, blurred vision, rash, hair loss, stuffy nose, facial swelling, aggravation of lupus erythematosus, itching, chest pain, back or joint pain, colitis, drug allergy (symptoms include fever and sore throat), and liver toxicity.

Drug Interactions

- Bisoprolol may interact with surgical anesthetics to increase the risk of heart problems during surgery. Some anesthesiologists recommend gradually stopping the drug by 2 days before surgery.
- Bisoprolol may interfere with the normal signs of low blood sugar and with the action of oral antidiabetes drugs.
- Bisoprolol increases the blood-pressure-lowering effects of other blood-pressure-reducing agents, including clonidine, guanabenz, and reserpine, and calcium channel blockers, such as nifedipine.
- Aspirin-containing drugs, indomethacin, sulfinpyrazone, and estrogen drugs may interfere with the blood-pressure-lowering effect of bisoprolol.
- Cocaine may reduce the effectiveness of all beta blockers.
- Bisoprolol may worsen the problem of cold hands and feet associated with taking ergot alkaloids, used to treat migraine. Gangrene is possible in people taking both an ergot and bisoprolol.
- Calcium channel blockers, diphenhydramine, flecainide, contraceptive drugs, quinolone antibacterials, and quinidine may increase the amount of bisoprolol in the bloodstream and lead to increased bisoprolol effects.
- Bisoprolol may increase the effects of ephedrine. Initially, high blood pressure and then a slow heart rate may result.
- Combining beta blockers with lidocaine can increase lidocaine levels, possibly leading to toxicity.
- Beta blockers taken with prazosin may increase the side effect of lightheadedness upon standing up that prazosin can produce.
- Beta blockers may block the effects of epinephrine.

- Smoking makes the liver break this drug down more quickly. If you stop smoking while taking bisoprolol, your daily dose may have to be reduced.

Food Interactions

This drug may be taken without regard to food or meals.

Usual Dose

Adult: starting dose—5 mg once daily. The daily dose may be gradually increased up to 20 mg. Maintenance dose—5–10 mg once daily. People with kidney or liver disease may need only 2.5 mg a day to start. Seniors should be treated cautiously; they may respond to lower doses.

Child: not recommended.

Overdosage

Symptoms of overdose include changes in heartbeat—unusually slow, unusually fast, or irregular—severe dizziness or fainting, breathing difficulties, bluish fingernails or palms, low blood pressure, heart failure, shock, and seizures. The victim should be taken to a hospital emergency room. ALWAYS bring the prescription bottle or container.

Special Information

Do not stop taking bisoprolol unless directed to do so by your doctor. It is meant for continuous use. Abrupt withdrawal may cause chest pain, breathing difficulties, increased sweating, and unusually fast or irregular heartbeat. Dosage should be reduced gradually over a period of about 2 weeks when bisoprolol treatment is stopped.

Call your doctor at once if you develop back or joint pain, breathing difficulties, cold hands or feet, depression, rash, or changes in heartbeat. Bisoprolol may produce an undesirable lowering of blood pressure, leading to dizziness or fainting; call your doctor if this happens to you. Also call your doctor if you experience persistent or bothersome anxiety, diarrhea, constipation, impotence, headache, itching, nausea or vomiting, nightmares or vivid dreams, upset stomach, trouble sleeping, stuffed nose, frequent urination, unusual tiredness, or weakness.

Bisoprolol may cause drowsiness, dizziness, blurred vision, or lightheadedness. Be careful when driving or performing complex tasks.

It is best to take bisoprolol at the same time every day. If you forget a dose, take it as soon as you remember. If it is within 8 hours of your next dose, skip the dose you forgot and continue with your regular schedule. Do not take a double dose.

Special Populations

Pregnancy/Breast-feeding: Infants born to women who took a beta blocker while pregnant had lower birth weights, low blood pressure, and reduced heart rates. Bisoprolol should be avoided by pregnant women and women who might become pregnant while taking it.

It is not known if bisoprolol passes into breast milk. Nursing mothers taking bisoprolol should use infant formula.

Seniors: Seniors taking bisoprolol may be more likely to suffer from cold hands and feet, reduced body temperature, chest pain, general feelings of ill health, sudden breathing difficulties, increased sweating, or changes in heartbeat.

Type of Drug

Bisphosphonates (bis-FOS-fun-ates)

Brand Names

Generic Ingredient: Alendronate Sodium
Fosamax

Generic Ingredients: Alendronate Sodium + Cholecalciferol
Fosamax Plus D

Generic Ingredient: Etidronate Disodium Ⓖ
Didronel

Generic Ingredient: Ibandronate Sodium
Boniva

Generic Ingredient: Risedronate Sodium Ⓖ
Actonel

Generic Ingredients: Risedronate Sodium + Calcium Carbonate
Actonel with Calcium

Generic Ingredient: Tiludronate Disodium
Skelid

Prescribed For

Prevention and treatment of osteoporosis (a condition characterized by loss of bone mass due to calcium depletion) in postmenopausal women and in older men; Paget's disease of bone;
and high blood calcium associated with high dosages of corticosteroid treatments and cancer.

General Information

Bisphosphonates have been used for many years to treat a variety of conditions associated with low bone mass caused by calcium depletion. They work on cells called osteoclasts that normally
break down bone tissue, making bones stronger by preventing
loss of bone mass. In osteoporosis, bones become weak and brittle, increasing the risk of spine, hip, and other bone fractures that
are a major cause of death and disability in older women. Etidronate has been used occasionally in children, but these drugs generally are not considered safe for use in children.

Cautions and Warnings

Do not use any bisphosphonate if you are **allergic** or **sensitive** to
any of its ingredients.

Do not use bisphosphonates if you have severe **kidney disease**
or active **stomach or intestinal disease** such as difficulty swallowing, ulcers, or stomach irritation. Notify your doctor if you experience any gastrointestinal problems while taking bisphosphonates.

Osteonecrosis of the jaw (ONJ), a condition in which bones of
the jaw lose their blood supply and eventually collapse, has been
reported in people treated with bisphosphonates. Most cases of
ONJ have been in cancer patients having dental procedures such
as tooth extractions. People at risk may be those with **cancer** and
those taking **corticosteroids** or those with **poor oral hygiene**.

Do not use ibandronate, alendronate, or risedronate if you cannot stand or sit upright for 30 minutes (see "Special Information").

Bisphosphonates can cause **low blood calcium** and should
not be used by people whose blood calcium is already low.

Bisphosphonates can cause severe and sometimes incapacitating bone, joint, and/or muscle pain.

Possible Side Effects

Side effects are generally mild and similar to those reported
by people taking an inactive placebo (sugar pill).

Possible Side Effects *(continued)*

Alendronate
▼ Most common: pain.
▼ Common: abdominal pain and discomfort, gas, stomach ulcers, and back pain.
▼ Less common: upset stomach, constipation, diarrhea, nausea, difficulty swallowing, muscle pain, headache, flu-like symptoms, accidents, and swelling in the arms or legs.
▼ Rare: vomiting and changes in taste. Contact your doctor if you experience any side effect not listed above.

Etidronate
▼ Most common: fever.
▼ Common: nausea, excess fluids, and flu-like symptoms.
▼ Less common: convulsions, constipation, inflammation of the lining of the mouth, changes in liver function, low blood levels of magnesium or phosphate, breathing difficulties, and changes in sense of taste.
▼ Rare: allergic reactions. Contact your doctor if you experience any side effect not listed above.

Ibandronate
▼ Most common: upper respiratory infection, back pain, bronchitis, and upset stomach.
▼ Common: arm or leg pain, muscle pain, headache, pneumonia, and urinary infections.
▼ Less common: dizziness, fainting, pain due to nerve lesions, weakness, allergic reactions, diarrhea, vomiting, dental problems, stomach pain, low blood cholesterol, joint problems, arthritis, and sore throat.
▼ Rare: eye problems have occurred with other drugs in this group but not with ibandronate. Contact your doctor if you experience any side effect not listed above.

Risedronate
▼ Most common: headache, diarrhea, abdominal pain, rash, and severe joint pain.
▼ Common: chest pain, dizziness, swelling in the arms or legs, constipation, nausea, sinus irritation, and bone pain.
▼ Less common: leg cramps, weakness, bronchitis, poor vision in one eye, dry eyes, ringing or buzzing in the ears,

Possible Side Effects *(continued)*

parathyroid gland problems, infection, rash and other skin problems, tooth problems, and vitamin D deficiency.

▼ Rare: fatigue and drug reactions, including swelling of the tongue and throat with difficulty breathing, generalized rash, and some blisters. Contact your doctor if you experience any side effect not listed above.

Tiludronate

▼ Most common: diarrhea and nausea.

▼ Common: headache, upset stomach, respiratory infection, runny nose, fluid in the lungs, and sinus irritation.

▼ Less common: vomiting, dizziness, tingling in the hands or feet, coughing, sore throat, gas, aches and pains, cataracts, eye redness, glaucoma, rash, skin disorders, tooth problems, swelling, infection, vitamin D deficiency, and muscle aches.

▼ Rare: tiredness, high blood pressure, fainting, appetite loss, constipation, abdominal pain, and sleeplessness. Contact your doctor if you experience any side effect not listed above.

Drug Interactions

- Antacids, calcium, and iron-containing supplements and foods can interfere with the absorption of bisphosphonates. Separate doses of these drugs and foods and a bisphosphonate by at least 30 minutes.
- Separate doses of tiludronate and aluminum-containing antacids by 1 hour.
- Aspirin can interfere with the absorption of tiludronate.
- Indomethacin can increase the amount of tiludronate absorbed into the blood by 2–4 times.
- Bisphosphonates may increase the gastrointestinal-irritating effects of aspirin, ibuprofen, and other NSAIDs.
- Drugs that reduce the amount of stomach acid, including ranitidine, cimetidine, and omeprazole, may increase the amount of ibandronate in the blood, but the degree of increase is not clinically important.
- Etidronate may affect the action of warfarin.
- Bisphosphonates reduce the ability of teriparatide to build new bone.

Food Interactions

Take these medicines with plain water. Food and drink—even mineral water, orange juice, or coffee—interfere with the absorption of these drugs. Take alendronate or risedronate every morning at least 30 minutes before eating, drinking, or taking other medications. Etidronate should be taken on an empty stomach 2 hours before a meal. Ibandronate should be taken as soon as you wake up and 1 hour before you eat or take any other medications, vitamins, or supplements. Tiludronate should be taken when you first wake up; wait 4 hours before eating breakfast.

Usual Dose

Alendronate
Adult: 10–40 mg a day; or 35–75 mg once weekly.
Child: not recommended.

Alendronate + Calcium
Adult: 70 mg/2800 IU once weekly.
Child: not recommended.

Etidronate
Adult: up to 4.5 mg per lb. a day to start, gradually increasing to no more than 9 mg per lb. per day.
Child: not recommended.

Ibandronate
Adult: 2.5 mg once a day; or one 150 mg tablet once a month.
Child: not recommended.

Risedronate
Adult: 5–30 mg a day; or 35 mg once weekly.
Child: not recommended.

Tiludronate
Adult: 400 mg a day.
Child: not recommended.

Overdosage

Little is known about the effects of bisphosphonate overdose. Very low blood calcium is the most serious symptom and requires emergency treatment. Other symptoms include upset stomach, heartburn, ulcer, and irritation of the esophagus. Milk or antacids may reverse these effects. These drugs can irritate the esophagus. Do not let the victim lie down or vomit. Overdose victims should be taken to a hospital emergency room. ALWAYS bring the prescription bottle or container.

Special Information

Food interferes with the effectiveness of these drugs. Carefully follow the directions in "Food Interactions" above.

Do not suck on any of these tablets or allow them to dissolve in your mouth because they can cause mouth sores.

To reduce the risk of stomach and throat irritation, do not lie down for at least 30 minutes after taking alendronate or risedronate. Do not lie down for 60 minutes after taking ibandronate.

Separate doses of calcium, iron, and vitamin D supplements from those of a bisphosphonate by at least 2 hours. If you forget a dose, take it as soon as you remember. If it is almost time for your next dose, skip the dose you forgot and continue with your regular schedule. If you forget a morning dose and take it later in the day, you must still follow the instructions in "Food Interactions" about avoiding food.

Special Populations

Pregnancy/Breast-feeding: Bisphosphonates cause abnormal bone development in animal fetuses and are toxic to pregnant animals. When any of these drugs is considered crucial by your doctor, its potential benefits must be carefully weighed against its risks.

It is not known if bisphosphonates pass into breast milk. Since these drugs affect bone formation, nursing mothers who must take a bisphosphonate should use infant formula.

Seniors: Seniors may use these drugs without special restriction.

Boniva   *see **Bisphosphonates**, page 164*

Generic Name

Bosentan   (boh-SEN-tan)

Brand Name

Tracleer

The information in this profile also applies to the following drug:

Generic Ingredient: Ambrisentan
Letairis

Type of Drug

Endothelin receptor antagonist.

Prescribed For

Pulmonary arterial hypertension.

General Information

These drugs lower blood pressure by working on the endothelin system. Endothelin is a hormone that plays an important role in maintaining blood pressure. It is normally found in blood vessels, but endothelin levels are very high in the blood and lungs of people with pulmonary arterial hypertension. People with this condition have high blood pressure, trouble breathing, and get very tired even when walking or doing other moderate exercising. Pulmonary arterial hypertension can be fatal.

Cautions and Warnings

These drugs should not be used by those who are **allergic** or **sensitive** to any of their ingredients.

Bosentan can cause liver injury. People taking these drugs should have their liver enzymes checked monthly. Enzyme increases can be a sign of liver injury and may be a reason to stop taking bosentan.

These drugs are broken down in the liver. People with **liver damage** should take them with caution.

These drugs should not be taken during **pregnancy** as they are likely to cause birth defects (see "Special Populations").

These drugs cause a reduction in **red blood cells,** leading to anemia. Larger doses of bosentan cause a greater loss of red blood cells.

Possible Side Effects

Ambrisentan

Most side effects are mild. Only stuffy nose increases with increased dosage.

▼ Most common: swelling in arms or legs, stuffy nose, sinusitis, flushing, heart palpitations, abdominal pain, constipation, difficulty breathing, and headache.

Bosentan

▼ Most common: headache and sore throat and nose.

Possible Side Effects *(continued)*

▼ Common: flushing, abnormal liver function, leg swelling,
low blood pressure, and heart palpitations.
▼ Less common: upset stomach, swelling, itching, anemia,
and tiredness.

Drug Interactions

- It is possible that bosentan may cause failure of hormonal
contraceptives.
- Cyclosporine, used to prevent transplant rejection, increases
blood levels of bosentan and ambrisentan. Do not combine
these drugs.
- Mixing glyburide, an antidiabetes drug, with bosentan increases the risk of elevated liver enzyme levels. Do not combine these drugs.
- Ketoconazole greatly increases blood levels of bosentan by
slowing its breakdown in the liver.
- Combining bosentan with a statin-type cholesterol-lowering
drug such as simvastatin, lovastatin, or atorvastatin reduces
the amount of statin drug in the blood. Dose increases may
be needed.
- Bosentan can reduce the amount of warfarin in the blood by
about $\frac{1}{3}$. Changes in warfarin dosage may be needed.
- Combining ambrisentan with atanazavir, clarithromycin,
indinavir, itraconazole, ketoconazole, nelfinavir, ritonavir,
omeprazole, saquinavir,or telithromycin may increase the
amount of ambrisentan in the blood. Caution is advised.
- Combining ambrisentan with rifampin may reduce the
amount of ambrisentan in the blood. Caution is advised.

Food Interactions

These drugs may be taken with or without food.

Usual Dose

Ambrisentan

   Adult (age 18 and over): 5–10 mg once a day. Do not crush, split,
or chew these tablets.
   Child: not recommended.

Bosentan

Adult (age 18 and over): 62.5 mg twice a day for 4 weeks, then 125 mg twice a day.

Child: not recommended.

Overdosage

Massive overdose may result in severe lowering of blood pressure, requiring emergency attention. The most common effects associated with overdosage are headache, low blood pressure, increased heart rate, and nausea and vomiting. Overdose victims should be taken to a hospital emergency room for treatment. ALWAYS bring the prescription bottle or container.

Special Information

Do not stop taking these drugs without gradually reducing the dosage as instructed by your doctor.

If you forget to take a dose, take it as soon as you remember. If it is almost time for your next dose, skip the dose you forgot and continue with your regular schedule. Do not take a double dose.

Contact your doctor at once if you develop severe itching, yellowing of the skin or eyes, tiredness, swelling in the arms or legs, nausea, vomiting, fever, or abdominal pain.

Doctors must enroll in special restricted distribution programs before they can prescribe these medicines, because of the risks of liver injury and birth defects associated with them. These medicines are not available in regular pharmacies but are mailed to you from a central pharmacy only after the testing and other program requirements have been met by your doctor.

Special Populations

Pregnancy/Breast-feeding: These medicines are very likely to cause major birth defects and should not be taken by pregnant women. Women must be sure they are not pregnant before beginning these treatments.

Women should also use non-hormone contraceptives while on these drugs. Hormone-based contraceptives such as birth control pills, injections, and implants may not work in women taking bosentan or ambrisentan.

It is not known if either of these medicines passes into breast milk. Nursing mothers should use infant formula.

Seniors: The greater chance of kidney, liver, and cardiac function side effects in seniors may affect drug dosage. Seniors may also experience more swelling in the arms or legs.

Type of Drug

Bowel Anti-Inflammatory Drugs (5-ASA Type)

Brand Names

Generic Ingredient: Balsalazide
Colazal

Generic Ingredient: Mesalamine [G]
Asacol   Pentasa
Canasa   Rowasa
Lialda

Generic Ingredient: Olsalazine
Dipentum

Prescribed For

Ulcerative colitis; rectal products prescribed for distal ulcerative colitis, proctitis, and proctosigmoiditis.

General Information

Chemical cousins of aspirin, these bowel anti-inflammatory drugs (5-ASA type) are used to treat symptoms of bowel inflammation. No one knows exactly how they work, but they are believed to have a local effect on the bowel. The tablet forms are made to delay drug release until they reach the colon. Little of the drug is absorbed into the blood; 70–90% remains in the colon.

Cautions and Warnings

Do not take bowel anti-inflammatories if you are **allergic** or **sensitive** to any of their ingredients or to aspirin. Although people who are sensitive or allergic to sulfasalazine have generally been able to tolerate mesalamine—which is an active agent in sulfasalazine—they should be cautious.

Bowel anti-inflammatories may worsen **colitis** or cause cramping, sudden abdominal pain, bloody diarrhea, fever, headache, or rash. Stop taking the drug at once and call your doctor if any of these symptoms develop.

Some people taking mesalamine have developed kidney problems. People who have or have had **kidney disease** should be cautious about using these drugs. All people taking mesalamine should have kidney function tests before and during drug therapy.

Possible Side Effects

Bowel anti-inflammatories are generally well tolerated. Tablets and capsules have the most side effects, suppositories the least.

Tablets

▼ Most common: headache; abdominal pain, cramps, or discomfort; belching; nausea; sore throat; and generalized pain.

▼ Common: constipation, diarrhea, upset stomach, vomiting, muscle weakness, dizziness, fever, runny nose, rash, skin spots, achy joints, back pain, and stiff muscles.

▼ Less common: worsening of colitis, gas, runny nose, chills, sweating, feeling unwell, tiredness, acne, itching, arthritis, chest pain, conjunctivitis (pinkeye), painful menstruation, swelling, and flu-like symptoms.

▼ Rare: sleeplessness, hair loss, leg or joint pain, and urinary burning or infection. Other rare side effects can occur in almost any part of the body. Contact your doctor if you experience any side effect not listed above.

Capsules

▼ Less common: abdominal pain, cramps, or discomfort; diarrhea; nausea; headache; respiratory infection; rash; and skin spots.

▼ Rare: worsening of colitis, constipation, gas, vomiting, dizziness, fever, sleeplessness, belching, upset stomach, sweating, feeling unwell, tiredness, itching, acne, achy joints, leg or joint pain, muscle aches, conjunctivitis (pinkeye), swelling, and hair loss. Other rare side effects can occur in almost any part of the body. Contact your doctor if you experience any side effect not listed above.

Suppositories

▼ Common: headache.

▼ Less common: abdominal pain, cramps, or discomfort; diarrhea or frequent stools; worsening of colitis; flatulence or gas; nausea; rectal pain, soreness, or burning; dizziness; dry mouth; fever; sore throat; cold symptoms; acne; rash; skin spots; and swelling.

Possible Side Effects *(continued)*

Rectal Suspension

▼ Common: abdominal pain, cramps, or discomfort; gas; nausea; headache; and flu-like symptoms.

▼ Less common: bloating; diarrhea; hemorrhoids; pain on enema insertion; rectal pain, soreness, or burning; dizziness; fever; feeling unwell; tiredness; cold symptoms; sore throat; itching; rash; skin spots; back pain; leg pain; and joint pain.

▼ Rare: constipation, muscle weakness, sleeplessness, swelling, hair loss, and urinary burning or infection. Contact your doctor if you experience any side effect not listed above.

Drug Interactions

None known.

Food Interactions

Take the tablet and capsule with food.

Usual Dose

Balsalazide

Tablets: 2250 mg 3 times a day for 8 weeks.

Mesalamine

Tablets: 800 mg 3 times a day for 6 weeks.

Once-daily tablets: 2–4 (1.2 mg each) once a day with a meal.

Capsules: 1000 mg 4 times a day for up to 8 weeks.

Suppositories: one 500-mg suppository twice a day for 3–6 weeks. Retain the suppository for 1–3 hours for maximum benefit.

Rectal Suspension: 1 bottle of suspension taken as an enema at bedtime every night for 3–6 weeks. The enema liquid should be retained for about 8 hours.

Olsalazine

Tablets: 1000 mg a day in 2 divided doses.

Overdosage

Symptoms are likely to include: ringing or buzzing in the ears, fainting or dizziness, headache, lethargy, confusion, drowsiness, sweating, rapid breathing, vomiting, and diarrhea. In case of overdose, call your local poison control center or hospital emergency room. You may be told to induce vomiting with ipecac syrup—available at any pharmacy—before taking the victim to the emergency room. If you seek treatment, ALWAYS bring the prescription bottle or container.

Special Information

The tablets and capsules must be swallowed whole. Call your doctor if they are visible in your stool. When using suppositories, handle them as little as possible to prevent melting.

Call your doctor if you develop chest pain, breathing or urinary difficulties, fever, unusual bleeding or bruising, worsening of colitis, or any bothersome or persistent side effects.

If you forget to administer a dose, do so as soon as you remember. If you take a tablet or capsule and it is within 4 hours of your next dose, skip the dose you forgot and continue with your regular schedule. If you take the suppositories or rectal solution and you do not remember until it is almost time for the next dose, skip the one you forgot and continue with your regular schedule. Do not take a double dose.

Special Populations

Pregnancy/Breast-feeding: Bowel anti-inflammatories can pass into the fetal circulation. When your doctor considers these drugs crucial, their potential benefits must be carefully weighed against their risks.

Small amounts of these drugs can pass into breast milk. Nursing mothers who must take these drugs should consider using infant formula.

Seniors: Seniors may use these drugs without special restriction.

Generic Name

Brimonidine (brim-ON-ih-dene) Ⓖ

Brand Name

Alphagan P

Type of Drug

Alpha agonist.

Prescribed For

Glaucoma and ocular hypertension (high pressure inside the eye).

General Information

Brimonidine tartrate stimulates alpha-2 receptors in the eye and lowers pressure there. The maximum effect occurs 2 hours after the drops are administered. Brimonidine reduces the amount of aqueous humor (liquid) produced inside the eye and increases the rate at which fluid flows out of the eyeball. That portion of brimonidine that finds its way into the bloodstream is broken down by the liver.

Cautions and Warnings

Do not use brimonidine if you are **allergic** or **sensitive** to any of its ingredients.

People with **kidney or liver disease** should use this drug with caution. People with **cardiovascular disease** should exercise caution with this medication because it can affect blood pressure. It should be used with caution in people with **depression, cerebral or coronary insufficiency,** and **Raynaud's disease.** Brimonidine may cause fatigue, drowsiness, and dizziness or fainting when rising from a sitting or lying position.

Brimonidine's effectiveness may decrease over time. Your doctor should check your eye pressure periodically to make sure the drug is still working.

Possible Side Effects

▼ Most common: dry mouth; redness, burning, and stinging of the eye; headache; blurred vision; sensation of something in the eye; drowsiness; and eye allergy and itching.

▼ Common: staining or erosion of the cornea, unusual sensitivity to bright light, eyelid redness or swelling, eye pain or ache, dry eye, respiratory symptoms, dizziness, eye irritation, upset stomach, weakness, abnormal vision, and muscle pain.

▼ Less common: crusty deposit on the eyelid, eye bleeding, abnormal taste sensation, sleeplessness, eye discharge, high blood pressure, anxiety, depression, heart palpitations, dry nose, and fainting.

Drug Interactions

- Brimonidine may enhance the effects of alcohol, barbiturates, sedatives, anesthetics, beta-blocking drugs, blood-pressure-lowering drugs, and cardiac glycosides.
- Tricyclic antidepressants can increase the breakdown of brimonidine.
- Do not combine brimonidine with monoamine oxidase inhibitor antidepressants.

Usual Dose

Adult and Child (age 2 and older): 1 drop in the affected eye every 8 hours, 3 times a day.

Child (under age 2): not recommended.

Overdosage

Little is known about the effects of accidental ingestion. Victims should be taken to a hospital emergency room for treatment. ALWAYS bring the prescription bottle or container.

Special Information

If you wear soft contact lenses, wait at least 15 minutes between the time you put the drops in your eye and when you put your lenses in.

To prevent possible infection, do not allow the dropper to touch your fingers, eyelids, or any surface. Wait at least 5 minutes before using any other eyedrops.

Brimonidine may make you drowsy. Be careful while driving or doing anything else that requires concentration while you are taking this drug.

It is important that brimonidine be used according to your doctor's directions. If you forget to administer a dose of brimonidine, do so as soon as you remember. If it is almost time for your next dose, skip the dose you forgot and continue with your regular schedule. Do not take a double dose.

Special Populations

Pregnancy/Breast-feeding: A small amount of brimonidine may pass into the circulation of the fetus. Pregnant women should use this drug with care.

It is not known if this drug passes into breast milk. Nursing mothers who must use this drug should consider using infant formula.

Seniors: Seniors may use brimonidine without special precaution.

Budeprion *see Bupropion, below*

Generic Name

Bupropion (bue-PROE-pee-on) Ⓖ

Brand Names

Budeprion	Wellbutrin SR
Budeprion XL	Wellbutrin XL
Wellbutrin	Zyban

Type of Drug

Antidepressant and smoking deterrent.

Prescribed For

Depression, seasonal affective disorder, and nicotine addiction.

General Information

Bupropion is used for major depression and seasonal affective disorder, and may work as a smoking deterrent by acting on key hormone systems in the brain. It works primarily on dopamine and noradrenaline, unlike the SSRI antidepressants, which primarily work on serotonin. Bupropion may not act until you have taken it for 2–4 weeks. The drug clears your system about 2 weeks after you stop taking it.

Cautions and Warnings

Do not take bupropion if you are **allergic** or **sensitive** to any of its ingredients.

Antidepressants have been associated with an increased risk of suicide, especially in **children** and **teenagers**. Suicide is always a risk in depressed people, who should only be allowed to have minimal quantities of medication in their possession. Clinical worsening of a depressed person's condition may also occur early in therapy with antidepressants.

People with **seizure disorders,** people who have had a seizure in the past, and people with **bulimia** or **anorexia nervosa** should be very careful about taking bupropion because they are at a higher risk of having a seizure. About 4 in 1000 people taking bupropion in dosages up to 450 mg a day develop a seizure. The risk of developing a seizure increases by about 10 times with dosages between 450 and 600 mg a day. About half of the people who developed a seizure on bupropion had a risk factor such as a history of head injury, a previous seizure, or a nervous system tumor, or were taking another drug associated with increased seizure risk.

People with unstable **heart disease** or those who have had a recent **heart attack** should take this drug with caution because of possible side effects.

Many people taking bupropion experience some restlessness, agitation, anxiety, and sleeplessness, especially soon after they start taking the drug. Some even require sleeping pills to counter this effect, and others find the stimulation so severe that they have to stop taking bupropion.

Bupropion may trigger a manic episode in those with depression or **bipolar disorder**.

People taking bupropion may experience hallucinations, delusions, or psychotic episodes. Dosage reduction or drug withdrawal is usually necessary to manage these reactions.

One-quarter of those who take bupropion lose their appetite and 5 or more lbs. of body weight. People who have lost weight due to their depression should be cautious about taking bupropion.

People switching from bupropion to a **monoamine oxidase inhibitor (MAOI) antidepressant**, or vice versa, should allow at least 2 weeks to pass between stopping one drug and starting the other.

People with **kidney or liver disease** require less bupropion at the beginning of treatment. Dosage should be increased cautiously.

An antidepressant other than bupropion should be seriously considered for people with a **history of drug abuse** because of the mild stimulation bupropion causes. These people may require larger-than-usual dosages, but they are still susceptible to seizures at these higher dosages.

Possible Side Effects

About 10% of people stop taking bupropion due to side effects.

▼ Most common: dry mouth; dizziness; rapid heartbeat; headache, including migraine; excessive sweating; nausea; vomiting; constipation; appetite loss; weight changes; sedation; agitation; sleeplessness; and tremors.

Possible Side Effects (continued)

▼ Less common: upset stomach, diarrhea, increased appetite, menstrual complaints, impotence, urinary difficulties, slowness of movement, salivation, muscle spasms, warmth, uncontrolled muscle movement, compulsion to move around or change positions, abnormal heart rhythms, blood-pressure changes, heart palpitations, fainting, itching, redness and rash, confusion, hostility, loss of concentration, reduced sex drive, anxiety, delusions, euphoria (feeling "high"), fatigue, joint pain, fever or chills, respiratory infection, and visual, taste, and hearing disturbances.

Drug Interactions

- Phenelzine (an MAOI) increases the risk of bupropion side effects. Allow at least 2 weeks to pass between stopping an MAOI and starting bupropion. Serious side effects can occur.
- Carbamazepine may reduce blood concentrations of bupropion.
- People taking both bupropion and levodopa + carbidopa or amantadine experience increased side effects. People taking these drugs should have their bupropion dosage increased gradually.
- Ritonavir may significantly increase bupropion blood levels and the risk of side effects.
- Don't mix bupropion with other drugs that increase the risk of seizures—including tricyclic antidepressants, haloperidol, lithium, loxapine, molindone, phenothiazine sedatives, and thioxanthene sedatives.
- Combining bupropion with a nicotine replacement drug can cause high blood pressure.
- Combining bupropion with warfarin can increase the risk of side effects.
- Do not combine Wellbutrin and Zyban, as they contain the same active ingredient.
- Alcohol should be avoided by people taking bupropion.

Food Interactions

Bupropion may be taken with food if it upsets your stomach.

Usual Dose

Depression
Adult: 200–450 mg a day; normal daily dosage is 300 mg.
Child (under age 18): not recommended.

Smoking Cessation
Adult: 150 mg twice a day. Begin treatment while you are still smoking.
Child (under age 18): not recommended.

Overdosage

Symptoms of overdose are likely to include severe side effects, such as seizures—present in a third of overdoses—hallucinations, loss of consciousness, and abnormal heart rhythms. Overdose victims should be taken to a hospital emergency room at once. ALWAYS bring the prescription bottle or container.

Special Information

Do not stop taking bupropion without your doctor's knowledge. Suddenly stopping the drug may cause withdrawal reactions and side effects.

Call your doctor if you experience agitation or excitement, restlessness, confusion, difficulty sleeping, anxiety, panic attacks, sleeplessness, irritability, hostility, aggressiveness, acting impulsively, a manic reaction, deepening depression, suicidal thinking, fast or abnormal heart rhythm, severe headache, seizure, rash, fainting, or any unusual or persistent side effect.

Bupropion may make you tired, dizzy, or lightheaded. Be careful when driving or doing any task that requires concentration.

Alcohol, sedatives, and other nervous system depressants increase the depressant effects of this drug. Alcohol also increases the risk of a seizure.

If you forget a dose, take it as soon as you remember. If it is almost time for your next dose and you take it several times a day, take 1 dose as soon as you remember and another in 3 or 4 hours, then go back to your regular schedule. Do not take a double dose.

Special Populations

Pregnancy/Breast-feeding: The safety of using bupropion during pregnancy is not known. When your doctor considers this drug crucial, its potential benefits must be carefully weighed against its risks. Pregnant women trying to quit smoking should use non-drug methods until their pregnancy is completed.

Bupropion passes into breast milk. Nursing mothers who must use bupropion should use infant formula.

Seniors: Seniors with reduced kidney or liver function may require reduced dosage.

Generic Name

Buspirone (bue-SPYE-rone) Ⓖ

Brand Name
BuSpar

Type of Drug
Minor sedative and antianxiety drug.

Prescribed For
Anxiety and generalized anxiety disorders; also prescribed for the aches, pains, fatigue, and cramps of premenstrual syndrome (PMS).

General Information
Buspirone hydrochloride has a potent antianxiety effect. It is approved by the Food and Drug Administration (FDA) for short-term relief of anxiety, but it may apparently be used safely for more than 4 weeks. The exact way in which buspirone works is not known, but it seems to lack the addiction dangers associated with other antianxiety drugs, including benzodiazepines. It neither severely depresses the nervous system nor acts as an anticonvulsant or muscle relaxant, as other antianxiety drugs do. Minor improvement will be apparent after only 7–10 days of drug treatment, but the maximum effect does not occur for 3 or 4 weeks.

Cautions and Warnings
Do not take buspirone if you are **allergic** or **sensitive** to any of its ingredients.

Buspirone should be used cautiously by people with **liver or kidney disease**.

Buspirone does not have any antipsychotic effect and should not be taken for symptoms of **psychosis.**

Although buspirone has not shown a potential for drug abuse, you should be aware of this possibility.

Buspirone should not be used with **monamine oxidase inhibitor (MAOI) antidepressants**.

Possible Side Effects

▼ Most common: dizziness, drowsiness, nausea, and headache.
▼ Common: fatigue, nervousness, lightheadedness, excitement, dry mouth, and insomnia.
▼ Less common: heart palpitations, muscle aches and pains,
tremors, rash, sweating, clamminess, rapid heartbeat, difficulty concentrating, anger or hostility, depression, loss of
interest, diarrhea, constipation, vomiting, and blurred vision.
▼ Rare: Rare side effects can occur in almost any part of the
body. Contact your doctor if you experience any side effect not listed above.

Drug Interactions

- Combining buspirone with an MAOI antidepressant may produce severe hypertension and may be dangerous.
- The effects of combining buspirone with other drugs that
work in the central nervous system (CNS) are not known. Do
not take other sedatives or antianxiety or psychoactive drugs
with buspirone unless prescribed by a doctor familiar with
your complete medical history.
- Erythromycin, itraconazole, ketoconazole, clarithromycin, diltiazem, verapamil, fluvoxamine, and ritonavir may increase
blood levels of buspirone. When used in combination, your
buspirone dosage may need to be adjusted.
- Buspirone may increase the side effects of haloperidol and
diazepam.
- Studies show that buspirone is not affected by alcohol, but
this combination should still be used with caution because
buspirone causes drowsiness and dizziness.
- The combination of buspirone and trazodone may cause liver
inflammation.
- Combining rifampin with buspirone may decrease buspirone's effectiveness.

Food Interactions

This drug may be taken either with or without food, but for the
most consistent results, always take your dose at the same time
of day in the same way—that is, with or without food. Avoid drinking large amounts of grapefruit juice with this drug.

Usual Dose

Adult: starting dosage—7.5 mg twice a day. Dosage may be increased gradually to 60 mg a day.

Overdosage

Symptoms of overdose are nausea, vomiting, dizziness, drowsiness, pinpointed pupils, and upset stomach. The overdose victim should be taken to a hospital emergency room. ALWAYS bring the prescription bottle or container.

Special Information

Buspirone may cause CNS depression, drowsiness, and dizziness. Be careful while driving or operating hazardous equipment. Avoid other CNS drugs and alcoholic beverages because they will enhance buspirone's effects.

Contact your doctor if you become restless, develop uncontrolled or repeated movements of the head, face, or neck, or have any intolerable side effects.

If you forget a dose, take it as soon as you remember. If it is almost time for your next dose, skip the dose you forgot and go back to your regular schedule. Do not take a double dose.

Special Populations

Pregnancy/Breast-feeding: Though buspirone has not been found to cause birth defects, be sure to inform your doctor if you are or might be pregnant while taking this drug. When this drug is considered crucial by your doctor, its potential benefits must be carefully weighed against its risks.

It is not known how much buspirone passes into breast milk. Nursing mothers who must take this drug should use infant formula.

Seniors: Several hundred seniors participated in drug evaluation studies without any unusual problems. However, the effect of this drug in seniors is not well known, and special problems may surface, particularly in those with kidney or liver disease.

Generic Name

Butenafine (bue-TEN-uh-fene)

Brand Names

Mentax   Mentax-TC

Type of Drug
Antifungal.

Prescribed For
Athlete's foot, jock itch, and ringworm.

General Information
Butenafine hydrochloride works by blocking the natural synthesis of a chemical—ergosterol—essential to the cell membrane (outer skin) of the fungus cell. Butenafine may actually kill the fungus if enough of it is present. Some butenafine is absorbed into the bloodstream.

Cautions and Warnings
Do not use butenafine if you are **allergic** or **sensitive** to any of its ingredients.

Possible Side Effects

▼ Common: rash, burning, stinging, worsening of the infection, swelling, irritation, and itching.

Drug Interactions
When you apply butenafine to the skin, do not combine it with any other topical medication.

Usual Dose
Adult and Child (age 12 and over): Apply enough to cover the affected area and surrounding skin once a day for 2–4 weeks, or twice a day for one week. Wash your hands after each application.
Child (under age 12): not recommended.

Overdosage
Little is known about the effects of accidental ingestion. Call your local poison control center or hospital emergency room for more information. ALWAYS bring the prescription bottle or container.

Special Information
This drug may irritate sensitive skin. Call your doctor if this happens—another medication may be more appropriate. Also call your doctor if you experience redness, itching, burning, blistering, swelling, or oozing.

Athlete's foot is relatively common and may be caused by a number of different kinds of fungi. Do not use this drug without your doctor's knowledge.

Butenafine is to be applied only to your skin. It should not be applied to other areas, including the eyes, nose, mouth, or vagina.

Do not bandage the area where the medication has been applied unless otherwise directed by your doctor.

If you apply the cream after bathing, be sure that your feet are completely dry, especially the areas between your toes. Do not wear socks made from wool or synthetic material or shoes that do not have adequate ventilation.

As is often the case when using an anti-infective, your symptoms may begin to improve before you have completed the full course of treatment. Be sure to use all of the medication as directed. If you are taking butenafine for jock itch or ringworm, wear loose-fitting clothing and keep the area cool and dry.

Call your doctor if the condition does not improve after 4 weeks of using the cream.

Special Populations

Pregnancy/Breast-feeding: Butenafine should only be used during pregnancy if absolutely necessary.

It is not known if this drug passes into breast milk. Nursing mothers who must use this drug should consider using infant formula.

Seniors: Seniors may use this medication without special precaution.

Generic Name

Calcitonin (kal-sih-TOE-nin)

Brand Names

Fortical   Miacalcin

Type of Drug

Polypeptide hormone.

Prescribed For

Osteoporosis (condition characterized by loss of bone mass due to depletion of minerals, especially calcium) in postmenopausal women.

General Information

Calcitonin helps to strengthen bone by adding more calcium to it and slowing the natural process by which bone is broken down. The calcitonin used in this drug is essentially identical to human calcitonin except that it is more potent. It is a synthetic version of the natural calcitonin found in salmon. Calcitonin can increase bone density and reduce the risk of fractures of the vertebrae (bones that comprise the spinal column), which are associated with back pain and loss of height. Calcitonin has been available for years as an injection, but the development of the nasal spray makes the drug easier to use.

Cautions and Warnings

Do not use calcitonin if you are **allergic** or **sensitive** to any of its ingredients. Although serious allergic reactions were reported with the injectable form, none have occurred with the nasal spray.

　　Changes in the tissues lining your nose are possible with long-term use of this product. An initial nasal examination and then periodic examinations are recommended.

Possible Side Effects

▼ Most common: stuffy nose, runny nose, and other nasal symptoms; and back pain.
▼ Less common: joint pain, nosebleed, and headache.

Drug Interactions

None known.

Food Interactions

None known.

Usual Dose

Adult: 1 spray (200 IU) a day.
Child: not recommended.

Overdosage

Little is known about the effects of calcitonin overdose or accidental ingestion. Nausea and vomiting have been reported after high doses. Call your local poison control center for more information. Overdose victims should be taken to a hospital emergency room. ALWAYS bring the prescription bottle or container.

Special Information

Alternate nostrils daily when using the nasal spray.

Before you take your first dose, you must activate the pump. Hold the bottle upright and press the two white arms toward the bottle 6 times until a faint spray is emitted. Once this occurs, the pump is activated and ready for use. It is not necessary to reactivate the pump every day.

Store new, unassembled bottles in the refrigerator. Keep the bottle in use at room temperature and discard after 30 days.

If you forget to administer a dose of the nasal spray, do so as soon as you remember. If it is almost time for the next dose, skip the dose you forgot and continue with your regular schedule. Call your doctor if you forget 2 or more doses.

Call your doctor if you develop severe nose irritation or any unusual or intolerable symptom. Follow your doctor's recommendations regarding calcium and vitamin D supplements. This drug is not intended to replace the need for dietary calcium.

Special Populations

Pregnancy/Breast-feeding: Calcitonin does not cross into the fetal circulation, though animal studies have associated the injectable form of the drug with low birth weight. This drug is recommended for use during pregnancy only if its possible benefits outweigh its risks.

It is not known if calcitonin passes into breast milk, though animal studies have shown that it reduces the amount of milk produced. Nursing mothers who must use calcitonin should consider using infant formula.

Seniors: Seniors may use this product without special precaution.

Generic Name

Capecitabine (cape-SE-tah-been)

Brand Name

Xeloda

Type of Drug

Antimetabolite.

Prescribed For

Breast cancer and colorectal cancer.

General Information

Capecitabine is prescribed for stages of breast and colorectal cancer in place of 5-FU, an injected drug that has been the basis for many chemotherapy programs. Capecitabine is converted in the body to 5-FU. Unlike many anticancer medications, capecitabine can be taken by mouth and has relatively few serious side effects.

Cautions and Warnings

Do not take capecitabine if you are **allergic** or **sensitive** to any of its ingredients or to 5-FU.

People taking **warfarin** or certain other **blood-thinning medications** are at risk of potentially fatal bleeding when capecitabine is added to their therapy. People taking these medications together should be closely monitored for changes in their response to the blood thinner.

People with **liver disease** should be carefully monitored by their doctors because capecitabine's effect on the liver is not known.

This drug is largely eliminated through the kidneys. People with severe **kidney disease** should not take it. Dose adjustments are required for those with moderate kidney disease.

Capecitabine may reduce fertility.

Capecitabine use is associated with heart and blood-vessel disease.

Capecitabine may cause severe diarrhea. Call your doctor if you experience symptoms (see "Special Information").

Jaundice has occurred in patients taking capecitabine requiring an interruption of medication until symptoms resolved.

Possible Side Effects

▼ Most common: diarrhea, constipation, nausea, vomiting, mouth sores, abdominal pain, hand-and-foot syndrome (see "Special Information"), inflammation of the skin, tingling or pain in the hands or feet, fatigue, loss of appetite, low blood-cell counts, eye irritation, and fever.

▼ Common: upset stomach, nail problems, headache, dizziness, sleeplessness, dehydration, swelling, muscle aches, and pain in the arms or legs.

▼ Less common and rare side effects can affect the stomach and intestines, skin, nervous system, tear ducts, lungs and

Possible Side Effects (continued)

respiratory system, heart and blood vessels, blood, urinary and reproductive tracts, liver, and other organs. Contact your doctor if you experience any side effect not listed above.

Drug Interactions

- Combining antacids and capecitabine can increase the amount of drug absorbed by about 20%. Separate doses of antacids and capecitabine by 2 hours.
- Leucovorin (a drug used in cancer treatment) increases the side effects of 5-FU. This combination has caused death in several seniors.
- Combining capecitabine with warfarin can cause excessive bleeding.
- When combining capecitabine with phenytoin, doses of phenytoin may need to be reduced due to an increase in side effects.

Food Interactions

Capecitabine should be taken within 30 minutes of a meal to avoid stomach problems.

Usual Dose

Adult (age 18 and over): 3000–5600 mg a day, depending on height and weight, in 2 doses. Capecitabine is used in 3-week cycles: 2 weeks on the drug, followed by 1 week off. Dosage may be reduced by 50% in people who experience severe side effects.

Child (under age 18): not recommended.

Overdosage

Symptoms include nausea, vomiting, diarrhea, bleeding and reduced blood-cell counts, and stomach irritation. Overdose victims should be taken to a hospital emergency room. ALWAYS bring the prescription bottle or container.

Special Information

Stop taking capecitabine and call your doctor if you have 4–6 more bowel movements a day than normal, vomit 2–5 times in 1 day, or become very nauseous. Depending on the severity of your symptoms, your doctor may reduce your dosage.

Capecitabine has caused hand-and-foot syndrome. Symptoms of this condition include numbness, tingling, pain, swelling, redness, and skin loss and blistering of the hands or feet. Stop taking the drug and call your doctor if you experience any of these symptoms.

People who develop stomatitis (symptoms include swelling, pain, or sores in the area of the mouth or tongue) should stop taking the drug and call their doctor at once.

Call your doctor, but do not stop taking the drug, if you develop a fever of 100.5°F or higher or other signs of infection.

If you forget a dose, take it as soon as you remember. If it is almost time for your next dose, take 1 dose right away and space the remaining daily dosage evenly throughout the day. Go back to your regular schedule the next morning. Call your doctor if you miss more than 2 doses in a row.

Special Populations

Pregnancy/Breast-feeding: Capecitabine can harm the fetus. Its potential benefits must be carefully weighed against its risks when capecitabine is considered crucial by your doctor. Effective contraception is absolutely necessary while taking this drug.

It is not known if capecitabine passes into breast milk. Nursing mothers who must take this drug should use infant formula.

Seniors: Seniors may be more sensitive to side effects, especially diarrhea and other stomach problems.

Generic Name

Captopril (KAP-toe-pril) Ⓖ

Brand Name
Capoten

Combination Products
Generic Ingredients: Captopril + Hydrochlorothiazide Ⓖ
Capozide

Type of Drug
Angiotensin-converting enzyme (ACE) inhibitor.

Prescribed For
High blood pressure and heart failure; diabetic kidney damage and post–heart attack management; also used for kidney hyperten-

sion, the management of people with a high risk of heart disease, chronic kidney disease, the prevention of a second stroke, and high blood pressure associated with other medical conditions, such as scleroderma and Takayasu's disease.

General Information

Captopril and other ACE inhibitors work by preventing the conversion of a hormone called angiotensin I to another hormone called angiotensin II, a potent blood-vessel constrictor. Preventing this conversion relaxes blood vessels, helps to reduce blood pressure, and relieves the symptoms of heart failure. Captopril also affects the production of other hormones and enzymes that participate in the regulation of blood-vessel dilation. Captopril usually begins working about 1 hour after it is taken.

In addition to its labeled uses, captopril has been studied in the diagnosis of certain kidney diseases and of primary aldosteronism; in the treatment of rheumatoid arthritis; in swelling and fluid accumulation; in Bartter's syndrome; in Raynaud's disease; and in post–heart attack treatment when the function of the left ventricle is affected.

Cautions and Warnings

Do not take captopril if you are **allergic** or **sensitive** to any of its ingredients. Severe sensitivity reactions can occur in **hemodialysis patients** or in those undergoing **venom immunization.**

People with **impaired kidney function** should not take captopril unless other antihypertensives have not worked or have had unacceptable side effects.

Swelling of the face, extremities, or throat has been known to occur with captopril, which can be dangerous (see "Special Information").

Although not common, captopril may cause very low blood pressure. It may also affect your kidneys, especially if you have **congestive heart failure.** Your doctor should check your urine for protein content during the first few months of captopril treatment. Captopril may cause a decline in kidney function.

Captopril may affect white-blood-cell counts, possibly increasing your susceptibility to infection. Your doctor should monitor your blood counts periodically.

Captopril can cause serious injury or death to the fetus if taken during **pregnancy**. Pregnant women should not take captopril.

ACE inhibitors may be less effective in some **black patients** with high blood pressure, especially when dietary salt intake is high. Nevertheless, they should still be considered useful blood pressure treatments. Swelling beneath the skin to form welts is more common among black patients.

Possible Side Effects

▼ Most common: rash, itching, and cough that usually goes away a few days after you stop taking the drug.

▼ Less common: dizziness, tiredness, sleep disturbances, headache, tingling in hands or feet, chest pain, heart palpitations, feeling unwell, abdominal pain, nausea, vomiting, diarrhea, constipation, appetite loss, dry mouth, breathing difficulties, and hair loss.

▼ Rare: Rare side effects can occur in almost any part of the body. Contact your doctor if you experience any side effect not listed above.

Drug Interactions

- The blood-pressure-lowering effect of captopril is additive with diuretic drugs and beta blockers. Any other drug that causes a rapid blood-pressure drop should be used with caution if you are taking captopril.
- Combining 325 mg of aspirin a day with captopril carries a higher risk of death than taking lower doses (less than 160 mg a day). People taking aspirin to prevent a heart attack should use the lower dose.
- Captopril may increase the effects of lithium; this combination should be used with caution.
- Mixing any ACE inhibitor with an NSAID pain reliever can increase the chances of kidney failure.
- Severe sensitivity reactions can occur in those taking allopurinol.
- Captopril may increase blood-potassium levels, especially when taken with dyazide or other potassium-sparing diuretics.
- Antacids and captopril should be taken at least 2 hours apart.
- Capsaicin may trigger or aggravate the cough associated with captopril.
- Indomethacin may reduce the blood-pressure-lowering effect of captopril.
- Phenothiazine sedatives and antivomiting agents may increase the effects of captopril.

- Probenecid increases captopril's effect as well as the chance of side effects.
- The combination of allopurinol and captopril increases the chance of an adverse drug reaction.
- Captopril may affect blood levels of digoxin. More digoxin in the blood increases the chance of digoxin-related side effects, while less digoxin in the blood can compromise its effectiveness.

Food Interactions

Captopril should be taken 1 hour before a meal.

Usual Dose

Adult: 25 mg 2 or 3 times a day to start. Dosage may be increased to 450 mg a day in divided doses, if needed. Dosage must be tailored to your needs. People with poor kidney function must take lower doses.

Child: 0.14–0.28 mg per lb. of body weight, 3 times a day.

Infant: 0.07–0.14 mg per lb. of body weight.

Overdosage

The principal effect of captopril overdose is a rapid drop in blood pressure, which may lead to dizziness or fainting. Take the overdose victim to a hospital emergency room immediately. ALWAYS bring the prescription bottle or container.

Special Information

Captopril may cause swelling of the face, lips, hands, and feet. This swelling may also affect the larynx (throat) and tongue and interfere with breathing. If this happens, go to a hospital emergency room at once. Call your doctor if you develop a sore throat, mouth sores, abnormal heartbeat, chest pain, a persistent rash, or losses in the sense of taste.

People who are already taking a diuretic (an agent that increases urination) may experience a rapid blood-pressure drop after their first dose of captopril or when their captopril dose is increased. To prevent this, your doctor may tell you to stop taking your diuretic or to increase your salt intake 2 or 3 days before starting captopril. The diuretic may then be restarted gradually.

You may get dizzy if you rise to your feet too quickly from a sitting or lying position when taking captopril.

Avoid strenuous exercise or very hot weather because heavy sweating or dehydration may lead to a rapid drop in blood pressure.

Avoid over-the-counter stimulants that can raise blood pressure while taking captopril, including diet pills and decongestants. Also, do not use potassium supplements or salt substitutes containing potassium without consulting your doctor.

If you forget to take a dose of captopril, take it as soon as you remember. If it is within 4 hours of your next dose, take 1 dose immediately and another in 5 or 6 hours, then go back to your regular schedule. Do not take a double dose.

Special Populations

Pregnancy/Breast-feeding: ACE inhibitors can cause fetal injury or death. Women who are or might be pregnant should not take ACE inhibitors. If you become pregnant, stop taking captopril and call your doctor immediately.

Small amounts of captopril pass into breast milk. Nursing mothers who must take this drug should consider using infant formula.

Seniors: Seniors may be more sensitive to the effects of captopril due to age-related declines in kidney or liver function.

Generic Name

Carbamazepine (car-bam-A-zuh-pene) Ⓖ

Brand Names

Atretol	Tegretol
Carbatrol	Tegretol-XR
Epitol	Teril
Equetro	

Type of Drug

Anticonvulsant.

Prescribed For

Seizure disorders as well as trigeminal and other neuralgias; also used to treat severe pain; psychiatric disorders including depression, bipolar disorder, intermittent explosive disorder, borderline personality disorder, post-traumatic stress disorder, psychotic disorders, and schizophrenia; withdrawal from alcohol, cocaine, or benzodiazepine-type drugs; restless leg syndrome; hereditary and non-hereditary chorea in children; and diabetes insipidus.

General Information

Carbamazepine was first approved for relief of the severe pain of trigeminal neuralgia. Over the years, it has gained wide use in seizure control, especially in people whose seizures are uncontrolled with phenytoin, phenobarbital, or primidone, or who have suffered severe side effects from these drugs. Carbamazepine is not a simple pain reliever and should not be taken for everyday aches and pains. It is associated with potentially fatal side effects.

Cautions and Warnings

Carbamazepine should not be used if you are **allergic** or **sensitive** to any of its ingredients or to any tricyclic antidepressant.

Carbamazepine should not be used if you have had **bone marrow depression.**

Carbamazepine may cause severe, possibly life-threatening blood reactions. People who have had **blood reactions to other drugs** are at particular risk for another reaction with carbamazepine. Your doctor should have a complete blood count done before you start taking this drug and repeat these tests weekly during the first 3 months of treatment, and then every month for the next 2–3 years. Unexplained fever or infection may be a sign of a blood reaction.

Monoamine oxidase inhibitor (MAOI) antidepressants should be discontinued 2 weeks before starting carbamazepine.

Rarely, severe, possibly fatal skin reactions can develop in a few people taking carbamazepine. **Asians** are 10 times more likely to develop these reactions than non-Asians.

Carbamazepine may aggravate **glaucoma** and should be used with caution by people with this condition. This drug may activate underlying **psychosis,** and, in older adults, **confusion** or **agitation**.

This drug is not for the relief of minor aches or pains.

Possible Side Effects

▼ Most common: dizziness, drowsiness, unsteadiness, nausea, and vomiting. Other common side effects are blurred or double vision, confusion, hostility, headache, and severe water retention.

▼ Less common: mood and behavioral changes, especially in children. Hives, itching, rash, and other allergic reactions may also occur.

Possible Side Effects *(continued)*

▼ Rare: Rare side effects can affect your breathing, speech, emotions, liver function, urinary function, and many other parts of the body. Contact your doctor if you experience any side effect not listed above.

Drug Interactions

- Carbamazepine blood levels may be increased by azoles (e.g. ketoconazole), acetazolamide, cimetidine, dalfopristin, danazol, delavirdine, diltiazem, haloperidol, isoniazid, propoxyphene, erythromycin-type antibiotics (except azithromycin), fluoxetine, fluvoxamine, loratadine, levetiracetam, macrolides, MAOIs, nefazodone, niacinamide, nicotinamide, protease inhibitors, quinine, quinupristin, terfenadine, tricyclic antidepressants, valproate, verapamil, or zileuton, leading to possible carbamazepine toxicity.
- Carbamazepine may reduce the effectiveness of contraceptive drugs and cause breakthrough bleeding.
- Charcoal tablets or powder, clozapine, methsuximide phenobarbital and other barbiturates, phenytoin, primidone and theophylline may decrease the absorption of carbamazepine. Levels of phenobarbital, a breakdown product of primidone, may be increased by combining primidone and carbamazepine.
- Carbamazepine reduces the effects of acetaminophen, the anticoagulant (blood thinner) warfarin, and theophylline (prescribed for asthma). Increased dosage of these drugs may be necessary. Other drugs counteracted by carbamazepine are antipsychotics (e.g. aripiprazole, clozapine, olanzapine, quetiapine, risperidone, and ziprasidone), benzodiazepines (e.g. diazepam and lorazepam), bupropion, cyclosporine, digitalis drugs, doxycycline, felodipine, lamotrigine, levothyroxine, methadone, mirtazapine, certain muscle relaxants, oxcarbazepine, praziquantel, statin drugs, tiagabine, topiramate, tramadol, and zonisamide.
- Combining carbamazepine and other antiseizure drugs, including felbamate, hydantoins, succinimides, and valproic acid, may cause unpredictable results. Combination treatments to control seizures must be customized to each person.

- Combining carbamazepine and lithium may increase nervous system side effects such as muscular twitching or impaired consciousness.
- Carbamazepine suspension should not be combined with other liquid medicines or diluents.

Food Interactions

Take carbamazepine with food if it causes stomach upset. Avoid taking carbamazepine with grapefruit products.

Usual Dose

Adult and Child (age 13 and over): 400–1200 mg a day, depending on the condition. Usual maintenance dose is 400–800 mg a day in 2 divided doses.

Child (age 6–12): 200–1000 mg a day, or 22–24 mg per lb. of body weight 2–3 times a day for suspension or 4 times a day for tablets. Do not exceed 1000 mg a day.

Child (under age 6): 22–24 mg per lb. of body weight 2–3 times a day for suspension or 4 times a day for tablets; dosage should not exceed 77 mg per lb. of body weight a day.

Dosage varies according to form. Liquid carbamazepine must be taken 3 times a day, regular carbamazepine tablets twice a day, and sustained-release tablets once daily. Never change your dosage schedule without first checking with your doctor.

Overdosage

Carbamazepine is a potentially lethal drug. Overdose symptoms appear in 1–3 hours. These include irregularity or difficulty in breathing, rapid heartbeat, changes in blood pressure, shock, loss of consciousness or coma, convulsions, muscle twitching, restlessness, uncontrolled body movements, drooping eyelids, psychotic mood changes, nausea, vomiting, and reduced urination. Induce vomiting right away with ipecac syrup—available at any pharmacy. Then take the victim to a hospital emergency room. ALWAYS bring the prescription bottle or container.

Special Information

Carbamazepine may cause dizziness and drowsiness. Take care while driving or doing any task that requires concentration.

Call your doctor at once if you experience yellowing of the skin or whites of the eyes, unusual bleeding or bruising, abdominal pain, pale stools, dark urine, impotence, mood changes, nervous system symptoms, swelling, fever, chills, sore throat, or mouth sores. These may be signs of a potentially fatal drug reaction.

If you forget a dose, skip it and go back to your regular schedule. If you miss more than 1 dose in a day, call your doctor. Do not stop taking this drug without first consulting your doctor.

Special Populations

Pregnancy/Breast-feeding: Carbamazepine caused birth defects in animal studies. Seizure disorder itself also increases the risk of birth defects. Pregnant women should take carbamazepine only after discussing with their doctors its potential benefits and risks.

Carbamazepine passes into breast milk. Nursing mothers who must take carbamazepine should use infant formula.

Seniors: Seniors taking this drug are more likely to develop heart problems, confusion, or agitation.

Type of Drug

Carbonic-Anhydrase Inhibitors, Eyedrops (kar-BON-ik an-HYE-drase)

Brand Names

Generic Ingredient: Dorzolamide
Trusopt

Generic Ingredient: Brinzolamide
Azopt

Combination Product
Generic Ingredients: Dorzolamide + Timolol
Cosopt

Prescribed For
Glaucoma.

General Information
These drugs are similar to acetazolamide, a carbonic-anhydrase inhibitor taken by mouth. Carbonic anhydrase is an enzyme found in many parts of the body, including the eyes. By blocking the effects of this enzyme, dorzolamide and brinzolamide slow the production of fluid inside the eye, reducing pressure. This effect is useful in treating open-angle glaucoma because the disease is

characterized by elevated eye pressure. Dorzolamide and brinzolamide are sulfonamides, or sulfa drugs, and although they are administered topically, they affect the body systemically.

Cautions and Warnings

Do not use these drugs if you are **allergic** or **sensitive** to any of their ingredients or to other sulfa drugs. Small amounts of these drugs enter the bloodstream. Rarely, people using them experience side effects or allergies associated with sulfa drugs.

These drugs have not been studied in people with very **poor kidney or liver function**. Since these drugs are eliminated via the kidneys, people with impaired kidney function should use an alternate glaucoma medication.

These drugs have not been studied in people with **acute angle-closure glaucoma**.

See Timolol, page 1129, for more information on the combination product Cosopt.

Possible Side Effects

Dorzolamide

▼ Most common: eye burning, stinging, or discomfort and a bitter taste in the mouth immediately after administering the eyedrops.

▼ Less common: allergic reactions, conjunctivitis (pinkeye), blurred vision, tearing, dry eye, and increased sensitivity to bright light.

▼ Rare: headache, nausea, weakness, tiredness, rash, and kidney stones. Dorzolamide can cause the same types of side effects as other sulfa drugs, but this is very unlikely. Contact your doctor if you experience any side effects not listed above.

Brinzolamide

▼ Common: blurred vision and a bitter, sour, or unusual taste in the mouth.

▼ Less common: eyelid inflammation; conjunctivitis (pinkeye); rash; dry eye; sensation of something in the eye; headache; eye redness, itching, discharge, or pain; and runny nose.

▼ Rare: allergic reactions, hair loss, chest pain, diarrhea, nausea, sore throat, tearing, itchy rash, double vision, dizziness,

Possible Side Effects *(continued)*

dry mouth, breathing difficulties, upset stomach, tired eyes, kidney pain, cornea problems, and formation of a crust or sticky sensation around the eyelid. Brinzolamide can cause the same types of side effects as other sulfa drugs, but this is very unlikely. Contact your doctor if you experience any side effect not listed above.

Drug Interactions

- If you are using more than 1 eyedrop product, separate doses of these drugs by at least 10 minutes.

Usual Dose

Adult: 1 drop in the affected eye 3 times a day.

Overdosage

Accidental ingestion of a bottle of dorzolamide or brinzolamide may affect blood levels of potassium and other electrolytes. The victim should be taken to a hospital emergency room. ALWAYS bring the prescription bottle or container.

Special Information

Call your doctor and stop using your eyedrops if you develop any unusual eye reaction or condition, including swollen eyelids and conjunctivitis (pinkeye).

Vision may be temporarily blurred when using the eyedrops. Use caution when driving or operating machinery.

If you wear soft contact lenses, take them out before using the eyedrops and put them back in 15 minutes after a dose.

To prevent infection, do not allow the eyedropper tip to touch your fingers, eyelids, or any surface. Wait at least 10 minutes before using any other eyedrops.

If you forget to administer a dose, do so as soon as you remember. If it is almost time for your next dose, skip the one you forgot and continue with your regular schedule. Do not take a double dose.

Special Populations

Pregnancy/Breast-feeding: Very high dosages of dorzolamide or brinzolamide caused birth defects in animal studies. While the risks of using these drugs during pregnancy are small in people, pregnant women should use dorzolamide or brinzolamide only after discussing its potential benefits and risks with their doctors.

It is not known if these drugs pass into breast milk. Nursing mothers who must use either drug should use infant formula.

Seniors: Seniors may be more sensitive to side effects.

Generic Name

Carvedilol (car-VAY-dih-lol) Ⓖ

Brand Names

Coreg   Coreg CR

Type of Drug

Alpha-beta-adrenergic blocker.

Prescribed For

Heart failure, high blood pressure, angina pain, and cardio-myopathy.

General Information

Carvedilol was the first beta blocker approved for heart failure. It is also the only beta blocker approved for severe heart failure.

Carvedilol blocks both the alpha- and beta-adrenergic portions of the central nervous system. This dual action reduces the amount of blood pumped with each heartbeat and also decreases the risk of tachycardia (very rapid heartbeat). Carvedilol's beta-blocking effects begin within an hour of taking the first dose; maximum blood-pressure-lowering occurs after 1 or 2 weeks. The drug also causes blood vessels to dilate (widen), allowing the heart to pump blood more efficiently.

Cautions and Warnings

Do not take carvedilol if you are **allergic** or **sensitive** to any of its ingredients, or if you have **AV block, sick sinus syndrome** or **severe bradycardia** (slow heart rate) without the use of a pacemaker.

Carvedilol should not be taken by patients with **bronchial disease,** such as **chronic bronchitis, emphysema,** or **asthma**.

Carvedilol therapy should not be stopped suddenly due to the risk of worsening the heart condition.

In studies, carvedilol caused mild and reversible liver injury in about 1 of every 100 people who took it. Those with severe **liver disease** should not take this medication. Call your doctor at once if you develop signs of liver damage (symptoms include severe itching, dark-colored urine, flu-like symptoms, appetite loss, and yellowing of the skin or whites of the eyes).

Check with your doctor about continuing carvedilol if you are to receive **general anesthesia**; heart function that is depressed by anesthetics can worsen if carvedilol is used at the same time.

Make sure your doctor knows if you have **diabetes.** Carvedilol can mask signs of **low blood sugar** and may increase the effects of insulin or oral antidiabetes drugs, making it more difficult to recover from the effects of low blood sugar.

Carvedilol can mask symptoms of an **overactive thyroid gland.** Abruptly stopping carvedilol can trigger an attack of hyperthyroidism.

Possible Side Effects

Most side effects are considered mild or moderate.

▼ Most common: dizziness, sleepiness or sleeplessness, diarrhea, abdominal pain, slow heartbeat, dizziness when rising from a sitting or lying position, swelling of the hands or feet, sore throat, breathing difficulties, tiredness, back pain, urinary infection, and viral infection.

▼ Less common: extra heartbeats; palpitations; blood-pressure changes; fainting; reduced blood supply to the arms and legs (symptoms include aches, cramps, pain, or tiredness on walking, or pain in the foot, thigh, hip, or buttocks); tingling in the hands or feet; reduced sensation; depression; nervousness; constipation; gas; liver irritation; cough; impotence and reduced sex drive in men; itching; rash; visual difficulties; ringing or buzzing in the ears; high blood cholesterol, sugar, or uric acid; anemia; weakness; hot flushes; leg cramps; dry mouth; not feeling well; sweating; and muscle ache.

▼ Rare: Rare side effects can affect the heart, mental status, the respiratory tract, the urinary tract, and the kidney. It can also cause hair loss, weight gain, high blood-triglyceride levels, low blood-platelet counts, and sugar in the urine. Contact your doctor if you experience any side effect not listed above.

Drug Interactions

• Carvedilol increases the effects of insulin and oral antidiabetes drugs. People taking this combination must monitor

their blood sugar levels regularly. Call your doctor if there is any change from your normal pattern.
- Carvedilol increases the effects of verapamil, diltiazem, and similar calcium-channel blocking drugs.
- Monoamine oxidase inhibitor antidepressants may increase the effects of carvedilol.
- Carvedilol increases the blood-pressure-lowering effect of clonidine. People taking this combination may need less clonidine to control their pressure.
- Carvedilol increases the amount of digoxin in the blood by about 15%. Your digoxin dosage may have to be adjusted.
- Cimetidine increases the amount of carvedilol absorbed into the blood by about 30%, but the importance of this interaction is not clear.
- Rifampin reduces the amount of carvedilol in the blood by about 70%. Dosage adjustment is necessary.
- Do not consume alcohol (including medicines that contain alcohol) within 2 hours of taking carvedilol.

Food Interactions
Take carvedilol with food to reduce the risk of dizziness or fainting.

Usual Dose
Heart Failure
Adult: 3.125 mg twice a day for 2 weeks. Dose may be doubled every 2 weeks to the highest level tolerated. Maximum daily dosage is 25 mg twice a day in people weighing less than 187 lbs., and 50 mg twice a day in people who weigh more.

High Blood Pressure and Cardiomyopathy
Adult: 6.25 mg twice a day to start, increased to 25 mg twice a day if needed.
Senior: Seniors may require smaller doses than younger adults.
Child (under age 18): not recommended.

Overdosage
Overdose may lead to very low blood pressure (symptoms include dizziness and fainting), slow heartbeat and other cardiac symptoms, including shock and heart attack, breathing difficulties, bronchial spasm, vomiting, periods of unconsciousness, and seizures. Overdose victims must be taken to a hospital emergency room. ALWAYS bring the prescription bottle or container.

Special Information

Carvedilol should be taken continuously. Do not stop taking it without your doctor's knowledge, because abrupt withdrawal may cause chest pain, breathing difficulties, increased sweating, and unusually fast or irregular heartbeat. The dose should be gradually reduced over a period of about 2 weeks.

People taking carvedilol may become dizzy or faint when rising quickly from a sitting or lying position. If this happens to you, sit or lie down until you feel better. Carvedilol can also cause drowsiness, lightheadedness, or blurred vision. Be careful when driving or doing any task that requires concentration.

Contact lens wearers are more likely to experience dry eyes with carvedilol.

Swallow extended-release tablets whole; do not crush or break them.

It is best to take carvedilol at the same time each day. If you forget a dose, take it as soon as you remember. If it is within 4 hours of your next dose, skip the dose you forgot and continue with your regular schedule. Do not take a double dose.

Special Populations

Pregnancy/Breast-feeding: Animal studies indicate that carvedilol passes into the fetal bloodstream and may interfere with pregnancy. When this drug is considered crucial by your doctor, its potential benefits must be carefully weighed against its risks.

It is not known if carvedilol passes into human breast milk, though it passes into rat breast milk. Beta-blocking drugs like carvedilol may affect babies' hearts. Nursing mothers who must take this drug should use infant formula.

Seniors: Seniors are more likely to develop dizziness and may require reduced dosage.

Celebrex   *see Celebrex, below*

Celecoxib (sel-eh-KOX-ib)

Brand Name

Celebrex

Type of Drug

Cyclooxygenase-2 (COX-2) inhibitor nonsteroidal anti-inflammatory drug (NSAID).

Prescribed For

Osteoarthritis, rheumatoid arthritis, juvenile rheumatoid arthritis, acute pain, some colon polyps (FAP), menstrual pain, and arthritis of the spine (ankylosing spondylitis).

General Information

Traditional NSAIDs work primarily by blocking the effects of COX-2, a body enzyme that plays an important role in regulating pain and inflammation. But these NSAIDs also have an unwanted effect: They interfere with cyclooxygenase-1 (COX-1), a related enzyme that helps to maintain the stomach's protective lining. NSAIDs that block the effects of this enzyme may produce side effects such as stomach irritation, gas, and stomach ulcers.

COX-2 inhibitors such as celecoxib are a class of NSAIDs that work about as well as the older NSAIDs. In fact, both 200 mg a day and 400 mg a day of celecoxib work as well as naproxen 500 mg twice a day. They interfere primarily with COX-2, leaving the stomach-protecting COX-1 relatively unaffected. This means that COX-2 inhibitor NSAIDs can relieve pain and inflammation just like traditional NSAIDs but are less likely to cause gastrointestinal (GI) side effects. Another advantage of celecoxib is that it does not cause thinning of the blood or affect blood platelets as can happen with older NSAIDs. Celecoxib is broken down in the liver.

Black patients absorb about 40% more celecoxib than Caucasians; its importance is unclear. Celecoxib is the first drug proven effective in reducing the number of intestinal polyps in people with the rare genetic disorder FAP.

Cautions and Warnings

Do not take celecoxib if you are **allergic** or **sensitive** to any of its ingredients or to sulfa drugs. NSAIDs should not be taken by people with **asthma** or by those who have had an **allergic reaction to aspirin or another NSAID.** They can develop a group of symptoms (runny nose with or without nasal polyps and a severe bronchial spasm) known as the aspirin triad.

COX-2 inhibitors, including celecoxib, have been associated with high blood pressure, kidney damage, heart attacks, and stroke. It should not be used to treat pain associated with **heart bypass surgery**. Two other COX-2 inhibitors were taken off the market because of safety concerns. Rofecoxib was removed because safety issues were noted after people had taken it for 18 months or more. Valdecoxib was taken off the market because of the lack of safety data, severe skin rashes, and concerns raised in people taking the drug after having had heart surgery.

NSAIDs can cause GI bleeding and ulcers and stomach perforation. This can occur at any time, with or without warning, in people who take NSAIDs regularly. Celecoxib should be used with caution by people who have had **stomach ulcers** or **GI bleeding.** Minor upper GI problems, such as upset stomach, are common and may occur at any time during NSAID therapy. People who develop bleeding or ulcers and continue NSAID treatment should be aware of the risk of developing more serious side effects. Risk of GI bleeding and ulcers is increased with longer duration of therapy as well as treatment with oral corticosteroids and anticoagulants, smoking, alcoholism, older age, and general poor health.

Children taking celecoxib may be more likely to vomit blood, suffer acute kidney failure, or develop rashes.

Celecoxib has not been studied in people with severe **kidney disease**. They should not use this drug unless their doctors closely monitor their kidney function.

Celecoxib can cause liver irritation and should be used with caution by people with **hepatitis** or **cirrhosis.** People with moderate **liver disease** can have twice as much celecoxib in their blood and require a reduced dosage. The effect of celecoxib in people with severe **liver failure** is not known.

Possible Side Effects

Side effects are similar to those of traditional NSAIDs. Stomach and intestinal side effects are about half as common.
- ▼ Most common: headache.
- ▼ Common: diarrhea, upset stomach, sinus irritation, and respiratory infection.
- ▼ Less common: abdominal pain, gas, nausea, back pain, swelling in the legs or arms, accidental injuries, sleeplessness, dizziness, sore throat, runny nose, and rash.
- ▼ Rare: Rare side effects can occur in almost any part of the body. Contact your doctor if you experience any side effect not listed above.

Drug Interactions

- Alcohol may increase the risk of serious GI-related side effects. Avoid alcohol.
- Combining celecoxib with an aluminum and magnesium antacid slightly reduces the amount of drug absorbed. Separate doses of these antacids and celecoxib by 1–2 hours.
- Fluconazole and lithium may raise celecoxib blood levels and increase the risk of side effects.
- While celecoxib may be combined with low dosages of aspirin, taking these drugs together can increase the risk of stomach or intestinal ulcers or other complications. The ulcer risk associated with this combination is less than that posed by single-drug therapy with a traditional NSAID.
- Celecoxib can reduce the blood-pressure-lowering effect of angiotensin-converting enzyme (ACE) inhibitors and diuretic drugs. This combination can also increase the risk of kidney damage after chronic celecoxib use.
- Celecoxib may affect lithium blood levels.
- NSAIDs can reduce the effect of furosemide and thiazide-type diuretics.
- Celecoxib should be used cautiously with warfarin. Concurrent use of these drugs may cause an increased risk of bleeding complications.

Food Interactions

Celecoxib can be taken without regard to food or meals. For optimal effectiveness, avoid taking this drug with high-fat meals.

Usual Dose

Adult (age 18 and over): arthritis—100–200 mg once or twice a day. FAP—400 mg twice a day.

Child (age 2 and over): juvenile rheumatoid arthritis—22–55 lbs: 50 mg twice a day; over 55 lbs: 100 mg twice a day.

Child (under age 2): not recommended.

Overdosage

Overdosage symptoms include lethargy, drowsiness, nausea, vomiting, and stomach pain. Stomach or intestinal bleeding or severe allergic reactions can occur. High blood pressure, kidney failure, breathing difficulties, and coma are rare.

The victim should be taken to a hospital emergency room. ALWAYS bring the prescription bottle or container.

Special Information

Call your doctor if you develop rash, itching, unexplained weight gain, nausea, fatigue, jaundice (yellowing of the skin or whites of the eyes), flu-like symptoms, lethargy, swelling, black stools, severe stomach pain, persistent headache, or any bothersome or persistent side effect.

If you forget a dose and remember within 1 or 2 hours of your scheduled time, take it right away. If you do not remember until later, skip the forgotten dose and continue with your regular schedule.

Special Populations

Pregnancy/Breast-feeding: Celecoxib has caused birth defects in animal studies. Any NSAID may affect fetal heart development during the second half of pregnancy. Pregnant women should not take celecoxib without their doctor's approval. When this drug is considered crucial by your doctor, its potential benefits must be carefully weighed against its risks.

NSAIDs may pass into breast milk. There is a possibility that a nursing mother taking celecoxib could affect her baby's heart or cardiovascular system. Nursing mothers who must take this drug should use infant formula.

Seniors: Generally, seniors can take this drug without special precaution. Those who weigh less than 110 lbs. should begin with the lowest possible dosage.

Type of Drug

Cephalosporin Antibiotics
(CEF-uh-loe-SPOR-in)

Brand Names

Generic Ingredient: Cefaclor 🅖
Raniclor

Generic Ingredient: Cefadroxil 🅖
Duricef

Generic Ingredient: Cefdinir
Omnicef

Generic Ingredient: Cefditoren Pivoxil
Spectracef

Generic Ingredient: Cefixime
Suprax

Generic Ingredient: Cefpodoxime Proxetil 🄖
Vantin

Generic Ingredient: Cefprozil 🄖
Cefzil

Generic Ingredient: Ceftibuten
Cedax

Generic Ingredient: Cefuroxime Axetil 🄖
Ceftin

Generic Ingredient: Cephalexin 🄖
Panixine Disperdose   Keflex

Prescribed For

Bacterial infections.

General Information

These antibiotics are related to cephalosporin C, which is similar to penicillin and is isolated from the *Cephalosporium acremonium* fungus. Of the more than 20 different antibiotic drugs derived from cephalosporin C, only those that are taken by mouth are included in *The Pill Book.* Most common infections can be treated with these antibiotics, but they are not interchangeable. Your doctor must select the appropriate antibiotic for a particular infection.

Cautions and Warnings

Do not take cephalosporin antibiotics if you are **allergic** or **sensitive** to any of their ingredients. Up to 15% of people allergic to penicillin may also be allergic to cephalosporins. The most common cephalosporin allergic reaction is a hive-like rash condition with redness over large areas of the body. Other sensitivity reactions include general rash, fever, and joint aches or pain. Such reactions generally begin after a few days of taking the antibiotic and resolve within a few days after the antibiotic is stopped.

Prolonged or repeated use of a cephalosporin may lead to a secondary infection not susceptible to the antibiotic.

Occasionally, people taking a cephalosporin develop colitis. Call your doctor if you develop severe diarrhea while taking one of these drugs.

People with **poor kidney function** may require less medicine to treat their infections. Rarely, people taking a cephalosporin have had a seizure, especially those with kidney disease whose dose was not reduced.

Some injectable cephalosporins have caused blood-clotting problems. This has not occurred in people taking an oral drug.

Rarely, severe anemia occurs in people taking cephalosporin antibiotics. Report any signs of anemia (such as pale skin color, weakness, tiredness, difficulty breathing, and abnormal heart rhythms) to your doctor.

Cefprozil oral suspension contains phenylalanine and cannot be taken by people with **phenylketonuria (PKU disease).**

Possible Side Effects

Most side effects are mild.
▼ Most common: diarrhea, headache, abdominal pain, constipation, gas, upset stomach, nausea, vomiting, itching, and rash.
▼ Less common: dizziness, tiredness, weakness, tingling in the hands or feet, confusion, appetite loss, changes in taste perception, and genital and anal itching. Colitis may develop.
Cefaclor may cause serum sickness (symptoms include fever, joint pain, and rash). Cephalosporins may cause changes in blood cells, kidney problems, liver inflammation, and jaundice, but these side effects are rarely a problem with oral cephalosporins.

Drug Interactions
- Antacids can reduce the amounts of cefaclor, cefdinir, cefditoren pivoxil, and cefpodoxime proxetil in the blood. Do not take antacids within 2 hours of these antibiotics.
- Cimetidine, famotidine, ranitidine, or nizatidine can reduce the effectiveness of cefpodoxime proxetil, cefditoren pivoxil, and cefuroxime axetil—do not combine these drugs.
- Iron and iron-fortified foods may interfere with the absorption of cefdinir. Separate your iron dose from the antibiotic by at

least 2 hours. Iron-fortified infant formula does not have this effect.

- Probenecid may increase blood levels of some cephalosporins.
- Potent (loop-type) diuretics can lead to kidney damage if mixed with a cephalosporin antibiotic.

Food Interactions

Generally, cephalosporins may be taken with food or milk if they upset your stomach. Cefditoren pivoxil should be taken with a meal. Food increases the absorption of cefpodoxime proxetil and cefuroxime axetil.

Usual Dose

Cefaclor
Adult: 250 mg every 8 hours, or 375–500 mg every 12 hours.
Child: 9 mg per lb. of body weight a day, in 2–3 equal doses.

Cefadroxil
Adult: 1–2 g a day, in 1–2 doses.
Child: 13 mg per lb. of body weight a day, in 1–2 doses.

Cefdinir
Adult and Child (age 13 and over): 600 mg a day, in 1–2 doses.
Child (age 6 months–12 years): 6.5 mg per lb. of body weight a day in 1–2 doses.

Cefditoren Pivoxil
Adult and Child (age 12 and over): 200–400 mg twice a day for 10 days.

Cefixime
Adult: 400 mg a day, in 1–2 doses.
Child: 3.5 mg per lb. of body weight a day, in 1–2 doses.

Cefpodoxime Proxetil
Adult and Child (age 13 and over): 200–400 mg a day, in 1–2 doses.
Child (age 5 months–12 years): 5 mg per lb. of body weight a day in 1–2 doses. Maximum daily dose for middle-ear infections is 400 mg; 200 mg for sore throat or tonsillitis.

Cefprozil
Adult and Child (age 13 and over): 500–1000 mg a day.
Child (age 6 months–12 years): 7–13 mg per lb. of body weight a day in 1–2 doses.

Ceftibuten

Adult and Child (age 12 and over): 400 mg once a day for 10 days.
Child: 4 mg per lb. of body weight, up to 400 mg, once a day.

Cefuroxime Axetil

Adult and Child (age 13 and over): 250–1000 mg a day in 1–2 doses.
Child (age 3 months–12 years): tablets—125–250 mg every 12 hours. Liquid—9–13 mg per lb. of body weight every 12 hours.

Cephalexin

Adult: 1000–4000 mg a day in divided doses, usually 250 mg every 6 hours, or 500 mg every 12 hours.
Child: 11–23 mg per lb. of body weight a day in divided doses. The dose may be increased to 46 mg per lb. of body weight for middle-ear infections.

Overdosage

Common symptoms of overdose are nausea, vomiting, and upset stomach. These can often be treated with milk or an antacid. Cephalosporin overdoses are generally not serious; contact a hospital emergency room or local poison control center for more information. If you seek treatment, ALWAYS bring the prescription bottle or container.

Special Information

Call your doctor if you develop severe abdominal cramps or diarrhea. Stop taking this drug and immediately call your doctor if you experience fever, chest tightness, breathing difficulties, redness, muscle aches, or swelling.

You must take the full course of treatment prescribed—even if you feel better in 2 or 3 days—to obtain the maximum benefit from any antibiotic.

Proper diagnosis is key to the effectiveness of an antibiotic: Do not take any antibiotic without consulting your doctor.

You should be aware that all cephalosporins may cause false results for certain urine tests for sugar. Cefuroxime may cause false results for blood sugar. Diabetics taking cephradine should not change their diet or diabetes medication without consulting their doctor.

If you miss a dose that you take once a day, take it as soon as you remember. If it is almost time for your next dose, take the dose you forgot right away and your next one 10–12 hours later. Then go back to your regular schedule. If you take the medication twice a day, take the dose you forgot right away and the next dose 5–6 hours later. Then go back to your regular schedule. If you take the medication 3 or more times a day, take the dose you missed right away and your next dose 2–4 hours later. Then go back to your regular schedule.

Most cephalosporin liquids must be kept in the refrigerator to maintain their strength. Only cefixime liquid does not require refrigeration. All of the liquid cephalosporins have a very limited shelf life. Do not keep any of these liquids beyond the 10 days–2 weeks specified on the label. Follow your pharmacist's storage instructions.

Special Populations

Pregnancy/Breast-feeding: These drugs are considered relatively safe during pregnancy, though small amounts pass into the fetus. Little information is available about the newer members of the group. Also, cephalosporins pass more quickly out of the bodies of pregnant women. Cephalosporins should only be used during pregnancy after carefully weighing their potential benefits against their risks.

Small amounts of most cephalosporin antibiotics pass into breast milk. Nursing mothers who must take a cephalosporin should use infant formula.

Seniors: Seniors may require a lower dosage if they have reduced kidney function.

Generic Name

Cetirizine (seh-TERE-ih-zene)

Brand Name

Zyrtec

The information in this profile also applies to the following drugs:

Generic Ingredient: Azelastine
Astelin

Generic Ingredient: Fexofenadine [G]
Allegra

Generic Ingredient: Levocetirizine [G]
Xyzal

Type of Drug

Antihistamine.

Prescribed For

Azelastine: runny nose, sneezing, nasal itching, and post-nasal drip. Cetirizine: stuffy and runny nose, itchy eyes, and scratchy throat caused by seasonal and year-round allergy, and for other symptoms of allergy such as rash, itching, and hives; also prescribed for chronic itching and for asthma. Fexofenadine: sneezing, stuffy and runny nose; scratchy throat and mouth; and itchy, watery, and red eyes caused by seasonal allergies. Levocetirizine: stuffy and runny nose, itchy eyes, and scratchy throat caused by seasonal and year-round allergy, and for other symptoms of allergy such as rash, itching, and hives; also prescribed for chronic itching.

General Information

Antihistamines generally work by blocking the release of histamine (a chemical released by body tissue during an allergic reaction) from the cell at the H_1 histamine receptor site, drying up secretions of the nose, throat, and eyes. Cetirizine causes less sedation than older antihistamines and appears to be just as effective. Levocetirizine is the active portion of the cetirizine molecule and is as effective as cetirizine with a similar side effect profile.

Cautions and Warnings

Do not take cetirizine if you are **allergic** or **sensitive** to any of its ingredients.

People with **kidney disease** should receive reduced dosages of cetirizine and levocetirizine. Do not take these drugs if kidney disease is severe. **Children** with kidney disease should not receive levocetirizine.

Possible Side Effects

▼ Common: headache, drowsiness, fatigue, dry mouth, bitter taste in the mouth, dizziness, runny nose, and sore throat.

▼ Less common: nosebleeds, stuffy nose, sneezing, cough, nausea, upset stomach, changes in bowel habits, nervousness, and fever (children).

▼ Rare: fainting and weight gain. Contact your doctor if you experience any side effect not listed above.

Drug Interactions

- Cimetidine may increase the level of azelastine in the blood.
- Cetirizine is less likely than other antihistamines to interact with drugs.
- Ritonavir increases the amount of levocetirizine and slows its breakdown in the body. This may result in increased levocetirizine side effects.

Food Interactions

- Ceterizine and levocetirizine may be taken without regard to food or meals.

Usual Dose

Azelastine Nasal Spray

Adult and Child (age 12 and over): 1–2 sprays in each nostril twice a day.

Child (age 5–11): 1 spray in each nostril twice a day.

Cetirizine

Adult and Child (age 6 and over): 5–10 mg once a day depending on symptoms. Reduce dosage in people with kidney disease.

Child (age 1–5): 2.5–5 mg a day.

Child (age 6 months–1 year): 2.5 mg a day.

Fexofenadine

Adult (age 12 and over): 60 mg twice a day or 180 mg once a day. People with kidney disease should take 60 mg a day.

Child (age 6–11): 30 mg twice a day.

Levocetirizine

Adult and Child (age 12 and over): 5 mg every evening.

Child (age 6–11): 2.5 mg (½ tablet) every evening. Dosage for children should not exceed 2.5 mg a day.

Child (under age 6): not recommended.

Overdosage

Drug overdose is likely to cause severe side effects. Overdose victims should be given ipecac syrup—available at any pharmacy—to make them vomit and be taken to a hospital emergency room. ALWAYS bring the prescription bottle or container.

Special Information

Use extra caution while doing anything that requires concentration, such as driving a car or operating hazardous machinery.

Report sore throat, unusual bleeding, bruising, tiredness, weakness, or any other unusual side effect to your doctor. Do not combine these drugs with alcohol or other nervous system depressants. Do not put azelastine nasal solution into your eyes.

If you forget to take a dose of cetirizine, take it as soon as you remember. If it is almost time for your next dose, skip the one you forgot and continue with your regular schedule. Do not take a double dose.

Special Populations

Pregnancy/Breast-feeding: Oral antihistamines are generally considered safe for use during pregnancy. But do not take any antihistamine without your doctor's knowledge if you are or might become pregnant—especially during the last 3 months of pregnancy, because newborns may have severe reactions to antihistamines.

Small amounts of antihistamine pass into breast milk. Nursing mothers who must take cetirizine should use infant formula.

Seniors: Antihistamines are more likely to cause dizziness, sleepiness, and confusion in seniors. Dosage reduction may be recommended depending on kidney function.

Generic Name

Cevimeline (seh-VIM-ih-lene) Ⓖ

Brand Name

Evoxac

Type of Drug

Cholinergic.

Prescribed For

Dry mouth in people with Sjögren's syndrome.

General Information

Sjögren's syndrome is a group of symptoms related to a lack of bodily secretions. People with this condition have very dry eyes and mucous membranes, facial lesions, and neck swelling. It often occurs in menopausal woman and is often associated with rheumatoid arthritis, poor blood circulation in the legs, and tooth decay. Cevimeline increases secretions in the mouth by binding to specific nervous system receptors and causing the release of more saliva.

Cautions and Warnings

Do not take cevimeline if you are **allergic** or **sensitive** to any of its ingredients.

This drug may make breathing more difficult and worsen **lung conditions** such as asthma, chronic bronchitis, or chronic obstructive pulmonary disease (COPD).

Eye conditions like **glaucoma** or **inflammation of the iris** may be worsened by cevimeline.

Cevimeline may affect the heart, and some people with **severe heart disease**, including those with a history of severe angina or heart attack, may not be able to compensate for this effect.

Cevimeline may worsen **gallstones** and **kidney stones** and should be avoided by people with a history of these conditions.

Cevimeline may cause visual blurring, especially at night.

Possible Side Effects

▼ Most common: excessive sweating, headache, nausea, sinus irritation, respiratory infection, runny nose, and diarrhea.

▼ Common: upset stomach, abdominal pains, urinary infection, coughing, and sore throat.

▼ Less common: vomiting, back pain, injury, rash, conjunctivitis (pinkeye), dizziness, bronchitis, severe joint pain, fatigue, bone pain, sleeplessness, hot flushes, excess salivation, chills, and anxiety.

▼ Rare: frequent urination, weakness, and flushing. Other rare side effects can occur in almost any part of the body. Contact your doctor if you experience any side effect not listed above.

Drug Interactions

- Combining cevimeline with a beta blocker can lead to heart rhythm disturbances.
- Cevimeline may interfere with the effects of anticholinergics, found in some medications for abdominal or stomach spasms or cramps.
- Cholinergics such as bethanechol, donepezil, physostigmine, pilocarpine, and pyridostigmine can add to the effects of cevimeline.
- Some drugs may interfere with the breakdown of cevimeline in the liver, increasing the chance of drug side effects. These

include amiodarone, celecoxib, chlorpheniramine, cimetidine, ciprofloxacin, clarithromycin, clomipramine, cocaine, diltiazem, erythromycin, fluconazole, fluoxetine, halofantrine, indinavir, itraconazole, ketoconazole, methadone, mibefradil, nelfinavir, paroxetine, quinidine, ranitidine, ritonavir, saquinavir, and terbinafine.

Food Interactions

Grapefruit juice may interfere with the breakdown of cevimeline in the liver, increasing the chance of drug side effects. Food interferes with the absorption of cevimeline into the bloodstream. Take this drug on an empty stomach.

Usual Dose

Adult: 30 mg 3 times a day.
Child: not recommended.

Overdosage

Overdose symptoms can include exaggerated drug side effects including headache, visual impairment, excess tearing and/or sweating, difficulty breathing, stomach or intestinal spasms, nausea, vomiting, diarrhea, changes in heart rhythm, blood pressure changes, shock, mental confusion, and tremors. Overdose victims should be taken to a hospital emergency room. ALWAYS bring the prescription bottle or container.

Special Information

Cevimeline may cause blurred vision, possibly interfering with driving or performing tasks that require reliable vision, especially at night or in low light.

If you sweat excessively while taking cevimeline, be sure to drink a lot of water. Excessive sweating can lead to dehydration.

If you miss a dose, take it as soon as you remember. If it is almost time for your next dose, skip the missed dose and continue with your regular schedule. Do not take a double dose.

Special Populations

Pregnancy/Breast-feeding: Pregnant women should take cevimeline only if it is considered crucial by your doctor, since its effect on the developing fetus is not known.

It is not known if cevimeline passes into breast milk, but nursing mothers who must take this drug should consider using infant formula.

Seniors: Older adults should be cautious about using this drug because of its possible effects on the kidney, liver, and heart, and on other diseases or medications.

Generic Name

Chlordiazepoxide (klor-dye-az-uh-POX-ide) Ⓖ

Brand Name
Librium

Type of Drug
Benzodiazepine sedative.

Prescribed For
Anxiety, tension, fatigue, agitation, and withdrawal symptoms of alcoholism; also prescribed for irritable bowel syndrome and panic attacks.

General Information
Chlordiazepoxide is a member of the group of drugs known as benzodiazepines.

Benzodiazepines work by a direct effect on the brain. They can relax you and make you more tranquil or sleepier, or they can slow nervous system transmissions in such a way as to act as an anticonvulsant. Many doctors prefer benzodiazepines to other drugs that can be used to similar effect because they tend to be safer, have fewer side effects, and are usually as effective, if not more so.

Cautions and Warnings
Do not take chlordiazepoxide if you are **allergic** or **sensitive** to any of its ingredients or to another benzodiazepine, including clonazepam.

Chlordiazepoxide can aggravate narrow-angle **glaucoma,** but you may take it if you have open-angle glaucoma and are receiving therapy for it.

Other conditions in which chlordiazepoxide should be used with caution are severe **depression,** especially with suicidal tendencies, severe **lung disease, sleep apnea** (intermittent cessation of breathing during sleep), **liver disease, drunkenness,** and **kidney disease.**

Chlordiazepoxide should not be taken by **psychotic patients** because it is not effective for them and can trigger unusual excitement, stimulation, and rage. It has also produced similar reactions among hyperactive and aggressive pediatric patients.

Chlordiazepoxide is not intended for more than 3–4 months of continuous use. Your condition should be reassessed before continuing chlordiazepoxide beyond that time.

Chlordiazepoxide may be addictive. Drug withdrawal may develop if you stop taking it after only 4 weeks of regular use, but is more likely after longer use. It may start with anxiety and progress to tingling in the hands or feet, sensitivity to bright light, sleep disturbances, cramps, tremors, muscle tension or twitching, poor concentration, flu-like symptoms, fatigue, appetite loss, sweating, and changes in mental state.

Dosage of chlordiazepoxide should be decreased gradually over 4–8 weeks after prolonged use.

Possible Side Effects

Weakness and confusion may occur, especially in seniors and in those who are sickly.

▼ Most common: mild drowsiness during the first few days of therapy.

▼ Less common: depression, lethargy, disorientation, edema, headache, inactivity, slurred speech, stupor, dizziness, tremor, constipation, dry mouth, nausea, inability to control urination, sexual difficulties, irregular menstrual cycle, changes in heart rhythm, low blood pressure, fluid retention, blurred or double vision, itching, rash, hiccups, nervousness, inability to fall asleep, and occasional liver dysfunction. If you experience any of these symptoms, stop taking the medicine and contact your doctor immediately.

▼ Rare: Rare side effects can occur in almost any part of the body. Contact your doctor if you experience any side effect not listed above.

Drug Interactions

- Chlordiazepoxide is a central-nervous-system depressant. Avoid alcohol, other sedatives, narcotics, barbiturates, monoamine oxidase inhibitor and other antidepressants, and antihistamines. Taking chlordiazepoxide with these drugs may result in excessive depression, tiredness, sleepiness, breathing difficulties, or related symptoms.

- Smoking may reduce the effectiveness of chlordiazepoxide by increasing the rate at which it is broken down by the body.
- The effects of chlordiazepoxide may be prolonged when it is taken with cimetidine, contraceptive drugs, disulfiram, fluoxetine, isoniazid, ketoconazole, metoprolol, probenecid, propoxyphene, propranolol, rifampin, or valproic acid.
- Theophylline may reduce chlordiazepoxide's sedative effects.
- If you take antacids, separate them by at least 1 hour from your chlordiazepoxide dose to prevent them from interfering with the passage of chlordiazepoxide into the bloodstream.
- Chlordiazepoxide may increase blood levels of digoxin and the chances for digoxin toxicity.
- Levodopa + carbidopa's effectiveness may be reduced by chlordiazepoxide.
- Phenytoin blood concentrations may be increased when taken with chlordiazepoxide, resulting in possible phenytoin toxicity.

Food Interactions

Chlordiazepoxide is best taken on an empty stomach but may be taken with food if it upsets your stomach.

Usual Dose

Adult: 5–100 mg a day. This range is due to individual response related to age, weight, disease severity, and other characteristics.

Child (age 6 and over): may be given if deemed appropriate by a doctor. Starting dose—5 mg 2–4 times a day. Maintenance dose—up to 30 mg a day for some children, but must be individualized to obtain maximum benefit.

Child (under age 6): not recommended.

Overdosage

Symptoms of overdose are confusion, sleepiness, poor coordination, lack of response to pain such as a pin prick, loss of reflexes, shallow breathing, low blood pressure, and coma. The victim should be taken to a hospital emergency room. ALWAYS bring the prescription bottle or container.

Special Information

Chlordiazepoxide can cause tiredness, drowsiness, inability to concentrate, or similar symptoms. Be careful if you are driving, operating machinery, or performing other activities that require concentration.

If you forget a dose of chlordiazepoxide, take it as soon as you remember. If it is almost time for your next dose, skip the dose you forgot and continue with your regular schedule. Do not take a double dose.

Special Populations

Pregnancy/Breast-feeding: Chlordiazepoxide may cause birth defects if taken during the first 3 months of pregnancy. Avoid chlordiazepoxide while pregnant.

Chlordiazepoxide may pass into breast milk. Nursing mothers who must take chlordiazepoxide should use infant formula.

Seniors: Seniors, especially those with liver or kidney disease, are more sensitive to the effects of chlordiazepoxide and generally require smaller doses to achieve the same effect.

Generic Name

Chlorpheniramine Maleate
(KLOR-fen-ERE-uh-mene MAL-ee-ate) [G]

Brand Names

Aller-Chlor	Efidac 24
Chlor-Trimeton	Pediox S
Chlor-Trimeton Allergy 8 Hour	Prohist+8
Chlor-Trimeton Allergy 12 Hour	QDALL AR

The information in this profile also applies to the following drugs:

Generic Ingredient: Cyproheptadine Hydrochloride [G]

Generic Ingredient: Dexchlorpheniramine Maleate [G]

Type of Drug

Antihistamine.

Prescribed For

Stuffy and runny nose, itchy eyes, and scratchy throat caused by seasonal allergy, and other symptoms of allergy such as rash, itching, and hives.

General Information

Antihistamines generally work by blocking the release of histamine (a chemical released by body tissue during an allergic reaction) from body cells at the H_1 histamine receptor site, drying up secretions of the nose, throat, and eyes.

Cautions and Warnings

Do not use this drug if you are **allergic** or **sensitive** to any of its ingredients.

Use chlorpheniramine maleate with care if you have a history of **thyroid disease, heart disease, high blood pressure,** or **diabetes**. This drug should be avoided or used with extreme care if you have **narrow-angle glaucoma, stomach ulcer** or other **stomach problems, enlarged prostate,** or **problems passing urine**. It should not be used by people who have **deep-breathing problems** such as asthma, emphysema, or chronic bronchitis.

Possible Side Effects

▼ Less common: rash or itching, sensitivity to bright light, increased sweating, chills, lowered blood pressure, headache, rapid heartbeat, sleeplessness, dizziness, disturbed coordination, confusion, restlessness, nervousness, irritability, euphoria (feeling "high"), tingling in the hands or feet, blurred or double vision, ringing in the ears, upset stomach, appetite loss, nausea, vomiting, constipation, diarrhea, urinary difficulties, chest tightness, wheezing, stuffy nose, and dryness of the mouth, nose, or throat. Young children may also develop nervousness, irritability, tension, and anxiety.

Drug Interactions

- Chlorpheniramine maleate should not be taken with a monoamine oxidase inhibitor antidepressant, because the combination may cause severe side effects.
- The effects of sedatives, benzodiazepines such as diazepam, and sleeping medications will be increased when any of these drugs is combined with chlorpheniramine maleate. It is extremely important for your doctor to know if you are taking

any other medication with chlorpheniramine maleate so that the dosage of that medication can be properly adjusted.

- Anticholinergenics may cause an increase in side effects of chlorpheniramine maleate.
- Be extremely cautious when drinking alcoholic beverages while taking this drug, which enhances the intoxicating and sedating effects of alcohol.

Food Interactions

You may take this drug with food if it upsets your stomach.

Usual Dose

Chlorpheniramine

Adult and Child (age 13 and over): 4 mg every 4–6 hours; do not take more than 24 mg a day.

Child (age 6–12): 2 mg every 4–6 hours; do not take more than 12 mg a day.

Child (age 2–5): 1 mg every 4–6 hours; do not take more than 4 mg a day.

Chlorpheniramine, Sustained-Release

Adult and Child (age 13 and over): 8–12 mg at bedtime, or every 8–12 hours during the day; do not take more than 24 mg a day.

Child (age 6–12): 8 mg during the day or at bedtime.

Child (under age 6): not recommended.

Cyproheptadine

Adult and Child (age 15 and over): 4–20 mg a day; do not exceed 32 mg a day.

Child (age 7–14): 4 mg 2–3 times a day; do not exceed 16 mg a day.

Child (age 2–6): 2 mg 2–3 times a day; do not exceed 12 mg a day.

Dexchlorpheniramine

Adult and Child (age 12 and over): 2 mg every 4–6 hours.

Child (age 6–11): 1 mg every 4–6 hours.

Child (age 2–5): 0.5 mg every 4–6 hours.

Dexchlorpheniramine, Sustained-Release

Adult and Child (age 12 and over): 4–6 mg every 8–10 hours and at bedtime.

Child (age 6–11): 4 mg once a day and at bedtime.
Child (under age 6): not recommended.

Tripelennamine
Adult and Child (age 12 and over): 25–50 mg every 4–6 hours; do not take more than 600 mg a day. Adults may take up to 3 100-mg, sustained-release tablets a day, although this much is not usually needed.
Child (under age 12): 2 mg per lb. of body weight a day in divided doses; no more than 300 mg a day should be given.

Overdosage

Symptoms of overdose include depression or stimulation, especially in children; dry mouth; fixed or dilated pupils; flushing of the skin; upset stomach; unsteadiness; and convulsions. Overdose victims should be made to vomit as soon as possible with ipecac syrup—available at any pharmacy—to remove excess drug from the stomach. Take the victim to a hospital emergency room immediately if the victim is unconscious or if you cannot induce vomiting. ALWAYS bring the prescription bottle or container.

Special Information

This drug may cause tiredness or loss of concentration: Be extremely cautious when driving or doing anything that requires close attention.

If you forget a dose of this drug, take it as soon as you remember. If it is almost time for your next dose, skip the one you forgot and continue with your regular schedule. Do not take a double dose.

Special Populations

Pregnancy/Breast-feeding: Animal studies have shown that some antihistamines may cause birth defects. Do not take any antihistamine without your doctor's knowledge if you are or might be pregnant—especially during the last 3 months of pregnancy, because newborns may have severe reactions to antihistamines.

Small amounts of some antihistamines pass into breast milk. Nursing mothers who must take chlorpheniramine maleate should use infant formula.

Seniors: Seniors are more sensitive to antihistamine side effects. Dosage reduction may be needed.

Generic Name

Chlorpromazine (klor-PROE-muh-zene) [G]

Brand Names

Sonazine   Thorazine*

The information in this profile also applies to the following drugs:

Generic Ingredient: Fluphenazine Hydrochloride [G]

Generic Ingredient: Thioridazine Hydrochloride [G]

Generic Ingredient: Trifluoperazine Hydrochloride [G]

Some products in this brand-name group are alcohol- or sugar-free. Consult your pharmacist.

Type of Drug

Phenothiazine antipsychotic.

Prescribed For

Psychotic disorders; moderate to severe depression with anxiety; agitation or aggressiveness in disturbed children; intractable pain; and senility. May also be used to relieve nausea, vomiting, hiccups, restlessness, acute intermittant porphyria, and apprehension before surgery or other procedures.

General Information

Chlorpromazine and other phenothiazines act upon a portion of the brain called the hypothalamus. Phenothiazines affect parts of the hypothalamus that control metabolism, body temperature, alertness, muscle tone, hormone balance, and vomiting. Chlorpromazine is available in suppositories and as liquid for those who have trouble swallowing tablets.

Cautions and Warnings

Do not take chlorpromazine if you are **allergic** or **sensitive** to any of its ingredients or to any phenothiazine drug. Do not take it if you have very **low blood pressure, Parkinson's disease,** or **blood, liver, kidney, or heart disease.**

Chlorpromazine may depress the cough reflex. People have accidentally choked to death because the cough reflex failed to protect them. Because of its effect in reducing vomiting, chlorpromazine may obscure symptoms of disease or toxicity due to over-dose of another drug.

Use chlorpromazine under your doctor's strict supervision if you have **glaucoma, epilepsy, ulcers,** or **urinary difficulties.**

Avoid exposure to extreme heat, because this drug may upset your body's temperature-control mechanism. Do not allow the liquid forms of this drug to come in contact with your skin because they are highly irritating.

Chlorpromazine may cause unusually high or low levels of cholesterol.

Possible Side Effects

▼ Most common: drowsiness, especially during the first or second week of therapy. If drowsiness becomes troublesome, contact your doctor.

▼ Less common: changes in blood components, including anemias, raised or lowered blood pressure, abnormal heart rate, heart attack, sensitivity to light, and faintness or dizziness.

▼ Rare: Rare side effects can occur in almost any part of the body. Contact your doctor if you experience any side effect not listed above.

Jaundice (symptoms include yellowing of the whites of eyes or skin) may appear; when it does, it is usually within the first 2–4 weeks of treatment. Normally the jaundice goes away when the drug is discontinued, but there have been cases when it has not.

Phenothiazines may produce extrapyramidal side effects, including spasm of the neck muscles, rolling back of the eyes, convulsions, difficulty swallowing, and symptoms associated with Parkinson's disease. These side effects seem very serious but usually disappear after the drug has been withdrawn; however, symptoms affecting the face, tongue, or jaw may persist for as long as several years, especially in older adults with a history of brain damage.

Chlorpromazine may cause an unusual increase in psychotic symptoms or may cause paranoid reactions, tiredness, lethargy, restlessness, hyperactivity, confusion at night, bizarre dreams, sleeplessness, depression, decreased sex drive, increased appetite, or euphoria (feeling "high").

Drug Interactions

- Be cautious about taking chlorpromazine with over-the-counter cough, cold, or allergy medications, barbiturates, alcohol, sleeping pills, narcotics or other sedatives, or any other drug that may produce a depressive effect.
- Aluminum antacids may reduce the effectiveness of phenothiazine drugs.
- Chlorpromazine may reduce the effectiveness of bromocriptine and appetite suppressants.
- Anticholinergic drugs may reduce the effectiveness of chlorpromazine and increase the chance of side effects.
- Phenothiazine drugs may counter the blood-pressure-lowering effect of guanethidine.
- Taking lithium together with a phenothiazine drug may lead to disorientation, loss of consciousness, or uncontrolled muscle movements.
- Combining propranolol and a phenothiazine drug may lead to unusually low blood pressure.
- Combining tricyclic antidepressants with a phenothiazine drug can lead to antidepressant side effects.
- Chlorpromazine may reduce the effectiveness of epinephrine and norepinephrine.
- Cigarette smoking reduces the amount of chlorpromazine in your blood. Smokers may need larger doses.

Food Interactions

Take liquid chlorpromazine with fruit juice or other liquids. You may also take it with food if it upsets your stomach.

Usual Dose

Adult: 30–1000 mg or more a day, individualized according to your disease and response.

Child (age 6 months and over): 0.25 mg per lb. of body weight every 4–6 hours, up to 200 mg or more a day, depending on disease, age, and response.

Child (under 6 months): not recommended.

Overdosage

Overdose symptoms include depression, extreme weakness, tiredness, lowered blood pressure, agitation, restlessness, uncontrolled muscle spasms, convulsions, fever, dry mouth, abnormal heart rhythms, and coma. The victim should be taken to a hospital emergency room immediately. ALWAYS bring the prescription bottle or container.

Special Information

Call your doctor at once if you develop sore throat, fever, rash, weakness, visual problems, tremors, muscle movements or twitching, yellowing of the skin or whites of the eyes, or darkening of the urine.

Do not stop taking chlorpromazine without your doctor's knowledge. It may take several weeks before this drug takes effect.

This drug may cause drowsiness. Use caution when driving or operating hazardous equipment. Avoid alcoholic beverages.

Chlorpromazine may cause unusual sensitivity to the sun and may turn your urine reddish brown to pink.

If dizziness occurs, avoid rising quickly from a sitting or lying position and avoid climbing stairs. Use caution in hot weather, because this drug may make you more prone to heat stroke.

If you are using sustained-release capsules, do not chew them or break them—swallow them whole. Liquid forms of phenothiazines must be protected from light. Do not take them out of their opaque bottles.

If you take chlorpromazine more than once a day and forget to take a dose, take it right away if you remember within an hour. If you do not remember within an hour, skip the dose you forgot and continue with your regular schedule. If you take 1 dose a day and forget a dose, skip the dose you forgot and continue your regular schedule the next day. Never take a double dose.

Special Populations

Pregnancy/Breast-feeding: Infants born to women taking this drug have experienced side effects—including jaundice and nervous system effects. Check with your doctor about taking chlorpromazine if you are or might be pregnant.

This drug may pass into breast milk. Nursing mothers who must take chlorpromazine should use infant formula .

Seniors: Seniors are more sensitive to the effects of this drug and usually achieve desired results with lower dosages. Some experts feel that seniors should receive ½–¼ the usual adult dose.

Generic Name

Chlorzoxazone (klor-ZOX-uh-zone) Ⓖ

Brand Names

Parafon Forte DSC   Strifon Forte DSC

Type of Drug

Skeletal muscle relaxant.

Prescribed For

Pain and spasm of muscular conditions, including strain, sprain, bruising, and lower back problems.

General Information

Chlorzoxazone works primarily on the spinal cord level and on the brain, acting as a mild sedative. This results in fewer spasms, less pain, and greater mobility. Chlorzoxazone provides only temporary relief and is not a substitute for other types of therapy, such as rest, surgery, and physical therapy.

Cautions and Warnings

Do not take chlorzoxazone if you are **allergic** or **sensitive** to any of its ingredients, or if you have a condition known as **porphyria**.

People with **poor liver or kidney function** should take this drug with caution because serious liver toxicity has rarely occurred in people using chlorzoxazone.

Chlorzoxazone may interact with other drugs that cause nervous system depression (see "Drug Interactions").

Because it is possible to become dependent on this drug, people with a history of substance abuse should take chlorzoxazone with caution.

Possible Side Effects

▼ Most common: dizziness, drowsiness, lightheadedness, malaise, and overstimulation.

▼ Less common: headache, stomach cramps or pain, diarrhea, constipation, heartburn, nausea, and vomiting.

▼ Rare: internal bleeding, liver problems, severe allergic-type skin reactions, and breathing problems. Contact your doctor if you experience any side effect not listed above.

Drug Interactions

- The depressive effects of chlorzoxazone may be enhanced by taking it with alcohol, sedatives, sleeping pills, or other nervous system depressants. Avoid these combinations.

Food Interactions

Take this drug with food if it upsets your stomach. The tablets may be crushed and mixed with food.

Usual Dose

Adult: 250–750 mg 3–4 times a day.
Child: 125–500 mg 3–4 times a day.

Do not take more medication than is prescribed.

Overdosage

Early signs of chlorzoxazone overdose may include nausea, vomiting, diarrhea, drowsiness, dizziness, lightheadedness, and headache. Victims may also feel sluggish or sickly and lose the ability to move their muscles. Breathing may become slow or irregular, and blood pressure may drop. Contact a doctor immediately or go to a hospital emergency room for treatment. ALWAYS bring the prescription bottle or container.

Special Information

Chlorzoxazone may make you drowsy or reduce your ability to concentrate. Be extremely careful while driving or operating hazardous equipment. Avoid alcoholic beverages.

Chlorzoxazone may turn your urine orange to purple-red; this is not dangerous.

Call your doctor if you develop drowsiness, weakness, an allergic reaction, skin rash or itching, breathing difficulties, black or tarry stools, vomiting of material that resembles coffee grounds, liver problems, or any other severe or bothersome side effect.

If you miss a dose of chlorzoxazone by more than an hour, skip the dose you forgot and continue with your regular schedule. Do not take a double dose.

Special Populations

Pregnancy/Breast-feeding: The safety of chlorzoxazone in pregnant women has not been established. Pregnant women should only take chlorzoxazone after carefully weighing its potential benefits against its risks.

It is not known if chlorzoxazone passes into breast milk. Nursing mothers should consider using infant formula.

Seniors: Seniors, especially those with severe liver disease, are more sensitive to the effects of chlorzoxazone.

Generic Name

Cholestyramine (kol-es-TYE-rah-meen) Ⓖ

Brand Names

LoCHOLEST	Questran
LoCHOLEST Light	Questran Light
Prevalite	

The information in this profile also applies to the following drugs:

Generic Ingredient: Colesevelam Hydrochloride
WelChol

Generic Ingredient: Colestipol Hydrochloride Ⓖ
Colestid

Type of Drug

Anti-hyperlipidemic (blood-fat reducer).

Prescribed For

High blood-cholesterol levels; generalized itching associated with bile duct obstruction—cholestyramine only; colitis; digitalis or thyroid overdose; and pesticide poisoning.

General Information

Cholestyramine resin lowers blood-cholesterol levels by absorbing bile acids in the bowel. Since the body uses cholesterol to make the bile acids—needed to digest fat—fat digestion can only continue by making more bile acid from blood cholesterol. This results in lower blood-cholesterol levels 4–7 days after starting cholestyramine.

Cholestyramine works entirely within the bowel and is never absorbed into the bloodstream. Though usually given 3–4 times a day, there appears to be no advantage to taking it more often than twice a day. The cholesterol-lowering effect of cholestyramine may be increased when it is taken with an HMG-CoA inhibitor or nicotinic acid. In some kinds of hyperlipidemia, colestipol may be more effective in lowering total blood cholesterol than clofibrate.

Cautions and Warnings

Do not use cholestyramine if you are **allergic** or **sensitive** to any of its ingredients or if your **bile duct is blocked.** The powder form should not be taken dry; doing so may result in the inhalation of powder into your lungs or a clogged esophagus.

If you are being treated for **hypothyroidism, diabetes, kidney or blood vessel disorder, obstructive liver disease,** or **alcholism,** consult your doctor before taking cholestyramine.

Cholestyramine may cause or worsen **constipation** and **hemorrhoids.** Most constipation is mild, but some people may need to stop the medication or take less of it.

Possible Side Effects

▼ Most common: constipation, which may be severe and in rare cases result in bowel impaction. Hemorrhoids may be worsened.

▼ Less common: abdominal pain and bloating, and bleeding disorders or black-and-blue marks due to interference with the absorption of vitamin K, a necessary factor in the blood clotting process. One person developed night-blindness because the medication interfered with vitamin A absorption into the blood. Other side effects include belching, gas, nausea, vomiting, diarrhea, heartburn, and appetite loss. Your stool may have an unusual appearance because of a high fat level.

▼ Rare: Rare side effects can affect your mouth, stomach and intestines, muscles and joints, mental status, urinary tract, and breathing. Contact your doctor if you experience any side effect not listed above.

Drug Interactions

● Cholestyramine interferes with the absorption of virtually all oral drugs, including acetaminophen, amiodarone, aspirin, cephalexin, chenodiol, clindamycin, clofibrate, contraceptive drugs, corticosteroids, diclofenac, iopanoic acid, iron, digitalis drugs, furosemide, gemfibrozil, glipizide, hydrocortisone, imipramine (an antidepressant), methyldopa, mycophenolate, nicotinic acid, penicillin, phenobarbital, phenytoin, piroxicam, propranolol, tetracycline, thiazide diuretics, thyroid drugs, tolbutamide, trimethoprim, ursodiol, warfarin and other anticoagulant (blood-thinning) drugs, and vitamins A, D, E, and K. Take other medications at least 1 hour before or 4–6 hours after taking cholestyramine.

Food Interactions

Take this medication before meals. The powder may be mixed with soda, water, juice, cereal, or pulpy fruits, such as applesauce or crushed pineapple. Cholestyramine bars should be thoroughly chewed and taken with plenty of fluids. Colestipol pills are swallowed whole.

Usual Dose

Cholestyramine: 4 g (1 packet) or 1 level scoopful taken 1–2 times a day or up to 6 times a day.

Colesevelam: 6 tablets once a day or in 2 divided doses.

Colestipol: 2–16 g (1–6 packets) once a day or in divided doses.

Overdosage

The most severe effect of overdose is obstruction of the gastrointestinal tract. Take the overdose victim to a hospital emergency room. ALWAYS bring the prescription bottle or container.

Special Information

Do not swallow the granules or powder in their dry form. Prepare each packet of powder by mixing it with soup, cereal, or pulpy fruit or by adding the powder to a 6-oz. glass of liquid, such as a carbonated beverage. If some of the drug sticks to the sides of the glass, rinse it with liquid and drink the remainder.

Constipation, gas, nausea, and heartburn may occur and then disappear with continued use of this medication. If constipation is a problem, your doctor may recommend drinking more fluids and taking a fiber supplement. Call your doctor if these side effects persist or if you develop unusual problems such as bleeding from the gums or rectum.

If you miss a dose of cholestyramine, skip it and continue with your regular schedule. Do not take a double dose.

Special Populations

Pregnancy/Breast-feeding: While cholestyramine does not affect the fetus directly, it may prevent the absorption of vitamins A, D, and E and other nutrients essential to the fetus' proper development—even when you take a prenatal vitamin supplement.

When this drug is considered crucial by your doctor, its potential benefits must be carefully weighed against its risks.

Cholestyramine is not absorbed into the body. However, reduced absorption of vitamins A, D, and E and other nutrients may make your milk less nutritious. Nursing mothers who must take cholestyramine should use infant formula.

Seniors: Seniors are more likely to experience side effects, especially those relating to the bowel.

Type of Drug

Cholinesterase Inhibitors
(KO-lin-ESS-tuh-rase)

Brand Names

Generic Ingredient: Donepezil

Aricept   Aricept ODT

Generic Ingredient: Galantamine

Razadyne   Razadyne ER

Generic Ingredient: Rivastigmine

Exelon   Exelon Transdermal System

Generic Ingredient: Tacrine

Cognex

Prescribed For

Alzheimer's disease. Also used for vascular dementia, dementia associated with Parkinson's disease, poststroke aphasia (problems with language), and improvement of memory in multiple sclerosis patients.

General Information

Cholinesterase inhibitors work by increasing the function of certain receptors in the brain that are stimulated by the hormone acetylcholine. They do this by interfering with cholinesterase, the enzyme that breaks down acetylcholine. People with Alzheimer's disease (a degenerative condition of the central nervous system) develop a shortage of this brain chemical early in the disease. There is no evidence that cholinesterase inhibitors reverse the degenerative effects of Alzheimer's, but they may slow the rate at which the disease worsens.

Cautions and Warnings

Do not take cholinesterase inhibitors if you are **allergic** or **sensitive** to any of their ingredients.

Cholinesterase inhibitors must be discontinued before **surgery** because they increase the effects of anesthetic drugs.

People with **heart disease** should use cholinesterase inhibitors with caution because they may slow heart rate and cause fainting. Two studies of people with mild symptoms of Alzheimer's disease taking **galantamine** revealed a higher rate of death from heart attack, stroke, or sudden death.

Cholinesterase inhibitors may be expected to cause increased stomach acid production and increased activity of the gastrointestinal tract. Possible complications include **ulcers** or **bleeding. Alcohol** and **nonsteroidal anti-inflammatory drugs** (NSAIDs) such as aspirin or ibuprofen may worsen this effect.

Using cholinesterase inhibitors may also lead to urinary blockage, increase the risk of generalized **seizures,** and worsen **asthma or other pulmonary diseases.** Use with caution if you have these conditions.

People with severe **liver dysfunction** should not take galantamine or tacrine.

Possible Side Effects

People taking cholinesterase inhibitors generally experience side effects at about the same rate as those taking a placebo (sugar pill).
▼ Most common: headache, general pain, accidents, nausea, diarrhea, sleeplessness, and dizziness.
▼ Common: tiredness, vomiting, appetite loss, and muscle cramps.
▼ Less common: arthritis, depression, abnormal dreams, fainting, black-and-blue marks, and weight loss.
▼ Rare: Rare side effects can occur in almost any part of the body. Contact your doctor if you experience any side effect not listed above.

Drug Interactions

- Cholinesterase inhibitors interfere with anticholinergic drugs (often prescribed for stomach disorders).

- Cholinesterase inhibitors can be expected to increase the effects of cevimeline, surgical anesthetic drugs, and drugs that irritate the stomach and intestines, such as aspirin, ibuprofen, and other NSAIDs.
- The breakdown of cholinesterase inhibitors (except rivastigmine) in the liver can be slowed by ketoconazole, itraconazole, quinidine, delavirdine, indinavir, nelfinavir, ritonavir, saquinavir, amiodarone, cimetidine, ciprofloxacin, norfloxacin, clarithromycin, diltiazem, erythromycin, fluconazole, fluvoxamine, celecoxib, chlorpheniramine, clomipramine, cocaine, doxorubicin, fluoxetine, halofantrine, haloperidol, levopromazine, methadone, mibefradil, paroxetine, ranitidine, terbinafine, mifepristone, nefazodone, and grapefruit juice.
- The breakdown of cholinesterase inhibitors (except rivastigmine) in the liver can be increased by efavirenz, nevirapine, barbiturates, carbamazepine, corticosteroids, phenytoin, pioglitazone, and rifampin.

Food Interactions

Donepezil can be taken with or without food.

Galantamine and rivastigmine should be taken with morning and evening meals.

The rivastigmine transdermal system patch can be used without regard to meals.

Food reduces the absorption of tacrine into the blood. It is best taken on an empty stomach, but you can take it with food if it upsets your stomach.

Usual Dose

Donepezil
Adult: 5 or 10 mg once a day.

Galantamine
Adult: 8–32 mg a day.

Rivastigmine
Adult: 3–12 mg a day, divided into 2 doses.

Rivastigmine Transdermal patch
Adult: Apply one 4.6-mg patch every day to start. Dose may be increased to one 9.5-mg patch every day.

Tacrine
Adult: 40–160 mg a day, divided into 4 doses.

Overdosage

Cholinesterase inhibitor overdose can be very serious. Symptoms include severe nausea, vomiting, salivation, sweating, slow heart rate, low blood pressure, slow breathing rate, convulsions, muscle weakness, and collapse. Take the overdose victim to a hospital emergency room at once. ALWAYS bring the prescription bottle or container.

Special Information

Donepezil should be taken just before bedtime.

Follow the special package directions for rivastigmine solution.

Do not remove the rivastigmine patch from its packaging until just before you are ready to apply it. Apply the patch to clean, dry, and hairless skin on the upper or lower back, upper arm, or chest that is also free of any powder, oil, moisturizer, or lotion that could keep the patch from sticking to your skin properly; skin should also be free of cuts, rashes, and irritations. Avoid places where the patch can be rubbed off by tight clothing. When changing your patch, apply your new patch to a different spot of skin (for example, on the right side of your body one day, then on the left side the next day). Do not use the same spot more than once every 14 days. Wear only one patch at a time and change it every 24 hours. If the patch falls off, apply a new patch for the rest of the day, then replace the patch the next day at the same time as usual.

Tobacco or nicotine use increases the rate at which tacrine and rivastigmine are cleared from the body.

If you forget a dose and take your medication once a day, take it as soon as you remember. If it is almost time for your next dose, skip the dose you forgot and continue with the regular schedule. If you take your medication 2 or more times a day, take your dose as soon as you remember. If it is almost time for your next dose, skip the dose you forgot and continue with your regular schedule. Do not take a double dose.

Special Populations

Pregnancy/Breast-feeding: One animal study of a cholinesterase inhibitor indicated a small risk of birth defects. When your doctor considers this drug crucial, its potential benefits must be carefully weighed against its risks.

It is not known if cholinesterase inhibitors pass into breast milk. Nursing mothers who must take this drug should use infant formula.

Seniors: Seniors with moderate kidney function loss should not take galantamine. Dosage adjustments are not needed for donepezil, tacrine, or rivastigmine.

Cialis   *see Erectile Dysfunction Drugs, page 426*

Generic Name

Ciclopirox   (sye-kloe-PERE-ox)   Ⓖ

Brand Names
Loprox   Penlac

Type of Drug
Antifungal.

Prescribed For
Fungus and yeast infections of the nails and skin, including athlete's foot, candida, and dandruff.

General Information
Ciclopirox slows the growth of a variety of fungus organisms and yeasts and kills many others. The drug penetrates the skin, hair, hair follicles, and sweat glands. Ciclopirox nail lacquer is used for toenail and fingernail fungus infections. Ciclopirox shampoo is used for dandruff.

Cautions and Warnings
Do not use this product if you are **allergic** or **sensitive** to any of its ingredients.

Possible Side Effects

▼ Common: burning, itching, stinging, or oozing at the application site.

Drug Interactions
None known.

Usual Dose

Cream/Lotion

Adult and Child (age 10 and over): Massage into cleansed affected skin and surrounding area twice a day.

Nail Lacquer

Adult: Apply to infected nails once a day. Use in conjunction with monthly visits to a health care professional.

Child (under age 10): not recommended.

Shampoo

Adult: Wet hair and apply 1–2 tsp to the scalp. Lather and leave on hair and scalp for 3 minutes, then rinse. Avoid contact with eyes. Repeat twice weekly for 4 weeks.

Child (under age 16): not recommended.

Overdosage

Accidental ingestion may cause nausea and upset stomach. Call your local poison control center or hospital for more information. If you seek treatment, ALWAYS bring the prescription container.

Special Information

This product can be expected to relieve symptoms within the first week of use. Follow your doctor's directions for the complete 2–4 week course of treatment with the cream or lotion to gain maximum benefit. The nail lacquer may be used for up to 48 weeks. Stopping the medication too soon can lead to a relapse.

When using ciclopirox nail lacquer, do not apply it to any skin other than that which surrounds the infected nails, because of possible irritation. Do not apply nail polish or any other nail lacquer to infected nails while you are using this product.

Avoid using ciclopirox nail lacquer near an open flame, since the product is flammable.

Do not cover cream or lotion with a bandage.

Call your doctor if the affected area burns, stings, or becomes red after you use this product, or if your symptoms do not clear up after 4 weeks of treatment; by then it is unlikely that this product will be effective.

If you forget a dose of ciclopirox, apply it as soon as you remember. Do not apply more than the amount prescribed to make up for the missed dose.

Special Populations

Pregnancy/Breast-feeding: Ciclopirox may pass to the fetus in very small amounts. In animal studies, high doses of ciclopirox given by mouth did not harm the fetus. Caution should be exercised when using ciclopirox during pregnancy.

It is unknown if ciclopirox passes into breast milk. Nursing mothers who must use this drug should consider using infant formula.

Seniors: Seniors may use this drug without special restriction.

Generic Name

Cilostazol (sil-oe-STAY-zol) Ⓖ

Brand Name
Pletal

Type of Drug
Antiplatelet.

Prescribed For
Intermittent claudication.

General Information
In intermittent claudication, leg muscles go into spasm due to reduced blood flow. This occurs when plaque buildup narrows blood vessels leading to the calf or other leg muscles. People with this condition often develop leg pain after walking only a short distance. Cilostazol prevents blood platelets from "clumping together" to begin the process of forming a blood clot, which can further obstruct arteries and worsen intermittent claudication. This drug is broken down in the liver.

Cautions and Warnings
Do not take this drug if you are **allergic** or **sensitive** to any of its ingredients.

People with **congestive heart failure** (CHF) should not take cilostazol. Some studies indicate that long-term use of this drug may cause cardiovascular problems.

People with **hemostatic disorders** or **active pathologic bleeding** should not take cilostazil.

Possible Side Effects

The risk of side effects increases with dosage.
▼ Most common: headache, infection, abdominal pain, abnormal stool, and diarrhea.
▼ Common: heart palpitations, rapid heartbeat, dizziness, upset stomach, nausea, sore throat, runny nose, back pain, and swelling in the arms or legs.
▼ Less common: gas, cough, fainting, and muscle aches.
▼ Rare: Rare side effects can occur in almost any part of the body. Contact your doctor if you experience any side effect not listed above.

Drug Interactions

- Avoid mixing cilostazol with ketoconazole, itraconazole, fluconazole, miconazole, fluvoxamine, fluoxetine, nefazodone, or sertraline because this interaction may slow the breakdown of cilostazol, prolonging its effects. Cilostazol dosage is reduced by 50% when it is combined with any of these drugs.
- Aspirin can increase the anticoagulant (blood-thinning) effect of cilostazol, but this combination has not caused serious bleeding problems. There is no information on the effect of combining cilostazol and other antiplatelet or anticoagulant drugs. Cilostazol dosage is reduced by 50% when it is combined with any of these drugs.
- Diltiazem increases cilostazol blood levels by about 50%. Cilostazol dosage is reduced by 50% when it is combined with diltiazem.
- Erythromycin and similar antibiotics increase cilostazol blood levels. Take half the regular dose of cilostazol when combining it with any of these drugs.
- Combining cilostazol and omeprazole increases the effects of cilostazol. Cilostazol dosage is reduced by 50% when it is combined with omeprazole.
- Smoking reduces the effectiveness of cilostazol by causing the liver to break it down faster.

Food Interactions

Take this drug on an empty stomach at least 30 minutes before or 2 hours after meals. Do not drink grapefruit juice at any time while taking cilostazol because it can interfere with the breakdown of the drug.

Usual Dose

Adult: 100 mg twice a day. 50 mg twice a day when combined with other drugs that may increase the effect of cilostazol.

Child: not recommended.

Overdosage

Symptoms of overdose are likely to be the most common side effects. Overdose victims should be taken to a hospital emergency room. ALWAYS bring the prescription bottle or container.

Special Information

Several weeks of cilostazol treatment may be necessary before you notice any improvement in symptoms. Maximum benefit usually occurs after 12 weeks.

If you forget a dose, take it as soon as you remember. If it is almost time for your next dose, skip the forgotten dose and continue with your regular schedule. Do not take a double dose.

Special Populations

Pregnancy/Breast-feeding: Animal studies suggest that cilostazol may harm the fetus, but there is no information on the effect of cilostazol in pregnant women. When this drug is considered crucial by your doctor, its potential benefits must be carefully weighed against its risks.

Cilostazol may pass into breast milk. Nursing mothers who must take this drug should use infant formula.

Seniors: Seniors can take this drug without special precaution.

Generic Name

Cimetidine (sih-MET-ih-dene) Ⓖ

Brand Names

Tagamet   Tagamet HB Ⓢ

Type of Drug

Histamine H_2 antagonist.

Prescribed For

Ulcers of the stomach and duodenum (upper intestine); also used for upset stomach, gastroesophageal reflux disease (GERD), benign stomach ulcer, bleeding in the stomach and duodenum, colorectal cancer, prevention of stress ulcer, hyperparathyroidism, fungal infections of the hair and scalp, herpes virus infection, excessive hairiness in women, chronic itching of unknown cause, skin reactions, warts, acetaminophen overdose, and other conditions characterized by the production of large amounts of gastric fluids. Cimetidine may be prescribed to stop the production of stomach acid during surgery.

General Information

Histamine H_2 antagonists work by turning off the system that produces stomach acid and other secretions. Cimetidine is effective in treating the symptoms of ulcer and preventing complications of the disease, although an ulcer that does not respond to another histamine H_2 antagonist will probably not respond to cimetidine. Histamine H_2 antagonists differ only in their potency. Cimetidine is the least potent; 1000 mg are roughly equal to 300 mg of either nizatidine or ranitidine, or 40 mg of famotidine. These drugs are roughly equal in their ability to treat ulcer disease and their risk of side effects.

Cautions and Warnings

Do not take cimetidine if you are **allergic** or **sensitive** to any of its ingredients or any histamine H_2 antagonist. Cimetidine has a mild antiandrogen effect, which probably causes the painful, swollen breasts that some people experience after taking this drug for a month or more.

People with **kidney or liver disease** should take cimetidine with caution because ⅓ of each dose is broken down in the liver and passes out of the body through the kidneys.

Do not self-treat with over-the-counter forms of cimetidine without the advice and supervision of your doctor.

The fact that symptoms are alleviated by cimetidine does not preclude the possibility of stomach cancer, which can have symptoms similar to other gastrointestinal (GI) disorders. Make sure your doctor screens for possible malignancy.

Some people—mostly the very ill—experience confusion, agitation, psychosis, hallucinations, depression, anxiety, or disorientation, usually within 2–3 days of starting cimetidine. Normally these symptoms stop 3–4 days after discontinuing the drug. Call your doctor if this happens to you.

Possible Side Effects

Serious side effects are uncommon.

▼ Most common: mild diarrhea, dizziness, rash, painful breast swelling, nausea and vomiting, headache, confusion, drowsiness, hallucinations, and impotence.

▼ Less common: liver inflammation, peeling or red and swollen rash, breathing difficulties, tingling in the hands or feet, delirious feelings, and oozing from the nipples.

▼ Rare: Cimetidine may affect white blood cells or blood platelets. Some symptoms of these effects are unusual bleeding or bruising, unusual tiredness, and weakness. Other rare side effects are inflammation of the pancreas, hair loss (reversible), abnormal heart rhythms, heart attack, muscle or joint pains, and drug reactions. Contact your doctor if you experience any side effect not listed above.

Drug Interactions

- Separate cimetidine from antacid doses by about 3 hours to avoid reducing cimetidine's effectiveness. Other drugs that may reduce the absorption of cimetidine are metoclopramide and anticholinergic drugs, including trihexyphenidyl hydrochloride, oxybutynin, and benztropine mesylate.

- Cigarette smoking reverses the healing effect cimetidine has on ulcers.

- Cimetidine may increase the side effects of a variety of drugs, possibly leading to drug toxicity. These drugs include alcohol; aminophylline; oral antidiabetes drugs; benzodiazepine sedatives, except lorazepam, oxazepam, and temazepam; caffeine; calcium channel blockers; carbamazepine; carmustine; chloroquine; flecainide; fluorouracil; labetalol; lidocaine; metoprolol; metronidazole; moricizine; mexiletine; narcotic pain relievers; nifedipine; ondansetron; pentoxifylline; phenytoin; procainamide; propafenone; propranolol; quinine; quinidine; tacrine; theophylline drugs, except dyphylline; triamterene; tricyclic antidepressants; valproic acid; and warfarin (a blood-thinner).

- Drugs whose absorption may be decreased by cimetidine are iron, indomethacin, fluconazole, ketoconazole, and tetracycline antibiotics.
- Enteric-coated tablets should not be taken with cimetidine. The change in stomach acidity causes the tablets to disintegrate prematurely in the stomach.
- Cimetidine may decrease the effects of digoxin and tocainide.

Food Interactions

None known.

Usual Dose

Adult: 400–800 mg at bedtime; 300 mg 4 times a day with meals and at bedtime; or 400 mg twice a day. To treat GERD—400 mg 4 times a day. Do not exceed 2400 mg a day. Users of Tagamet HB should not take more than 400 mg a day. Smaller doses may be as effective for seniors or those with impaired kidney function.

Overdosage

Little is known about the effects of cimetidine overdose, but victims may experience exaggerated side effects. Two deaths have occurred. Your local poison control center may advise giving ipecac syrup—available at any pharmacy—to induce vomiting and remove any drug remaining in the stomach. Victims who have definite symptoms should be taken to a hospital emergency room. ALWAYS bring the prescription bottle or container.

Special Information

Take cimetidine exactly as directed and follow your doctor's instructions regarding diet and other treatment in order to get the maximum benefit from the drug.

Do not take the maximum dose continuously for more than 2 weeks without the consent and supervision of your doctor.

Cigarette smoking is associated with stomach ulcers and reduces cimetidine's effectiveness.

Call your doctor at once if you develop any unusual side effects such as bleeding or bruising, tiredness, diarrhea, dizziness, rash, or hallucinations. Black, tarry stools or vomiting material that resembles coffee grounds may indicate your ulcer is bleeding.

If you miss a dose of cimetidine, take it as soon as possible. If it is almost time for your next dose, skip the dose you forgot and continue with your regular schedule. Do not take a double dose.

Special Populations

Pregnancy/Breast-feeding: Animal studies reveal no damage to the fetus, although cimetidine does pass into the fetal blood. When this drug is considered crucial by your doctor, its potential benefits must be carefully weighed against its risks.

Large amounts of cimetidine pass into breast milk. Nursing mothers who must take this drug should use infant formula.

Seniors: Seniors may need less medication due to loss of kidney function and be more susceptible to side effects, especially confusion and other nervous system effects (see "Cautions and Warnings").

Clarinex   *see Loratadine, page 660*

Generic Name

Clarithromycin   (klah-rith-roe-MYE-sin)   Ⓖ

Brand Names

Biaxin   Biaxin XL

Type of Drug

Macrolide antibiotic.

Prescribed For

Mild to moderate infections of the upper and lower respiratory tract, tonsillitis, pharyngitis, sinusitis, exacerbation of chronic bronchitis, middle-ear infections, and for duodenal ulcers; also used for skin and other infections, including membrane attack complex (MAC) in people with advanced HIV infection.

General Information

Clarithromycin and other macrolide antibiotics are either bactericidal (bacteria-killing) or bacteriostatic (inhibiting bacterial growth), depending on the organism in question and amount of antibiotic present. In ulcer disease, clarithromycin is used to fight *Helicobacter pylori* infection, which is present in almost all ulcers and most cases of stomach inflammation.

Cautions and Warnings

Do not take clarithromycin if you are **allergic** or **sensitive** to any of its ingredients or to any macrolide antibiotic.

Clarithromycin should not be used during **pregnancy**.

Clarithromycin is primarily eliminated from the body through the liver and kidneys. People with severe **kidney disease** may require dose adjustments. Liver disease generally does not require an adjustment.

Colitis (bowel inflammation) has been associated with all antibiotics (see "Possible Side Effects"). If colitis does develop, your doctor should start appropriate treatment. Mild cases of colitis usually respond to the discontinuation of the medicine.

Possible Side Effects

Most side effects are mild and go away once you stop taking clarithromycin.

▼ Most common: nausea, upset stomach, changes in sense of taste, headache, diarrhea, abdominal pain, vomiting, and rash in children. Colitis (symptoms include severe abdominal cramps and severe, persistent, and possibly bloody diarrhea) may develop.

▼ Rare: serious abnormal heart rhythms. Contact your doctor if you experience any side effect not listed above.

Drug Interactions

- Clarithromycin may increase the anticoagulant (blood-thinning) effects of warfarin in people who take it regularly, especially older adults. This combination requires careful monitoring by your doctor.
- Do not combine clarithromycin with astemizole or terfenadine.
- Combining clarithromycin and omeprazole raises the amount of both drugs in the blood.
- Two deaths have been reported in people combining clarithromycin and pimozide. Pimozide should not be used by people taking a macrolide antibiotic.
- Clarithromycin may raise blood levels of theophylline, possibly leading to a theophylline overdose. It can also increase the effects of caffeine.
- Combining clarithromycin and digoxin, cyclosporine, ergot alkaloids, or tacrolimus may lead to serious side effects.

- Combining clarithromycin and a statin cholesterol-lowering drug increases the risk of developing a painful and potentially fatal condition involving severe muscle degeneration.
- Combining clarithromycin and rifabutin or rifampin can interfere with the antibiotic's effect and increase the risk of intestinal side effects.
- Combining clarithromycin and ranitidine bismuth sulfate (for ulcers) can raise the amount of both drugs in the blood, but these effects are not considered important.
- Clarithromycin can increase the effects of alprazolam, diazepam, midazolam, and triazolam, causing excessive central-nervous-system (CNS) depression.
- Clarithromycin increases the effects of buspirone and can lead to buspirone side effects.
- Clarithromycin can raise blood levels of carbamazepine. People combining these drugs should be checked for changes in blood carbamazepine levels.
- Fluconazole increases the amount of clarithromycin in the blood.
- Combining zidovudine (an HIV drug—also known as AZT) and clarithromycin may affect the amount of zidovudine in the bloodstream.

Food Interactions

Clarithromycin can be generally taken without regard to food or meals; however, Biaxin XL should be taken with food.

Usual Dose

Adult: infections—250–500 mg every 12 hours (once a day for Biaxin XL) for 7–14 days. Dosage must be reduced in people with severe kidney disease. Ulcer—500 mg 3 times a day plus 40 mg omeprazole in the morning or ranitidine bismuth citrate 400 mg twice a day for 14 days, then omeprazole 20 mg every morning or ranitidine bismuth citrate 400 mg twice a day, for 15–28 days.

Child (age 6 months and over): 3.4 mg per lb. of body weight every 12 hours (once a day for Biaxin XL), up to 250–500 mg a dose, depending on the infecting organism, for 10 days.

Overdosage

Overdose may cause severe side effects, especially nausea, vomiting, stomach cramps, and diarrhea. Call your local poison control center or hospital emergency room for more information. If you seek treatment, ALWAYS bring the prescription bottle or container.

Special Information

Call your doctor if you develop nausea, vomiting, diarrhea, stomach cramps, or severe abdominal pain. Stop taking this medication and immediately call your doctor if you experience breathing difficulties, chest pain, hives, rash, itching, mouth sores, or unusual sensitivity to light.

Clarithromycin suspension must be shaken well before each dose. Do not store it in the refrigerator.

Clarithromycin may be gentler on the digestive tract than erythromycin.

Remember to complete the full course of treatment exactly as prescribed, even if you feel well sooner. Clarithromycin's effectiveness may be severely reduced otherwise.

Take clarithromycin at the same time each day. If you forget a dose, take it as soon as you remember. If it is within 4 hours of your next dose, skip the one you forgot and go back to your regular schedule.

Special Populations

Pregnancy/Breast-feeding: Clarithromycin affected the fetus in animal studies. This drug should not be used during pregnancy.

It is not known if clarithromycin passes into breast milk, but other macrolide antibiotics do. Nursing mothers who must take this drug should use infant formula.

Seniors: Seniors with severe kidney disease require a dosage adjustment.

Generic Name

Clemastine (KLEH-mas-tene) Ⓖ

Brand Names

DayHist-1   Tavist-1
Tavist   Tavist Allergy

Combination Product
*Generic Ingredients: Acetaminophen + Clemastine +
Pseudoephedrine*
Tavist Allergy/Sinus/Headache

Type of Drug

Antihistamine.

Prescribed For

Sneezing, stuffy and runny nose, itchy eyes, and scratchy throat caused by seasonal allergies and for other symptoms of allergies such as rash, itching, and hives.

General Information

Antihistamines generally work by blocking the release of naturally occuring histamine (a chemical released by body tissue during an allergic reaction) from cells at the H_1 histamine receptor site, drying up secretions of the nose, throat, and eyes. Clemastine fumarate is less sedating than most antihistamines, but not less sedating than astemizole, cetirizine, or loratadine.

Cautions and Warnings

Clemastine should not be taken if you are **allergic** or **sensitive** to any of its ingredients.

People with **asthma** or other **deep-breathing problems**, **heart disease**, **high blood pressure**, **diabetes**, **enlarged prostate**, **glaucoma**, **stomach ulcers** or other **stomach problems**, and **hyperthyroidism** should use clemastine with caution because its side effects can aggravate these problems.

Possible Side Effects

▼ Most common: drowsiness; headache; weakness; nervousness; stomach upset; nausea; vomiting; cough; stuffy nose; diarrhea; constipation; sore throat; nosebleeds; and dry mouth, nose, or throat.

▼ Less common: allergic reaction (symptoms include rash, itching, hives, and breathing difficulties), sleeplessness, menstrual irregularities, muscle aches, sweating, tingling in the hands or feet, frequent urination, visual disturbances, and ringing or buzzing in the ears.

Drug Interactions

- Combining clemastine with alcohol, sedatives, sleeping pills, or other nervous system depressants may increase the depressant effects of clemastine. Do not combine these drugs.
- The effects of oral anticoagulant (blood-thinning) drugs may be decreased by clemastine. Do not take this combination without your doctor's knowledge.

- Monoamine oxidase inhibitor antidepressants may increase the drying and other effects of clemastine. This combination can also worsen urinary difficulties.
- When taking antihistamines on a regular basis, notify your doctor if you are taking large amounts of aspirin. Effects of too much aspirin may be masked by the antihistamine.

Food Interactions

Clemastine is best taken on an empty stomach at least 1 hour before or 2 hours after eating; it may be taken with food if it upsets your stomach.

Usual Dose

Adult and Child (age 12 and over): 1.34 mg twice a day up to 8.04 mg of the syrup or 2.68 mg of the tablets in 24 hours.

Child (age 6–12) (syrup only): 0.67 mg twice a day or up to 4.02 mg a day.

Overdosage

Overdose is likely to cause severe side effects. Overdose victims should be given ipecac syrup—available at any pharmacy—to induce vomiting and should then be taken to a hospital emergency room for treatment. ALWAYS bring the prescription bottle or container.

Special Information

Clemastine may make it difficult for you to concentrate or perform complex tasks such as driving a car. Be sure to report any unusual side effects to your doctor.

Antihistamines may occasionally produce excitability, particularly in children.

If you forget to take a dose of clemastine, take it as soon as you remember. If it is almost time for your next dose, skip the one you forgot and continue with your regular schedule. Do not take a double dose.

Special Populations

Pregnancy/Breast-feeding: Do not take any antihistamines without your doctor's knowledge if you are or might be pregnant—especially during the last 3 months of pregnancy, because newborns may have severe reactions to antihistamines.

Small amounts of clemastine pass into breast milk. Nursing mothers who must take clemastine should use infant formula.

Seniors: Seniors are more sensitive to side effects.

Generic Name

Clindamycin (klin-duh-MYE-sin) Ⓖ

Brand Names

Cleocin	Clindesse
Cleocin T	Clindets
Clinda-Derm	Evoclin
Clindagel	

Type of Drug

Antibiotic.

Prescribed For

Serious bacterial infections. The vaginal cream is used to treat bacterial vaginosis. Topical clindamycin is used to treat acne and rosacea.

General Information

Clindamycin is one of the few oral drugs that is effective against anaerobic bacteria, which grow only in the absence of oxygen and are often found in infected wounds, lung abscesses, abdominal infections, and infections of the female genital tract. It also works against bacteria usually treated with penicillin or erythromycin, including serious respiratory tract infections. Clindamycin may be useful for treating certain skin or soft tissue infections. It kills the bacteria that frequently cause acne.

Clindamycin is not used to treat vaginal fungus or yeast infections.

Cautions and Warnings

Do not take clindamycin if you are **allergic** or **sensitive** to any of its ingredients or to lincomycin, another antibiotic.

People with **asthma** or a history of **allergies** should use clindamycin capsules with caution.

Clindamycin can cause a severe intestinal irritation called colitis, which can be fatal. Signs of colitis are diarrhea, blood in the stool, and abdominal cramps. Any form of this drug, including products applied to the skin and the vaginal cream, can provoke colitis. Because of this, clindamycin should be reserved for serious infections or those that cannot be treated with other drugs.

Clindamycin should be used with caution if you have **gastrointestinal disease** or **kidney or liver disease**.

Possible Side Effects

Capsules
▼ Most common: stomach pain; nausea; vomiting; diarrhea, in up to 20% of people; and pain when swallowing.
▼ Less common: itching; rash; signs of serious drug sensitivity, such as difficulties breathing and yellowing of the skin or the whites of the eyes; colitis (see "Cautions and Warnings"); effects on blood components; and joint pain.

Topical Lotion
▼ Most common: dry skin, redness, burning, peeling, oily skin, and itching.
▼ Less common: diarrhea, abdominal pain, upset stomach, and colitis (see "Cautions and Warnings").

Vaginal Cream
▼ Most common: vaginal itching or irritation; thick, white vaginal discharge; and pain during intercourse.
▼ Less common: nausea, vomiting, diarrhea, constipation, abdominal pain, dizziness, headache, vertigo, and colitis (see "Cautions and Warnings").

Drug Interactions
- Do not combine clindamycin and erythromycin.
- The absorption of clindamycin capsules into the bloodstream is delayed by Kaolin-Pectin Suspension (prescribed for diarrhea). Separate these drugs by at least 1 hour.
- Clindamycin should be used with caution by people also using neuromuscular agents.

Food Interactions
Take the oral medication with a full glass of water or with food to prevent irritation of the stomach and intestine.

Usual Dose

Capsules
Adult: 150–450 mg every 6 hours.

Child (under age 16): 3.5–11 mg per lb. of body weight a day, in 3–4 doses. For severe infections, at least 37.5 mg 3 times a day, regardless of weight.

Foam: Dispense enough to cover the affected area(s) onto a cool surface (the foam will melt on contact with warm skin). Use fingertips to massage small amounts into the affected area(s) until the foam disappears.

Suppositories: Insert 1 suppository a day for 3 consecutive days.

Topical Lotion: Wash the skin and pat dry before application. Apply enough to cover the affected area(s) with a thin coat twice a day.

Vaginal Cream: Insert 1 applicator's worth at bedtime for 7 consecutive days, except for Clindesse, which requires one applicator's worth once at any time of day.

Overdosage

Clindamycin overdose may lead to severe diarrhea and other drug side effects. Do not treat this diarrhea on your own. Discontinue use of this drug and call your local poison center for information. If you go to an emergency room for treatment, ALWAYS bring the prescription bottle or container.

Special Information

Prolonged or unsupervised use of clindamycin may lead to secondary infections from susceptible organisms, such as fungi. Take this drug for the full course of therapy as indicated by your physician.

If you develop severe diarrhea or abdominal pain, call your doctor at once. Call your doctor immediately if you experience breathing difficulties or jaundice (yellowing of the skin or whites of the eyes).

Women using the vaginal cream should not have vaginal intercourse or use other vaginal products such as tampons or douches until treatment is complete.

Use of latex condoms or diaphragms within 72 hours following treatment with the vaginal creams or suppositories is not recommended. These products may decrease the efficacy of condoms or diaphragms.

The topical lotion is for external use only. Avoid contact with your eyes or mucous membranes.

If you miss a dose of oral clindamycin, take it as soon as you remember. If it is almost time for your next dose of clindamycin, double that dose and go back to your regular dosage schedule.

Special Populations

Pregnancy/Breast-feeding: This drug crosses into fetal blood circulation. When the drug is considered crucial by your doctor, its potential benefits must be carefully weighed against its risks.

Clindamycin passes into breast milk. Nursing mothers who must take oral clindamycin should use infant formula.

Seniors: Seniors with other illnesses may be unable to tolerate diarrhea and other clindamycin side effects.

Generic Name

Clonazepam (klon-A-zeh-pam) Ⓖ

Brand Name
Klonopin

Type of Drug
Anticonvulsant.

Prescribed For
Petit mal and other seizures and panic attacks; also prescribed for periodic leg movements during sleep, speaking difficulty associated with Parkinson's disease, acute manic episodes, nerve pain, and schizophrenia.

General Information
Clonazepam is a benzodiazepine drug. Clonazepam is not used as a sedative or hypnotic. It is used only for the uses described above in people who have not responded to other drug treatments. Tolerance to the effects of clonazepam commonly develops within about 3 months of use. Your doctor may raise your clonazepam dosage periodically to maintain the drug's effect.

Cautions and Warnings
Do not take clonazepam if you are **allergic** or **sensitive** to any of its ingredients or any other benzodiazepine.

When stopping clonazepam treatments, the drug must be discontinued gradually. Abrupt discontinuance of clonazepam may lead to drug **withdrawal symptoms** including severe seizures, tremors, abdominal or muscle cramps, vomiting, and increased sweating.

Use clonazepam with caution if you have a chronic **respiratory illness**, since the drug tends to increase salivation and other respiratory secretions and can make breathing more labored.

Avoid using clonazepam if you have severe **depression**, severe **lung disease**, **sleep apnea** (intermittent cessation of breathing during sleep), **liver disease**, **alcoholism**, or **kidney disease**. These conditions may exacerbate the depressive effects of benzodiazepines, and such effects may be detrimental to your overall condition.

Clonazepam can aggravate **narrow-angle glaucoma**, but if you have open-angle glaucoma, you may take it.

Possible Side Effects

▼ Most common: drowsiness, poor muscle control, and behavioral changes.

▼ Rare: Rare side effects can occur in almost any part of the body but are most likely to affect mental function, stomach and intestines, urinary function, blood, and liver. Contact your doctor if you experience any side effect not listed above.

Drug Interactions

- The depressant effects of clonazepam are increased by sedatives, sleeping pills, narcotic pain relievers, antihistamines, alcohol, monoamine oxidase inhibitor antidepressants, tricyclic antidepressants, and other anticonvulsants.
- Mixing valproic acid and clonazepam may produce severe petit mal seizures.
- Smoking, phenobarbital, phenytoin, carbamazapine, and rifampin may reduce clonazepam's effectiveness.
- Clonazepam may increase the requirement for other anticonvulsant drugs in people who suffer from multiple types of seizures.
- The effects of clonazepam may be prolonged when it is taken with cimetidine, contraceptive drugs, disulfiram, fluvoxamine, isoniazid, oral antifungal medications (e.g. ketoconazole), metoprolol, probenecid, propoxyphene, or propranolol.
- Theophylline may reduce clonazepam's sedative effects.
- Separate antacids from your clonazepam dose by at least 1 hour to prevent them from interfering with clonazepam being absorbed into the bloodstream.
- Clonazepam may increase blood levels of digoxin and the risk of digoxin toxicity.
- Clonazepam may decrease the effect of levodopa + carbidopa.

Food Interactions

Clonazepam is best taken on an empty stomach but may be taken with food if it upsets your stomach.

Usual Dose

Clonazepam is available in either tablets or orally disintegrating tablets, called wafers. Wafers should not be opened until immediately before the dose is to be taken. Do not push the wafer through the foil. Use dry hands to remove the wafer. The wafer will disintegrate quickly in saliva.

Seizures

Adult and Child (age 10 and over): starting dose—0.5 mg 3 times a day. The dose is increased by 0.5–1 mg every 3 days until seizures are controlled or side effects develop. The maximum daily dose is 20 mg.

Panic attacks

Adult and Child (age 10 and over): starting dose—0.25 mg twice daily. The dose is increased to 1 mg a day after 3 days. Most people do not require a higher dose.

Child (under age 10 or below 66 lbs.): starting dose—0.022–0.066 mg per lb. of body weight a day in divided doses. Dosage can be increased gradually to a daily dose of 0.22–0.44 mg per lb. of body weight.

Other uses for clonazepam involve doses from 0.5–16 mg a day, depending on the condition and its severity. Clonazepam dosage must be reduced in people with impaired kidney function.

Overdosage

Overdose may cause confusion, coma, poor reflexes, sleepiness, low blood pressure, labored breathing, and other depressive effects. If the overdose is discovered within a few minutes and the victim is still conscious, it may be helpful to induce vomiting with ipecac syrup—available at any pharmacy. Overdose victims must be taken to a hospital emergency room. ALWAYS bring the prescription bottle or container.

Special Information

Clonazepam may interfere with your ability to drive or perform other complex tasks because it can cause drowsiness and difficulty in concentrating.

Your doctor should perform periodic blood counts and liver function tests while you are taking this drug to check for possible side effects.

Do not suddenly stop taking clonazepam—severe seizures may result. The dosage must be discontinued gradually by your doctor.

If you miss a dose by 1 hour or less, take it right away. Otherwise, skip the dose you forgot and go back to your regular schedule. Do not take a double dose.

Carry identification or wear a bracelet indicating that you have a seizure disorder for which you take clonazepam.

Special Populations

Pregnancy/Breast-feeding: Clonazepam crosses into the fetal circulation and can affect the fetus. Women who are or might be pregnant should avoid it. When the drug is considered crucial by your doctor, its potential benefits must be carefully weighed against its risks.

Some reports suggest a strong link between anticonvulsant drugs and birth defects, though most of the information pertains to phenytoin and phenobarbital, not clonazepam. It is also possible that the epileptic condition itself or genetic factors common to people with seizure disorders may figure in the higher incidence of birth defects.

Clonazepam may pass into breast milk. Nursing mothers who must take this drug should use infant formula.

Seniors: Seniors, especially those with liver or kidney disease, are more sensitive to the effects of this drug—especially dizziness and drowsiness—and may require smaller doses.

Generic Name

Clonidine (KLAH-nih-dene) Ⓖ

Brand Names

Catapres
Catapres-TTS-1

Catapres-TTS-2
Catapres-TTS-3

Type of Drug

Alpha receptor stimulant.

Prescribed For

High blood pressure, including hypertensive emergency (diastolic blood pressure over 120); also used for excess sweating, childhood growth delay, attention-deficit hyperactivity disorder (ADHD), Tourette's syndrome, restless leg syndrome, schizophrenic psychosis, migraine, ulcerative colitis, painful or difficult menstruation, hot flashes related to menopause, diagnosis of pheochromocytoma (adrenal-gland tumor), kidney poisoning associated with cyclosporine, diabetic diarrhea, smoking cessation, methadone and opiate detoxification, withdrawal from alcohol and benzodiazepines such as Valium, nerve pain following herpes attack, and allergic reactions in the presence of asthma triggered by external sources.

General Information

Clonidine stimulates nerve endings in the brain called alpha-adrenergic receptors. It reduces blood pressure by dilating (widening) blood vessels. Clonidine works quickly, decreasing blood pressure within 1 hour. The other uses of clonidine relate to its stimulation of alpha receptors in the body.

Cautions and Warnings

Do not take clonidine if you are **allergic** or **sensitive** to any of its ingredients.

People who have had a **stroke** or recent **heart attack** or who have **cardiac insufficiency** or **chronic kidney failure** should avoid taking clonidine.

Some people develop a tolerance of their clonidine dosage. If this happens, your blood pressure may increase and your doctor may prescribe a higher dose.

Never stop taking clonidine without your doctor's knowledge. If you abruptly stop taking clonidine, you may experience an unusual increase in blood pressure accompanied by agitation, headache, nervousness, and severe reactions, possibly death. Restarting clonidine therapy or taking another antihypertensive can reverse these effects.

Clonidine may cause degeneration of the retina. See your eye doctor for regular check-ups if you are taking this drug.

If you require surgery, your doctor will continue your clonidine therapy until about 4 hours before surgery and resume it as soon as possible afterward.

People who develop skin sensitivity (symptoms include rash, itching, and swelling) to Catapres-TTS, the transdermal patch form of clonidine, may experience the same reactions with oral clonidine.

Possible Side Effects

Tablets

▼ Most common: dry mouth, drowsiness, dizziness, constipation, and sedation.

▼ Common: headache and fatigue. These effects tend to diminish within 4–6 weeks.

▼ Less common: appetite loss, swelling or pain in the glands of the throat, nausea, vomiting, weight gain, blood-sugar elevation, breast pain or enlargement, worsening of congestive heart failure, heart palpitations, rapid heartbeat, painful blood-vessel spasm, abnormal heart rhythms, electrocardiogram changes, feeling unwell, changes in dream patterns, nightmares, difficulty sleeping, hallucinations, delirium, anxiety, depression, nervousness, restlessness, rash, hives, thinning or loss of scalp hair, difficult or painful urination, nighttime urination, retaining urine, decrease or loss of sex drive, weakness, muscle or joint pain, leg cramps, increased alcohol sensitivity, dryness and burning of the eyes, dry nose, loss of color, and fever.

Transdermal Patch

▼ Most common: dry mouth and drowsiness.

▼ Less common: constipation, nausea, changes in sense of taste, dry throat, fatigue, headache, lethargy, changes in sleep patterns, nervousness, dizziness, impotence, sexual difficulties, and mild skin reactions including itching, swelling, contact dermatitis, discoloration, burning, peeling, throbbing, white patches, and generalized rash. Rashes of the face and tongue have also occurred but cannot be specifically tied to transdermal clonidine.

Drug Interactions

• Combining clonidine and a beta-adrenergic blocker may increase the severity of a drug-withdrawal reaction and rebound high blood pressure. This reaction may be very serious.

• Combining verapamil and clonidine may lead to very low blood pressure and atrioventricular (AV) block (abnormality in heartbeat patterns). This reaction may be very serious.

• Avoid alcohol, barbiturates, and sedatives because they increase the depressive effects of clonidine.

- Tricyclic and other antidepressants, appetite suppressants, estrogens, stimulants, indomethacin and other nonsteroidal anti-inflammatory drugs (NSAIDs), and prazosin may counteract the effects of clonidine.
- Clonidine may reduce the therapeutic effects of levadopa + carbidopa.

Food Interactions

The tablets are best taken on an empty stomach but may be taken with food if they upset your stomach.

Usual Dose

Tablets

Adult: high blood pressure—100 mcg twice a day to start; may be raised by 100 mcg a day until maximum control is achieved. Take no more than 2400 mcg a day. Other uses—100–900 mcg a day, or up to 0.8 mcg per lb. of body weight in divided doses. Seniors should start with a lower dose and increase more slowly.

Child: 50–400 mcg orally twice a day.

Transdermal Patch

Adult: 100 mcg delivered daily from a patch applied once every 7 days. Up to two 300-mcg patches may be needed to control blood pressure. Transdermal dosage exceeding 600 mcg a day has not been shown to increase effectiveness.

Child: not recommended.

Overdosage

Symptoms of overdose are slow heartbeat, central-nervous-system depression, very slow breathing, low body temperature, pinpoint pupils, seizures, lethargy, agitation, irritability, nausea, vomiting, abnormal heart rhythms, mild increases in blood pressure followed by a rapid drop in blood pressure, dizziness, weakness, loss of reflexes, and vomiting. Victims should be taken to a hospital emergency room immediately. ALWAYS bring the prescription bottle or container.

Special Information

Clonidine causes drowsiness in about ⅓ of people who take it. Be extremely careful while driving or performing any task that requires concentration. This effect is prominent during the first few weeks of clonidine therapy and then tends to decrease.

Do not take over-the-counter cough and cold medications unless directed by your doctor.

Call your doctor if you become depressed or have vivid dreams or nightmares while taking clonidine, or if you develop swelling in your feet or legs, paleness or coldness in your fingertips or toes, or any persistent or bothersome side effect.

Apply the transdermal patch to a hairless area of skin such as the upper arm or torso. Use a different skin site each time. If the patch becomes loose, apply the supplied adhesive directly over it. If the patch falls off before 7 days are up, apply a new one. Do not remove the patch while bathing.

If you forget a dose of oral clonidine, take it as soon as possible and then go back to your regular schedule. If you miss 2 or more consecutive doses, consult your doctor; missed doses may cause blood pressure increases and severe adverse effects. Do not take a double dose.

Special Populations

Pregnancy/Breast-feeding: Clonidine passes into the fetal bloodstream. Animal studies show that clonidine may damage the fetus in doses as low as ⅓ the maximum dose. When this drug is considered crucial by your doctor, its potential benefits must be carefully weighed against its risks.

Clonidine passes into breast milk. Nursing mothers who must take this drug should use infant formula.

Seniors: Seniors are more susceptible to the effects of this drug and should begin with lower doses.

Generic Name

Clopidogrel (kloe-PID-oe-grel) Ⓖ

Brand Name
Plavix

Type of Drug
Antiplatelet.

Prescribed For
Heart attack and stroke prevention; also used for blood thinning after placement of a vascular stent.

General Information

Artery-clogging blood clots are often the cause of heart attacks and strokes. Clopidogrel reduces the risk of both by helping prevent blood-clot formation. This drug thins the blood by making platelets—the cells that aggregate to form clots—less "sticky." It starts working in as little as 2 hours after taking a single tablet. The drug's blood-thinning effect lasts until inactivated platelets are replaced by the body. Studies suggest that clopidogrel is more effective than aspirin in preventing heart attack and stroke in people at risk. People taking clopidogrel after stent surgery usually take it for a relatively short period. Those taking it to prevent a heart attack or stroke must take it for life.

Cautions and Warnings

Do not take clopidogrel if you are **allergic** or **sensitive** to any of its ingredients or to ticlopidine, a related antiplatelet. These drugs can rarely cause a rapid drop in white-blood-cell count.

People with **bleeding ulcers, brain hemorrhages,** or **other bleeding problems** should use clopidogrel with caution.

Thrombotic thrombocytopenic purpura (TTP) is a rare but serious complication of clopidogrel, sometimes reported after less than 2 weeks of treatment. See your doctor right away if you develop a sudden fever, unusual bruising, nosebleeds, bleeding gums, or any other unusual symptoms. TTP reduces your platelet count, interfering with blood clotting, and affects white-blood-cell count.

People with **liver problems** should use clopidogrel with caution.

Possible Side Effects

▼ Most common: rash and other skin problems.

▼ Common: chest pain, accidents, flu-like symptoms, pain, headache, dizziness, abdominal pain, upset stomach, joint pain, back pain, black-and-blue marks, and respiratory infection.

▼ Less common: tiredness, swollen arms or legs, high blood pressure, diarrhea, nausea, bleeding, nosebleeds, breathing difficulties, runny nose, coughing, bronchitis, high blood cholesterol, urinary infection, and depression.

▼ Rare: bleeding in the brain and stomach ulcer. Contact your doctor if you experience any side effect not listed above.

Drug Interactions

- Clopidogrel may interfere with the body's ability to break down fluvastatin, nonsteroidal anti-inflammatory drugs (NSAIDs), phenytoin, tamoxifen, tolbutamide, torsamide, and warfarin.
- Combining clopidogrel and NSAIDs may increase blood loss and bleeding in the stomach and intestines.
- Do not combine clopidogrel and other antiplatelet drugs or the anticoagulant (blood thinner) warfarin unless you are under your doctor's direct supervision. This interaction may prevent normal blood clotting and lead to severe bleeding problems.

Food Interactions

Clopidogrel may be taken without regard to food or meals.

Usual Dose

Adult: 75 mg a day.

Overdosage

Little is known about the effects of clopidogrel overdose aside from reduced blood clotting. Overdose victims should be taken to a hospital emergency room. ALWAYS bring the prescription bottle or container.

Special Information

Minor cuts may take longer to stop bleeding during treatment with clopidogrel. If you are having surgery, make sure your doctor knows you are taking clopidogrel. You may have to stop taking the drug 1 week before surgery.

If you forget a dose, take it as soon as you remember. If it is almost time for your next dose, skip the forgotten dose and continue with your regular schedule.

Special Populations

Pregnancy/Breast-feeding: The safety of using clopidogrel during pregnancy is not known. Other antiplatelet drugs, like aspirin, are not used during pregnancy due to their possible effects on mother and fetus. When this drug is considered crucial by your doctor, its benefits must be carefully weighed against its risks.

Clopidogrel may pass into breast milk. Nursing mothers who must take this drug should use infant formula.

Seniors: Seniors may take this drug without special precaution.

Generic Name

Clorazepate (klor-AZ-uh-pate) Ⓖ

Brand Names

Gen-Xene   Tranxene-SD
Tranxene   Tranxene T-Tab

Type of Drug

Benzodiazepine sedative.

Prescribed For

Anxiety, tension, fatigue, and agitation; symptoms of acute alcohol withdrawal; partial seizures; also prescribed for irritable bowel syndrome and panic attacks.

General Information

Clorazepate dipotassium is a benzodiazepine. Benzodiazepines directly affect the brain. They can relax you and make you more tranquil or sleepier, or they can slow nervous system transmissions in such a way as to act as an anticonvulsant. Many doctors prefer benzodiazepines to other drugs that can be used to similar effect because they tend to be safer, have fewer side effects, and usually work as well, if not better.

Cautions and Warnings

Do not take clorazepate if you are **allergic** or **sensitive** to any of its ingredients or to another benzodiazepine drug, including clonazepam.

Clorazepate can aggravate narrow-angle **glaucoma**, but you may take it if you have open-angle glaucoma and are receiving therapy for it.

Other conditions in which clorazepate should be avoided are: severe **depression**, severe **lung disease**, **sleep apnea** (intermittent cessation of breathing during sleep), **liver disease**, **drunkenness**, and **kidney disease**. In each of these conditions, the depressive effects of clorazepate may be enhanced or could be detrimental to your overall condition.

Clorazepate should not be taken by **psychotic patients** because it is not effective for them and can trigger unusual excitement, stimulation, and rage.

Clorazepate is not intended to be used for more than 3–4 months at a time. Your doctor should reassess your condition before continuing your prescription beyond that time.

Clorazepate may be addictive. It should be used with caution in people with a history of **drug dependence**.

Drug withdrawal may develop if you stop taking it after as few as 4 weeks of regular use but is more likely after longer use. It may start with anxiety and progress to tingling in the hands or feet, sensitivity to bright light, sleep disturbances, cramps, tremors, muscle tension or twitching, poor concentration, flu-like symptoms, fatigue, appetite loss, sweating, and changes in mental state. Your dosage should always be reduced gradually to prevent drug withdrawal symptoms.

Possible Side Effects

Weakness and confusion may occur, especially in seniors and in those who are more sickly.

▼ Most common: mild drowsiness during the first few days of therapy.

▼ Less common: confusion, depression, lethargy, disorientation, headache, inactivity, slurred speech, stupor, dizziness, tremors, constipation, dry mouth, nausea, inability to control urination, sexual difficulties, irregular menstrual cycle, changes in heart rhythm, low blood pressure, fluid retention, blurred or double vision, itching, rash, hiccups, nervousness, inability to fall asleep, and occasional liver and kidney dysfunction. If you have any of these symptoms, stop taking the medicine and contact your doctor immediately.

▼ Rare: Rare side effects can affect your heart, stomach and intestines, urinary tract, blood, muscles and joints. Contact your doctor if you experience any side effects not listed above.

Drug Interactions

- Clorazepate is a central-nervous-system depressant. Don't mix it with alcohol, other sedatives, narcotics, barbiturates, monoamine oxidase inhibitor and other antidepressants, and antihistamines. Taking clorazepate with these drugs may result in excessive depression, tiredness, sleepiness, breathing difficulties, or related symptoms.

- Smoking may reduce clorazepate's effectiveness by increasing the rate at which it is broken down by the body.
- Clorazepate's effects may be prolonged when it is mixed with cimetidine, contraceptive drugs, disulfiram, fluoxetine, isoniazid, ketoconazole, metoprolol, probenecid, propoxyphene, propranolol, rifampin, or valproic acid. Theophylline may reduce clorazepate's sedative effects.
- If you take antacids, separate them from your clorazepate dose by at least 1 hour to prevent them from interfering with the absorption of clorazepate into the bloodstream.
- Clorazepate may increase blood levels of digoxin and the chances of digoxin toxicity.
- The effect of levodopa + carbidopa may be decreased if it is taken together with clorazepate.
- Combining clorazepate with phenytoin may increase phenytoin blood concentrations and the chances of phenytoin toxicity.

Food Interactions

Clorazepate is best taken on an empty stomach, but it may be taken with food if it upsets your stomach.

Usual Dose
Immediate-Release

Adult and Child (age 9 and over): 15–60 mg daily. The average dose is 30 mg in divided quantities, but dosage must be adjusted to individual response for maximum effect. Maximum recommended daily dose is 90 mg. For treatment of anxiety, clorazepate may be taken as a single dose at bedtime.

Child (under age 9): not recommended.

Sustained-Release

Adult: The sustained-release form of clorazepate may be given as a single dose, either 11.25 or 22.5 mg, once every 24 hours. Sustained-release tablets are not recommended for the initial dosage.

Child: not recommended.

Overdosage

Symptoms of overdose are confusion, sleepiness, poor coordination, lack of response to pain such as a pin prick, loss of reflexes, shallow breathing, low blood pressure, and coma. The victim should be taken to a hospital emergency room. ALWAYS bring the prescription bottle or container.

Special Information

Clorazepate can cause tiredness, drowsiness, inability to concentrate, or similar symptoms. Be careful if you are driving, operating machinery, or performing other activities that require concentration.

People taking clorazepate for more than 3 or 4 months at a time may develop drug withdrawal reactions if the medication is stopped suddenly (see "Cautions and Warnings"). Do not stop taking clorazepate or increase or decrease your dosage without first consulting your doctor.

If you forget a dose of clorazepate, take it as soon as you remember. If it is almost time for your next dose, skip the dose you forgot and continue with your regular schedule. Do not take a double dose.

Special Populations

Pregnancy/Breast-feeding: Clorazepate may cause birth defects if taken during the first 3 months of pregnancy. Avoid this drug if you are or might be pregnant.

Clorazepate may pass into breast milk. Nursing mothers who must take clorazepate should use infant formula.

Seniors: Seniors, especially those with liver or kidney disease, are more sensitive to the effects of clorazepate and generally require smaller doses to achieve the same effect.

Generic Name

Clotrimazole (kloe-TRIM-uh-zole) Ⓖ

Brand Name

Mycelex

The information in this profile also applies to the following drug:

Generic Ingredient: Sertaconazole
Ertaczo

Type of Drug

Antifungal.

Prescribed For

Fungal infections of the mouth, skin, and vaginal tract.

General Information

Clotrimazole is useful against a variety of fungal organisms that other drugs do not affect. The exact way in which clotrimazole works is unknown. Sertaconazole is used for athlete's foot in people age 12 and older with compromised immune systems.

Cautions and Warnings

Do not use this product if you are **allergic** or **sensitive** to any of its ingredients.

If clotrimazole causes local itching or irritation, stop using it.

Do not use clotrimazole in your eyes.

Proper diagnosis is essential for effective treatment. Do not use this product without first consulting your doctor.

Possible Side Effects

Side effects are infrequent and usually mild.

Cream and Solution
▼ Most common: redness, stinging, blistering, peeling, itching, and swelling of local areas.

Vaginal Tablets
▼ Most common: mild burning, rash, mild cramps, and frequent urination. Your sexual partner may also experience some burning or itching.

Lozenges
▼ Most common: stomach cramps or pain, diarrhea, nausea, and vomiting.

Drug Interactions

None known.

Food Interactions

The oral form of clotrimazole is best taken on an empty stomach, at least 1 hour before or 2 hours after meals. However, you may take it with food as long as you allow the lozenge to dissolve fully in your mouth.

Usual Dose

Topical Cream and Solution

Adult and Child (over age 2): Apply to clean, dry, affected areas morning and night for 7 consecutive days or as needed. For athlete's foot and ringworm, use daily for 4 weeks. For jock itch, use daily for 2 weeks.

Vaginal Cream

Adult: 1 applicator's worth at bedtime for 3–7 consecutive days.

Vaginal Tablet

Adult: 1 tablet inserted into the vagina at bedtime for 3 days, or 2 tablets a day for 3–7 consecutive days.

Lozenge

Adult and Child (over age 3): 1 lozenge 5 times a day for 2 weeks or more.

Overdosage

Little is known about the effects of clotrimazole overdose or accidental ingestion. Call your local poison control center for more information. If you seek treatment, ALWAYS bring the prescription bottle or container.

Special Information

If treating a vaginal infection, you should refrain from sexual activity. Call your doctor if burning or itching develops or if the condition does not improve within 7 days.

If you are using the vaginal cream, you may want to wear a sanitary napkin to avoid staining your clothing. Do not use a tampon during treatment.

Dissolve the lozenge slowly in the mouth. This may take up to 30 minutes.

This medicine must be taken on consecutive days. If you forget a dose of oral clotrimazole, take it as soon as you remember. Do not double your dose.

When using clotrimazole for skin infections, do not cover the area with any kind of bandage unless directed to do so by your doctor. For athlete's foot, wear well-fitting, ventilated shoes, and change your socks at least once a day.

Clotrimazole is not effective on scalp or nails.

Special Populations

Pregnancy/Breast-feeding: Women who are or might be pregnant should talk to their doctor about the medication's risks and benefits. Women who are in the first 3 months of pregnancy should use this drug only if directed to do so by their doctor. If you are pregnant, your doctor may want you to insert vaginal tablets by hand rather than use a vaginal applicator.

It is unknown whether the drug passes into breast milk. Use with caution or use infant formula.

Seniors: Seniors may use this medication without special precaution.

Generic Name

Clozapine (KLOE-zuh-pene) G

Brand Names
Clozaril   FazaClo Orally Disintegrating Tablets

Type of Drug
Antipsychotic.

Prescribed For
Severe schizophrenia.

General Information
Clozapine is a unique antipsychotic that has the capacity to treat people who do not respond to or cannot tolerate other drugs. It works by a mechanism that differs from those of other antipsychotic drugs.

A very small number of people who take clozapine develop a rapid drop in their white-blood-cell count, known as agranulocytosis. This effect usually reverses itself when the drug is stopped, but the drug must be stopped as soon as it is discovered. An unusually large number of people who have developed clozapine agranulocytosis in the United States are of Eastern European Jewish descent, but the association is not very strong. Most cases of agranulocytosis occur between week 4 and week 10 of treatment. It is essential that blood samples be taken approximately every week and for 4 weeks after the drug is stopped to watch for this effect. Because of the risk of agranulocytosis, clozapine should not be tried until at least 2 other antipsychotic medicines have failed.

Some people taking antipsychotic drugs develop tardive dyskinesia, a potentially irreversible condition marked by uncontrollable movements. Tardive dyskinesia has not been seen in patients taking clozapine, a major advantage of this drug over other antipsychotic medicines. However, there is still a risk that this set of symptoms could occur with clozapine.

Cautions and Warnings

Do not take clozapine if you are **allergic** or **sensitive** to any of its ingredients.

Women, seniors, people with **serious illnesses**, those who are **emaciated**, those with a history of **diseases affecting the white blood cells**, or those who are taking other **medication that could affect white blood cells** may be more susceptible to clozapine agranulocytosis.

Clozapine has been associated with increased mortality in seniors with **dementia** or **Alzheimer's disease**. The specific causes of death related to clozapine and other atypical antipsychotic drugs were either due to a heart-related event or infection, mostly pneumonia. Clozapine should not be taken by those with dementia-related psychosis.

About 5% of people taking the drug experience a **seizure** in the first year of treatment. Seizure is most likely to occur at higher drug doses.

People with **heart disease** should be carefully monitored while on clozapine because of possible cardiac risks.

Clozapine may cause low blood pressure, especially at the beginning of therapy.

Clozapine has been associated with obesity, high cholesterol, high blood sugar, and diabetes. **Diabetics** and **pre-diabetics** (people with elevated blood sugar and a family history of diabetes) should be carefully monitored.

A serious set of side effects, known as neuroleptic malignant syndrome (NMS), includes a high fever and has been associated with clozapine when it is used together with lithium or other drugs. The symptoms that constitute NMS include muscle rigidity, mental changes, irregular pulse or blood pressure, increased sweating, and abnormal heart rhythm. NMS is potentially fatal and requires immediate medical attention.

Use this drug with caution if you have **glaucoma, prostate problems,** or **liver or kidney disease.**

Clozapine may interfere with mental or physical abilities because of the sedation it usually causes during the first few weeks of treatment.

Possible Side Effects

▼ Most common: rapid heartbeat, low blood pressure, dizziness, fainting, drowsiness or sedation, salivation, and constipation.

▼ Less common: headache, tremor, sleep disturbance, restlessness, slow muscle motions, absence of movement, agitation, convulsions, rigidity, restlessness, confusion, sweating, dry mouth, visual disturbances, high blood pressure, nausea, vomiting, heartburn or abdominal discomfort, fever, and weight gain.

▼ Rare: agranulocytosis (symptoms include fever with or without chills, sore throat, and sores or white spots on the lips or mouth), tardive dyskinesia (symptoms include lip smacking or puckering, puffing of the cheeks, rapid or wormlike tongue movement, uncontrolled chewing motions, and uncontrolled arm and leg movements), and NMS (see "Cautions and Warnings"). Other rare side effects can occur in almost any part of the body. Contact your doctor if you experience any side effect not listed above.

Drug Interactions

- Clozapine's anticholinergic effects—blurred vision, dry mouth, and confusion—may be enhanced by interaction with other anticholinergics, such as tricyclic antidepressants like amitriptyline.
- Drugs that reduce blood pressure may enhance the blood-pressure-lowering effects of clozapine.
- Alcohol and other nervous system depressants, including benzodiazepines and other antianxiety drugs, may enhance clozapine's sedative action. At least 1 person has died as a result of combining diazepam and clozapine.
- Combination contraceptive drugs may increase blood levels of clozapine leading to toxic side effects. Women starting on a combination contraceptive may need to have their clozapine dose adjusted.

- Clozapine should not be used with ritonavir.
- Cimetidine, caffeine, citalopram, ciprofloxacin, erythromycin, and ketoconazole may increase blood levels of clozapine resulting in increased side effects. Caution should be used with combining clozapine with paroxetine, fluvoxamine, or sertraline as similar reactions may occur, although these interactions are less well-defined.
- Clozapine may increase blood levels of digoxin, warfarin, heparin, and phenytoin.
- Use of clozapine with phenytoin, carbamazepine, and rifampin may cause decreases in blood levels of clozapine, reducing its effectiveness.
- The combination of lithium and clozapine may cause seizures, confusion, and NMS (see "Cautions and Warnings").
- Cigarette smoking may alter clozapine dosage requirements.
- Combining selective serotonin receptor inhibitors (SSRIs) with clozapine may require a lower clozapine dosage.

Food Interactions

None known.

Usual Dose

Tablets

Starting dose: 25 mg in divided doses twice a day; maintenance dose—generally, 300–450 mg a day in divided doses. Dosage may be increased gradually to a daily maximum of 900 mg in divided doses if required.

Orally Disintegrating Tablets

Starting dose: 12.5 mg once or twice a day increasing to 300–450 mg a day in divided doses by the end of 2 weeks. Dosage may then be increased up to 900 mg a day in divided doses if required.

Overdosage

Symptoms of overdose are delirium, drowsiness, changes in heart rhythm, unusual excitement, nervousness, restlessness, hallucinations, excessive salivation, dizziness or fainting, slow or irregular breathing, and coma. Overdose victims must be taken to a hospital emergency room immediately. ALWAYS bring the prescription bottle or container.

Special Information

Clozapine may cause a fever during the first few weeks of treatment. Generally, the fever is not important, but it may occasionally be necessary to stop treatment due to a persistent fever.

Regular blood tests are necessary to monitor blood composition for any changes that might be caused by clozapine.

Call your doctor at once if you develop lethargy or weakness, a flu-like infection, sore throat, feelings of ill health, fever, sweating, muscle rigidity, mental changes, irregular pulse or blood pressure, mouth ulcers, or dry mouth that lasts for more than 2 weeks.

Dry mouth, a common side effect of clozapine, may be countered by using gum, candy, ice, or a saliva substitute such as Orex or Moi-Stir.

Do not stop taking clozapine without your doctor's knowledge and approval, because a gradual dosage reduction may be necessary to prevent side effects.

Avoid alcohol or any other nervous system depressants while taking clozapine.

Some of the side effects of clozapine—drowsiness, blurred vision, and seizures—may interfere with the performance of complex tasks like driving or operating hazardous equipment.

While taking clozapine, rapidly rising from a sitting or lying position may cause you to become dizzy or faint.

If you take clozapine twice a day and forget a dose, take it as soon as you remember. If it is almost time for your next dose, take 1 dose as soon as you remember and another in 5 or 6 hours, then go back to your regular schedule. If you take clozapine 3 times a day and forget a dose, take it as soon as you remember. If it is almost time for your next dose, take 1 dose as soon as you remember and another in 3 or 4 hours, then go back to your regular schedule. Never take a double dose.

Orally disintegrating tablets should be left in the unopened blister until time of use. They should not be pushed through the foil. Just prior to use, peel the foil from the blister and gently remove the orally disintegrating tablet. Immediately place the tablet in the mouth, allow it to disintegrate and then swallow with saliva. No water is needed.

Special Populations

Pregnancy/Breast-feeding: This drug should be used during pregnancy only if your doctor determines that it is absolutely necessary.

Clozapine may pass into breast milk. Nursing mothers who must take this drug should use infant formula.

Seniors: Seniors may be more sensitive to the side effects of clozapine, such as dizziness on rapidly rising from a sitting or lying position, confusion, and excitability. Older men are also more likely to have prostate problems, a reason to be cautious with clozapine. Seniors with psychosis due to dementia who take clozapine are more likely to die from heart disorders and infections than those not taking it.

Generic Name

Codeine (KOE-deen) G

Brand Name

Only available in generic form.

The information in this profile also applies to the following drugs:

Generic Ingredient: Fentanyl G

Actiq Lozenge on a Stick	Fentora Buccal Tablet
Duragesic (Patch)	Ionsys (Patch)

Generic Ingredient: Morphine Sulfate G

Avinza	Oramorph SR
Kadian	RMS Suppositories
MS Contin	Roxanol
MSIR	

Generic Ingredient: Oxycodone Hydrochloride G

Combunox	OxyFAST
Endocodone	OxyIR
M-Oxy	Percolone
OxyContin	Roxicodone
Oxydose	

Generic Ingredient: Oxymorphone
Opana

Type of Drug

Narcotic.

Prescribed For

Mild to severe pain, breakthrough cancer pain, and cough. Long-acting narcotics are meant only for people with chronic pain. Also prescribed for pain and anxiety in pediatric burn patients.

General Information

Codeine relieves pain and suppresses cough. The pain-relieving effect of 30–60 mg of codeine is equal to approximately 650 mg, or 2 tablets, of aspirin. Codeine may be less effective than aspirin for pain associated with inflammation because aspirin reduces inflammation and codeine does not. Codeine suppresses the cough reflex but does not cure the underlying cause of the cough. Other narcotic cough suppressants are stronger pain relievers, but codeine remains the best cough medication available.

Morphine sulfate is a pure narcotic that has been in use for many years. In addition to pain relief, morphine's effects include drowsiness, mood changes, breathing difficulty, slowed movement of the gastrointestinal tract, nausea, vomiting, and changes in the endocrine and autonomic nervous systems. Morphine sulfate liquid, immediate-release tablets, and suppositories must be taken several times a day. The medication they contain is released immediately for absorption into the bloodstream. Extended- and controlled-release morphine products are designed to release some of the narcotic right away and the rest over a 24-hour period, allowing for less-frequent dosage.

Fentanyl is a potent pain reliever that can be substituted for other narcotic drugs. The patch form, which must be replaced about every 3 days, delivers fentanyl to the bloodstream at a steady rate. The lozenge has a shorter length of action than any other narcotic pain reliever, which makes it useful when given to children before surgery because it provides doctors with the flexibility to obtain maximum benefit with minimal side effects. The lozenge on a stick is used for breakthrough cancer pain as a booster for people already taking narcotic pain relievers. These forms should only be used under controlled circumstances because of the risk of side effects or overdose. Low dosages of fentanyl relieve pain—larger amounts cause loss of consciousness and breathing difficulties.

Oxycodone is a narcotic used to control moderate to severe pain. Most people take it together with aspirin (Percodan) or acetaminophen (Percocet), but it can be used by itself. This is a potent pain reliever that carries a risk of addiction with continued use.

Cautions and Warnings

Do not take narcotics if you are **allergic** or **sensitive** to any of their ingredients.

Long-term use of narcotics may cause drug dependence or **addiction**.

Use narcotics with extreme caution if you suffer from **asthma** or other **breathing problems.**

Narcotics may make it difficult to monitor the progress of people who have suffered **head injuries** and **acute abdominal conditions**.

Actiq contains fentanyl in an amount that can be fatal to children. Keep used and unused lozenges and lozenges on a stick out of reach of children.

Possible Side Effects

▼ Most common: lightheadedness, dizziness, sleepiness, nausea, vomiting, appetite loss, and sweating. If these occur, ask your doctor about lowering your dosage. Most of these side effects disappear if you lie down.

▼ Less common: euphoria (feeling "high"), headache, agitation, uncoordinated muscle movement, minor hallucinations, disorientation and visual disturbances, dry mouth, constipation, flushing of the face, rapid heartbeat, palpitations, faintness, urinary difficulties or hesitancy, reduced sex drive or impotence, itching, rash, anemia, lowered or raised blood sugar, and yellowing of the skin or whites of the eyes. Narcotic analgesics may aggravate convulsions in those who have had them.

More serious side effects of codeine are shallow breathing or breathing difficulties.

Drug Interactions

- Avoid combining narcotics with alcohol, sleeping medications, sedatives, other depressant drugs, or non-prescription drugs that have alcohol as an ingredient. Alcohol speeds the release of morphine from Avinza. The mixture can result in a deadly narcotic overdose.

- Narcotic analgesics should not be used at the same time as monoamine oxidase inhibitor antidepressants. Separate usage by at least 14 days.

- Combining a narcotic pain reliever with an anticholinergic medication may result in severe constipation.

- Combining a narcotic pain reliever with any other medication that lowers blood pressure can lead to excessive blood-pressure lowering. Avoid this combination.

- Combining cimetidine with a narcotic pain reliever may cause confusion, disorientation, breathing difficulties, and seizure.
- Reserpine, rifampin, and remifentanil may decrease the pain-relieving effects of morphine.
- Fentanyl should be used with caution with azole antifungals (e.g. ketoconazole).

Food Interactions

Codeine may be taken with food to reduce upset stomach. Morphine capsules and the fentanyl patch may be used without regard to food.

Usual Dose

Dosing of narcotic pain medications is highly individualized based on patient tolerance and response to medication.

Codeine

Adult: 15–60 mg every 4–6 hours for relief of pain; 10–20 mg every few hours as needed to suppress cough.

Child: 1 mg per lb. of body weight every 4–6 hours for relief of pain; 2.5–10 mg every 4–6 hours to suppress cough.

Fentanyl Lozenge and Lozenge on a Stick

Adult: 200–1600 mcg. Dosage may be repeated up to 4 times daily. Allow the lozenge to dissolve in your mouth. DO NOT CHEW.

Child: not recommended.

Fentanyl Patch: Apply to a clean and non-irritated patch of skin as directed, usually once every 3 days.

Morphine Extended-release and Controlled-release
Tablets and Capsules

Adult: 1–3 capsules a day, depending on the specific product and individual need.

Morphine Oral Liquid and Immediate-release Tablets

Adult: 5–30 mg every 4 hours.

Morphine Suppositories

Adult: 5–30 mg several times a day.

Oxycodone

Adult: 10–30 mg every 4 hours as needed. OxyContin should be swallowed whole and not broken.

Child: not recommended.

Overdosage

Symptoms include breathing difficulties or slowing of respiration, extreme tiredness progressing to stupor and then coma, pinpointed pupils, no response to pain stimulation, cold and clammy skin, slowing of heartbeat, lowering of blood pressure, convulsions, and cardiac arrest. The victim should be taken to a hospital emergency room immediately. ALWAYS bring the prescription bottle or container.

Special Information

Codeine is a respiratory depressant and affects the central nervous system (CNS), producing sleepiness, tiredness, or inability to concentrate. Be careful when driving or doing any task that requires concentration. Avoid alcohol.

Call your doctor if you develop breathing difficulties, constipation, dry mouth, or any bothersome or persistent side effect.

Apply the fentanyl patch only to non-irritated skin on a flat surface of the upper body. Hair at the application site should be clipped or cut, not shaved, before applying the patch. Do not use oils, soaps, lotions, alcohol, or anything else that might irritate the skin before applying the patch.

If you are taking a controlled-release narcotic product, do not crush, chew, or break the tablet or lozenge. Rapid release may result in a potentially fatal dose of the drug.

If you forget a dose of codeine, take it as soon as you remember. If it is almost time for your next dose, skip the one you forgot and continue with your regular schedule. Never take a double dose.

Special Populations

Pregnancy/Breast-feeding: Narcotics pass into the fetal circulation. Excessive use of them during pregnancy may cause drug dependence in newborns. Narcotics may also cause breathing difficulties in infants during delivery. Animal studies show that codeine may cause fetal harm. If given to a pregnant woman before cesarean section, fentanyl may cause drowsiness in newborns. When either of these drugs is considered crucial by your doctor, its potential benefits must be carefully weighed against its risks.

Narcotics pass into breast milk. Nursing mothers who must take codeine should use infant formula.

Seniors: Seniors are more likely to be sensitive to side effects and should be treated with the smallest effective dosage.

Generic Name

Colchicine (KOLE-chih-sene) Ⓖ

Type of Drug
Antigout medication.

Prescribed For
Prevention and treatment of gouty arthritis; also prescribed for Mediterranean fever; chronic progressive multiple sclerosis; cirrhosis of the liver; biliary cirrhosis; Behçet's disease; pseudogout (a condition caused by calcium deposits); amyloidosis; very low blood-platelet count (also known as ITP); skin reactions, including scleroderma, psoriasis, Sweet Syndrome, and other conditions; and nerve disability associated with chronic progressive multiple sclerosis.

General Information
While no one knows exactly how colchicine works, it appears to help people with gout by reducing the inflammatory response to uric acid crystals that form inside joints and by interfering with the body's mechanism for making uric acid. Unlike drugs that affect uric acid levels, colchicine does not block the progression of gout to chronic gouty arthritis; it will, however, relieve the pain of acute attacks and lessen the frequency and severity of attacks. It has no effect on other kinds of pain.

Cautions and Warnings
Do not use colchicine if you are **allergic** or **sensitive** to any of its ingredients or you suffer from any serious **blood, kidney, liver, stomach,** or **cardiac condition**.

Vomiting, abdominal pain, diarrhea, nausea, kidney damage, and blood in the urine may occur with colchicine, especially at maximum doses. This can worsen existing gastrointestinal (GI) or other conditions. Stop taking the medication and call your doctor if you develop one of these symptoms.

The weakness that people develop while taking colchicine is frequently related to high levels of colchicine in the blood caused by poor kidney function and improves without treatment 3–4 weeks after the drug is stopped. This reaction is often mistaken for other conditions.

Periodic blood counts should be done if you are taking colchicine for long periods of time.

Colchicine interferes with the absorption of **vitamin B$_{12}$** by affecting the lining of the GI tract.

Colchicine may affect the process of sperm generation in men.

The safety and effectiveness for use by **children** have not been established.

Possible Side Effects

▼ Common: vomiting, diarrhea, and abdominal pain may occur if you take maximum doses of colchicine for an acute gout attack. You may also experience severe diarrhea, kidney and blood-vessel damage, blood in the urine, and reduced urination.

▼ Less common: hair loss, rash, appetite loss, and muscle and nerve weakness.

▼ Rare: with long-term colchicine therapy—reduced white-blood-cell and platelet counts, nerve inflammation, blood-clotting problems, rash, unusual bleeding or bruising, tingling in the hands or feet, red or purple spots under the skin, and other reactions. Colchicine may interfere with sperm formation. Contact your doctor if you experience any side effect not listed above.

Drug Interactions

- Colchicine interferes with the absorption of vitamin B$_{12}$.
- Colchicine may increase sensitivity to central-nervous-system depressants, such as sedatives and alcohol.
- The following drugs may reduce colchicine's effectiveness: anticancer drugs, bumetanide, diazoxide, thiazide diuretics, ethacrynic acid, furosemide, mecamylamine, pyrazinamide, and triamterene.
- Taking phenylbutazone with colchicine increases the risk of side effects.
- Mixing the antibiotic clarithromycin with colchicine can lead to colchicine toxicity, especially in the elderly and those with kidney disease.

Food Interactions

None known.

Usual Dose

Acute Gout Attack: 1–1.2 mg. This dose may be followed by 0.5–1.2 mg every 1–2 hours until pain is relieved or nausea, vomiting, or diarrhea occurs. The total dose needed to control pain and inflammation during an attack varies from 4–8 mg.

Gout Prevention: 0.5–1.8 mg daily. In mild cases, 0.5 mg or 0.6 mg may be taken 3–4 days a week.

Familial Mediterranean Fever: 1–2 mg a day.

Cirrhosis of the Liver: 1 mg a day for 5 days each week.

Biliary Cirrhosis: 0.6 mg twice a day.

Amyloidosis: 0.5 mg 1–2 times a day.

Behçet's Disease: 0.5–1.5 mg a day.

Pseudogout: 0.6 mg twice a day.

ITP: 1.2–1.8 mg a day for 2 weeks or more.

Scleroderma: 1 mg a day.

Sweet Syndrome: 0.5 mg 1–3 times a day.

Other Skin Disorders: up to 1.8 mg a day, depending on the specific condition.

Overdosage

The lethal dose is estimated at 65 mg, although people have died after taking as little as 7 mg at once. Usually 1–3 days pass between the time that an overdose is taken and symptoms begin. Overdose symptoms start with nausea, vomiting, stomach pain, diarrhea—which may be severe and bloody—and burning sensations in the throat or stomach or on the skin. If you think you are experiencing overdose symptoms, contact your doctor immediately, or go to a hospital emergency room. ALWAYS bring the prescription bottle or container.

Special Information

Call your doctor if you develop rash, sore throat, fever, unusual bleeding or bruising, tiredness, weakness, numbness, or tingling. Seniors are more likely to develop drug side effects and should use this drug with caution.

Stop taking maximum doses of colchicine as soon as gout pain is relieved and reduce your dose to a maintenance level if your doctor has prescribed it for gout prevention. Stop taking the drug entirely and contact your doctor at the first sign of nausea, vomiting, stomach pain, or diarrhea.

If you forget a dose of colchicine, take it as soon as possible. If it is almost time for your next dose, skip the dose you forgot and continue with your regular schedule. Do not take a double dose.

Special Populations

Pregnancy/Breast-feeding: Colchicine can harm the fetus. Pregnant women should not take it unless the potential benefits clearly outweigh the risks.

It is not known if colchicine passes into breast milk. No problems with nursing infants are known, but nursing mothers who must take colchicine should consider using infant formula.

Seniors: Seniors, especially those with renal, hepatic, gastrointestinal, or heart disease, are more likely to develop side effects and should use colchicine with caution.

Combivent *see **Ipratropium**, page 597*

Concerta *see **Methylphenidate**, page 706*

Type of Drug

Contraceptives

Brand Names

Generic Ingredients: Low-Dose Estrogen + Low-Dose Progestin + Low Androgen Activity (Single-Phase Combination) Ⓖ

Alesse
Aviane
Levlite

Lutera
Lybrel

Generic Ingredients: Low-Dose Estrogen + High-Dose Progestin + Intermediate Androgen Activity (Single-Phase Combination)

Junel Fe 1/20
Loestrin 21 1/20
Loestrin 24-Fe

Loestrin Fe 1/20
Microgestin Fe 1/20

Generic Ingredients: Low-Dose Estrogen + Intermediate-Dose Progestin + Intermediate Androgen Activity (Single-Phase Combination) G

Cryselle	Nordette
Levian	Seasonale
Levlen	Seasonique
Lo/Ovral	

Generic Ingredients: Low-Dose Estrogen + High-Dose Progestin + Low Androgen Activity (Single-Phase Combination) G

Demulen 1/35	Mircette
Junel Fe 1.5/30	Zovia 1/35E
Kariva	

Generic Ingredients: Low-Dose Estrogen + High-Dose Progestin + High Androgen Activity (Single-Phase Combination)

Loestrin 21 1.5/30	Loestrin Fe 1.5/30

Generic Ingredients: Intermediate-Dose Estrogen + Low-Dose Progestin + Low Androgen Activity (Single-Phase Combination) G

Ortho-Cyclen

Generic Ingredients: Intermediate-Dose Estrogen + Intermediate-Dose Progestin + Intermediate Androgen Activity (Single-Phase Combination) G

Norinyl 1 + 50	Ortho-Novum 1/50

Generic Ingredients: Intermediate-Dose Estrogen + High-Dose Progestin + Low Androgen Activity (Single-Phase Combination) G

Demulen 1/50E	Ortho-Cept
Desogen	Zovia 1/50E

Generic Ingredients: Intermediate-Dose Progestin + Low-Dose Estrogen + No Androgen Activity (Single-Phase Combination)

Yaz

Generic Ingredients: Intermediate-Dose Progestin + Intermediate-Dose Estrogen + No Androgen Activity (Single-Phase Combination)

Yasmin

*Generic Ingredients: Intermediate-Dose Progestin + High-Dose
Estrogen + Intermediate Androgen Activity (Single-Phase
Combination)* 🄖

Norinyl 1 + 35	Ortho-Novum 1/35
Nortrel 1/35	Ovcon-50

*Generic Ingredients: High-Dose Estrogen + High-Dose Progestin
+ High Androgen Activity (Single-Phase Combination)* 🄖
Ovral

*Generic Ingredients: High-Dose Estrogen + Low-Dose Progestin
+ Low Androgen Activity (Single-Phase Combination)*

Brevicon	Nortrel 0.5/35
Modicon	Ovcon-35
Neocon 0.5/35	

*Generic Ingredients: Low-Dose Progestin + High-Dose Estrogen
+ Low Androgen Activity (3-Phase Combination)* 🄖
Tri-Norinyl

*Generic Ingredients: High-Dose Estrogen + Intermediate-Dose
Progestin + Low Androgen Activity (2-Phase Combination)*

Necon 10/11	Ortho-Novum 10/11

*Generic Ingredients: Low-Dose Estrogen + Low-Dose Progestin
+ Low Androgen Activity (3-Phase Combination)*
Ortho Tri-Cyclen Lo

*Generic Ingredients: Low-Dose Estrogen + High-Dose Progestin
+ Intermediate Androgen Activity (3-Phase Combination)* 🄖

Estrostep 21	Tilia Fe
Estrostep Fe	TriLegest Fe

*Generic Ingredients: Low-Dose Estrogen + High-Dose Progestin
+ Low Androgen Activity*
Cyclessa

*Generic Ingredients: Intermediate-Dose Estrogen + Low-Dose
Progestin + Low Androgen Activity (3-Phase Combination)* 🄖

Aranelle	Triphasil
Ortho Tri-Cyclen	Tri-Sprintec
Tri-Levlen	Trivora
TriNessa	Velivet

Generic Ingredients: High-Dose Estrogen + Intermediate-Dose Progestin + Low Androgen Activity (3-Phase Combination) [G]
Ortho-Novum 7/7/7

Generic Ingredient: High-Dose Progestin (Mini-Pill) [G]
Nor-Q.D.   Ortho–Micronor

Generic Ingredients: Low-Dose Estrogen + Low-Dose Progestin (Patch)
OrthoEvra

Generic Ingredients: Low-Dose Estrogen + Low-Dose Progestin (Vaginal Ring)
NuvaRing

Generic Ingredient: Etonorgestrel (Implant)
Implanon

Generic Ingredient: Progestin (Implant)
Norplant II

Generic Ingredient: Progestin (Intrauterine Insert)
Mirena

Generic Ingredient: High-Dose Progestin (Emergency Contraceptive)
Plan B

Prescribed For

Prevention of pregnancy, endometriosis, excessive menstruation, and cyclic withdrawal bleeding. Ortho Tri-Cyclen and Estrostep may be prescribed for moderate acne in women over age 15.

General Information

Contraceptive drugs are synthetic hormones containing either progestin or a progestin-estrogen combination. The overall effects of any contraceptive are influenced by the interaction of all active ingredients, including those with androgenic and anti-estrogenic activity. These drugs are similar to natural female hormones, which cannot be used as contraceptives because very large dosages would be required. Synthetic hormones are more potent and are effective at smaller dosages. Contraceptive drugs work by preventing sperm from reaching the unfertilized egg, preventing the implantation of a fertilized egg in the uterus, or preventing ovulation (the release of an unfertilized egg from the ovaries). They prevent acne by balancing hormone levels.

When properly used, hormonal contraceptives can be 97–99% effective at preventing pregnancy. These products vary in their effectiveness and in the amount and type of estrogen or progestin used. The side effects of these drugs tend to increase with the amount of hormone they contain. While low hormone dosages are preferred, contraceptives with the smallest amounts of estrogen may be less effective in some women than others.

Single-phase products provide constant levels of estrogen and progestin throughout the entire month-long pill cycle. In 2-phase combinations, the amount of estrogen remains at a steady low level throughout the cycle, while progestin levels increase and then decrease. This variation in progestin allows normal changes to take place in the uterus. Three-phase products are meant to simulate the normal hormone cycle and reduce breakthrough bleeding. Throughout the cycle, estrogen levels remain the same while those of progestin change to create a 3-part wave pattern. The amount of estrogen in 3-phase products is considered low. Breakthrough bleeding may occur with the older combination products from day 8 through 16 of the cycle.

The mini-pill, a progestin-only product, may cause irregular menstrual cycles and may be less effective than estrogen-progestin combinations. Mini-pills may be recommended to older women or women who should avoid estrogens (see "Cautions and Warnings").

The contraceptive patch releases small amounts of progestin and estrogen continuously over 3 weeks. The medication is absorbed into the blood vessels just below the skin. The patch works in the same way as contraceptive pills do.

The vaginal ring releases small amounts of etonogestrel, a progestin, and estradiol, an estrogen, in the vaginal canal over 3 weeks. The combination prevents pregnancy in the same way as combination pills do but may be less effective than contraceptive pills because some people find them harder to use.

Most contraceptive drugs are designed to simulate a normal menstrual cycle. By not taking the hormones 1 week out of the month, you continue to have your regular period. In fact, these products are often used to stabilize a woman's period. Two products, Seasonale and Seasonique, come in an 84-pill packet and are taken once a day for 3 months. This means you will only have your period once every 3 months. Another, Lybrel, is designed to be taken every day, eliminating monthly menstruation. Drosperi-none, the progestin found in Yasmin and Yaz, has been found to relieve Premenstrual Syndrome (PMS) symptoms in addition to acting as an effective contraceptive hormone.

Levonorgestrel, a progestin, is used in implants that provide ef-fective contraception for up to 5 years after surgical implantation under the skin of the upper arm or inside the uterus. Levonorgestrel implants should be replaced at least once every 5 years. Etonorgestrel implants are effective for 3 years. Implants can be removed at any time, reversing the contraceptive effect. The prog-estin intrauterine inserts provide effective contraception for about 1 year. The implant and intrauterine systems contain the same hor-mone found in the mini-pill and are associated with many of the same side effects and precautions as oral contraceptives.

Emergency contraceptives (sometimes referred to as the "morning-after pill") contain high doses of estrogen and progestin. They are intended for use only after contraceptive failure or un-protected intercourse. They should never be taken by a pregnant woman.

Contraceptive drugs in any form are associated with risks. These risks are greatest in women over age 35 who smoke and have high blood pressure.

Cautions and Warnings

Do not take contraceptives if you are **allergic** or **sensitive** to them or any of their ingredients.

The risk of breast cancer may be slightly higher among current and recent users of combination oral contraceptives. This risk ap-pears to decline after contraceptive use is stopped and is gone by 10 years after stopping combination contraceptive products. Breast cancers found in contraceptive users tend to be less ad-vanced than those in non-contraceptive users.

You should not use contraceptive drugs if you are or might be **pregnant,** have had **blood clots** in veins or arteries, **stroke,** any **blood-coagulation disorder,** known or suspected **cancer** of the breast, sex organs, or liver. Products with more estrogen, or those that provide higher sustained blood levels of estrogen, such as the contraceptive patch, are more likely to be associated with an increased risk of life-threatening blood clots.

Contraceptive drugs may cause eye lesions. Call your doctor at once if you develop visual difficulties of any kind.

Women taking the combination products Seasonale and Seasonique will have their period only once every 3 months and those taking Lybrel will not have a regular monthly period. It is absolutely essential for you to verify you are not pregnant if you think you may be pregnant for any reason.

The risks of contraceptive drugs increase if you are **physically immobile** or have **asthma; cardiac insufficiency; epilepsy; migraine; kidney problems;** a strong family history of **breast cancer; benign breast disease; diabetes; endometriosis; gallbladder disease or gallstones; liver problems,** including jaundice; **high blood cholesterol; high blood pressure; estrogen or progestin intolerance; depression; tuberculosis;** or **varicose veins**.

There is an increased risk of heart attack in women who have used contraceptive drugs for more than 5 years, or who are **between age 40 and 49** and have other coronary risk factors such as **smoking, obesity, high blood pressure, diabetes,** and **high blood cholesterol**. This risk remains even after the medication is stopped.

Smokers in their mid-30s or older who use contraceptive drugs are 5 times more likely to have a heart attack than nonsmokers taking contraceptives and 10–12 times more likely to have a heart attack than nonsmokers who do not use the pill. Death due to circulatory disease also increases substantially in smokers taking contraceptive drugs, especially in women at least 35 years old. The risk of stroke is also increased in this group. **Heavy smokers** (more than 15 cigarettes a day) should not use hormonal contraceptives.

Women with a history of **headaches, high blood pressure,** or **varicose veins** should avoid estrogen-containing products, as should older women and those who have experienced estrogen side effects.

Contraceptive drugs may mask the onset of **menopause**.

Progestin-only products are associated with an increased risk of blood-clotting problems.

The progestin in Yasmin and Yaz raises blood potassium levels. Women with **kidney, liver, or adrenal gland disease** should use either product with caution.

Intrauterine inserts have been associated with an increased risk of pelvic inflammatory disease (PID). The highest risk usually occurs within the first 20 days after insertion. Do not use intrauterine inserts if you have had an **ectopic pregnancy**.

Toxic Shock Syndrome has been associated with tampons, some barrier contraceptives, and the vaginal ring, although there is no proof that the product was the cause of the infection.

Possible Side Effects

▼ Common: Common side effects often result from using a product that is poorly suited to your body chemistry. Determining the right amount and type of hormone often minimizes these effects. If you are taking too much estrogen, you may experience nausea, bloating, high blood pressure, migraine, excess cervical mucous, skin discoloration, colon polyps, water retention, and swelling, or breast fullness or tenderness. Too little estrogen may cause early or midcycle breakthrough bleeding, spotting, or reduced periodic flow. Too much progestin is associated with weight gain and increased appetite, tiredness or fatigue, low periodic flow, acne, depression, breast regression, and androgen-related side effects (acne, oily scalp, hair loss, or excess hair growth). Too little progestin may cause late breakthrough bleeding, excessive periodic bleeding, or missed periods.

▼ Less common: abdominal cramps, infertility after discontinuance of the drug, breast tenderness, weight change, headache, rash, vaginal itching and burning, general vaginal infection, nervousness, dizziness, depression, cataracts, changes in sex drive, hair loss, and increased sensitivity to the sun.

▼ Rare: Women who use contraceptive drugs are more likely to develop several serious conditions, including blood clots in the deep veins, stroke, heart attack, liver cancer, gallbladder disease, and high blood pressure. Women who smoke cigarettes are at much higher risk for some of these adverse effects. Contact your doctor if you experience any side effect not listed above.

Drug Interactions

- Ampicillin, barbiturates, bexarotene, bosentan, carbamazepine, chloramphenicol, efavirenz, fluconazole, griseofulvin, ketoconazole, neomycin, nelfinavir, nitrofuratoin, oxcarbazepine, phenylbutazone, phenytoin, penicillin drugs, protease inhibitor drugs for HIV, rifampin, rifapentine, statin drugs (atorvastatin and rosuvastatin), St. John's wort, sulfa drugs, tetracycline products, and sedatives can make all contraceptive drugs less effective. Use backup birth control while taking these medications together.

- Contraceptive drugs may elevate blood levels of benzodiazepine sedatives and sleeping pills (midazolam, lorazepam, oxazepam, and temazepam), caffeine, cyclosporine, imatinib, metoprolol, corticosteroids, theophylline drugs, tizanidine, triptan-type migraine drugs, and tricyclic antidepressants, increasing the risk of side effects. Discuss mixing these medicines with your doctor. Dosage reductions may be needed.

- Contraceptive drugs may increase the toxic liver effects of acetaminophen and reduce the drug's effectiveness. Contraceptive drugs may increase or decrease the effect of anticoagulant (blood-thinning) drugs. Discuss the risks of this combination with your doctor.

- Mycophenolate interferes with only those contraceptives that contain levonorgestrel (Alesse, Aviane, Lessina, Levora, Levlite, Lutera, Lybrel, Mirena, Nordette, Norplant II, Portia, Plan B, Seasonale, Seasonique, and Triphasil). Backup contraception is recommended.

- Exenatide may reduce the effectiveness of contraceptive pills. Take them at least 1 hour before an injection of exenatide.

- Contraceptive drugs may reduce the effectiveness of clofibrate for elevated blood triglycerides, sulfonylurea drugs for diabetes, ursodiol for gallbladder disease, and pain relievers, including salicylates (aspirin).

- Contraceptive drugs may increase blood-cholesterol levels and interfere with blood tests for thyroid function and blood sugar.

- Acetaminophen may increase blood levels of ethinyl estradiol, a common contraceptive drug ingredient, increasing side effects and reducing contraceptive effectiveness.

- Since Yasmin and Yaz raise blood potassium levels, neither should be used if you are taking spironolactone or another potassium-sparing diuretic, potassium supplements, angiotensin-converting enzyme (ACE) inhibitors, angiotensin receptor antagonists, aldosterone antagonists, heparin, nonsteroidal anti-inflammatory drugs (NSAIDs), or other medications on a long-term basis that may further increase potassium levels.

- Contraceptive drugs may interfere with the effects of insulin for diabetes.
- Acitretin interferes with the contraceptive effect of progestin-only mini-pills. It is not known if it also interferes with combination contraceptive drugs.

Food Interactions

None known.

Usual Dose

Single-Phase, 2-Phase, and 3-Phase Combinations: The first day of bleeding is day 1 of the menstrual cycle. Beginning on the first day of the cycle, take 1 pill a day for 20–21 days according to the number of pills supplied by the manufacturer. If menstrual flow has not begun 7 days after taking the last pill, begin the next month's cycle of pills. Some manufacturers recommend starting the pills on a Sunday to make it easy to remember to take them. In this case, start taking your pills on the first Sunday after your period begins. If menstruation begins on a Sunday, take the first pill that day.

Seasonale: Take 1 pink tablet every day for 84 consecutive days. Do not skip a day. Then, take 1 white pill a day for 7 days. Then, start a new pill cycle. You may be pregnant if you do not have a period while you are taking the white pills.

Seasonique: Take 1 light blue-green tablet containinng levonorgestrel and ethinyl estradiol daily for 84 consecutive days, followed by 7 days of ethinyl estradiol tablets. Do not stop if spotting or breakthrough bleeding occurs. Report prolonged bleeding to your doctor.

Progestin-Only Mini-Pill: Take 1 pill every day.

Contraceptive Patch: Apply a new patch to the thigh, abdomen, or arm. Remove the patch after 3 weeks and then reapply a new patch after 1 week. Be sure to always apply a new patch on the same day of the week. If you are switching from birth control pills, apply the first patch on the same day you would start a new cycle of pills.

Vaginal Ring: Keep the vaginal ring in the vaginal canal for 3 weeks. Remove it and put a new one in 1 week later. If you did not use a hormonal contraceptive in the previous month, insert the ring between day 1 and day 5 of your cycle.

If you are switching from a combination birth control pill, insert the ring anytime during the week after you took your last pill but before you would have started your next cycle of pills. No additional contraception is necessary.

If you are switching from a mini-pill, insert the ring on the day after you take your last mini-pill.

If you are switching from a progestin implant or an IUD, insert the ring on the same day your implant or IUD is removed.

If you are switching from a progestin injection, insert the ring on the same day you would have received your next injection.

If you are switching from a progestin-only mini-pill, implant, injection, or IUD, use another form of contraception for the first 7 days after you insert the ring.

Emergency Contraception: Emergency contraceptive kits have only a few pills. They should be taken with a full meal. Take half the pills (1 or 2 depending on the brand you use) within 72 hours of unprotected sex, however they are most effective when taken within the first 24 hours. Take the rest of the pills 12 hours after the first dose. Emergency contraceptives reduce the risk of pregnancy by 75%.

The pregnancy test in the kit can be used to determine if you became pregnant earlier in your cycle or during a previous cycle. If the test is positive, consult your doctor before taking emergency contraception. If you vomit within one hour of taking either dose, contact your doctor.

Overdosage

An overdose may cause nausea and withdrawal bleeding in adult women. Overdose victims should be taken to a hospital emergency room. ALWAYS bring the prescription package.

Special Information

Use backup birth control to prevent pregnancy in the first 3 weeks after you begin taking contraceptive drugs.

Contraceptive drugs do not protect against sexually transmitted diseases.

Take your pill at the same time each day to establish a routine and ensure maximum contraceptive protection.

Call your doctor immediately if you experience severe abdominal pain; severe or sudden headache; pain in the chest, groin, or leg, especially the calf; sudden slurring of speech; changes in vision;

weakness, numbness, or pain in the arms or legs; coughing up of blood; loss of coordination; or shortness of breath. These symptoms may require emergency treatment.

Other problems that may require medical attention are bulging eyes; changes in vaginal bleeding; fainting; frequent or painful urination; a gradual increase in blood pressure; breast lumps or secretions; depression; yellowing of the skin or whites of the eyes; rash; redness or irritation; upper abdominal swelling, pain, or tenderness; an unusual or dark-colored mole; thick, white vaginal discharge; or vaginal itching or tenderness.

See your doctor for a check-up every 6–12 months.

Some manufacturers include 7 inert or iron pills in their packaging to be taken on days when the drug is not taken. This makes it easier for women to stay on schedule with their pills. The 7 pills bridge the gap between contraceptive cycles and allow women to take 1 pill every day without stopping.

For single- or 2-phase combinations: If you forget to take a pill for 1 day, take 2 pills the following day. If you miss 2 consecutive days, take 2 pills for the next 2 days. Then return to your schedule of 1 pill a day. If you miss 3 consecutive days, do not take any pills for the next 7 days and use another form of contraception; then start a brand new cycle.

Seasonale: The risk of pregnancy increases with each pink tablet you forget. Use another method of non-hormonal backup contraception any time you miss 2 or more pink tablets until you have taken a pink tablet every day for 7 consecutive days. You are protected against pregnancy if you miss 1 or more white tablets, as long as you begin taking the pink tablets again on the proper day.

Seasonique: The risk of ovulation and pregnancy increases with each forgotten light blue-green pill. If you miss 1 light blue-green pill, take it as soon as you remember and take the next pill at your regular time. This may mean you will take 2 pills on the same day. You don't need to use a backup birth control method if you forget only 1 pill. If you forget 2 light blue-green pills in a row, take 2 pills on the day you remember and take 2 pills the next day. Then go back to taking 1 pill a day until you finish your pack. If you miss 2 or more light blue-green pills in a row, you must use non-hormonal backup contraception until you have taken a light blue-green pill daily for 7 days in a row. If you miss 1 or more yellow tablets, you are still protected against pregnancy provided you begin taking light blue-green pills again on the proper day.

For 3-phase combinations: If you forget to take a pill for 1 day, take 2 pills the following day. If you miss 2 consecutive days, take 2 pills for the next 2 days. Then return to your schedule of 1 pill a day. If you forget to take a pill for 3 days in a row, stop taking the drug and use an alternate means of contraception until your period starts. ALWAYS use a backup contraceptive method for the remainder of your cycle if you forget even 1 pill of a 3-phase combination.

If you forget to apply the contraceptive patch on the same day of the week once every 4 weeks, you risk a loss of effectiveness on the days after you should have applied it. If the patch comes off or is partially detached in mid-cycle, you must start a new 3-week cycle at once by removing the old patch and applying a new one.

If the vaginal ring is accidentally expelled during the 3 weeks it is normally retained, rinse it off with water and replace it within 3 hours. Do not use hot water. If the ring is not reusable, insert a new ring and continue with your regular schedule. If you do not replace the ring within 3 hours, its effectiveness may be reduced. If you are in week 3 of the cycle, throw the ring away; you may insert a new one immediately, which will begin a new 3-week cycle and cause you to skip a period. Or, you may wait a week, during which time you will have periodic bleeding, and insert a new ring no later than 7 days after the vaginal ring was expelled. This option should be chosen if you had used the ring for 7 days in a row before it was expelled.

If, when it is expelled, you are in week 1 or 2 of your cycle and the ring is out for more than 3 hours, reinsert it and use an additional form of contraceptive until the ring has been worn for 7 consecutive days. A vaginal ring may break and then slip out or cause discomfort. Throw the ring away if this happens.

Missing a pill reduces your protection. If you keep forgetting to take your pills, you must use another birth control method.

If you take drugs that reduce the effectiveness of contraceptive drugs (see "Drug Interactions"), use a backup contraceptive method during that cycle to prevent accidental pregnancy.

Good dental hygiene is essential while taking contraceptive drugs. See your dentist regularly and brush and floss carefully because contraceptive drugs may increase the risk of an oral infection.

Contraceptive drugs may increase your sensitivity to the sun.

Wearing contact lenses may be uncomfortable while taking contraceptive drugs because the pills can cause minor changes in the shape of your eyes.

All contraceptive prescriptions come with a "patient package insert." Read it thoroughly as it gives detailed information about the drug and is required by federal law.

Special Populations

Pregnancy/Breast-feeding: Contraceptive hormones cause birth defects and may interfere with fetal development. They are not safe for use during pregnancy. If you think you are pregnant, use another form of contraception and stop taking your birth control pills.

Contraceptive hormones pass into breast milk. Combination contraceptive products reduce the amount of milk produced. Nursing mothers who must use any of these drugs should use infant formula.

Seniors: These products are not intended for women who have completed menopause.

Coreg   *see Carvedilol, page 203*

Type of Drug

Corticosteroids, Eye Products
(kor-tih-koe-STER-oids)

Brand Names

Generic Ingredient: Dexamethasone Ⓖ
Maxidex

Generic Ingredients: Dexamethasone + Ciprofloxacin
Ciprodex

Generic Ingredients: Dexamethasone + Tobramycin
Tobradex

Generic Ingredients: Dexamethasone + Neomycin Sulfate + Polymixin B Sulfate
Maxitrol

Generic Ingredient: Fluorometholone
Flarex   FML Forte
FML

Generic Ingredients: Fluorometholone + Tobramycin
Tobrasone

Generic Ingredient: Loteprednol Etabonate
Alrex   Lotemax

Generic Ingredients: Loteprednol Etabonate + Tobramycin
Zylet

Generic Ingredient: Prednisolone Acetate [G]
Econopred Plus   Pred Forte
Omnipred   Pred Mild

Generic Ingredients: Prednisolone Acetate + Gentamicin Sulfate
Pred G

Generic Ingredients: Prednisolone Acetate + Sulfacetamide Sodium
Blephamide   Blephamide S.O.P.

Generic Ingredients: Prednisolone Acetate + Neomycin Sulfate + Polymyxin B Sulfate
Poly-Pred

Generic Ingredient: Prednisolone Sodium Phosphate [G]

Generic Ingredients: Prednisolone Sodium Phosphate + Sulfacetamide Sodium
Vasocidin

Generic Ingredient: Rimexolone
Vexol

Prescribed For

Allergic and inflammatory eye conditions, and to speed healing after eye surgery or injury.

General Information

Corticosteroid eye products are prescribed for general relief of inflammation due to allergy and other causes. They are also used after eye surgery or serious eye injury to aid the healing process by reducing the natural inflammatory process. Very severe eye conditions that do not respond to these products may require treatment with corticosteroid drugs taken by mouth. Fluorometholone, medrysone, and prednisolone (up to 0.125%) are preferred for long-term treatment because they are least likely to raise the fluid pressure inside the eye. Corticosteroid eye products have not been widely studied in children, though fluorometholone has been proven safe for use in children age 2 and over.

Cautions and Warnings

Do not use a corticosteroid eye product if you are **allergic** or **sensitive** to corticosteroids. These products should be used with caution if you have a **fungal, herpes, tuberculosis, or viral infection of the eye,** or have **cataracts, glaucoma,** or **diabetes**. Do not use any of these products without your doctor's knowledge.

Long-term use of these products can lead to eye damage, including glaucoma, infection, and nerve damage.

Do not use any of these products in **children** without consulting a doctor.

Possible Side Effects

▼ Rare: watery eyes; glaucoma; optic nerve damage; gradual blurring, reduction, or loss of vision; eye pain or infections; drooping eyelid; eye burning, stinging, or redness; nausea; and vomiting. Contact your doctor if you experience any side effect not listed above.

Drug Interactions

- Corticosteroids applied to the eye may interfere with the effect of antiglaucoma drugs.
- The risk of raising fluid pressure inside the eye is increased when corticosteroid eye products are taken with anticholinergic drugs, especially atropine, over a long period of time.

Food Interactions

None known.

Usual Dose

Eyedrops: 1–2 drops several times a day.

Eye Ointment: Place a thin strip of ointment into the affected eye several times a day.

Overdosage

Swallowing a container of corticosteroid eyedrops or ointment usually does not produce serious effects. Call your local poison center or a hospital emergency room for more information. ALWAYS bring the prescription container.

Special Information

If you forget to administer a dose, do so as soon as you remember. If it is almost time for your next dose, skip the one you forgot and continue with your regular schedule.

To prevent infection, keep the eyedropper from touching your fingers, eyelids, or any surface. Wait at least 5 minutes before using any other eyedrops.

If the brand you are taking contains benzalkonium chloride, wait at least 15 minutes before inserting contact lenses. In some cases, you may be instructed not to wear contact lenses for the duration of treatment.

Special Populations

Pregnancy/Breast-feeding: Using large amounts of corticosteroid eyedrops during pregnancy may affect the adrenal gland of the fetus. When your doctor considers one of these products crucial, its potential benefits must be carefully weighed against its risks.

Oral corticosteroids pass into breast milk, but it is not known if this is also true of corticosteroid eyedrops. Nursing mothers who must use one of these medications should use infant formula.

Seniors: Seniors may use these products without special precaution.

Type of Drug

Corticosteroids, Inhalers
(kor-tih-koe-STER-oids)

Brand Names

Generic Ingredient: Beclomethasone Dipropionate

QVAR 40   QVAR 80

Generic Ingredient: Budesonide

Pulmicort Flexhaler   Pulmicort Respules

Generic Ingredients: Budesonide + Formoterol
Symbicort

Generic Ingredient: Ciclesonide
Alvesco

Generic Ingredient: Flunisolide
AeroBid   Aerospan HFA

Generic Ingredients: Fluticasone Propionate
Flovent Diskus   Flovent HFA

Generic Ingredients: Fluticasone Propionate + Salmeterol Xinafoate
Advair Diskus   Advair HFA

Generic Ingredient: Mometasone Furoate
Asmanex Twisthaler

Generic Ingredient: Triamcinolone Acetonide
Azmacort

Prescribed For

Chronic asthma and bronchial disease.

General Information

Corticosteroid inhalers relieve the symptoms associated with asthma and bronchial disease by reducing inflammation of bronchial mucous membranes, making it easier to breathe. Corticosteroid inhalers produce the same treatment effect as oral corticosteroids, with some important differences. Because inhalers deliver the drug directly to the lungs, smaller dosages can be used. They also have fewer side effects because little of the drug reaches the bloodstream. Corticosteroid inhalers can prevent asthma attacks if used regularly but do not relieve them once they start.

Cautions and Warnings

Do not use a corticosteroid inhaler if you are **allergic** or **sensitive** to any of its ingredients.

Corticosteroid inhalers should not be used as the primary treatment of **severe asthma.** They are recommended only for people who take prednisone or another oral corticosteroid, or for people who do not respond to other asthma drugs. These drugs cannot relieve asthma attacks once they start.

In people with asthma, death from adrenal gland failure has occurred during and after switching from an oral corticosteroid to an inhaler. Adrenal function is impaired for several months after the switch.

Those who use any corticosteroid product, including inhalation, are more likely to have reduced immune system function. This reduces the body's ability to fight infection from any source, including **chicken pox, shingles,** and **measles**. Adults who have not had these viral infections should take care to avoid becoming infected while using any corticosteroid product. Do not receive a **live virus vaccine** while taking corticosteroids of any kind, as they interfere with the body's reaction to the vaccine.

Combining an oral corticosteroid with a corticosteroid inhaler may cause pituitary gland suppression.

During a period of **severe stress,** you may have to switch to an oral corticosteroid if the inhaler does not control your asthma. During periods of stress or a severe asthmatic attack, people who have stopped using an inhaler should ask their doctors about taking an oral corticosteroid.

Corticosteroid inhalers may be associated with immediate or delayed drug reactions, including breathing difficulties, rash, and bronchospasm.

Use corticosteroids with caution if you have respiratory **tuberculosis, herpes** of the eye, a **bacterial, fungal,** or **parasitic infection**, or any other untreated **systemic infection**.

The combination products Advair and Symbicort both contain beta-2 agonists. In some asthma patients, beta-2 agonists may increase the risk of asthma-related death. See Formoterol, page 509, and Salmeterol, page 1013, for more information on these drugs.

Possible Side Effects

▼ Most common: dry mouth, hoarseness, rash, bronchospasm, respiratory infections, fungal infection of the mouth, runny nose, headache, upset stomach, and palpitations.

▼ Rare: depression, cough, wheezing, infection, and facial swelling. Cough and wheezing are probably caused by an ingredient in the inhaler other than the corticosteroid itself. Contact your doctor if you experience any side effect not listed above.

Drug Interactions

• Ketoconazole may increase blood levels of budesonide and fluticasone.

- Using an inhaled corticosteroid and an oral corticosteroid together may increase the effect of both drugs. Use with caution.
- See Formoterol, page 509, for further drug interactions for the combination product Symbicort.
- See Salmeterol, page 1013, for further drug interactions for the combination product Advair.

Food Interactions
None known.

Usual Dose

Beclomethasone
Adult and Child (age 13 and over): 2 inhalations (84 mcg) 3–4 times a day, or 4 inhalations twice a day. People with severe asthma may take up to 16 inhalations a day.

Child (age 6–12): 1–2 inhalations 3–4 times a day.

Child (under age 6): not recommended.

Budesonide
Adult: starting dose—200–400 mcg (1–2 inhalations) twice a day. Do not exceed 800 mcg a day.

Child (age 6 and over): 200 mcg (1 inhalation) twice a day. Do not exceed 400 mcg a day.

Child (under age 6): not recommended.

Budesonide Respules
Child (age 1–8): 1–2 ml once or twice a day via jet nebulizer connected to an air compressor.

Child (under age 1): consult your doctor.

Budesonide and Formoterol Inhalation
Adult and Child (age 12 and over): 2 inhalations morning and evening.

Child (under age 12): not recommended.

Ciclesonide
Adult and Child (age 12 and over): 1–2 inhalations once a day.

Child (under age 12): not recommended.

Flunisolide
Aerobid
Adult and Child (age 16 and over): 2 inhalations (500 mcg) morning and evening. Do not exceed 8 inhalations a day.

Child (age 6–15): 2 inhalations (500 mcg) morning and evening. Do not exceed 4 inhalations a day.

Child (under age 6): not recommended.

Aerospan HFA

Adult and Child (age 12 and over): 160–320 mcg morning and evening.

Child (age 6–11): 80–160 mcg morning and evening.

Child (under age 6): not recommended.

Fluticasone Inhalation

Adult and Child (age 12 and over): 88–660 mcg twice a day.

Child (6–12): 88–440 mcg twice a day.

Child (under age 6): not recommended.

Fluticasone Diskus

Adult and Child (age 12 and over): 100–1000 mcg twice a day.

Child (age 4–11): 50–100 mcg twice a day.

Child (under age 4): not recommended.

Fluticasone and Salmeterol

Advair Diskus

Adult and Child (age 12 and over): 1 inhalation morning and evening.

Child (under age 12): not recommended.

Advair HFA

Adult and Child (age 12 and over): 2 inhalations morning and evening.

Child (under age 12): not recommended.

Mometasone Furoate

Adult and Child (age 12 and older): 1–4 inhalations a day. If you take this drug only once a day, it should be taken in the afternoon or evening. Otherwise, doses should be divided between the morning and evening.

Child (under age 12): not recommended.

Triamcinolone

Adult and Child (age 13 and over): 2 inhalations (200 mcg) 3–4 times a day. Do not exceed 16 inhalations a day without your doctor's knowledge.

Child (age 6–12): 1–2 inhalations (100–200 mcg) 3–4 times a day. Do not exceed 12 inhalations a day.

Child (under age 6): not recommended.

Overdosage

Serious adverse effects are unlikely. Excessive use of large amounts of an inhaled corticosteroid may cause overdose symptoms and require gradually stopping the drug. Call your local poison control center or a hospital emergency room for more information.

Special Information

People using both a corticosteroid inhaler and a bronchodilator, such as albuterol, should use the bronchodilator first, wait a few minutes, and then use the corticosteroid inhaler. This allows more corticosteroid to be absorbed.

These drugs are for preventive therapy only and will not affect an asthma attack. Inhaled corticosteroids must be taken regularly, as directed. Wait at least 1 minute between inhalations.

To properly take this medication, thoroughly shake the inhaler if it is one that must be shaken. Take a drink of water to moisten your throat. Place the inhaler 2 finger-widths away from your mouth and tilt your head back slightly. While activating the inhaler, take a slow, deep breath for 3–5 seconds, then hold your breath for about 10 seconds, and finally breathe out slowly. Allow at least 1 minute between puffs. Rinse your mouth after each use to reduce dry mouth and hoarseness.

If you forget to administer a dose, do so as soon as you remember. If it is almost time for your next dose, skip the dose you forgot and continue with your regular schedule. Do not take a double dose. Tell your doctor or pharmacist if you forget to take more than 1 dose.

Special Populations

Pregnancy/Breast-feeding: Corticosteroids may cause birth defects or interfere with fetal development. When any of these drugs is considered crucial by your doctor, its potential benefits must be carefully weighed against its risks.

It is not known if inhaled corticosteroids pass into breast milk, though oral corticosteroids do. Nursing mothers who must take an inhaled corticosteroid should use infant formula.

Seniors: Seniors may use corticosteroid inhalers without special restriction. Tell your doctor if you have bone or bowel disease, colitis, diabetes, glaucoma, fungal or herpes infections, high blood pressure, high blood cholesterol, an underactive thyroid, or heart, kidney, or liver disease.

Type of Drug

Corticosteroids, Nasal
(kor-tih-koe-STER-oids)

Brand Names

Generic Ingredient: Beclomethasone Dipropionate
Beconase AQ

Generic Ingredient: Budesonide
Rhinocort

Generic Ingredient: Ciclesonide
Omnaris

Generic Ingredient: Flunisolide Ⓖ
Nasarel

Generic Ingredient: Fluticasone Furoate
Veramyst

Generic Ingredient: Fluticasone Propionate Ⓖ
Flonase

Generic Ingredient: Mometasone Furoate Monohydrate
Nasonex

Generic Ingredient: Triamcinolone Acetonide
Nasacort AQ

Prescribed For

Rhinitis (nasal inflammation) associated with seasonal or chronic allergy and other causes; also used to prevent recurrence of nasal polyps.

General Information

Nasal corticosteroids are used to treat severe symptoms of seasonal allergy that have not responded to other drugs such as decongestants. They work by reducing inflammation of the mucous membranes that line the nasal passages, making it easier to breathe. These drugs may take several days to produce an effect. Some nasal corticosteroids are approved for both allergic and non-allergic rhinitis.

Cautions and Warnings

Do not use a nasal corticosteroid if you are **allergic** or **sensitive** to corticosteroids. Rarely, serious and life-threatening drug-sensitivity reactions have occurred.

Very rarely, deaths caused by failure of the adrenal gland have occurred in people taking adrenal corticosteroid tablets or syrup who were switched to a nasal corticosteroid. This is a rare complication and usually results from stopping the liquid or tablets suddenly instead of gradually.

Combining prednisone or another oral corticosteroid with a nasal corticosteroid may cause **pituitary gland suppression,** although nasal corticosteroids alone rarely cause this problem.

Use nasal corticosteroids with caution if you have **tuberculosis, chicken pox, measles, shingles,** or any serious **fungal, bacterial, or viral infection.**

Do not receive a **live virus vaccine** while taking corticosteroids of any kind, as they interfere with the body's reaction to the vaccine.

Rarely, nasal Candida infections develop in people using a nasal corticosteroid. These infections may require treatment with an antifungal drug, as well as the discontinuance of the nasal corticosteroid.

During a period of severe **stress,** you may have to switch to an oral corticosteroid drug if the nasal form does not control your symptoms.

Children using nasal corticosteriods may experience reduction in growth velocity.

Possible Side Effects

▼ Most common: mild irritation of the nose, nasal passages, and throat; burning; stinging; dryness; and headache.

▼ Less common: lightheadedness, nausea, nosebleed or bloody mucous, unusual nasal congestion, bronchial asthma, sneezing attacks, runny nose, sore throat, and loss of the sense of taste.

▼ Rare: ulcers of the nasal passages, watery eyes, vomiting, hypersensitivity reactions (symptoms include itching, rash, swelling, bronchospasms, and breathing difficulties), nasal infection, wheezing, perforation of the wall between the nostrils, and increased eye pressure. Contact your doctor if you experience any side effect not listed above.

Drug Interactions

- Do not use fluticasone propionate with ritonavir.
- Ephedrine, phenobarbital, and rifampin may decrease the effect of nasal corticosteroids.
- Use caution when combining ketoconazole with any nasal corticosteroid.

Usual Dose

Beclomethasone

Adult and Child (age 13 and over): 1 spray (42 mcg) in each nostril 2–4 times a day.

Child (age 6–12): 1 spray (42 mcg) in each nostril 3 times a day.

Child (under age 6): not recommended.

Budesonide

Adult and Child (age 6 and over): 2 sprays (64 mcg) in each nostril morning and evening, or 4 sprays in the morning.

Child (under age 6): not recommended.

Ciclesonide

Adult and Child (age 12 and over): 2 sprays (50 mcg/spray) in each nostril once a day.

Child (under age 12): not recommended.

Flunisolide

Adult and Child (age 15 and over): 2 sprays (50 mcg) in each nostril twice a day to start; may be increased up to 8 sprays a day in each nostril.

Child (age 6–14): 1 spray (25 mcg) in each nostril 3 times a day, or 2 sprays in each nostril twice a day.

Child (under age 6): not recommended.

Fluticasone Furoate

Adult and Child (age 12 and over): 2 sprays in each nostril once a date to start. Dose may be reduced to 1 spray in each nostril afer symptoms are controlled.

Child (age 2–11): 1 spray in each nostril once a day.

Child (under age 2): not recommended.

Fluticasone Propionate

Adult: 2 sprays (100 mcg) in each nostril once a day or divided in 2 doses, to start. Dosage may be reduced in half in a few days, if tolerated.

Child (age 4 and over): 1 spray (50 mcg) in each nostril once a day; may be increased to 2 sprays a day in each nostril, if needed.

Child (under age 4): not recommended.

Mometasone

Adult and Child (age 12 and over): 2 sprays (100 mcg) in each nostril once a day; may be increased to 4 sprays a day in each nostril.

Child (under age 12): not recommended.

Triamcinolone

Adult and Child (age 13 and over): 2 sprays (220 mcg) in each nostril once a day; may be increased to 4 sprays a day in each nostril.

Child (age 6–12): 1 spray in each nostril once a day; may be increased to 2 sprays a day in each nostril, if needed.

Child (under age 6): not recommended.

Overdosage

Serious adverse effects are unlikely after accidental ingestion. Rarely, excessive use of large amounts of nasal corticosteroids may cause overdose symptoms such as irregular menses, acne, facial puffiness, and weight gain. These symptoms require gradual, not immediate, discontinuation of the drug. Call your local poison control center or a hospital emergency room for more information. ALWAYS bring the presciption container.

Special Information

It may be necessary to clear your nasal passages with a nasal decongestant before using a nasal corticosteroid to allow it to reach the mucous membranes.

Some of these drugs take 10–14 days to start working. Beclomethasone, budesonide, and triamcinolone work faster, in 3–7 days; ciclesonide starts working within 1 or 2 days and shows additional benefits after several weeks of use; in some cases, triamcinolone and budesonide provide relief in 12 hours. Flunisolide may take up to 2 weeks. Do not use any of these drugs continuously for more than 3 weeks unless you have experienced a definite benefit.

If you are using more than one spray at a time, wait at least 1 minute between sprays.

Nasal corticosteroids may cause irritation and drying of mucous membranes in the nose. Call your doctor if this effect persists or if symptoms get worse.

Call your doctor if you are exposed to measles or chicken pox while using any of these medicines.

People using a nasal corticosteroid to prevent the return of nasal polyps after surgery may experience nosebleeds because the drug can slow healing of the wound.

If you forget to administer a dose, do so as soon as you remember. If it is almost time for your next dose, skip the dose you forgot and continue with your regular schedule. Do not take a double dose.

Special Populations

Pregnancy/Breast-feeding: Taking large amounts of corticosteroids during pregnancy may slow fetal growth. While the small amount of drug absorbed into the blood after nasal application is unlikely to have any effect, consult your doctor before taking any corticosteroid if you are or might be pregnant.

Dexamethasone passes into breast milk. Nursing mothers who must use this drug should use infant formula. It is not known if other nasal corticosteroids pass into breast milk, though oral corticosteroids do. Nursing mothers should consider using infant formula.

Seniors: Seniors may use nasal corticosteroids without special restriction. Tell your doctor if you have bone or bowel disease, colitis, diabetes, glaucoma, fungal or herpes infections, high blood pressure, high blood cholesterol, an underactive thyroid, or heart, kidney, or liver disease.

Type of Drug

Corticosteroids, Oral (kor-tih-koe-STER-oids)

Brand Names

Generic Ingredient: Betamethasone
Celestone

Generic Ingredient: Budesonide
Entocort EC

Generic Ingredient: Cortisone Acetate Ⓖ

Generic Ingredient: Dexamethasone Ⓖ
Mymethasone

Generic Ingredient: Fludrocortisone Ⓖ

Generic Ingredient: Hydrocortisone Ⓖ
Cortef

Generic Ingredient: Methylprednisolone Ⓖ
Medrol

Generic Ingredient: Prednisolone Ⓖ
Orapred   Pediapred
Orapred ODT   Prelone

Generic Ingredient: Prednisone Ⓖ
Prednisone Intensol   Sterapred

Prescribed For

A wide variety of disorders from rash to cancer, including adrenal disease, adrenal hormone replacement, bursitis, arthritis, severe skin diseases including psoriasis and other rashes, severe or disabling allergies, asthma, drug or serum sickness, attacks of multiple sclerosis, severe respiratory diseases including pneumonitis, blood disorders, gastrointestinal (GI) disease including ulcerative colitis and Crohn's disease, and inflammation of the nerves, heart, or other organs. Dexamethasone is also used to treat mountain sickness, vomiting, bronchial disease in premature babies, excessive hairiness, and hearing loss associated with bacterial meningitis. Fludrocortisone is used to treat Addison's disease and for symptomatic orthostatic hypotension. Prednisone is used to improve strength and function of some muscular dystrophy patients. Methylprednisolone is used to decrease mortality in some patients suffering from severe alcoholism and chronic active hepatitis.

General Information

Produced by the adrenal gland, natural corticosteroids are hormones that affect almost every body system. The major differences among corticosteroid drugs are potency and variation in secondary effects. Doctor preference and past experience with a corticosteroid usually determine which drug to prescribe for a specific disease.

Cautions and Warnings

Do not use an oral corticosteroid if you are **allergic** or **sensitive** to any of its ingredients.

Corticosteroids may mask symptoms of an **infection.** Because these drugs compromise the immune system, new infections may occur during corticosteroid treatment; when this happens, a relatively minor infection that would respond to ordinary treatment can turn serious. Corticosteroids may impair immune response to **hepatitis B,** prolonging recovery. They may reactivate dormant **amebiasis** (a parasitic infection). Corticosteroids should not be taken if you have a **fungal blood infection,** because they can allow the infection to spread more easily. They should be used with caution by people with **herpes eye infection, tuberculosis** or in any other **bacterial, fungal, or viral infections.**

Long-term use of any corticosteroid may increase the risk of developing cataracts, glaucoma, or eye infections, especially viral or fungal.

When stopping a corticosteroid, dosage must be reduced gradually under a doctor's supervision—otherwise you may experience adrenal gland failure.

If you are taking large corticosteroid doses, you should not receive any **live virus vaccine** because corticosteroids interfere with the body's reaction to the vaccine.

Hydrocortisone and cortisone may lead to high blood pressure. Other corticosteroids are less likely to affect blood pressure.

Corticosteroids should be used with caution if you have severe **kidney disease.**

High-dose or long-term corticosteroid therapy may aggravate or worsen **stomach ulcers.** This may occur when total dosage reaches 1000 mg of prednisone, 150 mg of betamethasone or dexamethasone, 5000 mg of cortisone, 4000 mg of hydrocortisone, 1000 mg of prednisolone, or 800 mg of methylprednisolone.

People who have recently stopped taking a corticosteroid and are going through a period of **stress** may need small doses of a rapid-acting corticosteroid, such as hydrocortisone, to get them through this period. Call your doctor if you think you might be experiencing this kind of stress reaction.

Use corticosteroids with caution if you have had a recent **heart attack** or have **ulcerative colitis, heart failure, high blood pressure, blood-clotting tendencies, thrombophlebitis, osteoporosis, antibiotic-resistant infections, Cushing's disease, myasthenia gravis, metastatic cancer, diabetes, underactive thyroid disease, cirrhosis of the liver,** or **seizure disorders.**

Corticosteroid psychosis (symptoms include euphoria or feeling "high," delirium, sleeplessness, mood swings, personality changes, and severe depression) may develop in people taking dosages greater than 40 mg a day of prednisone. These symptoms may also develop with other corticosteroids taken in equivalent doses (see "Usual Dose" for relative equivalencies). Symptoms of corticosteroid psychosis usually develop within 15–30 days of beginning treatment. These symptoms may also be linked to other factors—women and those with a family history of psychosis are more at risk.

Corticosteroids can cause loss of calcium, which may result in bone fractures and aseptic necrosis of the femoral and humoral heads (a condition in which the large bones in the hip degenerate from loss of calcium).

Prednisone may aggravate **emotional instability.**

Corticosteroids do not cure **multiple sclerosis (MS)** or slow its progression, though they may speed recovery from attacks of the disease.

Corticosteroid products often contain **tartrazine dyes** and **sulfite preservatives.** Many people are allergic to these chemicals.

Possible Side Effects

▼ Most common: headache, respiratory infections, acne, and bruising.

▼ Common: water retention (swollen ankles), back pain, heart failure, upset stomach (possibly leading to stomach or duodenal ulcer), potassium loss, dizziness, fatigue, insomnia, weight gain, increased appetite, nausea, stomach gas, abdominal pain, general pain, muscle weakness, loss of muscle mass, slowed healing of wounds, increased sweating, allergic rash, itching, convulsions, excess hair growth, and worsening of a pre-existing psychiatric condition.

▼ Less common: irregular menstruation; slowed growth in children, particularly after lengthy periods of corticosteroid treatment; adrenal or pituitary gland suppression; diabetes; drug sensitivity or allergic reactions; blood clots; moon face; feeling unwell; euphoria; mood swings; personality changes; and severe depression.

▼ Rare: Rare side effects can appear in any part of the body. Contact your doctor if you experience any side effect not listed above.

Drug Interactions

- Tell your doctor if you are taking any oral anticoagulant (blood-thinning) drug. If you begin taking a corticosteroid, your anticoagulant dosage may have to be adjusted.
- Combining a corticosteroid and a diuretic such as hydrochlorothiazide may cause loss of blood potassium. Low blood potassium may increase the side effects of digitalis drugs.
- Contraceptive drugs, estrogen, erythromycin, azithromycin, clarithromycin, and ketoconazole may increase the risk of corticosteroid side effects.
- Barbiturates, aminoglutethimide, phenytoin and other hydantoin anticonvulsants, rifampin, ephedrine, colestipol, and cholestyramine may reduce the effectiveness of corticosteroids.
- Corticosteroids may decrease the effects of aspirin and other salicylates, growth hormones, and isoniazid.
- Combining a corticosteroid and a theophylline drug may require a dosage adjustment of either or both drugs.
- Corticosteroids may interfere with laboratory tests. Tell your doctor if you are taking any of these drugs so that tests are properly analyzed.
- Limit your intake of alcohol while on oral corticosteroids.

Food Interactions

Take corticosteroids with food or a small amount of antacid to avoid stomach upset. If stomach upset continues, notify your doctor. Grapefruit juice doubles the amount of some oral corticosteroids absorbed into the blood.

Usual Dose

Once-daily doses should be taken in the morning. Dosages vary greatly and depend upon the specific disease being treated. Dosages for infants and children should be individualized according to severity of disease and response to treatment.

Betamethasone: starting dosage—0.6–7.2 mg a day. Maintenance dosage—0.6–7.2 mg a day.

Budesonide: 9 mg a day.

Cortisone: starting dosage—25–300 mg a day. Maintenance dosage—25–300 mg a day.

Dexamethasone: 0.75–9 mg a day. Daily dosage sometimes exceeds 9 mg. A temporary dosage increase may be necessary if you are experiencing emotional stress. In alternate-day therapy, twice the usual daily dose is taken every other day.

Hydrocortisone: 20–240 mg a day.

Methylprednisolone: starting dosage—4–48 mg or more a day. Maintenance dosage varies. A temporary dosage increase may be necessary if you are experiencing emotional stress. In alternate-day therapy, twice the usual daily dose is taken every other day.

Prednisone and Prednisolone: 5–60 mg a day. Daily dosage sometimes exceeds 60 mg. A temporary dosage increase may be necessary if you are experiencing emotional stress. In alternate-day therapy, twice the usual daily dose is taken every other day.

Equivalent doses: Using 5 mg of prednisone as the basis for comparison, equivalent doses of other corticosteroids are 0.6 mg–0.75 mg of betamethasone, 25 mg of cortisone, 0.75 mg of dexamethasone, 20 mg of hydrocortisone, 4 mg of methylprednisolone, and 5 mg of prednisolone.

Overdosage

Symptoms of overdose are anxiety, depression or stimulation, joint or muscle pain, blurred vision, stomach bleeding, increased blood sugar, high blood pressure, and water retention. The victim should be taken to a hospital emergency room immediately. ALWAYS bring the prescription bottle or container.

Special Information

Do not stop taking this medication without your doctor's knowledge. Suddenly stopping any corticosteroid drug may have severe consequences; the dosage must be gradually reduced by your doctor.

Call your doctor if you develop unusual weight gain, black or tarry stools, swelling of the feet or legs, muscle weakness, vomiting of blood, menstrual irregularity, prolonged sore throat, fever, cold or infection, appetite loss, nausea and vomiting, diarrhea, weight loss, weakness, dizziness, or low blood sugar.

If you take several doses a day and forget a dose, take the dose you forgot as soon as possible. If it is almost time for your next dose, skip the one you forgot and double the next dose. If you take 1 dose a day and forget a dose, skip the dose you forgot and continue with your regular schedule. Do not take a double dose.

If you take a corticosteroid every other day and forget a dose, take it immediately if you remember it in the morning of your regularly scheduled day. If it is much later in the day, skip the dose you forgot and take it the following morning, then go back to your regular schedule. Do not take a double dose.

Special Populations

Pregnancy/Breast-feeding: Studies have shown that long-term corticosteroid therapy at high dosages may cause birth defects, as may chronic corticosteroid use during the first 3 months of pregnancy. When this drug is considered crucial by your doctor, its potential benefits must be carefully weighed against its risks.

Corticosteroids taken by mouth may pass into breast milk. Most nursing mothers who must take a corticosteroid should use infant formula, though low dosages of some of these drugs may be taken for short periods while breast-feeding. Consult your doctor.

Seniors: Seniors are more likely to develop high blood pressure while taking an oral corticosteroid. Older women are more susceptible to osteoporosis (a condition characterized by loss of bone mass due to depletion of minerals, especially calcium) associated with high dosages of oral corticosteriods. Lower dosages are just as effective in seniors and cause fewer side effects.

Type of Drug

Corticosteroids, Topical
(kor-tih-koe-STER-oids)

Brand Names

CLASS 1—Super-potent topical products
*Generic Ingredient: Betamethasone Dipropionate gel,
ointment 0.05%* [G]
Diprolene gel/ointment

Generic Ingredient: Clobetasol Propionate 0.05% cream, foam, gel, lotion, shampoo, ointment Ⓖ

Clobex	Olux
Cormax	Olux E
Embeline	Temovate
Embeline E	

Generic Ingredient: Diflorasone Diacetate ointment 0.05% Ⓖ

Olux-E Foam   Psorcon E

Generic Ingredient: Fluocinonide cream 0.1% Ⓖ

Vanos

Generic Ingredient: Flurandrenolide tape 4 mcg/cm^2 Ⓖ

Cordran Tape

Generic Ingredient: Halobetasol Propionate cream/ ointment 0.05% Ⓖ

Ultravate

CLASS 2—High-potency topical products
Generic Ingredient: Amcinonide ointment 0.1% Ⓖ

Generic Ingredient: Betamethasone Dipropionate cream 0.05% Ⓖ

Diprolene AF

Generic Ingredients: Betamethasone Dipropionate (0.064%) + Calcipotriene (0.005%) ointment

Taclonex

Generic Ingredient: Desoximetasone Cream, ointment 0.25% and 0.05%; 0.05% gel Ⓖ

Topicort   Topicort LP

Generic Ingredient: Diflorasone Diacetate cream, ointment 0.05% Ⓖ

Apexicon	Florone E
Apexicon E	Maxiflor
Florone	Psorcon

Generic Ingredient: Fluocinonide cream, gel, ointment, solution 0.05% Ⓖ

Lidex   Lidex E

Generic Ingredient: Halcinonide cream, ointment, solution 0.1%

Halog

Generic Ingredient: Mometasone Furoate ointment 0.1% Ⓖ

Elocon

Generic Ingredient: Triamcinolone Acetonide ointment 0.5% Ⓖ

CLASS 3—Upper mid-strength topical products

Generic Ingredient: Amcinonide lotion 0.1% Ⓖ

Generic Ingredient: Betamethasone Dipropionate cream 0.05% Ⓖ

Diprolene   Teladar
Maxivate

Generic Ingredient: Betamethasone Valerate ointment 0.1% Ⓖ

Generic Ingredient: Fluocinolone Acetonide Ⓖ

Capex Shampoo

Generic Ingredient: Fluticasone Propionate cream 0.05% Ⓖ

Cutivate

Generic Ingredient: Triamcinolone Acetonide cream 0.5% Ⓖ

Delta-Tritex   Kenonel
Flutex   Triacet
Kenalog Cream   Triderm
Kenalog-H

CLASS 4—Mid-strength topical products

Generic Ingredient: Amcinonide cream 0.1% Ⓖ

Generic Ingredient: Betamethasone Dipropionate lotion 0.05% and foam 0.12% Ⓖ

Diprosone   Maxivate Lotion
Luxiq Foam

Generic Ingredient: Desoximetasone cream 0.05% [G]
Topicort

Generic Ingredient: Fluocinolone Acetonide [G]
Synalar Ointment 0.025%   Synalar-HP Cream 0.2%

Generic Ingredient: Flurandrenolide ointment 0.05% [G]
Cordran

Generic Ingredient: Fluticasone Propionate lotion 0.05% [G]
Cutivate

Generic Ingredient: Hydrocortisone Valerate ointment 0.2% [G]
Westcort

Generic Ingredient: Mometasone Furoate cream, lotion, solution 0.1% [G]
Elocon

Generic Ingredient: Prednicarbate ointment 0.1% [G]
Dermatop E

Generic Ingredient: Triamcinolone Acetonide 0.1% [G]

Aristocort A	Delta-Tritex Cream
Aristocort Cream and Ointment	Kenalog
	Triderm

CLASS 5—*Lower mid-strength topical products*
Generic Ingredient: Betamethasone Valerate cream, lotion 0.1% [G]

Beta-Val	Dermabet
Betatrex	Valnac

Generic Ingredient: Clocortolone Pivalate cream 0.1%
Cloderm

Generic Ingredient: Desonide ointment 0.05% [G]

Desonate	Tridesilon
DesOwen	Verdeso Foam
Lokara	

Generic Ingredient: Fluocinolone Acetonide cream 0.025% [G]
Synalar

Generic Ingredient: Flurandrenolide cream, lotion G
Cordran Lotion 0.05%   Cordran SP 0.05%
Cordran Ointment 0.25%

Generic Ingredient: Fluticasone Propionate ointment 0.005% G
Cutivate

Generic Ingredient: Hydrocortisone Butyrate Cream, ointment, solution 0.1% G
Locoid

Generic Ingredient: Hydrocortisone Probutate 0.1%
Pandel

Generic Ingredient: Hydrocortisone Valerate cream 0.2% G
Westcort

Generic Ingredient: Prednicarbate Cream 0.1% G
Dermatop E

CLASS 6—Mild topical products
Generic Ingredient: Alclometasone Dipropionate cream, ointment 0.05% G
Aclovate

Generic Ingredient: Desonide cream, lotion 0.05% G
DesOwen   Tridesilon
Lokara

Generic Ingredient: Fluocinolone Acetonide cream, shampoo, solution 0.01% G
Derma-Smoothe/FS Oil   FS Shampoo
Flurosyn   Synalar

Generic Ingredient: Flurandrenolide cream G
Cordran SP 0.025%

Generic Ingredient: Triamcinolone Acetonide cream 0.1%
Aristocort

Generic Ingredient: Triamcinolone Acetonide cream 0.025% G
Flutex   Triacet
Kenalog

CLASS 7—Least potent topical products

Generic Ingredient: Hydrocortisone G

1% HC
Ala-Cort
Ala-Scalp
Alcortin
Analpram-HC
Anusol-HC
Cetacort
Cortaid Intensive Therapy
Cortizone-5
Cortizone-10
Cortizone-10 Plus
Cortizone-10 Quickshot
Cortizone for Kids
Delcort
Extra Strength CortaGel
Hemril
Hi-Cor 1.0
Hi-Cor 2.5
Hycort
HydroSkin
HydroTex
Hytone
Ivy Soothe
Maximum Strength Bactine
Maximum Strength Cortaid
Maximum Strength Cortaid Faststick
Maximum Strength KeriCort-10
Nutracort
Procort
Proctocream-HC
Proctofoam-HC
Stie-cort
Synacort
Tegrin HC
Texacort

Generic Ingredient: Hydrocortisone Acetate cream, ointment 0.5% and 1% G

Cortef Feminine Itch
Corticaine
Cortifoam
Dricort
Gynecort Female Creme
Lanacort
Maximum Strength Caldecort
Micort-HC
U-Cort

Prescribed For

Inflammation, itching, eczema, dermatitis, vitiligo (patchy loss of skin color), blistering skin diseases, lupus and other connective tissue diseases, psoriasis, and many other specialized skin problems; may also be used to treat severe diaper rash.

General Information

Topical corticosteroids do not cure the underlying cause of skin problems, but they can relieve symptoms of rash, itching, or inflammation by interfering with the body mechanisms that produce them. You should never use a topical corticosteroid without your doctor's knowledge because it could mask a symptom important in diagnosing your condition. Also, improper use of a topical corticosteroid could lead to unwanted and sometimes permanent side effects. In general, ointment forms of topical steroids are more potent and usually more effective than cream or lotion forms. Ointments are also less likely to cause allergic reactions because they contain fewer inactive ingredients.

Generic products in this group can vary in potency and produce different results from their brand-name counterparts, even though they contain the identical quantity of active ingredient. Topical steroids are rated from 1 (most potent) to 7 (least potent). Generally, products within a potency class are interchangeable. Ask your doctor or pharmacist which products are interchangeable. The lowest potency products are available without a prescription. Ointments tend to be more potent than creams and solutions and different product concentrations affect their classification.

Super-potent topical corticosteroids (class 1) should not be used on the face, neck, under the arms, or in the groin area. These products are generally reserved for situations in which less potent products have not worked. They should be used with caution, and should only be applied to the areas that are affected with the rash. Using a product in this category for longer than 2 weeks at a time increases the risk of permanent skin damage.

High-potency topical corticosteroids (classes 2 and 3) are best for the trunk, arms, and legs, but should not be used on the face, neck, under the arms, or in the groin area. Using a product in this category for longer than 2 weeks at a time increases the risk of permanent skin damage.

Intermediate-potency topical corticosteroids (classes 4 and 5) can be used in children for up to 1–2 weeks at a time. This type of medication is best for the trunk and extremities. It is safer for use on thin skin, and less effective on thicker skin.

Low-potency topical corticosteroids (classes 6 and 7) can be used on any part of the body, and can be used in children. They are the best choice for the face, underarm area, groin, neck, and other occluded areas such as skin folds.

Cautions and Warnings

Do not use a topical corticosteroid if you are **allergic** or **sensitive** to corticosteroids or to any ingredients of the aerosol, cream, gel, lotion, ointment, or solution. Do not use a topical corticosteroid as the sole treatment for **bacterial skin infections** such as impetigo, **viral skin diseases** such as herpes, **fungal skin infections** such as athlete's foot, or known **tuberculosis** of the skin. These drugs should not be used in the **ear** if the eardrum is perforated. Do not use a topical corticosteroid on **ulcerated skin**, or to treat **acne**.

Skin problems can become less responsive with time if a product is applied continuously over a long period of time. This can result in a flare-up of the problem when the medication is stopped. Using a less potent product may avoid this problem.

Rectal corticosteroid products should not be used if you have any serious **bowel condition,** including bowel perforation, obstruction, abscess, and systemic fungal infection.

The rectal foam is not expelled after it has been applied and may result in higher drug blood levels than those associated with rectal enema products. The risk of systemic (whole-body) side effects is greater when more of the drug enters the blood. If there is no improvement after 2 or 3 weeks of using a rectal corticosteroid, contact your doctor.

Using a topical corticosteroid around the eyes for prolonged periods may cause cataracts, glaucoma and/or permanent thinning and fragility of skin around the eyes where the corticosteroid is being applied.

Children may be more susceptible to serious systemic side effects from topical corticosteroids, including growth retardation, Cushing's syndrome, and suppression of natural corticosteroid production, requiring a tapering of the medication, especially if the medications are applied to large areas over long periods. Superpotent topical corticosteroids are not recommended for children.

Possible Side Effects

▼ Most common: burning; itching; irritation; "steroid" acne; skin thinning, tightening, or discoloration; stretch marks; dry cracked skin; bruising; and secondary infection. These effects are more likely when the treated area is covered with an occlusive bandage (one that prevents contact with water and air). Side effects are more likely with extended use of high-potency topical corticosteroid products and when the treated area is covered with a bandage that completely prevents skin contact with.water and air.

Possible Side Effects (continued)

▼ Significant amounts of corticosteroids may be absorbed into the bloodstream if large amounts are used for long periods. This can result in systemic effects and may cause serious problems, particularly in people with liver disease. Systemic side effects include lightheadedness, hives, growth suppression, and adrenal suppression.

Drug Interactions
None known.

Usual Dose
Adult

Cream, Ointment, Solution, Foam, and Aerosol: Apply a thin film to the skin 2–3 times a day. High- and super-potent products should be applied no more than twice a day, and should be used for short-term treatment, usually 2–3 weeks at a time. Some may have to be applied only once a day.

Rectal Enema: 100 mg nightly for 21 days.

Rectal Foam: 1 applicator's worth, 1–2 times a day for 2–3 weeks.

Child: Dosages for children should be limited to the lowest possible potency.

Overdosage
Serious adverse effects are unlikely after accidental ingestion. Excessive use of large amounts of topical corticosteroids may cause overdose symptoms and require gradual discontinuation of the drug. Call your local poison control center or a hospital emergency room for more information. ALWAYS bring the prescription bottle or container.

Special Information
To prevent secondary infection, clean the skin before applying the drug. Apply a very thin film and rub in gently—effectiveness depends on contact area, not the thickness of the layer applied.

Do not wash, rub, or put clothing on the area until the medication has dried.

Topical corticosteroids have an additive effect: with continuous use, 1 or 2 applications a day may be as effective as 3 or more. Once the drug begins to take effect, your doctor may recommend reducing the dose to the minimum level needed to control the condition.

Flurandrenolide tape comes with specific directions for use; follow them carefully.

If your doctor instructs you to apply plastic wrap or any other occlusive dressing, follow directions carefully. These dressings can increase the penetration of the drug into your skin by as much as 10 times, which may be a crucial element in the medication's effectiveness. Occlusive dressings should not be used with any of the super-potent topical products.

If you are using one of these products for diaper rash, do not use tight-fitting diapers or plastic pants, which can cause too much drug to be absorbed into the blood.

Your doctor may prescribe a specific form of the product with good reason. Do not change forms without your doctor's knowledge; a different form may not be as effective.

If you forget to administer a dose, do so as soon as you remember. If it is almost time for your next dose, skip the one you forgot and continue with your regular schedule. Do not administer a double dose.

Special Populations

Pregnancy/Breast-feeding: Large amounts of corticosteroids applied to the skin for long periods of time may increase the risk of birth defects. When your doctor considers any of these drugs crucial, its potential benefits must be carefully weighed against its risks. Do not use any over-the-counter hydrocortisone product for more than a few days without your doctor's knowledge.

Nursing mothers who must use a topical corticosteroid should consider using infant formula. If you apply a corticosteroid to the nipple area, be sure to completely clean the area prior to nursing. Nursing mothers should never use the highest potency corticosteroids (classes 1, 2 or 3) because of the risk of absorbing large amounts of drug into the system that could find its way into breast milk. Nursing mothers should discuss topical corticosteroid use with their doctor before applying any product.

Seniors: Seniors are more susceptible to high blood pressure and osteoporosis (a condition characterized by loss of bone mass due to depletion of minerals, especially calcium) associated with large dosages. These effects are unlikely with topical corticosteroids unless a high-potency medication is used over a large area for an extended period.

Brand Name

Cortisporin Otic

Generic Ingredients
Hydrocortisone + Neomycin Sulfate + Polymyxin B Sulfate Ⓖ

Other Brand Names
AK-Spore H.C. Otic
AntibiOtic
Cortatrigen Ear Drops
Drotic
Ear-Eze
LazerSporin-C

Octicair
Otic-Care
Otocort
Pediotic
UAD

Type of Drug
Antibiotic and corticosteroid combination.

Prescribed For
Superficial ear infection, ear inflammation or itching, and other outer ear problems.

General Information
Cortisporin Otic contains a corticosteroid to reduce inflammation and 2 antibiotics to treat local ear infections. This combination can be quite useful for local ear problems because of its dual method of action and its relatively broad applicability.

Cautions and Warnings
Do not use Cortisporin Otic if you are **allergic** or **sensitive** to any of its ingredients.

Cortisporin Otic is designed for use in the ear. It can be very damaging if placed into the eye.

Cortisporin should not be used if you have **herpes simplex**, **vaccinia**, or **chickenpox**. It also should not be used by patients sensitive to **sulfite**.

Cortisporin Otic should not be used if you have a **perforated eardrum.**

Possible Side Effects
▼ Local irritation, such as itching or burning, may occur as a drug sensitivity or allergic reaction.

Drug Interactions

None known.

Usual Dose

3–4 drops in the affected ear 3–4 times a day. Treatment should not last beyond 10 days.

Overdosage

The amount of drug contained in each bottle is too small to cause serious problems. Call a hospital emergency room or your local poison control center for more information. If you seek treatment, ALWAYS bring the prescription bottle or container.

Special Information

Use only when prescribed by a physician. Overuse of this or similar products can result in the growth of new organisms, such as fungi. If new infections or problems appear, stop using the drug and contact your doctor.

Before administering drops, wash your hands, then hold the closed bottle in your hand for a few minutes to warm it to body temperature. Shake well for 10 seconds. For best results, drops should not be self-administered, but given by another person. The person receiving the drops should lie on his or her side with the affected ear facing upward. Fill the dropper and instill the required number of drops directly in the ear canal.

If the drops are being given to an infant, hold the earlobe down and back to allow the drops to run in. If the drops are being given to an older child or adult, hold the earlobe up and back to allow them to run in. Do not put the dropper into the ear or allow it to touch any part of the ear or bottle. Keep the ear tilted for about 5 minutes after the drops have been put in or insert a soft cotton plug, whichever is recommended by your doctor.

If you forget to administer a dose of Cortisporin Otic, do so as soon as you remember. If it is almost time for your next dose, skip the dose you forgot and continue with your regular schedule. Do not apply a double dose.

Special Populations

Pregnancy/Breast-feeding: There are no studies of Cortisporin Otic in pregnant women but it does contain a corticosteroid, which when used over long periods of time in other formulations may increase the risk of birth defects. This drug should only be used during pregnancy after carefully weighing it potential benefits against its risks. Nursing mothers who must take this drug should use infant formula.

Seniors: Seniors may use this product without special restriction.

Brand Name

Cosopt

Generic Ingredients
Dorzolamide + Timolol

Type of Drug
Carbonic anhydrase inhibitor and beta blocker combination.

Prescribed For
Open-angle glaucoma and ocular hypertension.

General Information
Cosopt contains 2 glaucoma drugs that work in different ways. It is intended for people whose glaucoma does not respond to either drug used alone. Small amounts of dorzolamide and timolol—the active ingredients in Cosopt—enter the bloodstream.

Cautions and Warnings
Do not use Cosopt if you are **allergic** or **sensitive** to any of its ingredients or cannot take sulfa drugs or beta blockers. Cosopt should not be used by people with bronchial **asthma,** severe **chronic obstructive pulmonary disease, slow heart rate** or **heart block, heart failure,** or who are in **shock.**

People with **diabetes** or an **overactive thyroid** should use Cosopt with caution since beta blockers can mask the signs of low blood sugar or hyperthyroidism.

Small amounts of both ingredients enter the bloodstream and can produce the same kinds of systemic (whole-body) reactions associated with larger dosages of either a sulfa drug or beta blocker. Stop using the drug at once and call your doctor if a serious reaction develops.

Beta blockers may have to be discontinued prior to **major surgery** because they can affect the heart's ability to respond normally. Some people taking a beta blocker experience severe reductions in blood flow while undergoing general anesthesia.

Dorzolamide should not be used by people with **kidney disease** and has not been studied in people with **liver disease.**

People with a history of **severe allergic reactions** who take a beta blocker may be at increased risk of experiencing a reaction because the drug blocks part of the body's natural allergic response.

Timolol can worsen the muscle weakness that accompanies **myasthenia gravis**.

Possible Side Effects

▼ Most common: changes in sense of taste, especially bitterness or sourness; increased sensitivity to light; and a burning or stinging sensation in the eye.

▼ Common: eye redness, irritation, or itching, and blurred vision.

▼ Less common: abdominal pain, back pain, eyelid inflammation, bronchitis, cloudy vision, eye discharge or swelling, conjunctivitis (pinkeye), corneal erosion, corneal staining, lens cloudiness, cough, dizziness, dry eye, upset stomach, drug particles in the eye, eye pain, tearing, eyelid scaling, eyelid pain or discomfort, sensation of something in the eye, headache, high blood pressure, influenza, lens discoloration, nausea, sore throat, cataracts, sinus irritation, respiratory infection, urinary infection, visual problems, and retinal detachment.

▼ Rare: slow heartbeat, heart block or failure, chest pain, stroke, depression, diarrhea, dry mouth, breathing difficulties, low blood pressure, stuffy nose, rash, tingling in the hands or feet, kidney stones, and vomiting. Contact your doctor if you experience any side effect not listed above.

See Dorzolamide, page 200, and Timolol, page 1129, for further side effect information.

Drug Interactions

● If you use more than 1 eyedrop medication, separate doses of these drugs by at least 10 minutes.

● Cosopt can increase the effect of other carbonic anhydrase inhibitors.

● Combining Cosopt with an oral beta blocker or another calcium antagonist may increase the risk of side effects, especially changes in heart rhythm and low blood pressure.

- Do not combine Cosopt and another beta-blocking eyedrop.
- Combining Cosopt and reserpine can lead to low blood pressure, slowing of heartbeat, and dizziness or fainting.
- Combining Cosopt with digitalis and a calcium antagonist, or with quinidine, can slow heartbeat.

See Dorzolamide, page 200, and Timolol, page 1129, for further drug interactions.

Usual Dose

Adult: 1 drop in the affected eye twice a day.
Child: not recommended.

Overdosage

Little is known about the effects of Cosopt overdose or accidental ingestion. Possible overdose symptoms include dizziness, headache, shortness of breath, slow heartbeat, breathing difficulties, heart attack, and nervous system effects. Call your local poison control center or a hospital emergency room for more information. If you seek treatment, ALWAYS bring the prescription bottle or container.

Special Information

Conjunctivitis (pinkeye) and eyelid reactions can occur due to an allergic reaction or as the result of local irritation. If you experience either of these problems, stop using the drug and call your doctor so that your condition can be evaluated.

To prevent infection, do not allow the eyedropper to touch your fingers, eyelids, or any surface. Wait at least 10 minutes before using any other eyedrops.

Cosopt contains benzalkonium chloride (a preservative), which may be absorbed by soft contact lenses. Remove your soft contact lenses before using the eyedrops; you may put them back in 15 minutes after a dose.

If you forget a dose of Cosopt, take it as soon as you remember. If it is almost time for your next dose, skip the forgotten dose and continue with your regular schedule.

Store Cosopt away from sunlight.

Special Populations

Pregnancy/Breast-feeding: The safety of using Cosopt is not known. When this drug is considered crucial by your doctor, its potential benefits must be carefully weighed against its risks.

It is not known if dorzolamide passes into breast milk, though timolol does. Nursing mothers who must use Cosopt should use infant formula.

Seniors: Seniors may use Cosopt without precaution.

Coumadin   *see Warfarin, page 1212*

Cozaar   *see Angiotensin II Blockers, page 80*

Crestor   *see Statin Cholesterol-Lowering Agents,* page 1052

Generic Name

Cromolyn   (KROE-muh-lin) Ⓖ

Brand Names

Crolom	Intal
Gastrocrom	Opticrom

The information in this profile also applies to the following drugs:

Generic Ingredient: Nedocromil

Alocril	Tilade

Type of Drug

Allergy preventive and antiasthmatic.

Prescribed For

Prevention of severe allergic reactions, including asthma, runny nose, and mastocytosis; also prescribed for food allergies, eczema, dermatitis, chronic itching, and hay fever. It may be used to treat and prevent chronic inflammatory bowel disease. The eyedrops are used to treat conjunctivitis (pinkeye) and other eye irritations.

General Information

Unlike antihistamines, which work against histamine that has been released into the system, cromolyn sodium prevents allergy, asthma, and other conditions by stabilizing mast cells, a key component in any allergic reaction because they release histamine. Cromolyn prevents the release of histamine and other chemicals from mast cells. The drug works only in the areas to which it is applied; only 7–8% of an inhaled dose and 1% of a swallowed capsule is absorbed into the blood. Even the oral capsules, which one would normally expect to be absorbed into the blood, treat only gastrointestinal-tract allergies. Cromolyn products must be used on a regular basis to be effective in reducing the frequency and intensity of allergic reactions.

Cautions and Warnings

Do not take cromolyn if you are **allergic** or **sensitive** to any of its ingredients. Rarely, people have experienced severe allergic attacks after taking cromolyn.

Cromolyn should never be used to treat an acute allergy attack. It is intended only to prevent or reduce the number of allergic attacks and their intensity. Once the proper dosage level has been established for you, reducing that level may result in a recurrence of attacks.

People with **kidney or liver disease** require reduced dosage.

Cough or bronchial spasm may occasionally occur after the inhalation of a cromolyn dose. Severe bronchospasm is rare.

Cromolyn aerosol should be used with caution in people with **abnormal heart rhythm** or **diseased coronary blood vessels** because of a possible reaction to the propellants used in the product.

Possible Side Effects

▼ Most common: rash and itching. Headache and diarrhea (for capsules). Watery, itchy, dry, or puffy eyes; and styes (for eyedrops). Most capsule and eyedrop side effects are minor and may be attributable to the underlying condition; a variety have been reported but cannot be tied conclusively to the drug.

▼ Less common: local irritation, including nasal stinging, sneezing, tearing, cough, and stuffy nose; urinary difficulty or frequency; dizziness; headache; joint swelling; muscle

---

Possible Side Effects *(continued)*

pain; a bad taste in the mouth; sore throat; nosebleeds; abdominal pain; and nausea.

▼ Rare: severe drug reactions, consisting of coughing, difficulty in swallowing, hives, itching, breathing difficulties, or swelling of the eyelids, lips, or face. Contact your doctor if you experience any side effect not listed above.

Drug Interactions
None known.

Food Interactions
Inhaled or swallowed cromolyn products should not be mixed with any food, juice, or milk. The nasal and eye products may be taken without regard to food or meals.

Usual Dose
Inhaled Capsules or Solution
Adult and Child (age 2 and over): starting dose—20 mg 4 times a day. Children under age 5 may inhale cromolyn powder if their allergies are severe. The solution must be given with a power-operated nebulizer and face mask. Handheld nebulizers are not adequate. To prevent exercise asthma, 20 mg may be inhaled up to 1 hour before exercise.

Aerosol
Adult and Child (age 5 and over): up to 2 sprays 4 times a day, spaced equally throughout the day. To prevent exercise asthma, 2 puffs may be inhaled up to 1 hour before exercise.

Nasal Solution
Adult and Child (age 6 and over): 1 spray in each nostril 3–6 times a day at regular intervals. First blow your nose, and then inhale the spray.

Oral Capsules
Adult and Child (age 12 and over): 2 dissolved capsules 4 times a day taken a half hour before meals and at bedtime.

Child (age 2–12): 1 dissolved capsule (100 mg) 4 times a day a half hour before meals and at bedtime. Dosage may be increased to about 13–18 mg per lb. of body weight in 4 equal doses.

Child (under age 2): about 10 mg per lb. of body weight a day divided into 4 equal doses. This product is recommended in infants and young children only if absolutely necessary.

Eyedrops

Adult and Child (age 4 and over): 1–2 drops in each eye 4–6 times a day at regular intervals.

Overdosage

No action is necessary other than medical observation. Call your local poison control center or a hospital emergency room for more information. ALWAYS bring the prescription bottle or container.

Special Information

Cromolyn is taken to prevent or minimize severe allergic reactions. It is imperative that you take cromolyn products on a regular basis to provide equal protection throughout the day.

If you are taking cromolyn to prevent seasonal allergies, it is essential that you start taking the medication before you come into contact with the cause of the allergy and that you continue treatment while you are exposed to it.

Cromolyn oral capsules should be opened and their contents mixed with about 4 oz. of hot water. Stir until the powder completely dissolves and the solution is completely clear, then fill the rest of the glass with cold water. Drink the entire contents of the glass. Do not mix the solution with food, juice, or milk.

Do not wear soft contact lenses while using cromolyn eyedrops. The lenses may be replaced a few hours after you stop taking the drug. To prevent contamination, do not touch the applicator tip to any surface including the eyes or fingers.

Call your doctor if you develop wheezing, coughing, a severe drug reaction (see "Possible Side Effects"), rash, or any bothersome or persistent side effect.

Call your doctor if your symptoms do not improve or if they worsen.

If you forget to administer a dose, do so as soon as you remember and space the remaining daily dosage evenly throughout the day. Do not take a double dose.

Special Populations

Pregnancy/Breast-feeding: In animal studies, very large dosages of cromolyn administered by vein have affected the fetus, though no birth defects were reported. When this drug is considered crucial by your doctor, its potential benefits must be carefully weighed against its risks.

It is not known if cromolyn passes into breast milk. Nursing mothers who must use cromolyn should use infant formula.

Seniors: Older adults with reduced kidney or liver function may require lower dosages.

Generic Name

Cyclobenzaprine (sye-cloe-BEN-zuh-prene) Ⓖ

Brand Names

Amrix   Flexeril

Type of Drug

Skeletal muscle relaxant.

Prescribed For

Serious muscle spasm and acute muscle pain; also used to treat fibrositis (muscular rheumatism).

General Information

Cyclobenzoprine hydrochloride is used to treat severe muscle spasms; it is prescribed as part of a coordinated program of rest, physical therapy, and other measures.

Cautions and Warnings

Do not take cyclobenzaprine if you are **allergic** or **sensitive** to any of its ingredients.

This drug should not be taken for several weeks following a **heart attack** or by people with **abnormal heart rhythms, heart failure, heart block** (disruption of the electrical impulses that control heart rate), or **hyperthyroidism** (overactive thyroid gland).

Cyclobenzaprine should be avoided by people with **urinary retention, glaucoma,** or **increased eye pressure**.

This drug may increase the chances of cavities or gum disease.

Cyclobenzaprine is intended only for short-term use of 2–3 weeks.

Cyclobenzaprine is chemically similar to tricyclic antidepressants and may produce some of the more serious side effects associated with those drugs. Abruptly stopping cyclobenzaprine may cause nausea, headache, and feelings of ill health; this is not a sign of addiction.

Possible Side Effects

▼ Most common: dry mouth, drowsiness, and dizziness.

▼ Less common: muscle weakness, fatigue, nausea, constipation, upset stomach, unpleasant taste, blurred vision, headache, nervousness, and confusion.

▼ Rare: Rare side effects can occur in almost any part of the body. Contact your doctor if you experience any side effect not listed above.

Drug Interactions

- The effects of alcohol, sedatives, or other nervous system depressants may be increased by cyclobenzaprine.
- Cyclobenzaprine may increase some side effects of atropine, ipratropium, and other anticholinergic drugs.
- The combination of cyclobenzaprine and a monoamine oxidase inhibitor antidepressant may produce very high fever, convulsions, and possibly death. Do not take these drugs within 14 days of each other.
- Cyclobenzaprine may increase the effects of haloperidol, loxapine, molindone, pimozide, anticoagulant (blood-thinning) drugs, anticonvulsants, thyroid hormones, antithyroid drugs, phenothiazines, thioxanthenes, and nasal decongestants such as naphazoline, oxymetazoline, phenylephrine, and xylometazoline.
- Barbiturates and carbamazepine may counteract the effects of cyclobenzaprine.
- Fluoxetine, ranitidine, cimetidine, methylphenidate, estramustine, estrogens, and contraceptive drugs may increase the effects and side effects of cyclobenzaprine.
- Cyclobenzaprine may counteract the effects of clonidine, guanadrel, and guanethidine.

Food Interactions

None known.

Usual Dose

Adult and Child (age 15 and over): 5–10 mg 3 times a day.

Child (under age 15): not recommended.

Overdosage

Cyclobenzaprine overdose may cause confusion, loss of concentration, hallucinations, agitation, overactive reflexes, fever or vomiting, rigid muscles, and other side effects of the drug. It may also cause drowsiness, low body temperature, rapid or irregular heartbeat and other kinds of abnormal heart rhythms, heart failure, dilated pupils, convulsions, very low blood pressure, stupor, coma, and sweating. Overdose victims must be taken to a hospital emergency room. ALWAYS bring the prescription bottle or container.

Special Information

Cyclobenzaprine causes drowsiness, dizziness, or blurred vision in more than 40% of people who take it, which may interfere with the ability to perform complex tasks like driving or operating equipment. Avoid alcohol, sedatives, and other nervous system depressants because they can enhance sedative effects of cyclobenzaprine.

Call your doctor if you develop rash; hives; itching; urinary difficulties; clumsiness; confusion; depression; convulsions; difficulty breathing; irregular heart rate; chest pain; fever; yellowing of the skin or whites of the eyes; swelling of the face, lips, or tongue; or any other persistent or bothersome side effect.

If you forget a dose of cyclobenzaprine, take it as soon as you remember. If you take cyclobenzaprine once a day and it is almost time for your next dose, skip the one you forgot and continue with your regular schedule. If you take cyclobenzaprine twice a day and it is almost time for your next dose, take 1 dose as soon as you remember, another in 5 or 6 hours, and then go back to your regular schedule. If you take cyclobenzaprine 3 times a day and it is almost time for your next dose, take 1 dose as soon as you remember, another in 3 or 4 hours, and then go back to your regular schedule. Never take a double dose.

Special Populations

Pregnancy/Breast-feeding: The safety of cyclobenzaprine in pregnant women has not been established. Cyclobenzaprine should only be used if the potential benefits outweigh the risks.

It is not known if cyclobenzaprine passes into breast milk, but antidepressants with a similar chemical structure do pass into breast milk. Nursing mothers who must take this drug should consider using infant formula.

Seniors: Seniors are more likely to be sensitive to the effects of cyclobenzaprine. Use of Amrix in particular is not recommended in the elderly.

Generic Name

Cyclosporine (sye-kloe-SPOR-in) Ⓖ

Brand Names

Gengraf
Neoral

Restasis Ophthalmic Emulsion
Sandimmune

Type of Drug

Immunosuppressant.

Prescribed For

Kidney, heart, or liver transplantation; also used for bone-marrow, heart-lung, and pancreas transplants; also prescribed for patchy hair loss, rheumatoid arthritis, aplastic anemia, atopic dermatitis, Behçet's disease, cirrhosis of the liver, ulcerative colitis, dermatomyositis, eye symptoms of Graves' disease, insulin-dependent diabetes, kidney inflammation, multiple sclerosis (MS), severe psoriasis and psoriasis-related arthritis, myasthenia gravis, pemphigus, sarcoidosis of the lung, and pyoderma gangrenosum. Cyclosporine eye emulsion is prescribed for dry eyes.

General Information

Cyclosporine is used to prevent rejection of transplanted organs. It works by blocking the activity of T-cells, which protect the body against invading microorganisms or foreign substances. Cyclosporine also prevents the production of a substance known as interleukin-II that activates T-cells. In 1995, a new form of cyclosporine called Neoral, a microemulsion, was introduced by its manufacturer. This form is as safe and effective as the original product but is better absorbed into the bloodstream and requires less medication to achieve the same effect. Cyclosporine eye emulsion treats dry eye caused by inflammation of the cornea and tissue that covers the white part of the eye. It reduces inflammation and allows tears to form and flow.

Cautions and Warnings

Cyclosporine should be prescribed only by doctors experienced in immunosuppressive therapy and the care of organ-transplant patients. Sandimmune is always used with corticosteroid drugs like prednisone. Neoral and Gengraf have been used with a corticosteroid and azathioprine, an immune suppressant. When **combined with other immune suppressants,** cyclosporine must be used with great care because oversuppression of the immune system may lead to lymphoma or extreme susceptibility to infection.

Sandimmune, the original oral form of cyclosporine, is poorly absorbed into the bloodstream; it must be taken in a dosage that is 3 times greater than the injectable dosage. People taking this drug by mouth for a long period of time should have their blood checked for cyclosporine levels so that the dosage may be adjusted if necessary. Since more of both Gengraf and Neoral is absorbed into the blood you will probably need less of it. Do not substitute Neoral or Gengraf for Sandimmune; they are not equivalent to each other.

Cyclosporine causes kidney toxicosis (kidney poisoning)—different from transplant rejection—in 25–35% of people taking it to prevent organ rejection. Mild symptoms usually start after about 2 or 3 months of treatment. Reducing drug dosage may control this effect. In one study, clonidine skin patches used before and after surgery decreased toxic risks to the kidney.

Liver toxicosis is seen in about 5% of transplant patients taking cyclosporine. It usually appears in the first month and may be controlled by reducing dosage.

Convulsions may develop, especially in people also taking **high dosages of corticosteroids**. Other nervous system side effects are listed below (see "Possible Side Effects").

In one study, cyclosporine increased cholesterol and other blood-fat levels. It is not known how this affects people who take the drug on a long-term basis.

There is conflicting information on how cyclosporine affects blood sugar. **Kidney-transplant patients** taking the drug have developed insulin-dependent diabetes, which is related to the dosage of cyclosporine and reverses itself when you stop taking the drug. On the other hand, cyclosporine preserves the function of insulin-producing cells in the pancreas and has allowed many insulin-dependent diabetics to live without taking insulin.

Live vaccines should not be given to people taking cyclosporine.

Do not use cyclosporine eye drops if you have an eye infection.

Small amounts of cyclosporine eye emulsion may be absorbed into the bloodstream, but the risk of body-wide side effects is small.

Possible Side Effects

▼ Most common: Cyclosporine is known to be toxic to the kidneys. Your doctor will carefully monitor your kidney function while you are taking it. Other side effects are high blood pressure, increased hair growth, infection, and enlargement of the gums. Lymphoma may develop in people whose immune systems are excessively suppressed.

▼ Less common: tremors, cramps, acne, brittle hair or fingernails, convulsions, headache, confusion, diarrhea, nausea or vomiting, tingling in the hands or feet, facial flushing, reduced white-blood-cell and platelet counts, sinus inflammation, swollen and painful male breasts, drug allergy (symptoms include rash, itching, hives, and breathing difficulties), conjunctivitis (pinkeye), fluid retention and swelling, ringing or buzzing in the ears, hearing loss, high blood sugar, and muscle pain.

▼ Rare: blood in the urine, heart attack, itching, anxiety, depression, lethargy, weakness, mouth sores, difficulty swallowing, intestinal bleeding, constipation, pancreas inflammation, night sweats, chest pain, joint pain, visual disturbances, and weight loss. Contact your doctor if you experience any side effect not listed above.

Cyclosporine Eye Drops

▼ Most common: burning sensation.

▼ Less common: red-eye, discharge from the eye, overflow of tears, eye pain, a feeling of something in the eye, itching, stinging, and visual disturbances, usually blurring.

Drug Interactions

• Cyclosporine should be used carefully with other kidney-toxic drugs including nonsteroidal anti-inflammatory drugs (NSAIDs) such as ibuprofen, naproxen, and sulindac; ciprofloxacin; gentamicin; tobramycin; vancomycin; trimethoprim-sulfamethoxazole; melphalan; amphotericin B; ketoconazole; azapropazon; colchicine; diclofenac; cimetidine; ranitidine; and tacrolimus.

• Drugs that may increase blood levels of cyclosporine include contraceptive drugs; amiodarone; diltiazem; nicardipine;

verapamil; fluconazole; itraconazole; ketoconazole; azithromycin; clarithromycin; erythromycin; quinapristin and dalfopristin; methylprednisolone—this combination also causes convulsions; allopurinol; bromocriptine; colchicine; imatinib; danazol; and metoclopramide. With ketoconazole, your doctor may use this drug interaction to reduce your cyclosporine dosage.

- Drugs that decrease cyclosporine levels and may lead to organ rejection include octreotide, orlistat, sulfinpyrazone, ticlopidine, terbinafine, nafcillin, rifampin, carbamazepine, phenobarbital, phenytoin, and St. John's wort. Rifabutin may also decrease concentrations of cyclosporine and should be used with caution.

- Cyclosporine interferes with the body's ability to clear digoxin, prednisolone, and statin drugs. People taking any of these drugs who start on cyclosporine must have their drug dosage reduced.

- Combining cyclosporine and nifedipine may lead to gum overgrowth.

- Cyclosporine increases blood potassium. Excessive blood-potassium levels may be reached if cyclosporine is taken with enalapril, lisinopril, a potassium-sparing diuretic such as spironolactone, salt substitutes, potassium supplements, or high potassium—low sodium—food.

- Psoriasis patients using other immunosuppressant drugs or receiving radiation therapy should not take cyclosporine due to the danger of infection.

- Cyclosporine prevents the normal body response to live vaccines. People taking cyclosporine should be vaccinated only after specific discussions with their doctors. You must wait for a period of several months to several years after stopping the medication before vaccination may be considered again.

Food Interactions

Cyclosporine may be taken with food if it upsets your stomach. For optimal effectiveness, avoid eating a fatty meal within half an hour of taking Neoral.

You may mix Neoral in a glass—not a paper or plastic cup—with room-temperature orange or apple juice or chocolate milk to make it taste better. Do not drink grapefruit juice because it speeds the breakdown of cyclosporine. Drink immediately after mixing, then put more juice or chocolate milk in the glass and drink it to be sure that the entire dose has been taken. Neoral should not be taken with unflavored milk because it may be unpalatable.

Usual Dose

In general, the usual dosage of Neoral is lower than Sandimmune, but dosage must be individualized for you by your doctor. Do not substitute one brand for the other.

Sandimmune

Adult: The usual oral dosage of cyclosporine is 6–8 mg per lb. of body weight a day. The first dose, typically 15 mg per lb., is given 4–12 hours before the transplant operation or immediately after surgery. This dosage is slowly reduced to 11–22 mg per lb. of body weight.

Child: Similar dosages are usually prescribed, but because children tend to release the drug from their bodies faster than adults, larger and more frequent doses may be needed.

Neoral and Gengraf

Adult: In newly transplanted patients, the usual oral dosage of Neoral is 3–4 mg per lb. of body weight a day divided into 2 doses. The initial oral dose of Gengraf is the same as for Sandimmune. The first dose is given 4–12 hours before the transplant operation or immediately after surgery. This dosage is continued after the operation for 1–2 weeks and then slowly reduced to maintain a target amount of cyclosporine in the body. Dosage may vary according to the organ transplanted.

In people being treated for rheumatoid arthritis or psoriasis, the initial dose of Neoral and Gengraf is 1.13 mg per lb. of body weight increased gradually to a maximum of 1.8 mg per lb. of body weight.

Child: Similar dosages are usually prescribed but, because children tend to release the drug from their bodies faster than adults, larger and more frequent doses may be needed.

Cyclosporine Eye Emulsion

One drop in the affected eye(s) every 12 hours. Before using, rotate and turn the vial over a few times until you have a uniform, white, opaque fluid inside. If you use artificial tears, allow 15 minutes between products. Discard the open vial immediately after use.

Overdosage

Overdose victims may be expected to develop side effects and symptoms of extreme immunosuppression. Induce vomiting with ipecac syrup—available at any pharmacy—which is recommended up to 2 hours after the overdose was taken. Call your doctor or local poison control center before inducing vomiting. If you must go to a hospital emergency room, ALWAYS bring the prescription bottle or container.

Special Information

Call your doctor at the first sign of fever; sore throat; tiredness; weakness; nervousness; unusual bleeding or bruising; tender or swollen gums; convulsions; irregular heartbeat; confusion; numbness or tingling of your hands, feet, or lips; breathing difficulties; severe stomach pain with nausea; or blood in the urine. Other side effects such as shaking or trembling of the hands, increased hair growth, acne, headache, leg cramps, nausea, or vomiting are less serious but should be brought to your doctor's attention, particularly if they are bothersome or persistent.

Maintain good dental hygiene while taking cyclosporine and use extra care when brushing and flossing because the drug increases your risk of oral infection. Cyclosporine may also cause swollen gums. See your dentist regularly.

Continue taking your medication as long as your doctor prescribes it. Do not stop taking it without your doctor's knowledge. If you cannot take one of the oral forms, cyclosporine can be given by injection.

Do not keep either brand of the oral liquid in the refrigerator. After the bottle is opened, use the medication within 2 months. At temperatures below 68°F, Neoral can form a gel and a light sediment can form in Sandimmune. These do not affect the potency of either product. They can still be used and are effective.

If you forget a dose, take it as soon as you remember if it is within 12 hours of your regular dose. If not, skip the dose you forgot and continue with your regular schedule. Do not take a double dose.

For cyclosporine eye emulsion, each small plastic container is meant to be used once and then thrown away along with any remaining medication. Do not allow the tip of the disposable vial to touch the eye or any surface, as this may contaminate the emulsion.

Patients with decreased tear production typically should not wear contact lenses. But those that do must remove them before using cyclosporine eye emulsion. Lenses may be reinserted 15 minutes after using the medicine.

Special Populations

Pregnancy/Breast-feeding: In animal studies cyclosporine damages the fetus. Though a small number of pregnant women have taken cyclosporine without major problems, it is recommended that pregnant women avoid cyclosporine. When this drug is considered crucial by your doctor, its potential benefits must be carefully weighed against its risks.

Cyclosporine passes into breast milk. Nursing mothers who must take cyclosporine should use infant formula.

Seniors: Due to decreased kidney function, seniors are more susceptible to kidney toxicosis.

Cymbalta   *see Venlafaxine, page 1200*

Generic Name

Darunavir   (dah-ROON-uh-vere)

Brand Name

Prezista

Type of Drug

Protease inhibitor.

Prescribed For

Advanced human immunodeficiency virus (HIV) infection that has not responded to other protease inhibitors.

General Information

Part of the multidrug "cocktail" responsible for important gains in the fight against acquired immunodefiency syndrome (AIDS), darunavir is a member of a group of anti-HIV drugs called protease inhibitors. These drugs work at the end of the HIV reproduction process, when proteins are "cut" into strands of exactly the correct size to duplicate HIV. An enzyme known as protease cuts the protein. Protease inhibitors prevent the mature HIV virus from being formed by inhibiting this cutting process. Proteins that are cut to the wrong length or that remain uncut are inactive.

Darunavir must be taken with a low dose of ritonavir, another protease inhibitor, to extend the action of darunavir in the body.

Without ritonavir, darunavir would be eliminated too rapidly to be effective. Darunavir must also be accompanied by at least 2 other AIDS antivirals. Protease inhibitors revolutionized HIV treatment because, when taken in combination, they reduce the amount of HIV virus in the bloodstream to levels that are often undetectable by current methods—CD4 (immune system) cell counts and viral load (amount of virus in the blood) measurements. Multiple-drug therapy has transformed HIV from a fatal disease to a manageable chronic illness.

Cautions and Warnings

Do not take darunavir if you are **allergic** or **sensitive** to any of its ingredients, to sulfa drugs, or to ritonavir.

Darunavir can cause a severe or life-threatening rash.

If a serious toxic reaction occurs while taking darunavir, you should stop the drug until your doctor can determine the cause or until the reaction resolves itself. Then treatment can be resumed.

This drug is primarly broken down in the liver. Use caution if you have moderate to severe **liver disease.**

Darunavir may raise your blood sugar, worsen your **diabetes,** or bring out latent diabetes. People with diabetes who take darunavir may need the dosage of their antidiabetes medication adjusted.

People with **hemophilia** may be more likely to bleed while taking a protease inhibitor.

The HIV virus may become resistant to darunavir or other protease inhibitors. For this reason it is essential that you take darunavir exactly according to your doctor's directions.

Protease inhibitors can cause body fat redistribution, including increased fat deposits in the upper back and neck, breast and around the back, chest, and stomach. Fat may be lost from the legs, arms, and face. Some people with HIV and a history of an opportunistic infection may develop signs and symptoms of the infection soon after anti-HIV treatment is started. This is called immune reconstitution syndrome.

Darunavir is involved in many drug interactions. Check with your doctor before adding anything new to your treatment program.

Possible Side Effects

▼ Most common: diarrhea, nausea, headache, and common cold symptoms.

Possible Side Effects *(continued)*

▼ Less common: vomiting, abdominal pain, and constipation.
▼ Rare: Rare side effects can occur in almost any part of the body. Contact your doctor if you experience any side effect not listed above.

Drug Interactions

- Do not take any of the following medicines with darunavir + ritonavir: astemizole, terfenidine, ergot-based drugs for migraine headache, cisapride, pimozide, midazolam, or triazolam. Mixing these drugs with darunavir + ritonavir can result in very high blood levels and serious side effects.
- Carbamazepine, phenobarbital, phenytoin, rifampin, and St. John's wort can substantially reduce blood levels of darunavir. Do not mix these medicines.
- Lopinavir + ritonavir and saquinavir can significantly reduce blood levels of darunavir. Darunavir significantly increases blood levels of lopinavir + ritonavir. Do not mix these drugs.
- Mixing darunavir with indinavir can increase blood levels of both drugs.
- Darunavir + ritonavir does not appear to affect blood levels of atazanavir, nor does atazanavir appear to affect blood levels of darunavir + ritonavir. It may be possible to combine these two protease inhibitors.
- Taking darunavir with tenofovir can increase blood levels of both drugs. These drugs can be combined with no dose adjustments, though it is necessary to watch carefully for kidney damage related to tenofovir.
- Darunavir can increase blood levels of efavirenz and efavirenz reduces darunavir levels. These medicines should be mixed with caution.
- Darunavir increases nevirapine blood levels but the combination can be taken with no dose adjustment.
- If didanosine is a part of a darunavir + ritonavir treatment program, it must be taken on an empty stomach, 1 hour before or 2 hours after darunavir + ritonavir, which should be taken with food.
- Darunavir increases blood levels of clarithromycin, itraconazole, and ketoconazole. Daily dosage of itraconazole and ketoconazole should not exceed 200 mg. No clarithromycin

adjustment is necessary in people with normal kidney function.

- Darunavir + ritonavir may reduce voriconazole levels in the blood. Do not mix these medicines.
- Darunavir + ritonavir can increase rifabutin levels in the bloodstream. Rifabutin can also reduce darunavir levels in the bloodstream. If rifabutin is mixed with darunavir + ritonavir, the rifabutin dose should be 150 mg every other day.
- Caution should be exercised when combining darunavir + ritonavir with calcium channel blockers such as felodipine, nifedipine, and nicardipine.
- Darunavir increases blood levels of the heart antiarrhythmic drugs bepridil, lidocaine, and quinidine. These drugs should be used together with caution and only in situations where blood levels of the heart drugs can be monitored regularly.
- Darunavir + ritonavir can reduce blood levels of warfarin. It is necessary to monitor warfarin levels while taking this combination.
- Darunavir + ritonavir can raise blood levels of the tricyclic antidepressant desipramine and the tetracyclic antidepressant trazodone. Dosage reduction is recommended.
- Darunavir + ritonavir may reduce blood levels of the SSRI antidepressants sertraline and paroxetine. SSRI doses may have to be increased to account for this effect.
- Darunavir + ritonavir can drastically increase the blood levels of some statin-type cholesterol-lowering drugs, substantially increasing the risk of statin side effects. Simvastatin, pravastatin, and lovastatin should not be mixed with darunavir + ritonavir. It is also possible to take darunavir + ritonavir with atorvastatin, although it can increase the level of atorvastatin in the bloodstream. If atorvastatin is prescribed, it is best to begin with 10 mg a day and slowly increase the dose as necessary. Little is known about how darunavir + ritonavir affects rosuvastatin. The safest statin to take with darunavir + ritonavir is fluvastatin.
- Darunavir + ritonavir can increase blood levels of inhaled corticosteroids dexamethasone and fluticasone, the anti-rejection drugs cyclosporine, tacrolimus, and sirolimus. The corticosteroids reduce darunavir blood levels, interfering with its effectiveness.
- Darunavir + ritonavir can reduce methadone levels in the bloodstream. Methadone dose adjustment may be needed.

- Darunavir + ritonavir reduces the effectiveness of some contraceptive drugs by decreasing the amount of the hormones ethinyl estradiol and norethindrone in the bloodstream. Women mixing these medicines should use additional contraceptive measures (e.g., condoms).
- Protease inhibitors may drastically increase blood levels of erectile dysfunction drugs sildenafil, vardenafil, and tadalafil, increasing the risk of side effects including low blood pressure, visual changes, and persistent, painful erection.
- Dexamethasone may reduce blood levels of darunavir.

Food Interactions

Take darunavir with food. The amount of darunavir absorbed into the blood is vastly reduced when it is taken on an empty stomach, thus negating its antiviral effects.

Usual Dose

Adult: 600 mg (2 300-mg tablets) with 100 mg ritonavir twice a day. Do not chew these tablets.

Child: not recommended.

Overdosage

Little is known about the effects of darunavir overdose, but 3200 mg of darunavir has been given to study volunteers with no adverse effects. Call your local poison center or hospital emergency room for more information. If you take the victim to a hospital emergency room, ALWAYS bring the prescription bottle or container.

Special Information

Darunavir is not a cure for HIV. It will not prevent you from transmitting the HIV virus to another person; you must still practice safe sex. You may still develop opportunistic infections or other complications associated with advanced HIV disease.

The long-term effects of this drug are not known.

It is imperative for you to take this medication exactly according to your doctor's instructions. Do not skip any doses. Skipping doses of darunavir increases the risk that you will become resistant to the drug. If you forget a dose of darunavir or ritonavir and remember within 6 hours, take it as soon as you remember and then continue with your regular schedule. If 6 hours have passed since the time when you should have taken your medicine, skip the forgotten dose and take your next dose at the regular time. Do not take a double dose.

Special Populations

Pregnancy/Breast-feeding: Animal studies with darunavir reveal no damage to the fetus, but there are no data on how this drug affects pregnant women. Darunavir should only be used during pregnancy after carefully weighing its potential benefits against its risks.

It is not known if darunavir passes into breast milk. Nursing mothers with HIV should use infant formula, regardless of whether they take this drug, to avoid transmitting the virus.

Seniors: Seniors can take this drug without special precaution.

Generic Name

Deferasirox (deh-fur-ASS-sih-rox)

Brand Name

Exjade

Type of Drug

Iron chelating agent.

Prescribed For

Chronic iron overload.

General Information

Deferasirox binds with iron in stored in the liver. It can also bind small amounts of zinc and copper but the importance of these effects are not known. Almost ¾ of every dose is absorbed into the bloodstream. Most of the drug is broken down in the liver and passes out of the body in the feces. Women clear this drug from their bodies 17.5% slower than men, but this has not affected how it is used or the doses given.

Cautions and Warnings

Do not take deferasirox if you are **allergic** or **sensitive** to any of its ingredients. Most reactions occur within the first month of treatment.

People with **liver disease** should have monthly blood tests while taking deferasirox.

Kidney failure has developed in people taking deferasirox with fatal results in some cases. People with or those who are at risk of kidney failure should have routine kidney monitoring while taking this medication. People who are at risk for kidney failure includes seniors, those with kidney disease, and people taking medicines that affect kidney function. Dose adjustment may be needed.

Deferasirox has been associated with potentially severe reduced white-blood-cell and platelet counts, usually in people with pre-existing **blood disorders**.

Rarely, deferasirox has caused hearing loss and eye problems. You should have a full hearing and eye exam before starting on this drug and once a year thereafter.

Skin rash can occur with this medicine. If it is severe, the drug may have to be temporarily stopped. It may be restarted at a lower dosage.

Possible Side Effects

▼ Most common: fever, headache, abdominal pain, cough, sore throat, nasal irritation, diarrhea, flu symptoms, nausea, and vomiting.

▼ Common: respiratory infections, bronchitis, runny nose, rash, upper abdominal pain, joint pain, back pain, tonsillitis, and ear infection.

▼ Less common: itching.

▼ Rare: stomach pain, swelling in the arms or legs, sleep disorder, skin color changes, dizziness, anxiety, gallstones, fatigue, early cataract and hearing loss, some visual haziness, and other eye disorders. Contact your doctor if you experience anything unusual.

Drug Interactions

● Do not mix antacids containing aluminum with deferasirox. They can prevent it from being absorbed.

Food Interactions

This drug should be taken at the same time every day on an empty stomach, 30 minutes before eating.

Usual Dose

Adult and Child (age 2 and over): 9–13.6 mg per lb. of body weight once a day. Dose adjustments will be made according to your response. See "Special Information" for a specific instructions on how to take these tablets.

Overdosage

Large doses of 2–3 times the prescribed amount taken for several weeks with no adverse effects have occurred. Overdose symptoms include hepatitis (mild fever, muscle or joint aches, nausea, vomiting, appetite loss, slight abdominal pain, diarrhea, and fatigue) and some drug side effects. Take the victim to a hospital emergency room for treatment because the heart may be affected. ALWAYS bring the prescription bottle or container.

Special Information

Call your doctor at once if you develop a severe skin rash.

You must have regular vision and hearing tests while taking deferasirox.

Deferasirox tablets should not be chewed or swallowed whole. They must first be mixed completely in ½–1 glass of water, orange juice, or apple juice. The tablet will not dissolve but tablet particles will become suspended in the liquid. Drink the resulting suspension immediately. If there is anything left in the glass after drinking the suspension, add a small amount of liquid, mix it with the remaining tablet particles and drink it.

This drug can cause dizziness. Be cautious while driving, operating machinery, or doing anything that requires intense concentration.

If you forget a dose, take it as soon as you remember. If it is almost time for the next dose, skip the one you forgot and continue with your regular schedule. Do not take a double dose.

Special Populations

Pregnancy/Breast-feeding: There are no studies of ranolazine in pregnant women or of its effect on the developing fetus. Pregnant women should take this drug only if its potential benefits outweigh the risks.

This drug may pass into breast milk. Nursing mothers should consider using infant formula.

Seniors: Seniors may experience more drug side effects than younger adults due to greater chances of reduced kidney, liver, and heart function; other diseases; or drug side effects.

Depakote see **Valproic Acid,** page 1194

Generic Name

Desmopressin (dez-moe-PRES-in) Ⓖ

Brand Names
DDAVP   Stimate
Minirin

Type of Drug
Pituitary hormone replacement.

Prescribed For
Nighttime bed-wetting and diabetes insipidus (central or cranial diabetes); also used to control bleeding in certain forms of hemophilia A and von Willebrand's disease.

General Information
Desmopressin acetate is a synthetic version of antidiuretic hormone (ADH). When ADH is lacking, the body has difficulty retaining fluid. People lacking ADH experience excessive thirst, increased urination, and dehydration; desmopressin controls these symptoms. When used for nighttime bed-wetting, desmopressin should be used in conjunction with behavioral or other non-drug therapies.

Cautions and Warnings
Do not take desmopressin if you are **allergic** or **sensitive** to any of its ingredients.

People, especially **children** and **seniors** and people with **cystic fibrosis** and **electrolyte imbalances,** should only drink enough fluid to satisfy their thirst while taking desmopressin because of the risk of water intoxication, which can result in seizures that could lead to coma. People with **coronary artery disease, heart disease,** or **high blood pressure** should use this drug with caution.

Heart attacks and **strokes** after treatment with desmopressin have been reported in people at risk for them, but there is no definite link to desmopressin use.

People using desmopressin should have their urine checked regularly by their doctor. Your doctor should also check for nasal swelling, congestion, and scarring.

Possible Side Effects

▼ Rare: slight increases in blood pressure, loss of sodium, water intoxication (symptoms include coma, confusion, drowsiness, continuing headache, decreased urination, rapid weight gain, and seizures), edema, stomach or abdominal cramps, nausea, redness or flushing of the skin, passing headaches, vulvar pain, and stuffy or runny nose. Contact your doctor if you experience any side effect not listed above.

Drug Interactions

- Desmopressin may increase the effects of other drugs that raise blood pressure. This only happens with large dosages.
- Chlorpropamide and carbamazepine may increase the effects of desmopressin.

Food Interactions

None known.

Usual Dose

Nasal Solution—Nighttime Bed-Wetting
Adult and Child (age 6 and over): 20 mcg (0.2 mL) at bedtime.
Child (under age 6): not recommended.

Nasal Solution—Diabetes Insipidus
Adult: 0.1–0.4 mL a day in 1–3 doses.
Child (age 3 months–12 years): 0.05–0.3 mL a day in 1–2 doses.

Tablets—Nighttime Bed-wetting
Adult and Child (age 6 and over): Begin with 0.2 mg at bedtime, adjusting to individual need up to 0.6 mg.
Child (under age 6): not recommended.

Tablets—Diabetes Insipidus
Adult: Begin with 0.05 mg twice a day. Daily dosage should be increased according to individual need, up to 1.2 mg a day divided into 2–3 doses.
Child (age 4 and over): Begin with 0.05 mg and adjust according to individual need.
Child (under age 4): not recommended.

Overdosage

Symptoms include headache, difficulty breathing, abdominal cramps, nausea, and facial flushing. Call your doctor or a hospital emergency room if you suspect an overdose. Because there is no known antidote to desmopressin, your dosage may be temporarily reduced until overdose symptoms subside. If you seek treatment, ALWAYS bring the prescription bottle or container.

Special Information

Call your doctor if you develop headache, breathing difficulties, heartburn, nausea, abdominal or stomach cramps, or vulvar pain.

The Stimate Nasal Solution spray pump and Minirin spray must be primed before its first use. To prime the pump, press down 4 times. Stimate delivers 25 doses per bottle. Throw away the bottle after 25 doses have been used, because anything remaining after the 25th dose is likely to deliver less drug than is needed.

If you forget a dose of desmopressin, take it as soon as you remember. If you don't remember until your next dose, skip the forgotten dose and continue with your regular schedule. Do not take a double dose.

Special Populations

Pregnancy/Breast-feeding: The safety of using desmopressin during pregnancy is not known, though it has been used to treat diabetes insipidus in pregnant women without apparent harm to the fetus. When this drug is considered crucial by your doctor, its potential benefits must be carefully weighed against its risks.

Desmopressin may pass into breast milk. Nursing mothers who must use this drug should use infant formula.

Seniors: Seniors should avoid drinking too much fluid while taking desmopressin.

Detrol LA   see *Tolterodine*, page 1144

Generic Name

Diazepam (dye-AZ-uh-pam) G

Brand Names

Diastat	Valium
Diazepam Intensol	Valrelease

The information in this profile also applies to the following drugs:

Generic Ingredient: Lorazepam Ⓖ

Ativan   Lorazepam Intensol

Generic Ingredient: Oxazepam Ⓖ

Type of Drug

Benzodiazepine sedative.

Prescribed For

Anxiety, tension, fatigue, agitation (particularly due to alcohol withdrawal), muscle spasm, and seizures; also prescribed for irritable bowel syndrome and panic attacks.

General Information

Diazepam and other benzodiazepines directly affect the brain. They can relax you and make you more tranquil or sleepy, or they can slow nervous system transmissions in such a way as to act as an anticonvulsant.

Cautions and Warnings

Do not take diazepam if you know you are **allergic** or **sensitive** to any of its ingredients or to another benzodiazepine drug, including clonazepam.

Diazepam can aggravate narrow-angle **glaucoma,** but you may take it if you have open-angle glaucoma and are receiving therapy for it.

Other conditions in which diazepam should be avoided are severe **depression,** severe **lung disease, sleep apnea** (intermittent cessation of breathing during sleep), **liver disease, drunkenness,** and **kidney disease**. In all of these conditions, the depressive effects of diazepam may be enhanced or could be detrimental to your overall condition.

Diazepam should not be taken by **psychotic patients**. It is not effective for them and can trigger unusual excitement, stimulation, and rage.

Diazepam is not intended for more than 3–4 months of continuous use. Your condition should be reassessed before continuing your medication beyond that time.

Diazepam may be addictive. It should be used with caution in people with a history of **drug dependence**.

Drug withdrawal may develop if you stop taking it after only 4 weeks of regular use but is more likely after longer use. It may start with anxiety and progress to tingling in the hands or feet, sensitivity to bright light, sleep disturbances, cramps, tremors, muscle tension or twitching, poor concentration, flu-like symptoms, fatigue, appetite loss, sweating, and changes in mental state. Your dosage should always be reduced gradually to prevent drug withdrawal symptoms.

Possible Side Effects

▼ Most common: mild drowsiness during the first few days of therapy. Weakness and confusion may occur, especially in seniors and in those who are sickly. If these effects persist, contact your doctor.

▼ Less common: depression, lethargy, disorientation, headache, inactivity, slurred speech, stupor, dizziness, tremors, constipation, dry mouth, nausea, inability to control urination, sexual difficulties, irregular menstrual cycle, changes in heart rhythm, low blood pressure, fluid retention, blurred or double vision, itching, rash, hiccups, nervousness, hysteria, psychosis, inability to fall asleep, and occasional liver dysfunction. If you have any of these symptoms, stop taking the drug and contact your doctor at once.

▼ Rare: Rare side effects can affect your heart, stomach and intestines, urinary tract, blood, muscles, and joints. Contact your doctor if you experience any side effect not listed above.

Drug Interactions

- Diazepam is a central-nervous-system depressant. Avoid alcohol, other sedatives, narcotics, barbiturates, monoamine oxidase inhibitor antidepressants, antihistamines, and antidepressants. Taking diazepam with these drugs may lead to excessive depression, drowsiness, or difficulty breathing.
- Smoking may reduce diazepam's effectiveness by increasing the rate at which it is broken down by the body.
- Effects of diazepam may be prolonged when taken with cimetidine, contraceptive drugs, disulfiram, fluoxetine, isoniazid, ketoconazole, rifampin, metoprolol, probenecid, propoxyphene, propranolol, and valproic acid.
- Theophylline may reduce the sedative effects of diazepam.
- If you take antacids, separate them from your diazepam dose by at least 1 hour to prevent them from interfering with the passage of diazepam into the bloodstream.

- Diazepam may increase blood levels of digoxin and the chances for digoxin toxicity.
- Levodopa + carbidopa's effects may be decreased if it is taken with diazepam.
- Combining diazepam and phenytoin may increase phenytoin blood concentrations and the risk of phenytoin toxicity.

Food Interactions

Diazepam is best taken on an empty stomach, but it may be taken with food if it upsets your stomach.

Usual Dose

Solution or Tablets

Adult: 2–40 mg a day. Dosage must be adjusted to individual response for maximum effect. In seniors, less of the drug is usually required to control tension and anxiety.

Child (6 months and over): 1–2.5 mg 3 or 4 times a day; more may be needed to control anxiety and tension.

Child (under 6 months): not recommended.

Rectal Gel

Adult and Child (age 12 and over): 0.09 mg per lb. of body weight. Approximate dosage: 5 mg if 31–60 lbs., 10 mg if 61–110 lbs., 15 mg if 111–165 lbs., or 20 mg if 166–244 lbs.

Child (age 6–11): 0.14 mg per lb. of body weight. Approximate dosage: 5 mg if 22–40 lbs., 10 mg if 41–82 lbs., 15 mg if 83–121 lbs., or 20 mg if 122–163 lbs.

Child (age 2–5): 0.23 mg per lb. of body weight. Approximate dosage: 5 mg if 13–24 lbs., 10 mg if 25–49 lbs., 15 mg if 50–73 lbs., or 20 mg if 74–97 lbs.

An extra 2.5 mg of the rectal gel may be given if a more precise dosage is needed or as a partial replacement for people who do not retain the full dosage after it is first inserted rectally.

Overdosage

Symptoms of overdose include confusion, sleepiness, poor coordination, lack of response to pain, loss of reflexes, shallow breathing, low blood pressure, and coma. The victim should be taken to a hospital emergency room. ALWAYS bring the prescription bottle or container.

Special Information

Diazepam can cause tiredness, drowsiness, inability to concentrate, or similar symptoms. Be careful if you are driving, operating machinery, or performing other activities that require concentration.

People taking diazepam for more than 3 or 4 months at a time may develop drug withdrawal reactions if the medication is stopped suddenly (see "Cautions and Warnings"). Do not stop taking diazepam or decrease the dosage without first consulting your doctor.

If you forget a dose of diazepam, take it as soon as you remember. If it is almost time for your next dose, skip the one you forgot and continue with your regular schedule. Do not take a double dose.

Special Populations

Pregnancy/Breast-feeding: Diazepam may cause birth defects if taken during the first 3 months of pregnancy. Avoid taking any benzodiazepine if you are or might be pregnant.

Diazepam may pass into breast milk. Nursing mothers who must take this drug should use infant formula.

Seniors: Seniors, especially those with liver or kidney disease, are more sensitive to the effects of diazepam and generally require smaller doses to achieve the same effect.

Generic Name

Dicyclomine (dih-SYE-kloe-meen) Ⓖ

Brand Names

Bemote	Dilomine
Bentyl	Di-Spaz
Byclomine	Or-Tyl
Dibent	

Type of Drug

Antispasmodic and anticholinergic.

Prescribed For

Irritable bowel, spastic colon, and similar digestive problems; also prescribed for colic in children over age 6 months.

General Information

Dicyclomine hydrochloride has been used for many years to calm "nervous stomach." It and other anticholinergics work by blocking the effects of the neurohormone acetylcholine in the gastrointestinal (GI) tract. This reduces the mobility of the GI tract and slows the production of enzymes and other secretions.

Cautions and Warnings

Do not take dicyclomine if you are **allergic** or **sensitive** to any of its ingredients.

Dicyclomine should not be used by those with **obstructive disease of the GI or urinary tract, severe ulcerative colitis, reflux esophagitis, acute bleeding with unstable heart function, myasthenia gravis,** or **glaucoma.**

Dicyclomine should not be used in **infants less than age 6 months** or by **breastfeeding mothers.**

This drug should be used with caution if you have **heart disease, Down's syndrome, spastic paralysis, reduced mobility of the stomach and lower esophagus, fever, urinary difficulties, enlarged prostate, hiatal hernia, intestinal paralysis, kidney or liver disease, rapid heartbeat, hyperthyroidism (overactive thyroid gland), high blood pressure,** or **ulcerative colitis.**

Dicyclomine reduces your ability to sweat and may lead to heat exhaustion and heatstroke, which can be life-threatening. Avoid extended heavy exercise and limit your exposure to high temperatures.

Anticholinergenic psychosis has been reported by those taking anticholinergenics, but it usually resolves within 24 hours after discontinuation of the drug.

Possible Side Effects

▼ Common: dry mouth, dizziness, blurred vision, nausea, and lightheadedness.

▼ Less common: drowsiness, weakness, nervousness, constipation, and decreased sweating.

Possible Side Effects (continued)

▼ Rare: drug allergy (symptoms include rash, itching, hives, and breathing difficulties), confusion, eye pain, dizziness when rising quickly from a sitting or lying position, a bloated feeling, difficult or painful urination, headache, memory loss, and vomiting. Contact your doctor if you experience any side effect not listed above.

Drug Interactions

- Antacids containing calcium or magnesium, citrates, sodium bicarbonate, and carbonic anhydrase inhibitor drugs may increase dicyclomine's therapeutic effect and side effects.
- Combining dicyclomine with other anticholinergic drugs including atropine, belladonna, clidinium, glycopyrrolate, hyoscyamine, isopropamide, propantheline, and scopolamine may intensify side effects.
- Dicyclomine may reduce stomach acidity and blood levels of oral ketoconazole (an antifungal).
- Dicyclomine may decrease the therapeutic effects of antiglaucoma medications. Taking dicyclomine with corticosteroids used to treat glaucoma may be hazardous.
- Dicyclomine may counteract the effect of metoclopramide in reducing nausea and vomiting.
- Taking dicyclomine with a narcotic pain reliever may cause severe constipation.
- Taking this or any drug that slows the movement of stomach and intestinal muscles with a potassium chloride supplement —especially one in wax-matrix tablet form—may lead to excessive irritation of the stomach.
- Combining dicyclomine with amantadine, certain drugs to control heart rhythm, antihistamines, nitrates or nitrites, may increase dicyclomine side effects.
- Dicyclomine may increase the effects of atenolol and digoxin.
- Phenothiazine drugs, monoamine oxidase inhibitor antidepressants, benzodiazepines, and tricyclic antidepressants may increase side effects of dicyclomine. The effectiveness of phenothiazines to control psychotic symptoms may be decreased.

Food Interactions

Take dicyclomine on an empty stomach, a half hour before or 2 hours after a meal.

Usual Dose

Adult: 80–160 mg a day in 4 divided doses. Seniors should receive the lowest possible dosage and increase only as needed.

Child (age 2 and over): 5–10 mg 3–4 times a day.

Child (age 6 months–2 years): 5–10 mg of syrup 3–4 times a day.

Child (under 6 months): not recommended.

Overdosage

Symptoms include blurred vision; clumsiness; confusion; breathing difficulties; dizziness; drowsiness; dry mouth, nose, or throat; rapid heartbeat; fever; hallucinations; weakness; slurred speech; excitement, restlessness, or irritability; warmth; and dry or flushed skin. Take the victim to a hospital emergency room at once. ALWAYS bring the prescription bottle or container.

Special Information

Children taking dicyclomine may be more likely to develop high body temperature in hot weather and other side effects and should be carefully watched for side effects. Dicyclomine should not be given to infants or children unless the doctor decides that its use is absolutely necessary.

Call your doctor if you develop diarrhea, rash, flushing, eye pain, dry mouth, urinary difficulties, constipation, increased sensitivity to light, or any bothersome or persistent side effect.

Brush and floss your teeth regularly while taking this drug. Because dicyclomine may cause dry mouth, you may be more likely to develop cavities or other dental problems. Ice or hard candy may relieve dry mouth.

Constipation may be treated by using a laxative.

Dicyclomine may make you drowsy or tired and cause blurred vision. Be careful when driving or doing any task that requires concentration.

If you forget a dose, take it as soon as you remember. If it is almost time for your next dose, skip the dose you forgot and continue with your regular schedule. Do not take a double dose.

Special Populations

Pregnancy/Breast-feeding: A few cases of human malformation were linked to dicyclomine, but studies have shown that the drug has no effect on the fetus. When this drug is considered crucial by your doctor, its potential benefits must be carefully weighed against its risks.

Dicyclomine can reduce the amount of milk produced. Infants given dicyclomine may faint, go limp, and develop breathing problems and seizures. Nursing mothers who must take this drug should use infant formula.

Seniors: Seniors may be more susceptible to side effects, especially memory loss, changes in mental state, and glaucoma. Seniors may obtain maximum benefit with smaller dosages.

Digitek *see **Digoxin**, below*

Generic Name

Digoxin (dih-JOX-in) Ⓖ

Brand Names

Digitek

Lanoxin

Lanoxicaps

Type of Drug

Cardiac glycoside.

Prescribed For

Congestive heart failure (CHF) and other heart conditions involving a very rapid heartbeat.

General Information

Digoxin works directly on heart muscle. It improves the heart's pumping ability or helps to control its beating rhythm. People with heart failure often develop swelling of the lower legs, feet, and ankles; digoxin improves these symptoms by improving blood circulation. Digoxin is generally used as part of the lifelong treatment of CHF.

Cautions and Warnings

Do not use digoxin if you are **allergic** or **sensitive** to it. Digoxin allergies are rare.

Digoxin should not be used in people with **ventricular fibrillation.**

Digoxin should be used with caution in people with **sick sinus syndrome** or incomplete **AV block**, as it may cause a worsening of these conditions.

Digoxin has been used to treat **obesity**. The risk of fatal heart rhythms associated with such treatment makes it extremely dangerous as weight-loss medication. Many heart disease symptoms may be associated with digoxin. Report any unusual side effects to your doctor at once.

Kidney disease may increase blood levels of digoxin. Your dosage may need adjustment.

Long-term use of digoxin may cause the body to lose potassium, especially since it is generally used in combination with diuretics (agents that increase urination). For this reason, be sure to eat a balanced diet and high-potassium foods—bananas, citrus fruits, melons, and tomatoes.

Digoxin should be used with caution in people with **electrolyte disorders**.

Digoxin requirements vary with **thyroid status**. If you are taking digoxin and your thyroid status changes, your doctor will have to alter your digoxin dosage.

Possible Side Effects

Adult and Senior

▼ Common: dizziness, headache, nausea, and diarrhea.

▼ Less common: appetite loss, vomiting, weakness, apathy, drowsiness, blurred or yellow-tinted vision, seeing halos around bright lights, depression, psychoses, confusion or disorientation, restlessness, hallucinations, delirium, seizure, nerve pain, abnormal heart rhythms, and slow pulse.

▼ Rare: Enlargement of the breasts has been reported after long-term use of digoxin. Contact your doctor if you experience any side effect not listed above.

Child

▼ Children are more likely to develop abnormal heart rhythms before they see yellow or green halos or spots and before they develop nausea, vomiting, diarrhea, or stomach pain. Any abnormal heart rhythms that develop while a child is taking digoxin should be assumed to be a side effect.

Drug Interactions

- Drugs that may increase the effect of digoxin are alprazolam, amiloride aminoglycoside antibiotics, amiodarone, anticholinergic drugs, benzodiazepines, captopril, clarithromycin, diltiazem, diphenoxylate, dipyridamole, erythromycin, esmolol, felodipine, flecainide, hydroxychloroquine, ibuprofen, indomethacin, itraconazole, nifedipine, nitrendipine, omeprazole, propafenone, propantheline, quinidine, quinine, spironolactone, tetracycline, tolbutamide, triamterene, and verapamil.
- Drugs that may decrease blood levels of digoxin include aminoglutethimide, aminoglycosides, aminosalicylic acid, antacids, anti-cancer combinations, antidiabetes medication, antihistamines, barbiturates, cholestyramine, colestipol, cyclosporine, kaolin-pectin mixtures, metoclopramide, oral kanamycin, oral neomycin, oral sulfonylureas, phenylbutazone, phenytoin and related anti-seizure drugs, rifampin, St. John's wort, sucralfate, and sulfasalazine.
- Disopyramide may alter the effects of digoxin, although the exact interaction is not well understood.
- Thiazide and loop diuretics, furosemide, ethacrynic acid, and bumetanide increase digoxin's effect and increase the risk of side effects.
- Spironolactone may increase or decrease the side effects of digoxin; amiloride may reduce the effect of digoxin on the force of heart contraction.
- The effects of digoxin on the heart may be additive to those of ephedrine, epinephrine and other stimulants, beta blockers, calcium salts, procainamide, and rauwolfia drugs.
- Digoxin dosage must be adjusted when it is combined with a thyroid drug.

Food Interactions

These drugs may generally be taken without regard to meals. Taking your medication after a high-fiber meal reduces the amount of drug absorbed into your blood.

Usual Dose

Adult and Child (age 10 and over): starting dosage—known as the digitalizing or loading dose—is about 4–7 mcg per lb. of body weight. Digitalization may also be accomplished with a lower dosage over 7 days. Maintenance dosage—0.125–0.5 mg; it must be corrected for kidney function. For seniors, a lower dosage is required.

Child (under age 10): starting dosage—5–30 mcg per lb. of body weight. Maintenance dosage—20–35% of the starting dosage. Careful measurement of your child's digoxin dosage is crucial to safe and effective treatment.

Overdosage

Adult: Symptoms include appetite loss, nausea, vomiting, diarrhea, headache, weakness, apathy, blurred vision, yellow or green spots or halos before the eyes, yellowing of the skin or whites of the eyes, and changes in heartbeat.

Senior: Vomiting, diarrhea, and eye trouble are frequently seen.

Child: An early sign is a change in heart rhythms.

Call your doctor immediately if any of these symptoms appear. Take the victim to a hospital emergency room. ALWAYS bring the prescription bottle or container.

Special Information

Take each day's dose at the same time of day.

Do not stop taking digoxin without your doctor's knowledge.

Lanoxicaps are better absorbed than tablet forms of digoxin. For this reason, each dose of Lanoxicaps is slightly lower than the corresponding digoxin tablet.

Avoid over-the-counter diet and cold medications containing stimulants.

Call your doctor at once if you develop side effects.

There may by some variation between digoxin tablets from different manufacturers. Do not change drug brands without telling your doctor.

Check your pulse every day—your doctor will teach you how—and call your doctor if it drops below 60 beats per minute.

If you forget a dose and remember at least 12 hours before your next dose, take it right away. If you do not remember until it is less than 12 hours before your next dose, skip the one you forgot and continue with your regular schedule. Do not take a double dose. Call your doctor if you miss a dose for 2 or more days.

Special Populations

Pregnancy/Breast-feeding: Digoxin crosses into the fetal circulation. While digoxin is sometimes used during pregnancy to treat fetal heart disease, women who are or might be pregnant should not take digoxin without their doctor's approval. When your doctor considers this drug crucial, its potential benefits must be carefully weighed against its risks.

Small amounts of digoxin pass into breast milk. Nursing mothers who take digoxin should use infant formula.

Seniors: Seniors are more sensitive to digoxin's effects, especially appetite loss. Seniors with impaired renal function may need lower dosages.

Generic Name

Diltiazem (dil-TYE-uh-zem) Ⓖ

Brand Names

Cardizem	Dilt-CD
Cardizem CD	Diltia XT
Cardizem LA	Diltzac
Cartia XT	Taztia XT
Dilacor XR	Tiazac

Type of Drug

Calcium channel blocker.

Prescribed For

Angina pectoris, chronic stable angina, Raynaud's disease, prevention of second heart attacks, tardive dyskinesia (severe side effects associated with antipsychotic and other drugs), and hypertension (high blood pressure).

General Information

Diltiazem hydrochloride is one of many calcium channel blockers available in the U.S. These drugs block the passage of calcium, an essential factor in muscle contraction, into the heart and smooth muscles. Such blockage of calcium interferes with the contraction of these muscles, which in turn dilates (widens) the veins and vessels that supply blood to them. This dilating effect reduces blood pressure, the amount of oxygen used by the heart muscle, and the risk of blood vessel spasm. Diltiazem is therefore useful in treating not only hypertension but also angina pectoris, a condition related to poor oxygen supply to the heart muscle and characterized by brief attacks of chest pain.

Diltiazem affects the movement of calcium only into muscle cells; it has no effect on calcium in the blood.

Cautions and Warnings

Do not take diltiazem if you are **allergic** or **sensitive** to any of its ingredients.

Diltiazem can slow your heart and interfere with normal electrical conduction. For people with a condition called **sick sinus syndrome,** this can result in temporary heart stoppage.

Diltiazem should not be taken if you are having a **heart attack** or if you have **lung congestion**. Diltiazem should be taken with caution by people with **heart failure** because it can worsen that condition.

Low blood pressure may occur, especially in people also taking a beta blocker.

Studies have shown that people taking calcium channel blockers—usually those taken several times a day, not those taken once daily—have a greater chance of having a heart attack than people taking beta blockers or another medicine for the same purposes. Discuss this with your doctor to be sure you are receiving the best possible treatment.

Diltiazem can cause severe **liver damage** and should be taken with caution if you have had hepatitis or any other liver condition.

Caution should also be exercised if you have a history of **kidney problems,** although no clear tendency toward causing kidney damage is seen with this drug.

Possible Side Effects

▼ Common: dizziness, lightheadedness, weakness, headache, and fluid accumulation in the hands, legs, or feet.

▼ Less common: low blood pressure, fainting, increase or decrease in heart rate, abnormal heart rhythm, heart failure, nervousness, fatigue, nausea, rash, tingling in the hands or feet, hallucinations, temporary memory loss, difficulty sleeping, diarrhea, vomiting, constipation, upset stomach, itching, unusual sensitivity to sunlight, painful or stiff joints, liver inflammation, and increased urination, especially at night.

Drug Interactions

● Diltiazem taken with a beta-blocking drug for hypertension is usually well tolerated, but may lead to heart failure in people with already weakened hearts.

- Calcium channel blockers, including diltiazem, may add to the effects of digoxin. This effect is not observed with any consistency, however, and only affects people with a large amount of digoxin already in their systems.
- Cimetidine and ranitidine increase the amount of diltiazem in the bloodstream and may account for a slight increase in the drug's effect.
- Diltiazem may increase blood levels of cyclosporine, carbamazepine, encainide, and theophylline, and thus increase the chance of side effects from these drugs.
- Diltiazem may cause a decrease in blood lithium levels, possibly undermining lithium's antimanic effect.
- Calcium channel blockers may cause bleeding when taken alone or combined with aspirin.

Food Interactions

Diltiazem is best taken on an empty stomach, at least 1 hour before or 2 hours after meals.

Usual Dose

Immediate-Release Products
30–60 mg 4 times a day.

Sustained-Release/Extended-Release Products
Cardizem CD: 120–480 mg once a day.
Cardizem LA: 120–540 mg once a day.
Cartia XT: 120–300 mg once a day.
Dilacor XR: 180–480 mg once a day.
Dilt-CD: 120–360 mg once a day.
Diltia XT: 180–480 mg once a day.
Diltzac: 120–360 mg once a day.
Taztia XT: 120–150 mg once a day.
Tiazac: 120–360 mg once a day.

Overdosage

Symptoms of diltiazem overdose are very low blood pressure and reduced heart rate. Overdose victims must be made to vomit with ipecac syrup—available at any pharmacy—within 30 minutes of taking the overdose. Do not induce vomiting if the victim has fainted or is convulsing. If overdose symptoms have developed or more than 30 minutes have passed, vomiting is of little value. Take the victim to a hospital emergency room immediately. ALWAYS bring the prescription bottle or container.

Special Information

Call your doctor if you develop any of the following symptoms: swelling of the hands, legs, or feet; severe dizziness; constipation or nausea; or very low blood pressure.

Do not open, chew, or crush sustained-release capsules of diltiazem.

If you take your diltiazem 3 or 4 times a day and forget a dose, take it as soon as you remember. Space the remaining doses throughout the rest of the day. If you take diltiazem 1 or 2 times a day and forget to take a dose, take it as soon as you remember. If it is almost time for your next dose, skip the one you forgot and continue with your regular schedule. Never take a double dose.

Special Populations

Pregnancy/Breast-feeding: In animal studies, high doses of diltiazem interfered with the development of the fetus. Diltiazem should not be taken by women who are or might be pregnant. When your doctor considers this drug crucial, its potential benefits must be carefully weighed against its risks.

Because diltiazem passes into breast milk, nursing mothers taking this drug should use infant formula.

Seniors: Seniors may be more sensitive to the effects of this drug because it takes longer to pass out of their bodies.

Generic Name

Dimenhydrinate (dye-men-HYE-drih-nate) Ⓖ

Brand Names

Calm-X	Dramamine
Dimetabs	Triptone

The information in this profile also applies to the following drugs:

Generic Ingredient: Meclizine Ⓖ

Antivert	Bonine
Antivert 25	Meni-D
Antivert 50	Ru-Vert-M
Antrizine	

Type of Drug

Antihistamine and antiemetic (an agent that prevents or relieves nausea and vomiting).

Prescribed For

Nausea, vomiting, vertigo, and dizziness associated with motion sickness.

General Information

Dimenhydrinate, which depresses middle ear function, is a mixture of diphenhydramine—an antihistamine believed to be the active ingredient—and another ingredient. Meclizine is an antihistamine. It takes a little longer to start working than dimenhydrinate, but its effects last much longer. Meclizine does a better job of preventing motion sickness than treating its symptoms. It takes 30 minutes to 1 hour to work and lasts for 12–24 hours.

Cautions and Warnings

Do not take dimenhydrinate if you are **allergic** or **sensitive** to any of its ingredients. Newborn babies should not be given this drug.

People with a **prostate condition, stomach ulcer, intestinal obstruction, bladder problems, difficulty urinating, glaucoma, asthma,** or **abnormal heart rhythms** should use dimenhydrinate only while under a doctor's care.

Because it controls nausea and vomiting, dimenhydrinate may hide the symptoms of **appendicitis** or **overdoses of other drugs.**

Possible Side Effects

▼ Most common: drowsiness.
▼ Less common: confusion; nervousness; excitation; restlessness; headache; sleeplessness, especially in children; tingling; heavy or weak hands; fainting; dizziness; tiredness; rapid heartbeat; low blood pressure; heart palpitations; blurred or double vision; difficult or painful urination; increased sensitivity to the sun; appetite loss; nausea; vomiting; diarrhea; upset stomach; constipation; nightmares; rash; drug reaction (symptoms include rash, itching, hives, and breathing difficulties); ringing or buzzing in the ears; dry mouth, nose, or throat; stuffy nose; wheezing; and increased chest phlegm or chest tightness.

Drug Interactions

- This drug should not be taken with a monoamine oxidase inhibitor antidepressant.
- Taking dimenhydrinate with an alcoholic beverage, other antihistamine, sedative, or other central-nervous-system (CNS)

depressant may cause excessive dizziness, drowsiness, or other signs of depression.
- Side effects of anticholinergics may be increased when taken with dimenhydrinate.
- Combining dimenhydrinate and certain antibiotics that cause dizziness or other ear-related side effects may mask early signs of these side effects, especially in infants and children.

Food Interactions

Take dimenhydrinate with food or milk if it upsets your stomach.

Usual Dose

Dimenhydrinate

Adult and Child (age 13 and over): 50–100 mg—1 or 2 tablets or 4–8 tsp.—30 minutes prior to travel; then every 4–6 hours; do not take more than 400 mg a day.

Child (age 6–12): 25–50 mg—½ or 1 tablet or 2–4 tsp.—every 6–8 hours; do not take more than 150 mg a day.

Child (age 2–5): up to 25 mg—½ or 1 tablet or 2 tsp.—every 6–8 hours; do not take more than 75 mg a day.

Child (under age 2): Consult your doctor.

Meclizine

Adult and Child (age 13 and over): 25–50 mg 1 hour before travel; repeat every 24 hours for duration of journey. Up to 100 mg a day in divided doses may be needed to control dizziness from other causes.

Child: not recommended.

Overdosage

Symptoms of overdose include drowsiness, clumsiness, unsteadiness, feeling faint, facial flushing, and dry mouth, nose, or throat. Convulsions, coma, and breathing difficulties may also develop. Overdose victims should be taken to a hospital emergency room for treatment. ALWAYS bring the prescription bottle or container.

Special Information

For maximum effectiveness against motion sickness, take dimenhydrinate 1–2 hours before traveling; it may still be effective if taken 30 minutes before traveling.

This drug may cause drowsiness: Be extremely cautious when driving, operating hazardous machinery, or doing anything that requires concentration.

Dimenhydrinate may cause dry mouth, nose, or throat. Sugarless candy, gum, or ice chips can usually relieve these symptoms. Constant dry mouth may increase the likelihood of developing tooth decay or gum disease. Pay special attention to oral hygiene while you are taking dimenhydrinate, and contact your doctor if dry mouth lasts more than 2 weeks.

If you forget to take a dose of dimenhydrinate, take it as soon as you remember. If it is almost time for your next dose, skip the one you forgot and continue with your regular schedule. Do not take a double dose.

Special Populations

Pregnancy/Breast-feeding: Animal studies suggest that meclizine may cause birth defects. Do not take any antihistamine without your doctor's knowledge if you are or might be pregnant —especially during the last 3 months of pregnancy, because newborns may have severe reactions to antihistamines.

Small amounts of dimenhydrinate may pass into breast milk. Dimenhydrinate may also slow milk production. Nursing mothers who must take dimenhydrinate should use infant formula.

Seniors: Seniors are more sensitive to antihistamine side effects and should take the lowest effective dose.

Diovan   *see Angiotensin II Blockers, page 80*

Generic Name

Diphenhydramine Hydrochloride
(dye-fen-HYE-druh-mene hye-droe-KLOR-ide) Ⓖ

Brand Names

40 Winks
AllerMax
AllerMax Maximum Strength
Altaryl Children's Allergy
Banophen
Banophen Allergy
Benadryl Allergy

Benadryl Children's Allergy*
Benadryl Children's Dye Free
Benadryl Dye Free Allergy
   Liquid Gels
Children's Pediacare Nighttime
   Cough*
Compoz Gel Caps

Compoz Nighttime Sleep Aid
Diphen AF
Diphenhist
Dormin
Dytuss
Genahist
Midol PM
Miles Nervine
Nytol Quick Caps
Nytol Quick Gels Maximum
    Strength
Scot-Tussin Allergy*
Siladryl

Simply Sleep
Sleep-Eze 3
Sleepinol Maximum Strength
Sleepwell 2-Nite
Snoozefast
Sominex Original Formula
Sylphen Cough
TheraFlu Thin Strips Multi
    Symptom
Triaminic Thin Strips Cough
    and Runny Nose
Tusstat
Unisom

*Some products in this brand-name group are alcohol- or sugar-free.

Type of Drug
Antihistamine.

Prescribed For
Stuffy and runny nose, itchy eyes, and scratchy throat caused by seasonal allergy and for other symptoms of allergy such as itching, rash, and hives; also prescribed for motion sickness, insomnia, and Parkinson's disease.

General Information
Antihistamines generally work by blocking the release of histamine (a chemical released by body tissue during an allergic reaction), drying the nose, throat, and eye secretions. Diphenhydramine is the most common active ingredient found in nonprescription sleep aids.

Cautions and Warnings
This drug should not be used if you are **allergic** or **sensitive** to any of its ingredients. It should be avoided or used with extreme care if you have **narrow-angle glaucoma, stomach ulcer, intestinal obstruction, other stomach problems, difficulty urinating,** or **enlarged prostate**. It should not be used by people who have **sleep apnea** or **deep-breathing problems** such as **asthma**. Use with care if you have a history of **thyroid disease, heart disease, emphysema, chronic bronchitis,** or **high blood pressure**.

Possible Side Effects

▼ Common: drowsiness and weakness.

▼ Less common: itching, rash, sensitivity to bright light, perspiration, fever, chills, lowering of blood pressure, headache, rapid heartbeat, sleeplessness, dizziness, disturbed coordination, confusion, restlessness, nervousness, irritability, euphoria (feeling "high"), tingling and weakness of the hands or feet, blurred or double vision, ringing in the ears, upset stomach, appetite loss, nausea, vomiting, constipation, diarrhea, urinary difficulties, thickening of lung secretions, tightness of the chest, wheezing, nasal stuffiness, and dry mouth, nose, or throat.

Drug Interactions

- This drug should not be taken with a monoamine oxidase inhibitor antidepressant.
- The effects of sedatives, sleeping medications, and other central-nervous-system (CNS) depressants will be intensified when combined with diphenhydramine hydrochloride; it is extremely important that doses of these drugs are properly adjusted.
- This drug increases the intoxicating and sedating effects of alcohol.

Food Interactions

Take this drug with food if it upsets your stomach.

Usual Dose

Allergy

Adult: 25–50 mg 3–4 times a day.

Child (over 20 lbs.): 12.5–25 mg 3–4 times a day.

Nighttime Sedation

Adult and Child (age 12 and over): 25–50 mg at bedtime.

Cough Syrup

Adult and Child (age 12 and over): 25 mg every 4 hours; do not take more than 150 mg in 24 hours.

Child (age 6–12): 12.5 mg every 4 hours; do not take more than 75 mg in 24 hours.

Child (age 2–6): 6.25 mg every 4 hours; do not take more than 25 mg in 24 hours.

Child (under age 2): not recommended.

Thin Strips
TheraFlu
    Adult and Child (age 12 and over): 1 strip every 4 hours; do not take more than 6 strips in 24 hours.

Triaminic
    Child (age 6–12): 1 strip every 4 hours; do not take more than 6 strips in 24 hours.

Overdosage

Symptoms of overdose include depression or stimulation—especially in children; dry mouth; fixed or dilated pupils; flushing; and upset stomach. Overdose victims should be made to vomit with ipecac syrup—available at any pharmacy. Take the overdose victim to a hospital emergency room immediately if you cannot induce vomiting. ALWAYS bring the prescription bottle or container.

Special Information

This drug may cause drowsiness. Be extremely cautious when driving or operating hazardous equipment.

If you are taking this medication for motion sickness, take the first dose at least 30 minutes prior to exposure.

If you forget to take a dose of diphenhydramine hydrochloride, take it as soon as you remember. If it is almost time for your next dose, skip the one you forgot and continue with your regular schedule. Do not take a double dose.

Special Populations

Pregnancy/Breast-feeding: Animal studies have shown that some antihistamines may cause birth defects. Do not take any antihistamine without your doctor's knowledge if you are or might be pregnant—especially during the last 3 months of pregnancy—because newborns may have severe reactions to antihistamines.

Small amounts of antihistamine pass into breast milk. Nursing mothers who must take this drug should use infant formula.

Seniors: Seniors are more sensitive to antihistamine side effects and may require lower dosages.

Generic Name

Disopyramide (die-soe-PIE-rah-mide) Ⓖ

Brand Names

Norpace   Norpace CR

Type of Drug

Antiarrhythmic.

Prescribed For

Abnormal heart rhythms.

General Information

Disopyramide phosphate slows the rate at which nerve impulses are carried through heart muscle, reducing the response of heart muscle to those impulses. It acts on the heart similarly to the more widely used antiarrhythmic medications procainamide hydrochloride and quinidine sulfate. Disopyramide is often prescribed for people who do not respond to other antiarrhythmic drugs.

Cautions and Warnings

Do not take disopyramide if you are **allergic** or **sensitive** to any of its ingredients or if you have **heart block**, unless you have a cardiac pacemaker.

This drug can worsen **heart failure** or trigger severely **low blood pressure**. It should be used in combination with another antiarrhythmic agent or beta blocker with caution.

In rare instances, disopyramide has caused a reduction in blood-sugar levels. Therefore, the drug should be used with caution by **diabetics, older adults**—who are more susceptible to this effect—and people with **poor kidney or liver function.** Ask your doctor if you should have your blood-sugar levels checked while taking this drug.

Because of its anticholinergic effects, men with a severe **prostate condition** and people who have **glaucoma, myasthenia gravis,** or severe **difficulty urinating** should use disopyramide with caution.

People with **liver or kidney disease** must take a reduced dose of disopyramide.

Potassium levels affect the action of disopyramide. People with **blood potassium levels** that are out of the normal range must correct this imbalance before starting disopyramide.

Possible Side Effects

▼ Most common: dry mouth, urinary difficulty, and constipation.

▼ Common: blurred vision; dry eyes, nose, and throat; frequent urination; nausea; stomach pain or bloating; gas; dizziness; fatigue; headache; and nervousness.

▼ Less common: itching, rashes, muscle weakness, generalized aches and pains, not feeling well, low blood-potassium levels, increases in blood-cholesterol and triglyceride levels, heart failure, and low blood pressure.

▼ Rare: Rare side effects can occur in almost any part of the body. Contact your doctor if you experience any side effect not listed above.

Drug Interactions

- Phenytoin and rifampin may increase the rate at which the body removes disopyramide from the blood. Your disopyramide dose may need alteration if this combination is used. Other drugs known to increase drug breakdown by the liver, such as barbiturates and primidone, may also have this effect.

- Other antiarrhythmic drugs, such as procainamide and quinidine, may increase the effect of disopyramide, making dosage reduction necessary. At the same time, disopyramide may reduce the effectiveness of quinidine.

- When disopyramide is combined with a beta-blocking drug, increased disopyramide effects, additive effects, or depression of heart function may result.

- Azole antifungals, clarithromycin, diclofenac, doxycycline, erythromycin, imatinib, isoniazid, nefazodone, nicardipine, propofol, protease inhibitors, telithromycin, and verapamil may increase the amount of disopyramide in your blood, causing abnormal heart rhythms or other cardiac effects.

- Disopyramide may reduce the effectiveness of oral anticoagulant (blood-thinning) drugs. Your doctor should check your anticoagulant dosage to be sure you are getting the right amount.

- Hydantoins may cause a decrease in the effectiveness of disopyramide.

- Disopyramide may increase the amount of digoxin in your blood, though the amount of the increase is not likely to affect your heart.
- St. John's wort may decrease disopyramide levels.

Food Interactions

Disopyramide should be taken on an empty stomach at least 1 hour before or 2 hours after meals.

Usual Dose

Adult: 400–800 mg a day (divided into 2 or 4 doses for the immediate-release form). In severe cases, 400 mg every 6 hours may be required. This level of dosage should be monitored in the hospital. The sustained-release preparation is taken every 12 hours. People with reduced kidney function should receive a lower dosage, depending on the degree of kidney function present. People with liver failure should take 400 mg a day.

Child (age 13–18): 2.5–7 mg a day per lb. of body weight.

Child (age 5–12): 4.5–7 mg a day per lb. of body weight.

Child (age 1–4): 4.5–9 mg a day per lb. of body weight.

Child (under age 1): 4.5–13.5 mg a day per lb. of body weight.

Overdosage

Overdose symptoms are breathing difficulties, abnormal heart rhythms, and unconsciousness. In severe cases, overdosage can lead to death. Overdose victims should be made to vomit with ipecac syrup—available at any pharmacy—to remove any remaining drug from the stomach. Call your doctor or poison control center before doing this. If you must go to a hospital emergency room, ALWAYS bring the prescription bottle or container. Prompt and vigorous treatment can mean the difference between life and death in severe overdosage.

Special Information

Disopyramide may cause symptoms of low blood sugar: anxiety, chills, cold sweats, drowsiness, excessive hunger, nausea, nervousness, rapid pulse, shakiness, unusual weakness, tiredness, or cool, pale skin. If this happens to you, eat some chocolate, candy, or other high-sugar food, and call your doctor at once.

Disopyramide can cause dry mouth, urinary difficulty, constipation, or blurred vision. Call your doctor if these symptoms become severe or intolerable, but do not stop taking the medication without your doctor's approval.

If disopyramide is required for a child and capsules are not appropriate, your pharmacist can make a liquid product. Do not do this at home: This medication requires special preparation. The liquid should be refrigerated and protected from light and should be thrown away after 30 days.

Do not crush, chew, or open sustained-release capsules.

If you forget to take a dose of disopyramide, take it as soon as possible. However, if it is within 4 hours of your next dose, skip the dose you forgot and go back to your regular schedule. Do not take a double dose.

Special Populations

Pregnancy/Breast-feeding: Do not take this drug if you are pregnant or planning to become pregnant while using it, because it will pass into the fetus and may affect its development. When disopyramide is considered crucial by your doctor, its potential benefits must carefully be weighed against its risks.

Disopyramide passes into breast milk. Nursing mothers who must take this drug should use infant formula.

Seniors: Seniors, especially those with liver or kidney disease, are more sensitive to the effects of this drug.

Generic Name

Dofetilide (DOH-fet-a-lyed)

Brand Name

Tikosyn

Type of Drug

Antiarrhythmic.

Prescribed For

Specific abnormal heart rhythms.

General Information

Dofetilide is used to establish and maintain normal sinus rhythm in the heart. Dofetilide is available only to hospitals and doctors who receive specific training and education on how to use this drug because of the risks associated with using it.

Cautions and Warnings

Do not take dofetilide if you are **allergic** or **sensitive** to any of its ingredients.

Dofetilide is reserved for people whose abnormal heart rhythms have not responded to other drugs. People taking dofetilide must be in a hospital or other facility for at least 3 days where appropriate blood tests can be performed to monitor kidney and heart function.

This drug is cleared through the kidneys. **Poor kidney function** increases the amount of dofetilide in the body. Liver disease has no effect on dofetilide blood levels.

Dofetilide, like other antiarrhythmic drugs, can cause severe and sometimes fatal abnormal rhythms of its own.

Do not take dofetilide without first talking to your doctor if you have a **low blood level of potassium or magnesium**.

Women may be at a greater risk for some arrhythmias caused by dofetilide.

Possible Side Effects

Serious heart arrhythmias can develop in up to 3½% of patients taking up to 1000 mcg a day of dofetilide. People taking daily doses above 1000 mcg a day are at up to 5 times greater risk for arrhythmias.

▼ Most common: headache, chest pain, and respiratory infection.

▼ Common: difficulty breathing, nausea, and dizziness.

▼ Less common: flu; sleeplessness; accidental injury; back pain; diarrhea; abdominal pain; angina; anxiety; joint pain; weakness; atrial and ventricular arrhythmia; high blood pressure; pain; heart palpitations; swollen legs, ankles, or arms; sweating; and urinary infections.

▼ Rare: some arrhythmias, heart attack, hives, slow heartbeat, stroke, facial or other paralysis, tingling in the hands or feet, cough, liver damage, migraine, fainting, and sudden death. Contact your doctor if you experience any side effect not listed above.

Drug Interactions

Dofetilide should not be given with drugs that are known to interact with it. Dofetilide must be stopped at least 2 days before any potentially interacting drug is taken.

● Do not mix dofetilide with any product containing verapamil, a calcium channel blocker, or trimethoprim, used for urinary infections. These combinations can substantially raise the amount of dofetilide in the blood.

- Some drugs may increase the amount of dofetilide in the blood by inhibiting enzymes that break it down in the liver. They include delavirdine, indinavir, ritonavir, saquinavir, amiodarone, cimetidine, ciprofloxacin, clarithromycin, cannabis, diltiazem, erythromycin, fluconazole, fluvoxamine, itraconazole, ketoconazole, mifepristone, nefazodone, norfloxacin, mibefradil, selective serotonin reuptake inhibitors (SSRIs), troleandomycin, and zafirlukast.

- Some drugs may reduce the amount of dofetilide in the blood by stimulating enzymes that break it down in the liver, including efavirenz, nevirapine, carbamazepine, corticosteroids, modafinil, phenobarbital and other barbiturates, phenytoin, pioglitazone, and rifampin. Amiloride, metformin, megestrol, and triamterene can interfere with the elimination of dofetilide via the kidney, raising blood levels of the drug.

- Other drugs that can increase the effects of dofetilide are other antiarrhythmic drugs, bepridil, phenothiazines, and tricyclic antidepressants.

- Mixing dofetilide with digoxin may lead to a ventricular arrhythmia called torsade de pointes. Thiazides, furosemide, and other potassium-depleting diuretics can also increase the risk of this arrhythmia.

Food Interactions

Grapefruit juice may increase dofetilide blood levels.

Usual Dose

Adult: 125–500 mcg twice a day.
Child (under 18 years): not recommended.

Overdosage

Dofetilide overdose is likely to cause significant heart rhythm problems. Overdose victims must be treated symptomatically by their cardiologist.

Special Information

Read all information supplied to you before you begin taking this medication and read it again if anything in your treatment program changes.

Tell your doctor about any changes in your prescription or non-prescription drug use or in your use of vitamins, minerals, and other dietary supplement products.

Be sure that any other doctor or hospital that treats you and might prescribe another drug knows you are taking dofetilide.

Call your doctor at once if you develop any signs of altered electrolyte balance including excessive or prolonged diarrhea, sweating, vomiting, appetite changes, or excessive thirst.

If you forget to take a dose, take it as soon as you remember. If it is almost time for your next dose, skip the dose you forgot and continue with your regular schedule. Do not take a double dose.

Special Populations

Pregnancy/Breast-feeding: Dofetilide causes birth defects in animal studies. Pregnant women should take this drug only after discussing with their doctors its potential benefits and risks.

It is unknown whether dofetilide passes into breast milk. Nursing mothers who take it should consider using infant formula.

Seniors: Older adults may take this drug without special restriction.

Brand Name

Donnatal

Generic Ingredients

Atropine Sulfate + Hyoscyamine Sulfate + Phenobarbital + Scopolamine Hydrobromide Ⓖ

Other Brand Names

Antispas	Donnapine
Antispasmodic	Donnatal Extentabs
Barbidonna	Hyosophen
Bellatal	Spasmolin

The information in this profile also applies to the following drugs:

Generic Ingredient: Hyoscyamine Sulfate Ⓖ

Anaspaz	ED-SPAZ
A-Spas S/L	Hyosol
Cytospaz	Hyosyne
Donnamar	IB-Stat

Levbid　　　　　　　　Neosol
Levsin　　　　　　　　NuLev
Levsinex Timecaps　　Spasdel
Medispaz　　　　　　　Symax

Generic Ingredient: Propantheline Ⓖ
Pro-Banthine

Type of Drug

Anticholinergic combination.

Prescribed For

Stomach spasm and gastrointestinal (GI) cramps; also used to treat motion sickness.

General Information

Donnatal is a mild antispasmodic sedative. Its principal action is to counteract the effect of acetylcholine, an important neurohormone. Donnatal is used only to relieve symptoms, not to treat the underlying condition, and there is considerable doubt among medical experts that this drug lives up to its claims. In addition to the brand names listed above, there are about 50 other anticholinergic combinations with similar properties. All are used to relieve cramps and all are about equally effective. Some have additional ingredients to reduce or absorb excess gas in the stomach, to coat the stomach, or to control diarrhea. Donnatal and products like it should not be used for more than the temporary relief of symptoms.

Cautions and Warnings

Do not take Donnatal if you are **allergic** or **sensitive** to any of its ingredients.

Donnatal should not be used by people with **glaucoma, rapid heartbeat,** severe **intestinal disease** such as **ulcerative colitis, intestinal obstruction, urinary difficulties, asthma, myasthenia gravis, acute intermittent porphyria, acute bleeding** with unstable heart function, or **hiatal hernia**.

Phenobarbital may be habit-forming and should not be administered to people with a history of **drug dependence**.

Donnatal should be used with caution in **children** and in people with **brain damage, spastic paralysis, Down's syndrome, heart disease, high blood pressure, hyperthyroidism** (overactive thyroid gland), **kidney or liver disease, autonomic neuropathy,** or **gastric ulcer**.

Donnatal can reduce your ability to sweat and may lead to heat exhaustion. Avoid extended heavy exercise and limit your exposure to high temperatures.

Possible Side Effects

▼ Most common: blurred vision, dry mouth, urinary difficulties, flushing, and dry skin.

▼ Less common: rapid or unusual heartbeat, increased sensitivity to bright light, loss of the sense of taste, headache, nervousness, tiredness, weakness, dizziness, sleeplessness, nausea, vomiting, fever, stuffy nose, heartburn, loss of sex drive, decreased sweating, constipation, feeling bloated, and allergic reactions such as fever and rash.

Drug Interactions

- Although Donnatal contains only a small amount of phenobarbital, it is wise to avoid alcohol or other sedative drugs. Although unlikely, phenobarbital interactions are possible with anticoagulants, adrenal corticosteroids, narcotics, sleeping pills, digitalis or other cardiac glycosides, and antihistamines.
- Some phenothiazine drugs, sedatives, tricyclic antidepressants, and narcotics may increase the side effects of the atropine sulfate ingredient in Donnatal, causing dry mouth, urinary difficulties, and constipation. The effectiveness of phenothiazines to control psychotic symptoms may be decreased.
- Combining Donnatal and the antiviral amantadine may increase the side effects of Donnatal.
- Donnatal may increase the side effects of atenolol and digoxin.
- Antacids may decrease Donnatal's effectiveness; do not take antacids within 1 hour of taking Donnatal.

Food Interactions

Take Donnatal 30–60 minutes before meals.

Usual Dose

Donnatal

Adult (age 13 and over): 1–2 tablets, capsules, or tsp. 3–4 times a day, or 1 extended-release tablet every 12 hours.

Child (age 2–12): ½ the adult dosage.
Child (under age 2): not recommended.

Propantheline
Adult: 15 mg 3 times a day before meals, and 30 mg at bedtime.
Senior: 7.5 mg 3 times a day.
Child (under age 12): not recommended.

Overdosage

Symptoms of overdose include dry mouth; difficulty swallowing; thirst; blurred vision; sensitivity to bright light; flushed, hot, or dry skin; rash; fever; abnormal heart rate; high blood pressure; urinary difficulties; restlessness; confusion; delirium; and breathing difficulties. The victim should be taken to a hospital emergency room immediately. ALWAYS bring the prescription bottle or container.

Special Information

Call your doctor if you experience persistent diarrhea, bloating, fever, heart palpitations, rash, flushing, or eye pain.

Do not crush or chew Donnatal tablets.

Dry mouth usually can be relieved by chewing gum or sucking hard candy or ice chips. Constipation can be treated with a stool-softening laxative.

Donnatal may reduce the amount of saliva in your mouth, making it easier for bacteria to grow there. Pay special attention to dental hygiene while taking this medication to prevent cavities and gum disease.

Donnatal may cause drowsiness and blurred vision. Be careful when driving or operating hazardous equipment.

If you forget to take a dose of Donnatal, take it as soon as you remember. If it is almost time for your next dose, skip the one you forgot and continue with your regular schedule. Do not take a double dose.

Special Populations

Pregnancy/Breast-feeding: Donnatal may cause drug dependency or breathing problems in newborns and may interfere with labor and delivery. When this drug is considered crucial by your doctor, its potential must be carefully weighed against its risks.

Donnatal may pass into breast milk and may reduce the amount of milk produced. It may cause tiredness, shortness of breath, and a slower-than-normal heartbeat in infants. Nursing mothers who must take this medication should consider using infant formula.

Seniors: Seniors are often more sensitive to the side effects of Donnatal, such as excitement, confusion, drowsiness, agitation, constipation, dry mouth, and urinary difficulties. Memory may be impaired and glaucoma worsened.

Generic Name

Doxazosin (dok-SAY-zoe-sin) G

Brand Names
Cardura   Cardura XL

Type of Drug
Antihypertensive.

Prescribed For
High blood pressure and benign prostatic hyperplasia (BPH); also used with digoxin and diuretic drugs to treat congestive heart failure.

General Information
Doxazosin mesylate and other alpha-adrenergic blocking agents, or alpha blockers, reduce blood pressure by dilating (widening) blood vessels. They achieve this effect by blocking nerve endings known as alpha$_1$ receptors. The maximum blood-pressure-lowering effect of doxazosin is seen between 2 and 6 hours after taking a dose. In BPH treatment, doxazosin works by relaxing smooth muscles in the prostate and neck of the bladder. Doxazosin helps the symptoms of BPH, and taking it for several years may eliminate the need for surgery or allow the use of a less invasive type of surgery. Doxazosin's effect lasts for 24 hours. It is mostly broken down in the liver; little passes out of the body via the kidneys.

Doxazosin may slightly reduce cholesterol levels and improve the ratio of high-density lipoprotein (HDL)—"good" cholesterol—and low-density lipoprotein (LDL)—"bad cholesterol"—a positive step for people with a blood-cholesterol problem.

Cautions and Warnings
Do not take doxazosin if you are **allergic** or **sensitive** to any of its ingredients or to any alpha blocker.

Doxazosin may cause dizziness and fainting, especially the first few doses. This is known as a first-dose effect, which can be minimized by limiting the first dose to 1 mg at bedtime. First-dose effects occur in about 1% of people taking an alpha blocker and may recur if the drug is stopped for a few days and then started again.

Doxazosin should be taken with caution if you have **liver disease**.

White-blood-cell counts may be slightly decreased in people taking doxazosin.

Rarely, alpha blockers, including doxazosin, have led to priapism (painful and prolonged erection). Call your doctor immediately if this happens. If not treated promptly, this condition can lead to impotence.

Possible Side Effects

▼ Most common: headache, dizziness, and weakness.

▼ Less common: heart palpitations, abnormal heart rhythms, chest pain, nausea, diarrhea, constipation, abdominal pain or discomfort, gas, breathing difficulties, nosebleed, sore throat, runny nose, muscle or joint pain, visual disturbances, conjunctivitis (pinkeye), ringing in the ears, fainting, depression, decreased sex drive or sexual function, tingling in the hands or feet, nervousness, tiredness, anxiety, sleeplessness, poor muscle coordination, muscle stiffness, poor bladder control, frequent urination, itching, rash, sweating, fluid retention, facial swelling and flushing, and back, neck, shoulder, arm, or leg pain.

▼ Rare: vomiting, dry mouth, sinus irritation, bronchitis, cold or flu symptoms, worsening of asthma, coughing, hair loss, weight gain, and fever. Contact your doctor if you experience any side effect not listed above.

Drug Interactions

- Doxazosin may interact with beta blockers to increase the risk of dizziness or fainting after the first dose of doxazosin.
- The blood-pressure-lowering effect of doxazosin may be reduced by indomethacin.
- When taken with other blood-pressure-lowering drugs, doxazosin produces a severe reduction of blood pressure.
- The blood-pressure-lowering effect of clonidine may be reduced by doxazosin.

- Doxazosin should be taken with caution in combination with clarithromycin, ketoconazole, and itraconazole.

Food Interactions

None known.

Usual Dose

Adult: 1 mg morning or evening to start; may be increased to a total of 16 mg, taken once a day. Extended-release tablets—4 mg once daily at breakfast; may be increased to a total of 8 mg. Do not chew, cut, or crush extended-release tablets.

Child: not recommended.

Overdosage

Overdose may produce drowsiness, poor reflexes, and very low blood pressure. Overdose victims should be taken to a hospital emergency room at once. ALWAYS bring the prescription bottle or container.

Special Information

Take doxazosin exactly as prescribed. Do not stop taking it unless directed to do so by your doctor. Avoid over-the-counter drugs that contain stimulants because they may increase your blood pressure.

Doxazosin may cause dizziness, headache, and drowsiness, especially 2–6 hours after you take your first dose, although these effects can persist after the first few doses. Use caution when getting up from a sitting or lying position.

Call your doctor if you develop severe dizziness, heart palpitations, or any bothersome or persistent side effect.

Wait 12–24 hours after taking your first dose of doxazosin before driving or doing anything that requires concentration. Take your dose at bedtime to minimize this problem.

If you forget a dose, take it as soon as you remember. If it is almost time for your next dose, skip the dose you forgot and continue with your regular schedule. Do not take a double dose.

Special Populations

Pregnancy/Breast-feeding: The safety of using doxazosin during pregnancy is not known, although animal studies have shown that alpha blockers may affect fetal development. When this drug is considered crucial by your doctor, its potential benefits must be carefully weighed against its risks.

Small amounts of doxazosin pass into breast milk. Nursing mothers who must take this drug should use infant formula.

Seniors: Seniors, especially those with liver disease, may be more sensitive to the effects and side effects of doxazosin.

Generic Name

Doxercalciferol (dox-er-kal-SIH-fer-ahl) G

Brand Names

Drisdol Liquid   Hectorol Capsules

Type of Drug

Vitamin D supplement.

Prescribed For

Elevated parathyroid hormone levels in patients undergoing kidney dialysis.

General Information

Doxercalciferol is a synthetic form of vitamin D that is processed in the body to form active vitamin D. Vitamin D, along with parathyroid hormone, are key elements of the calcium-regulating system in the body. Normally, your body releases parathyroid hormone if blood calcium levels are too low. Parathyroid hormones move calcium from the place where it is found in greatest quantity—your bones—into the bloodstream. This can have disastrous effects for a wide variety of body functions where calcium is crucial including muscle contraction, nervous system function, bone fragility, and blood clotting. Doxercalciferol helps to stabilize the system and normalize parathyroid hormone levels that can be artificially elevated in dialysis patients.

Cautions and Warnings

Do not use doxercalciferol if you are **allergic** or **sensitive** to any of its ingredients.

Do not take any other vitamin D supplement while taking this drug.

People with a tendency toward **high calcium or vitamin D levels** should not take doxercalciferol.

Before taking this medication, tell your doctor if you have **liver disease**. You may not be able to take doxercalciferol, or you may require a dosage adjustment or special monitoring during treatment.

Dialysis patients experience increases in blood calcium and phosphate while taking this drug.

Possible Side Effects

▼ Common: swelling, headache, general discomfort, nausea, vomiting, dizziness, difficulty breathing, and itching.
▼ Less common: loss of appetite, indigestion, weight gain, joint pain, constipation, sleepiness, and slowed heart rate.

Drug Interactions

- Do not take antacids that contain magnesium while you are taking doxercalciferol.
- Cholestyramine may reduce the absorption of doxercalciferol.
- Prolonged use of mineral oil may reduce the absorption of doxercalciferol.
- Do not combine any other over-the-counter or prescription medicines, or vitamin supplements with doxercalciferol without first talking with your doctor.
- The following medicines can slow the transformation of doxercalciferol to its active form in the body, reducing its effectiveness: ketoconazole, erythromycin, delaviridine, indinavir, nelfinavir, ritonavir, amiodarone, aprepitant, chloramphenicol, cimetidine, ciprofloxacin, clarithromycin, diltiazem, fluconazole, fluvoxamine, gestodene, itraconazole, mifepristone, nefazodone, norfloxacin, mibefradil, and verapamil.
- The following drugs can increase the breakdown of doxercalciferol in the liver, possibly reducing its effectiveness: efavirenz, nevirapine, barbiturates, carbamazepine, glucocorticoids, modafinil, phenobarbital, phenytoin, rifampin, St. John's wort, oxcarbazepine, pioglitazone, and rifabutin. Dosage adjustment may be needed.
- Digoxin may cause symptoms of alcohol intolerance when combined with disulfiram or metronidazole.

Food Interactions

Avoid grapefruit products as they can slow the transformation of doxercalciferol to its active form in the body, reducing its effectiveness.

You may need to limit your consumption of foods containing vitamin D. Consult your doctor.

Usual Dose

Adult: starting dose—10 mcg 3 times a week during kidney dialysis treatment. Dosage may be adjusted to 2.5 mcg at 8-week intervals if necessary.

Child: not recommended.

Overdosage

Symptoms include weakness, headache, drowsiness, nausea, vomiting, dry mouth, metallic taste in mouth, constipation, muscle pain, bone pain, and irregular heartbeat. Call your local poison control center or a hospital emergency room for more information. If you seek treatment, ALWAYS bring the prescription bottle or container.

Special Information

Compliance with dosage instruction, diet, and calcium supplementation is important while taking doxercalciferol.

Lab tests are required to monitor therapy while taking doxercalciferol.

Doxercalciferol may cause dizziness. Use caution while driving or performing other tasks requiring alertness, coordination, or physical dexterity.

Special Populations

Tell your doctor or pharmacist if you are pregnant, planning on becoming pregnant, or breast-feeding.

The safety of using doxercalciferol during pregnancy is not known. When this drug is considered crucial by your doctor, its potential benefits must be carefully weighed against its risks.

It is not known if doxercalciferol passes into breast milk. Nursing mothers who must use this drug should use infant formula.

Seniors: Seniors may use this drug without special precaution.

Generic Name

Dronabinol (droe-NAB-ih-nol)

Brand Name

Marinol

Type of Drug

Antinauseant.

Prescribed For

Nausea and vomiting associated with cancer chemotherapy, and appetite stimulation and weight-loss prevention in people with acquired immunodeficiency syndrome (AIDS).

General Information

Dronabinol is a legal form of marijuana. The psychoactive chemical in marijuana is delta-9-THC. Dronabinol has all of the psychological effects of marijuana and is therefore considered to be a highly abusable drug. It can cause personality changes, feelings of detachment, hallucinations, and euphoria (feeling "high"). Younger adults have reported a greater success rate with dronabinol, probably because they are better able to tolerate these effects.

Most people start taking dronabinol while in the hospital so their response to the drug and its possible adverse effects can be monitored. Dronabinol has also been studied as a glaucoma treatment.

Cautions and Warnings

Do not take dronabinol if you are **allergic** or **sensitive** to any of its ingredients, to marijuana, or to sesame oil.

Dronabinol should not be used to treat nausea and vomiting caused by anything other than cancer chemotherapy.

Dronabinol should be used with caution in those with a history of **seizure disorders** or **substance abuse.**

Dronabinol has a profound effect on mental states; it will impair your ability to operate complex equipment or engage in any activity that requires intense concentration, sound judgment, or coordination—such as driving a car.

Dronabinol produces withdrawal symptoms when the drug is stopped. These may develop within 12 hours of the drug's discontinuation and include restlessness, sleeplessness, and irritability. Within a day after the drug has been stopped, stuffy nose, hot flashes, sweating, loose stools, hiccups, or appetite loss may occur. The symptoms usually subside within a few days.

Dronabinol should be used with caution by people with **heart disease** or **high blood pressure**. Dronabinol should be used with caution by people with a **manic-depressive or schizophrenic history** because it may aggravate the underlying disease.

Possible Side Effects

▼ Most common: drowsiness, euphoria, dizziness, anxiety, muddled thinking, perceptual difficulties, poor coordination, irritability, a separation in time and space, depression, weakness, sluggishness, nausea and vomiting, headache, hallucinations, memory lapses, loss of muscle coordination, unsteadiness, paranoia, depersonalization, disorientation, confusion, rapid heartbeat, and dizziness when rising from a sitting or lying position.

▼ Less common: difficulty talking or slurred speech, facial flushing, excessive perspiration, nightmares, ringing or buzzing in the ears, fainting, diarrhea, loss of bowel control, and muscle pain.

Drug Interactions

- Dronabinol increases the effects of alcohol, sleeping pills, sedatives, and other depressants. It also enhances the effects of psychoactive drugs including tricyclic antidepressants, amphetamines, cocaine, and other stimulants.
- Dronabinol may increase the effects of fluoxetine and disulfiram.
- The effects of theophylline drugs are reduced by dronabinol.
- Combining dronabinol and antihistamines or anticholinergic drugs may cause either rapid heartbeat or excessive drowsiness.

Food Interactions

This drug may be taken without regard to food or meals; as an appetite stimulant, it is often taken before meals.

Usual Dose

Antiemetic: 5 mg 1–3 hours before starting chemotherapy treatment and repeated every 2–4 hours after treatment, for a total of 4–6 doses a day. Dosage may be increased up to 15 mg per dose if needed; psychiatric side effects increase greatly at higher dosages.

Appetite Stimulant: 2.5 mg before lunch or dinner, or 2.5 mg at bedtime. Dosage may be increased to 20 mg a day.

Overdosage

Overdose symptoms may occur at usual dosages or at higher dosages if the drug is being abused. The primary symptoms of overdose are the psychological symptoms listed above (see "Possible Side Effects"). In some cases, overdose may lead to panic reactions or seizure. Contact a hospital or local poison center for more information. If you seek treatment, ALWAYS bring the prescription bottle or container.

Special Information

Be careful when driving or performing any task that requires concentration. Avoid alcohol and other central nervous system (CNS) depressants.

Dronabinol may cause acute psychiatric or psychological side effects. Call your doctor if any develop.

The capsules must be stored in the refrigerator.

If you forget a dose, take it as soon as you remember. If it is almost time for your next dose, skip the one you forgot and continue with your regular schedule. Do not take a double dose.

Special Populations

Pregnancy/Breast-feeding: Animal studies have shown adverse effects on the fetus. When this drug is considered crucial by your doctor, its benefits must be carefully weighed against its risks.

Dronabinol passes into breast milk. Nursing mothers who must take this drug should use infant formula.

Seniors: Seniors may be more sensitive to this drug, especially its psychological effects.

Brand Name

Dyazide

Generic Ingredients

Hydrochlorothiazide + Triamterene Ⓖ

Other Brand Names

Maxzide   Maxzide-25

The information in this profile also applies to the following drugs:

Generic Ingredients: Amiloride + Hydrochlorothiazide Ⓖ
Hydro-Ride   Moduretic

Generic Ingredients: Spironolactone + Hydrochlorothiazide Ⓖ
Aldactazide   Spironazide
Alzide Novo-Spirozine   Spirozide

Type of Drug

Diuretic (an agent that increases urination).

Prescribed For

Hypertension (high blood pressure) or any condition where it is desirable to eliminate excess water from the body.

General Information

Dyazide combines a thiazide diuretic and a potassium-sparing diuretic. The latter, triamterene, helps the body retain potassium while producing a diuretic effect. This balances the other ingredient, hydrochlorothiazide, which normally causes a loss of potassium. Different products contain differing concentrations of these 2 drugs. Dyazide should be used only when you need its exact proportion of ingredients, and should not be used for initial therapy of hypertension or edema. It may be used alone or with other antihypertensive drugs such as beta blockers. Dosage adjustment may be necessary.

Cautions and Warnings

Do not use dyazide if you are **allergic** or **sensitive** to any of its ingredients or to any sulfa drug or if you have a history of allergy.

Do not use Dyazide if you have **nonfunctioning kidneys, bronchial asthma,** or **hyperkalemia** (high blood potassium levels).

Do not combine any **potassium supplement** and Dyazide without your doctor's knowledge. Dyazide may reduce blood levels of sodium and potassium and raise blood calcium levels.

Dyazide should be used with caution in people with **diabetes, liver disease,** or an **electrolyte imbalance.**

Possible Side Effects

▼ Most common: appetite loss, drowsiness, lethargy, headache, gastrointestinal upset, cramping, and diarrhea.

▼ Less common: rash—possibly severe, mental confusion, fever, feeling unwell, impotence, bright red tongue, burning sensation in the tongue, tingling in the toes and fingers, restlessness, anemia or other effects on blood components, increased sensitivity to sunlight, and dizziness when rising quickly from a sitting position. Dyazide may also produce muscle spasms, gout, weakness, and blurred vision.

Drug Interactions

- Dyazide increases the effect of other blood-pressure-lowering drugs. This is why other blood-pressure drugs are often prescribed with Dyazide, but dosage adjustments may be required.
- Combining Dyazide and digitalis drugs, amphotericin B, or adrenal corticosteroids increases the risk of body-fluid imbalance. If you are taking insulin or an oral antidiabetic drug and begin taking Dyazide, the insulin or antidiabetic dosage may have to be modified.
- Dyazide may increase the risk of allopurinol side effects.
- Dyazide may decrease the effects of oral anticoagulant (blood-thinning) drugs.
- Antigout drug dosage may have to be modified since Dyazide raises uric-acid levels.
- Dyazide may prolong the effects of chemotherapy drugs on reducing white-blood-cell counts.
- Dyazide may increase the effects of diazoxide, which may lead to symptoms of diabetes.
- Dyazide should not be taken with loop diuretics because the combination can lead to an extreme diuretic effect and an extreme effect on blood-sodium levels.
- Dyazide may increase the effect of vitamin D, which may cause high blood-calcium levels.
- Propantheline and other anticholinergics may increase the diuretic effect of Dyazide.
- Lithium carbonate taken with Dyazide should be monitored carefully by a doctor due to an increased risk of lithium side effects.
- Cholestyramine and colestipol prevent Dyazide from being absorbed. Dyazide should be taken at least 2 hours before cholestyramine or colestipol.
- Methenamine and other urinary agents may reduce the effect of Dyazide.
- Some nonsteroidal anti-inflammatory drugs (NSAIDs), particularly indomethacin, may reduce the effect of Dyazide. Sulindac, another NSAID, may increase its effect.
- Potassium-sparing diuretics should be used with caution in combination with ACE inhibitors.

Food Interactions

Take this drug with food if it upsets your stomach.

Usual Dose

Adult

Amiloride combination: 1–2 tablets daily with meals.

Spironolactone combination: 1–8 tablets daily.

Triamterene combination: 1–2 capsules or tablets a day.

Child: not recommended.

Overdosage

Symptoms may include tingling in the arms or legs, weakness, fatigue, changes in heartbeat, a sickly feeling, dry mouth, restlessness, muscle pain or cramps, urinary difficulties, nausea, and vomiting. In some cases, low blood pressure and decreased respiration may occur. Take the victim to a hospital emergency room immediately. ALWAYS bring the prescription bottle or container.

Special Information

Dyazide causes excess urination at first, but this subsides after several weeks of use. Diuretics are usually taken early in the day to prevent excessive nighttime urination that may interfere with sleep.

Dyazide may make you drowsy. Be careful when driving or performing any task that requires concentration.

Call your doctor if you develop muscle pain, sudden joint pain, weakness, cramps, nausea, vomiting, restlessness, excessive thirst, tiredness, drowsiness, increased heart or pulse rate, diarrhea, dizziness, headache, or rash.

People with diabetes may experience an increased blood-sugar level and require dosage adjustments of their antidiabetic medications.

Avoid other drugs while taking Dyazide unless otherwise directed by your doctor. Avoid alcohol.

If you are taking Dyazide for the treatment of hypertension or congestive heart failure (CHF), avoid over-the-counter cough, cold, or allergy medications, which may contain stimulants.

Take Dyazide exactly as prescribed. Be aware that all triamterene-hydrochlorothiazide products are not equal to each other and should not be freely substituted. Check with your doctor and pharmacist before switching brands.

If you forget a dose, take it as soon as you remember. If it is almost time for your next dose, skip the dose you forgot and continue with your regular schedule. Do not take a double dose.

Special Populations

Pregnancy/Breast-feeding: Dyazide may enter the fetal circulation, though it is sometimes used to treat specific conditions in pregnant women. When this drug is considered crucial by your doctor, its potential benefits must be carefully weighed against its risks.

The thiazide diuretic in Dyazide passes into breast milk. Nursing mothers who must take Dyazide should use infant formula.

Seniors: Seniors are more sensitive to the effects of Dyazide.

Generic Name

Econazole (ee-KON-uh-zole) G

Brand Name

Spectazole

Type of Drug

Antifungal.

Prescribed For

Fungal infections of the skin, including athlete's foot, jock itch, and ringworm.

General Information

Econazole nitrate can kill fungal organisms that may have penetrated to deep layers of the skin. Very small amounts of econazole are absorbed into the bloodstream.

Cautions and Warnings

Do not use econazole if you are **allergic** or **sensitive** to any of its ingredients.

Do not apply econazole cream in or near your eyes.

Long-term application of this product to large areas of skin may cause liver damage.

Possible Side Effects

▼ Most common: burning, itching, stinging, and redness in the areas to which the cream has been applied.

Drug Interactions

None known.

Usual Dose

Adult: Apply enough of the cream to cover affected areas with a thin layer 1–2 times a day.

Overdosage

Accidental ingestion may cause nausea, upset stomach, drowsiness, and liver inflammation or damage. Call your local poison control center for more information. If you seek treatment, ALWAYS bring the prescription container.

Special Information

Clean the affected areas before applying econazole cream, unless otherwise directed by your doctor. Dry the infected area thoroughly and wear loose-fitting clothes to keep the area cool and dry.

Call your doctor if the treated area burns, stings, or becomes red.

This product can be expected to relieve symptoms within 1 or 2 days after you begin using it. Follow your doctor's directions for the complete 2–4-week course of treatment to gain maximum benefit. Stopping the drug too soon can lead to a relapse.

If you forget a dose of econazole, apply it as soon as you remember. If it is almost time for your next dose, skip the one you forgot and continue with your regular schedule. Do not apply a double dose.

Special Populations

Pregnancy/Breast-feeding: When given by mouth to pregnant animals in high doses, econazole was toxic to the fetus. It should be strictly avoided during the first 3 months of pregnancy. During the last 6 months of pregnancy, it should be used only if absolutely necessary.

Econazole may pass into breast milk. Nursing mothers who must take this drug should consider using infant formula.

Seniors: Seniors may take this drug without special restriction.

Generic Name

Efalizumab (ef-ah-LIZ-u-mab)

Brand Name

Raptiva

Type of Drug

Immune system suppressant.

Prescribed For

Chronic to severe plaque psoriasis.

General Information

Efalizumab is a manmade antibody that works by binding to specific areas of certain white blood cells called *leukocytes*. This prevents the leukocytes from interacting with other cells and interrupts inflammation that is involved in the development of patches of psoriatic skin. The molecule that efaluzimab interacts with is found on many other key cells found in the immune system, and this is the source of many of the drug's more serious side effects.

Cautions and Warnings

Do not use this drug if you are **allergic** or **sensitive** to any of its ingredients.

People taking efalizumab are at a greater risk of infection because it suppresses the immune system. Contact your doctor if you develop any kind of infection, including a common cold. Serious infections may require hospitalization.

The chances of malignancy may be increased by efalizumab because it suppresses the immune system. People with **any type of cancer** should not use this drug.

Efalizumab may lead to bleeding because it can cause a drastic reduction in blood-platelet counts. People with a history of **low blood-platelet counts** should be extremely cautious about using efalizumab.

Psoriasis can get worse or recur during or after efalizumab treatment in a small number of people. Call your doctor immediately if your condition worsens while you are taking efalizumab.

Possible Side Effects

Headache, fever, nausea, and vomiting are common after taking the very first dose of efalizumab. A "conditioning" dose of about 0.3 mg per lb. of body weight is often given to minimize these reactions.

▼ Most common: headache, infections, chills, nausea, and pain.

▼ Common: muscle aches, flu-like symptoms, itching, and fever.

Possible Side Effects *(continued)*

▼ Less common: back pain, arthritis, lung inflammation, and acne.

▼ Rare: psoriasis, arthritis, joint pain, malignancy, low blood-platelet count, and drug allergy or sensitivity. Other rare side effects can occur in almost any part of the body. Contact your doctor if you experience any side effect not listed above.

Drug Interactions

• Efalizumab is an immune system suppressant and should not be combined with other immune suppressant drugs because of the increased risk of infection and malignancy.

• Combining vaccines (live and acellular) with efalizumab may exaggerate the body's response to the vaccine and increase the risk of developing the disease against which the vaccination is being administered. People taking efalizumab should not receive vaccines.

Food Interactions

None known.

Usual Dose

Adult: 0.3 mg per lb. of body weight to start. Then about 0.5 mg per lb. of body weight once a week on the same day. The maximum dose is 200 mg by subcutaneous injection. Mix your dose immediately before it is to be injected and throw away any unused medicine.

Child: not recommended.

Overdosage

Doses up to 4 times the recommended dose have been taken for 10 weeks without additional side effects. However, overdose victims should be taken to a hospital emergency room for observation. ALWAYS bring the prescription bottle or container.

Special Information

See your doctor regularly while you are taking efaluzimab. Regular blood tests are required to make sure your blood platelets are not unusually low.

Tell your doctor if you gain or lose weight, since doses of efaluzimab are based on how much you weigh.

Tell your doctor about all medicines you are taking including other medicines for psoriasis, non-prescription drugs, vitamins, and herbal supplements.

Store unused medicine in the refrigerator. Throw away medicine that has been mixed but not used.

Call your doctor immediately if you develop bleeding gums, black-and-blue marks, any kind of infection, begin to bruise easily, or if you are told by another doctor that you have any kind of cancer.

This drug is given by injection under the skin. For more information on how to properly administer this drug, see page 1242.

Special Populations

Pregnancy/Breast-feeding: It is not known how efaluzimab will affect a growing fetus. Animal studies using doses equal to 30 times the human dose showed no adverse effects. While animal studies of efaluzimab reveal no damage to the fetus, this drug should be used only during pregnancy after carefully weighing its potential benefits against its risks.

It is not known if efaluzimab passes into breast milk, although it might affect the nursing infant's developing immune system. Nursing mothers who must take this drug should use infant formula.

Seniors: Seniors should be cautious about using efaluzimab because of the increased risk of infection.

Effexor *see Venlafaxine, page 1200*

Generic Name

Eflornithine (eh-FLOOR-nih-thene)

Brand Name
Vaniqa

Type of Drug
Hair growth retardant.

Prescribed For
Removal of unwanted facial hair by women.

General Information

This drug has only been studied for its ability to prevent hair growth on the face and chin and should not be used on other body areas. It works by interfering with enzymes in the skin necessary for hair growth, slowing the rate at which hair will grow. Improvement may be seen as soon as 4–8 weeks after you start using eflornithine, but the condition will return within 8 weeks after you stop using it.

Cautions and Warnings

Do not use eflornithine if you are **allergic** or **sensitive** to any of its ingredients.

For external use only; do not ingest.

Possible Side Effects

Eflornithine side effects are similar to those of a placebo (sugar pill).

▼ Most common: acne, bumps, or small pustules on the skin.
▼ Common: stinging.
▼ Less common: headache, dizziness, burning, itching, redness, tingling, irritation, rash, hair loss, upset stomach, and appetite loss.
▼ Rare: fainting, ingrown hairs, inflamed hair follicles, facial swelling, nausea, bleeding, contact dermatitis, inflammation of one or both lips, herpes breakout, numbness, and dilated blood vessels and pores on the nose and cheeks. Contact your doctor if you experience any side effect not listed above.

Food and Drug Interactions

None known.

Usual Dose

Adult and Child (age 12 and over): Apply a thin layer of cream to affected areas and rub in thoroughly 2 times a day at least 8 hours apart. Do not wash your face until at least 4 hours after you have applied eflornithine cream. Wait at least 5 minutes after hair removal to apply eflornithine.

Child (under age 12): not recommended.

Overdosage

Little is known about the effects of eflornithine overdose or accidental ingestion. Call your local poison control center for more information. ALWAYS bring the prescription container.

Special Information

If you forget to apply a dose of eflornithine, apply it as soon as you remember. Bear in mind that at least 8 hours must elapse between doses and you cannot wash the area for another 4 hours after application. If it is almost time for your next dose, skip the dose you forgot and continue with your regular schedule.

This product slows hair growth. It is not a depilatory. You will have to continue shaving, tweezing, or using another hair removal technique.

Wait several minutes after application of eflornithine before applying cosmetics or sunscreen.

Use only on your face and neck.

Call your doctor if your skin becomes irritated or if you develop other side effects. If skin irritation continues, you may have to stop using eflornithine.

Special Populations

Pregnancy/Breast-feeding: Eflornithine cream may cause birth defects. When this drug is considered crucial by your doctor, its potential benefits must be carefully weighed against its risks.

It is not known if this drug passes into breast milk. Nursing mothers should use infant formula.

Seniors: Seniors may use eflornithine without special restriction.

Generic Name

Enalapril (uh-NAL-uh-pril) G

Brand Name

Vasotec

Combination Product

Generic Ingredients: Enalapril + Hydrochlorothiazide G
Vaseretic

Type of Drug

Angiotensin-converting enzyme (ACE) inhibitor.

Prescribed For

Hypertension (high blood pressure), heart failure, diabetic kidney disease, and heart attack treatment when the function of the left ventricle has been affected. Also prescribed for kidney failure, kidney hypertension, managing people with a high risk of heart disease, chronic kidney disease, and preventing a second stroke.

General Information

Enalapril maleate and other ACE inhibitors work by preventing the conversion of a hormone called angiotensin I to another hormone called angiotensin II, a potent blood-vessel constrictor. Preventing this conversion relaxes blood vessels, thus reducing blood pressure and relieving symptoms of heart failure. Enalapril also affects the production of other hormones and enzymes that participate in the regulation of blood-vessel dilation. Enalapril begins working about 1 hour after you take it and continues to work for 24 hours.

Cautions and Warnings

Do not take enalapril if you are **allergic** or **sensitive** to any of its ingredients. Severe sensitivity reactions can occur in **hemodialysis** patients taking enalapril or those undergoing **venom immunization**.

Swelling of the face, extremities, or throat has been known to occur with enalapril, which can be dangerous (see "Special Information").

Enalapril occasionally causes very low blood pressure.

Enalapril may affect your kidney function, especially if you have **congestive heart failure**. Your doctor should check your urine for protein content during the first few months of treatment. Dosage adjustment of enalapril is necessary if you have **reduced kidney function**.

Enalapril can affect white-blood-cell counts, possibly increasing your susceptibility to infection. Your doctor should monitor your blood counts periodically.

Enalapril may cause serious injury or death to the fetus if taken during **pregnancy**. Pregnant women should not take enalapril.

ACE inhibitors may be less effective in some **black patients** with high blood pressure, especially when dietary salt intake is high. Nevertheless, they should still be considered useful blood pressure treatments. Swelling beneath the skin to form welts is more common among black patients.

Possible Side Effects

▼ Most common: dizziness, fatigue, headache, and chronic cough. The cough usually goes away a few days after you stop taking the medication.

▼ Less common: chest tightness or pain, dizziness when rising from a sitting or lying position, fainting, abdominal pain, nausea, vomiting, diarrhea, bronchitis, urinary tract infection, breathing difficulties, weakness, and rash.

▼ Rare: Rare side effects can occur in almost any part of the body. Contact your doctor if you experience any side effect not listed above.

For additional information about enalapril + felodipine, see Felodipine, page 471.

Drug Interactions

- The blood-pressure-lowering effect of enalapril is additive with diuretic drugs and beta blockers. Any other drug that causes a rapid drop in blood pressure should be used with caution if you are taking enalapril.
- Enalapril may increase the effects of lithium; this combination should be used with caution.
- Aspirin and other nonsteroidal anti-inflammatory drugs (NSAIDs) reduce the blood-pressure-lowering effects of enalapril and other ACE inhibitors. The combination may cause reductions in kidney function.
- Enalapril may increase blood-potassium levels, especially when taken with dyazide or other potassium-sparing diuretics.
- Antacids and enalapril should be taken at least 2 hours apart.
- Capsaicin may trigger or aggravate the cough associated with enalapril therapy.
- Indomethacin may reduce the blood-pressure-lowering effects of enalapril.
- Phenothiazine sedatives and antiemetics may increase the effects of enalapril.
- Rifampin may reduce the effects of enalapril.
- The combination of allopurinol and enalapril increases the chance of side effects. Avoid this combination.
- Enalapril affects blood levels of digoxin. More digoxin in the blood increases the chance of digoxin-related side effects,

while less digoxin in the blood can compromise its effectiveness.
- Severe sensitivity reactions can occur in those taking allopurinol.

For additional information about enalapril + felodipine, see Felodipine, page 471.

Food Interactions
You may take enalapril with food if it upsets your stomach.

Usual Dose
Enalapril
Adult: 5–40 mg a day in 1 or 2 doses. People with poor kidney function need less medication.

Enalapril + Felodipine
Adult: 1–2 tablets a day.

Overdosage
The principal effect of enalapril overdose is a rapid drop in blood pressure, as evidenced by dizziness or fainting. Take the overdose victim to a hospital emergency room immediately. ALWAYS bring the prescription bottle or container.

Special Information
Enalapril can cause swelling of the face, lips, hands, or feet. This swelling can also affect the larynx (throat) or tongue and interfere with breathing. If this happens, go to a hospital emergency room at once. Call your doctor if you develop a sore throat, mouth sores, abnormal heartbeat, chest pain, persistent rash, or loss of taste perception.

Some people who start taking enalapril after they are already on a diuretic (an agent that increases urination) experience a rapid drop in blood pressure after their first doses or when their dosage is increased. To prevent this from happening, your doctor may tell you to stop taking your diuretic 2 or 3 days before starting enalapril or to increase your salt intake during that time. The diuretic may then be restarted gradually.

You may get dizzy if you rise to your feet too quickly from a sitting or lying position when taking enalapril.

Avoid strenuous exercise or very hot weather because heavy sweating or dehydration can cause a rapid drop in blood pressure.

While taking enalapril, avoid over-the-counter diet pills, decongestants, and other stimulants that can raise blood pressure. Also, do not take potassium supplements or salt substitutes containing potassium without consulting your doctor.

If you take enalapril once a day and forget to take a dose, take it as soon as you remember. If it is within 8 hours of your next dose, skip the one you forgot and continue with your regular schedule. If you take enalapril twice a day and miss a dose, take it right away. If it is within 4 hours of your next dose, take 1 dose immediately and another in 5 or 6 hours, then go back to your regular schedule. Never take a double dose.

Special Populations

Pregnancy/Breast-feeding: ACE inhibitors can cause fetal injury or death. Women who are or might become pregnant should not take ACE inhibitors. Sexually active women of childbearing age who must take enalapril must use an effective contraceptive method to prevent pregnancy. If you become pregnant, stop taking the medication and call your doctor immediately.

Small amounts of enalapril pass into breast milk. Nursing mothers who must take this drug should use infant formula.

Seniors: Seniors may be more sensitive to the effects of this drug due to age-related losses in kidney or liver function.

Endocet see *Percocet,* page 863

Generic Name

Enfuvirtide (en-FUV-ir-tide)

Brand Name

Fuzeon

Type of Drug

Antiviral fusion inhibitor.

Prescribed For

Human immunodeficiency virus (HIV) infection.

General Information

Enfuvirtide is the first of a new class of anti-HIV drugs. Unlike all other anti-HIV medicines, it works by preventing the HIV virus from fusing to healthy CD4 cells, a key part of the human immune system. This helps fight HIV by having fewer HIV-infected cells as well as a healthier immune system to fight off the HIV virus. Enfuvirtide is always prescribed in combination with other antiviral medicines. It is possible for the HIV virus to become resistant to enfuvirtide, but this drug can work against types of the virus that have become resistant to other anti-HIV therapies.

Cautions and Warnings

Do not take enfuvirtide if you are **allergic** or **sensitive** to any of its ingredients. Symptoms of drug allergy can include generalized itching, rash, severe chills, and low blood pressure. In rare cases, enfuvirtide triggers severe hypersensitivity. Patients experiencing symptoms (a combination of rash, fever, nausea, and/or respiratory distress) should stop using enfuvirtide and seek medical attention immediately.

People taking enfuvirtide may be more likely to develop bacterial pneumonia. See your doctor regularly and report any difficulty breathing or unusual respiratory reactions.

Enfuvirtide may raise blood sugar levels, worsen diabetes, or trigger latent diabetes. People with diabetes who take this drug may need to have the dosage of their anti-diabetes medication adjusted.

Possible Side Effects

▼ Most common: allergic skin reaction at the site of injection (symptoms include itching, rash, and swelling of tissue under the skin), diarrhea, nausea, fatigue, and sleeplessness.

▼ Common: tingling in the hands or feet, depression, anxiety, cough, sinusitis, herpes infection, weight loss, appetite loss, weakness, itching, and muscle ache.

▼ Less common: taste changes, small skin tumors, flu infection, constipation, abdominal pain, pancreas inflammation, conjunctivitis (pinkeye), and lymph gland inflammation.

▼ Rare: Rare side effects can affect the blood, immune system, kidneys, urinary tract, and central nervous system. Contact your doctor if you experience any side effect not listed above.

Drug Interactions

Enfuvirtide is not broken down in the liver and does not affect liver enzyme systems, so it is not likely to be involved in common drug interactions.

Food Interactions

None known.

Usual Dose

Adult and Child (age 17 and over): 90 mg injected under the skin into the upper arm, thigh, or abdomen twice a day.

Child (age 6–16): 0.91 mg per lb. of body weight twice a day, up to 90 mg per injection. Be sure to increase enfuvirtide dosage as your child's weight increases.

Child (under age 6): not recommended.

Overdosage

Little is known about the effects of enfuvirtide overdose. Take the victim to a hospital emergency room. ALWAYS bring the prescription bottle or container.

Special Information

Enfuvirtide is not a cure for HIV. It will not prevent you from transmitting the HIV virus to another person; you must still practice safe sex. People taking this drug may still develop opportunistic infections and other complications associated with HIV infection.

This drug is given by injection under the skin. For information on how to properly administer this drug, see page 1242.

Do not use a vial of enfuvirtide if the final solution has particles floating in it. It should be completely clear, colorless, and have no bubbles in the vial.

You may keep solutions of enfuvirtide in the refrigerator and use them for up to 24 hours after they have been mixed. After that, they must be thrown away.

Tell your doctor if you are pregnant, become pregnant, or plan to become pregnant.

Do not stop taking this, or any other anti-HIV medicine, without first consulting your doctor.

Special Populations

Pregnancy/Breast-feeding: While animal studies of enfuvirtide reveal no damage to the fetus, this drug should only be used during pregnancy after carefully weighing its potential benefits against its risks. A national registry has been established to gather information on pregnant women who take this drug.

It is not known if enfuvirtide passes into breast milk. Nursing mothers with HIV should always use infant formula, regardless of whether they take this drug, to avoid transmitting the virus to their child.

Seniors: The effects of enfuvirtide in seniors is unknown.

Generic Name

Entacapone (in-TACK-a-pohn)

Brand Name
Comtan

Type of Drug
Antiparkinsonian.

Prescribed For
Parkinson's disease patients for whom levodopa + carbidopa loses its effectiveness between doses.

General Information
Entacapone is always used in combination with levodopa + carbidopa. Some patients experience signs and symptoms of an end-of-dose "wearing-off" effect with these drugs. Entacapone enhances the effect of levodopa + carbidopa by reversing the action of an enzyme known as catechol-O-methyltransferase (COMT), which is primarily responsible for breaking down levodopa in the body.

Cautions and Warnings
Do not take entacapone if you are **allergic** or **sensitive** to any of its ingredients.

Do not take entacapone with phenelzine or tranyleypromine, as a very serious reaction may occur.

People with **liver disease** should use entacapone with caution as they may accumulate twice as much of this drug in their blood as people with normal liver function.

Entacapone has been rarely associated with the formation of fibrous tissues in unusual places such as the urinary tract and lungs. It has also caused fluid in the lungs.

Entacapone may cause kidney toxicity.

Entacapone may increase the risk of dizziness or fainting when rising from a sitting or lying down position.

Hallucinations have been reported with other Parkinson's disease drugs.

Possible Side Effects

▼ Most common: difficulty performing voluntary muscle functions, excessive muscle activity, nausea, urine discoloration, and diarrhea.

▼ Common: reduced muscle activity, dizziness, fatigue, constipation, and abdominal pain.

▼ Less common: low blood pressure and fainting when rising from a sitting or lying position, hallucinations, anxiety, agitation, gastritis or other stomach disorders, dry mouth, vomiting, increased sweating, back pain, taste changes, shortness of breath, easy bruising, weakness, and bacterial infection.

▼ Rare: muscle damage or death, high fever, and confusion. Contact your doctor if you experience any side effect not listed above.

Drug Interactions

- Do not mix entacapone with the monoamine oxidase inhibitor (MAOI) antidepressants phenelzine or tranylcypromine. Entacapone may be taken with the MAOI selegiline.
- Other drugs broken down by COMT will also be affected by entacapone. Isoproterenol, epinephrine, ephedrine, norepinephrine, isoetharine, and others will interact with entacapone, even when taken by inhalation. The result may be increased heart rate, arrhythmias, and excessive changes in blood pressure.
- Cholestyramine, probenecid, erythromycin, rifampin, ampicillin, and chloramphenicol may interfere with the elimination of entacapone from the body.
- Entacapone may enhance the effects of sedatives and other nervous system depressants.

Food Interactions

This drug may be taken with or without food.

Usual Dose

Adult: 200 mg with each levodopa + carbidopa dose, up to 1600 mg a day.

Child: not recommended.

Overdosage

Theoretically, a massive entacapone overdose could prove lethal by completely inhibiting COMT throughout the body. There have been no reports of significant entacapone overdose. Doses up to 800 mg have been taken and side effects were mainly abdominal pain and loose stools. Other effects that might be expected include difficulty breathing, loss of muscle coordination, reduced level of activity, and convulsions. Overdose victims should be taken to a hospital emergency room as soon as possible. ALWAYS bring the prescription bottle or container.

Special Information

Always take your entacapone dose together with your levodopa + carbidopa dose. If you forget a dose, take it as soon as you remember. If it is within 2 hours of your next dose, skip the dose you forgot and continue with your regular schedule.

This drug can cause dizziness, nausea, sweating, or fainting when rising quickly from a sitting or lying position, especially at the beginning of treatment.

Increased body movements and twitching, twisting, or uncontrolled tongue, lip, face, arm, or leg movement may occur. If this happens, your doctor may need to adjust your dose of levodopa + carbidopa.

Exercise caution when performing tasks, such as driving, that require coordination and concentration until your body has become accustomed to the effects of entacapone.

Gradually reducing the dose of entacapone decreases some drug side effects.

Rapid withdrawal can cause high fever, sweating, unstable blood pressure, stupor, and muscular rigidity. Patients who stop using entacapone should be monitored.

Entacapone can cause your urine to turn a brownish-orange color. This change is harmless.

Special Populations

Pregnancy/Breast-feeding: Entacapone causes birth defects, miscarriage and abortion in pregnant animals. When this drug is considered crucial by your doctor, its potential benefits must be weighed against its risks.

Entacapone passes into the breast milk of animals but no information on humans is available. Nursing mothers who must take this drug should use infant formula.

Seniors: Seniors may take this drug without special precaution.

Generic Name

Entecavir (en-TEK-ah-veer)

Brand Name

Baraclude

Information in this monograph also applies to:

Generic Ingredient: Telbivudine
Tyzeka

Type of Drug

Antiviral.

Prescribed For

Chronic hepatitis B infection in adults.

General Information

Entecavir is a prescription medicine for adults with chronic hepatitis B virus (HBV) infection in which the virus is multiplying and damaging the liver. Entecavir can reduce the amount of virus in the body, make it harder for new liver cells to be infected by the virus, and improve the general condition of the liver. They work by attacking HBV polymerase, an enzyme essential to the reproduction of the hepatitis B virus inside an infected cell. These drugs are eliminated from the body via the kidney. Telbivudine does not work against HIV infection and can be taken together with HIV drug therapy. These medicines do not cure HBV or stop you from spreading HBV to others, generally through sexual contact or exposure to infected blood. The HBV virus can live outside the body for one week.

Cautions and Warnings

Do not take these medicines if you are **allergic** or **sensitive** to any of their ingredients.

Entecavir should be used with caution in people who have both **HIV** and **HBV** because of possible HIV resistance developing after entecavir is taken.

Severe worsening of **HBV** has occurred in people who stopped taking this medication.

These drugs can lead to further **liver damage**. In rare cases, they have been associated with liver failure that resulted in death. The safety of this drug in people who have had a **liver transplant** is not known.

These drugs are eliminated through the kidneys. People with **kidney disease** may require lower doses.

Telbivudine has also been associated with lactic acidosis, a condition in which excess lactic acid in the body causes the blood to become acidic. Feeling very weak or tired, experiencing unusual muscle pain, difficulty breathing, stomach pain with nausea and vomiting, feeling cold—especially in your arms and legs, feeling dizzy or lightheaded, and a fast or irregular heartbeat may be signs of lactic acidosis. It is a medical emergency and must be treated in the hospital. This has happened in some people taking these medications.

Possible Side Effects

Entecavir
▼ Most common: headache, fatigue, dizziness, and nausea.
▼ Less common: diarrhea, upset stomach, vomiting, tiredness, and sleeplessness.
▼ Rare: Rare side effects may affect almost any part of the body. Contact your doctor if you experience any side effect not listed above.

Telbivudine
▼ Most common: upper respiratory infection, fatigue, not feeling well, muscle tenderness or weakness, abdominal pain, nasal irritation, and sore throat.
▼ Common: flu or flu-like symptoms, diarrhea or loose stools, and throat pain.
▼ Less common: fever, joint pain, rash, back pain, dizziness, muscle ache, sleeplessness, and upset stomach.

Drug Interactions

- These drugs do not affect liver enzymes and have a low interaction potential.
- Drugs that affect kidney function may affect blood concentrations of entecavir and telbivudine.
- Other hepatitis B treatments (lamivudine, adefovir, cyclosporine, and pegylated interferon-alpha 2a) do not affect either entecavir or telbivudine and are not affected by them.

Food Interactions

Take entecavir at least 2 hours after a meal and 2 hours before the next meal. Telbivudine may be taken without regard to food or meals.

Usual Dose

Entecavir

Adult and Child (age 16 and over): 0.5–1 mg once daily. People with kidney failure may be treated with as little as 0.05–0.1 mg a day.
Child (under age 16): not recommended.

Telbivudine

Adult and Child (age 16 and over): 600 mg once daily. People with moderate to severe kidney failure may be treated with a single 600 mg dose every 2, 3, or 4 days depending on the seriousness of kidney disease.
Child (under age 16): not recommended.

Overdosage

There are no reports of entecavir overdose. People taking single doses up to 40 mg or multiple doses up to 20 mg per day for up to 14 days had no unusual side effects. One person accidentally took an overdose with no consequences. People taking up to 1800 mg a day of telbivudine had no increase in side effects. Overdose victims should be taken to a hospital emergency room for treatment, where dialysis may be necessary to remove the drug from the blood. ALWAYS bring the prescription bottle or container.

Special Information

Call your doctor if you develop muscle aches, pains, or weakness; if your skin or the white part of your eyes turns yellow; if your urine becomes dark; if your bowel movements turn light in color; if you don't feeling like eating food for several days or longer; if you become nauseous; or if you have lower stomach pain. These can be signs of a serious liver problem called hepatotoxicity, which has occurred in some people taking these medications.

Your hepatitis B may get worse or become very serious if you stop taking these medications. Do not stop taking them or change your daily dose without talking to your doctor.

If you forget to take your daily entecavir dose, take it as soon as you remember but do not take a double dose. Call your doctor if you forget to take 2 or more doses in a row.

Entecavir oral solution is a ready-to-use product and should not be mixed with water or any other liquid product. Each bottle of the oral solution comes with a dosing spoon that is calibrated in 1-mL increments, up to 10 mL. Hold the spoon upright and gradually fill it to the mark next to the prescribed dose. Drink the liquid directly from the dosing spoon. Your pharmacist can help you properly measure your medication dose. Rinse the dosing spoon with water after each daily dose and allow it to air dry.

Special Populations

Pregnancy/Breast-feeding: Animal studies of entecavir revealed slowed development of the skeleton. Animal studies of telbivudine did not reveal any effects on the developing fetus. However, it is not known if either medicine is safe to use during pregnancy or if it helps prevent the hepatitis B virus from passing on to a developing fetus. If your doctor considers entecavir or telbivudine crucial for you, potential benefits must be carefully weighed against their risks. A data bank has been established to collect information from doctors on pregnant women who do take these medicines.

These medicines may pass into breast milk. Nursing mothers who must take these drugs should use infant formula.

Seniors: Dosage reduction may be needed in seniors because of normal declines in kidney function.

Brand Name

Entex PSE

Generic Ingredients

Guaifenesin + Pseudoephedrine Hydrochloride Ⓖ

Other Brand Names

Anatuss LA	Coldmist Jr.
Aquatab D Dosepack	Coldmist LA
Coldmist	Congess Jr.

Congess SR
Congestac
Deconsal LA
D-Feda II
Durasal II
Duratuss AM/PM
Dynex
Endal-SR
Guaifed
Guaifed-PD
Guaifed-PSE
Guaifed SR
Guaifenex GP
Guaifenex PSE 60
Guaifenex PSE 80
Guaifenex PSE 85
Guaifenex PSE 120
Guaifenex RX
Guaimax-D
Guaipax PSE
Guaitab
Guaituss PE
Guai-Vent PSE
Iosal II
Maxifed
Maxifed G
Med-RX
Miraphen PSE

Nasabid
Nasabid-SR
Nasatab LA
PanMist
PanMist-Jr.
PanMist LA
Profen II
Pseudovent
Pseudovent-PED
Respa-1st
Respaire-60 SR
Respaire-120 SR
Robitussin PE
Ru-Tuss DE
Rymed
Sinufed Timecelles
Sinutab
Stamoist E
Sudal 60/500
Sudal120/600
Sudal SR
Syn-RX
Touro LA
Tuss-LA
V-Dec-M
Versacaps
Zephrex
Zephrex LA

The information in this profile also applies to the following drugs:

Generic Ingredients: Guaifenesin + Ephedrine Hydrochloride Ⓖ
Broncholate   Bronkaid

Generic Ingredients: Guaifenesin + Phenylephrine Hydrochloride Ⓖ

Deconsal II
Deconsal Pediatric
Endal
Entex LA
Liquibid D
Liquibid-D 1200
Liquibid-PD

PhenaVent
PhenaVent D
PhenaVent LA
PhenaVent PED
Rescon GG
Sinupan
Sinuvent PE

Type of Drug

Decongestant and expectorant combination.

Prescribed For

Cold or allergy and for nasal congestion, runny nose and cough associated with other upper respiratory conditions.

General Information

The decongestant ingredient in Entex PSE, pseudoephedrine, dramatically reduces congestion and stuffiness. The decongestant ingredients ephedrine and phenylephrine act similarly. The expectorant, guaifenesin, is used to help loosen thick mucus that may contribute to chest congestion; the effectiveness of guaifenesin and other expectorants has not been established. There are other drugs on the market using this same general formula—an expectorant plus a decongestant—but they use different decongestant ingredients or a combination of decongestants plus guaifenesin. Nothing cures a cold or allergy, but Entex PSE may provide relief from symptoms.

Cautions and Warnings

Do not take Entex PSE if you are **allergic** or **sensitive** to any of its ingredients.

Entex PSE may cause anxiety or nervousness or interfere with sleep.

Do not use Entex PSE if you have **ventricular tachycardia** (quickened heartrate), or **hypertension** (high blood pressure).

Entex PSE should be used with extreme caution in those with **heart disease,** other **heart rhythm disorders, thyroid disease, diabetes, glaucoma, stomach ulcer, urinary blockage,** or a **prostate condition.**

Entex PSE should not be used over extended periods of time to treat **persistent or chronic cough** especially one that may be caused by cigarette smoking, asthma, or emphysema.

Possible Side Effects

▼ Most common: anxiety, restlessness, sleeplessness, tension, excitation, dizziness, drowsiness, and headache.
▼ Less common: nausea, vomiting, upset stomach, low blood pressure, heart palpitations, chest pain, rapid or slow heartbeat, abnormal heart rhythms, irritability, euphoria (feeling

---

Possible Side Effects *(continued)*

"high"), eye irritation and tearing, hysterical reaction, appetite loss, kidney stones, urinary difficulties in men with a prostate condition, weakness, loss of facial color, and breathing difficulties.

Drug Interactions

- Entex PSE should be avoided if you are taking a monoamine oxidase inhibitor (MAOI) antidepressant for depression or hypertension because the MAOI may cause a very rapid rise in blood pressure or increase side effects such as dry mouth or nose, blurred vision, and abnormal heart rhythms.
- The decongestant in Entex PSE may interfere with blood-pressure-lowering medication.

Food Interactions

Take Entex PSE with food if it upsets your stomach.

Usual Dose

Adult and Child (age 12 and over): 1 tablet or capsule twice a day or 2 tsp. of liquid 4 times a day.

Child (age 6–11): ½–1 tablet or 1 capsule twice a day or 1 tsp. of liquid 4 times a day.

Overdosage

Most cases of overdose are not severe. Symptoms include sedation, sleepiness, increased sweating, and increased blood pressure. Hallucinations, convulsions, nervous system depression, and breathing difficulties are more prominent in older adults. Most cases of overdose are not severe. Induce vomiting with ipecac syrup—available at any pharmacy. Call your local poison control center or a hospital emergency room before doing this. If you seek treatment, ALWAYS bring the prescription bottle or container.

Special Information

Call your doctor if your side effects are severe or gradually become intolerable.

If you forget a dose, take it as soon as you remember. If it is almost time for your next dose, skip the one you forgot and continue with your regular schedule. Do not take a double dose.

Special Populations

Pregnancy/Breast-feeding: Women who are or might be pregnant should avoid Entex PSE. When your doctor considers this drug crucial, its potential benefits must be carefully weighed against its risks.

The decongestant in Entex PSE may pass into breast milk. Nursing mothers who must take Entex PSE should consider using infant formula.

Seniors: Seniors are more sensitive to the effects of Entex PSE.

Generic Name

Epoetin (EE-poh-eh-tin)

Brand Names

Epogen   Procrit

Type of Drug

Red-blood-cell growth stimulator.

Prescribed For

Anemia; may also be used for reducing the need for blood or red-blood-cell transfusions.

General Information

Epoetin is a natural hormone that stimulates the bone marrow to produce red blood cells. It is used for anemia that does not respond to iron supplements. In most cases of anemia, there are plenty of red blood cells circulating, but they lack iron. People who need epoetin do not have enough red blood cells. Epoetin stimulates the production of new red blood cells to carry needed oxygen.

Cautions and Warnings

Do not use epoetin if you are **allergic** or **sensitive** to albumin or products manufactured from animal cells.

People with **uncontrolled high blood pressure** should not use epoetin.

Some people with **chronic kidney failure** and **severe anemia** should not take epoetin. Epoetin is not a replacement for emergency blood transfusion.

Epoetin is not intended for **anemia caused by folate or iron deficiency, hemolysis, or gastrointestinal bleeding.**

People using epoetin may require anticoagulant medicine to prevent **blood clotting** during treatment. Tell your doctor if you have any blood-clotting disorders.

In rare cases, people taking epoetin may have seizures. Avoid driving or any other activities where a sudden seizure could be dangerous. Do not take epoetin if you have a history of **seizures** or **strokes.**

Epoetin should be avoided in patients with **blood cancers** such as lymphoma, because it can act as a growth factor for the tumor.

If your hemoglobin levels become too high, your chance of heart attack, stroke, heart failure, blood clots, and death is increased. It is important to have your blood tested and adjust dosage of epoetin accordingly throughout treatment.

Possible Side Effects

Side effects reported in studies of epoetin were similar to those reported with an inactive placebo (sugar pill).

▼ Most common: high blood pressure, headache, constipation, diarrhea, nausea, joint pain, fever, fatigue, itching, rash, and difficulty breathing.

▼ Common: swelling, vomiting, chest pain, skin reactions at the site of injection, weakness, dizziness, urinary infections, diarrhea, upset stomach, blood clots, anxiety, tingling in the hands or feet, and trunk pain.

▼ Rare: stroke and heart attack. Contact your doctor if you experience any side effect not listed above.

Food and Drug Interactions

None known.

Usual Dose

Adult: starting dose—23–69 units per lb. of body weight 3 times a week by intravenous or subcutaneous injection. Final dose is based on response and need. Surgery patients take 138 units per lb. for 10 days before surgery or 276 units once a week for 3 weeks before surgery and another dose on the day of surgery. Dialysis patients take epoetin once a week.

Child (under age 12): 23 units per lb. of body weight 3 times a week by intravenous or subcutaneous injection. Final dose is based on response and need.

Child (under 1 month): not recommended.

Overdosage

Little is known about the effects of epoetin overdose. Call your local poison control center or a hospital emergency room for information. If you seek treatment, ALWAYS bring the prescription container.

Special Information

People taking epoetin should have regular blood tests to assure the drug is working well. Your doctor may want to take blood samples twice a week for several weeks and then test your blood regularly.

Epoetin has been used by athletes to enhance physical performance. This is called blood doping and has resulted in several deaths because the percentage of red blood cells in a blood sample can reach hazardous levels.

Epoetin must be stored in a refrigerator.

Most patients will need to take iron supplements with this drug.

This drug can be given by injection under the skin. For more information on how to properly administer this drug, see page 1242.

Special Populations

Pregnancy/Breast-feeding: Animal studies suggest that epoetin may enter fetal circulation. When this drug is considered crucial by your doctor its potential benefits must be carefully weighed against its risks.

It is not known if epoetin passes into breast milk. Nursing mothers who must take it should use infant formula.

Seniors: Seniors may use this product without special precaution.

Type of Drug

Erectile Dysfunction Drugs

Generic Ingredient: Sildenafil Citrate
Viagra   Revatio

Generic Ingredient: Tadalafil
Cialis

Generic Ingredient: Vardenafil
Levitra

Prescribed For

Erectile dysfunction (ED). Sildenafil is also prescribed for pulmonary hypertension.

General Information

The chemical nitric oxide is released in the penis during sexual stimulation. Nitric oxide causes the release of an enzyme called cyclic guanosine monophosphate (cGMP), which increases blood flow into the penis, producing an erection. cGMP is broken down by the enzyme phosphodiesterase type 5 (PDE5). In men with low levels of cGMP, these medicines help achieve and maintain an erection by inhibiting PDE5, thus causing higher levels of cGMP. ED can be the result of nerve, blood vessel, or psychological problems. These drugs, which are effective in about 70% of men, only help when poor blood flow is the cause of the dysfunction. Women have reported some benefit from sildenafil, although it has been widely studied only in men. Vardenafil and tadalafil are intended only for men. These medicines start working in 30–60 minutes and their effects usually last from 2–4 hours, although some have noted an effect for 24 hours or more. Some drug interactions and kidney or liver diseases extend this time. Tadalafil begins working in 30–60 minutes and can remain in the body for more than 2 days, much longer than the other medicines in this group. Low-dose tadalafil may be taken every day for chronic ED.

Pulmonary hypertension, a rare disease in which high pressure in the blood vessels moves from the heart to the lungs, is sometimes treated with sildenafil.

Cautions and Warnings

Do not take ED drugs if you are **allergic** or **sensitive** to any of their ingredients.

These medicines **lower blood pressure** and should be avoided if you have high (greater than 170/100) or low (less than 90/50) blood pressure. Several people have died from a sudden blood-pressure drop after combining erectile dysfunction medications with other medications that can reduce blood pressure.

These medicines should never be taken by those taking heart medications called **nitrates,** as fatal reactions have occurred.

People with **heart disease** may experience heart problems with sildenafil or vardenafil, including a heart attack. These reactions can occur during or shortly after sexual activity.

Avoid these medicines if you have had a **heart attack, stroke,** or life-threatening **abnormal heart rhythms** in the past 6 months, or if you have **heart failure,** unstable **angina pectoris, damage to the penis,** or a progressive eye disease called **retinitis pigmentosa.** Blindness is a rare side effect of sildenafil and may be a problem with all of these medications.

People taking sildenafil or vardenafil have experienced difficulties seeing blue or green colors and may see things with a blue tinge surrounding them. This happens because they affect an enzyme in the eye. The effect clears up after the drug passes out of the body.

People with **kidney or liver damage** retain these medicines in their bodies longer than people whose kidneys and liver function normally. People with kidney or liver problems should always begin with the lowest possible dosage.

People with **priapism** (painful erection lasting more than 6 hours) or a condition that predisposes them to priapism—such as **leukemia, multiple myeloma,** or **sickle cell anemia**—should be cautious about taking these medicines.

Vardenafil and sildenafil should be avoided by people with **stomach or bleeding ulcers** because its effect on these conditions is not known.

Possible Side Effects

Sildenafil
▼ Most common: headache and flushing.
▼ Less common: upset stomach, stuffy nose, urinary tract infection, diarrhea, rash, dizziness, seizure, anxiety, prolonged and possibly painful erection, double vision, visual changes, bloodshot eyes, burning eyes, swelling in the eye, and blood vessel diseases in the retina.
▼ Rare: Rare side effects can occur in almost any part of the body. Contact your doctor if you experience any side effect not listed above.

Tadalafil
▼ Most common: headache.
▼ Common: upset stomach. Back pain and muscle aches can develop 12–24 hours after taking tadalafil and go away on their own after 2 days.

Possible Side Effects *(continued)*

▼ Less common: flushing, nasal congestion, and arm or leg pain.

▼ Rare: prolonged or painful erections. Other rare side effects can occur in almost any part of the body. Contact your doctor if you experience any side effect not listed above.

Vardenafil

▼ Most common: headache and flushing.

▼ Less common: upset stomach, sinus infection, flu-like symptoms, dizziness, and nausea.

▼ Rare: prolonged or painful erection. Other rare side effects can occur in almost any part of the body. Contact your doctor if you experience any side effect not listed above.

Drug Interactions

- Do not combine any of these drugs with nitrates (such as nitroglycerin) and other drugs that lower blood pressure. The combination can cause a sudden, rapid drop in blood pressure.

- Do not take vardenafil if you are taking an alpha blocker (such as alfuzosin, doxazosin, prazosin, tamsulosin, or terazosin). Tadalafil may be taken only with tamsulosin. You may take sildenafil at its lowest possible dose with an alpha blocker, but you must separate the doses by at least 4 hours.

- Combining cimetidine and sildenafil leads to a substantial (more than 50%) increase in the amount of sildenafil in the blood.

- Erythromycin, itraconazole, ketoconazole, and protease inhibitors (used to combat HIV) can cause sildenafil blood levels to almost double. Vardenafil levels can increase by 400–1000% when combined with these medicines. If you are taking one of these medicines, do not take more than the lowest possible dose of your ED drug. Do not take tadalafil more than once every 3 days if you are also taking one of these medicines.

- Rifampin can be expected to reduce the effect of ED medicines by reducing the amount of drug in the blood. Other drugs that may reduce the effects of these drugs are carba-mazepine, phenobarbital, and phenytoin.

- Dihydrocodeine—a widely used prescription pain reliever—may increase the effects of sildenafil, yielding substantially prolonged erections, sometimes lasting for hours.
- Do not combine sildenafil, tadalafil, and vardenafil. The effects of combining these drugs are not known.
- Do not take vardenafil if you are taking any medicine to treat an abnormal heartbeat, including amiodarone, procainamide, quinidine, and sotalol.
- Combining sildenafil with selective serotonin reuptake inhibitors (SSRIs) or tacrolimus may increase the risk of silde-nafil side effects.
- Alcohol adds to the blood-pressure-lowering effects of these medicines.

Food Interactions

Grapefruit juice may increase the amount of these drugs in the blood. Taking sildenafil with a high-fat meal reduces the amount of drug absorbed. Tadalafil and vardenafil may be taken without regard to food or meals.

Usual Dose

Sildenafil

Adult: 50 mg taken about 1 hour before sexual activity. Individual doses can range from 25–100 mg. The maximum dosing frequency is once a day.

Senior: Begin with 25 mg and gradually increase dosage as needed.

Tadalafil

Adult: 10 mg taken about 1 hour before sexual activity. Individual doses can range from 2.5–20 mg. Do not take more than 1 dose of tadalafil a day.

Senior: Begin with 5 mg and gradually increase dosage as needed.

Vardenafil

Adult: 10 mg taken about 1 hour before sexual activity. Individual doses can range from 5–20 mg.

Senior: Begin with 5 mg and gradually increase dosage as needed.

Overdosage

Sildenafil and tadalafil overdose are likely to produce exaggerated drug side effects. Vardenafil overdose may cause neck pain, muscle aches, or vision changes. Call your local poison control center or hospital emergency room for more information. If you seek treatment, ALWAYS bring the prescription bottle or container.

Special Information

Call your doctor and do not engage in sexual activity if the erection produced by ED drugs is painful or lasts 4 or more hours, or if you experience dizziness, nausea, or chest pain after taking an ED drug. In rare cases, men taking ED drugs have reported a sudden decrease or loss of vision and/or hearing. Call your doctor right away if you experience this adverse side effect.

People who use organic nitrates for gardening or other purposes can experience a severe and dangerous blood pressure drop if they take sildenafil or vardenafil. It is not known how long you have to wait to resume nitrate use.

These drugs do not protect against sexually transmitted diseases.

Special Populations

Pregnancy/Breast-feeding: There is no evidence that sildenafil or vardenafil harm the fetus; however, they are not intended for pregnant women or nursing mothers.

Seniors: Men age 65 and over eliminate these drugs more slowly than younger men and should begin with the lowest possible dosage.

Generic Name

Ergoloid Mesylates (ER-goe-loid MES-il-ates) Ⓖ

Brand Names

Gerimal   Hydrogenated Ergot Alkaloids
Hydergine

Type of Drug

Psychotherapeutic agent.

Prescribed For

Age-related decline in mental capacity.

General Information

Ergoloid mesylates are used to treat decreased mental capacity of unknown cause in people over age 60. These drugs should not be used for any condition that is treatable with another drug or that may be reversible. People who respond to ergoloid mesylates are likely to have Alzheimer's disease or some other cause of dementia. Nobody knows exactly how ergoloid mesylates produce their effect, but they improve the supply of blood to the brain in test animals, reduce their heart rate, and improve muscle tone in blood vessels. Some studies show the drugs to be very effective in relieving mild symptoms of mental impairment, while others find it to be only moderately effective. They are most beneficial in people whose symptoms are due to the effects of high blood pressure in the brain.

Cautions and Warnings

Do not take ergoloid mesylates if you are **allergic** or **sensitive** to any of their ingredients or you have **psychotic symptoms** or **psychosis**.

Ergoloid mesylates should be used with caution in people with **liver disease, low blood pressure,** or **slow heartbeat.**

Possible Side Effects

Ergoloid mesylates do not produce serious side effects.

▼ Common: When taken under the tongue, these drugs may cause irritation, nausea, or upset stomach. Other side effects are drowsiness, slow heartbeat, and rash.

Drug Interactions

None known.

Food Interactions

Do not eat, drink, or smoke while you have an ergoloid mesylates pill under your tongue.

Usual Dose

Starting dose is 1–2 mg 3 times a day. Increase as needed. Do not exceed 12 mg a day.

Overdosage

Symptoms include blurred vision, dizziness, fainting, flushing, headache, appetite loss, nausea, vomiting, stomach cramps, and stuffy nose. Take the victim to a hospital emergency room. ALWAYS bring the prescription bottle or container.

Special Information

The effects of ergoloid mesylates are gradual and frequently not seen for up to 6 months. A 6-month period of treatment with ergoloid mesylates is recommended before your doctor can fully evaluate your response to the drug. Your doctor should periodically reevaluate your condition to determine if ergoloid mesylates treatment is still needed and that it is working for you.

Dissolve sublingual tablets under the tongue. Do not chew or crush them; they are not effective if swallowed whole.

If you forget a dose, skip it and go back to your regular schedule. Do not take a double dose. Call your doctor if you miss 2 or more consecutive doses.

Special Populations

Pregnancy/Breast-feeding: Ergoloid mesylates may interfere with fetal development. When these drugs are considered crucial by your doctor, their potential benefits must be carefully weighed against their risks.

Ergoloid mesylates pass into breast milk. Nursing mothers who must take these drugs should use infant formula.

Seniors: Seniors are more likely to develop side effects, especially hypothermia (low body temperature).

Generic Name

Erythromycin (eh-rith-roe-MYE-sin) Ⓖ

Brand Names

Akne-mycin	Eryderm
A/T/S	Erygel
E-Base	Ery-Tab
E-Glades	Erythra-derm
E-Mycin	PCE
Eryc	

The information in this profile also applies to all forms of erythromycin:

Generic Ingredient: Erythromycin Estolate Ⓖ

Generic Ingredient: Erythromycin Ethylsuccinate Ⓖ
E.E.S.   Pediamycin
EryPed

*Generic Ingredients: Erythromycin Ethylsuccinate +
Sulfisoxasole* Ⓖ
Eryzole   Pediazole

Generic Ingredient: Erythromycin Stearate Ⓖ
Erythrocin Stearate

Type of Drug

Macrolide antibiotic.

Prescribed For

Infections of virtually any part of the body: upper and lower respiratory tract infections; sexually transmitted diseases; urinary tract infections; infections of the mouth, gums, or teeth; and infections of the nose, ears, or sinuses. It is prescribed for acne and may be used for mild to moderate skin infections. Erythromycin is effective against diphtheria and dysentery. It is also prescribed for legionnaires' disease, rheumatic fever, whooping cough, and bacterial endocarditis. It is prescribed to patients with pelvic inflammatory disease as an alternative to penicillin. The eye ointment is used to prevent newborn gonococcal or chlamydial eye infections.

General Information

Erythromycin and other macrolide antibiotics are either bactericidal (bacteria-killing) or bacteriostatic (inhibiting bacterial growth), depending on the organism in question and amount of antibiotic present. Erythromycin is deactivated by stomach acid, so the tablet form is made to bypass the stomach and dissolve in the intestine.

Since the action of this antibiotic depends on its concentration in the invading bacteria, it is crucial that you follow your doctor's directions regarding the spacing of doses as well as the number of days you must take the medication—otherwise, this antibiotic may be much less effective.

Cautions and Warnings

Do not take erythromycin if you are **allergic** or **sensitive** to any of its ingredients or to any macrolide antibiotic.

Erythromycin is excreted primarily through the liver. People with **liver disease or damage** should consult their doctors. Those on long-term therapy with erythromycin should have periodic blood tests. If you restart erythromycin after having experienced liver damage, it is likely that symptoms will recur within 48 hours.

Erythromycin estolate has occasionally produced liver problems (symptoms include fatigue, nausea, vomiting, abdominal cramps, and fever). If you are susceptible to **stomach problems**, erythromycin may cause mild to moderate stomach upset; discontinuing the drug will reverse this condition.

Colitis (bowel inflammation) has been associated with all antibiotics and can range from mild to life-threatening (see "Possible Side Effects").

Possible Side Effects

▼ Most common: nausea, vomiting, stomach cramps, and diarrhea. Colitis (symptoms include severe abdominal cramps and severe, persistent, and possibly bloody diarrhea) may develop. Side effects of the topical erythromycin include peeling, dryness, itching, and oiliness.

▼ Less common: hairy tongue, itching, irritation of the anal or vaginal region, eye irritation, and skin tenderness. If any of these symptoms appear, call your physician immediately.

▼ Rare: hearing loss—which reverses itself after the drug is stopped and occurs most often in people with liver and kidney problems—and abnormal heart rhythms. Contact your doctor if you experience any side effect not listed above.

Drug Interactions

- Antacids may slightly affect the release of erythromycin from your body. This effect is not considered important.
- Do not combine erythromycin with astemizole or terfenadine.
- Erythromycin may slow the breakdown of carbamazepine (an anticonvulsant prescribed for seizures). Avoid this combination.
- Mixing erythromycin with rifabutin or rifampin can interfere with the antibiotic's effect and increase the risk of intestinal side effects.
- Do not combine erythromycin and pimozide. Two people died after combining pimozide and a macrolide antibiotic.

- Erythromycin may neutralize penicillin. It may also neutralize the antibiotics lincomycin and clindamycin.
- Erythromycin interferes with the elimination of theophylline from the body, possibly leading to theophylline overdose.
- Mixing erythromycin with a statin cholesterol-lowering drug increases the risk of developing a potentially fatal condition involving severe muscle pain and destruction.
- Do not mix erythromycin with sparfloxacin, ketoconazole, itraconazole, fluconazole, diltiazem, verapamil, troleando-mycin, mibefradil, nefazodone, or clarithromycin. These mixtures can lead to severe, possibly fatal, abnormal heart rhythms. Grepafloxacin (another fluoroquinolone) should only be mixed with erythromycin in hospitalized patients whose hearts can be monitored during treatment.
- Combining erythromycin and alfentanil (an injectable pain reliever), bromocriptine, buspirone, digoxin, disopyramide, ergotamine, cyclosporine, methylprednisolone (a corticosteroid), tacrolimus, vinblastine, or benzodiazepines (such as alprazolam, diazepam, midazolam, and triazolam) increases the risk of drug side effects.
- Erythromycin estolate may increase the liver side effects of other drugs that affect the liver.
- Erythromycin may increase the anticoagulant (blood-thinning) effects of warfarin in people who take it regularly, especially older adults. People taking this combination should be tested regularly.
- Erythromycin may increase the effects of caffeine.

Food Interactions

Grapefruit juice slows the breakdown of erythromycin, increasing the amount of drug in the blood. For optimum effectiveness, take erythromycin base and erythromycin stearate on an empty stomach with a 6–8 oz. glass of water 1 hour before or 2 hours after meals. Other forms of erythromycin can be taken without regard to food or meals.

Usual Dose

Tablet and Suspension

Adult: 250–400 mg every 6 hours, taken 1 hour before meals, or 500 mg every 12 hours. Maximum dose is 4 g a day.

Child: 15–25 mg per lb. of body weight a day in divided doses depending on age, weight, and severity of infection.

Eye Ointment: ½ inch 2–6 times a day.

Topical Solution: Apply morning and night.

Doses of erythromycin ethylsuccinate are 60% higher due to differences in chemical composition.

Overdosage

Overdose may cause severe side effects, especially nausea, vomiting, stomach cramps, and diarrhea. Mild hearing loss, ringing or buzzing in the ears, or fainting may also occur. Call your local poison control center or a hospital emergency room for more information. ALWAYS bring the prescription bottle or container.

Special Information

Erythromycin is used instead of penicillin for mild to moderate infections in people who are allergic to penicillin. Erythromycin is not the antibiotic of choice for severe infections.

Erythromycin products should be stored at room temperature, except for oral and topical liquids, which should be kept in the refrigerator.

Call your doctor if you develop nausea; vomiting; diarrhea; stomach cramps; severe abdominal pain; rash, itching, or redness; dark or amber-colored urine; yellowing of the skin or whites of the eyes; or any severe or persistent side effect.

If you forget a dose of oral erythromycin, take it as soon as you remember. If it is almost time for your next dose, space the next 2 doses over 4–6 hours, then continue with your regular schedule. Do not take a double dose.

Remember to complete the full course of therapy prescribed even if you feel well before you finish the medication.

Special Populations

Pregnancy/Breast-feeding: Erythromycin passes into the fetal circulation. Erythromycin estolate has caused mild liver inflammation in about 10% of pregnant women who took it and should not be used if you are or might be pregnant. Other forms of erythromycin have been used safely without difficulty.

Erythromycin passes into breast milk. Nursing mothers who must take erythromycin should use infant formula.

Seniors: Seniors with liver disease should use caution. Seniors taking high doses of erythromycin may be at an increased risk of hearing loss.

Generic Name

Estazolam (es-TAZ-oe-lam) Ⓖ

Type of Drug

Benzodiazepine sedative.

Prescribed For

Insomnia and sleep disturbances.

General Information

Estazolam is a member of the group of drugs known as benzodiazepines. They work by a direct effect on the brain. Benzodiazepines make it easier to go to sleep and decrease the number
of times you wake up during the night. Estazolam is considered an
intermediate-acting sedative and generally remains in your body
long enough to give you a good night's sleep with minimal "hangover."

Cautions and Warnings

Do not take estazolam if you are **allergic** or **sensitive** to any of its
ingredients. Severe allergic reactions may occur. People with **respiratory disease** taking estazolam may experience **sleep apnea**
(intermittent cessation of breathing during sleep). People who
already have, or suspect they have, sleep apnea should not take
estazolam.

People with **kidney or liver disease** should be carefully monitored while taking estazolam. Take the lowest possible dose to
help you sleep.

Clinical **depression** may be increased by estazolam, which can
depress the nervous system. Intentional overdose is more common among depressed people who take sleeping pills than among
those who do not.

All benzodiazepines can be addictive if taken for long periods
of time and can cause drug withdrawal symptoms if discontinued
suddenly. It should be used with caution in people with a history
of **drug dependence**. Withdrawal symptoms include tremors,
muscle cramps, insomnia, agitation, diarrhea, vomiting, sweating,
and convulsions.

People with a history of **seizures** should not abruptly stop taking estazolam.

Possible Side Effects

▼ Common: drowsiness, headache, dizziness, talkativeness, nervousness, apprehension, poor muscle coordination, light-headedness, daytime tiredness, muscle weakness, slowness of movement, hangover, and euphoria (feeling "high").

▼ Less common: nausea, vomiting, rapid heartbeat, confusion, temporary memory loss, upset stomach, stomach cramps and pain, depression, blurred or double vision and other visual disturbances, constipation, changes in sense of taste, appetite changes, stuffy nose, nosebleeds, common cold symptoms, asthma, sore throat, cough, breathing difficulties, diarrhea, dry mouth, allergic reaction, fainting, abnormal heart rhythm, itching, acne, dry skin, sensitivity to bright light or to the sun, rash, nightmares or strange dreams, sleeplessness, tingling in the hands or feet, ringing or buzzing in the ears, ear or eye pain, menstrual cramps, frequent urination and other urinary difficulties, blood in the urine, discharge from the penis or vagina, lower back and joint pain, muscle spasms and pain, fever, swollen breasts, and weight changes.

▼ Rare: Rare side effects can affect your heart, stomach and intestines, urinary tract, blood, muscles, and joints. Contact your doctor if you experience any side effect not listed above.

Drug Interactions

● As with all benzodiazepines, the effects of estazolam are enhanced if it is taken with an alcoholic beverage, antihistamine, sedative, barbiturate, anticonvulsant medication, antidepressant, or monoamine oxidase inhibitor antidepressant.

● Carbamazepine and phenytoin may reduce blood levels and the effectiveness of estazolam by stimulating liver enzymes responsible for its breakdown.

● Ketoconazole, itraconazole, nefazodone, fluvoxamine, diltiazem, isoniazid, some macrolide antibiotics, contraceptive drugs, cimetidine, and disulfiram may increase the effect of estazolam by interfering with the drug's breakdown in the liver. Probenecid also increases estazolam's effects by interfering with it passing through the kidneys into urine.

- Cigarette smoking, rifampin, and theophylline may reduce the effect of estazolam.
- Levodopa + carbidopa's effectiveness may be decreased by estazolam.
- Estazolam may increase the amount of zidovudine (an HIV drug—also known as AZT), phenytoin, or digoxin in your bloodstream, increasing the chances of side effects.
- The combination of clozapine and benzodiazepines has led to respiratory collapse in a few people. Estazolam should be stopped at least 1 week before starting clozapine treatment.

Food Interactions

Estazolam may be taken with food if it upsets your stomach.

Usual Dose

Adult (age 18 and over): 1–2 mg at bedtime.

Senior: 1 mg at bedtime. Small or frail patients should start on 0.5 mg. Dosage should be increased cautiously.

Child (under age 18): not recommended.

Overdosage

The most common overdose symptoms are confusion, sleepiness, depression, loss of muscle coordination, and slurred speech. Coma and death may also occur. People who take an estazolam overdose must be made to vomit with ipecac syrup—available at any pharmacy—to remove any remaining drug from the stomach: Call your doctor or a poison control center before doing this. The victim must be taken to a hospital emergency room for treatment if 30 minutes have passed since the overdose was taken or if symptoms have begun to develop. ALWAYS bring the prescription bottle or container.

Special Information

Never take more estazolam than your doctor has prescribed.

Avoid alcoholic beverages and other nervous system depressants while taking estazolam.

Exercise caution while performing tasks that require concentration and coordination, such as driving; estazolam may make you tired, dizzy, or lightheaded. People taking estazolam or any other sleeping medicine may experience unusual and complex reactions while asleep, such as driving, making phone calls, and cooking with no memory of the event.

If you take estazolam daily for 3 or more weeks, you may experience some withdrawal symptoms when you stop taking the drug, especially temporary sleep disturbance. In rare cases, patients discontinuing estazolam have suffered seizures or delirium. Patients with a history of seizures should taper when stopping use of this drug.

If you forget to take a dose of estazolam and remember within about 1 hour of your regular time, take it right away. If you do not remember until later, skip the dose you forgot and go back to your regular schedule. Do not take a double dose.

Special Populations

Pregnancy/Breast-feeding: Estazolam absolutely should not be used by pregnant women or by women who may become pregnant.

Estazolam passes into breast milk. The drug should not be taken by nursing mothers.

Seniors: Seniors are more susceptible to the effects of estazolam.

Type of Drug

Estrogens (ES-troe-jens)

Brand Names

Generic Ingredient: Conjugated Estrogens
Premarin   Premarin Cream

Generic Ingredient: Conjugated Estrogens (Synthetic)
Cenestin   Enjuvia

Generic Ingredients: Conjugated Estrogens + Medroxyprogesterone
Premphase   Prempro

Generic Ingredient: Esterified Estrogens
Menest

Generic Ingredients: Esterified Estrogens + Methyltestosterone
Estratest

Generic Ingredient: Estradiol 🅖

Alora	Estring
Climara	Estrogel
Divigel	Evamist Transdermal Spray
Elestrin	Femring
Estrace	Femtrace
Estraderm	Gynodiol

Innofem   Vivelle
Menostar   Vivelle-Dot
Vagifem

Generic Ingredients: Estradiol + Drospirenone
Angeliq

Generic Ingredients: Estradiol + Levonorgestrel
Climara Pro   Nuvaring

Generic Ingredients: Estradiol + Norgestimate [G]
Prefest

Generic Ingredient: Estropipate
Ogen Cream   Ortho-Est

Generic Ingredients: Ethinyl Estradiol + Norethindrone [G]
Activella Combipatch.   FemHRT 1/5

Prescribed For

Moderate to severe menopausal symptoms such as hot flashes, night sweats and sleep problems, vaginal dryness and irritation (creams and gels); also prescribed for ovarian failure, osteoporosis prevention, male breast cancer, advanced prostate cancer, abnormal bleeding of the uterus, female castration, Turner's syndrome, and birth control.

General Information

Six estrogens have been identified in women but only 3 are present in large amounts: estradiol, estrone, and estriol. Estradiol is the most potent and most important. Other estrogens are produced by chemical conversions in the body. Estradiol, for example, is transformed into estrone, which in turn becomes estriol. Estrogens all have the same actions and side effects; only potency varies. More potent types require smaller dosages to produce the same effect.

Millions of women have taken hormone replacement therapy (HRT) to manage menopausal symptoms, but studies show that HRT does not improve quality of life for most. Women who experience severe menopause symptoms must weigh the benefits of prolonged hormone replacement therapy against its risks.

Estrogens are largely responsible for the growth and maintenance of the female reproductive system and sex characteristics. They affect the release of hormones from the pituitary gland (controller of hormone production and regulator of basic bodily functions). These hormones control the functioning of capillaries (smallest blood vessels), may cause fluid retention, affect protein breakdown in the body, prevent ovulation and breast engorgement after childbirth, and influence the shaping and maintenance of the skeleton through an effect on calcium.

Estrogen products differ in their hormone content and dosage. Some may affect one part of the body more than another. Generally, though, estrogens are interchangeable as long as dosage differences are taken into account.

Cautions and Warnings

Do not take estrogens if you are **allergic** or **sensitive** to any of their ingredients.

Products containing an estrogen and a progestin should not be used for the prevention or treatment of **bladder-control problems, heart disease**, or **mental decline (dementia)**.

Women with an intact uterus who choose hormone replacement therapy for menopausal symptoms should take the lowest effective dose for the shortest possible time to minimize the risks associated with these medicines. The results of a very large study called the Women's Health Initiative (WHI) first published in 2002 and updated with new reports, have drastically changed the face of estrogen replacement therapy. The study found a small but insignificant increase in the risk of non-fatal heart attacks. There was no increase in heart disease in the estrogen plus progestin part of the WHI. Early results of the WHI found 4–6 more cases of invasive breast cancer for every 10,000 women in the study and tumors were harder to detect. But this result was not confirmed after more than 7 years of additional study. Estrogens may also lead to abnormal mammograms. An increased risk of a stroke was found in the WHI study. The risk of blood clots forming in the body was doubled in women taking hormone therapy. This study did show some benefits of long-term hormone replacement in colon cancer and osteoporosis, but these benefits may not outweigh the risks of hormone replacement therapy.

Women with **liver damage or disease, blood-clotting problems,** or **abnormal vaginal bleeding** whose cause is unknown, should not take estrogens.

Women who smoke cigarettes and take estrogen have a greater risk of cardiovascular side effects, including stroke and blood clotting.

Estrogens may increase the risk of endometrial cancer by 4.5–14 times in postmenopausal women taking them without progestin for prolonged periods of time; the risk depends on duration of treatment and dosage. Women who have a strong **family history of breast cancer** or who have **breast nodules or cysts** or an **abnormal mammogram** should be cautious about using estrogens. Women with **estrogen-dependent cancer** or **breast cancer** should not take estrogens, except some being treated for **breast cancer that has spread**. Women taking an estrogen for **breast cancer that has spread to their bones** can develop large increases in blood calcium.

Postmenopausal women taking estrogen are 2–3 times more likely to develop gallbladder disease.

Estrogens can raise blood pressure. Pressure usually returns to normal when the drug is stopped.

People with **thrombophlebitis** should avoid these drugs. The risk is greatest with very high dosages. Lower hormone dosages may not be a problem.

Estrogens should not be used to treat painful **breast enlargement** that sometimes develops after giving birth.

Estrogens can cause significant increases in blood triglycerides and cause pancreas inflammation in women with **inherited blood-fat disorders**.

Vaginal estrogen cream may stimulate bleeding of the uterus. It may also cause breast tenderness, vaginal discharge, and withdrawal bleeding if the product is suddenly stopped. Women with **endometriosis** may experience heavy vaginal bleeding.

Women taking hormone replacement therapy are at a 50% greater than normal risk of senile dementia.

Drospirenone, a progestin and an ingredient in Angeliq, can raise blood potassium levels in some people because it opposes the hormone aldosterone. It should not be used in people with conditions that can lead to high blood potassium such as **kidney disease** or a **poorly functioning adrenal gland**. Drosperinone should be used with caution by women who are also taking other medicines that raise blood potassium, such as nonsteroidal anti-inflammatory drugs (NSAIDs), potassium-sparing diuretics, potassium supplements, angiotensin-converting enzyme (ACE) inhibitors, AII receptor antagonists, and heparin. Your doctor may want to check your blood potassium level if you might be at risk of high blood potassium.

Possible Side Effects

▼ Most common: breast enlargement or tenderness, ankle and leg swelling, appetite loss, weight changes, water retention and bloating, nausea, vomiting, and abdominal cramps. The estrogen patch may cause rash, irritation, and redness where it is applied.

▼ Less common: bleeding gums, breakthrough vaginal bleeding, vaginal spotting or discharge, changes in menstrual flow, painful menstruation, premenstrual syndrome (PMS), absence of menstrual periods during and after estrogen use, uterine fibroid enlargement, vaginal *Candida* infection, a cystitis-like condition, mild diarrhea, yellowing of the skin or whites of the eyes, eye lesions, contact-lens intolerance, rash, hair loss, development of new hairy patches, migraine, mild dizziness, depression, increased sex drive (women), and decreased sex drive (men).

▼ Rare: stroke, blood-clot formation, dribbling or sudden passage of urine, loss of coordination, chest pain, leg pain, breathing difficulties, slurred speech, and changes in vision. Men who take large estrogen dosages for prostate cancer have a greater risk of heart attack, phlebitis, and blood clots in the lungs. Contact your doctor if you experience any side effect not listed above.

Drug Interactions

- Phenytoin, ethotoin, mephenytoin, and topiramate may interfere with estrogen's effects.
- Estrogens may reduce the effect of oral anticoagulant (blood-thinning) drugs. Your anticoagulant dosage may need an adjustment.
- Estrogens may increase the side effects of antidepressants and phenothiazine sedatives.
- Low estrogen dosages may increase phenothiazine's effectiveness.
- Estrogens may increase cyclosporine and corticosteroid blood levels. Dosage adjustments of the non-estrogen drugs may be needed.
- Estrogens may reduce the effectiveness of thyroid replacement therapy.

- Rifampin, barbiturates, carbamazepine, St. John's wort, and other drugs that stimulate the liver to break down drugs may reduce estrogen blood levels.
- Estrogens may interfere with tamoxifen and bromocriptine.
- Women, especially those over age 35, who smoke cigarettes and take estrogen have a much greater risk of developing stroke, hardening of the arteries, or blood clots in the lungs. The risk increases with age and tobacco use.
- Estrogens interfere with many diagnostic tests. Make sure your doctor knows you are taking estrogen before conducting any blood tests or other diagnostic procedures.

Food Interactions

Estrogens may be taken with food to reduce nausea and upset stomach. Avoid drinking grapefruit juice if you are taking this drug.

Usual Dose

Dosage varies. All of these products, including the transdermal skin patch, may be taken continuously or on a cyclic schedule of 3 weeks on, 1 week off.

Tablets

Chlorotrianisene: 12–200 mg.
Conjugated estrogens: 0.3–30 mg.
Conjugated estrogens, synthetic: 0.625–1.25 mg.
Esterified estrogens: 0.3–30 mg.
Estradiol: 0.5–30 mg.
Estropipate: 0.625–7.5 mg.
Ethinyl estradiol: 0.02–3.0 mg.

Estradiol Transdermal Patch (0.025, 0.0375, 0.05, 0.075, or 0.1 mg)

Alora, Estraderm, and Esclim: 1 patch twice a week; or use 1 patch twice a week for 3 weeks, stop for 1 week, then start again.

Climara and Fempatch: 1 patch every week; or use 1 patch once a week for 3 weeks, stop for 1 week, then start again.

Estradiol Transdermal Spray: 1–3 sprays (1.53 mg estradiol in each spray) applied next to each other every morning on the inner surface of the forearm, starting near the elbow. Do not allow the sprays to overlap each other. Allow the spray to dry for about 2 minutes and do not wash the arm for 30 minutes. Do not apply the spray to any other part of the body.

Estradiol Gel: Spread 1 pumpful of the gel as thinly as possible over the entire area on the inside and outside of your arm from wrist to shoulder, once a day at the same time every day.

Vaginal Cream

Conjugated estrogens: 0.52 g a day for 3 weeks; stop for 1 week, then start again.

Dienestrol: 1 applicatorful 12 times a day for 12 weeks, half the original dosage for another 12 weeks, then 1 applicatorful 13 times a week.

Estradiol: 24 g a day for 2 weeks, half the starting dosage for another 2 weeks, then 1 g 13 times a week.

Estropipate: 24 g a day for 3 weeks; stop for 1 week, then start again.

Estradiol Ring

Insert once every 3 months.

Overdosage

Symptoms may include nausea and vaginal bleeding in adult women. Call your local poison control center or a hospital emergency room for information. If you seek treatment, ALWAYS bring the prescription bottle or container.

Special Information

Call your doctor if you develop breast pain or tenderness, swelling of the feet and lower legs, rapid weight gain, chest pain, breathing difficulties, pain in the groin or calves, unusual or persistent vaginal bleeding, missed menstrual period, lumps in the breast, sudden severe headache, dizziness or fainting, disturbances in speech or vision, weakness or numbness in the arms or legs, abdominal pain, sudden severe vomiting, depression, yellowing of the skin or whites of the eyes, or jerky or involuntary muscle movement.

Women taking estrogens or combined estrogen and progestin therapy should have yearly breast exams, perform monthly breast self-examinations, and have regular mammograms.

Talk to your health care provider about ways to reduce risk factors for heart disease (blood-pressure control, improving your diet, stopping tobacco use) and osteoporosis (an appropriate diet, vitamin D and calcium supplements, weight-bearing exercise).

Tell your doctor if you are having surgery or require bedrest; your doctor may have you stop taking estrogen 4–6 weeks beforehand to prevent the risk of blood clots.

Your doctor should reevaluate your need for estrogen vaginal cream every 36 months. Do not stop using the drug suddenly because this may increase your risk of developing unpredicted or breakthrough vaginal bleeding.

Women using the cream who develop breast tenderness, start to bleed, or have other vaginal discharge should contact their doctors at once.

Estrogen skin patches should be applied to a clean, dry, non-oily, hairless area of intact skin, preferably on the abdomen. Do not apply it to your breasts or waist, or to any area where tight-fitting clothes may loosen the patch from your skin. The application site should be rotated to prevent irritation, and each site should have a patch-free period for 7 days.

Good dental hygiene is important while taking estrogen because estrogen may increase your risk of oral infection. Dental work should be completed prior to starting estrogen, if possible.

Vaginal estrogen cream should be inserted high into the vagina, about $\frac{2}{3}$ of the length of the applicator.

Press the vaginal ring into an oval and insert as deeply as possible in the upper $\frac{1}{3}$ of the vagina.

Some of these products contain tartrazine (a commonly used orange dye and food coloring). If you are allergic to tartrazine or have asthma, check with your pharmacist to find out if your estrogen product contains this coloring agent.

If you forget a dose, take it as soon as you remember. If it is almost time for your next dose, skip the one you forgot and continue with your regular schedule. Do not take a double dose.

Authorities note that the risk of serious complications for an individual woman taking hormone replacement therapy is very small. Thus, you may decide to take hormones but your decision should be based on a complete discussion of the facts and your individual situation with your doctor. Continue to talk with your doctor regularly about weighing the risks against the benefits of taking estrogen.

Special Populations

Pregnancy/Breast-feeding: Estrogens harm the fetus and should never be used during pregnancy for any reason.

Estrogens pass into breast milk and reduce its flow. Nursing mothers who must take them should use infant formula.

Seniors: The risk of side effects increases with age, especially if you smoke. Women age 65 or older taking estrogens may be more likely to develop a stroke, blood clot, or dementia, a condition where people suddenly or gradually lose normal mental function and intellectual capacity.

Generic Name

Eszopiclone (ess-oh-PIK-lone)

Brand Name
Lunesta

Type of Drug
Sedative.

Prescribed For
Insomnia.

General Information
Eszopiclone is a nonbenzodiazepine sleeping pill that is believed to work in much the same way as the drug zolpidem and as benzodiazepine-type sleeping pills and sedatives. Unlike the benzodiazepines, however, eszopiclone has little muscle-relaxing or antiseizure effects. This drug is rapidly absorbed and usually starts working within a few minutes. Eszopiclone causes little or no "hangover," and there are no rebound effects after stopping the drug. In studies of eszopiclone, tolerance to its effects did not develop even after 6 months of continued use. Eszopiclone is broken down in the liver, and the level of this drug in the body does not increase after you take it for several days.

Cautions and Warnings
Do not take eszopiclone if you are **allergic** or **sensitive** to any of its ingredients.

People with severe **liver disease** should use eszopiclone with caution and must take less of this medication than those with normal liver function or mild liver disease.

Sleeping problems often result from a **physical or psychological illness.** Eszopiclone does not affect the underlying causes of insomnia. It should be taken only with your doctor's knowledge. If you cannot sleep even after 7–10 days of taking eszopiclone, contact your doctor.

Eszopiclone has caused amnesia (memory loss), but this happens mostly at dosages larger than 2 mg per night.

Suddenly stopping eszopiclone after having taken it for some time may produce drug withdrawal (symptoms include fatigue, nausea, flushing, lightheadedness, crying, vomiting, stomach cramps, panic, nervousness, and general discomfort).

People with a history of **substance abuse** may be more likely to develop drug dependence on eszopiclone. Eszopiclone doses of 6–12 mg are similar to 20 mg of diazepam in their potential for abuse.

Eszopiclone is a nervous system depressant and may cause loss of coordination and concentration. It should be taken just before bedtime. People taking sleep medicine may experience unusual and complex reactions while asleep, such as driving, making phone calls, or cooking with no memory of the event. Eszopiclone may also interfere with normal activities the next day, especially if taken with alcohol.

Eszopiclone should be avoided by people with severe **depression,** severe **lung disease,** and **sleep apnea** (intermittently stopping breathing when you are asleep). You should not take this drug if you are **drunk.**

Possible Side Effects

Adults

Some side effects are more likely with larger doses (viral infection, dry mouth, dizziness, hallucinations, infections, rash, and unpleasant taste).

▼ Most common: headache, drowsiness, unpleasant taste, and lung infections.

▼ Common: dry mouth, dizziness, and nausea.

▼ Less common: nervousness, vomiting, viral infections, anxiety, confusion, depression, hallucinations, reduced sex drive, rash, male breast enlargement and/or pain, painful menstruation, chest pain, migraines, and swelling of the arms or legs.

▼ Rare: Rare side effects can occur in almost any part of the body. Contact your doctor if you experience any side effect not listed above.

Possible Side Effects *(continued)*

Seniors

Some side effects are more common with larger doses, including dry mouth, pain, and unpleasant taste.

▼ Most common: headache.

▼ Common: pain, dry mouth, diarrhea, and upset stomach.

▼ Less common: accidental injury, abnormal dreaming, nervousness, nerve pain, itching, and urinary infection.

▼ Rare: Rare side effects can occur in almost any part of the body. Contact your doctor if you experience any side effect not listed above.

Drug Interactions

- Mixing eszopiclone with olanzapine can affect your coordination and ability to perform tasks.
- Mixing eszopiclone with ketoconazole more than doubles blood levels of eszopiclone. Other drugs that may have a similar interaction include itraconazole, clarithromycin, nefazodone, troleandomycin, ritonavir, and nelfinavir.
- Rifampin can be expected to drastically reduce the effectiveness of eszopiclone because it increases levels of liver enzymes that break down eszopiclone.
- Avoid combining eszopiclone with alcohol and other nervous system depressants, including sedatives, narcotics, barbiturates, antidepressants, and antihistamines.

Food Interactions

For the most rapid and complete effect, take eszopiclone on an empty stomach at least 2 hours after a meal. It will take longer for eszopiclone to work if you have had a high-fat meal immediately before taking it.

Usual Dose

Adult (age 18 and over): 2–3 mg immediately before bedtime or after you are in bed and have trouble falling asleep. Eszopiclone can act very quickly.

Child (up to age 17): not recommended.

Senior: 1–2 mg immediately before bedtime.

People with liver disease: 1 mg.

Overdosage

Overdose can result in nervous system depression, from unconsciousness to light coma. Combining eszopiclone with alcohol or other nervous system depressants may be fatal or affect other body organs. One person took up to 36 mg of eszopiclone and fully recovered. Take the victim to a hospital emergency room at once. ALWAYS bring the prescription bottle or container.

Special Information

Eszopiclone may cause tiredness, drowsiness, and an inability to concentrate. Be careful when driving or performing any task that requires concentration on the day following a dose. Make sure you get 7–8 hours of sleep after taking eszopiclone.

People taking eszopiclone on a regular basis may develop a drug withdrawal reaction if the medication is stopped suddenly (see "Cautions and Warnings").

Do not take a double dose of this medication.

Special Populations

Pregnancy/Breast-feeding: Some animal studies with doses of eszopiclone up to 800 times the human equivalent showed it did not affect a developing fetus, and other studies showed some modest effects. However, there is no information on the use of eszopiclone in pregnant women. If your doctor considers eszopiclone crucial for you, its potential benefits must be carefully weighed against its risks.

It is not known if eszopiclone passes into breast milk. Nursing mothers who must take this drug should use infant formula.

Seniors: Seniors, who are likely to be more sensitive to eszopiclone and its side effects, should start on a 1-mg dose and take the lowest effective dosage.

Generic Name

Etanercept (eh-TAN-er-sept)

Brand Name

Enbrel

Type of Drug

Immune system modulator.

Prescribed For

Rheumatoid arthritis, juvenile rheumatoid arthritis, psoriatic arthritis, ankylosing spondylitis, and psoriasis.

General Information

Etanercept binds to a specific protein in the body known as tumor necrosis factor (TNF) and blocks it from interacting with cell surfaces. TNF is involved in normal inflammatory and immune responses and the inflammatory processes of rheumatoid arthritis, juvenile rheumatoid arthritis, and other conditions. Etanercept can also interfere with biological actions that are either caused or regulated by TNF.

Cautions and Warnings

Do not use etanercept if you are **allergic** or **sensitive** to any of its ingredients.

Serious infections and malignancies are possible in people using etanercept because of its ability to suppress the immune response. This may be more common in people with other conditions that predispose them to infections such as advanced or uncontrolled **diabetes**.

Levels of blood platelets and some white blood cells may be reduced in rare cases, leading to persistent fever, bruising, bleeding, and pale skin. Contact your doctor if any of these symptoms develop.

Etanercept may increase the risk of some nervous system disorders including multiple sclerosis.

Etanercept may cause or worsen **congestive heart failure.**

In rare cases people taking etanercept have developed a lupus-like syndrome which may disappear when the drug is discontinued.

People taking etanercept should not receive any **live vaccines,** because the body may not be able to respond as expected to the vaccine.

Possible Side Effects

Reactions may develop at the site where etanercept is injected. Injection sites should be rotated among the thigh, abdomen, and upper arm to avoid excessive bruising or other skin damage.

Possible Side Effects *(continued)*

▼ Most common: infection, injection-site reactions, upper respiratory infection, headache, and runny nose.

▼ Common: nausea, dizziness, sore throat, cough, weakness, abdominal pain, rash, and respiratory problems.

▼ Less common: upset stomach, sinus irritation, vomiting, swelling in the legs or feet, mouth sores, and hair loss.

▼ Rare: malignancy, stroke, seizure, tingling in the hands or feet, nervous system irritation similar to multiple sclerosis, eye inflammation, joint pain, generalized pain, appetite loss, blood vessel inflammation in the skin, dry eyes, lumps under the skin, fever, flu-like symptoms, weight gain, chest pain, flushing, diarrhea, taste changes, difficulty breathing, worsening of existing lung conditions, itching, and skin reactions. Contact your doctor if you experience any side effect not listed above.

Drug Interactions

- Do not mix etanercept in the same syringe as another drug.
- Using etanercept with anakinra increases the risk of serious infections.

Food Interactions

None known.

Usual Dose

Adult: rheumatoid arthritis, psoriatic arthritis, ankylosing spondylitis—50 mg a week. Plaque psoriasis: 50 mg twice a week, reducing to 50 mg a week after 3 months.

Child (age 4–17): 0.36 mg per lb. of body weight, up to 50 mg a week, 3–4 days apart.

Child (under age 4): not recommended.

Overdosage

In one study, a patient accidentally self-administered 62 mg of etanercept twice a week for 3 weeks with no ill effects. Call your local poison control center or a hospital emergency room for more information. If you seek treatment, ALWAYS bring the prescription container.

Special Information

Etanercept is taken by injection under the skin. Be sure you understand how to measure the proper dose of etanercept and how to self-inject it.

To mix and inject etanercept: Withdraw all the water supplied with the medicine into a syringe and slowly inject it into the vial containing etanercept. Swirl the mixture gently to avoid excess foaming in the vial. *Do not shake the vial.*

Do not combine etanercept with any other injectable drug.

Etanercept may be stored in a refrigerator for up to 14 days after it is mixed.

Single-use pre-filled syringes must be refrigerated. Do not use past the provided expiration date.

If you forget to administer a dose, do so as soon as you remember. Remember that etanercept doses must be administered at least 3 days apart. Call your doctor or pharmacist if you have any questions about how to time your etanercept doses.

Special Populations

Pregnancy/Breast-feeding: The safety of using etanercept during pregnancy is not known. When this drug is considered crucial by your doctor, its potential benefits must be carefully weighed against its risks.

It is not known if this drug passes into breast milk. Nursing mothers who must take it should use infant formula.

Seniors: Seniors are more likely to develop infections while using etanercept.

Evista   *see Raloxifene, page 954*

Generic Name

Exemestane   (ex-eh-MES-tane)

Brand Name

Aromasin

Type of Drug

Aromatase inhibitor.

Prescribed For

Breast cancer. Also prescribed for prostate cancer prevention.

General Information

Some breast cancers depend on the presence of the hormone estrogen to stimulate their growth. Depriving these cancers of estrogen is an effective way of treating the condition. Exemestane significantly reduces the amount of estrogen in the blood by binding permanently to an enzyme called aromatase, an essential element in the conversion of androgen (male hormones) to estrogen in premenopausal and postmenopausal women. Exemestane does not affect other hormones in the body. Exemestane is broken down in the liver.

Cautions and Warnings

Do not take exemestane if you are **allergic** or **sensitive** to any of its ingredients.

Exemestane may be prescribed for men and postmenopausal women only.

Possible Side Effects

▼ Most common: fatigue, hot flashes, pain, depression, sleeplessness, anxiety, nausea, and breathing difficulties.

▼ Common: flu-like symptoms, leg swelling, high blood pressure, dizziness, headache, vomiting, abdominal pain, leg swelling or other fluid retention, sweating, appetite loss, constipation, and coughing.

▼ Less common: increased appetite, diarrhea, fever, weakness, tingling in the hands or feet, broken bones, bronchitis, sinusitis, rash, itching, urinary infection, and swollen lymph glands.

▼ Rare: chest pain; confusion; reduced sensitivity to stimulation; upset stomach; joint, back, or other bone pain; respiratory infection; sore throat; runny nose; and hair loss. Contact your doctor if you experience any side effect not listed above.

Drug Interactions

- Estrogen-containing drugs reduce the effectiveness of exemestane. Do not combine these drugs.

- Rifampin, phenytoin, carbamazepine, phenobarbital, and St. John's wort may potentially reduce the effectiveness of exemestane.

Food Interactions

Take this drug with a meal. The amount of exemestane absorbed into the blood is increased by 40% when taken with a high-fat meal.

Usual Dose

Adult: 25 mg once a day with or just after a meal. Dose adjustment is not needed in people with kidney or liver disease.

Child: not recommended.

Overdosage

Doses as large as 600 mg have been well tolerated by women with advanced breast cancer. Overdose victims should be taken to a hospital emergency room for evaluation and treatment. ALWAYS bring the prescription bottle or container.

Special Information

If you forget a dose, skip the forgotten dose and continue with your regular schedule. Contact your doctor if you skip more than one dose.

Special Populations

Pregnancy/Breast-feeding: Exemestane is intended only for postmenopausal women. It can cause birth defects and miscarriage and should not be used by pregnant women or women who may become pregnant.

Exemestane may pass into breast milk. Nursing mothers who must take it should use infant formula.

Seniors: Seniors may take this drug without special precaution.

Generic Name

Exenatide (ex-EN-ah-tide)

Brand Name

Byetta

Type of Drug

Incretin mimetic.

Prescribed For

Type 2 diabetes.

General Information

Exenatide is a unique drug that improves blood sugar control in people with type 2 diabetes who have been unsuccessful with diabetes pills. It is added to existing therapy and does not replace other treatments. Exenatide has many of the same actions as GLP-1, a natural incretin hormone. It differs chemically and works differently from other diabetes medications, including insulin.

Exenatide begins working about 30 minutes after injection and continues to work for at least 8 hours. It helps the pancreas to release insulin into the blood in response to sugar levels, so insulin rises when blood sugar is high and declines as blood sugar declines. It reduces the production of a hormone called *glucagon,* which raises blood sugar. Exenatide also keeps food in the stomach longer, which in turn helps reduce the amount of sugar absorbed from dietary sources. Exenatide increases the number of beta cells (that produce insulin) in animals and may have the same effect in humans. This could help reduce the need for other medicines and improve diabetes control.

Cautions and Warnings

Do not take exenatide if you are **allergic** or **sensitive** to any of its ingredients.

This drug is not a substitute for insulin. Exenatide has only been studied together with metformin, glitazones, and/or sulfonylureas. It has not been studied with other diabetes pills or insulin.

People with severe **kidney disease** should not use exenatide.

People with severe **stomach or intestinal disease** should not use exenatide.

Inflammation of the pancreas can occur with this drug. Symptoms include nausea, vomiting, fever, rapid pulse, and painful and swollen abdomen that may develop slowly and worsen when you eat or may be severe and constant.

Low blood sugar may occur if you are taking exenatide with a sulfonylurea-type antidiabetes drug or with a glitazone.

Antibodies to exenatide may develop, but antibody levels generally go down with time. Most patients who develop antibodies still have good sugar control and similar types of side effects as people who do not develop exenatide antibodies.

Possible Side Effects

▼ Most common: nausea, vomiting, diarrhea, and low blood sugar (when mixed with a sulfonylurea-type drug or metformin plus a sulfonylurea).

▼ Less common: low blood sugar (when mixed with a glitazone), feeling jittery, dizziness, headache, and upset stomach.

▼ Rare: rash, abdominal swelling and pain, constipation, and kidney failure. Contact your doctor if you experience any side effect not listed above.

Drug Interactions

- Exenatide has been studied with a number of other medications commonly taken by people with diabetes (digoxin, lovastatin, lisinopril, and acetaminophen) and no significant interactions were noted.
- Combining exenatide with a sulfonylurea-type drug may lead to hypoglycemia (low blood sugar). Your doctor may change your sulfonylurea dose to solve this problem.
- Take all oral medicines at least 1 hour before you inject exenatide to ensure maximum absorption. If you must take oral drugs with food or meals, take them with a snack or meal when exenatide is not being injected. Exenatide extends the time that drugs remain in the stomach and may reduce the amount of medication absorbed when taken by mouth.
- Exenatide may reduce the effectiveness of oral contraceptive pills. Take them at least 1 hour before an injection of exenatide.
- Exenatide may increase the amount of warfarin in the body and increase the risk of bleeding.

Food Interactions

None known.

Usual Dose

Adult: 5 or 10 mcg twice a day by subcutaneous injection within an hour before breakfast and dinner.

Child: Exenatide has not been studied in children.

Overdosage

The effects of an exenatide overdose are severe nausea, severe vomiting, and severe, rapid drops in blood sugar levels. An oral sugar source may help, but overdose victims should be taken to a hospital emergency room for evaluation and treatment. ALWAYS bring the exenatide pen with you.

Special Information

Each dose of exenatide must be given as an injection under the skin of the thigh, abdomen, or upper arm within 1 hour before your breakfast and dinner meals. For information on how to properly administer this drug, see page 1242.

If you forget a dose of exenatide, skip the dose you forgot and continue with your regular schedule. Do not take a double dose.

Exenatide injection is clear and colorless. Do not use if it has any color, is cloudy, or if there are any particles floating in it.

Keep this drug in the refrigerator, and do not use it after the expiration date has passed.

This drug may lead to a loss of appetite and loss of body weight. Do not change your regular dosage if this happens to you.

Special Populations

Pregnancy/Breast-feeding: In animal studies using doses equal to 3 times the usual human dose, exenatide was shown to affect the growth of the fetus. If you are or might be pregnant and your doctor considers this drug crucial, its potential benefits must be weighed against its risks.

Small amounts of exenatide may pass into breast milk and may affect a nursing infant. Nursing mothers taking this drug should use infant formula.

Seniors: Seniors may take this drug without special restriction.

Generic Name

Ezetimibe (eh-ZEH-tim-ibe)

Brand Name

Zetia

Combination Product

Generic Ingredients: Ezetimibe + Simvastatin

Vytorin

Type of Drug

Cholesterol-lowering agent.

Prescribed For

High cholesterol, high LDL ("bad") cholesterol, high triglycerides, and low HDL ("good") cholesterol; also prescribed for two rare genetic disorders called homozygous familial hypercholesterolemia and homozygous sitosterolemia.

General Information

Unlike statin drugs, ezetimibe interferes with the absorption of cholesterol through the intestine and into the bloodstream. Ezetimibe may be helpful for people whose LDL ("bad") cholesterol remains high despite treatment with a statin drug. Cholesterol-lowering medicines should always be used together with appropriate diet and exercise.

Ezetimibe may be taken alone but is often taken in combination with a statin drug (generally simvastatin). Vytorin is a brand-name combination of these 2 medications. See Statin Cholesterol-Lowering Agents, page 1052.

Cautions and Warnings

Do not take this drug if you are **allergic** or **sensitive** to any of its ingredients.

People with **liver disease** or **elevated liver enzyme** measurements should not take ezetimibe because its effects on the liver are not known.

Ezetimibe does not slow hardening of the arteries.

There may be a risk of myopathy (skeletal muscle disorder) with ezetimibe; contact your doctor if you experience any unexplained muscle pain, tenderness, or weakness. Ezetimibe + simvastatin has the same effect as simvastatin alone; see Statin Cholesterol-Lowering Agents, page 1052.

Possible Side Effects

Ezetimibe side effects are similar to those reported by people taking a placebo (sugar pill).

▼ Most common: headache, back pain, joint pain, and abdominal pain.

▼ Common: muscle ache and respiratory infection.

▼ Less common: fatigue, chest pain, diarrhea, sore throat, and cough.

For additional information about ezetimibe + simvastatin, see Statin Cholesterol-Lowering Agents, page 1052.

Drug Interactions

- Cholestyramine reduces the amount of ezetimibe absorbed in the blood. Separate these drugs by 2 hours or more.
- Cyclosporine (to prevent organ transplant rejection) may substantially increase the amount of ezetimibe in the blood. This combination must be monitored closely by your doctor.
- Gemfibrozil (another blood-fat reducer) can increase the amount of ezetimibe in the blood.
- Fenofibrate may increase the effects of ezetimibe. Fibrates other than fenofibrate should not be used with ezetimibe due to the risk of gallbladder complications. For additional information about ezetimibe + simvastatin, see Statin Cholesterol-Lowering Agents, page 1052.

Food Interactions

This drug can be taken without regard to food or meals.

Usual Dose

Ezetimibe
    Adult and Child (age 10 and over): 10 mg once a day.
    Child (age 9 and under): not recommended.

Ezetimibe + Simvastatin
    Adult: 10 mg ezetimibe plus 10–80 mg simvastatin once a day in the evening. The simavastatin dose depends on individual need.

Overdosage

Little is known about the effects of ezetimibe overdose. Call your local poison control center or a hospital emergency room for information. If you seek treatment, ALWAYS bring the prescription bottle or container.

Special Information

If you are taking more than one drug to lower cholesterol or another blood fat, consider the side effects of all of those drugs combined.

Special Populations

Pregnancy/Breast-feeding: Little is known about the effects of ezetimibe during pregnancy. When this drug is considered crucial by your doctor, its potential benefits must be carefully weighed against its risks. Statin drugs should never be taken by a pregnant woman or nursing mother.

It is not known if ezetimibe passes into breast milk. Nursing mothers who must take it should use infant formula.

Seniors: Seniors may use this drug without special precaution.

Generic Name

Famciclovir (fam-SYE-kloe-vere)

Brand Name

Famvir

Type of Drug

Antiviral.

Prescribed For

Herpes zoster (shingles), genital herpes, herpes labilalis (cold sores), and herpes simplex in HIV-infected people.

General Information

Famciclovir is absorbed into the body and converted to the antiviral penciclovir, the drug that actually works against shingles by interfering with the reproduction of DNA in the herpes virus. Famciclovir does not affect DNA in uninfected body cells. Famciclovir is broken down by the liver and eliminated from the body through the kidneys.

Cautions and Warnings

Do not take famciclovir if you are **allergic** or **sensitive** to any of its ingredients.

Those with **reduced kidney function** should have their dosage adjusted accordingly.

Severe liver disease reduces the maximum possible concentration of famciclovir in the blood and increases the time it takes to reach this maximum level; however, dosage adjustment is not normally required.

Possible Side Effects

▼ Most common: headache, nausea, and diarrhea.
▼ Less common: fever, fatigue, pain, vomiting, constipation, appetite loss, dizziness, tingling in the hands or feet, sleepiness, sore throat, sinus irritation, itching, gas, dysmemorrhea, and signs of shingles.

Possible Side Effects (continued)

▼ Rare: chills, abdominal pain, back or joint pain, and upset stomach. Contact your doctor if you experience any side effect not listed above.

Drug Interactions

● Probenecid, cimetidine, and theophylline interfere with the elimination of famciclovir from the body, possibly leading to higher levels of famciclovir in the blood.

● People who took famciclovir and digoxin together experienced increased digoxin in their blood.

Food Interactions

None known.

Usual Dose

Shingles

Adult (age 18 and over): 500 mg every 8 hours for 1 week. People with reduced kidney function may require a reduced dose taken as infrequently as once a day.

Genital Herpes

Adult (age 18 and over): 1000 mg twice daily for 1 day; or 250 mg twice a day for up to 1 year for suppression; or 250 mg 3 times a day for 7 days for initial episode. People with reduced kidney function take the same dose but less often, as infrequently as once every 2 days. HIV-infected people should take 500 mg twice a day for 7 days.

Cold Sores

Adult (age 18 and over): 1500 mg as a single dose. Initiate therapy at the earliest sign or symptom of a cold sore (tingling, itching, or burning).

Overdosage

Little is known about the effects of famciclovir overdose. Overdose victims should be taken to a hospital emergency room for treatment. ALWAYS bring the prescription bottle or container.

Special Information

Famciclovir treatment should be started as soon as shingles is diagnosed. For maximum benefit, be sure to complete the full week of treatment.

Famciclovir is not a cure for genital herpes and it is not known if it will prevent the transmission of the herpes virus to another person. Avoid sexual intercourse when herpes lesions are present even while taking famciclovir for genital herpes.

Begin taking famciclovir at the first sign of a herpes attack (symptoms include pain, tenderness, burning, itching, tingling, ulcers, or scabs). The effectiveness of starting famciclovir 6 hours or more after symptoms or lesions appear has not been established.

Call your doctor if you experience any unusual or intolerable side effects.

If you forget a dose of famciclovir, take it as soon as you remember. If it is almost time for your next dose, skip the dose you forgot. Do not take a double dose. Call your doctor if you forget more than 2 doses in a row.

Special Populations

Pregnancy/Breast-feeding: Famciclovir should only be taken by a pregnant woman if it is absolutely necessary and the possible benefits outweigh the risks to the fetus.

In animal studies, penciclovir (the active form of famciclovir) passed into breast milk in high concentrations but it is not known if this holds true for humans. Nursing mothers who must take this drug should use infant formula.

Seniors: Seniors clear famciclovir from the bloodstream more slowly than younger people and should have their dosage adjusted according to their level of kidney function.

Generic Name

Famotidine (fam-OE-tih-dine) Ⓖ

Brand Names

Fluxid	Pepcid AC
Pepcid	Pepcid Complete

Type of Drug

Histamine H_2 antagonist.

Prescribed For

Ulcers of the stomach and duodenum (upper intestine). This drug is also used to treat gastroesophageal reflux disease (GERD), stress ulcer, and other conditions characterized by the production of large amounts of gastric fluids; to prevent stress ulcer and stomach and upper intestinal bleeding; and to stop the production of stomach acid during surgery. Pepcid AC is approved for heartburn.

General Information

Histamine H_2 antagonists work by turning off the system that produces stomach acid and other secretions. Famotidine is effective in treating the symptoms of ulcer and preventing complications of the disease, although an ulcer that does not respond to another histamine H_2 antagonist will probably not respond to famotidine. Histamine H_2 antagonists differ only in their potency. Cimetidine is the least potent; 1000 mg are roughly equal to 300 mg of either nizatidine or ranitidine, or 40 mg of famotidine. All these drugs have roughly equivalent success rates in treating ulcer disease and comparable risk of side effects.

Cautions and Warnings

Do not take famotidine if you are **allergic** or **sensitive** to any of its ingredients or to any histamine H_2 antagonist.

People with **kidney or liver disease** should take famotidine with caution because $\frac{1}{3}$ of each dose is broken down in the liver and the rest passes out of the body through the kidneys.

Do not self-treat with over-the-counter (OTC) forms of famotidine without the advice and supervision of your doctor.

Possible Side Effects

▼ Most common: headache.

▼ Less common: dizziness, mild diarrhea, and constipation.

▼ Rare: Rare side effects can occur in almost any part of the body. Contact your doctor if you experience any side effect not listed above.

Drug Interactions

- Enteric-coated tablets should not be taken with famotidine. The change in stomach acidity that famotidine produces causes the tablets to disintegrate prematurely in the stomach.
- Antacids, anticholinergics, and metoclopramide may slightly reduce the amount of famotidine absorbed into the blood. No special precaution is needed.

Food Interactions

Famotidine may be taken without regard to food or meals.

Usual Dose

Adult: 20–40 mg at bedtime, or 20 mg twice a day for 4–8 weeks. Dosage should be reduced in people with severe kidney disease.

Child (age 1–16): 0.23–0.45 mg per lb. of body weight, at bedtime or in 2 divided doses, up to 40 mg a day.

Child (under age 1): Consult your doctor.

Over-the-counter forms of famotidine such as Pepcid AC or Pepcid Complete should only be used for the temporary relief of heartburn, and are not recommended for children under 12 years of age. Do not take more than 2 capsules or chewable tablets in 24 hours.

Overdosage

Little is known about the effects of famotidine overdose, but victims may experience exaggerated side effects. Your local poison control center may advise giving ipecac syrup—available at any pharmacy—to induce vomiting and remove any remaining drug from the stomach. Victims who have definite symptoms should be taken to a hospital emergency room. ALWAYS bring the prescription bottle or container.

Special Information

Take famotidine exactly as directed and follow your doctor's instructions regarding diet and other treatment in order to get the maximum benefit from the drug. Antacids may be taken together with famotidine if needed.

Do not take the maximum dose continuously for more than 2 weeks without the consent and supervision of your doctor.

Cigarettes worsen stomach ulcers and may reduce famotidine's effectiveness.

Call your doctor at once if you develop any unusual side effects such as bleeding or bruising, tiredness, diarrhea, dizziness, or rash. Black, tarry stools or vomiting material that resembles coffee grounds may indicate your ulcer is bleeding.

If you forget a dose of famotidine, take it as soon as you remember. If it is almost time for your next dose, skip the one you forgot and continue with your regular schedule. Do not take a double dose.

Special Populations

Pregnancy/Breast-feeding: Although animal studies revealed no damage to the fetus, famotidine should be avoided by women who are or might be pregnant. When this drug is considered crucial by your doctor, its possible benefits must be carefully weighed against its risks.

Famotidine may pass into breast milk. Nursing mothers who must take this drug should use infant formula.

Seniors: Seniors may need lower doses due to loss of kidney function and may be more susceptible to side effects.

Generic Name

Felbamate (FEL-bam-ate)

Brand Name

Felbatol

Type of Drug

Anticonvulsant.

Prescribed For

Partial seizures and Lennox-Gastaut syndrome in children.

General Information

Felbamate is related to the older sedative meprobamate. Exactly how felbamate works is not known, but it raises the seizure threshold and prevents the seizure impulse from spreading in the brain, as do other anticonvulsants. Felbamate should only be used when other seizure drugs have failed because of the risks associated with it. About half of each dose passes out of the body through the kidneys; the other half is broken down and eliminated by the liver.

Cautions and Warnings

Do not take felbamate if you are **allergic** or **sensitive** to any of its ingredients or to any related drugs such as meprobamate.

Felbamate is associated with an increase in the risk of aplastic anemia, a potentially fatal condition.

Possibly fatal liver failure occurs in people taking felbamate much more often than normal. Regular liver function tests are recommended. People with **liver disease** should not take felbamate.

Felbamate is not recommended as first-line epilepsy treatment. Felbamate should be used only by those with severe epilepsy for whom the benefits outweigh the risks. Doctors prescribing felbamate should be thoroughly familiar with the drug and must obtain written, informed consent from patients before prescribing.

Felbamate should never be suddenly stopped or seizures may become more frequent. Dosage should be gradually reduced or replaced by another anticonvulsant.

Felbamate may cause increased sensitivity to the sun. Wear protective clothing and use sunscreen while taking this drug.

People with **kidney disease** may require lower doses.

Possible Side Effects

Adult

▼ Most common: sleeplessness, sleepiness, fatigue, headache, dizziness, nervousness, upset stomach, vomiting, constipation, nausea, and appetite loss.

▼ Common: anxiety, tremors, walking unusually, depression, tingling in the hands or feet, diarrhea, liver inflammation, abdominal pains, respiratory infections, abnormal vision, and taste changes.

▼ Less common: weakness, dry mouth, stupor, abnormal thinking, rash, sinus irritation, sore throat, muscle aches, fever, and chest pain.

▼ Rare: Rare side effects can occur in almost any part of the body. Contact your doctor if you experience any side effect not listed above.

Child

▼ Most common: abdominal pain, fever, respiratory infections, sleeplessness, sleepiness, nervousness, vomiting, constipation, and black-and-blue marks.

▼ Common: headache, appetite loss, hiccups, sore throat, coughing, middle ear infections, fatigue, weight loss, temporary loss of urine control, pain, walking unusually, weakness, abnormal thinking, emotional instability, pinpoint pupils, rash, upset stomach, and low white-blood-cell count.

▼ Rare: Rare side effects can occur in almost any part of the body. Contact your doctor if your child experiences any side effect not listed above.

Drug Interactions

- Combining felbamate and other antiseizure drugs usually requires dosage adjustments due to the risk of drug interaction. Dosage of felbamate should be reduced by 20–33% to reduce the risks of associated side effects.
- Combining felbamate and carbamazepine reduces blood levels of both drugs by roughly half. Dosage adjustments are necessary.
- Combining phenobarbital and felbamate increases the amount of phenobarbital in the blood and decreases felbamate levels. Dosage adjustments are necessary.
- If you combine felbamate and phenytoin, your phenytoin dosage may have to be reduced by as much as 40%. This combination also decreases felbamate blood levels by almost 50%.
- Felbamate increases blood levels of valproic acid and methsuximide.

Food Interactions

Felbamate is best taken on an empty stomach but may be taken with food if it causes upset stomach.

Usual Dose

Adult and Child (age 14 and over): 1200–3600 mg a day, divided into 3–4 doses.

Child (age 2–13): 6.8–20.5 mg per lb. a day, divided into 3–4 doses.

Overdosage

Overdose symptoms may include upset stomach, increased heart rate, and felbamate side effects. Call your local poison control center or a hospital emergency room for more information. If you seek treatment, ALWAYS bring the prescription bottle or container.

Special Information

Do not take more felbamate than your doctor has prescribed.

Felbamate can cause drowsiness; be careful when driving or performing tasks that require concentration.

Avoid prolonged exposure to the sun while taking felbamate.

Call your doctor if you develop any bothersome or persistent side effect.

Maintain good dental hygiene while taking felbamate and use extra care when brushing or flossing because this drug can cause swollen gums. See your dentist regularly.

If you forget a dose, take it as soon as you remember. If it is almost time for your next dose, take 1 dose right away and another in 3 or 4 hours, then go back to your regular schedule. Do not take a double dose.

Special Populations

Pregnancy/Breast-feeding: This drug may cross into fetal circulation. When the drug is considered crucial by your doctor, its potential benefits must be carefully weighed against its risks.

Felbamate passes into breast milk. Nursing mothers who must take this drug should consider using infant formula.

Seniors: Seniors, especially those with liver, kidney, or heart disease, may be more sensitive to the effects of this drug and should receive lower doses.

Generic Name

Felodipine (feh-LOE-dih-pene) Ⓖ

Brand Name
Plendil

Combination Product
Generic Ingredients: Enalapril + Felodipine
Lexxel

Type of Drug
Calcium channel blocker.

Prescribed For
High blood pressure.

General Information
Felodipine is one of many calcium channel blockers available in the U.S. Its once-daily dosage schedule makes it particularly suited to treating high blood pressure. Felodipine blocks the passage of calcium, an essential factor in muscle contraction, into the heart and smooth muscles. Such blockage interferes with the contraction of these muscles, which in turn dilates (widens) the veins and vessels that supply blood to them. This dilating effect reduces blood pressure, the amount of oxygen used by the heart muscle, and the risk of blood vessel spasm. Felodipine is therefore useful in

treating not only high blood pressure but also angina pectoris (brief attacks of chest pain), a condition related to poor oxygen supply to the heart muscles.

Felodipine only affects the movement of calcium into muscle cells; it has no effect on calcium in the blood.

Lexxel is a combination of felodipine and enalapril, an angiotensin converting enzyme (ACE) inhibitor.

Cautions and Warnings

Do not take felodipine if you are **allergic** or **sensitive** to any of its ingredients.

On rare occasions, felodipine may cause very low blood pressure that may lead to stimulation of the heart and rapid heartbeat and can worsen **angina**. This reaction may happen when treatment is first started, when dosage is increased, or if the drug is rapidly withdrawn; it may be avoided by reducing dosage gradually.

Studies have shown that people taking calcium channel blockers—usually those taken several times a day, not those taken only once daily—have a greater chance of having a heart attack than do people taking beta blockers or other medications for the same purpose. Discuss this with your doctor to be sure you are receiving the best possible treatment.

Patients taking a beta-blocking drug who begin taking felodipine may develop heart failure or increased angina.

People with severe **liver disease** may require dosage adjustments.

People taking felodipine who have had a **heart attack** and have **lung congestion** may experience worsened heart failure, since this drug can actually reduce the force of each heartbeat.

Possible Side Effects

Side effects produced by calcium channel blockers are generally mild and rarely cause people to stop taking them. Side effects are more common with higher doses and in older patients.

▼ Most common: swelling in the ankles, feet, or legs; dizziness; lightheadedness; muscle weakness or cramps; facial flushing; and headache.

▼ Less common: respiratory infections, cough, tingling in the hands or feet, upset stomach, abdominal pains, chest pains,

---

Possible Side Effects (*continued*)

nausea, constipation, diarrhea, heart palpitations, sore throat, runny nose, back pain, and rash.

▼ Rare: Rare side effects can affect the heart, stomach, blood, and joints. It can affect your mood, sex drive, and urinary tract. Contact your doctor if you experience any side effect not listed above.

Drug Interactions

- Felodipine may increase the amount of beta-blocking drugs in the bloodstream. This can lead to heart failure, very low blood pressure, or an increased incidence of angina. However, in many cases these drugs have been taken together with no problem.
- Felodipine increases the effects of other blood-pressure-lowering drugs. Such drug combinations are often used to treat hypertension.
- Cimetidine, ranitidine, and azole antifungals such as ketoconazole and itraconazole increase the amount of felodipine in the blood and may account for a slight increase in the drug's effect.
- Phenytoin and other hydantoin antiseizure medicines, carbamazepine, and barbiturate sleeping pills and sedatives may decrease the amount of felodipine in the blood, reducing its effect on the body.
- Erythromycin and cyclosporine may increase the side effects of felodipine.
- Felodipine may increase the effects of digoxin, theophylline (prescribed for asthma and other respiratory problems), and oral anticoagulant (blood-thinning) drugs.
- Felodipine may also interact with quinidine (prescribed for abnormal heart rhythm) to produce low blood pressure, very slow heart rate, abnormal heart rhythms, and swelling in the arms or legs.
- Calcium channel blockers may cause bleeding when taken alone or combined with aspirin.

Food Interactions

You may take felodipine with food if it upsets your stomach. Avoid taking felodipine with grapefruit juice—it doubles the amount of drug absorbed.

Usual Dose

2.5–10 mg a day. No patient should take more than 20 mg a day. Do not stop taking felodipine abruptly. The dosage should be reduced gradually over a period of time.

Overdosage

Felodipine overdose can cause low blood pressure. If you think you have taken an overdose of felodipine, call your doctor or go to a hospital emergency room. ALWAYS bring the prescription bottle or container.

Special Information

Call your doctor if you develop constipation, nausea, very low blood pressure, breathing difficulties, increased heart pain, dizziness, or lightheadedness, or if other side effects are bothersome or persistent.

Swelling of the hands or feet may develop within 2 or 3 weeks of starting felodipine. The chances of this happening depend on age and dosage. It occurs in less than 10% of people under age 50 taking 5 mg a day and in more than 30% of those over age 60 taking 20 mg a day.

Be sure to continue taking your medication even if you feel well, and follow any instructions for diet restriction or other treatments to help maintain lower blood pressure.

Do not break or crush felodipine tablets.

It is important to maintain good dental hygiene while taking felodipine and to use extra care when using your toothbrush or dental floss because of the chance that the drug will make you more susceptible to certain infections.

If you forget to take a dose of felodipine, take it as soon as you remember. If it is almost time for your next dose, skip the dose you forgot and continue with your regular schedule. Do not take a double dose.

Special Populations

Pregnancy/Breast-feeding: Animal studies of felodipine have shown that it crosses into the fetal circulation and causes birth defects. Women who are or who might become pregnant while taking this drug should not take it without their doctor's approval. The potential benefit of taking felodipine must be carefully weighed against its risks.

It is not known if felodipine passes into breast milk. Nursing mothers who take felodipine should use infant formula.

Seniors: Seniors, especially those with liver disease, are more sensitive to the effects of this drug.

Generic Name

Fenofibrate (fen-oe-FIH-brate) G

Brand Names

Antara   TriCor
Lipoten   Triglide
Lofibra

Type of Drug

Anti-hyperlipidemic (blood-fat reducer).

Prescribed For

High blood cholesterol and/or triglycerides; also prescribed for syndrome X, a condition which increases the risk of type 2 diabetes.

General Information

Fenofibrate works by interfering with the body's ability to make triglyceride and by increasing its breakdown by enzymes in the body. It also reduces levels of uric acid, total cholesterol, low-density lipoprotein (LDL) cholesterol—the "bad" cholesterol—and other blood lipids. High-density lipoprotein (HDL) cholesterol—the "good" cholesterol—levels are increased. This drug should only be used in people with very high triglyceride levels who are at risk for pancreatitis (inflammation of the pancreas) and have not responded to other treatments, including statin drugs. Generic fenofibrate is not equivalent to the TriCor brand because of a new product formulation and should not be substituted for the brand unless your doctor approves of the switch.

Cautions and Warnings

Do not take fenofibrate if you are **allergic** or **sensitive** to any of its ingredients.

People taking fenofibrate and other triglyceride-lowering drugs are more likely to die from causes unrelated to triglyceride levels. Fenofibrate reduces the risk of a heart attack or other cardiac event in people with high triglyceride levels and low levels of HDL cholesterol, especially among people with diabetes. The evidence for this benefit is not as strong as it is for the statin drugs.

People taking fenofibrate and gemfibrozil may develop pancreatitis (inflammation of the pancreas).

People with **liver or severe kidney disease** should avoid fenofibrate. People with less severe kidney disease require reduced dosage.

People taking fenofibrate are more likely to develop gallstones.

Fenofibrate can destroy muscle cells, leading to kidney failure, especially when combined with a statin cholesterol-lowering drug (see "Drug Interactions").

Possible Side Effects

▼ Most common: abnormal liver function, abdominal pain, and respiratory disorders.

▼ Common: rash, headache, upset stomach, pain, weakness, tiredness, and flu-like symptoms.

▼ Less common: joint pain, abnormal heart rhythms, reduced sex drive, dizziness, increased appetite, sleeplessness, tingling in the hands or feet, nausea, vomiting, diarrhea, abdominal pain, constipation, stomach noise or gas, frequent urination, vaginal irritation, runny nose, cough, sinus irritation, eye irritation, blurred vision, conjunctivitis (pinkeye), earache, and tiny particles inside the eye ("floaters").

▼ Rare: allergic reactions including severe rash, itching, liver inflammation or enlargement, gallstones, gallbladder disease, muscle aches, and increased sensitivity to the sun. Contact your doctor if you experience any side effect not listed above.

Drug Interactions

• Combining fenofibrate and a statin cholesterol-lowering drug (atorvastatin, cerivastatin, fluvastatin, lovastatin, pravastatin, or simvastatin) can lead to severe muscle pain, muscle cell destruction, and kidney failure. If you have extremely high blood-fat levels, the potential benefits of this combination may outweigh the risks. In people taking this combination, the health of muscles and kidneys must be monitored regularly via blood tests.

• Fenofibrate increases the effects of anticoagulant (blood-thinning) drugs. Your anticoagulant dosage may need an adjustment.

• Combining fenofibrate and cyclosporine can increase the risk of kidney toxicity. This combination should only be used if it is absolutely necessary and the lowest possible dosage is taken.

- If you are taking cholestyramine or colestipol (both are used to reduce blood-fat levels) as well as fenofibrate, take the fenofibrate at least 1 hour before or 4–6 hours after these drugs.

Food Interactions

All forms of fenofibrate, except TriCor, should be taken with food to get the best effect. TriCor may be taken without regard to food or meals.

Usual Dose

These products may not be substituted for each other because of important dosage differences.

Antara

Adult: 43–130 mg a day with food.

Senior: Begin with 43 mg a day. This dosage also applies to people with kidney disease.

Child: not recommended.

Lofibra

Adult: 67–200 mg a day with food.

Senior: Begin with 67 mg a day. This beginning dosage also applies to people with kidney disease.

Child: not recommended.

Lipofen

Adult: 50–150 mg a day with food.

Senior: Begin with 50 mg a day. This dosage also applies to people with kidney disease.

Child: not recommended.

TriCor

Adult: 48–145 mg a day.

Senior: Begin with 48 mg a day. This dosage also applies to people with kidney disease.

Child: not recommended.

Triglide

Adult: 50–160 mg a day.

Senior: Begin with 50 mg a day. This dosage also applies to people with kidney disease.

Child: not recommended.

Overdosage
Little is known about the effects of fenofibrate overdose. Victims should be taken to a hospital emergency room. ALWAYS bring the prescription bottle or container.

Special Information
People should take fenofibrate only after a triglyceride-lowering diet and other medications have failed. While taking fenofibrate, follow the diet recommended by your doctor.

If you forget a dose, take it as soon as you remember. If it is almost time for your next dose, skip the forgotten dose and continue with your regular schedule.

Special Populations
Pregnancy/Breast-feeding: Fenofibrate causes fetal injury and death in animal studies. When this drug is considered crucial by your doctor, its potential benefits must be carefully weighed against its risks.

This drug should not be taken by nursing mothers because of its potential to affect the nursing infant.

Seniors: Seniors are more likely to experience side effects and should never start with more than the lowest recommended dosage.

Generic Name

Finasteride (fin-ASS-ter-ide) Ⓖ

Brand Names
Proscar   Propecia

The information in this profile also applies to the following drug:

Generic Ingredient: Dutasteride
Avodart

Type of Drug
Alpha-reductase inhibitor and androgen hormone inhibitor.

Prescribed For
Benign prostatic hyperplasia (BPH) and male-pattern baldness. May also play a role in preventing prostrate cancer.

General Information
Finasteride works by interfering with the action of the enzyme alpha-reductase, which converts testosterone into 5-dihydrotestosterone

(DHT). By suppressing DHT levels, finasteride reduces the size of the prostate in most men who take the drug for BPH. You may need to take finasteride for 6–12 months before its effects can be assessed.

Urine flow improves in about 60% of men taking finasteride for BPH and symptoms improve in about 30%. In one study, men experienced a significant regression in prostate size after 3 months, and the reduction was maintained through the 12-month study period; these men experienced a significant improvement in urine flow that could be maintained up to 36 months.

Studies of finasteride for hair loss on the top and back-middle of the scalp show new hair growth in 65–80% of men taking the drug continuously for 2 years. The drug must be taken for 3 months or more before it begins to have an effect and must be taken continuously to maintain hair growth. Once you stop taking this drug, any new hair you have grown is likely to fall out in the next 12 months. Between 14–17% of men taking the drug continued to lose hair throughout the study period.

Finasteride has been studied as therapy following radical prostatectomy surgery and in the prevention of first-stage prostate cancer, acne in women, and unusual hairiness.

Cautions and Warnings

Do not take finasteride if you are **allergic** or **sensitive** to any of its ingredients.

This drug should not be used in **women** or **children.** Pregnant women must not handle the tablets and capsules because of the risk to the fetus.

People who do not respond to finasteride may have a condition that causes BPH-like symptoms, such as prostate cancer, bladder or nerve disorders, or physical obstruction of the urinary tubes. Finasteride cannot be used to treat these conditions.

Because it is broken down in the liver, finasteride must be used with caution by people with **liver disease**.

Finasteride may mask symptoms of **prostate cancer** by causing a reduction in the level of prostate-specific antigen (PSA), an increasingly acknowledged indicator of prostate cancer.

Possible Side Effects

Side effects are generally mild and often subside with continued use of the drug.

Possible Side Effects (continued)

▼ Common: impotence, loss of sex drive, decreased amount of semen, breast tenderness and enlargement, testicular pain, and drug sensitivity reactions including lip swelling and rash.

Drug Interactions

- Finasteride may reduce the effectiveness of theophylline and aminophylline, although dosage adjustments usually are not required.
- Finasteride affects the PSA blood test used for prostate cancer screening. Be sure your doctor knows you are taking this drug if you have a PSA test done or are being tested for prostate cancer.
- Dustasteride blood levels may increase when mixed with ritonavir, ketoconazole, cimetidine, and ciprofloxacin, all of which are inhibitors of a liver enzyme called CYP3A4. Blood levels of dutasteride also increase with verapamil and diltiazem.

Food Interactions

You may take finasteride with food if it upsets your stomach.

Usual Dose

Dutasteride
Adult: 0.5 mg (1 capsule) once a day.
Child: not recommended.

Finasteride
Adult: BPH—5 mg once a day. Male-pattern baldness—1 mg once a day.
Child: not recommended.

Women should not take finasteride.

Overdosage

Side effects are unlikely. Doses of dutasteride as high as 400 mg a day have been taken with no adverse side effects. Call your local poison control center or a hospital emergency room for more information. If you seek treatment, ALWAYS bring the prescription bottle or container.

Special Information

Women who are or might be pregnant should not handle crushed finasteride tablets because small amounts of the drug may be absorbed into the blood, possibly affecting the fetus.

If your sexual partner is or might be pregnant and you start taking finasteride, you must wear a condom during sex to avoid directly exposing her to finasteride in the semen.

Semen volume may decrease while on finasteride. Impotence or reduced sex drive is also a risk.

If you forget a dose, take it as soon as you remember. If it is almost time for your next dose, skip the one you forgot and continue with your regular schedule. Do not take a double dose. Call your doctor if you miss a dose for 2 or more days.

Special Populations

Pregnancy/Breast-feeding: This drug is not intended for women. Finasteride will harm the fetus if taken during pregnancy. It is not known if finasteride passes into breast milk.

Seniors: Seniors with liver disease should use this drug with caution.

Brand Name

Fioricet

Generic Ingredients

Acetaminophen + Butalbital + Caffeine Ⓖ

Other Brand Names

Americet	Femcet
Dolgic LQ	Margesic
Dolgic Plus	Medigesic
Esgic	Repan
Esgic-Plus	Triad

Type of Drug

Barbiturate and analgesic (pain reliever) combination.

Prescribed For

Symptom relief of tension headache.

General Information

Fioricet is one of many combination products containing a barbiturate—butalbital—and an analgesic—acetaminophen. Products of this kind also often contain a sedative or a narcotic. Other analgesic combinations, such as Fiorinal, substitute aspirin for acetaminophen.

Cautions and Warnings

Do not take Fioricet if you are **allergic** or **sensitive** to any of its ingredients.

Use this drug with caution if you have **kidney or liver disease** or a history of **porphyria**.

Chronic (long-term) use of Fioricet may lead to drug dependence or addiction. It is not recommended for multiple or recurrent headaches.

Butalbital is a respiratory depressant and affects the central nervous system (CNS), producing drowsiness, tiredness, and an inability to concentrate. Alcohol increases the CNS depression caused by this drug.

The safety and effectiveness of these medications have not been established in children under age 12.

For additional information see "Cautions and Warnings" in Acetaminophen (page 7).

Possible Side Effects

▼ Most common: lightheadedness, dizziness, sedation, shortness of breath, nausea, vomiting, upset stomach and a feeling of intoxication.

▼ Less common: weakness, headache, agitation, tremor, uncoordinated muscle movement, disorientation, dry mouth, constipation, facial flushing, changes in heart rate, palpitations, feeling faint, urinary difficulties, rash, and itching.

For additional information see "Possible Side Effects" in Acetaminophen (page 7).

Drug Interactions

● Combining Fioricet with alcohol, sedatives, barbiturates, sleeping pills, antihistamines, monoamine oxidase inhibitor antidepressants, or other CNS depressants may cause tiredness, drowsiness, and trouble concentrating.

- These medications may reduce the effectiveness of corticosteroids, contraceptives containing estrogen, beta blockers (e.g. propranolol), doxycycline, felodipine, griseofulvin, nifedipine, phenylbutazone, quinine, theophylline, warfarin, and tricyclic antidepressants.

For additional information see "Drug Interactions" in Acetaminophen (page 7).

Food Interactions

Fioricet is best taken on an empty stomach but may be taken with food if it upsets your stomach.

Usual Dose

1–2 tablets or capsules every 4 hours or as needed; do not exceed 6 doses a day.

Overdosage

Symptoms include breathing difficulties, nervousness progressing to stupor or coma, pinpointed pupils, cold and clammy skin and lowered heart rate or blood pressure, nausea, vomiting, dizziness, ringing in the ears, facial flushing, sweating, and thirst. Take the victim to a hospital emergency room immediately. ALWAYS bring the prescription bottle or container.

Special Information

Fioricet may cause drowsiness. Be careful when driving or performing any task that requires concentration.

You should avoid alcohol while taking this medication.

Do not take Fioricet for longer or in amounts greater than prescribed.

If you have been taking this medication for more than a few weeks, do not stop taking it without your doctor's instruction. Suddenly stopping Fioricet may lead to withdrawal symptoms.

Call your doctor if your headache or pain persists or gets worse, or if you develop side effects that are bothersome or persistent.

If you forget a dose, take it as soon as you remember. If it is almost time for your next dose, skip the one you forgot and continue with your regular schedule. Do not take a double dose.

For additional information see "Special Information" in Acetaminophen (page 7).

Special Populations

Pregnancy/Breast-feeding: Fioricet should not be taken during pregnancy. It is associated with birth defects, prolonged labor and delayed delivery, and breathing problems in newborns. Regular use of Fioricet during the last 3 months of pregnancy may also cause drug dependency in the newborn.

Fioricet passes into breast milk. Breast-feeding while using Fioricet may cause babies to become tired, short of breath, or have a slow heartbeat. Nursing mothers who must take this drug should use infant formula.

Seniors: Fioricet may have a greater depressant effect on seniors. Seniors are also more likely to experience stimulation and disorientation.

Brand Name

Fiorinal

Generic Ingredients
Aspirin + Butalbital + Caffeine Ⓖ

Other Brand Names
Butalgen	Fiorimor
Farbital	Fortabs
Fiorigen	Lanorinal

Type of Drug
Barbiturate and analgesic (pain reliever) combination.

Prescribed For
Symptom relief of tension headache.

General Information
Pain relief products often combine an analgesic with a sedative. The analgesic ingredient in Fiorinal is aspirin; other brand-name products, such as Esgic and Fioricet, contain acetaminophen. The sedative ingredient in pain-relief combinations may be a barbiturate, narcotic, or other sedative. Fiorinal contains the barbiturate butalbital. Fiorinal also contains caffeine, which is often used in analgesic combinations that treat headache because it enhances the pain-relieving effect of aspirin.

Cautions and Warnings
Do not take Fiorinal if you are **allergic** or **sensitive** to any of its ingredients.

Do not give Fiorinal to **children** or **teenagers** with chickenpox or flu-like symptoms due to the aspirin content and danger of Reye's syndrome.

Use Fiorinal with extreme caution if you suffer from **peptic ulcer,** problems with **blood clotting** or other **bleeding disorders,** or are about to have **surgery.**

This drug should be used with caution if you have **kidney or liver disease, diabetes,** or a history of **porphyria**.

Long-term use of this drug may cause drug dependence and addiction. It is not recommended for the treatment of multiple recurrent headaches.

Butalbital is a respiratory depressant and affects the central nervous system (CNS), producing drowsiness, tiredness, and an inability to concentrate. Alcohol increases the CNS depression caused by butalbital.

The safety and efficacy of Fiorinal use in children under age 12 has not been established.

For additional information see "Cautions and Warnings" in Aspirin (page 110).

Possible Side Effects

▼ Most common: lightheadedness, dizziness, and sedation.
▼ Less common: nausea, vomiting, flatulence, and rash.
For additional information see "Possible Side Effects" in Aspirin (page 110).

Drug Interactions

- Combining Fiorinal with alcohol, sedatives, barbiturates, sleeping pills, antihistamines, monoamine oxidase inhibitor antidepressants, or other CNS depressants may cause tiredness, drowsiness, and trouble concentrating.
- Fiorinal may enhance the effects of oral anticoagulants (blood thinners), oral antidiabetes drugs, insulin, and nonsteroidal anti-inflammatory drugs (NSAIDs).
- Fiorinal may decrease the effectiveness of medications taken for gout, including probenicid and sulfinpyrazone.

For additional information see "Drug Interactions" in Aspirin (page 110).

Food Interactions

Fiorinal is best taken on an empty stomach but may be taken with food if it upsets your stomach.

Usual Dose

1–2 tablets or capsules every 4 hours or as needed. Do not exceed 6 doses a day.

Overdosage

Symptoms include breathing difficulties, nervousness progressing to stupor or coma, pinpointed pupils, cold and clammy skin, lowered heart rate or blood pressure, nausea, vomiting, stomach pain, dizziness, ringing in the ears, flushing, sweating, and thirst. Symptoms of mild overdose are rapid and deep breathing, nausea, vomiting, dizziness, ringing or buzzing in the ears, flushing, sweating, thirst, headache, drowsiness, diarrhea, and rapid heartbeat. Severe overdose may cause fever, excitement, confusion, convulsions, liver or kidney failure, coma, and bleeding. Take the victim to a hospital emergency room immediately. ALWAYS bring the prescription bottle or container.

Special Information

Fiorinal may cause drowsiness. Be careful when driving or performing any task that requires concentration.

Avoid alcohol while taking Fiorinal.

If you have been taking this medication for more than a few weeks, do not stop taking it without your doctor's instruction. Suddenly stopping this drug may lead to withdrawal symptoms.

Do not take Fiorinal for longer or in amounts greater than prescribed.

Call your doctor if your headache pain persists or gets worse, or if you develop any bothersome or persistent side effect.

If you forget a dose, take it as soon as you remember. If it is almost time for your next dose, skip the dose you forgot and continue with your regular schedule. Do not take a double dose.

For additional information see "Special Information" in Aspirin (page 110).

Special Populations

Pregnancy/Breast-feeding: Fiorinal should not be taken during pregnancy. Pregnant women taking it may experience prolonged labor, delayed delivery, and bleeding problems. Fiorinal increases the risk of birth defects and may cause breathing or bleeding problems in newborns. Regular use of Fiorinal during the last 3 months of pregnancy may also cause drug dependency in the newborn.

Fiorinal passes into breast milk. Breast-feeding while using Fiorinal may cause tiredness, shortness of breath, or slowed heartbeat in the baby. Nursing mothers who must take Fiorinal should use infant formula.

Seniors: Fiorinal may have a greater depressant effect on seniors. Seniors are also more likely to experience stimulation and disorientation.

Brand Name

Fiorinal with Codeine

Generic Ingredients
Aspirin + Butalbital + Caffeine + Codeine Phosphate Ⓖ

Type of Drug
Barbiturate, narcotic, and analgesic (pain reliever) combination.

Prescribed For
Symptom relief of tension headache.

General Information
Fiorinal with Codeine is one of many combination products containing a barbiturate, an analgesic, and a narcotic. In Fiorinal with Codeine, butalbital is the barbiturate, aspirin is the analgesic, and codeine is the narcotic. These products often also contain a sedative, and acetaminophen may be substituted for aspirin.

Cautions and Warnings
Do not take Fiorinal with Codeine if you are **allergic** or **sensitive** to any of its ingredients. Even recommended doses of aspirin can cause severe allergic reaction in those with an aspirin allergy.

Do not take this medication if you suffer from **peptic ulcer, bleeding disorders,** or a history of **porphyria**.

Use this medication with caution if you have **kidney or liver disease** or **diabetes**.

Fiorinal with Codeine may cause postural low blood pressure (symptoms include dizziness or fainting when rising from a sitting or lying position).

Long-term use of this drug may cause drug dependence or addiction.

It is not recommended for treatment of multiple, recurrent headaches.

Fiorinal with Codeine is a respiratory depressant and affects the central nervous system (CNS), producing sleepiness, tiredness, or inability to concentrate. Alcohol increases the depression caused by codeine and butalbital.

Do not give Fiorinal with Codeine to **children** or **teenagers** with chickenpox or flu-like symptoms. The aspirin content presents the danger of Reye's syndrome.

For additional information see "Cautions and Warnings" in Aspirin (page 110).

Possible Side Effects

▼ Most common: dizziness, sleepiness, nausea, and vomiting.
▼ Less common: dry mouth, difficulty swallowing, heartburn, rapid heart rate, leg pain and muscle fatigue, urinary problems, rash, fever, earache, stuffy nose, and ringing in the ears. Narcotic analgesics may aggravate convulsions in those who have had them.

For additional information see "Possible Side Effects" in Aspirin (page 110).

Drug Interactions

- Interaction with alcohol, sedatives, barbiturates, sleeping pills, antihistamines, or other drugs that produce sedation may cause tiredness, drowsiness, and trouble concentrating.
- Taking Fiorinal with Codeine with a monoamine oxidase inhibitor antidepressant may cause increased central nervous system effects.
- This medication may reduce the effectiveness of medications for the treatment of gout including probenicid and sulfapyrazone.
- Fiorinal with Codeine may enhance the effects of blood thinners, oral antidiabetes drugs, insulin, and nonsteroidal anti-inflammatory drugs (NSAIDs).

For additional information see "Drug Interactions" in Aspirin (page 110).

Food Interactions

Fiorinal with Codeine is best taken on an empty stomach but may be taken with food if it upsets your stomach.

Usual Dose

1–2 tablets or capsules every 4 hours or as needed; do not exceed 6 doses a day.

Overdosage

Usual overdose symptoms include breathing difficulties, nervousness progressing to stupor or coma, pinpointed pupils, cold clammy skin and lowered heart rate or blood pressure, nausea, vomiting, dizziness, ringing in the ears, flushing, sweating, and thirst. Symptoms of mild overdose include rapid and deep breathing, nausea, vomiting, dizziness, ringing or buzzing in the ears, flushing, sweating, thirst, headache, drowsiness, diarrhea, and rapid heartbeat. Severe overdose may cause fever, excitement, confusion, convulsions, liver or kidney failure, coma, or bleeding. Take the victim to a hospital emergency room immediately. ALWAYS bring the prescription bottle or container.

Special Information

This drug may cause drowsiness. Be careful when driving or performing any task that requires concentration.

Avoid alcohol while taking this drug.

If you have been taking this medication for more than a few weeks, do not stop taking it without your doctor's instruction. Suddenly stopping this drug may lead to withdrawal symptoms.

Do not take this drug for longer or in amounts greater than prescribed.

Call your doctor if you experience breathing difficulties, or persistent nausea, vomiting, or constipation.

If you forget a dose, take it as soon as you remember. If it is almost time for your next dose, skip the one you forgot and continue with your regular schedule. Do not take a double dose.

For additional information see "Special Information" in Aspirin (page 110).

Special Populations

Pregnancy/Breast-feeding: Fiorinal with Codeine should not be used during pregnancy. Pregnant women taking it may experience prolonged labor, delayed delivery, and bleeding problems. This drug increases the risk of birth defects and may cause breathing or bleeding problems in newborns. Regular use of Fiorinal with Codeine during the last 3 months of pregnancy may also cause drug dependency in the newborn.

Fiorinal with Codeine passes into breast milk. Breast-feeding while using this drug may cause tiredness, shortness of breath, or a slow heartbeat in the baby. Nursing mothers who must take this drug should use infant formula.

Seniors: This drug may have a greater depressant effect on seniors. Other effects that may be more prominent are stimulation, disorientation, lightheadedness, and dizziness or fainting when rising suddenly from a sitting or lying position.

Generic Name

Flecainide (FLEH-kan-ide) G

Brand Name
Tambocor

Type of Drug
Antiarrhythmic.

Prescribed For
Abnormal heart rhythm.

General Information
Flecainide is prescribed in situations where the abnormal heart rhythm is so severe as to be life-threatening and the patient does not respond to other drug treatments. Like other antiarrhythmic drugs, flecainide works by affecting the movement of nervous impulses within the heart. Flecainide's effects may not become apparent for 3–4 days after you start taking it.

Cautions and Warnings
Do not take flecainide if you are **allergic** or **sensitive** to any of its ingredients or if you have **heart block,** unless you have a cardiac pacemaker. As with other antiarrhythmic drugs, there is no proof that flecainide helps people live longer or avoid sudden death.

Flecainide causes or worsens **arrhythmias** in 7% of people who take it; this risk increases with certain kinds of underlying heart disease and higher doses of the drug. Flecainide causes or worsens **heart failure** in about 5% of people taking it because it tends to reduce the force and rate of each heartbeat.

Flecainide is extensively broken down in the liver. People with **poor liver function** should not take flecainide unless the benefits clearly outweigh the risks.

Changes in the pH of urine may affect the effectiveness of flecainide.

Possible Side Effects

▼ Most common: dizziness, fainting, lightheadedness, unsteadiness, visual disturbances including blurred vision and seeing spots before the eyes, breathing difficulties, headache, nausea, fatigue, heart palpitations, chest pain, tremors, weakness, constipation, bloating, a bad taste in your mouth, and abdominal pain.

▼ Less common: new or worsened heart arrhythmias or heart failure, heart block, slowed heart rate, vomiting, diarrhea, upset stomach, loss of appetite, stomach gas, dry mouth, tingling in the hands or feet, partial or temporary paralysis, loss of muscle control, flushing, sweating, ringing or buzzing in the ears, anxiety, sleeplessness, depression, not feeling well, twitching, weakness, convulsions, speech disorders, stupor, memory loss, personality loss, nightmares, apathy, eye pain, unusual sensitivity to bright light, sagging eyelids, reduced white-blood-cell or blood-platelet counts, impotence, reduced sex drive, frequent urination, urinary difficulty, itching, rash, fever, muscle ache, closing of the throat, and swollen lips, tongue, or mouth.

Drug Interactions

- The combination of propranolol and flecainide may cause an exaggerated lowering in heart rate. Other drugs that slow the heart may also interact with flecainide to produce an excessive slowing of heart rate.
- Avoid megadoses of vitamin C while taking this drug.
- The amount of flecainide in your blood and its effect on your heart may be increased if it is taken together with cimetidine, disopyramide, or verapamil.
- Your dose of flecainide should be halved when given with amiodarone.
- Smokers may need a larger dose of flecainide than nonsmokers.
- Flecainide may increase the amount of digoxin in the bloodstream, increasing the chance of side effects.

Food Interactions

A strict vegetarian diet and anything that makes urine less acid interferes with flecainide's elimination from the body, increasing drug toxicity.

Usual Dose

Adult: starting dose—50–100 mg every 12 hours. Maximum dosage is 400 mg a day.

Child (under 18 years): not recommended.

Overdosage

Flecainide overdose affects heart function, causing slower heart rate, low blood pressure, and possible death from respiratory failure. Victims of flecainide overdose should be taken to a hospital emergency room for treatment. ALWAYS bring the prescription bottle or container.

Special Information

Flecainide can make you dizzy, lightheaded, or disoriented. Take care while driving or performing complex tasks.

Call your doctor if you develop chest pains, an abnormal heartbeat, breathing difficulties, bloating in your feet or legs, tremors, fever, chills, sore throat, unusual bleeding or bruising, yellowing of the whites of your eyes, or any other intolerable side effect.

If you forget to take a dose of flecainide and remember within 6 hours, take it as soon as possible. If you do not remember until later, skip the dose you forgot and continue with your regular schedule. Do not take a double dose.

Special Populations

Pregnancy/Breast-feeding: At high doses, flecainide damages an animal fetus. When this drug is considered crucial by your doctor, its potential benefits must be weighed against its risks.

Flecainide passes into breast milk. Nursing mothers who must take this drug should use infant formula.

Seniors: Seniors with reduced kidney or liver function are more likely to develop side effects and require a lower dosage.

Flomax   *see Tamsulosin, page 1080*

Flonase *see Corticosteroids, Nasal, page 303*

Flovent *see Corticosteroids, Inhalers, page 309*

Generic Name

Flucytosine (floo-SYE-toe-sene)

Brand Name
Ancobon

Type of Drug
Antifungal.

Prescribed For
Serious blood-borne fungal infections.

General Information
Flucytosine is meant for fungal infections—*Candida, chromomycoses,* and *cryptococcus*—carried in the blood that affect the urinary tract, respiratory tract, central nervous system, heart, and other organs. It is not meant for fungal infections of the skin, such as common athlete's foot.

Cautions and Warnings
Do not take this drug if you are **allergic** or **sensitive** to any of its ingredients.

   People with **kidney disease** must be closely monitored by their doctors and should take this medication with extreme caution; daily dosage must be reduced.

   Flucytosine can worsen **bone-marrow depression** in people whose immune systems are already compromised. Liver and kidney function and blood composition should be monitored while you are taking this drug.

   The safety and efficacy of flucytosine have not been established in **children**.

Possible Side Effects

▼ Most common: unusual tiredness or weakness, liver inflammation, yellowing of the eyes or skin, abdominal pain, diarrhea, loss of appetite, nausea, vomiting, rash, redness, itching, sore throat, fever, and unusual bleeding or bruising.

▼ Less common: chest pains, breathing difficulties, sensitivity to the sun or bright light, dry mouth, duodenal ulcers, severe bowel irritation, stomach bleeding, interference with kidney function, kidney failure, reduced red- and white-blood-cell counts or other changes in blood composition, headache, hearing loss, confusion, dizziness, weakness, shaking, sedation, psychosis, hallucinations, heart attack, and low blood-sugar and potassium levels.

Drug Interactions

- Amphotericin B increases flucytosine's effectiveness; this combination is generally used to produce better results.
- Flucytosine may interfere with some routine blood tests.
- Cytosine may inactivate the antifungal activity of flucytosine.

Food Interactions

Take flucytosine with food if it upsets your stomach.

Usual Dose

22–66 mg per lb. a day, in divided doses.

Overdosage

Little is known about the effects of flucytosine overdose, but it may cause exaggerated drug side effects. If you seek treatment at a hospital, ALWAYS bring the prescription bottle or container.

Special Information

Take the capsules a few at a time over 15 minutes to avoid nausea and vomiting.

Call your doctor if you develop unusual tiredness or weakness; yellowing of the skin or whites of the eyes; rash, redness, or itching; sore throat or fever; unusual bleeding or bruising; or any persistent or intolerable side effect.

Maintain good dental hygiene while taking flucytosine. Use extra care when using your toothbrush or dental floss because of the risk that flucytosine will make you more susceptible to infection. Dental work should be completed prior to starting on this drug.

Exposure to sunlight may cause rash, itching, redness, discoloration of the skin, or severe sunburn. Stay out of direct sunlight when taking flucytosine.

If you forget a dose, take it as soon as you remember. If it is almost time for your next dose, take 1 dose right away and another in 3 or 4 hours, then go back to your regular schedule. Do not take a double dose.

Special Populations

Pregnancy/Breast-feeding: Flucytosine causes birth defects in animals and crosses the placenta. Flucytosine should be used by pregnant women only when its potential benefits clearly outweigh its risks.

It is not known if flucytosine passes into breast milk. Nursing mothers who must take this drug should use infant formula.

Seniors: Dosage adjustment may be required due to age-related loss of kidney function.

Type of Drug

Fluoroquinolone Anti-Infectives
(flor-oe-QUIN-oe-lone)

Brand Names

Generic Ingredient: Ciprofloxacin Ⓖ

Ciloxan Eyedrops   Cipro XR
Cipro   Proquin XR

Generic Ingredient: Gatifloxacin
Zymar Eyedrops

Generic Ingredient: Gemifloxacin
Factive

Generic Ingredient: Levofloxacin Ⓖ

Iquix Eyedrops   Quixin Eyedrops
Levaquin

Generic Ingredient: Lomefloxacin
Maxaquin

Generic Ingredient: Moxifloxacin

Avelox   Vigamox Eyedrops

Generic Ingredient: Norfloxacin
Noroxin

Generic Ingredient: Ofloxacin Ⓖ
Floxin   Ocuflox Eyedrops
Floxin Otic

Prescribed For

Infections of the lower respiratory system, sinuses, urinary tract, skin, bone and joints, lungs, and prostate; also prescribed for sexually transmitted diseases, prostatitis, infectious diarrhea, bronchitis, pneumonia, typhoid fever, anthrax, and traveler's diarrhea. The eyedrops are used to treat ocular infections, the eardrops for ear infections.

General Information

Fluoroquinolone anti-infectives work against many organisms that traditional antibiotics have trouble killing. They do not work against the common cold, flu, or other viral infections. The fluoroquinolones were first used as treatment for urinary infections and then other uses developed over the years. The new uses depend on how well the specific drug penetrates different body tissues as well as on how they have been tested in the laboratory. Individual fluoroquinolones are not all equally effective in treating all infections.

Cautions and Warnings

Do not take a fluoroquinolone if you are **allergic** or **sensitive** to any of its ingredients, or to any drug in this group, or have had a reaction to related medications such as nalidixic acid. Severe, possibly fatal, allergic reactions can occur even after the very first dose. These reactions include cardiovascular collapse, loss of consciousness, tingling, swelling of the face or throat, breathing difficulties, itching, and rash. Stop taking the drug if you experience allergic symptoms and seek medical help at once.

Fluoroquinolones may cause increased pressure on parts of the brain, leading to convulsions and psychotic reactions. Other possible effects include tremors, restlessness, lightheadedness, confusion, and hallucinations. Fluoroquinolones should be used with caution in people with **head trauma, seizure disorders,** or other **nervous system conditions**.

Moxifloxacin should not be used by people with **liver disease**.

Moxifloxacin should be avoided by people with **heart rhythm problems** or those taking drugs that can affect heart rhythm.

People with **kidney disease** require reduced dosage of these drugs, except in the case of moxifloxacin.

People taking fluoroquinolones may be unusually sensitive to the **sun**. Avoid the sun while taking this drug and for several days following therapy, even if you are using sunscreen.

People taking a fluoroquinolone may develop colitis that could range from mild to very serious. Contact your doctor if you develop diarrhea or cramps.

Fluroquinolones can worsen **myasthenia gravis**. Use with caution.

Prolonged fluoroquinolone use can lead to fungal overgrowth.

Patients taking a fluoroquinolone may experience ruptures of the shoulder, hand, Achilles tendon, or other tendons that may require surgery or lead to extended disability.

Possible Side Effects

Side effects are rarely serious.

▼ Common: nausea (most likely with ciprofloxacin and moxifloxacin), vomiting, and diarrhea (may be most likely with moxifloxacin and ofloxacin).

▼ Less common: dizziness, abdominal pain, headache, and liver inflammation.

▼ Rare: Rare side effects, including some severe drug reactions, can occur in almost any part of the body. In once-daily studies of ciprofloxacin eardrops, there were a few reports of nausea, formation of flaky scales, inflammation of the external ear, temporary hearing loss, ringing or buzzing in the ears, middle-ear inflammation, tremors, high blood pressure, and fungal infection. Contact your doctor if you experience any side effect not listed above.

Drug Interactions

- Separate your fluoroquinolone dose from that of antacids, didanosine, iron supplements, or zinc by 2–6 hours. These drugs decrease the amount of fluoroquinolone absorbed. Moxifloxacin must be taken 4 hours before or 8 hours after antacids, iron, or zinc.

- Nitrofurantoin may antogonize norfloxacin's antibacterial effects. Do not take these drugs together.
- Moxifloxacin can increase the risk of abnormal heart rhythms. Combining this drug with astemizole, erythromycin, tricyclic antidepressants, and antipsychotics increases the risk of abnormal heart rhythms associated with this drug.
- People taking drugs to correct abnormal heart rhythms should avoid fluoroquinolones.
- Nonsteroidal anti-inflammatory drugs (NSAIDs) and anti-inflammatory drugs should not be combined with fluoroquinolones because of the increased risk of stimulation and seizures.
- Sucralfate reduces the amount of fluoroquinolone absorbed in the blood. Take sucralfate at least 6 hours after taking a fluoroquinolone.
- Probenecid may increase the risk of some fluoroquinolone side effects. Cimetidine may also increase fluoroquinolone blood levels.
- Fluoroquinolones (except moxifloxacin) may increase the effect of oral anticoagulant drugs such as warfarin. Your anticoagulant dosage may have to be reduced.
- Fluoroquinolones may increase the toxic effects of cyclosporine (used for organ transplants) on your kidneys.
- Fluoroquinolones (except moxifloxacin) may increase theophylline blood levels and the risk of side effects.
- Azlocillin may increase the risk of ciprofloxacin side effects.
- Ciprofloxacin and norfloxacin may increase caffeine's effects.

Food Interactions

Levofloxacin, lomefloxacin, and moxifloxacin may be taken with or without food. Take ofloxacin and norfloxacin at least 2 hours before or 2 hours after meals or antacids. Ciprofloxacin is best taken 1 hour before or 2 hours after meals, but may be taken with food. Dairy products and calcium-fortified orange juice interfere with the absorption of ciprofloxacin and should be avoided.

Usual Dose

Check with your doctor if you suffer from kidney failure as your fluoroquinolone dosage may need to be reduced.

Tablets
    Adult
        Ciprofloxacin: 100–750 mg twice a day.
        Ciprofloxacin XR: 1000 mg once a day.

Gemifloxacin: 320 mg once a day.

Levofloxacin: 250–750 mg once a day.

Lomefloxacin: 400 mg a day.

Moxifloxacin: 400 mg a day.

Norfloxacin: 400 mg every 12 hours; a single dose of 800 mg may be taken for gonorrhea.

Ofloxacin: 200–400 mg every 12 hours.

Child: not recommended.

Eyedrops

Ciprofloxacin: 1–2 drops in the affected eye several times a day.

Gatifloxacin: days 1–2—2 drops in the affected eye every 2 hours while awake, up to 8 times a day, then 4 times a day for the next 5 days.

Levofloxacin: days 1–2—1–2 drops in the affected eye every 2 hours while awake, up to 8 times a day. Days 3–7—1–2 drops in the affected eye every 4 hours while awake, up to 4 times a day.

Moxifloxacin: 1 drop in the affected eye 3 times a day for 1 week.

Ofloxacin: bacterial conjunctivitis—days 1–2, place 1–2 drops in the affected eye every 2–4 hours while awake; days 3–7, place 1–2 drops in the affected eye every 4–6 hours while awake. Bacterial corneal ulcer—days 1–2, place 1–2 drops in the affected eye every 30 minutes while awake; awaken 4–6 hours after you go to sleep for one more dose; days 3–7 or 9, place 1–2 drops in the affected eye every hour while awake; days 7–9, or through the end of treatment, place 1–2 drops in the affected eye 4 times a day.

Eardrops

Ofloxacin: 5–10 drops in the affected ear twice a day.

Overdosage

Overdose symptoms generally mimic drug side effects. Overdose may cause kidney failure and, in the case of moxifloxacin, abnormal heart rhythms. Call your local poison control center or a hospital emergency room for more information. You may be told to induce vomiting with ipecac syrup—available at any pharmacy—before taking the victim to an emergency room. If you seek treatment, ALWAYS bring the prescription bottle or container.

Special Information

Take each dose with a full glass of water. Be sure to drink at least 8 glasses of water a day while taking any of these drugs to help avoid kidney side effects.

Drug sensitivity reactions can develop even after only 1 dose. Stop taking the drug and get immediate medical attention if you feel faint or develop itching, rash, facial swelling, breathing difficulties, convulsions, depression, visual disturbances, dizziness, headache, lightheadedness, or any sign of a drug reaction.

Colitis can be caused by any anti-infective medication. If diarrhea develops, call your doctor at once.

Avoid excessive sunlight. Call your doctor if you become sensitive to the sun.

Call your doctor if you experience pain, inflammation, or rupture of a tendon.

Follow your doctor's directions exactly. Complete the full course of drug therapy, even if you feel well.

Eyedrops

To avoid infection, do not let the eyedropper tip touch your finger, eyelid, or any surface. Wait 5 minutes before using another eyedrop or eye ointment.

Call your doctor at once if your vision declines or if eye stinging, itching or burning, redness, irritation, swelling, or pain worsens.

Fluoroquinolones can cause changes in vision, dizziness, drowsiness, and lightheadedness. Be careful when driving or performing any task that requires concentration.

If you forget to administer a dose, do so as soon as you remember. If it is almost time for your next dose, skip the missed dose and continue with your regular schedule. Do not take a double dose.

Special Populations

Pregnancy/Breast-feeding: Animal studies have shown that fluoroquinolones may damage the fetus or reduce the likelihood of a successful pregnancy. When a fluoroquinolone is considered crucial by your doctor, its potential benefits must be carefully weighed against its risks.

Fluoroquinolones pass into breast milk. Nursing mothers who must take them should use infant formula.

Seniors: With the exception of moxifloxacin, seniors may require reduced dosage due to age-related decreases in kidney function. The risk of a ruptured tendon may increase in seniors, especially those taking a corticosteroid. In the case of eyedrops, seniors may also need less medication.

Generic Name

Fluoxymesterone (flue-OX-ee-MES-ter-one) Ⓖ

Brand Name

Halotestin

Type of Drug

Androgen (male hormone).

Prescribed For

Men: hormone replacement or augmentation and male menopause; also prescribed as male contraception for up to 12 months, and for delayed puberty.

Women: breast pain and fullness in women who have given birth, and certain types of breast cancer.

General Information

Fluoxymesterone is an androgen. Androgens are responsible for the normal growth and development of male sex organs and for maintaining secondary sex characteristics including hair distribution, vocal cord thickening, muscle development, and fat distribution.

Cautions and Warnings

Do not use fluoxymesterone if you are **allergic** or **sensitive** to any of its ingredients.

Androgens do not improve athletic performance and may cause serious side effects.

Women taking any androgen may develop deepening of the voice, oily skin, acne, hairiness, increased sex drive, and menstrual irregularities.

Androgens should be avoided if possible by **young boys** who have not gone through puberty.

Fluoxymesterone worsens **gynecomastia** (a condition characterized by swollen male breast tissue).

Men with unusually **high blood levels of calcium,** known or suspected **prostate cancer** or **prostate destruction,** or **breast cancer** should not use fluoxymesterone, nor should anyone with **severe liver, heart, or kidney disease**.

Long-term, high-dose androgen therapy may cause severe liver disease, including hepatitis and cancer, reduced sperm count, and water retention.

Blood cholesterol may be raised by androgens. This can be a problem for people who have **heart disease**.

Androgens may cause or worsen **sleep apnea** (a condition characterized by intermittent cessation of breathing during sleep).

For patients with **diabetes,** this drug may affect blood sugar levels.

Possible Side Effects

Men
▼ Most common: inhibition of testicle function, impotence, chronic erection, and painful enlargement of breast tissue.

Women
▼ Most common: unusual hairiness, male-pattern baldness, deepening of the voice, and enlargement of the clitoris. These changes are usually irreversible once they occur. Increased blood calcium and menstrual irregularities may also develop.

Men and Women
▼ Most common: changes in sex drive, headache, anxiety, depression, a tingling feeling, sleep apnea, flushing, rash, acne, habituation (the drug may be habit-forming), excitation, chills, sleeplessness, water retention, nausea, vomiting, diarrhea, hepatitis (symptoms include yellowing of the skin or whites of the eyes), liver inflammation, and liver cancer. Symptoms resembling those of a stomach ulcer may also develop.

Drug Interactions

- Fluoxymesterone may increase the effect of an oral anticoagulant (blood-thinner); dosage of the anticoagulant may have to be reduced.
- Combining an androgen and imipramine or another tricyclic antidepressant may result in a severe paranoid reaction.
- Androgens may decrease insulin requirements.

Food Interactions

Take fluoxymesterone with meals if it upsets your stomach.

Usual Dose

Adult: 5–40 mg a day.
Child: not recommended.

Overdosage

Symptoms include nausea, vomiting, and diarrhea. Call your local poison control center or a hospital emergency room for more information. If you seek treatment, ALWAYS bring the prescription bottle or container.

Special Information

Androgens must be taken only under the close supervision of your doctor. The dosage and clinical effects of fluoxymesterone vary widely and require constant monitoring.

Call your doctor if you develop nausea or vomiting, swelling of the legs or feet, yellowing of the skin or whites of the eyes, or a painful or persistent erection. Women should call their doctors immediately if they develop a deep or hoarse voice, acne, hairiness, male-pattern baldness, or menstrual irregularities.

If you forget a dose, take it as soon as you remember. If it is almost time for your next dose, skip the one you forgot and continue with your regular schedule. Do not take a double dose.

Special Populations

Pregnancy/Breast-feeding: Fluoxymesterone should never be taken by pregnant or nursing women because it can affect the developing fetus and nursing infant.

Seniors: Seniors are more likely to develop prostate enlargement or prostate cancer. A marked increase in sex drive may also occur.

Generic Name

Flurazepam (fluh-RAZ-uh-pam) Ⓖ

Brand Name

Dalmane

Type of Drug

Benzodiazepine sedative.

Prescribed For

Insomnia and sleep disturbances.

General Information

Flurazepam is a member of the group of drugs known as benzo-diazepines. Benzodiazepines work by a direct effect on the brain. They make it easier to go to sleep and decrease the number of times you wake up during the night. Flurazepam and quazepam remain in your bloodstream longer than other drugs in this class, thus resulting in the greatest incidence of morning "hangover."

Cautions and Warnings

Do not use flurazepam if you are **allergic** or **sensitive** to any of its ingredients.

People with **kidney or liver disease** should be carefully moni-tored while taking flurazepam. Take the lowest possible dose to help you sleep.

People with **respiratory disease** may experience sleep apnea (intermittent cessation of breathing during sleep) while taking flurazepam.

Clinical **depression** may be increased by flurazepam, which can depress the nervous system. Intentional overdose is more common among depressed people who take sleeping pills than among those who do not.

Some people have experienced amnesia while taking fluraz-epam.

All benzodiazepines can be addictive if taken for long periods of time and can cause drug withdrawal symptoms if discontinued suddenly. It should be used with caution in people with a history of **drug dependence**. Withdrawal symptoms include tremors, muscle cramps, insomnia, agitation, diarrhea, vomiting, sweating, and convulsions.

Tapering the drug when stopping may help prevent withdrawal symptoms. People with a history of **seizures** should be particu-larly cautious when stopping use of this drug.

Possible Side Effects

▼ Common: drowsiness, headache, dizziness, talkativeness, nervousness, apprehension, poor muscle coordination, light-headedness, daytime tiredness, muscle weakness, slow-ness of movement, hangover, and euphoria (feeling "high").

▼ Less common: nausea, vomiting, rapid heartbeat, confu-sion, temporary memory loss, upset stomach, stomach cramps and pain, depression, blurred or double vision and

Possible Side Effects (*continued*)

other visual disturbances, constipation, changes in sense of taste, appetite changes, stuffy nose, nosebleeds, common cold symptoms, asthma, sore throat, cough, breathing difficulties, diarrhea, dry mouth, allergic reaction, fainting, abnormal heart rhythm, itching, rash, acne, dry skin, sensitivity to the sun, nightmares or strange dreams, sleeplessness, tingling in the hands or feet, ringing or buzzing in the ears, ear or eye pain, menstrual cramps, frequent urination and other urinary difficulties, blood in the urine, discharge from the penis or vagina, lower back and other pain, muscle spasms and pain, fever, swollen breasts, and weight changes.

▼ Rare: Rare side effects can affect your heart, stomach and intestines, urinary tract, blood, muscles, and joints. Contact your doctor if you experience any side effect not listed above.

Drug Interactions

- As with all benzodiazepines, the effects of flurazepam are enhanced if it is taken with an alcoholic beverage, antihistamine, sedative, barbiturate, anticonvulsant medication, antidepressant, or monoamine oxidase inhibitor antidepressant.
- Contraceptive drugs, cimetidine, disulfiram, and isoniazid may increase the effect of flurazepam by reducing the drug's breakdown in the liver. Probenecid also increases flurazepam's effects.
- Cigarette smoking, rifampin, and theophylline may reduce the effect of flurazepam on your body by increasing the rate at which it is broken down by the liver.
- Levodopa + carbidopa's effectiveness may be decreased by flurazepam.
- Flurazepam may increase the amount of zidovudine (an HIV drug—also known as AZT), phenytoin, or digoxin in your bloodstream, increasing the chances of side effects.
- Mixing clozapine with a benzodiazepine has led to respiratory collapse in a few people. Flurazepam should be stopped at least 1 week before starting clozapine treatment.

Food Interactions

Flurazepam may be taken with food if it upsets your stomach.

Usual Dose

Adult and Child (age 15 and over): 15–30 mg at bedtime. Dosage must be individualized for maximum benefit.

Senior: starting dose—15 mg at bedtime.

Child (under age 15): not recommended.

Overdosage

The most common overdose symptoms are confusion, sleepiness, depression, loss of muscle coordination, and slurred speech. Coma may also occur. Patients who overdose on this drug must be made to vomit with ipecac syrup—available at any pharmacy— to remove any remaining drug from the stomach. Call your doctor or a poison control center before doing this. If 30 minutes have passed since the overdose was taken or if symptoms have begun to develop, take the victim immediately to a hospital emergency room for treatment. ALWAYS bring the prescription bottle or container.

Special Information

Never take more flurazepam than your doctor has prescribed.

Avoid alcoholic beverages and other nervous system depressants while taking flurazepam.

Exercise caution while performing tasks that require concentration and coordination. Flurazepam may make you tired, dizzy, or lightheaded.

If you take flurazepam daily for 3 or more weeks, you may experience some withdrawal symptoms when you stop taking the drug. Do not stop taking flurazepam suddenly or increase or decrease your dosage without first consulting your doctor.

If you forget a dose and remember within 1 hour, take it as soon as you remember. If you do not remember until later, skip the dose you forgot and go back to your regular schedule. Do not take a double dose.

Special Populations

Pregnancy/Breast-feeding: Flurazepam absolutely should not be used by pregnant women or by women who may become pregnant.

Flurazepam passes into breast milk. The drug should not be taken by nursing mothers.

Seniors: Seniors are more susceptible to the effects of flurazepam.

Generic Name

Flutamide (FLUE-tuh-mide) Ⓖ

Type of Drug

Antiandrogen.

Prescribed For

Prostate cancer and excessive hairiness in women.

General Information

Prostatic cancer is sensitive to anything that removes the source of androgen (male hormone). Flutamide works by slowing the up-take of androgen or by interfering with the binding of androgen to body tissues. It is always prescribed together with a luteinizing hormone-releasing hormone (LHRH) drug.

Cautions and Warnings

Do not take flutamide if you are **allergic** or **sensitive** to any of its ingredients.

Severe liver injury may occur with flutamide; your doctor should monitor your liver function. People with severe **liver disease** should not take flutamide.

This drug may cause jaundice and severe blood conditions, including hemolytic anemia. People with certain **blood disorders** and people who **smoke** are at greater risk for these side effects.

A few men taking this drug have developed breast cancer. Flutamide may reduce sperm counts.

Possible Side Effects

▼ Most common: diarrhea, cystitis, and bleeding from the rectum.

▼ Common: rectal irritation, blood in the urine, hot flashes, loss of libido, impotence, nausea, rash, and swollen breasts.

▼ Less common: drowsiness, confusion, depression, anxiety, nervousness, appetite loss, stomach problems, anemia, low white-blood-cell and blood-platelet counts, arm or leg swelling, urinary and muscle problems, and high blood pressure.

Possible Side Effects (continued)

▼ Rare: hepatitis, jaundice, and breathing difficulties. Contact your doctor if you experience any side effect not listed above.

Drug Interactions

- Flutamide may increase the effects of blood-thinning drugs such as warfarin. Dosage adjustment may be necessary.

Food Interactions

None known.

Usual Dose

Adult: 250 mg (2 capsules) every 8 hours, 3 times a day. Total daily dose should be 750 mg.

Child: not recommended.

Overdosage

Overdose symptoms may include tiredness or low activity levels, slow breathing, weakness, tearing, appetite loss, vomiting, swollen and tender breasts, and liver inflammation. Overdose victims should be taken to a hospital emergency room. ALWAYS bring the prescription bottle or container.

Special Information

Report anything unusual to your doctor, especially pain or tenderness in the upper right abdomen, yellowing of the skin or whites of the eyes, severe itching, dark urine, persistent appetite loss, and unexplained flu-like symptoms. These may be signs of severe liver toxicity.

Flutamide can turn your urine amber or yellow-green and cause unusual sun sensitivity. Use sunscreen and wear long-sleeved protective clothing while you are taking flutamide.

Flutamide must be taken exactly as prescribed. Call your doctor if you miss a dose of this drug.

Special Populations

Pregnancy/Breast-feeding: This drug is not intended for use by women.

Seniors: Seniors may take this drug without special precaution.

Generic Name

Formoterol (for-MOH-ter-ol)

Brand Names

Foradil Aerolizer   Performist
Foradil Certihaler

Combination Product
Generic Ingredients: Formoterol + Budesonide
Symbicort

The information in this profile also applies to the following drug:

Generic Ingredient: Arformoterol
Brovana

Type of Drug

Bronchodilator.

Prescribed For

Maintenance of asthma, bronchospasm during exercise, and chronic obstructive pulmonary disorder, including chronic bronchitis, and emphysema.

General Information

Formoterol is a long-acting beta-2 agonist, used in the prevention of asthma attacks and bronchial spasms. It is not effective in stopping an asthma attack once it has begun. Patients suffering from severe asthma should always have a short-acting bronchodilator available in case of an acute attack.

Cautions and Warnings

Do not use formoterol if you are **allergic** or **sensitive** to any of its ingredients.

Formoterol should not be used by patients with **significantly or rapidly worsening asthma.** In some asthma patients, formoterol may increase the chance of death from asthma.

Formoterol is not a replacement for corticosteroid inhalers. Patients should continue to use their corticosteroid inhalers at the same dosage in conjunction with formoterol.

Patients who have been taking inhaled, short-acting beta-2 agonists should stop regular use of these, and use them only to treat acute asthma symptoms.

Formoterol can cause paradoxical bronchospasm, a potentially life-threatening condition. Patients who experience symptoms should discontinue use of formoterol immediately.

Formoterol can cause irregular heartbeat and should be used with caution by patients with a history of **heart disease** or **high blood pressure**. Patients with a history of **seizures**, **strokes**, or **diabetes** should also be carefully monitored for a recurrence or worsening of these conditions.

Possible Side Effects

▼ Most common: tremors, dizziness, insomnia, and chest pain.
▼ Common: restlessness, weakness, sore throat, and difficulty breathing.
▼ Less common: lightheadedness, angina, abnormal heart rhythm, heart palpitations, and bronchospasm.
▼ Rare: severe worsening of asthma, extreme allergic reaction, and angioedema (a potentially life-threatening swelling of the lips and throat). Contact your doctor if you experience any side effect not listed above.

Drug Interactions

- Formoterol's effects may be increased by monoamine oxidase inhibitor (MAOI) antidepressants, tricyclic antidepressants, thyroid drugs, other bronchodilators, and some antihistamines.
- The effect of formoterol may be lessened by beta-blocking drugs, such as propranolol.
- Formoterol may antagonize the effects of blood-pressure-lowering drugs, especially reserpine, methyldopa, and guanethidine.
- Using formoterol with antihistamines; disopyramide; phenothiazines; procainamide; quinidine and similar drugs; theophylline; and tricyclic antidepressants may increase the risk of heart damage and life-threatening cardiac arrhythmias.

Food Interactions

None known.

Usual Dose

Arformoterol
Adult: Inhale 15 mcg every 12 hours.
Child: not recommended.

Formoterol
Adult and Child (age 5 and over)
Foradil Aerolizer: Inhale 12 mcg every 12 hours.
Foradil Certihaler: Inhale 10 mcg every 12 hours.
Perforomist: Inhale 20 mcg every 12 hours.
Child (under age 5): not recommended.

Formoterol + Budesonide Combination
Adult: Inhale 1 puff every 12 hours.
Child: not recommended.

Overdosage

Formoterol overdose may cause nausea, vomiting, tremor, sleepiness, rapid or irregular heartbeat, low blood sugar, blood acidity, and life-threatening cardiac arrhythmias. Patients experiencing severe symptoms should go to a hospital emergency room. ALWAYS bring the prescription bottle or container.

Special Information

The drug should be inhaled during the second half of your inward breath. This will allow the medication to reach more deeply into your lungs.

Be sure to follow your doctor's directions for the use of formoterol. Using more than you need can increase the risk of side effects and worsen your symptoms. If your condition worsens after taking formoterol, stop taking it and call your doctor at once.

Call your doctor at once if you develop chest pains, rapid heartbeat, palpitations, muscle tremors, dizziness, headache, or swelling of the throat, or if you still have trouble breathing after using the medication.

If a dose of formoterol is forgotten, take it as soon as you remember. If it is almost time for your next dose, skip the dose you forgot and continue with your regular schedule. Do not take a double dose.

Formoterol capsules must only be used with the inhaler that is provided with this medicine. Do not use other medicines with the formoterol inhaler. Patients should be aware that the gelatin capsule may fragment, causing a risk that gelatin particles will be inhaled. This risk is minimized by being careful to pierce the gelatin capsule only once. Capsules should be used immediately after they are taken from the blister pack.

Special Populations

Pregnancy/Breast-feeding: The safety of formoterol in pregnant women has not been studied. The potential benefit of using this medication must be carefully weighed against its risks.

It is not known if formoterol passes into breast milk. Nursing mothers who take this should consider using infant formula.

Seniors: Seniors may be more sensitive to the effects of this drug. Follow your doctor's directions and report any side effects at once.

Fosamax   *see **Bisphosphonates,** page 164*

Generic Name

Fosfomycin   (fos-foe-MYE-sin)

Brand Name

Monurol

Type of Drug

Urinary anti-infective.

Prescribed For

Uncomplicated urinary infections.

General Information

Fosfomycin kills a variety of bacteria. It works by preventing bacteria from sticking to the wall of the urinary tract and by interfering with bacterial cell division. In the body, it is converted to its active form—free fosfomycin. Generally, bacteria that are resistant to other antibiotics are not resistant to fosfomycin, so this drug may work where others have failed.

Cautions and Warnings

Do not take fosfomycin if you are **allergic** or **sensitive** to any of its ingredients. Fosfomycin is meant to be taken once, in a single dose. Taking more than 1 packet of fosfomycin only increases side effects; it does not improve the drug's effectiveness.

Possible Side Effects

▼ Less common: diarrhea, vaginal irritation, runny nose, nausea, and headache.
▼ Rare: Rare side effects can occur in almost any part of the body. Contact your doctor if you experience any side effect not listed above.

Drug Interactions
- Metoclopramide reduces fosfomycin blood levels.

Food Interactions
You may take fosfomycin with or without food.

Usual Dose
Adult (age 12 and over): 1 packet mixed with water.
Child (under age 12): not recommended.

Overdosage
Little is known about the effects of fosfomycin overdose. Call your local poison control center or a hospital emergency room for more information. If you seek treatment, ALWAYS bring the prescription container.

Special Information
Do not take fosfomycin powder in its dry form. Mix the contents of the packet with 3–4 oz. of cool or cold water until it dissolves. Then drink the solution immediately.

Call your doctor if your infection does not improve within 2 or 3 days.

Special Populations
Pregnancy/Breast-feeding: The safety of using fosfomycin during pregnancy is not known. When this drug is considered crucial by your doctor, its potential benefits must be carefully weighed against its risks.

It is not known if fosfomycin passes into breast milk. Nursing mothers who must take this drug should use infant formula.

Seniors: Seniors may take fosfomycin without special restriction.

Generic Name

Fosinopril (fos-IN-oe-pril) Ⓖ

Brand Name

Monopril

Combination Product

Generic Ingredients: Fosinopril + Hydrochlorothiazide Ⓖ
Monopril HCT

Type of Drug

Angiotensin-converting enzyme (ACE) inhibitor.

Prescribed For

High blood pressure and heart failure. Also prescribed for renal failure, kidney hypertension, post–heart attack management, management of people with a high risk of heart disease, diabetes, chronic kidney disease, and preventing a second stroke.

General Information

Fosinopril sodium and other ACE inhibitors work by preventing the conversion of a hormone called angiotensin I to another hormone called angiotensin II, a potent blood-vessel constrictor. Preventing this conversion relaxes blood vessels, thus reducing blood pressure and relieving the symptoms of heart failure. Fosinopril also affects the production of other hormones and enzymes that participate in the regulation of blood vessel dilation. Fosinopril begins working 2–6 hours after you take it.

Cautions and Warnings

Do not take fosinopril if you are **allergic** or **sensitive** to any of its ingredients. Severe reactions may involve angioedema, a possibly life-threatening swelling of the face, throat, or intestines (see "Special Information"). These reactions are more likely in **hemodialysis** patients and those undergoing **venom immunization**.

Fosinopril occasionally causes very low blood pressure or affects your kidneys. Your doctor should check your urine for changes during the first few months of treatment.

ACE inhibitors can affect your white-blood-cell count, possibly increasing your susceptibility to infection. Blood counts should be checked periodically.

Fosinopril may cause serious injury or death to the fetus if taken during **pregnancy**. Pregnant women should not take fosinopril.

ACE inhibitors may be less effective in some **black patients** with high blood pressure, especially when dietary salt intake is high. Nevertheless, they should still be considered useful blood pressure treatments. Swelling beneath the skin to form welts is more common among black patients.

Possible Side Effects

▼ Most common: chronic cough and dizziness, especially when rising from a sitting or lying position. The cough usually goes away a few days after you stop taking the medicine.

▼ Less common: chest pain, low blood pressure, fatigue, diarrhea, headache, vomiting, and nausea.

▼ Rare: Rare side effects can affect your heart, sleeping, stomach and intestines, skin, sex drive, and joints. Contact your doctor if you experience any side effect not listed above.

Drug Interactions

- The blood-pressure-lowering effect of fosinopril is additive with diuretic drugs and beta blockers. Any other drug that causes a rapid drop in blood pressure should be used with caution if you are taking an ACE inhibitor.
- Fosinopril may increase the effects of lithium; this combination should be used with caution.
- Aspirin and other nonsteroidal anti-inflammatory drugs (NSAIDs) reduce the blood pressure-lowering effects of fosinopril and other ACE inhibitors. This may cause reductions in kidney function.
- Fosinopril may increase potassium levels in your blood, especially when taken with dyazide or other potassium-sparing diuretics.
- Antacids and fosinopril should be taken at least 2 hours apart.
- Capsaicin may trigger or aggravate the cough associated with fosinopril therapy.
- Indomethacin may reduce the blood-pressure-lowering effects of fosinopril.
- Phenothiazine sedatives and antivomiting drugs may increase the effects of fosinopril.
- Severe sensitivity reactions can occur in people taking allopurinol.

- Fosinopril may affect blood levels of digoxin. More digoxin in the blood increases the chance of digoxin-related side effects while less digoxin in the blood can compromise its effectiveness.

Food Interactions

You may take fosinopril with food if it upsets your stomach.

Usual Dose

Adult: 10–80 mg once a day. People with liver disease may require lower dosages.

Overdosage

The principal effect of ACE inhibitor overdose is a rapid drop in blood pressure, as evidenced by dizziness or fainting. Take the overdose victim to a hospital emergency room immediately. ALWAYS bring the prescription bottle or container.

Special Information

Call your doctor if you develop swelling of the face or throat, if you have sudden difficulty in breathing, or if you develop a sore throat, mouth sores, abnormal heartbeat, chest pain, persistent rash, or loss of taste perception. Unexplained swelling of the face, lips, hands, and feet can also affect the larynx (throat) and tongue and interfere with breathing. If this happens, the victim should be taken to a hospital emergency room at once.

Some people who start taking an ACE inhibitor after they are already on a diuretic (an agent that increases urination) experience a rapid drop in blood pressure after their first doses or when the dosage is increased. To prevent this from happening, you may be told to stop taking the diuretic 2 or 3 days before starting the ACE inhibitor or to increase your salt intake during that time. The diuretic may then be restarted gradually.

You may get dizzy if you rise to your feet quickly from a sitting or lying position when taking fosinopril.

Avoid strenuous exercise or very hot weather, because heavy sweating or dehydration can cause a rapid decrease in blood pressure.

Avoid over-the-counter diet pills, decongestants, and other stimulants that can raise blood pressure. Also, do not take potassium supplements or salt substitutes containing potassium without consulting your doctor.

If you forget to take a dose of fosinopril, take it as soon as you remember. If it is within 8 hours of your next dose, skip the one you forgot and continue with your regular schedule. Do not take a double dose.

Special Populations

Pregnancy/Breast-feeding: ACE inhibitors can cause fetal injury or death. Women who are or might be pregnant should not take ACE inhibitors. Stop taking the drug and contact your doctor if you become pregnant.

Large amounts of fosinopril pass into breast milk. Nursing mothers who must take this drug should use infant formula.

Seniors: Seniors may be more sensitive to the effects of fosinopril.

Brand Name

Fosrenol

Generic Ingredient
Lanthanum Carbonate

Type of Drug
Phosphate binder.

Prescribed For
High blood phosphate levels (hyperphosphatemia) in people with end-stage renal disease (ESRD).

General Information
People with ESRD, a form of kidney disease, tend to retain phosphorous. High phosphate levels, in turn, can affect calcium balance in the body and cause deposits of this mineral to build up in the wrong places. Lanthanum helps manage high blood phosphate levels by binding to phosphate in food before it can be absorbed into the blood. This is the same mechanism used by other phosphate-lowering drugs (sevelamer and the antacids aluminum hydroxide and calcium carbonate). Lanthanum, like other phosphate binders, must be taken with meals so that it can bind phosphate ions in the stomach before they can be absorbed into the blood. Very little of this drug is absorbed into the blood and it is not broken down in the body.

Cautions and Warnings

Do not take fosrenol if you are **allergic** or **sensitive** to any of its ingredients.

People with an **active peptic ulcer, ulcerative colitis, Crohn's disease,** or **bowel obstruction** should use this medication with caution.

Researchers found no difference in bone fracture rates or overall survival for lanthanum than for other phosphate-binding treatments over 3 years. The study period was too short to assume that it would improve bone fractures or survival beyond 3 years.

Possible Side Effects

Side effects primarily affect the digestive tract and are similar to other phosphate-lowering treatments in type and frequency.

▼ Most common: nausea, vomiting, complications with the dialysis graft, diarrhea, constipation, abdominal pains, and low blood pressure.

▼ Common: bronchitis and runny nose.

▼ Less common: high blood calcium levels.

▼ Rare: Other side effects may affect any organ or organ system. Contact your doctor if you experience any side effect not listed above.

Drug Interactions

- Lanthanum strongly binds to phosphate in the stomach and might also bind to other medications in the stomach. However, no interaction was found in tests conducted with warfarin, digoxin, enalapril, furosemide, metoprolol, or phenytoin.
- Compounds known to interact with antacids should not be taken within 2 hours of taking lanthanum.

Food Interactions

This drug must be taken with or immediately after meals.

Usual Dose

Adult: 750–1500 mg with or immediately after each meal. Completely chew each tablet before you swallow it. Do not swallow whole tablets.

Child: not recommended.

Overdosage

There have been no reports of lanthanum overdose, even with single doses up to 1000 mg per pound of body weight. Symptoms of overdose are likely to occur in the digestive tract. Overdose victims may be taken to a hospital emergency room for evaluation. ALWAYS bring the prescription bottle or container.

Special Information

If you forget to take lanthanum with or immediately after a meal, skip the forgotten dose and continue with your regular schedule.

Be sure to follow the low-phosphate diet your doctor prescribes. It is a key element in helping to manage your blood phosphate levels.

Special Populations

Pregnancy/Breast-feeding: Animal studies with doses several times the maximum human dose revealed some harm to the developing fetus. Pregnancy in a woman with end-stage renal disease, especially those on dialysis, is uncommon because of reduced fertility and carries serious risks for a woman and her baby, including anemia, uncontrolled high blood pressure, and infection. This drug is not recommended for pregnant women.

It is not known if lanthanum passes into breast milk. Nursing mothers who must take it should consider using infant formula.

Seniors: Seniors may use this medication without special restriction.

Generic Name

Ganciclovir (gan-SYE-kloe-vere) Ⓖ

Brand Name

Vitrasert

The information in this profile also applies to the following drug:

Generic Ingredient: Valganciclovir
Valcyte

Type of Drug

Antiviral.

Prescribed For

Cytomegalovirus (CMV) infections of the eye and CMV infections in other parts of the body, in people with compromised immune systems.

General Information

Ganciclovir works by preventing reproduction of the virus CMV. Unlike other antiviral drugs, it works only against this virus and herpes simplex virus. The drug is eliminated through the kidneys.

Though most often used for CMV retinitis (eye infection), ganciclovir has also been used for CMV infections of the urine, blood, throat, and semen. It is also used to prevent CMV infection. Ganciclovir is helpful in controlling CMV infection in heart, kidney, and kidney-pancreas transplant patients. Valganciclovir is not indicated for use in liver transplant patients.

Valganciclovir (Valcyte) is broken down by the body into ganciclovir, and all information in this profile applies to both drugs, unless otherwise noted.

Cautions and Warnings

Do not take ganciclovir if you are **allergic** or **sensitive** to any of its ingredients.

Ganciclovir causes anemia, reduced white-blood-cell count, and blood-platelet loss. Regular monitoring of blood and platelet counts is recommended while taking this drug.

Ganciclovir is intended only for people who are **immunocompromised**. It is not intended to treat or prevent CMV infections in **newborns**.

Detachment of the retina has been noted in people taking ganciclovir, as well as in people with CMV who have not taken the drug. The relationship between ganciclovir and this effect is not well known.

Ganciclovir causes increased sensitivity to the sun; use a sunscreen or wear protective clothes when you go outside.

People with **kidney disease** should use ganciclovir with caution, and may require treatment at a lower dosage.

Studies of ganciclovir in blacks, Hispanics, and Caucasians showed a trend toward higher blood levels among Caucasians than other groups.

Intravenous ganciclovir has been given to a small number of children under age 12 with mixed results. Side effects were similar to those experienced by adults taking the drug.

Possible Side Effects

▼ Most common: fever, diarrhea, abdominal pain, reduced white-blood-cell counts, anemia, rash, sweating, nausea, vomiting, and appetite loss.

▼ Common: infection; chills; stomach gas; low platelet counts (symptoms include bleeding or oozing blood); tingling; burning; numbness or pain in the hands, arms, legs, or feet; itching; pneumonia; weakness; and headache.

Drug Interactions

- Pentamidine, flucytosine, vincristine, vinblastine, adriamycin, amphotericin B, trimethoprim-sulfamethoxazole, and other cytotoxic drugs may increase the side effects of ganciclovir and should be used together only if absolutely necessary, and only if the potential benefits outweigh the risks.

- People taking imipenem-cilastatin together with ganciclovir have experienced seizures. Avoid this combination.

- Mixing ganciclovir with other drugs that can be damaging to the kidneys may increase the rate and extent of kidney damage.

- Probenecid interferes with ganciclovir release through the kidneys and substantially increases blood levels of ganciclovir.

- Mixing ganciclovir with the anti-HIV drugs didanosine or zidovudine (AZT) may increase didanosine or AZT levels and reduce ganciclovir levels. Because AZT and ganciclovir both cause anemia and low white-blood-cell counts, many people cannot tolerate this combination.

Food Interactions

High-fat, high-calorie meals can increase the amount of ganciclovir absorbed into the blood. Take this drug with food.

Usual Dose

Ganciclovir

Adult and Child (age 13 and over): 3000 mg a day, divided into 3 or 6 equal doses. People with reduced kidney function will need to have their dosage reduced accordingly, possibly to as little as 500 mg 3 times a week.

Child (under age 13): not recommended.

Valganciclovir

Adult and Child (age 13 and over): 900 mg a day, divided into 2 equal doses of 450 mg each. People with reduced kidney function will need to have their dosage reduced accordingly, possibly to as little as 500 mg 3 times a week.

Child (under age 13): not recommended.

Overdosage

Little is known about the effects of ganciclovir overdose. As much as 6000 mg a day has been taken with only temporary lowering of white-blood-cell count. Call your hospital emergency room for instructions in case of ganciclovir overdose.

Special Information

Ganciclovir does not cure CMV eye infection, and immunocompromised people taking this drug may find their disease worsening. Dosage reductions or discontinuation of the drug may be necessary if white-blood-cell or platelet counts get too low.

Ganciclovir may cause infertility in men and women. Women of child-bearing age should use effective contraception while taking this drug. Men should use a condom while taking the drug and for at least 90 days afterward to avoid passing the drug to their partners.

Good dental hygiene is important while taking ganciclovir to minimize the risk of infection. If you have dental work done while taking this drug, expect the healing process to take longer.

Regular blood tests are necessary to watch for white-blood-cell or platelet-level alterations.

It is very important to take ganciclovir exactly as directed. If you forget a dose, take it as soon as you remember and continue with your regular schedule.

Special Populations

Pregnancy/Breast-feeding: Animal studies showed ganciclovir to be toxic to the fetus. There is no reliable information about its effect in pregnant women, but it should be taken only when the possible benefits outweigh the risks. Women who are likely to become pregnant while taking this drug should use reliable contraception.

It is not known if ganciclovir passes into breast milk, but the possible side effects of this drug on a nursing infant should be kept in mind. Nursing mothers who must take this drug should use infant formula.

Seniors: Seniors often have reduced kidney function; dosage adjustments may be needed.

Generic Name

Gemfibrozil (jem-FI-broe-zil) Ⓖ

Brand Name
Lopid

Type of Drug
Anti-hyperlipidemic (blood-fat reducer).

Prescribed For
High blood triglycerides.

General Information
Gemfibrozil consistently reduces blood triglycerides and reduces the risk of heart disease in people with high levels of triglycerides, low levels of high-density lipoprotein (HDL) cholesterol, the "good" cholesterol, and high levels of low-density lipoprotein (LDL) cholesterol, the "bad" cholesterol. It works by affecting the breakdown of body fats and by reducing the amount of triglyceride manufactured by the liver. It is usually prescribed only for people with very high blood-fat levels who have not responded to dietary changes or other therapies. Gemfibrozil usually has little effect on blood-cholesterol levels, although it may reduce blood cholesterol in some people.

Cautions and Warnings
Do not take gemfibrozil if you are **allergic** or **sensitive** to any of its ingredients or have severe **liver or kidney disease**. Some people taking gemfibrozil have experienced worsening of kidney function.

Gemfibrozil users may have an increased risk of developing gallbladder disease and gallstones.

People taking gemfibrozil and fenofibrate may develop pancreatitis (inflammation of the pancreas).

People taking gemfibrozil may develop muscle aches and inflammation. Tell your doctor if you experience muscle tenderness or weakness.

Estrogen drugs may cause massive increases in triglyceride levels. Stopping estrogen therapy in these cases may reduce triglyceride levels to normal.

Gemfibrozil may cause a moderate rise in blood sugar and mild decreases in white-blood-cell counts.

Possible Side Effects

▼ Most common: abdominal and stomach pain, fatigue, heartburn, gas, diarrhea, nausea, and vomiting.

▼ Less common: rash, itching, dizziness, blurred vision, anemia, reduced levels of white blood cells, increased blood sugar, and muscle pain—especially in the arms or legs.

▼ Rare: dry mouth, constipation, appetite loss, upset stomach, sleeplessness, tingling in the hands or feet, ringing or buzzing in the ears, back pain, painful muscles or joints, swollen joints, feeling unwell, reduction in blood potassium, and abnormal liver function. Contact your doctor if you experience any side effect not listed above.

Drug Interactions

- Gemfibrozil increases the effects of oral anticoagulant (blood-thinning) drugs. Your anticoagulant dosage must be reduced when starting gemfibrozil.

- Combining gemfibrozil with a statin cholesterol-lowering drug (atorvastatin, fluvastatin, lovastatin, pravastatin, rosuvastatin, or simvastatin) has led to the destruction of skeletal muscles. This effect may begin as early as 3 weeks after you start taking the combination or may not appear for months.

- Combining gemfibrozil and sulfonylurea antidiabetes drugs or repaglinide may cause unexpectedly low blood sugar levels. The sulfonylurea drug dosage may need adjustment.

- Gemfibrozil can substantially increase the amount of glitazone antidiabetes drugs in the blood. Glitazone dosages may need to be adjusted.

- Combining gemfibrozil and cyclosporine may decrease the effectiveness of cyclosporine. This combination should only be used if it is absolutely necessary and the lowest possible dose of gemfibrozil is used.

Food Interactions

Gemfibrozil is best taken on an empty stomach 30 minutes before meals but may be taken with food if it upsets your stomach. It is important that you follow your doctor's dietary instructions.

Usual Dose
Adult: 1200 mg a day, divided into 2 doses taken 30 minutes before breakfast and dinner.
Child: not recommended.

Overdosage
There have been reported cases of overdosage with gemfibrozil. Symptoms reported with overdosage were abdominal cramps, abnormal liver function tests, diarrhea, joint and muscle pain, nausea, and vomiting. Induce vomiting with ipecac syrup—available at any pharmacy—but call your doctor or local poison control center before doing this. If you go to a hospital emergency room, ALWAYS bring the prescription bottle or container.

Special Information
Your doctor should perform periodic blood counts during the first year of gemfibrozil treatment to check for anemia or other changes in blood components. Liver-function tests are also necessary. Blood-sugar levels should be checked periodically while you are taking gemfibrozil, especially if you are diabetic or have a family history of diabetes.

Gemfibrozil may cause dizziness or blurred vision. Be careful when driving or doing any task that requires concentration.

Gemfibrozil is less effective if you are greatly overweight.

Call your doctor if side effects become severe or intolerable, especially diarrhea, nausea, vomiting, or stomach pain or gas. These may disappear if your doctor reduces the dosage.

If you forget a dose, take it as soon as you remember. If it is almost time for your next dose, skip the one you forgot and continue with your regular schedule. Do not take a double dose.

Special Populations
Pregnancy/Breast-feeding: The safety of using gemfibrozil during pregnancy is not known. When this drug is considered crucial by your doctor, its potential benefits must be carefully weighed against its risks.

It is not known if this drug passes into breast milk. Nursing mothers who must take it should use infant formula.

Seniors: Seniors are more likely to develop drug side effects due to normal declines in kidney function.

Generic Name

Glatiramer (glah-TYE-ram-er)

Brand Name

Copaxone

Type of Drug

Relapsing-remitting multiple sclerosis (MS) therapy.

Prescribed For

MS.

General Information

Glatiramer is a mixture of several amino acids. It is thought to work by modifying the immune processes responsible for MS. In studies, people who took the drug for over a year were twice as likely to be relapse-free as those who took a placebo (sugar pill).

Cautions and Warnings

Do not use this drug if you are **allergic** or **sensitive** to any of its ingredients or to mannitol.

About 10% of people who self-administer glatiramer experience a post-injection reaction with symptoms that include flushing, chest pain, heart palpitations, anxiety, breathing difficulties, closing of the throat, and an itchy rash. These symptoms usually go away without treatment. This reaction generally occurs after several months of drug therapy, though it may occur earlier.

About 21% of the people who took glatiramer in drug studies had chest pain, but the exact relationship of this pain to use of glatiramer could not be determined. Report any chest pain to your doctor at once.

Glatiramer may make you more sensitive to sunlight.

Because it interferes with immune response, glatiramer may increase your risk of developing infections and tumors.

Glatiramer may interfere with kidney function.

Possible Side Effects

▼ Most common: infections, weakness, pain, chest pain, flu-like symptoms, back pain, flushing, heart palpitations, anxiety, muscle stiffness or spasticity, an urgent need to urinate, swollen lymph glands, injection-site reactions

---

Possible Side Effects (continued)

(including pain, inflammation, itching, an unknown mass at the injection site, welts, skin marks, and bleeding), breathing difficulties, runny nose, and joint pain.

▼ Common: fever, neck pain, facial swelling, bacterial infection, migraine, rapid heartbeat, tremors, fainting, appetite loss, vomiting, general stomach disorders, vaginal infection, painful menstruation, black-and-blue marks, swelling in the arms or legs, bronchial irritation, spasm of the larynx, and ear pain.

▼ Less common: chills, cysts, agitation, foot drop, nervousness, rolling eyeballs, rapid eye movement, confusion, speech problems, cold sores, redness, itchy rash, skin nodules, stomach pain and irritation, and weight gain.

▼ Rare: Other side effects can occur in almost any part of the body, including the heart and blood vessels, digestive system, blood and lymph systems, muscles and bones, respiratory system, kidney, reproductive system, and eyes. Contact your doctor if you experience any side effect not listed above.

Food and Drug Interactions

None known.

Usual Dose

Adult (age 18 and over): 20 mg a day by injection under the skin.
Child (under age 18): not recommended.

Overdosage

Little is known about the effects of glatiramer overdose. Call you local poison control center or a hospital emergency room for information. If you seek treatment, ALWAYS bring the prescription bottle or container.

Special Information

This medication is given by injection. For information on how to properly administer this drug, see page 1242.

Store unused glatiramer in the refrigerator before it is mixed with the diluent supplied by the manufacturer. Do not use any other diluent. The mixed injection must be used right away.

Suggested injection sites are the arms, abdomen, hips, and thighs. Be sure to rotate injection sites.

Glatiramer works best if given at the same time each day.

If you forget to administer a dose, do so as soon as you remember. If it is almost time for your next dose, skip the dose you forgot and continue with your regular schedule. Do not take a double dose. Call your doctor if you miss more than 2 doses in a row.

Special Populations

Pregnancy/Breast-feeding: The safety of using glatiramer during pregnancy is not known. When this drug is considered crucial by your doctor, its potential benefits must be carefully weighed against its risks.

It is not known if glatiramer passes into breast milk. Nursing mothers who must take it should use infant formula.

Seniors: Seniors may use glatiramer without special restriction.

Type of Drug

Glitazone Antidiabetes Drugs
(GLIT-uh-zone)

Brand Names

Generic Ingredient: Pioglitazone Hydrochloride
Actos

Generic Ingredient: Rosiglitazone Maleate
Avandia

Combination Products
Generic Ingredients: Pioglitazone Hydrochloride + Metformin Hydrochloride
ACTOplus Met

Generic Ingredients: Pioglitazone Hydrochloride + Glimepiride
Duetact

Generic Ingredients: Rosiglitazone Maleate + Metformin Hydrochloride
Avandamet

Generic Ingredients: Rosiglitazone Maleate + Glimepiride
Avandaryl

Prescribed For

Type 2 diabetes.

General Information

The glitazones reduce the amount of sugar produced by the liver and increase insulin sensitivity of muscle, liver, and fat cells. They may also help to control blood-fat levels, which are often elevated in diabetes. Glitazones work by affecting genes responsible for controlling the use of sugar and fat in the body, making cells more sensitive to insulin. They are effective for people with type 2 diabetes, whose cells do not respond well to insulin. Glitazones only work when insulin is present. They do not increase the amount of insulin made in the pancreas. Glitazones can be used alone or combined with other diabetes drugs. Studies have indicated that taking rosiglitazone can delay or prevent type 2 diabetes in people with pre-diabetes.

Cautions and Warnings

Do not take these drugs if you are **sensitive** or **allergic** to any of their ingredients or to related drugs. Glitazones may cause fluid retention, worsening or leading to **heart failure**. Some studies have indicated the risk of **heart attack** may be increased in people taking rosiglitazone. Other studies have shown that pioglitazone decreases the risk of heart attack. The effects of these drugs on the heart are still being investigated.

Glitazones are broken down in the liver; people with **liver disease** should not take them. Liver enzyme monitoring is recommended for all people taking a glitazone. People taking pioglitazone and rosiglitazone have experienced liver failure, though no direct causal effect of the drug has been established.

Glitazones may raise blood levels of cholesterol and other blood fats.

These drugs can trigger ovulation. **Premenopausal women** who are not ovulating may be at risk of becoming pregnant.

Glitazones can cause weight gain, which increases with dosage.

Rosiglitazone may increase the risk of broken bones in the hands, arms, or feet.

Women may achieve maximum benefit with smaller dosages.

Possible Side Effects

Pioglitazone
In studies, the side effects of pioglitazone were about the same as those for a placebo (sugar pill).

Possible Side Effects *(continued)*

▼ Most common: upper respiratory infections, headaches, and sinus irritation.
▼ Common: muscle aches, tooth problems, and sore throat.
▼ Less common: anemia and swollen legs or arms.
▼ Rare: swelling below the surface of the skin, especially around the eyes and lips; yellowing of the skin or whites of the eyes, hepatitis, and liver failure. Contact your doctor if you experience any side effect not listed above.

For additional side effects of ACTOplus Met, see Metformin (page 696). For additional side effects of Duetact, see Sulfonylurea Diabetes Drugs (page 1065).

Rosiglitazone

▼ Common: upper respiratory infections, accidental injuries, and headache.
▼ Less common: swollen legs or arms, back pain.
▼ Rare: swelling below the surface of the skin, especially around the eyes and lips; may also affect the hands, feet and throat. Also, hives, anemia, blurry or distorted vision, and low blood sugar. Contact your doctor if you experience any side effect not listed above.

For additional side effects of Avandamet, see Metformin (page 696). For additional side effects of Avandaryl, see Sulfonylurea Diabetes Drugs (page 1065).

Drug Interactions

- Mixing gemfibrozil (for very high triglycerides) with a glitazone increases the amount of the glitazone absorbed into the body. A reduction in the dose of the glitazone may be needed if you start taking gemfibrozil.
- Rifampin can reduce the amount of a glitazone that is absorbed by the body, possibly leading to higher blood sugar levels.
- Ketoconazole may significantly increase the amount of pioglitazone in the body. Other drugs that may have a similar effect but have not yet been studied include itraconazole, erythromycin, calcium channel blockers, corticosteroids, cyclosporine, protease inhibitor anti-HIV drugs, tacrolimus, triazolam, and trimetrexate.

- Mixing pioglitazone with atorvastatin may reduce the amount of either drug in the body.
- Pioglitazone may reduce the effectiveness of contraceptive drugs containing norethindrone and ethinyl estradiol. Higher-dose contraceptives or another contraceptive method may be needed.
- Pioglitazone may stimulate the breakdown of other drugs also metabolized in the liver.
- Taking rosiglitazone and insulin may increase the risk of fluid retention and heart failure.

For additional drug interactions for Avandamet and ACTOplus Met, see Metformin (page 696). For additional drug interactions for Avandaryl and Duetact, see Sulfonylurea Diabetes Drugs (page 1065).

Food Interactions

Grapefruit juice may interfere with the breakdown of pioglitazone in the liver. Otherwise, these drugs may be taken with or without food, except for Avandaryl, which should be taken with the first meal of the day.

Usual Dose

Adult

Pioglitazone: 15–45 mg once a day.

Rosiglitazone: 8 mg once a day or in divided doses.

ACTOplus Met: 15/500 mg–45/2550 mg once or twice a day.

Avandamet: 2/500 mg–4/1000 mg twice a day.

Avandaryl: 4/1 mg–8/4 mg with the first meal of the day.

Duetact: 30/2 mg–30/4 mg once a day.

Child: not recommended.

Overdosage

Little is known about the effects of glitazone overdose. Take the victim to a hospital emergency room. ALWAYS bring the prescription bottle or container.

Special Information

Diet, calorie control, exercise, and weight loss are essential to controlling type 2 diabetes. Do not depend solely on this drug to manage your condition.

Alcohol, smoking, age, and race do not affect the way that glitazones are processed in the body.

Call your doctor if you develop symptoms of liver disease, including nausea, vomiting, abdominal pain, fatigue, appetite loss, or dark-colored urine.

See your doctor for regular monitoring of blood sugar, glycosylated hemoglobin (a more sensitive indicator of long-term diabetes control), and liver function.

If you forget a dose of any of these medicines, take it as soon as you remember. If it is almost time for your next dose, skip the dose you forgot and continue with your regular schedule.

Special Populations

Pregnancy/Breast-feeding: The safety of using glitazones during pregnancy is not known. Most experts recommend that diabetes be controlled with insulin during pregnancy.

It is not known if glitizones pass into breast milk. Nursing mothers who must take it should consider using infant formula.

Seniors: Seniors may take this drug without special restriction.

Glycolax   *see Polyethylene Glycol, page 895*

Generic Name

Guanabenz   (GWAN-uh-benz)   Ⓖ

Type of Drug
Antihypertensive.

Prescribed For
High blood pressure.

General Information
Guanabenz acetate works by depressing the central nervous system by stimulating certain receptors. Initially, guanabenz reduces blood pressure without a major effect on blood vessels; however, long-term use of guanabenz may result in the dilation (widening) of blood vessels and a slight slowing of pulse rate. Guanabenz may be taken alone or with a thiazide diuretic.

Cautions and Warnings
Do not take guanabenz if you are **allergic** or **sensitive** to any of its ingredients.

People with severe **kidney or liver disease** should take this drug with caution. Guanabenz should also be used with caution by people who have had a recent **heart attack** or **stroke.**

Possible Side Effects

Risk and severity of side effects increase with dosage.

▼ Most common: drowsiness, sedation, dry mouth, dizziness, weakness, and headache.

▼ Less common: chest pain; swelling in the hands, legs, or feet; heart palpitations or abnormal heart rhythms; stomach or abdominal pain or discomfort; nausea; diarrhea; vomiting; constipation; anxiety; poor muscle control; depression; difficulty sleeping; stuffy nose; blurred vision; muscle aches and pains; breathing difficulties; frequent urination; decreased sex drive; impotence; unusual taste in the mouth; and swollen and painful breasts in men.

Drug Interactions

- Other blood-pressure-lowering agents such as beta blockers increase the effect of guanabenz.
- The sedating effects of guanabenz are increased by combining it with sedatives, sleeping pills, or other central-nervous-system (CNS) depressants, including alcohol.
- People taking this drug for high blood pressure should avoid over-the-counter drugs that might aggravate their condition, including decongestants, cold and allergy remedies, and diet pills—all of which may contain stimulants.

Food Interactions

This drug is best taken on an empty stomach, but it may be taken with food if it upsets your stomach.

Usual Dose

Adult: 4 mg twice a day to start, increased gradually to a maximum dose of 32 mg twice a day—though doses this large are rarely needed.

Child (under age 12): not recommended.

Overdosage

Overdose causes sleepiness, lethargy, low blood pressure, irritability, pinpoint pupils, and reduced heart rate. Overdose victims should be made to vomit with ipecac syrup—available at any pharmacy—but call your doctor or poison control center first. If you must go to a hospital emergency room, ALWAYS bring the prescription bottle or container.

Special Information

Take guanabenz exactly as prescribed for maximum benefit. If any side effect becomes severe or intolerable, contact your doctor.

Guanabenz often causes tiredness or dizziness; avoid alcohol because it increases these effects. Take care when driving or doing anything that requires concentration.

Do not stop taking guanabenz without your doctor's approval. Suddenly stopping this drug may cause a rapid increase in blood pressure. Dosage must be gradually reduced by your doctor.

If you forget a dose, take it as soon as you remember. If it is almost time for your next dose, skip the one you forgot and continue with your regular schedule. Do not take a double dose. Call your doctor if you miss 2 or more consecutive doses.

Special Populations

Pregnancy/Breast-feeding: Guanabenz may affect the fetus. It should be avoided by women who are or might be pregnant. When guanabenz is considered crucial by your doctor, its potential benefits must be carefully weighed against its risks.

It is not known if guanabenz passes into breast milk. Nursing mothers who must take this drug should use infant formula.

Seniors: Seniors are more sensitive to the sedating and blood-pressure-lowering effects of guanabenz.

Generic Name

Haloperidol (hal-oe-PER-ih-dol) Ⓖ

Brand Name

Haldol

Type of Drug

Butyrophenone antipsychotic.

Prescribed For

Psychotic disorders, including Tourette's syndrome; severe behavioral problems in children; short-term treatment of hyperactive children; chronic schizophrenia; vomiting; treatment of acute psychiatric situations; and phencyclidine (PCP) psychosis.

General Information

Haloperidol is one of many nonphenothiazine agents used to treat psychosis. These drugs are equally effective when given in therapeutically equivalent doses. The major differences are in the type and severity of side effects. Some people may respond well to one and not at all to another. Haloperidol acts on a portion of the brain called the hypothalamus. It affects parts of the hypothalamus that control metabolism, body temperature, alertness, muscle tone, hormone balance, and vomiting. Haloperidol is available in liquid form for those who have trouble swallowing tablets.

Cautions and Warnings

Haloperidol should not be used by people who are **allergic** or **sensitive** to any of its ingredients.

People with very **low blood pressure, Parkinson's disease,** or **blood, liver, heart, or kidney disease** should avoid this drug.

If you have **glaucoma, epilepsy** or a history of **seizures, ulcers,** or **difficulty urinating,** haloperidol should be used with caution and under strict supervision of your doctor.

If haloperidol is used to control mania in bipolar disorder, a rapid depressive mood swing may occur.

Haloperidol can upset the body's temperature-regulating mechanism creating a risk for heat stroke or dehydration.

Haloperidol may cause dystonia, tardive dyskinesia, or neuroleptic malignant syndrome, all serious conditions.

Possible Side Effects

▼ Most common: drowsiness, blurred vision, constipation, diarrhea, dizziness, dry mouth, headache, loss of appetite, nausea, stomach pain, or sleeplessness.

▼ Less common: jaundice (yellowing of the whites of the eyes or skin), which may occur in the first 2–4 weeks. The jaundice usually goes away when the drug is discontinued, but there have been cases in which it did not. If you notice this effect, develop fever, or generally feel unwell, contact your doctor immediately. Other less common side effects are changes in components of the blood, including anemias; raised or lowered blood pressure; abnormal heartbeat; restlessness; anxiety; euphoria (feeling "high"); depression; confusion; acne-like skin reactions; excessive salivation;

Possible Side Effects *(continued)*

breast engorgement; development of breast tissue in males; vomiting; excessive sweating; menstrual irregularities; impotence; and breathing difficulties.

▼ Rare: neurological effects such as spasms of the neck muscles, severe stiffness of the back muscles, rolling back of the eyes, convulsions, difficulty in swallowing, and symptoms associated with Parkinson's disease. These effects usually disappear after the drug has been withdrawn; however, symptoms of the face, tongue, or jaw may persist for years, especially in seniors with a long history of brain disease. If you experience any of these effects, contact your doctor immediately. Other rare side effects can occur in almost any part of the body. Contact your doctor if you experience any side effect not listed above.

Drug Interactions

- Be cautious about taking haloperidol with barbiturates, sleeping pills, narcotics or other sedatives, tricyclic antidepressants, alcohol, or any other medication that may produce a depressive effect.
- Combining haloperidol with carbamazepine may decrease the effectiveness of haloperidol requiring a dosage adjustment.
- The use of azole antifungal agents (e.g. ketoconazole) may cause an increase in haloperidol side effects, possibly requiring adjustments in haloperidol doses.
- Anticholinergic drugs may reduce the effectiveness of haloperidol and increase the risk of side effects.
- Severe low blood pressure or heartbeat irregularities may occur if haloperidol is combined with epinephrine or dopamine.
- Taking lithium together with haloperidol may lead to disorientation, loss of consciousness, or uncontrolled muscle movements.
- Combining fluoxetine with haloperidol may increase the effects of haloperidol.
- Haloperidol may increase the effects of antihypertensive drugs.

- Haloperidol may affect phenytoin levels, as well as levels of other antipsychotic drugs.
- Careful dosage monitoring is required if haloperidol is taken with rifampin.

Food Interactions

Haloperidol is best taken on an empty stomach, but you may take it with food if it upsets your stomach.

Usual Dose

Psychotic disorders

Adult: starting dose—0.5–2 mg 2 or 3 times a day. Some patients may need 3–5 mg 2 or 3 times a day. Rarely, some patients may require up to 100 mg a day.

Child (age 3–12 or 33–88 lbs.): starting dose—0.5 mg a day. Dosage may be increased in 0.5-mg steps every 5–7 days.

Child (under age 3): not recommended.

Tourette's syndrome

Adult: starting dose—0.5–1.5 mg 3 times a day; up to 10 mg a day may be needed.

Child (age 3–12 or 33–88 lbs.): 0.02–0.03 mg per lb. a day. The same dosages apply to children with behavioral disorders or hyperactivity.

Overdosage

Symptoms of overdose are depression, extreme weakness, tiredness, desire to sleep, coma, lowered blood pressure, uncontrolled muscle spasms, agitation, restlessness, convulsions, fever, dry mouth, and abnormal heart rhythm. The patient should be taken to a hospital emergency room immediately. ALWAYS bring the prescription bottle or container.

Special Information

This medication may cause drowsiness. Use caution when driving or operating hazardous equipment; also, avoid alcoholic beverages while taking it.

Haloperidol may cause unusual sensitivity to the sun. It may also turn your urine reddish-brown or pink.

If dizziness occurs, avoid sudden changes in posture and avoid climbing stairs.

Avoid extreme heat while taking haloperidol. This medication may make you more prone to heat stroke.

If you forget to take a dose of haloperidol, take it as soon as you remember. Take the rest of the day's doses evenly spaced throughout the day. Do not take a double dose.

Special Populations

Pregnancy/Breast-feeding: Serious problems have been seen in pregnant animals given large amounts of haloperidol. Although haloperidol has not been studied in pregnant women, you should avoid this drug if you are or might be pregnant.

Haloperidol passes into breast milk. Nursing mothers who must use this medication should use infant formula.

Seniors: Seniors are more sensitive to the effects of this medication and usually require ¼–½ the usual adult dose. Seniors are also more likely to develop side effects.

Brand Name

Helidac

Generic Ingredients
Bismuth Subsalicylate + Metronidazole + Tetracycline

The information in this profile also applies to the following drug:

Generic Ingredients: Bismuth Subcitrate Potassium + Metronidazole + Tetracycline
Pylera

Type of Drug
Antibacterial combination.

Prescribed For
Duodenal ulcers.

General Information
Research has shown that the bacterium *Helicobacter pylori* is usually present in ulcer disease and some forms of gastritis. Drugs used to treat the *H. pylori* infection are prescribed along with a drug that alleviates ulcer symptoms by blocking stomach acid. There are a variety of approaches to treating ulcers by using combinations of various antibiotic and acid-blocking drugs. Helidac combines 3 drugs with antibacterial or antibiotic action. This combination generally works by disrupting the cell walls of the bacterium and interfering with its ability to make proteins or duplicate

itself. It is often prescribed together with ranitidine, cimetidine, or another acid blocker. Other treatments use other drug combinations.

Cautions and Warnings

Do not take Helidac if you are **allergic** or **sensitive** to any of its ingredients.

Do not take Helidac if you have severe **liver or kidney disease**. People with less severe liver disease may require a reduced dosage.

Rarely, bismuth causes severe nervous system toxicity. Symptoms go away after the drug is stopped.

Bismuth subsalicylate can cause dark stools or darkening of the tongue. This darkening of stools is not dangerous; however, be aware that blood in the stool often manifests as blackening of the stool.

Children or teenagers who have or are recovering from **chickenpox** should not use Helidac because it contains a small amount of salicylate, which is related to aspirin. Children or teenagers who take aspirin or a salicylate may develop Reye's syndrome; symptoms include nausea and vomiting.

Bismuth can also cause ringing in the ears, especially if taken along with another aspirin-containing drug.

Metronidazole can cause convulsive seizures and nervous system effects including numbness or tingling in the arms, legs, hands, or feet. The risk of developing these effects increases with dosage and duration of use. Call your doctor at once if you experience any of these effects.

Metronidazole should be taken with caution by people who have had **blood diseases** or **nervous system disorders,** such as seizure disorders.

Candida infections may worsen while you are taking metronidazole.

Other infections, called superinfections, can develop while you are taking tetracycline. If this happens, your doctor will discontinue Helidac and prescribe a different drug to treat your *H. pylori* infection, as well as another drug to treat the superinfection.

Tetracycline should not be used in children under age 8 due to the risk of tooth discoloration.

People taking tetracycline can develop pseudotumor cerebri (pressure inside the brain), the symptoms of which are usually headache and blurred vision. Symptoms usually go away when the drug is stopped, but permanent damage can result.

Tetracycline may increase your sensitivity to the sun; use sunscreen and wear protective clothing.

Tetracycline may make contraceptive drugs less effective. Another or additional forms of contraceptive should be used.

Possible Side Effects

▼ Most common: nausea and diarrhea.

▼ Less common: abdominal pain, blood in the stool, headache, anal discomfort, appetite loss, dizziness, tingling in the hands or feet, vomiting, muscle weakness, constipation, sleeplessness, pain, and respiratory infections.

For more information on possible side effects, see Metronidazole, page 718, and Tetracycline Antibiotics, page 1103.

Drug Interactions

- Tetracycline antibiotics, which are bacteriostatic, may interfere with the action of bactericidal (bacteria-killing) agents such as penicillin. You should not take both kinds of antibiotics for the same infection.
- Antacids, mineral supplements, and multivitamins containing bismuth, calcium, zinc, magnesium, and iron can reduce the effectiveness of tetracycline. Separate doses of your antacid, mineral supplement, vitamin with minerals, or sodium bicarbonate and Helidac by at least 2 hours.
- Tetracycline and metronidazole may each increase the effect of anticoagulant (blood-thinning) drugs such as warfarin. An adjustment in the anticoagulant dosage may be required.
- Cimetidine can increase metronidazole blood levels. Your metronidazole dosage may be reduced if you are also taking cimetidine.
- Tetracycline should not be used with methoxyflurane due to the risk of a toxic interaction.
- Tetracycline may increase blood levels of digoxin in a small number of people, leading to possible digoxin side effects. In some people this interaction with digoxin can occur for months after tetracycline has been stopped. If you are taking this combination, watch carefully for digoxin side effects and call your doctor if any develop.
- Tetracycline may reduce diabetic insulin requirements. If you are using this combination, be sure to carefully monitor your blood-sugar level.

- Tetracycline may increase or decrease lithium blood levels. Metronidazole raises lithium blood levels, effects, and toxicity.
- Combining alcohol and metronidazole may cause abdominal cramps, nausea, vomiting, headaches, and flushing. Modification of the taste of alcohol has also been reported. Metronidazole should not be used if you are taking disulfiram (a drug used to maintain alcohol abstinence) because the combination can cause confusion and psychotic reactions.
- Phenobarbital and other barbiturates can decrease metronidazole's effectiveness.
- Drugs that cause nervous system toxicity, such as mexiletine, ethambutol, isoniazid, lincomycin, lithium, pemoline, and long-term high-dose pyridoxine (vitamin B6) should not be taken with metronidazole because of the increased risk of nervous system side effects.
- Metronidazole may increase phenytoin blood levels and the risk of phenytoin side effects; your doctor may need to adjust your phenytoin dosage.

Food Interactions

Do not take this drug with milk or dairy products. Helidac should be taken with meals and at bedtime.

Usual Dose

Helidac

Adult: Each dose consists of 4 pills. Take all 4 pills, 4 times a day for 14 days with a full glass of water. Take your acid blocker according to your doctor's directions.

Child: not recommended.

Pylera

Adult: 3 pills 4 times a day for 10 days with a full glass of water. Take your acid blocker according to your doctor's directions.

Child: not recommended.

Overdosage

All 3 ingredients in Helidac can be dangerous if taken in overdose, but salicylate poisoning is the most threatening. Symptoms of salicylate toxicity are rapid or heavy breathing, nausea, vomiting, ringing or buzzing in the ears, high fever, lethargy, rapid heartbeat, and confusion. Other more serious symptoms may develop. Take the victim to a hospital emergency room at once. ALWAYS bring the prescription bottle or container.

Special Information

Tetracycline can reduce the effectiveness of contraceptive drugs; you should use backup contraception while taking Helidac. Breakthrough bleeding is also possible.

Bismuth can cause a temporary darkening of your tongue or stool. This is a harmless effect. Stool darkening should not be confused with blood in the stool, which turns it black.

Avoid alcohol while taking Helidac and for 1 day after you stop taking it.

Call your doctor if you develop ringing in the ears. This can be a sign of salicylate toxicity from the bismuth.

If you forget a dose, take it as soon as you remember. If it is almost time for your next dose, skip the dose you forgot and continue with your regular schedule. Never take a double dose.

Special Populations

Pregnancy/Breast-feeding: Helidac should not be taken by pregnant women. Tetracycline affects bone and tooth development in the fetus.

Tetracycline and metronidazole pass into breast milk. Tetracycline interferes with the development of the child's skull, bones, and teeth, and metronidazole also may cause side effects in the baby. Nursing mothers who must take Helidac should use infant formula.

Seniors: Seniors may take this drug without special restriction.

Type of Drug

HIV Antivirals

Brand Names

Generic Ingredient: Abacavir
Ziagen

Generic Ingredient: Delavirdine
Rescriptor

Generic Ingredient: Didanosine
Videx   Videx EC

Generic Ingredient: Efavirenz
Sustiva

Generic Ingredient: Emtricitabine
Emtriva

Generic Ingredient: Etravirine
Intelence

Generic Ingredient: Lamivudine
Epivir   Epivir-HBV

Generic Ingredient: Nevirapine
Viramune

Generic Ingredient: Stavudine
Zerit

Generic Ingredient: Tenofovir
Viread

Generic Ingredient: Zidovudine
Retrovir

Combination Products
Generic Ingredients: Abacavir + Lamivudine
Epzicom

Generic Ingredients: Abacavir + Lamivudine + Zidovudine
Trizivir

Generic Ingredients: Efavirenz + Emtricitabine + Tenofovir
Atripla

Generic Ingredients: Emtricitabine + Tenofovir
Truvada

Generic Ingredients: Lamivudine + Zidovudine
Combivir

Prescribed For

Human immunodeficiency virus (HIV) infection.

General Information

Zidovudine (also known as azidothymidine or AZT) was the first drug approved for treating HIV infection. Over the years, AZT use has been expanded from adults to children to the prevention of HIV transmission between a pregnant woman and her developing fetus.

These drugs, nucleoside and non-nucleoside antiviral agents, inhibit the reproduction of the HIV virus by interfering with and altering an enzyme called HIV reverse transcriptase, essential to the virus' ability to reproduce. When infected cells try to build more HIV virus with the altered reverse transcriptase, the result is an inactive molecule. This reduces the total viral load and helps the body's immune system deal with remaining HIV virus.

People with HIV infection always take these drugs in combination with at least one protease inhibitor and another antiviral. Combination pills of HIV antivirals have been developed because the combinations work better and reduce the number of required pills each day, making it easier to comply with an anti-HIV regimen. Some drugs, such as entecavir, are eliminated through the urine while others, such as abacavir and nevirapine, are broken down in the liver. This difference is important because it will affect how each drug interacts both with other antivirals and other medicines, and how it is affected by liver and kidney disease.

Cautions and Warnings

Do not take any of these drugs if you are **allergic** or **sensitive** to any of their ingredients. Stop taking abacavir at the first sign of drug allergy. Abacavir is associated with fatal sensitivity reactions (fever, skin rash, fatigue, nausea, vomiting, diarrhea, pain, sore throat, difficulty breathing, or cough). Call your doctor at once if you develop signs of a reaction. Abacavir, or the combination product Trizivir, should be discontinued and other treatment started immediately. People have died from abacavir sensitivity.

People with **kidney disease** require lower dosages of emtricitabine, lamivudine, stavudine, and tenofovir than people with normal kidney function. People with **liver disease** may require lower doses of abacavir, didanosine, efavirenz, and nevirapine.

People with **kidney or liver disease** should not use any fixed-dose combination antiviral product because the dosage of individual ingredients cannot be changed. Individual medicines must be used in this case. AZT should be used with caution by these patients.

Up to 50% of patients who take didanosine experience symptoms of nervous system inflammation and about 33% need to reduce their dosage to control these symptoms. Some symptoms are numbness, tingling, and pain in the hands and feet. People who already have signs of **nerve damage** should not take didanosine.

The HIV virus can become resistant to HIV antivirals. HIV strains that are resistant to emtricitabine can also be resistant to lamivudine, but often remain sensitive to many other antiviral drugs, including abacavir, delavirdine, didanosine, efavirenz, nevirapine, stavudine, tenofovir, and AZT. Resistance to abacavir has developed in laboratory versions of HIV also resistant to lamivudine and didanosine. HIV that is resistant to protease inhibitors is not likely to be resistant to abacavir.

People with both **HIV and hepatitis B** should not use emtricitabine due to a large increase in the risk of liver damage. These people should also use caution if discontinuing use of lamivudine; worsening of hepatitis B virus infection has been reported when lamivudine was stopped. Special monitoring and follow-up of anti-hepatitis B therapy may be necessary.

Efavirenz can raise blood cholesterol by 10–20%.

These drugs can rarely cause liver enlargement and lactic acidosis (a potentially fatal metabolic imbalance). People with a history of **alcohol abuse** or **hepatitis** should use these drugs with caution. This mainly occurs in **women** but **obesity** and long-term treatment may also be risk factors, however people with no known risk factors have also developed these problems. Symptoms of liver problems include yellow skin, dark urine, pale stool, lower abdominal pain, and loss of appetite. Symptoms of lactic acidosis include heart problems, bluish discoloration of the skin, cold hands or feet, rapid heartbeat, low blood pressure, dehydration, rapid or difficulty breathing, lethargy, stupor or coma, vomiting, and/or abdominal pain. Call your doctor immediately if you develop these or any other unusual symptoms.

Lamivudine and didanosine have rarely caused fatal inflammation of the pancreas. Symptoms include major changes in blood-sugar levels, increased triglyceride blood levels, a drop in blood calcium, nausea, vomiting, and abdominal pain. People who develop **pancreatic inflammation** must stop taking these drugs.

Trizivir is associated with liver toxicity. People with HIV who also have chronic **liver disease** due to **hepatitis B** infection are especially likely to be affected.

Trizivir and AZT may cause muscle irritation and abnormalities similar to those caused by HIV infection.

HIV antivirals can cause a significant reduction in bone mineral density, increasing the risk of bone fractures.

AZT has been associated with low white-blood-cell count and anemia.

People taking HIV antivirals may experience unusual fat accumulation or redistribution leading to buffalo hump, breast enlargement, abnormal thinness, or a round, moon-shaped face. The exact reasons for this are not known.

Possible Side Effects

Abacavir

Abacavir is always taken with other drugs, so the side effects listed here are those of the drugs in combination.

Adult

▼ Most common: nausea, headache, fatigue, vomiting, diarrhea, and appetite loss.
▼ Common: sleep disturbances.

Child

▼ Most common: nausea, vomiting, fever, headache, diarrhea, and rash.
▼ Common: appetite loss.

Delavirdine and Efavirenz

More than half of people who take these drugs experience some nervous system and psychiatric side effects and rash. About 2% have to stop treatment because of them. Children are more likely than adults to develop rash.

▼ Most common: nausea, dizziness, sleeplessness, headache, and temporary rash.
▼ Common: abnormal dreaming, poor concentration, tiredness, and diarrhea.
▼ Less common: itching, sweating, stomach pain or gas, upset stomach, reduced sensitivity to stimulation, depression, appetite loss, hallucinations, and nervousness.
▼ Rare: blisters, wet ulcers, peeling skin, blood in the urine, delusions, inappropriate behavior, and severe depression. Blood cholesterol can rise 10–20%. Other rare side effects can occur in almost any part of the body. Contact your doctor if you experience any side effect not listed above.

Didanosine

Adult

▼ Most common: diarrhea, nervous system inflammation, fever, chills, itching, rash, abdominal pain, weakness, headache, nausea, vomiting, infection, pneumonia, and pancreatic inflammation.
▼ Less common: tumors, muscle pain, appetite loss, dry mouth, convulsions, abnormal thought patterns, breathing difficulties, drug allergy, anxiety, nervousness, twitching,

Possible Side Effects (*continued*)

confusion, depression, and blood component abnormalities.

▼ Rare: Rare side effects can occur in almost any part of the body. Contact your doctor if you experience any side effect not listed above.

Child

Almost all children who take didanosine experience side effects. They are likely to experience many of the same reactions as adults, most commonly chills, fever, weakness, appetite loss, nausea and vomiting, diarrhea, liver dysfunction, headache, nervousness, sleeplessness, cough, runny nose, asthma or breathing difficulties, rash, and skin problems. Four children taking didanosine developed severe eye disease, resulting in some loss of sight. The progress of the eye disease slowed or stopped when dosage was reduced. Children taking this drug should have an eye examination every 6 months or if vision starts to worsen.

Emtricitabine

Because this drug is always taken with other antiviral drugs, the listed side effects are those of the drugs in combination. The risk of developing specific side effects can be different depending on the exact drug combination you are taking. The long-term effects of emtricitabine are not known.

▼ Most common: rash, itching, allergic reactions, cough, runny nose, nausea, weakness, diarrhea, abdominal pain, depression, and headache.

▼ Common: discoloration of the soles of the feet or palms of the hands, upset stomach, vomiting, joint or muscle pain, unusual dreams, dizziness, sleeplessness, and tingling or pain in the hands or feet.

▼ Rare: Rare side effects can occur in almost any part of the body. Contact your doctor if you experience any side effect not listed above.

Lamivudine

Because this drug is always taken with AZT, the listed side effects are those of the drugs in combination. The long-term effects of lamivudine are not known.

Possible Side Effects *(continued)*

▼ Most common: headache, not feeling well, fever, chills, rash, nausea, vomiting, diarrhea, appetite loss, abdominal pain or cramps, nervous system problems including tingling and poor coordination, sleeplessness, dizziness, depression, stuffy or runny nose, cough, and muscle pain.

▼ Common: upset stomach, joint pain, and tingling in the hands or feet in children. Lamivudine may affect the results of a variety of blood tests.

▼ Rare: pancreas irritation, more often seen in children than adults. Contact your doctor if you experience any side effect not listed above.

Nevirapine

▼ Most common: rash, fever, nausea, headache, hypersensitivity, and changes in liver function tests.

▼ Less common: abdominal pain, mouth or throat sores, tingling in the hands or feet, muscle aches, and liver inflammation.

▼ Rare: diarrhea, pain, and changes of sensation in the arms or legs. Contact your doctor if you experience any side effect not listed above.

Stavudine and Etravirine

Most common side effects apply to both stavudine and etravirine. Common and less common side effects apply to stavudine only.

▼ Most common: peripheral neuropathy, which can produce tingling, burning, numbness, or pain in the hands, arms, feet, or legs; diarrhea; nausea; vomiting; headache; fever; chills; weakness; abdominal pain; back pain; muscle or joint ache; generalized pain; not feeling well; sleeplessness; anxiety; depression; nervousness; breathing difficulties; appetite and weight loss; rash; itching; and sweating.

▼ Common: allergic reactions; flu-like symptoms; swollen lymph glands, usually felt under the arms or in the neck; chest pain; constipation; upset stomach; and dizziness.

▼ Less common: pelvic pain, tumors, hypertension (high blood pressure), swelling, flushing, stomach ulcers, confusion, migraine headache, sleepiness, tremors, nerve pain, asthma, pneumonia, skin tumors, conjunctivitis (pinkeye),

Possible Side Effects (*continued*)

visual disturbances, painful urination, genital pain, painful menstruation, and vaginitis.

▼ Rare: frequent urination, blood in the urine, impotence, fainting, paralysis, inflammation of the pancreas, nerve pain, and peeling skin. Contact your doctor if you experience any side effect not listed above.

Tenofovir
▼ Most common: nausea, diarrhea, weakness, and headache.

▼ Common: vomiting, stomach gas, abdominal pain, and loss of appetite.

Trizivir
▼ Most common: anemia, reduced white-blood-cell counts, chills, rash, nausea, vomiting, diarrhea, appetite loss, abdominal pain or cramps, nervous system problems, including tingling and poor coordination, sleeplessness, dizziness, depression, stuffy or runny nose, cough, muscle pain, fever, headache, feeling or being sick, and weakness.

▼ Common: sensitivity reaction (fever, skin rash, fatigue, and gastrointestinal symptoms, such as nausea, vomiting, diarrhea or abdominal pain, and respiratory symptoms such as sore throat, difficulty breathing, or cough), upset stomach, joint pain, tingling in the hands or feet, and sleep disturbances. Trizivir may affect the results of a variety of blood tests.

▼ Less common: blood infection, nervousness, and irritability.

▼ Rare: pancreas irritation, weight loss, seizures, heart failure and other cardiac abnormalities, blood in the urine, and bladder infections. Contact your doctor if you experience any side effect not listed above.

Zidovudine
Adult
▼ Most common: anemia, reduced white-blood-cell counts, headache, fatigue, loss of appetite, vomiting, nausea, sleeplessness, and muscle aches.

▼ Less common: Less common side effects can occur in almost any part of the body. Contact your doctor if you experience any side effect not listed above.

Possible Side Effects (continued)

Child

▼ Most common: anemia, reduced white-blood-cell counts, vomiting, abdominal pain, fever, cough, liver enlargement, skin rash, diarrhea, nausea, and sleeplessness.

▼ Less common: headache, blood infection, nervousness, and irritability.

▼ Rare: weight loss, seizures, heart failure and other cardiac abnormalities, blood in the urine, and bladder infections. Contact your doctor if you experience any side effect not listed above.

Drug Interactions

Abacavir

- Alcohol interferes with the elimination of abacavir through the liver and can lead to a 40% increase in the amount of drug in the blood.

- Abacavir can increase blood levels of acetaminophen, amitriptyline, bumetanide, chloral hydrate, chlorpheniramine, chlorpromazine, chlorzoxazone, doxepin, fluconazole, imipramine, ketoconazole, labetalol, lamotrigine, miconazole, morphine, naloxone, nonsteroidal anti-inflammatory drugs (NSAIDs), oxazepam, promethazine, propofol, propranolol, and valproic acid.

- Cigarette smoking and clofibrate may reduce the amount of abacavir in the blood.

- Combining abacavir with isoniazid may decrease abacavir levels and increase isoniazid levels in the blood.

- Abacavir levels in the blood may be decreased if you are also taking phenobarbital, phenytoin, or T3 thyroid hormone replacement.

- Abacavir may increase the speed with which methadone is cleared from the body. Changes in methadone dose are usually not required.

Delavirdine, Efavirenz, and Etravirine

- Combining delavirdine, efavirenz, or etravirine with astemizole; midazolam, triazolam, or other benzodiazepine drugs; or ergot-containing products can lead to life-threatening abnormal heart rhythms, excessive sedation, or severe breathing difficulties. Do not combine these drugs.

- Delavirdine, efavirenz, or etravirine increase the nervous system effects of alcohol, sedatives, antidepressants, and other psychoactive drugs.
- Combining delavirdine, efavirenz, or etravirine with ritonavir increases blood levels of both drugs. This interaction increases the effectiveness of anti-HIV therapy as well as the risk of side effects.
- Delavirdine, efavirenz, or etravirine reduce indinavir and amprenavir blood levels. Your indinavir or amprenavir dosage may need to be increased.
- Delavirdine, efavirenz, or etravirine significantly reduce saquinavir blood levels.
- The antifungal drugs ketoconazole, itraconazole, and voriconazole increase the amount of delavirdine, efavirenz, or etravirine in the blood by about 50% while the concentration of the antifungals is significantly reduced. These drugs should not be mixed.
- Combining delavirdine, efavirenz, or etravirine with clarithromycin, ethinyl estradiol, nelfinavir, or rifampin can alter blood levels of either drug. The importance of these interactions is unclear and dosage adjustments are unnecessary.
- Anticonvulsants and rifabutin decrease blood levels of delavirdine, efavirenz, or etravirine. Dosage adjustments may be necessary.
- Nevirapine decreases blood levels of delavirdine, efavirenz, or etravirine.
- Antacids and didanosine may reduce the amount of delavirdine, efavirenz, or etravirine in the blood by interfering with its absorption; take these drugs and delavirdine, efavirenz, or etravirine at least 1 hour apart.
- Delavirdine, efavirenz, or etravirine decrease blood levels of methadone.
- Combining delavirdine, efavirenz, or etravirine and warfarin may increase the risk of excessive bleeding.
- The effect of delavirdine, efavirenz, or etravirine on contraceptive drugs is not known. People combining these drugs should use an additional contraceptive method.
- Delavirdine, efavirenz, or etravirine should not be combined with St. John's wort.

Didanosine

- Other drugs that may cause inflammation of the nervous system such as chloramphenicol, cisplatin, disulfiram, ethionamide, glutethimide, gold, hydralazine, isoniazid, metronidazole, nitro-furantoin, ribavirin, and vincristine should be avoided while you are taking didanosine.

- Use extreme caution when combining didanosine with stavu-dine in pregnant women, as fatal lactic acidosis has been re-ported with this combination.
- Drugs that may cause inflammation of the pancreas, including intravenous pentamidine, should not be taken with didanosine.
- The use of allopurinol with didanosine is not recommended because it raises didanosine blood levels.
- Quinolone anti-infectives, tetracycline antibiotics, and other drugs whose absorption into the bloodstream may be af-fected by antacids should not be taken within 2 hours of tak-ing didanosine because of its high magnesium and aluminum content.

Emtricitabine

- Do not mix emtricitabine or an emtricitabine combination with lamivudine or any combination drug containing lamivudine.

Lamivudine

- Lamivudine increases maximum blood levels of AZT by 39%, which is helpful in fighting the HIV virus.
- Trimethoprim-sulfamethoxazole, taken for opportunistic AIDS-related infections, increases the amount of lamivudine in the blood.

Nelfinavir

- Anticonvulsant medication such as carbamazepine, pheny-toin, or phenobarbital may reduce the amount of nelfinavir in the blood.
- Nelfinavir interferes with the liver's ability to break down tri-azolam, midazolam, statin drugs (except pravastatin and sim-vastatin), ergot derivatives, amiodarone, and quinidine. Do not combine nelfinavir with any of these drugs as severe side effects may result.
- Combining nelfinavir with indinavir or saquinavir, other pro-tease inhibitors, results in large increases in the amounts of both drugs in the blood. Other drugs that increase the amount of nelfinavir in the blood are ketoconazole and ritonavir.
- Combining rifabutin with nelfinavir lowers the amount of nel-finavir in the blood and raises the amount of rifabutin. Ri-fabutin dosage should be cut in half when this combination is used.

- Do not combine rifampin or pimozide and nelfinavir. Combine nelfinavir and sildenafil or vardenafil with extreme caution.
- Nelfinavir reduces the amount of contraceptive hormones in your bloodstream (see "Special Information").
- If you combine nelfinavir, lamivudine, and zidovudine (an HIV drug—also known as AZT), your AZT dosage may have to be increased.
- St. John's wort may decrease the effectiveness of nelfinavir. Avoid this combination.

Nevirapine

- Rifampin and rifabutin may stimulate liver enzymes that break down nevirapine, reducing the amount of nevirapine in the blood. Neither of these drugs should be combined with nevirapine.
- Nevirapine may reduce the effectiveness of ketoconazole. Ketoconazole should not be combined with nevirapine.
- The enzyme systems that break down protease inhibitors are stimulated by nevirapine. Combining nevirapine and a protease inhibitor may reduce the amount of protease inhibitor in the blood, reducing its effectiveness and increasing the risk of protease inhibitor resistance.
- Combining nevirapine with a contraceptive drug may reduce the effectiveness of the contraceptive by lowering the amount of hormone in the blood.
- Nevirapine may interact with many medications, both prescription and over-the-counter, including herbal products such as St. John's wort.

Stavudine

- Combining stavudine with didanosine or hydroxyurea may increase the risk of lactic acidosis, peripheral neuropathy, inflamed pancreas, or liver toxicity.
- Methadone and AZT may reduce blood levels of stavudine by more than 25%.
- Doxorubicin and ribavirin may affect stavudine; use with caution.

Tenofovir

- Tenofovir may reduce the breakdown of acetaminophen, amitriptyline, caffeine, clomipramine, clozapine, cyclobenzaprine, estradiol, fluvoxamine, haloperidol, imipramine, mexiletine, naproxen, propranolol, riluzole, ropivacaine, tacrine, theophylline, verapamil, warfarin, zileuton, and zolmitriptan, modestly increasing the amount of these drugs in the blood.

- Tenofovir increases blood levels of didanosine, which increases the risk of side effects. People taking both of these drugs must take tenofovir either 2 hours before or 1 hour after taking didanosine.
- Tenofovir decreases the amount of ritonavir and lopinavir (with higher tenofovir doses) absorbed into the bloodstream.
- At higher tenofovir doses, the blood concentration of lamivudine may be reduced.
- The effect of tenofovir on contraceptive drugs is not known, but it can increase the amount of estradiol (a contraceptive hormone) in the blood. People combining these drugs should use an additional contraceptive method.
- Tenofovir may decrease blood levels of atazanavir.

Trizivir

- Trizivir slows the elimination of alcohol from the body and can lead to a large increase of alcohol in the blood.
- Interferon beta-1b, methadone, aspirin, indomethacin, probenecid, trimethoprim/sulfamethoxazole (an anti-infective combination), trimethoprim, and valproic acid increase the amount of Trizivir in the blood and the risk of Trizivir side effects.
- Cigarette smoking, clofibrate, phenobarbital, liothyronine, isoniazid, acetaminophen, and rifampin may reduce the amount of Trizivir in the blood.
- Trizivir should not be used with stavudine, doxorubicin, or ribavirin because the 2 drugs may antagonize each other.
- Mixing Trizivir with anti-cancer drugs or drugs that suppress the immune system increases the risk of blood toxicity.
- Mixing clarithromycin or fluconazole with Trizivir can increase the amount of Trizivir in the blood, but the importance of this interaction is not known.
- Atovaquone increases the amount of Trizivir in the blood by interfering with its breakdown in the liver. Trizivir dosage reduction may be necessary.
- Combining Trizivir with other drugs that can damage your kidneys, including pentamidine, amphotericin B, flucytosine, vincristine, vinblastine, adriamycin, and alpha- and beta-interferon, increases the risk of loss of some kidney function.
- Trizivir can increase blood levels of acetaminophen, amitriptyline, bumetanide, chloral hydrate, chlorpheniramine, chlorpromazine, chlorzoxazone, doxepin, fluconazole, imipramine,

ketoconazole, labetalol, lamotrigine, miconazole, morphine, naloxone, nonsteroidal anti-inflammatory drugs (NSAIDs), oxazepam, promethazine, propofol, and propranolol.

- Combining Trizivir and isoniazid may increase isoniazid levels in the blood.
- Acyclovir is used in combination with Trizivir to combat opportunistic infections in AIDS patients; however, this combination may cause severe drowsiness or lethargy.
- Other drugs that can cause anemia, including alpha-interferon and ganciclovir, should be used carefully in combination with Trizivir because of the risk of worsening drug-related anemia.
- Taking phenytoin and Trizivir together may affect the amounts of both drugs in the blood, usually increasing the amount of Trizivir. The effect on phenytoin blood levels varies. This combination can result in either too much phenytoin (leading to increased phenytoin side effects) or too little phenytoin (leading to a possible increase in the number of seizures). Your doctor should check your phenytoin levels if you are also taking Trizivir.

Zidovudine

- Combining AZT with other drugs that can damage your kidneys, such as pentamidine, amphotericin B, flucytosine, vincristine, vinblastine, adriamycin, alpha- and beta-interferon increases the risk of loss of some kidney function.
- Avoid using AZT with stavudine, ribavirin, and doxorubicin.
- Probenecid may reduce the rate at which your body eliminates AZT, increasing the amount of the drug in your blood and the risk for side effects. Other drugs that can reduce the liver's ability to break down AZT are acetaminophen, aspirin, indomethacin, and trimethoprim; combining any of these drugs with AZT may lead to increased side effects.
- Acyclovir is often used in combination with AZT to combat opportunistic infections in AIDS patients; however, this combination may cause lethargy or seizures.
- Other drugs that can cause anemia, including ganciclovir, should be used carefully in combination with AZT because of the risk of worsening drug-related anemia.
- Taking AZT together with rifampin may reduce the amount of AZT absorbed into the blood.
- Taking phenytoin and AZT together may affect the amounts of both drugs in the blood, usually increasing the amount of

AZT. The effect on phenytoin blood levels varies. This combination can result in either too much phenytoin (leading to phenytoin side effects) or too little phenytoin (leading to a possible increase in the number of seizures). Your doctor should check your phenytoin levels if you are also taking AZT.

- Atovaquone, fluconazole, methadone, probenecid, trimethoprim, and valproic acid may increase blood levels of AZT.

Food Interactions

Most of these drugs may be taken with or without food.

Food may prevent the absorption of a dose of didanosine by up to 50%. Take didanosine either 30 minutes before or 2 hours after eating. Efavirenz may be taken with or without food, but do not take efavirenz with a high-fat meal because it will increase the amount of efavirenz absorbed by about 50%, raising the risk of adverse effects. Symptoms may be more severe if taken with alcohol. Lamivudine is absorbed more slowly when taken with food, but not enough to affect the total amount of drug that reaches the blood.

Usual Dose

Abacavir

Adult (age 17 and over): 300 mg twice a day. For mild hepatic impairment—200 mg twice a day. Oral solution—15 mL twice a day.

Child (age 3 months–16 years): 3.6 mg per lb. of body weight twice a day, up to a maximum of 300 mg in each dose.

Child (under 3 months): not recommended.

Atripla

Adult (age 18 and over): 1 tablet a day on an empty stomach. Taking the combination at bedtime may make it easier to tolerate.

Child (under age 18): not recommended.

Combivir

Adult and Child (age 12 and over): 1 tablet—lamivudine 150 mg plus zidovudine 300 mg—twice a day. Poor kidney or liver function requires reducing the dosage of both drugs. In this situation, it is preferable to take the individual drugs separately so that you retain maximum dosage flexibility.

Child (under age 12): not recommended.

Delavirdine

Adult: 400 mg three times a day.

Didanosine
Adult: 250–400 mg a day (tablets); 167–250 mg every 12 hours (powder).

Child: 50–250 mg a day, based on weight and height.

Efavirenz
Adult: 600 mg once a day, preferably at bedtime at first.

Child (88 lbs. and over): 600 mg a day.

Child (71.5–87 lbs.): 400 mg a day.

Child (55–71.5 lbs.): 350 mg a day.

Child (44–54 lbs.): 300 mg a day.

Child (33–43 lbs.): 250 mg a day.

Child (22–32 lbs.): 200 mg a day.

Child (under age 3 or less than 22 lbs.): not recommended.

Emtricitabine
Capsules
Adult (age 18 and over): 200 mg once a day. People with reduced kidney function may take as little as 200 mg once every 4 days. Dialysis patients take 1 dose after dialysis is complete.

Child (over 68 lbs): 200 mg once a day.

Oral Solution
Adult: 240 mg (24 mL) once a day.

Child: 2.7 mg per lb. of child's body weight up to 240 mg a day.

Epzicom
Adult: 1 tablet—lamivudine 300 mg plus abacavir 600 mg—once a day.

Child (under age 18): not recommended.

Etravirine
Adult: 100 mg twice a day with food.

Child: not recommended.

Lamivudine
Adult and Child (age 16 and over): 150 mg twice a day combined with other antiretroviral agents. Adults who weigh less than 110 lbs. should receive about 1 mg per lb. of body weight twice a day. Dosage is reduced as kidney function decreases. For hepatitis B, take 100 mg once a day.

Child (age 3 months to 16 years): about 1.4–2 mg per lb. of body weight twice a day, no more than 150 mg per dose.

Child (under 3 months): not recommended.

Nevirapine

Adult: starting dose—200 mg a day for 2 weeks. Maintenance dose—200 mg twice a day in combination with a nucleoside type antiviral such as didanosine or AZT.

Child (age 2 months–8 years): starting dose—about 2 mg per lb. of body weight a day for 2 weeks. Maintenance dose—3 mg per lb. of body weight twice a day. The total daily dose should not exceed 400 mg.

Child (under 2 months): not recommended.

Stavudine

Immediate-release

Adult and Child (66 lbs. and over): 30–40 mg every 12 hours. Dosage reduction may be needed in seniors.

Child (under 66 lbs): 0.5 mg per lb. every 12 hours.

Extended-release

Adult: 75–100 mg once a day.

Child: not recommended.

Tenofovir

Adult (age 18 and over): 300 mg once a day. If you are taking tenofovir and didanosine, take your tenofovir 2 hours before or 1 hour after taking didanosine.

Child: not recommended.

Trizivir

Adult (88 lbs. and over): 1 tablet twice a day.

Adult (less than 88 lbs.): not recommended.

Child (age 13 and over, and 88 lbs. and over): 1 tablet twice a day.

Child (age 13 and over, but under 88 lbs.): not recommended.

Child (under age 13): not recommended.

Truvada

Adult: 1 tablet a day. People with mild kidney disease should take 1 tablet every other day.

Child: not recommended.

Zidovudine

Adult: symptomatic AIDS—100 mg every 4 hours around the clock, even if sleep must be interrupted. Dosage may be reduced if side effects develop. Asymptomatic AIDS—100 mg every 4 hours during waking hours.

Pregnancy: AZT is used to prevent transmission of HIV infection to the fetus. After 14 weeks of pregnancy—100 mg 5 times a day until labor starts. During labor and delivery—intravenously, until the umbilical cord is clamped.

Child (age 3 months–12 years): up to 100 mg every 6 hours.

Child (under age 3 months): about 1 mg per lb. of body weight every 6 hours by mouth, starting within 12 hours of birth and continuing through 6 weeks of age. The drug may be given intravenously if necessary.

Overdosage

Little is known about the effects of abacavir, emtricitabine, lamivudine, nelfinavir, nevirapine, and tenofovir overdose. Didanosine overdose will cause many of the drug's usual side effects, especially inflammation of the nervous system or pancreas, diarrhea, and liver failure. Efavirenz overdose may include dizziness, nausea, loss of concentration, and other nervous system effects. Chronic stavudine overdose can produce peripheral neuropathy (see "Special Information") and liver toxicity. The most serious effect of AZT overdose is suppression of the bone marrow and its ability to make red and white blood cells.

Call your local poison control center or a hospital emergency room for more information. Victims of an overdose of any combination HIV antiviral product should be taken to a hospital emergency room for treatment. ALWAYS bring the prescription bottle or container.

Special Information

These drugs are not a cure for HIV. They will not prevent you from transmitting the HIV virus to another person; you must still practice safe sex. People taking these drugs may still develop opportunistic infections and other complications associated with HIV infection. It is very important to take these drugs exactly as prescribed. Remember, every dose of HIV medication you forget or skip can make it more difficult for the drugs to do their job and can also lead to the development of HIV resistance.

People with HIV infection must take especially good care of their teeth and gums to minimize the risk of developing oral infections.

Abacavir

Stop taking this drug and call your doctor at the first sign of allergy or sensitivity. Symptoms include fever, rash, fatigue, nausea, vomiting, diarrhea, abdominal pain, sore throat, difficulty breathing, and coughing. Some patients who experienced a hypersensitivity reaction were thought to have a respiratory infection at first. If you continue to take abacavir and are allergic to it, more severe reactions including a life-threatening drop in blood pressure could develop within hours. Report anything unusual to your doctor.

If you forget to take a dose and remember within 2–3 hours, take the medication. If you forget until it is almost time for your next dose, skip the forgotten dose and continue with your regular schedule.

Delavirdine

Delavirdine solution is somewhat better absorbed than the tablets. The amount of drug absorbed from delavirdine tablets can be increased by allowing the 100 mg tablet to disintegrate in water and then swallowing the mixture. 200 mg tablets do not dissolve in water.

Didanosine

If you are taking didanosine chewable tablets, be sure to thoroughly chew each tablet. You may also completely dissolve them in about ¼ cup of water and drink the entire mixture immediately. Do not mix didanosine tablets with juice or any other acidic drink. If you are using the powdered form of didanosine, make a solution by pouring the entire contents of a packet into ½ cup of water. Stir until dissolved and drink immediately. Do not mix didanosine powder with juice or any other acidic drink. For children, your pharmacist will prepare a mixture of 10 mg per ml of didanosine and an equal amount of Mylanta Double Strength Antacid or Maalox TC Antacid. This mixture must be stored in a refrigerator and can be kept for 30 days. Shake well before using.

Spilled didanosine should be cleaned immediately to prevent accidental poisoning.

If you forget to take a dose of didanosine, take it as soon as you remember. If it is almost time for your next dose, allow 4–8 hours to pass between the dose you took late and your next dose, and then continue with your regular schedule. Call your doctor for more specific advice if you forget to take several doses.

Efavirenz

People with achlorhydria (absence of stomach acid) should take efavirenz with an acidic drink, such as orange or cranberry juice. About half of people taking efavirenz develop dizziness, loss of concentration, depression, delusions, or drowsiness. Call your doctor if this occurs or if strange behavior develops. Do not combine efavirenz with alcohol, sedatives, or other psychoactive drugs. Be careful when driving or performing any task that requires concentration. Take your medication at bedtime to better tolerate the depressant effects of efavirenz. If you forget a dose, take it as soon as you remember. Contact your doctor if you forget your medication for 1 day.

Emtricitabine

If you forget a dose, take it as soon as you remember. If it is almost time for your next dose, skip the dose you forgot and continue with your regular schedule. Call your doctor if you forget 2 or more doses in a row. Call your doctor immediately if your child develops signs of pancreas inflammation while taking emtricitabine. Symptoms include severe abdominal pain, tense abdominal muscles, sweating, feeling very ill, shallow and rapid breathing, fever, and possible fainting.

Lamivudine

Call your doctor at once if your child develops signs of pancreas inflammation while taking lamivudine. Symptoms include very severe abdominal pain, tense abdominal muscles, sweating, feeling very ill, shallow and rapid breathing, fever, and possible fainting.

If you forget a dose, take it as soon as you remember. If it is almost time for your next dose, skip the dose you forgot and continue with your regular schedule. Call your doctor if you forget 2 or more doses in a row.

Nevirapine

Call your doctor at once if you develop any rash or other skin side effect.

If you forget a dose of nevirapine, take it as soon as you remember. If it is almost time for your next dose, skip the dose you forgot and continue with your regular schedule. If you forget to take nevirapine for a week, you will have to start the treatment program all over again, beginning with 200 mg a day for 2 weeks.

Stavudine

Peripheral neuropathy (symptoms include tingling, pain, or numbness in the hands, arms, legs, or feet) occurs in 15–20% of people who take stavudine. If the drug is stopped, symptoms may disappear, although they can actually worsen for a time after you stop taking stavudine. If the symptoms do go away, your doctor may restart stavudine treatment at a lower daily dosage.

Your stavudine dosage will be reduced if you develop symptoms of neuropathy or if you have reduced kidney function.

Tell your doctor immediately if you have symptoms of extreme weakness, nausea, difficulty breathing, or weight loss.

If you forget a dose of stavudine, take it as soon as you remember. If it is almost time for your next dose, take the dose you forgot, take the next 2 doses 8 hours apart, and then go back to your regular schedule. Do not take a double dose. Call your doctor if you skip more than 2 consecutive doses.

Tenofovir

If you forget a dose of tenofovir, take it as soon as you remember. If it almost time for your next dose, skip the dose you forgot and continue with your regular schedule. Do not take a double dose. Skipping doses of this drug increases the risk that your HIV will become resistant to its effects.

Trizivir

Stop taking Trizivir and call your doctor at the first sign of allergy or drug sensitivity (fever, rash, fatigue, nausea, vomiting, diarrhea, or abdominal pain). See your doctor if any significant change in your health occurs. Periodic blood counts are very important while taking Trizivir to detect possibly serious side effects.

If you miss a dose of Trizivir, take it as soon as possible. If it is almost time for your next dose, skip the dose you forgot and continue with your regular schedule. Call your doctor if you forget 2 or more doses in a row. Do not take more Trizivir than your doctor prescribed.

Zidovudine (AZT)

If you miss a dose of AZT, take it as soon as possible. If it is almost time for your next dose, allow 2–4 hours to pass between the dose you took late and your next dose, and then continue with your regular schedule. Do not take a double dose.

Protect AZT capsules and liquid from light.

Special Populations

Pregnancy/Breast-feeding: When any of these drugs are considered necessary for you by your doctor, their potential benefits must be carefully weighed against their risks. Most of these drugs pass into breast milk. It is recommended that all nursing mothers who must take any HIV antiviral medicines use infant formula to avoid transmitting the virus to their child.

Abacavir
Abacavir passes into the fetal circulation. In animal studies, it caused low birth weight and increased the risk of stillbirth. The effect of abacavir in pregnant women is not known.

Didanosine
Didanosine was slightly toxic to pregnant animals receiving doses 12 times human levels. There are no studies of pregnant women taking this drug; however, women who are or might become pregnant should only take didanosine if absolutely necessary and should use effective contraception to avoid passing on the virus.

Efavirenz
This drug may cause birth defects if taken during the first 3 months of pregnancy. Women taking this medicine and its combinations should avoid becoming pregnant and should be tested to ensure they are not pregnant before starting treatment. Birth defects are much less likely if it is taken in the final 6 months of pregnancy. Your doctor may consider efavirenz if you are pregnant and have no other treatment options, but you should discuss the risks and benefits of treatment with him or her.

Emtricitabine
Emtricitabine enters the fetal circulation. A national registry has been established to gather information on pregnant women who must use this drug.

Lamivudine
Lamivudine passes into the blood circulation of the fetus. Some animal studies of lamivudine indicate that it may be dangerous to the fetus, but others showed no effect. There is no information about the effect of lamivudine in pregnant women.

Nevirapine
Studies of nevirapine in pregnant have shown a significant decrease in fetal body weight.

Stavudine
Animal studies show that stavudine passes to the fetus and causes birth defects, but there is no direct information on what happens in humans.

Tenofovir
Animal studies of tenofovir using up to 19 times the human dose have revealed no birth defects. There are no studies in pregnant women.

Trizivir
Animal studies of all 3 ingredients of Trizivir harmed developing fetuses. Notify your doctor at once if you do become pregnant.

Zidovudine (AZT)
If you are HIV-positive and pregnant, talk to your doctor about taking or continuing this drug. AZT treatment in HIV-positive women who are pregnant has been shown to sharply reduce the risk of transmitting the HIV virus to babies. Treatment should begin by the 14th week of pregnancy and continue through delivery. The baby should also be given AZT for the first 6 weeks of life. Studies have shown that the risk of birth defects is not increased by taking AZT during pregnancy.

Seniors: Seniors may require lower doses of these drugs because of reduced liver, kidney, or cardiac function.

Humalog   see *Insulin,* page 585

Generic Name

Hydralazine (hye-DRAL-uh-zene) Ⓖ

Brand Name
Apresoline

Type of Drug
Antihypertensive.

Prescribed for
High blood pressure, aortic insufficiency after heart valve replacement, and congestive heart failure (CHF).

General Information
Although its mechanism of action is not completely understood, hydralazine hydrochloride is believed to lower blood pressure by relaxing vascular smooth muscles throughout the body. This also helps to improve heart function and blood flow to the kidneys and brain.

Cautions and Warnings
Do not use hydralazine if you are **allergic** or **sensitive** to any of its ingredients.

Long-term administration of more than 200 mg a day of hydralazine may produce the symptoms of lupus erythematosus (a chronic condition affecting the body's connective tissue), including muscle and joint pain, skin reactions, fever, kidney inflammation, and anemia, although they usually disappear when the drug is discontinued. Report any fever, chest pain, feelings of ill health, or other unexplained symptoms to your doctor. The risk of developing lupus increases with higher dosages; approximately 5% of people taking 100 mg a day and 10% of people taking 200 mg a day of hydralazine develop lupus.

Hydralazine may actually improve kidney blood flow and kidney function in people who have below-normal function. It should be used with caution in people with advanced **kidney damage**.

Hydralazine may worsen heart problems and should be used with care in people with a history of **heart disease**. It can cause angina pain and may cause heart attacks. This medication should also be used with caution in people with **pulmonary hypertension**.

Tingling in the hands or feet caused by hydralazine may be relieved by taking pyridoxine (vitamin B_6).

People taking hydralazine may develop reduced hemoglobin and red-blood-cell counts. Reduced white-blood-cell and platelet counts may also occur. Periodic blood counts are recommended while taking hydralazine.

Possible Side Effects

▼ Most common: headache, appetite loss, nausea, vomiting, diarrhea, rapid heartbeat, and chest pain.

▼ Less common: stuffy nose; flushing; tearing, itching, or redness of the eyes; numbness or tingling in the hands or feet; dizziness; tremors; muscle cramps; depression; disorientation; anxiety; itching; rash; fever; chills; occasional hepatitis (symptoms include yellowing of the skin or whites of the eyes); constipation; urinary difficulties; and adverse effects on normal blood composition.

Drug Interactions

- Taking hydralazine with the beta blockers metoprolol or propranolol may result in increased blood levels of both hydralazine and the beta blocker.
- Indomethacin may reduce the effects of hydralazine.

- Do not use over-the-counter cough, cold, or allergy medications, or appetite suppressants. These products often contain stimulant ingredients that can increase blood pressure.

Food Interactions

Take hydralazine with food.

Usual Dose

Adult: 10 mg 4 times day for the first 2–4 days, increased to 25 mg 4 times a day for the rest of the first week. Dosage is then increased until the maximum effect is seen.

Child: 0.34 mg per lb. of body weight a day divided in 4 doses; increased up to 200 mg a day.

Overdosage

Symptoms include extreme lowering of blood pressure, rapid heartbeat, headache, flushing, chest pain, and abnormal heart rhythms. If you experience any of these symptoms, contact your doctor immediately. If you go to a hospital emergency room, ALWAYS bring the prescription bottle or container.

Special Information

Take hydralazine exactly as prescribed.

Call your doctor if you experience prolonged and unexplained tiredness, fever, muscle or joint aches, or chest pain while taking this drug.

If you forget a dose, take it as soon as you remember. If it is almost time for your next dose, skip the one you forgot and continue with your regular schedule. Do not take a double dose.

Special Populations

Pregnancy/Breast-feeding: High doses of hydralazine caused birth defects in animal studies, and temporary blood-related problems have been seen in newborns whose mothers took hydralazine during pregnancy. Women who are or might be pregnant should not take hydralazine unless its possible benefits have been carefully weighed against its risks.

Hydralazine passes into breast milk. Nursing mothers who must take this drug should consider using infant formula.

Seniors: Seniors are more sensitive to the blood-pressure-lowering effects of hydralazine and its side effects, especially low body temperature.

Generic Name

Hydroxyzine (hye-DROK-suh-zene) G

Brand Names

Atarax   Vistaril

Type of Drug

Antihistamine and antianxiety agent.

Prescribed For

Nausea, vomiting, anxiety, tension, agitation, itching caused by allergy, and sedation.

General Information

Hydroxyzine is an antihistamine with antianxiety, muscle-relaxing, antiemetic (antivomiting), bronchial-dilating, pain-relieving, and antispasmodic properties. Hydroxyzine has been used to treat a variety of problems including stress related to dental or other minor surgical procedures, acute emotional problems, anxiety associated with heart disease, skin problems, and behavioral difficulties in children.

Cautions and Warnings

Hydroxyzine should not be used if you are **allergic** or **sensitive** to any of its ingredients, or to cetirizene.

Changes in heart rhythm have occurred in people taking this drug to relieve anxiety.

Hydroxyzine may worsen **porphyria,** a rare condition. People with this condition should not take hydroxyzine.

Because hydroxyzine controls nausea and vomiting, it may hide the symptoms of **appendicitis** or **overdoses** of other drugs.

Possible Side Effects

Wheezing, chest tightness, and breathing difficulties are signs of a drug-sensitivity reaction.

▼ Most common: dry mouth and drowsiness. These usually disappear after a few days of continuous use or when the dose is reduced.

▼ Rare: occasional tremors or convulsions at higher doses. Contact your doctor if you experience any side effect not listed above.

Drug Interactions

- This drug should not be taken with a monamine oxidase inhibitor antidepressant.
- Hydroxyzine depresses the nervous system, producing drowsiness and sleepiness. Do not take this drug with alcohol, sedatives, or other antihistamines or central nervous system (CNS) depressants. When hydroxyzine is taken with one of these drugs, the dose of the latter should be cut in half.

Food Interactions

Take hydroxyzine with food if it upsets your stomach.

Usual Dose

Adult: 25–100 mg 3–4 times a day for anxiety and allergic reactions; 50–100 mg for sedation.

Child (age 6 and over): 50–100 mg 3–4 times a day for anxiety and allergic reactions; 0.27 mg per lb. of body weight for sedation.

Child (under age 6): 50 mg 3–4 times a day for anxiety and allergic reactions; 0.27 mg per lb. of body weight for sedation.

Overdosage

The most common sign of overdose is sleepiness. Overdose victims should be taken to a hospital emergency room for treatment. ALWAYS bring the prescription bottle or container.

Special Information

Hydroxyzine may cause drowsiness: Be careful when driving, operating hazardous machinery, or doing anything that requires concentration.

The dry mouth associated with taking hydroxyzine may increase your risk of dental cavities and decay. Pay attention to dental hygiene while taking this drug.

Call your doctor if you develop a drug-sensitivity reaction to hydroxyzine (symptoms include wheezing, chest tightness, and breathing difficulties).

If you forget a dose of hydroxyzine, take it as soon as you remember. If it is almost time for your next dose, skip the one you forgot and continue with your regular schedule. Do not take a double dose.

Special Populations

Pregnancy/Breast-feeding: Animal studies have shown that regular treatment with hydroxyzine during the first few months of pregnancy may cause birth defects. Do not take this drug without your doctor's knowledge if you are or might be pregnant.

Hydroxyzine may reduce the amount of breast milk you produce and may pass into breast milk. Nursing mothers who must take hydroxyzine should use infant formula.

Seniors: Seniors are more sensitive to side effects and may require lower dosages.

Hyzaar   *see Angiotensin II Blockers, page 80*

Generic Name

Iloprost (EYE-low-prahst)

Brand Name
Ventavis

Type of Drug
Synthetic prostacyclin.

Prescribed For
Pulmonary hypertension.

General Information
Pulmonary hypertension occurs when blood pressure rises in the arteries that supply blood to the lungs. This condition can develop by itself, but it also occurs among children with congenital heart problems, people with heart valve damage, and people with heart failure. People with pulmonary hypertension tend to become dizzy and tired, and easily lose their breath. Exercise becomes very difficult as the condition worsens. Iloprost improves the symptoms of pulmonary hypertension by dilating (opening) blood vessels in the lungs and throughout the body. It also affects the normal function of blood platelets in the clotting process. In clinical studies, many people taking iloprost were able to maintain their condition at an acceptable level while using the medicine.

Cautions and Warnings

Do not take iloprost if you are **allergic** or **sensitive** to any of its ingredients.

People with moderate to severe **liver disease** should be cautious about using this drug because it is eliminated from the body through the liver.

The effects of **dialysis** on iloprost are not known.

Dizziness or fainting may occur when you first start taking this medicine. Your doctor should monitor your blood pressure, heart rate, and breathing when you start using this medicine.

Do not swallow this medicine or allow it to get into your eyes.

This medicine has not been studied in people with **chronic obstructive pulmonary disease, severe asthma,** or **active lung infections**.

If signs of pulmonary edema occur (difficulty breathing, wheezing, cough, feeling of "drowning," or gurgling or grunting sounds with breathing) stop treatment immediately.

Possible Side Effects

▼ Most common: flushing, coughing, headache, nausea, and low blood pressure.
▼ Common: lock jaw, sleeplessness, vomiting, flu-like symptoms, back pain, heart palpitations, dizziness or fainting when rising from a lying or sitting position, muscle cramps, vomiting blood, and increased liver enzymes and other abnormal lab tests.
▼ Less common: tongue pain and pneumonia.
▼ Rare: Rare side effects can include congestive heart failure, chest pain discomfort or tightness, rapid heartbeat, difficulty breathing, swelling in the arms or legs, and kidney failure. Contact your doctor if you experience any side effect not listed above.

Drug Interactions

● Iloprost may increase the blood-pressure-lowering effects of some blood-pressure-lowering drugs, especially those that work by dilating (widening) blood vessels.
● Iloprost may increase the risk of bleeding in people taking oral blood-thinning (anticoagulant) drugs.

Food Interactions
None known.

Usual Dose
Adult: 2.5–5 mcg by inhalation 6–9 times a day while awake. Do not inhale this drug more than once every 2 hours even though its effect may not last for 2 hours.

Child: not recommended.

Overdosage
There are no known cases of iloprost overdose, but symptoms should mimic the known effects of this drug, including headache, flushing, nausea, vomiting, and diarrhea. Take the overdose victim to a hospital emergency room at once. ALWAYS bring the prescription bottle or container.

Special Information
This drug has only been studied with the nebulizer provided by its manufacturer. Using it with any other type or brand of nebulizer may result in the incorrect dose of iloprost being inhaled.

Do not mix any other drug with iloprost when you inhale it.

Do not allow this product to come into contact with your skin or eyes. Do not swallow it.

You must use a fresh ampule of iloprost for each inhalation. Place all the liquid in the ampule into the medication chamber, choose your inhaler dose (2.5 or 5 mcg), inhale the medicine, and throw away any remaining medication from that iloprost ampule.

Call your doctor at once if your symptoms get worse despite using this medicine. Other treatments may be needed.

Special Populations
Pregnancy/Breast-feeding: Animal studies indicate that iloprost given by intravenous injection may cause birth defects. Pregnant women should use this drug only if its potential benefits outweigh the risks.

It is not known if this drug passes into breast milk. Nursing mothers who must take it should use infant formula because of the possibility that it may be transmitted to their nursing infant.

Seniors: Seniors should use the lowest possible dose of this medicine because of normal declines in kidney and liver function.

Generic Name

Imiquimod (ih-MIH-kwih-mod)

Brand Name

Aldara

Type of Drug

Immune modifier.

Prescribed For

Genital warts, perianal warts, actinic keratosis, superficial Basal Cell Carcinoma (sBCC), and condyloma acuminata.

General Information

Imiquimod has no direct antiviral activity. Animal studies suggest that imiquimod stimulates the skin to produce cytokines, potent natural chemicals that fight the warts, but its actual effect on genital warts and condyloma is not known. In studies of the drug, 50% of people who used it had complete clearance of their warts. But imiquimod is not a cure for genital warts—new ones may develop while others are being treated. Only minimal amounts of imiquimod enter the bloodstream.

Cautions and Warnings

Do not use this product if you are **allergic** or **sensitive** to any of its ingredients.

Imiquimod has not been studied in other viral diseases of the skin, such as papilloma virus, and should not be used to treat them, since its effect is unknown.

Do not apply imiquimod to any area until it has healed from any previous drug or surgery. Imiquimod can worsen skin that is already inflamed or sunburnt.

Imiquimod may increase your sun sensitivity. Avoid exposure to sunlight.

Imiquimod is not recommended for patients with **lowered immune response**.

Possible Side Effects

▼ Most common: redness, itching, erosion of the skin, burning, flaking, abrasions, swelling, and fungal infections in women.

Possible Side Effects *(continued)*

▼ Common: pain, marks on the skin, ulcers, skin scabbing, and headache.
▼ Less common: skin soreness, flu-like symptoms, skin discoloration, muscle aches, fungal infections in men, and diarrhea.

Drug Interactions

- Do not apply imiquimod with other drugs that may cause skin irritation.

Usual Dose

Genital Warts

Adult: At bedtime, apply a thin layer of the cream to external warts and rub it in until the cream disappears. Do not bandage. Leave it on the skin for 6–10 hours, then remove the cream with mild soap and water. Do this 3 times a week—for example, Monday, Wednesday, and Friday. Continue treatment for up to 16 weeks or until the warts go away.

Child: not recommended.

Actinic Keratosis

Adult: Wash and let the treatment area dry thoroughly. Apply twice a week—for example, Monday and Thursday—before bedtime for 16 weeks to the face or neck, but not both. After 8 hours, remove the cream with mild soap and water.

Child: not recommended.

Superficial Basal Cell Carcinoma (sBCC)

Adult: Wash and let the treatment area dry thoroughly. Apply 5 times per week at bedtime for 6 weeks to the sBCC, including the 1 cm surrounding the tumor. After 8 hours, wash the areas with mild soap and water.

Child: not recommended.

Overdosage

Overdose is not likely because such a small amount of imiquimod is absorbed through the skin. Accidental ingestion of imiquimod may cause low blood pressure. Anyone who has swallowed imiquimod should be taken to a hospital emergency room. ALWAYS bring the prescription bottle or container.

Special Information

Wash your hands before each application of imiquimod.

Most skin reactions are mild. If you develop a severe skin reaction to imiquimod, call your doctor and remove the cream with a mild soap and water. You can resume treatment with imiquimod after the reaction has completely subsided.

Imiquimod may weaken condoms and vaginal diaphragms. These birth control methods may prove undependable while you are using imiquimod cream. Avoid sexual contact while the cream is on your skin.

Uncircumcised men who use imiquimod to treat warts under the foreskin should retract the foreskin and cleanse the area every day.

Imiquimod is meant to be applied to the skin only. Do not let it get into your eyes, mouth, nose, or other mucous membranes. If you forget to apply a dose of imiquimod, do it as soon as you remember. If you don't remember until your next scheduled application, space the remaining doses equally throughout the rest of the week and continue with your regular schedule.

Throw away unused and partially used packets.

Special Populations

Pregnancy/Breast-feeding: The safety of using imiquimod during pregnancy is not known. When this drug is considered crucial by your doctor, its potential benefits must be carefully weighed against its risks.

It is not known if imiquimod passes into breast milk. Nursing mothers who must use this drug should consider using infant formula.

Seniors: Seniors may use this drug without special precaution.

Imitrex see **Triptan-Type Antimigraine Drugs,** page 1178

Generic Name

Indinavir (in-DIN-uh-vere)

Brand Name

Crixivan

Type of Drug

Protease inhibitor.

Prescribed For

Human immunodeficiency virus (HIV) infection.

General Information

Part of the multidrug "cocktail" responsible for the most important gains in the fight against acquired immunodeficiency syndrome (AIDS), indinavir sulfate belongs to a group of anti-HIV drugs called protease inhibitors. Triple-drug cocktails were considered responsible for the first overall reduction in the AIDS death rate, recorded in 1996. Protease inhibitors work in a unique way but are not a cure for HIV infection or AIDS. When the HIV virus attacks a cell, it must be converted into viral DNA. Older drugs, known as reverse transcriptase inhibitors, interfere with this step, but they need help in fighting HIV. Protease inhibitors work at the end of the HIV reproduction process, when proteins are "cut" into strands of exactly the right size to duplicate HIV. The protein is cut by a protease enzyme. Protease inhibitors prevent the mature HIV virus from being formed by interfering with this cutting process. Proteins that are cut to the wrong length or that remain uncut are inactive.

Protease inhibitors are always taken with 1 or 2 other nucleoside antiviral drugs such as efavirenz, emtricitabine, lamivudine, tenofovir, or zidovudine (AZT). Protease inhibitors revolutionized HIV treatment because, when taken in combination, they reduce the amount of HIV virus in the bloodstream to levels that are undetectable by current methods—CD_4 cell (immune system cell) counts and viral load (amount of virus in the blood) measurements. Multiple-drug therapy has changed the current view of HIV from a fatal disease to a manageable chronic illness. Newer approaches are exploring multiple protease-inhibitor treatment.

People taking a protease inhibitor may still develop infections or other conditions associated with HIV disease. Because of this, it is very important for you to remain under the care of a doctor or other health care provider. The long-term effects of indinavir are not known. You may be able to pass the HIV virus to others even if you are on triple-drug therapy.

Cautions and Warnings

Do not take indinavir if you are **allergic** or **sensitive** to any of its ingredients. People with mild or moderate **liver disease** or **cirrhosis** break down indinavir more slowly than those with normal liver function and may be more likely to develop side effects. People with cirrhosis should receive a reduced dose of indinavir.

About 4 of every 100 people taking indinavir can develop a kidney stone, indicated by pain in the middle to lower abdomen or back, or painful urination. Drinking at least 6 full glasses of liquid—48 oz.—a day will reduce your risk of developing a stone.

Indinavir may raise blood sugar, worsen **diabetes,** or bring out latent diabetes. Diabetics who take indinavir may have to have the dose of their antidiabetes medication adjusted against this effect.

Possible Side Effects

▼ Most common: nausea, abdominal pain, and headache.
▼ Common: kidney stones, itching, weakness or fatigue, pain in the side, diarrhea, vomiting, changes in sense of taste, acid regurgitation, and sleeplessness.
▼ Less common: dizziness, drowsiness, and back pain.
▼ Rare: Rare side effects can occur in almost any part of the body. Contact your doctor if you experience any side effect not listed above.

Drug Interactions

- Rifampin reduces the amount of indinavir in the blood. Do not combine these drugs.
- Indinavir should not be used with amiodarone, as amiodarone toxicity may result.
- Indinavir interferes with the liver's ability to break down terfenadine, triazolam, and midazolam. Do not combine indinavir with any of these drugs, as severe side effects may result.
- Combining indinavir with clarithromycin or with zidovudine (AZT) increases the amount of each drug in the blood. Combining indinavir with isoniazid increases the amount of isoniazid in the blood.
- Combining indinavir with rifabutin can reduce the amount of indinavir absorbed into the blood by ⅓ and double the amount of rifabutin absorbed.
- Didanosine interferes with the absorption of indinavir into the body. If you need both of these medications, take them at least 1 hour apart.

- Combining fluconazole with indinavir reduces the amount of indinavir in the blood by about 20%.
- Combining indinavir with ketoconazole increases the amount of indinavir in the blood by about 65%.
- Combining indinavir with quinidine raises indinavir levels by about 10%.
- Taking indinavir with AZT and lamivudine results in ⅓ more AZT in the blood and small decreases in lamivudine blood levels.
- Indinavir raises the amount of stavudine absorbed into the blood by 25% and the amount of trimethoprim by about 20%.
- Delaviridine increases the effects of indinavir.
- St. John's wort and efavirenz decrease the effects of indinavir.
- Indinavir increases the effects of ritonavir, sildenafil, tadalafil, vardenafil, and fentanyl.
- Combining indinavir with contraceptive drugs can result in higher blood hormone levels. This may lead to an excess of hormone-related side effects. If this happens to you, your doctor may be able to lower the dose of your contraceptive drug.

Food Interactions

Indinavir is best taken with water—or liquids such as skim milk or juice—at least 1 hour before or 2 hours after a meal. You should not eat meals that are high in calories, fat, and protein from 1 hour before to 2 hours after taking indinavir. You may take indinavir with a light meal.

Usual Dose

Adult: 800 mg every 8 hours, around the clock. People with cirrhosis should take 600 mg every 8 hours.

Child: not recommended.

Overdosage

Little is known about the effects of indinavir overdose except that it may cause severe drug side effects. Take overdose victims to a hospital emergency room at once. ALWAYS bring the prescription bottle or container.

Special Information

Indinavir does not cure HIV. It will not prevent you from transmitting HIV to another person; you must still practice safe sex. You may still develop opportunistic infections or other complications associated with advanced HIV disease.

It is imperative to take your HIV medication exactly as prescribed. Missing doses of indinavir makes you more likely to become resistant to the drug and to lose the benefits of therapy.

Call your doctor if you develop pains in the middle to lower abdomen, back pain, or painful urination. Drink at least 48 oz. of liquid each day—for example, six 8-oz. glasses.

Stay in close touch with your doctor while taking indinavir and report anything unusual.

Some patients experience changes in body fat. The long-term effects of these changes are not known.

If you forget a dose of indinavir, take it as soon as you remember. If it is almost time for your next dose, skip the dose you forgot and continue with your regular schedule. Do not take a double dose.

Indinavir capsules are sensitive to moisture. Store them in the original container and leave the drying agent in the bottle.

Special Populations
Pregnancy/Breast-feeding
There is little information on how indinavir affects pregnant women and their fetuses. Pregnant women should take this drug with caution.

Indinavir passes into breast milk. Women with HIV and nursing mothers who must take indinavir should use infant formula.

Seniors: Seniors may take indinavir without special restriction.

Generic Name

Indomethacin (IN-doe-METH-uh-sin) G

Brand Names

Indochron E-R	Indocin SR	Indocin

Type of Drug
Nonsteroidal anti-inflammatory drug (NSAID).

Prescribed For
Rheumatoid arthritis; osteoarthritis; ankylosing spondylitis; menstrual pain; tendinitis; bursitis; painful shoulder; gout—except

Indocin SR; sunburn; migraine and cluster headache—except Indocin SR. Indomethacin has been used to prevent premature labor, to treat a rare condition in premature infants called *patent ductus arteriosus*, and (in eyedrop form) to treat a severe and unusual inflammation in the retina.

General Information

Indomethacin and other NSAIDs are used to relieve pain and inflammation. We do not know exactly how NSAIDs work, but they may achieve their effects by blocking the body's production of a hormone called prostaglandin and the action of other body chemicals. Pain relief comes about 30 minutes after taking the first dose of indomethacin and lasts for 4–6 hours, but its anti-inflammatory effect takes a week to become apparent and may take 2 weeks to reach maximum effect. Indomethacin is broken down in the liver and eliminated through the kidneys. Indomethacin is available in capsule, oral suspension, and rectal suppository forms. Because of its adverse effects, indomethacin should only be used at the lowest possible dosage and when other NSAID therapy has not been effective.

Cautions and Warnings

Do not take indomethacin if you are **allergic** or **sensitive** to any of its ingredients or to any other NSAID. Those with a history of **asthma** attacks brought on by an NSAID, iodides, or aspirin should not take indomethacin.

Indomethacin may cause gastrointestinal (GI) bleeding, ulcers, and stomach perforation, which can occur at any time, with or without warning, in people who take indomethacin regularly. People with **a history of active GI bleeding** should be cautious about taking any NSAID. People who develop bleeding or ulcers and continue NSAID treatment may develop more serious side effects. Indomethacin should not be used by people who have had **ulcers or other stomach lesions**.

Indomethacin may affect platelets and blood clotting at high doses and should be avoided by people with **clotting problems** and **those taking warfarin**.

People with **heart failure** who use indomethacin may experience swelling in their arms, legs, or feet.

Indomethacin may worsen **depression or other psychiatric disorders, epilepsy,** and **parkinsonism**.

Indomethacin should never be used as "first therapy" for any disorder, with the possible exception of ankylosing spondylitis, because of the severe side effects associated with this drug.

Indomethacin may cause severe toxic effects to the kidney. Report any unusual side effects to your doctor, who might need to periodically test your kidney function. People with advanced **kidney disease** should avoid taking indomethacin.

Indomethacin may make you unusually sensitive to the effects of the sun.

Possible Side Effects

▼ Most common: headache, dizziness, diarrhea, nausea, vomiting, constipation, stomach gas, stomach upset or irritation, and appetite loss, especially during the first few days of treatment.

▼ Less common: stomach ulcers, GI bleeding, hepatitis, gallbladder attacks, painful urination, poor kidney function, kidney inflammation, blood and protein in the urine, dizziness, fainting, nervousness, depression, hallucinations, confusion, disorientation, tingling in the hands or feet, lightheadedness, itching, increased sweating, dry nose and mouth, heart palpitations, chest pain, breathing difficulties, and muscle cramps.

▼ Rare: severe allergic reactions including closing of the throat, fever and chills, changes in liver function, jaundice (yellowing of the skin or whites of the eyes), and kidney failure. People who experience such effects must be promptly treated in a hospital emergency room or doctor's office. NSAIDs have caused severe skin reactions; if this happens to you, see your doctor immediately. Contact your doctor if you experience any side effect not listed above.

Drug Interactions

- Indomethacin may increase the effects of oral anticoagulant (blood-thinning) drugs such as warfarin. Your anticoagulant dose may need to be reduced.
- Combining diflunisal and indomethacin has resulted in fatal GI hemorrhage.
- Indomethacin may reduce the blood-pressure-lowering effect of beta blockers, angiotensin-converting enzyme (ACE)

inhibitor drugs, and loop, potassium-sparing, or thiazide diuretics.

- Taking indomethacin with cyclosporine may increase the kidney-related side effects of both drugs. Methotrexate side effects may be increased in people also taking indomethacin.
- Indomethacin may increase digoxin levels in the blood.
- Indomethacin may increase the body's absorption of penicillamine.
- Combining indomethacin with phenylpropanolamine—found in many over-the-counter (OTC) drug products—may cause an increase in blood pressure.
- Combining indomethacin and dipyridamole may increase water retention.
- Indomethacin may increase phenytoin's side effects.
- Lithium blood levels may be increased by indomethacin.
- Combining indomethacin with selective serotonin reuptake inhibitors (SSRIs) may increase the risk of GI bleeding.
- Indomethacin blood levels may be affected by cimetidine.
- Cholestyramine may decrease the effectiveness of indomethacin.
- Probenecid may increase the risk of indomethacin side effects.
- Aspirin and other salicylates should never be combined with indomethacin to treat arthritis.
- Do not take indomethacin and triamterene concurrently, as this combination may cause acute kidney failure.

Food Interactions

Take indomethacin with a glass of water, food, or a magnesium/aluminum antacid to avoid an upset stomach.

Usual Dose

Adult and Child (age 15 and over): 50–200 mg a day, individualized to your needs.

Child (under age 15): not recommended.

Overdosage

People have died from NSAID overdoses. Common signs of overdose are drowsiness, nausea, vomiting, diarrhea, abdominal pain, rapid breathing, rapid heartbeat, increased sweating, ringing or buzzing in the ears, confusion, disorientation, stupor, and coma. Take the victim to a hospital emergency room at once. ALWAYS bring the prescription bottle or container.

Special Information

Take each dose with a full glass of water and do not lie down for 15–30 minutes afterward.

Indomethacin can make you drowsy or tired: Be careful when driving or operating hazardous equipment. Do not take any OTC products containing acetaminophen or aspirin while taking indomethacin. Avoid alcohol.

Contact your doctor if you develop rash or itching, visual disturbances, weight gain, breathing difficulties, fluid retention, hallucinations, black or tarry stools, persistent headache, or any unusual or intolerable side effect.

If you forget a dose of indomethacin, take it as soon as you remember. If you take indomethacin once a day and it is within 8 hours of your next dose, or if you take several doses a day and it is within 4 hours of your next dose, skip the dose you forgot and continue with your regular schedule. Never take a double dose.

Special Populations

Pregnancy/Breast-feeding: Indomethacin may affect the developing fetal heart if used during the second half of pregnancy. Pregnant women should not take indomethacin without their doctor's approval. When the drug is considered crucial by your doctor, its potential benefits must be carefully weighed against its risks.

Indomethacin may pass into breast milk. There is a possibility that the heart of a nursing baby could be affected by indomethacin. Nursing mothers who must take indomethacin should use infant formula.

Seniors: Seniors may be more susceptible to side effects, especially ulcer disease.

Generic Name

Infliximab (in-FLIX-ih-mab)

Brand Name

Remicade

Type of Drug

Monoclonal antibody.

Prescribed For

Crohn's disease, ankylosing spondylitis, and rheumatoid arthritis. Infliximab may also be used for plaque psoriasis, ulcerative colitis, psoriatic arthritis, psoriasis, and juvenile arthritis.

General Information

High levels of tumor necrosis factor (TNFα), which plays an important role in the inflammatory process, are linked to the worsening of Crohn's disease and rheumatoid arthritis. Infliximab neutralizes TNFα so that it cannot exert its effects. TNFα levels have been found to correlate with the severity of Crohn's disease.

Cautions and Warnings

Do not take infliximab if you are **allergic** or **sensitive** to any of its ingredients or to any murine proteins.

The safety and effectiveness of more than 3 infliximab infusions are not known.

People taking infliximab may develop serious infections such as tuberculosis and fungal infections. Some of these infections have been fatal.

Infliximab may cause allergic reactions including itching, breathing difficulties, and low blood pressure (symptoms include dizziness and fainting). These reactions may require emergency treatment. Lupus erythematosus may develop but goes away once drug treatment is stopped.

People with **compromised immune systems** should be cautious about using this drug because it can suppress immune function and result in serious infections.

People with **congestive heart failure** should take infliximab with caution because it may worsen heart function.

People with **nervous system disorders** or **seizures** should take infliximab with caution.

Rarely, cases of T-cell lymphoma have been reported in adolescents and young adults with Crohn's disease treated with infliximab.

Possible Side Effects

Most people (8 of 10) experience more than 1 side effect. Sixteen percent develop a reaction to the drug within 2 hours. Those reactions include fever, chills, itching, rash, chest pain, changes in blood pressure, and breathing difficulties.

Possible Side Effects (continued)

▼ Most common: headache, nausea, upper respiratory infection, abdominal pain, fatigue, and fever.
▼ Common: sore throat, vomiting, pain, dizziness, bronchitis, rash, runny nose, chest pain, coughing, itching, sinus inflammation, muscle aches, back pain, and fungus infection.
▼ Less common: Less common side effects can occur in almost any part of the body.
▼ Rare: lymphoma, abnormal vision, lupus-like syndrome, liver failure, blood abnormalities, and seizure.

Child
Side effects also include blood in the stool, respiratory tract allergic reaction, anemia, and bone fracture.

Drug Interactions
• Infliximab should not be combined with any drug infused into the bloodstream.

Food Interactions
None known.

Usual Dose
Adult: 1.35–2.25 mg per lb. of body weight. Another dose may be given 2 and 6 weeks after the first injection, then every 8 weeks.
Child (age 6 and over): Crohn's disease treatment—2.25 mg per lb. of body weight. Another dose may be given 2 and 6 weeks after the first injection, then every 8 weeks.
Child (under age 6): not recommended.

Overdosage
Symptoms may include drug side effects. Take the victim to a hospital emergency room. ALWAYS bring the prescription bottle or container.

Special Information
Call your doctor at once if you develop chest pain, fever, chills, itching, hives, flushing of face, or troubled breathing within a few hours after receiving your medicine, or if you develop yellowing of the skin or eyes, dark brown urine, right-sided abdominal pain, fever, or severe tiredness.

This medication is given by injection. For information on how to properly administer this drug, see page 1242.

Special Populations

Pregnancy/Breast-feeding: The safety of taking infliximab during pregnancy is not known. When this drug is considered crucial by your doctor, its potential benefits must be carefully weighed against its risks.

It is not known if infliximab passes into breast milk. Nursing mothers who must take it should use infant formula.

Seniors: Seniors may be more likely to develop infections while taking this drug.

Generic Name

Insulin (IN-suh-lin)

Most Common Brand Names

Generic Ingredient: Regular Insulin

Humulin R   Novolin R

Generic Ingredient: Insulin Aspart

Novolog   Novolog Mix 70/30

Generic Ingredient: Insulin Detemir

Levemir

Generic Ingredient: Insulin Glargine

Lantus

Generic Ingredient: Insulin Glulisine

Apidra

Generic Ingredient: Insulin Lispro

Humalog   Humalog Mix 50/50
Humalog Mix 75/25

Generic Ingredient: NPH Insulin

Humulin N   Novolin N

Generic Ingredients: NPH Insulin + Insulin

Humulin 50/50   Novolin 70/30
Humulin 70/30

Type of Drug

Antidiabetic.

Prescribed For

Type 1 and type 2 diabetes mellitus; also prescribed for gestational diabetes and hyperkalemia (very high blood-potassium levels) and for severe complications of diabetes such as ketoacidosis or diabetic coma. Insulin may be prescribed in combination with oral antidiabetes drugs for people with type 2 diabetes who do not respond to pills alone.

General Information

Insulin, a hormone made in the pancreas, helps the body turn sugar into energy. Insulin works by helping sugar enter body cells. Also, insulin helps us store energy that we can use later. Between meals, insulin helps us use the fat, sugar, and protein we have stored. In type 1 diabetes, the body does not make any insulin naturally. Type 2 diabetics may actually produce more insulin than normal people, but because their bodies do not properly utilize it, they may require supplemental insulin. Without insulin, glucose cannot get into body cells and the cells will not work properly. Insulin dosage must be balanced against the amount and type of food eaten and the amount of exercise you do. Blood glucose can drop too low or rise too high if insulin dosage is not changed with diet and exercise patterns.

The most widely used variety is human insulin. It is identical to natural human insulin, but it is manufactured by semisynthetic or recombinant DNA methods. Older products were made with animal insulin but had some impurities. No animal-based products are currently available in the U.S. All types of insulin must be injected because insulin is destroyed by stomach acid.

Rapid-acting insulins: Regular insulin starts to work in 30–60 minutes and lasts only 8–12 hours. Insulin aspart, glulisine, and lispro are all very short-acting insulins designed to control mealtime blood sugar spikes in both type 1 and type 2 diabetes. They begin working in 15 minutes and last for 2–5 hours.

Intermediate-acting insulins: NPH insulin starts working in 60–90 minutes and lasts for 12–16 hours.

Long-acting insulins: Insulin glargine starts working in about an hour and lasts for at least 24 hours. Insulin detemir lasts between 6 and 24 hours, depending upon the dose. Larger doses last for longer periods of time. Other factors that influence insulin response include diet, exercise, and the use of other drugs.

Cautions and Warnings

Low blood sugar (see "Overdosage" for symptoms) can result from taking too much insulin, doing excess physical work or exercise without eating, not absorbing food normally because meals are postponed or skipped, or because of illness with vomiting, fever, or diarrhea. You may be able to correct the imbalance by eating sugar, food with sugar, or a commercial 40% glucose product.

Hypersensitivity reactions to injected insulin can develop at the site of injection, such as redness, swelling, and itching, and may indicate a need to change the type of insulin you use. Reactions such as difficulty catching your breath, feeling your throat closing, fast pulse, sweating, low blood pressure with or without fainting, and skin eruptions may be life-threatening.

Thyroid disease can affect the clearance of insulin from the body.

Possible Side Effects

▼ Most common: low blood sugar (see "Overdosage" for symptoms), weight gain, low blood potassium.

▼ Less common: high blood sugar, redness, swelling, itching or rash at the site of injection; changes in the distribution of body fat; allergic reactions, salt and water retention; and swelling.

▼ Rare: worsening of eyesight due to breakdown of the retina of the eye. Contact your doctor if you experience any side effect not listed above.

Drug Interactions

- Drugs that reduce the effect of insulin include acetazolamide, HIV antivirals, albuterol, asparaginase, atypical antipsychotics, calcitonin, contraceptive drugs, corticosteroids, cyclophosphamide, danazol, dextrothyroxine, diazoxide, diltiazem, dobutamine, epinephrine, estrogens, ethacrynic acid, isoniazid, lithium carbonate, morphine, niacin, nicotine, phenothiazines, phenytoin, somatropin, terbutaline, thiazide diuretics, and thyroid hormones. Dosage increases may be required.
- Drugs that increase the effects of insulin include oral antidiabetes drugs, ACE inhibitors, alcohol, anabolic steroids, beta blockers, calcium, chloroquine, clofibrate, clonidine, disopyramide, fluoxetine, guanethidine, lithium carbonate,

monoamine oxidase inhibitor antidepressants, mebendazole, pentamidine, phenylbutazone, propoxyphene, pyridoxine, salicylates, sulfinpyrazone, sulfa drugs, and tetracycline. Dosage reductions may be required.

- Beta-blocking drugs can mask the symptoms of low blood sugar and thus increase the risk of insulin side effects.
- Quitting smoking—regardless of whether you are using a nicotine patch or gum, or another smoking deterrent—can also lower blood sugar. A lower insulin dosage may be necessary if you stop smoking.
- Insulin may affect blood-potassium levels and digitalis drugs.

Food Interactions

Follow your doctor's instructions on diet.

Usual Dose

Dosage must be individualized. Regular insulin is generally injected 30 minutes before meals. Aspart, glulisine, and lispro are injected 15 minutes before meals or within 20 minutes after you start eating. NPH insulin may be taken a half hour before breakfast or at night, according to your doctor's instructions. Glargine is usually taken once a day at bedtime; detemir may be given once or twice daily. Premixed insulins are given twice a day, before the morning and evening meal.

Overdosage

Accidentally swallowing insulin has little or no effect. Injecting too much insulin causes an insulin reaction or low blood sugar. Symptoms occur suddenly and include weakness, fatigue, nervousness, confusion, headache, double vision, convulsions, dizziness, psychosis, unconsciousness, rapid and shallow breathing, numbness or tingling around the mouth, hunger, nausea, loss of skin color, dry skin, and pulse changes. Overdose victims should immediately eat high-sugar, low-fat foods such as fruit juice or a glucose product for diabetics to raise blood-sugar levels. If victims are unable to eat or drink (due to a seizure, unconsciousness, or other debilitating condition), they should be immediately given an injection of glucagon and taken to a hospital emergency room.

Special Information

Use the same brand and strength of insulin and insulin syringes or administration devices to avoid dosage errors. Rotate injection sites every 1–2 weeks. For information on how to properly administer injectable insulin, see page 1242.

Ketoacidosis develops over hours or days. Symptoms are drowsiness, dim vision, a feeling of not getting enough air, thirst, nausea, vomiting, breath that smells like acetone (nail polish remover), abdominal pain, loss of appetite, dry and red skin, and rapid pulse. Go to an emergency room or contact your doctor immediately if these symptoms develop.

Mix insulins only according to your doctor's directions; do not change the method or order of mixing. Insulin glargine and insulin detemir should not be mixed with anything else, including another insulin product. Your pharmacist may also mix your insulins to ensure accuracy.

Take the exact dose of insulin prescribed. Too much insulin will excessively lower blood sugar, and too little will not control diabetes. Follow the diet prescribed by your doctor and avoid alcohol.

You may develop low blood sugar suddenly (see "Overdosage" for symptoms) if you take too much insulin, work or exercise more strenuously than usual, skip a meal, take insulin too long before a meal, or vomit before a meal. To help raise low blood sugar, drink fruit juice or eat a glucose bar or lump of sugar, which you should carry with you at all times. If the signs of low blood sugar do not clear up within 30 minutes, call your doctor. You may need further treatment.

Your insulin requirements may change if you get sick, especially if you vomit or have a fever.

If your insulin is in suspension form, you must gently rotate the vial and turn it over several times to evenly distribute the particles throughout the liquid before withdrawing the dose. Do not shake the vial.

People with diabetes must maintain good dental hygiene because of their increased risk of developing oral infections. Be sure your dentist knows you have diabetes. Visit your doctor every 3–6 months and have your eyes checked annually.

Read and follow all patient information provided with insulin products. Monitor your blood and urine regularly for sugar and ketones.

Insulin products are generally stable at room temperature for about 2 years. They must be kept away from direct sunlight and extreme temperatures. Most manufacturers recommend that insulin be stored in a refrigerator or another cool place, although it should not be put in a freezer. Partly used vials of insulin should be thrown away after several weeks if not used. Do not use any insulin that looks different from the way it did when you purchased it.

If you forget a dose, take it as soon as you remember. If it is almost time for your next dose, or if you completely forget 1 or more doses, call your doctor for exact instructions.

Special Populations

Pregnancy/Breast-feeding: Pregnant women must follow their doctor's directions for insulin use exactly, because insulin requirements normally decrease during the first half of pregnancy and then increase during the second half.

Insulin does not pass into breast milk. Breast-feeding can reduce your insulin needs, so your doctor should closely monitor your insulin dosage during this period.

Seniors: Seniors may use insulin without special restriction.

Generic Name

Interferon Alpha (in-ter-FEER-on AL-fuh)

Brand Names

Alferon N	Pegasys
Infergen	PegIntron
Intron A	

Type of Drug

Antiviral.

Prescribed For

Chronic hepatitis B and C, hairy cell leukemia, malignant melanoma, and AIDS-related Kaposi's sarcoma; also used to treat laryngeal papillomatosis (growths in the respiratory tract) in children and genital warts, bladder cancer, carcinoid tumors, chronic myelocytic leukemia, kidney cancer, non-Hodgkin's lymphoma, multiple myeloma, mycosis fungoides, ovarian cancer, polycythemia vera (a cancer of the blood), skin cancer, and thrombocytosis.

General Information

Interferon alpha attaches to the surface of an infected cell and stimulates a complicated set of reactions. These reactions lead to the production of enzymes inside the cell that prevent the hepatitis C virus (HCV), for example, from reproducing. Other causes of hepatitis do not respond to interferon treatment. Hepatitis C infection can be especially serious in people with HIV. Interferon alpha or a long-acting (pegylated) interferon called Pegasys, taken either alone or in combination with the antiviral ribavirin, can be given to people coinfected with chronic HCV and HIV, who are at greatest risk for progression to serious disease. Treatment does not always work, but HIV-infected patients may benefit from treatment with this combination.

Cautions and Warnings

Do not take interferon alpha if you are **allergic** or **sensitive** to any of its ingredients. Serious and life-threatening allergic or drug-sensitivity reactions can develop including an itchy rash, swelling, and breathing difficulties.

People taking this drug must be closely monitored by their doctors and receive periodic blood tests and liver and thyroid function tests.

People with **kidney or heart disease** should use this drug with caution. If heart disease worsens during treatment, the drug should be discontinued.

Interferon alpha may worsen **liver disease**.

Interferon alpha can affect the nervous system in many ways, including causing seizures, coma, dizziness, memory loss, agitation, psychosis, and complete loss of sensation. These effects generally go away when the drug is stopped.

Interferon alpha may cause menstrual problems or interfere with ovulation.

Depression and suicidal behavior has been reported in association with interferon alpha treatment. People who develop severe side effects or become depressed while taking this drug should have their dosage temporarily lowered. The drug should be stopped if depression is severe. Patients with an existing **psychiatric condition,** or a history of depression or other psychiatric disorders, should not be treated with interferon alpha.

It is not known if this drug is safe for children.

Possible Side Effects

▼ Most common: anxiety, sleep disturbances, depression, hair loss, nausea, diarrhea, abdominal pain, muscle or joint

Possible Side Effects *(continued)*

pain, weakness, headache, fever, chills, injection-site reactions, back pain, and generalized pain.

▼ Common: dizziness, confusion, abnormal thought patterns,
memory loss, tingling in the hands or feet, rash, dry skin,
sweating, vomiting, appetite loss, weight loss, cough, bronchitis, breathing difficulties, pneumonia, pleurisy, lung problems, runny nose, and sore throat.

▼ Less common: poor vision, abnormal heart rhythms, high
blood pressure, chest pain, high blood sugar, thyroid problems, urinary infection, low sex drive, accidental injury, liver
problems, migraine, increased sensitivity to the sun, psoriasis, attempted suicide, seizures, and a ruptured spleen.

▼ Rare: blood in the urine, eye problems, rheumatoid arthritis, lupus and other autoimmune conditions, painful spasms
of blood vessels in the legs, and worsening of diabetes and
thyroid problems. Contact your doctor if you experience
any side effect not listed above.

Drug Interactions

● Interferon alpha may interfere with the breakdown of vinblastine, zidovudine (also known as AZT), and theophylline.

Food Interactions

None known.

Usual Dose

All dosages are for adults (age 18 and over). Administration in children is not recommended.

Alferon N: 0.05 ml (250,000 IU) per wart twice weekly for up to
8 weeks. The maximum recommended dose per treatment session
is 0.5 ml (2.5 million IU).

Infergen: 9 mcg in a single subcutaneous injection 3 times a week
for 24 weeks. Allow at least 2 days between doses.

Intron A: 2–5 million units by subcutaneous or intramuscular injection 3 times a week for 6–18 months. Larger doses (10–20 million
units) are given by intravenous infusion.

Pegasys: 180 mcg once a week for 48 weeks. Dosage reduction to 135 mcg may be necessary, depending on reaction.

PegIntron: 1–1.5 mcg for every 2.2 lbs. of body weight by subcutaneous injection once a week for 1 year.

Overdosage

Symptoms may include increased side effects and changes in lab test results. Seizures have occurred at high dosages. Repeated overdose may cause lethargy or coma. Call your local poison control center or a hospital emergency room for more information. If you seek treatment, ALWAYS bring the prescription bottle or container.

Special Information

This drug does not prevent you from giving hepatitis C to others through unprotected sex or contact with blood or other body fluids.

People who have a seizure disorder or other nervous system problem, low white-blood-cell or blood-platelet count, or asthma or other breathing problems, or who take drugs that depress bone marrow function may be especially sensitive to the effects of interferon alpha.

This medication is given by injection under the skin. For information on how to properly administer this drug, see page 1242.

Ibuprofen, aspirin, and other anti-inflammatory drugs may alleviate some of the discomfort associated with starting interferon alpha.

Your doctor may instruct you to drink extra fluids while taking interferon alpha. This will help prevent low blood pressure due to excess loss of water.

This drug must be stored in the refrigerator and protected from light. Do not shake or freeze it.

Special Populations

Pregnancy/Breast-feeding: Animal studies suggest that interferon alpha may harm the fetus and cause spontaneous abortion. When this drug is considered crucial by your doctor, its potential benefits must be carefully weighed against its risks.

It is not known if this drug passes into breast milk. Nursing mothers who must take it should use infant formula.

Seniors: Seniors with liver, kidney, or heart conditions should use this drug with caution.

Generic Name

Interferon Beta (in-ter-FEER-on BAY-tuh)

Brand Names

Avonex (interferon beta-1a)   Rebif (interferon beta-1a)
Betaseron (interferon beta-1b)

Type of Drug

Multiple sclerosis (MS) therapy; biological response modifier.

Prescribed For

MS; also used for HIV infection, AIDS-related Kaposi's sarcoma, metastic renal-cell carcinoma, herpes of the lips or genitals, malignant melanoma, cutaneous T-cell lymphoma, and acute non-A/non-B hepatitis.

General Information

The interferons are a family of natural proteins produced in response to viral infection and other biological inducers. Three major classes of interferons have been identified: alpha, beta, and gamma; they each have overlapping, yet distinct, biologic activities. Interferon beta has antiviral effects, slows cell growth, and helps regulate the immune system. The way it works in MS is not clearly understood. However, it is known that interferon beta interacts with specific receptors on the surface of human cells. Binding causes the production of a number of gene products believed to mediate the biological actions of interferon beta. People receiving this drug may be vaccinated, but the effectiveness of the vaccination is unpredictable.

Cautions and Warnings

Do not take interferon beta if you are **sensitive** or **allergic** to any of its ingredients or to human albumin. Rare severe allergic reactions have been reported.

The safety and benefit of interferon beta in **chronic progressive MS** is unproven.

Some people taking interferon beta in studies had severe depression and suicidal tendencies. People with **depression, suicidal ideation,** or **severe psychiatric symptoms** should use any interferon product with caution and report any changes in their emotions or behavior to a doctor.

People with **seizure disorders** may be more likely to develop a seizure while taking interferon beta.

Up to 75% of people who take interferon beta are likely to develop flu-like symptoms including fever, chills, muscle aches, sweating, and feeling unwell. These symptoms may prove stressful to people with **heart disease**.

Interferon beta may cause increased sensitivity to the sun. Wear protective clothing and use sunscreen.

In rare cases, severe liver disease has occurred while taking interferon beta. People with **liver or thyroid disease** should not use this drug.

Interferon beta can cause reductions in white-blood-cell and platelet counts.

People with a history of **latex allergy** should use caution, as some of this drug's packaging may contain latex.

Possible Side Effects

In general, interferon beta-1a has fewer side effects than interferon beta-1b.

Interferon Beta-1a

▼ Most common: respiratory infection, sinusitis, headache, fever, weakness, chills, dizziness, muscle aches, abdominal pain, flu-like symptoms, depression, painful menstruation, diarrhea, nausea, upset stomach, and sleeping difficulties. Pain, burning, or stinging at the injection site may also occur.

▼ Less common: swelling, pelvic pain, cyst, thyroid goiter, heart palpitations, bleeding, laryngitis, breathing difficulties, joint pain, stiffness, tiredness, speech problems, convulsions, uncontrolled movements, hair loss, urinary urgency, and cystitis.

▼ Rare: Rare side effects can occur in almost any part of the body. Contact your doctor if you experience any side effect not listed above.

Interferon Beta-1b

▼ Most common: pain, burning, or stinging at the injection site, sinusitis, headache, migraine, fever, weakness, chills, muscle ache, abdominal pain, flu-like symptoms, depression, menstrual disorders, painful menstruation, constipation,

Possible Side Effects *(continued)*

diarrhea, vomiting, liver inflammation, sweating, and reduced white-blood-cell count.

▼ Less common: itching, swelling, pelvic pain, cyst, thyroid goiter, heart palpitations, high blood pressure, rapid heartbeat, bleeding, laryngitis, breathing difficulties, muscle weakness, stiffness, tiredness, speech problems, convulsions, uncontrolled movements, visual disturbances or conjunctivitis (pinkeye), urinary urgency, cystitis, breast pain, cystic breast disease, breast cancer, and weight changes.

▼ Rare: Rare side effects can occur in almost any part of the body. Contact your doctor if you experience any side effect not listed above.

Food and Drug Interactions
None known.

Usual Dose
Adult
Avonex: 30 mcg into a large muscle once a week.

Betaseron: usual dose—0.25 mg injected under the skin every other day. Patients are started at ¼ of the usual dose and increased gradually over 7 weeks to the regular dose. Betaseron comes with a special solution with which to mix the product before injection.

Rebif: usual dose—44 mcg injected 3 times a week, 2 days apart, usually late in the day. Patients are started on injections of 8.8 mcg 3 times weekly. Dosage is increased over 4 weeks to the usual dose.

Child (under age 18): not recommended.

Overdosage
Little is known about the effects of interferon beta overdose. Symptoms may include exaggerated side effects. Call your local poison control center or a hospital emergency room for more information. If you seek treatment, ALWAYS bring the prescription bottle or container.

Special Information
Interferon beta-1a and interferon beta-1b may be associated with severe depression. Mood swings or changes, lack of interest in

daily activities, excessive sleep, and other possible signs of depression should be reported to your doctor at once.

This medication is given by injection. For information on how to administer this drug, see page 1242.

If you forget to administer a dose, do so as soon as you remember. If it is almost time for your next dose, skip the one you forgot and continue with your regular schedule. Do not take a double dose.

Special Populations

Pregnancy/Breast-feeding: Animal studies show that interferon beta may cause abortion. Women who are or might be pregnant should not use this drug.

It is not known if interferon beta passes into breast milk. Nursing mothers who must take it should consider using infant formula.

Seniors: Seniors may use this drug without special restriction.

Generic Name

Ipratropium (ipe-ruh-TROE-pee-um) [G]

Brand Name

Atrovent

Combination Products

Generic Ingredients: Ipratropium Bromide + Albuterol Sulfate

Combivent   DuoNeb

The information in this profile also applies to the following drugs:

Generic Ingredient: Tiotropium Bromide

Spiriva

Type of Drug

Anticholinergic.

Prescribed For

Bronchospasm associated with bronchitis, emphysema, and other chronic lung diseases; also prescribed for runny nose.

General Information

Ipratropium bromide is related to atropine sulfate, another anticholinergic drug. Ipratropium works against natural acetylcholine in the bronchial muscles, causing them to dilate. It has little effect on other parts of the body. Much of each inhaled dose is swallowed and passes out of the body in the stool. Like all anticholinergic drugs, ipratropium has a drying effect; the nasal spray provides relief from runny nose.

Cautions and Warnings

Do not use ipratropium if you are **allergic** or **sensitive** to any of its ingredients or to atropine, soya lecithin, or any related product.

Ipratropium should be used with caution if you have **glaucoma, prostate disease,** or **bladder obstruction**.

Ipratropium is not meant for the treatment of acute bronchospasm. This drug should be used only to prevent bronchospasm associated with chronic lung diseases.

Patients may experience a temporary blurring of vision or worsening of **narrow-angle glaucoma** if the solution comes into direct contact with the eyes.

Possible Side Effects

Generally, ipratropium side effects are infrequent and mild.

Inhalation

▼ Most common: bronchitis, upper respiratory infection, nervousness, dizziness, headache, nausea, upset stomach, blurred vision, sensitivity to bright light, dry mouth, throat irritation, cough, worsening of symptoms, rash, and mouth irritation.

▼ Less common: rapid heartbeat, heart palpitations, urinary difficulties, tingling in the hands or feet, poor coordination, itching, hives, flushing, loss of hair, constipation, tremors, fatigue or sleeplessness, and hoarseness.

▼ Rare: worsening of glaucoma, eye pain, low blood pressure, and severe skin reactions. Contact your doctor if you experience any side effect not listed above.

Nasal Spray

▼ Most common: headache, upper respiratory infection, nosebleeds, and nasal dryness.

▼ Less common: dry mouth or throat and stuffed nose.

▼ Rare: changes in sense of taste, nasal burning, red and itchy eyes, coughing, dizziness, hoarseness, heart palpitations, rapid heartbeat, thirst, ringing or buzzing in the ears, blurred vision, and difficulty urinating. Contact your doctor if you experience any side effect not listed above.

Drug Interactions

None known.

Food Interactions

Do not inhale a dose of ipratropium if you have any food in your mouth.

Usual Dose

Inhalation

Adult and Child (age 12 and over): 2 inhalations 4 times a day; no more than 12 inhalations every 24 hours. For DuoNeb, 1 vial 3–4 times a day, 6–8 hours apart.

Child (under age 12): not recommended.

Nasal Spray

Adult and Child (age 5 and over): 2 sprays of 0.03% solution per nostril up to 2–3 times a day; the 0.06% solution frequency is 3–4 times a day.

Overdosage

The risk of overdose is small because very little ipratropium is absorbed into the bloodstream. Ipratropium accidentally sprayed into the eye will cause blurred vision. ALWAYS bring the prescription bottle or container with you if you go to an emergency room for treatment.

Special Information

Use this product according to your doctor's instructions. Do not stop taking ipratropium without your doctor's approval even if you feel well.

Call your doctor if you develop rash or hives, sores on the mouth or lips, blurred vision, or other side effects that are bothersome or persistent.

Call your doctor if you stop responding to your usual dose of ipratropium: This may be a sign that your condition has worsened.

Prolonged use of ipratropium may decrease or stop the flow of saliva produced in your mouth. This can expose you to an increased chance of cavities, gum disease, oral infections, and other problems. Dry mouth can be relieved with hard candies or regular fluids. Increased attention to dental hygiene is important.

If, in addition to ipratropium, you use a corticosteroid inhaler or cromolyn sodium for lung disease, use ipratropium about 5 minutes before using the other inhaler.

If you take ipratropium and albuterol, metaproterenol, or another beta-stimulating aerosol product for bronchial disease, use the beta stimulator about 5 minutes before ipratropium unless otherwise instructed by your doctor. Ipratropium solution for inhalation can be mixed with albuterol or metaproterenol for inhalation as long as the mixture is used within 1 hour. The combination product Combivent (a mixture of ipratropium and albuterol) is also available.

The first use of each ipratropium nasal pump requires 2 pumps to prime the spray. Regular use of the spray should prevent the need to prime the pump again. If you do not use the spray for 3 days, you will have to prime the spray again with 2 pumps.

If you forget to administer a dose of ipratropium, do so as soon as you remember. If it is almost time for your next dose, skip the one you forgot and continue with your regular schedule. Do not take a double dose.

Store this product at room temperature—59°–86°F—and avoid freezing. Unused vials of the solution for inhalation should be stored in their foil wrapper.

Special Populations

Pregnancy/Breast-feeding: Massive oral doses of ipratropium have caused birth defects in animals. Ipratropium should be used during pregnancy only if clearly needed.

It is not known if ipratropium passes into breast milk. Nursing mothers who must take this drug should consider using infant formula.

Seniors: Seniors may use ipratropium without special precaution.

Type of Drug

Iron Supplements

Brand Names

Generic Ingredient: Carbonyl Iron, 100% Iron

Feosol	Ircon
Icar	

Generic Ingredient: Ferrous Fumarate **G**, *33% Iron*

Chromagen	Feostat
Femiron	Ferretts

Ferro-Sequels   Nephro-Fer $

Hemocyte   Vitron-C $

Generic Ingredient: Ferrous Gluconate G, *12% Iron*
Fergon

Generic Ingredient: Ferrous Sulfate G, *20–30% Iron*
ED-IN-SOL   Fer-Gen-Sol
Feosol   Fer-In-Sol
Feratab   Slow-FE

Generic Ingredient: Polysaccharide Iron Complex
Ferrex 150   Niferex-150
Fe-Tinie 150   Nu-Iron
Hytinic   Nu-Iron 150
Niferex $

Prescribed For

Iron-deficiency anemia.

General Information

Iron supplements are used to treat anemias that result from iron deficiency. Iron is incorporated into red blood cells, which carry oxygen throughout the body. Iron is absorbed only in a small section of the gastrointestinal (GI) tract called the duodenum, the upper part of the small intestine. Sustained-release iron products should be used only to help minimize the stomach discomfort that iron supplements can cause, as some of the drug in these forms may bypass the duodenum and not be absorbed. Other products combining iron with vitamins or special extracts may also be used to treat iron-deficiency anemia. Iron supplements are available in many different forms and they all have different amounts of iron. When choosing an iron supplement, you must be sure to take one that gives you the amount of elemental iron you need.

Cautions and Warnings

Do not take an iron supplement if you are **allergic** or **sensitive** to any of its ingredients or if you have **hemochromatosis, hemosiderosis,** or a **hemolytic anemia**.

Do not take iron supplements if you have a history of **stomach problems, peptic ulcer,** or **ulcerative colitis**. People with normal iron levels should not take any iron product on a regular basis.

Possible Side Effects

▼ Common: stomach upset or irritation, nausea, diarrhea, constipation, appetite loss, darkened stools, and leg cramps.

▼ Less common: heartburn, darkened urine, and staining of the teeth.

Drug Interactions

- Iron and tetracycline interfere with each other. Iron may also interfere with the absorption of cephalosporin-type antibiotics. Separate doses of these by at least 2 hours.
- Iron interferes with the absorption of levodopa + carbidopa, methyldopa, penicillamine, and quinolone antibacterials.
- Antacids, cimetidine, and other acid reducers interfere with iron absorption.
- Ascorbic acid (vitamin C) and chloramphenicol increase the amount of iron absorbed.
- Iron reduces the effectiveness of levothyroxine, a thyroid replacement hormone. Combining these 2 drugs may lead to symptoms of hypothyroidism (underactive thyroid gland).

Food Interactions

Iron supplements are best taken on an empty stomach, but they may be taken with food if they upset your stomach. Eggs and milk interfere with iron absorption. Coffee or tea consumed with a meal or within an hour of eating reduces the amount of iron absorbed into the blood. Do not take iron products together with calcium supplements and food. If you need both iron and calcium, take calcium carbonate (Tums) and use it between meals.

Usual Dose

Iron dosage is the same regardless of type. Read the product label to determine iron content.

Adult and Child (age 13 and over): 0.9–1.4 mg per lb. of body weight a day, divided in 3 doses.

Pregnant Women: 30 mg a day. Do not take with food or meals.

Child (age 3–12): 0.45–0.7 mg per lb. of body weight a day, divided in 3–4 doses.

Child (age 6 months–2 years): up to 2.7 mg per lb. of body weight a day, divided in 3–4 doses.

Child (under age 2): 10–25 mg a day, divided in 3–4 doses.

Overdosage

Iron overdosage can be fatal. Accidental overdose of iron-containing products is a leading cause of fatal poisoning in children under age 6. Always keep iron supplements out of the reach of children. Overdose symptoms usually appear after 30 minutes to several hours; they include tiredness, vomiting, diarrhea, upset stomach, weak and rapid pulse, and lowered blood pressure—or, after massive doses, shock, black and tarry stools due to massive bleeding in the stomach or intestine, and pneumonia. In case of overdose, call your local poison control center of a hospital emergency room. You may be told to induce vomiting with ipecac syrup—available at any pharmacy—and to give the victim eggs and milk before seeking treatment. Time is a critical factor in emergency care: Stomach pumping should not be performed after the first hour of iron ingestion due to the risk of stomach perforation. If you seek treatment, ALWAYS bring the prescription bottle or container.

Special Information

Iron often causes black discoloration of stools and is slightly constipating. However, stools that are black or tarry may also indicate bleeding in the stomach or intestine. If you experience this symptom, discuss it with your doctor at once.

Do not chew or crush sustained-release iron products. Liquid iron products may stain your teeth. Mix water or juice with them and sip the iron through a straw to prevent tooth contact.

Nausea may be minimized by slowly increasing to the recommended dosage.

If you forget a dose, take it as soon as you remember. If it is almost time for your next dose, skip the one you forgot and continue with your regular schedule. Do not take a double dose.

Special Populations

Pregnancy/Breast-feeding: This drug is safe for use during pregnancy and breast-feeding and is frequently prescribed for pregnant and nursing women. If you are pregnant, however, you should check with your doctor before taking any medication.

Seniors: Seniors may require larger dosages.

Generic Name

Isosorbide Dinitrate (eye-soe-SORE-bide dih-NYE-trate) G

Brand Names

Dilatrate-SR
Isochron
Isordil

Isordil Tembids
Isordil Titradose

The information in this profile also applies to the following drug:

Generic Ingredient: Isosorbide Mononitrate G

Imdur
ISMO

Isotrate ER
Monoket

Type of Drug

Antianginal agent.

Prescribed For

Heart or chest pain associated with angina pectoris; also pre-scribed in congestive heart failure (CHF) and similar conditions to prevent the recurrence of chest or heart pain and to reduce stress on the heart.

General Information

Isosorbide dinitrate and other nitrates are used to treat pain as-sociated with heart problems. While the exact nature of their ac-tion is not fully understood, they are believed to relax vascular smooth muscles. Isosorbide dinitrate sublingual tablets begin working in 2–5 minutes and last for 1–3 hours. The regular tablets begin working in 20–40 minutes and continue for 4–6 hours. The sustained-release form may take up to 4 hours to begin working and lasts for 6–8 hours. Isosorbide mononitrate begins working in 30–60 minutes and lasts for an undetermined period of time.

Cautions and Warnings

Do not take isosorbide dinitrate if you are **allergic** or **sensitive** to any of its ingredients or to another nitrate product, such as nitroglycerin.

If you have or recently have had a **head injury,** use this drug with caution.

This drug may be inappropriate for you if you have had a re-cent **heart attack** or have severe **anemia,** severe **kidney or liver** disease, **overactive thyroid, cardiomyopathy** (loss of blood-pumping ability due to damaged heart muscle), **glaucoma,** or **low blood pressure,** especially postural low blood pressure (symptoms include dizziness or fainting when rising from a sitting or lying position).

If you have been taking isosorbide for several weeks or longer, do not suddenly stop using it.

Possible Side Effects

▼ Common: headache and flushing, which should disappear after your body adjusts to the drug. You may experience lightheadedness, dizziness, and weakness during this process. There is a risk of blurred vision and dry mouth; if either occurs, stop taking the drug and call your doctor.

▼ Less common: rapid heartbeat, low blood pressure, fainting, nausea, vomiting, weakness, trouble urinating, bronchitis, sweating, and rash with itching, redness, and peeling. If these symptoms appear, discontinue the medication and consult your doctor.

Drug Interactions

- If you take isosorbide dinitrate, do not self-medicate with over-the-counter appetite suppressants and cough, cold, and allergy remedies, since many contain ingredients that may aggravate heart disease.
- Taking this drug with large amounts of alcohol may rapidly lower blood pressure, resulting in weakness, dizziness, and fainting.
- Nitrates raise dihydroergotamine blood levels, which may elevate blood pressure or block isosorbide's effects.
- Calcium channel blockers and large doses of aspirin can increase isosorbide blood levels and the risk of side effects.
- Do not take sildenafil, vardenafil, or taldenafil if taking isosorbide or another nitrate drug. The combination can result in a rapid and potentially fatal drop in blood pressure.

Food Interactions

Take isosorbide on an empty stomach with a glass of water unless you get a persistent headache. If this occurs, the drug can be taken with meals.

Usual Dose

Adult

Isosorbide Dinitrate: starting dosage—5–20 mg 2–3 times a day; maintenance dosage—10–40 mg every 6 hours. Sustained-release starting dosage—40 mg; maintenance dosage—40–80 mg every 8–12 hours. Sublingual tablets starting dosage—2.5–5 mg, increased gradually until angina is relieved. All dosing should include a daily dose-free interval of at least 14 hours to prevent the development of drug tolerance.

Isosorbide Mononitrate: 20 mg twice a day, with the 2 doses taken 7 hours apart. Usually, the first dose is taken upon waking and the second dose is taken 7 hours later. Extended-release tablets should begin with 30–60 mg once a day; after several days this may be increased to 120 mg once a day. Although it is rare, 240 mg may be required.

Child: not recommended.

Overdosage

Overdose can result in low blood pressure; very rapid heartbeat; flushing; perspiration followed by cold, bluish, and clammy skin; headache; heart palpitations; blurred vision and other visual disturbances; dizziness; nausea; vomiting; difficult, slow breathing; slow pulse; confusion; moderate fever; and paralysis. Take the victim to a hospital emergency room at once. ALWAYS bring the prescription bottle or container.

Special Information

If you take this drug sublingually (under the tongue), be sure the tablet is fully dissolved before you swallow the drug. Do not crush or chew sustained-release capsules or tablets. Avoid alcohol.

Do not switch brands of isosorbide without consulting your doctor or pharmacist—they may not be equivalent.

Call your doctor if you develop a persistent headache, dizziness, facial flushing, blurred vision, or dry mouth.

You may develop a tolerance to the effects of isosorbide, in which case you may have to schedule your doses so that there is no isosorbide in your body for a period of time every 24 hours. Follow your doctor's instructions.

If you take isosorbide on a regular schedule and forget a dose, take it as soon as you remember. If you take isosorbide more than once a day and it is within 2 hours of your next dose, skip the dose you forgot and continue with your regular schedule. If you take the sustained-release form once a day and it is within 6 hours of your next dose, skip the dose you forgot and continue with your regular schedule. Never take a double dose.

Special Populations

Pregnancy/Breast-feeding: Isosorbide crosses into the fetal circulation. When this drug is considered crucial by your doctor, its potential benefits must be carefully weighed against its risks.

This drug passes into breast milk. Nursing mothers who must take it should consider using infant formula.

Seniors: Seniors may be more sensitive to the effects and side effects of isosorbide because of the greater chance of reduced liver, kidney, or cardiac function, and the increased likelihood of concurrent diseases and drug therapies.

Generic Name

Isotretinoin (eye-soe-TRET-ih-noin)

Brand Names

Accutane   Claravis
Amnesteem   Sotret

Type of Drug

Anti-acne.

Prescribed For

Severe cystic acne that has not responded to other treatment.

General Information

It is not known exactly how isotretinoin, which is related to vitamin A, works in cases of severe cystic acne. It reduces the amount of sebum (the skin's natural oily lubricant), shrinks the skin glands that produce sebum, and inhibits keratinization (hardening of the skin cells)—key to the problem of severe acne because it leads to the buildup of sebum within skin follicles and causes the formation of closed comedones (whiteheads). Sebum production may be permanently reduced after isotretinoin treatment.

Isotretinoin is also being studied as a treatment for keratinization and mycosis fungoides.

Cautions and Warnings

Do not take isotretinoin if you are **allergic** or **sensitive** to any of its ingredients or to vitamin A (or any vitamin A product) or to paraben preservatives.

Isotretinoin greatly increases the risk of severe birth defects (including very low IQs as well as multiple physical defects), abortion, and premature birth. Not every fetus exposed to isotretinoin will be affected, but women who are **pregnant or nursing** must not take isotretinoin.

Isotretinoin has been associated with depression, psychosis, and suicidal thoughts or attempts. Use with caution if you have a history of **psychiatric disorders**.

Isotretinoin has been associated with pseudotumor cerebri (increased pressure in the brain). The symptoms of this condition include severe headaches, nausea, vomiting, and visual disturbances.

Isotretinoin may cause an increased risk for pancreatitis, sometimes fatal, and low white-blood-cell counts.

Diabetics taking isotretinoin may have to have their diabetes drugs re-evaluated by their doctors. Some new cases of diabetes were found in people taking isotretinoin, but no direct relationship to drug therapy has been found.

Isotretinoin may cause temporary opaque spots on the cornea of your eye, causing visual disturbances. These are usually gone by 2 months after the drug is stopped.

Difficulty seeing at night or in the dark can develop suddenly while taking isotretinoin.

Several cases of severe bowel inflammation (symptoms include abdominal discomfort and pain, severe diarrhea, or bleeding from the rectum) have developed in people taking isotretinoin.

About 25% of people who take isotretinoin develop high blood-triglyceride levels. Fifteen percent have lower high-density lipoprotein (HDL)—"good" cholesterol—and 7% have higher total cholesterol.

Several cases of hepatitis have been linked to this drug. Fifteen percent of people who take it develop signs of liver inflammation.

Isotretinoin may worsen **osteoporosis**, cause low bone density, and slow bone healing. Long-term treatment or multiple courses of therapy may worsen these problems.

Children age 13–17 may experience increased back pain while using isotretinoin. This drug has not been studied in children under age 12.

Isotretinoin causes extreme elevations of blood-triglyceride levels and milder elevations of other blood-fat levels including cholesterol. It also can raise blood-sugar or uric-acid levels and can increase liver-function-test values.

Possible Side Effects

Side effects increase with dosage.

▼ Most common: dry, chapped, or inflamed lips; dry mouth; dry nose; nosebleeds; eye irritation; conjunctivitis (pinkeye); dry or flaky skin; rash; itching; peeling skin on the face, palms, or soles; unusual sensitivity to the sun; temporary skin discoloration; brittle nails; inflammation of the nailbed or bone under toes or fingernails; temporary hair thinning; nausea; vomiting; abdominal pain; tiredness; lethargy; sleeplessness; headache; tingling in the hands or feet; dizziness; protein, blood, or white blood cells in the urine; urinary difficulties; blurred vision; bone and joint aches or pains; and muscle pain or stiffness.

▼ Less common: wound crusting caused by an exaggerated healing response stimulated by the drug, hair problems other than thinning, appetite loss, upset stomach or intestinal discomfort, severe bowel inflammation, stomach or intestinal bleeding, weight loss, visual disturbances, contact lens intolerance, pseudotumor cerebri, mild bleeding or easy bruising, fluid retention, and lung or respiratory system infection. Several people taking isotretinoin have developed widespread herpes simplex infections.

Drug Interactions

- Vitamin A supplements increase isotretinoin's side effects and must be avoided while taking this drug. Avoid alcohol because this combination can severely raise blood-triglyceride levels.
- Combining tetracycline antibiotics and isotretinoin may increase the risk of pseudotumor cerebri.
- Isotretinoin may reduce the amount of carbamazepine (an anticonvulsant) in the blood.
- Isotretinoin may decrease the effectiveness of contraceptive drugs. Use an additional form of contraception.

Food Interactions

Isotretinoin should be taken with food or meals. Avoid eating beef or chicken liver while taking isotretinoin, because liver contains very large amounts of vitamin A. Limit your intake of foods containing moderate to large amounts of vitamin A.

Usual Dose

Adult and Child (age 13 and over): 0.22–0.9 mg per lb. of body weight a day in 2 divided doses for 15–20 weeks. Lower doses may be effective, but relapses are more common. Isotretinoin, like vitamin A, dissolves in body fat. Individuals who weigh more than 155 lbs. may need doses at the high end of the usual range.

If the total acne lesion count drops by 70% in 15–20 weeks, the drug may be discontinued. Stop taking isotretinoin for 2 months after 15–20 weeks of treatment. A second course of treatment may be needed if the acne does not clear.

Overdosage

Isotretinoin overdose is likely to cause nausea, vomiting, facial flushing, abdominal pain, lethargy, and other common drug side effects. Overdose victims must be made to vomit with ipecac syrup—available at any pharmacy—to remove any remaining drug from the stomach. Call your doctor or poison control center before doing this. If you must go to a hospital emergency room, ALWAYS bring the prescription bottle or container.

Special Information

Women of childbearing age should not take isotretinoin unless their severe, disfiguring acne has not responded to any other treatment, they are using effective contraception, they understand that it causes serious birth defects, and they have had two negative pregnancy tests during the 2 cycles before taking isotretinoin and after the last incidence of unprotected sex. You may have to have a pregnancy test each month of your treatment before another prescription is written. You should start taking isotretinoin on day 2 or 3 of your next period. Be sure your doctor knows if you are breast-feeding, diabetic, taking a vitamin A supplement—as a multivitamin or vitamin A alone—or if you or any family member has a history of high blood-triglyceride levels. Continue using contraceptives for at least 1 month after stopping isotretinoin.

Your skin may become unusually sensitive to the sun while you are taking this drug. Use sunscreen and wear protective clothing

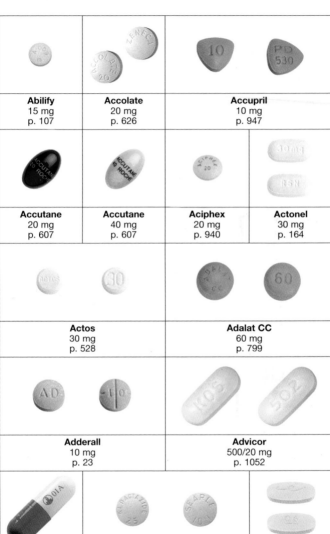

Abilify 15 mg p. 107	**Accolate** 20 mg p. 626	**Accupril** 10 mg p. 947
Accutane 20 mg p. 607	**Accutane** 40 mg p. 607	**Aciphex** 20 mg p. 940 **Actonel** 30 mg p. 164
Actos 30 mg p. 528	**Adalat CC** 60 mg p. 799	
Adderall 10 mg p. 23	**Advicor** 500/20 mg p. 1052	
Aggrenox 25/200 mg p. 30	**Aldactazide** 25/25 mg p. 397	**Allegra** 60 mg p. 215

A

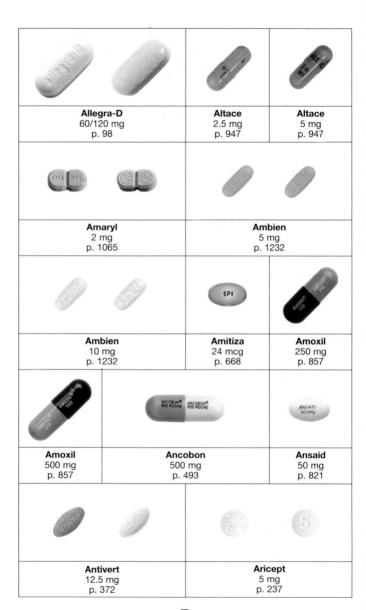

Allegra-D 60/120 mg p. 98	**Altace** 2.5 mg p. 947	**Altace** 5 mg p. 947
Amaryl 2 mg p. 1065	**Ambien** 5 mg p. 1232	
Ambien 10 mg p. 1232	**Amitiza** 24 mcg p. 668	**Amoxil** 250 mg p. 857
Amoxil 500 mg p. 857	**Ancobon** 500 mg p. 493	**Ansaid** 50 mg p. 821
Antivert 12.5 mg p. 372	**Aricept** 5 mg p. 237	

B

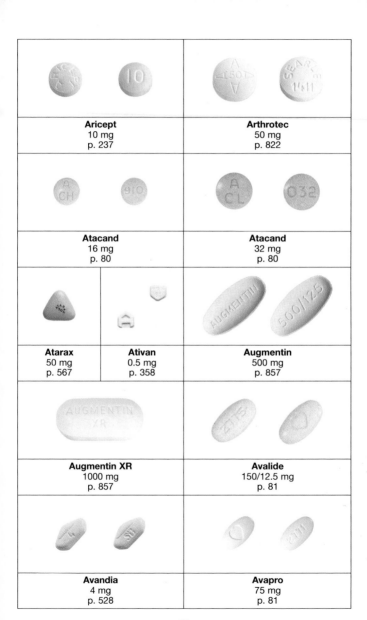

| **Aricept**
10 mg
p. 237 | **Arthrotec**
50 mg
p. 822 |
| **Atacand**
16 mg
p. 80 | **Atacand**
32 mg
p. 80 |

| **Atarax**
50 mg
p. 567 | **Ativan**
0.5 mg
p. 358 | **Augmentin**
500 mg
p. 857 |

| **Augmentin XR**
1000 mg
p. 857 | **Avalide**
150/12.5 mg
p. 81 |
| **Avandia**
4 mg
p. 528 | **Avapro**
75 mg
p. 81 |

C

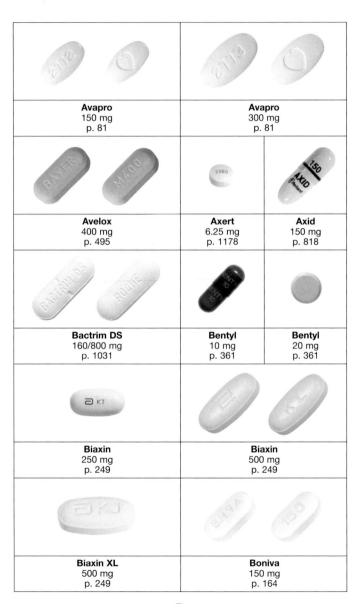

Avapro 150 mg p. 81	**Avapro** 300 mg p. 81	
Avelox 400 mg p. 495	**Axert** 6.25 mg p. 1178	**Axid** 150 mg p. 818
Bactrim DS 160/800 mg p. 1031	**Bentyl** 10 mg p. 361	**Bentyl** 20 mg p. 361
Biaxin 250 mg p. 249	**Biaxin** 500 mg p. 249	
Biaxin XL 500 mg p. 249	**Boniva** 150 mg p. 164	

D

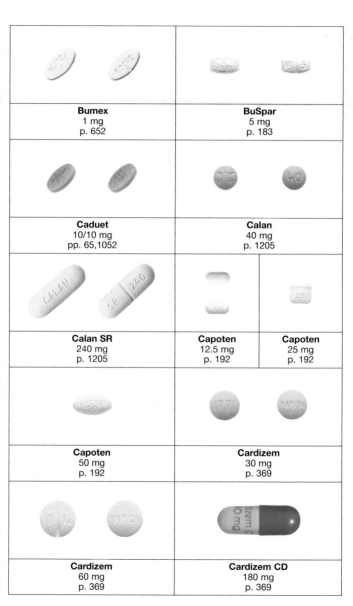

Bumex 1 mg p. 652	**BuSpar** 5 mg p. 183
Caduet 10/10 mg pp. 65,1052	**Calan** 40 mg p. 1205

Calan SR 240 mg p. 1205	**Capoten** 12.5 mg p. 192	**Capoten** 25 mg p. 192

Capoten 50 mg p. 192	**Cardizem** 30 mg p. 369
Cardizem 60 mg p. 369	**Cardizem CD** 180 mg p. 369

E

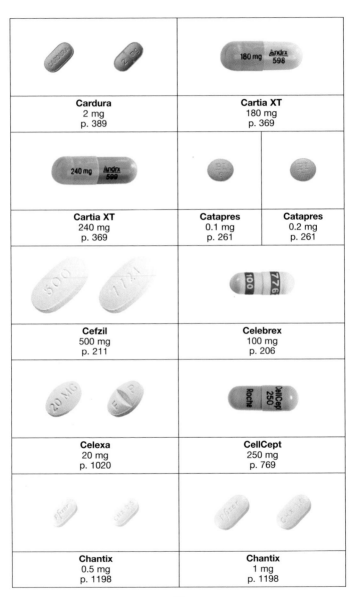

Cardura 2 mg p. 389	**Cartia XT** 180 mg p. 369
Cartia XT 240 mg p. 369	**Catapres** 0.1 mg p. 261	**Catapres** 0.2 mg p. 261
Cefzil 500 mg p. 211	**Celebrex** 100 mg p. 206
Celexa 20 mg p. 1020	**CellCept** 250 mg p. 769
Chantix 0.5 mg p. 1198	**Chantix** 1 mg p. 1198

F

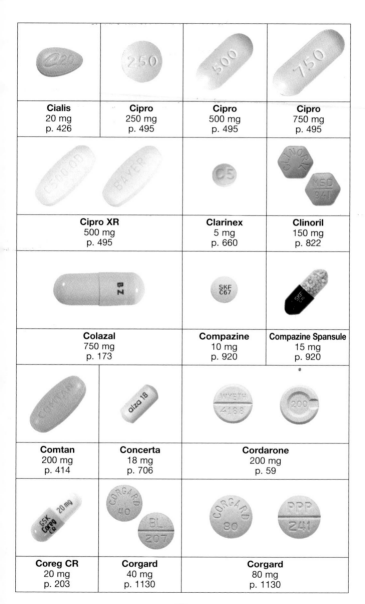

Cialis 20 mg p. 426	**Cipro** 250 mg p. 495	**Cipro** 500 mg p. 495	**Cipro** 750 mg p. 495
Cipro XR 500 mg p. 495		**Clarinex** 5 mg p. 660	**Clinoril** 150 mg p. 822
Colazal 750 mg p. 173		**Compazine** 10 mg p. 920	**Compazine Spansule** 15 mg p. 920
Comtan 200 mg p. 414	**Concerta** 18 mg p. 706	**Cordarone** 200 mg p. 59	
Coreg CR 20 mg p. 203	**Corgard** 40 mg p. 1130	**Corgard** 80 mg p. 1130	

G

Coumadin 5 mg p. 1212	**Covera-HS** 180 mg p. 1205	**Cozaar** 25 mg p. 81	**Cozaar** 50 mg p. 81
Cymbalta 20 mg p. 1200	**Dalmane** 30 mg p. 503	**Darvocet-N** 100 mg p. 929	
Daypro 600 mg p. 822		**Deconamine SR** 8/120 mg p. 97	
Demerol 50 mg p. 685		**Depakote** 125 mg p. 1194	**Depakote** 250 mg p. 1194
Depakote ER 500 mg p. 1194	**Depakote Sprinkle** 125 mg p. 1194	**Desyrel** 50 mg p. 1159	**Desyrel** 100 mg p. 1159

H

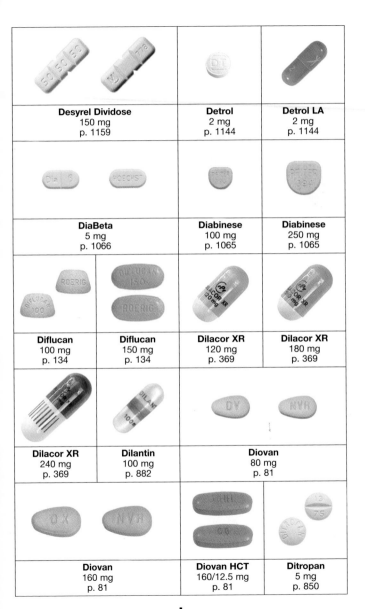

Desyrel Dividose 150 mg p. 1159	**Detrol** 2 mg p. 1144	**Detrol LA** 2 mg p. 1144
DiaBeta 5 mg p. 1066	**Diabinese** 100 mg p. 1065	**Diabinese** 250 mg p. 1065
Diflucan 100 mg p. 134	**Diflucan** 150 mg p. 134	**Dilacor XR** 120 mg p. 369	**Dilacor XR** 180 mg p. 369
Dilacor XR 240 mg p. 369	**Dilantin** 100 mg p. 882	**Diovan** 80 mg p. 81	
Diovan 160 mg p. 81		**Diovan HCT** 160/12.5 mg p. 81	**Ditropan** 5 mg p. 850

I

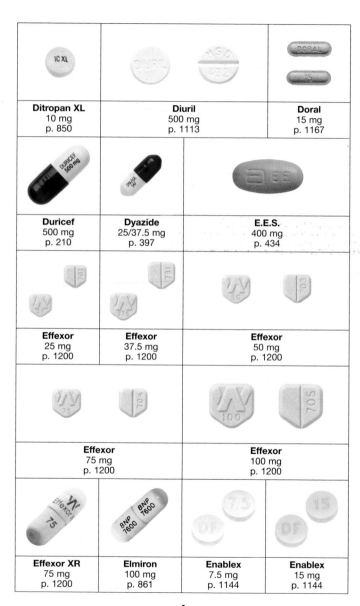

Ditropan XL 10 mg p. 850	**Diuril** 500 mg p. 1113	**Doral** 15 mg p. 1167
Duricef 500 mg p. 210	**Dyazide** 25/37.5 mg p. 397	**E.E.S.** 400 mg p. 434
Effexor 25 mg p. 1200	**Effexor** 37.5 mg p. 1200	**Effexor** 50 mg p. 1200
Effexor 75 mg p. 1200		**Effexor** 100 mg p. 1200
Effexor XR 75 mg p. 1200	**Elmiron** 100 mg p. 861	**Enablex** 7.5 mg p. 1144 — **Enablex** 15 mg p. 1144

J

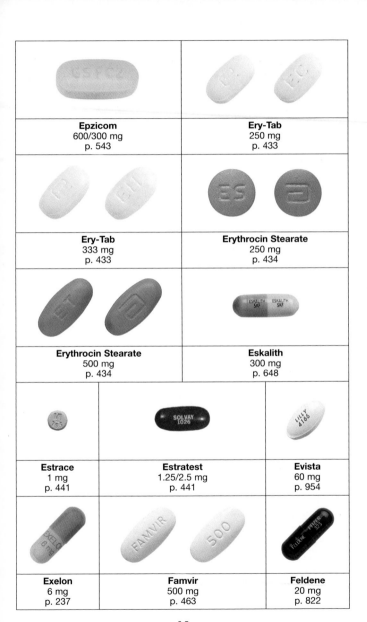

Epzicom
600/300 mg
p. 543

Ery-Tab
250 mg
p. 433

Ery-Tab
333 mg
p. 433

Erythrocin Stearate
250 mg
p. 434

Erythrocin Stearate
500 mg
p. 434

Eskalith
300 mg
p. 648

Estrace
1 mg
p. 441

Estratest
1.25/2.5 mg
p. 441

Evista
60 mg
p. 954

Exelon
6 mg
p. 237

Famvir
500 mg
p. 463

Feldene
20 mg
p. 822

K

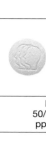

Fioricet
50/325/40 mg
pp. 481, 863

Flagyl
250 mg
p. 718

Flexeril
10 mg
p. 338

Flomax
0.4 mg
p. 1080

Floxin
400 mg
p. 496

Fosamax
10 mg
p. 164

Fosamax
40 mg
p. 164

Geodon
20 mg
p. 1228

Gleevec
100 mg
p. 754

Glucophage
500 mg
p. 696

Glucophage
850 mg
p. 696

Glucophage XR
500 mg
p. 696

L

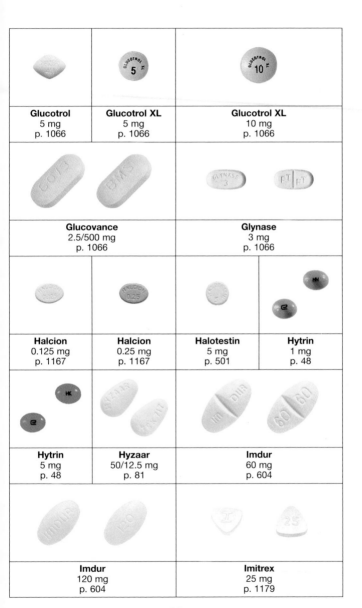

Glucotrol 5 mg p. 1066	**Glucotrol XL** 5 mg p. 1066	**Glucotrol XL** 10 mg p. 1066

Glucovance 2.5/500 mg p. 1066	**Glynase** 3 mg p. 1066

Halcion 0.125 mg p. 1167	**Halcion** 0.25 mg p. 1167	**Halotestin** 5 mg p. 501	**Hytrin** 1 mg p. 48

Hytrin 5 mg p. 48	**Hyzaar** 50/12.5 mg p. 81	**Imdur** 60 mg p. 604

Imdur 120 mg p. 604	**Imitrex** 25 mg p. 1179

M

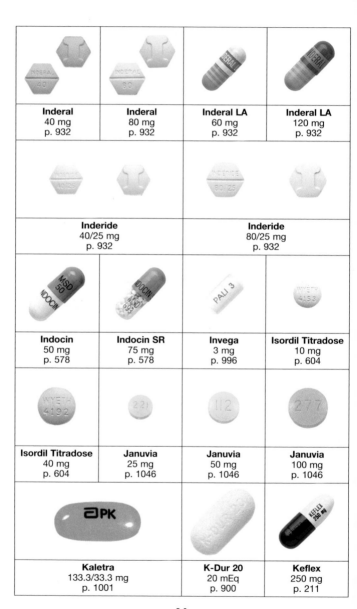

Inderal 40 mg p. 932	**Inderal** 80 mg p. 932	**Inderal LA** 60 mg p. 932	**Inderal LA** 120 mg p. 932
Inderide 40/25 mg p. 932		**Inderide** 80/25 mg p. 932	
Indocin 50 mg p. 578	**Indocin SR** 75 mg p. 578	**Invega** 3 mg p. 996	**Isordil Titradose** 10 mg p. 604
Isordil Titradose 40 mg p. 604	**Januvia** 25 mg p. 1046	**Januvia** 50 mg p. 1046	**Januvia** 100 mg p. 1046
Kaletra 133.3/33.3 mg p. 1001		**K-Dur 20** 20 mEq p. 900	**Keflex** 250 mg p. 211

N

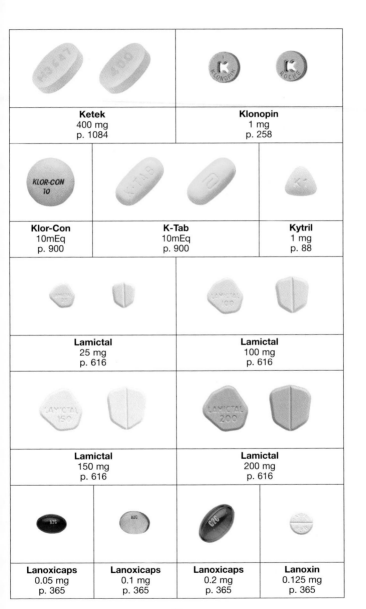

Ketek 400 mg p. 1084	**Klonopin** 1 mg p. 258

Klor-Con 10mEq p. 900	**K-Tab** 10mEq p. 900	**Kytril** 1 mg p. 88

Lamictal 25 mg p. 616	**Lamictal** 100 mg p. 616

Lamictal 150 mg p. 616	**Lamictal** 200 mg p. 616

Lanoxicaps 0.05 mg p. 365	**Lanoxicaps** 0.1 mg p. 365	**Lanoxicaps** 0.2 mg p. 365	**Lanoxin** 0.125 mg p. 365

Lanoxin 0.25 mg p. 365	**Lanoxin** 0.5 mg p. 365	**Lasix** 40 mg p. 653
Lasix 80 mg p. 653	**Lescol** 20 mg p. 1052	**Lescol** 40 mg p. 1052

Levaquin 500 mg p. 495	**Levatol** 20 mg p. 714	**Levitra** 10 mg p. 426

Levoxyl 25 mcg p. 1118	**Levoxyl** 50 mcg p. 1118	**Levoxyl** 100 mcg p. 1118	**Levoxyl** 125 mcg p. 1118

Levoxyl 175 mg p. 1118	**Lexapro** 10 mg p. 1020

P

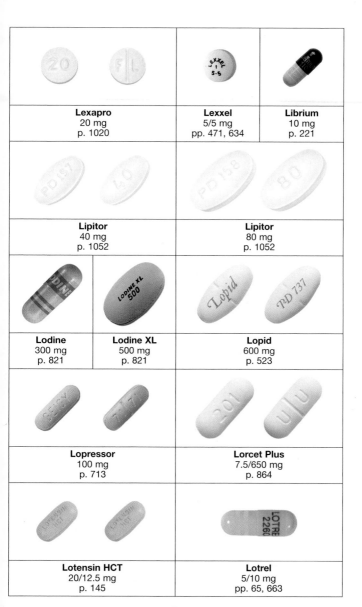

| **Lexapro** 20 mg p. 1020 | **Lexxel** 5/5 mg pp. 471, 634 | **Librium** 10 mg p. 221 |

| **Lipitor** 40 mg p. 1052 | **Lipitor** 80 mg p. 1052 |

| **Lodine** 300 mg p. 821 | **Lodine XL** 500 mg p. 821 | **Lopid** 600 mg p. 523 |

| **Lopressor** 100 mg p. 713 | **Lorcet Plus** 7.5/650 mg p. 864 |

| **Lotensin HCT** 20/12.5 mg p. 145 | **Lotrel** 5/10 mg pp. 65, 663 |

Q

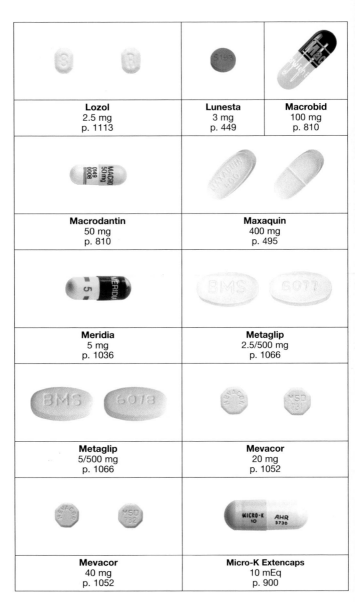

Lozol 2.5 mg p. 1113	**Lunesta** 3 mg p. 449	**Macrobid** 100 mg p. 810
Macrodantin 50 mg p. 810		**Maxaquin** 400 mg p. 495
Meridia 5 mg p. 1036		**Metaglip** 2.5/500 mg p. 1066
Metaglip 5/500 mg p. 1066		**Mevacor** 20 mg p. 1052
Mevacor 40 mg p. 1052		**Micro-K Extencaps** 10 mEq p. 900

R

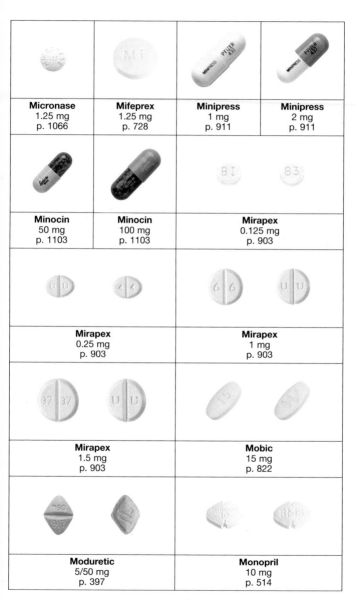

Micronase 1.25 mg p. 1066	**Mifeprex** 1.25 mg p. 728	**Minipress** 1 mg p. 911	**Minipress** 2 mg p. 911

Minocin 50 mg p. 1103	**Minocin** 100 mg p. 1103	**Mirapex** 0.125 mg p. 903

Mirapex 0.25 mg p. 903	**Mirapex** 1 mg p. 903

Mirapex 1.5 mg p. 903	**Mobic** 15 mg p. 822

Moduretic 5/50 mg p. 397	**Monopril** 10 mg p. 514

S

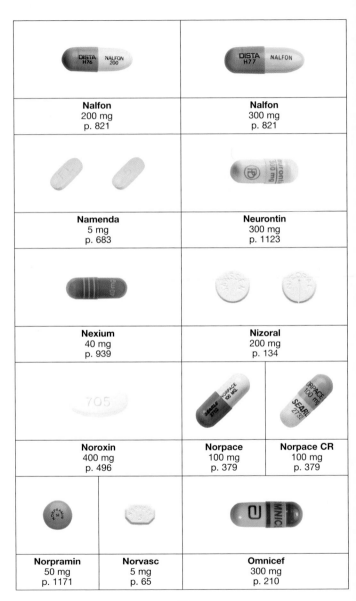

Nalfon 200 mg p. 821	**Nalfon** 300 mg p. 821
Namenda 5 mg p. 683	**Neurontin** 300 mg p. 1123
Nexium 40 mg p. 939	**Nizoral** 200 mg p. 134
Noroxin 400 mg p. 496	**Norpace** 100 mg p. 379 / **Norpace CR** 100 mg p. 379
Norpramin 50 mg p. 1171 / **Norvasc** 5 mg p. 65	**Omnicef** 300 mg p. 210

T

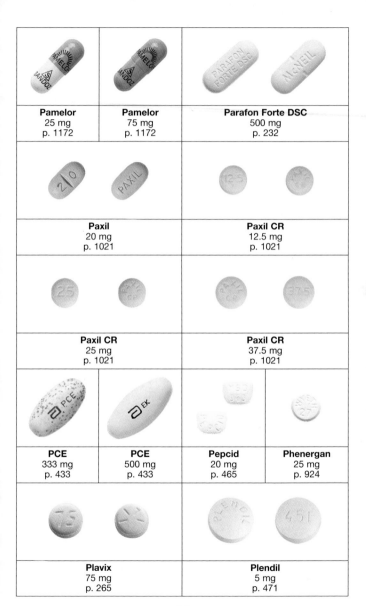

Pamelor 25 mg p. 1172	**Pamelor** 75 mg p. 1172	**Parafon Forte DSC** 500 mg p. 232

Paxil 20 mg p. 1021	**Paxil CR** 12.5 mg p. 1021

Paxil CR 25 mg p. 1021	**Paxil CR** 37.5 mg p. 1021

PCE 333 mg p. 433	**PCE** 500 mg p. 433	**Pepcid** 20 mg p. 465	**Phenergan** 25 mg p. 924

Plavix 75 mg p. 265	**Plendil** 5 mg p. 471

U

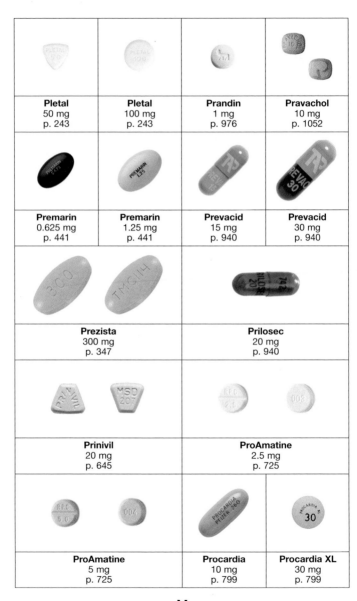

Pletal 50 mg p. 243	**Pletal** 100 mg p. 243	**Prandin** 1 mg p. 976	**Pravachol** 10 mg p. 1052
Premarin 0.625 mg p. 441	**Premarin** 1.25 mg p. 441	**Prevacid** 15 mg p. 940	**Prevacid** 30 mg p. 940

Prezista 300 mg p. 347	**Prilosec** 20 mg p. 940
Prinivil 20 mg p. 645	**ProAmatine** 2.5 mg p. 725

ProAmatine 5 mg p. 725	**Procardia** 10 mg p. 799	**Procardia XL** 30 mg p. 799

V

Procardia XL 60 mg p. 799	**Procardia XL** 90 mg p. 799	**Prograf** 1 mg p. 1071	**Prograf** 5 mg p. 1071
Prometrium 100 mg p. 680	**Proscar** 5 mg p. 478		**Protonix** 40 mg p. 940
Provera 2.5 mg p. 679	**Provera** 5 mg p. 679	**Prozac** 10 mg p. 1020	**Prozac** 20 mg p. 1020
Prozac Weekly 90 mg p. 1020	**Quinidex Extentabs** 300 mg p. 950	**Razadyne** 8 mg p. 237	
Reglan 10 mg p. 710		**Remeron** 30 mg p. 738	

W

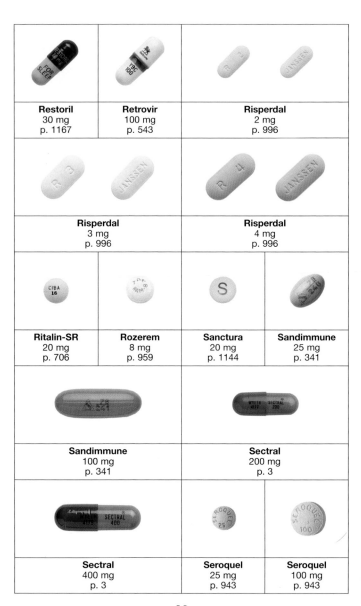

Restoril 30 mg p. 1167	**Retrovir** 100 mg p. 543	**Risperdal** 2 mg p. 996	
Risperdal 3 mg p. 996		**Risperdal** 4 mg p. 996	
Ritalin-SR 20 mg p. 706	**Rozerem** 8 mg p. 959	**Sanctura** 20 mg p. 1144	**Sandimmune** 25 mg p. 341
Sandimmune 100 mg p. 341		**Sectral** 200 mg p. 3	
Sectral 400 mg p. 3		**Seroquel** 25 mg p. 943	**Seroquel** 100 mg p. 943

X

	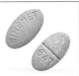	
Seroquel 200 mg p. 943	**Sinemet** 10/100 mg p. 1042	**Sinemet** 25/250 mg p. 1042

Sinemet CR 50/200 mg p. 1042	**Singulair** 10 mg p. 626

	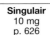
Skelaxin 400 mg p. 694	**Sonata** 5 mg p. 1223

Sprycel 70 mg p. 754	**Starlix** 60 mg p. 976

Strattera 10 mg p. 125	**Strattera** 25 mg p. 125

Y

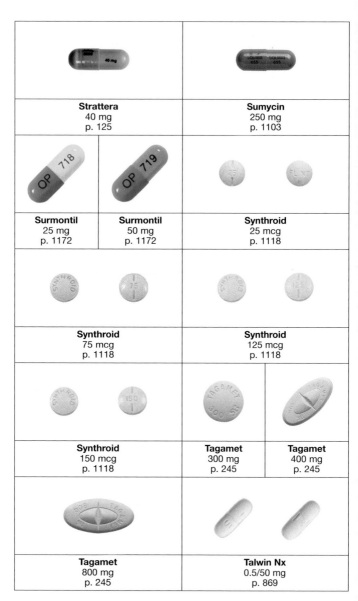

Strattera 40 mg p. 125	**Sumycin** 250 mg p. 1103
Surmontil 25 mg p. 1172 **Surmontil** 50 mg p. 1172	**Synthroid** 25 mcg p. 1118
Synthroid 75 mcg p. 1118	**Synthroid** 125 mcg p. 1118
Synthroid 150 mcg p. 1118	**Tagamet** 300 mg p. 245 **Tagamet** 400 mg p. 245
Tagamet 800 mg p. 245	**Talwin Nx** 0.5/50 mg p. 869

Z

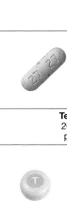	
Tegretol 200 mg p. 196	**Tegretol (Chewable)** 100 mg p. 196

Tegretol-XR 100 mg p. 196	**Tiazac** 240 mg p. 369	**Ticlid** 250 mg p. 1126

Tindamax 500 mg p. 718	**Tolectin** 600 mg p. 822

Tolinase 100 mg p. 1066	**Tolinase** 500 mg p. 1066	**Topamax** 25 mg p. 1148

		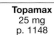
Toprol-XL 50 mg p. 713	**Toprol-XL** 100 mg p. 713	**Tranxene T-Tab** 15 mg p. 268

AA

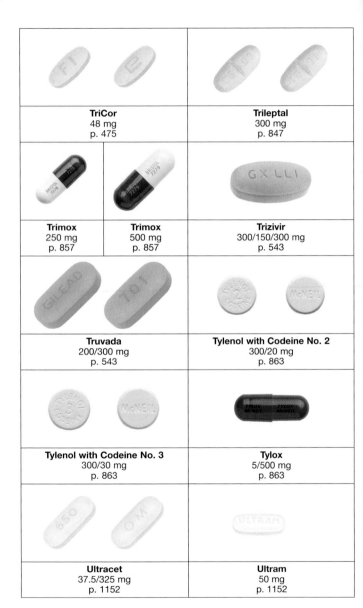

TriCor 48 mg p. 475	**Trileptal** 300 mg p. 847

Trimox 250 mg p. 857	**Trimox** 500 mg p. 857	**Trizivir** 300/150/300 mg p. 543

Truvada 200/300 mg p. 543	**Tylenol with Codeine No. 2** 300/20 mg p. 863

Tylenol with Codeine No. 3 300/30 mg p. 863	**Tylox** 5/500 mg p. 863

Ultracet 37.5/325 mg p. 1152	**Ultram** 50 mg p. 1152

BB

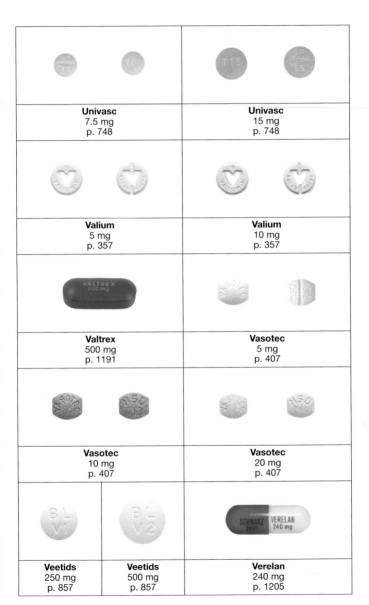

Univasc 7.5 mg p. 748	**Univasc** 15 mg p. 748
Valium 5 mg p. 357	**Valium** 10 mg p. 357
Valtrex 500 mg p. 1191	**Vasotec** 5 mg p. 407
Vasotec 10 mg p. 407	**Vasotec** 20 mg p. 407

Veetids 250 mg p. 857	**Veetids** 500 mg p. 857	**Verelan** 240 mg p. 1205

CC

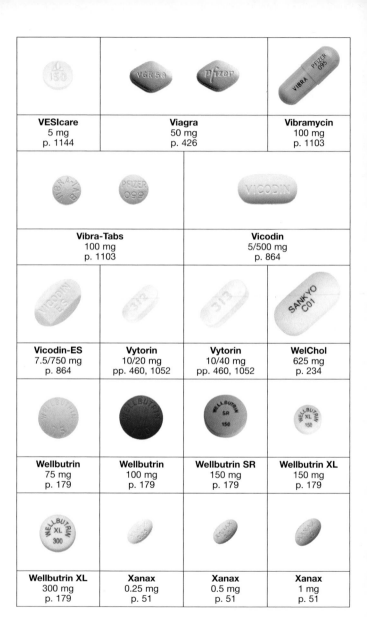

VESIcare 5 mg p. 1144	**Viagra** 50 mg p. 426	**Vibramycin** 100 mg p. 1103

Vibra-Tabs 100 mg p. 1103	**Vicodin** 5/500 mg p. 864

Vicodin-ES 7.5/750 mg p. 864	**Vytorin** 10/20 mg pp. 460, 1052	**Vytorin** 10/40 mg pp. 460, 1052	**WelChol** 625 mg p. 234
Wellbutrin 75 mg p. 179	**Wellbutrin** 100 mg p. 179	**Wellbutrin SR** 150 mg p. 179	**Wellbutrin XL** 150 mg p. 179
Wellbutrin XL 300 mg p. 179	**Xanax** 0.25 mg p. 51	**Xanax** 0.5 mg p. 51	**Xanax** 1 mg p. 51

DD

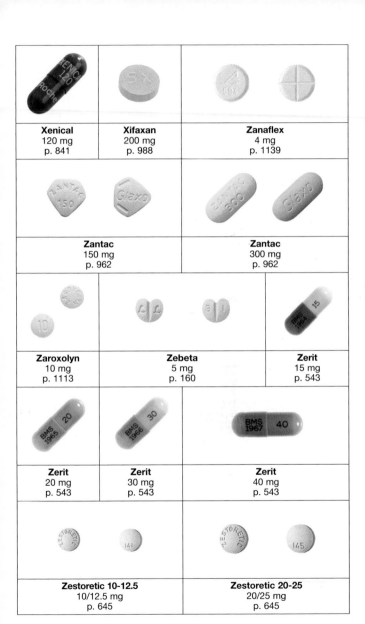

Xenical 120 mg p. 841	**Xifaxan** 200 mg p. 988	**Zanaflex** 4 mg p. 1139	
Zantac 150 mg p. 962		**Zantac** 300 mg p. 962	
Zaroxolyn 10 mg p. 1113	**Zebeta** 5 mg p. 160		**Zerit** 15 mg p. 543
Zerit 20 mg p. 543	**Zerit** 30 mg p. 543	**Zerit** 40 mg p. 543	
Zestoretic 10-12.5 10/12.5 mg p. 645		**Zestoretic 20-25** 20/25 mg p. 645	

EE

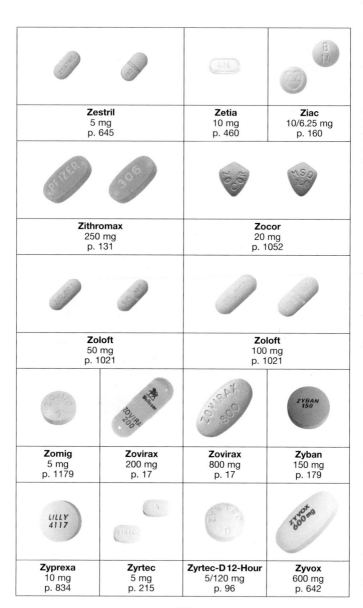

Zestril 5 mg p. 645	**Zetia** 10 mg p. 460	**Ziac** 10/6.25 mg p. 160
Zithromax 250 mg p. 131	**Zocor** 20 mg p. 1052	
Zoloft 50 mg p. 1021	**Zoloft** 100 mg p. 1021	

Zomig 5 mg p. 1179	**Zovirax** 200 mg p. 17	**Zovirax** 800 mg p. 17	**Zyban** 150 mg p. 179
Zyprexa 10 mg p. 834	**Zyrtec** 5 mg p. 215	**Zyrtec-D 12-Hour** 5/120 mg p. 96	**Zyvox** 600 mg p. 642

FF

until your doctor can determine if you are likely to develop this effect.

Call your doctor if you develop any severe or unusual side effects, such as abdominal pain; bleeding from the rectum; severe diarrhea; headache; nausea or vomiting; visual difficulties; severe muscle, bone, or joint aches or pains; or unusual sensitivity to sunlight or to ultraviolet light.

Your acne may worsen when isotretinoin treatment begins, but then it should improve. Do not be alarmed if this happens, but tell your doctor.

Avoid using depilatories or waxing while using isotretinoin, and for 6 months after treatment.

Do not donate blood during isotretinoin treatment—or for at least 30 days after you have stopped—because of the risk to the fetus of a pregnant woman who may receive the blood.

If you forget a dose of isotretinoin, take it as soon as you remember. If it is almost time for your next dose, skip the one you forgot and continue with your regular schedule. Do not take a double dose.

Special Populations

Pregnancy/Breast-feeding: Pregnant women should never take isotretinoin because it will injure the fetus. Your doctor will confirm that you are not pregnant before starting isotretinoin (see "Special Information"). Accidental pregnancy during isotretinoin therapy may be grounds for an abortion due to the severe birth defects this drug will cause. Call your doctor immediately.

It is not known if isotretinoin passes into breast milk. Nursing mothers who must take it should use infant formula.

Seniors: Seniors may take this medication without special restriction.

Kariva   *see **Contraceptives,** page 287*

Generic Name

Ketotifen   (kee-toe-TIH-fen) Ⓖ

Brand Names

Alaway Eyedrops   Zaditor Eyedrops

The information in this profile also applies to the following drug:

Generic Ingredient: Lodoxamide
Alomide Eyedrops

Type of Drug

Antihistamine.

Prescribed For

Conjunctivitis (pinkeye) caused by allergies and itching of the eyes caused by allergic reaction.

General Information

Ketotifen relieves and prevents eye itchiness and irritation associated with seasonal allergies. Lodoxamide only prevents itchiness and allergies. They achieve their effects by stabilizing mast cells in the eye, which prevents the release of chemicals such as histamine that cause redness and irritation during an allergic reaction. Ketotifen starts working within minutes after administering the drops. This drug has not been studied in children under age 3. Lodoxamide may be used in children age 2 and over.

Cautions and Warnings

Do not use this drug if you are **allergic** or **sensitive** to any of its ingredients.

Possible Side Effects

▼ Most common: eye redness, headache, and runny nose.
▼ Less common: a burning or stinging sensation in the eye, eye discharge, tearing, increased sensitivity to bright light, dilation of the pupil, allergic reactions, rash, flu-like symptoms, and sore throat.

Drug Interactions

If you use more than 1 eyedrop medication, separate doses of these drugs by at least 1 hour.

Usual Dose

Ketotifen

Adult and child (age 3 and over): 1 drop in the affected eye every 8–12 hours.

Lodoxamide

Adult and child (age 2 and over): 1–2 drops in affected eye 4 times a day.

Overdosage

Accidental ingestion of an entire bottle of ketotifen is unlikely to cause side effects since it contains less than 2 mg of medicine. Call your local poison control center or a hospital emergency room for more information. If you seek treatment, ALWAYS bring the prescription bottle or container.

Special Information

Do not wear contact lenses if your eyes are red because they may worsen the irritation.

Ketotifen does not alleviate eye irritation caused by contact lenses.

Remove your soft contact lenses before using ketotifen eyedrops; you may replace them 10 minutes after a dose.

To prevent contamination, do not allow the eyedropper to touch your fingers, eyelids, or any surface.

If you forget to administer a dose, do so as soon as you remember. If it is almost time for your next dose, skip the dose you forgot and continue with your regular schedule. Do not take a double dose.

Special Populations

Pregnancy/Breast-feeding: In animal studies, very large dosages of ketotifen caused bone malformations in the fetus. When this drug is considered crucial by your doctor, its potential benefits must be carefully weighed against its risks.

Though unlikely, ketotifen may pass into breast milk. Nursing mothers who must use this drug should use infant formula.

Seniors: Seniors may use this drug without special precaution.

Klor-Con   *see Potassium Replacements, page 899*

Generic Name

Labetalol   (luh-BET-uh-lol) Ⓖ

Brand Name

Trandate

Type of Drug

Adrenergic blocker and antihypertensive.

Prescribed For

Hypertension (high blood pressure).

General Information

Labetalol hydrochloride is unique because it selectively blocks both alpha- and beta-adrenergic impulses. This combination of actions contributes to its ability to reduce blood pressure. Other drugs can increase or decrease heart rate; labetalol has an advantage over other beta blockers because it rarely affects heart rate. Labetalol may be used alone or in combination with other antihypertensive drugs, especially loop and thiazide diuretics.

Cautions and Warnings

Do not take labetalol if you are **allergic** or **sensitive** to any of its ingredients. People with **asthma, chronic bronchitis, emphysema,** severe **heart failure, reduced heart rate,** and **heart block** (disruption of the electrical impulses that control heart rate) should not take labetalol. People with **angina** who take labetalol for hypertension risk aggravating their angina if they suddenly stop taking the drug. These people should have their dosage reduced gradually over 1–2 weeks. Labetalol should be used with caution if you have **liver disease**.

Possible Side Effects

Side effects develop early and increase with dosage.
▼ Most common: dizziness, tingling of the scalp, nausea, upset stomach, distortion in the sense of taste, fatigue, sweating, impotence, urinary difficulties, bile-duct blockage, bronchial spasm, breathing difficulties, muscle weakness, cramps, dry eyes, blurred vision, rash, facial swelling, and hair loss.
▼ Less common: aggravation of lupus erythematosus (chronic condition affecting the body's connective tissue), stuffy nose, headache, depression, confusion, disorientation, loss of short-term memory, emotional instability, colitis, drug allergy (symptoms include fever, sore throat, and breathing difficulties), and a reduction in levels of white blood cells and blood platelets.

Drug Interactions

- Labetalol may suppress normal signs of low blood sugar and interfere with the action of oral antidiabetes drugs.
- Combining labetalol and a tricyclic antidepressant may cause tremor.
- Labetalol may interfere with the effect of some antiasthma drugs, especially ephedrine, isoproterenol, and other beta stimulants.
- Cimetidine increases the amount of labetalol absorbed into the bloodstream from oral tablets.
- Glutethimide decreases the amount of labetalol in the blood.
- Labetalol may increase the blood-pressure-lowering effect of nitroglycerin.
- Use caution when combining labetalol with calcium channel blockers, especially verapamil.
- Labetalol should not be combined with halothane anesthesia.

Food Interactions

This drug may be taken with food if it upsets your stomach. Food increases the amount of labetalol absorbed into the blood.

Usual Dose

Adult: starting dosage—100 mg twice a day; may be increased gradually to as much as 1200 mg twice a day. Maintenance dosage—200–400 mg twice a day.

Seniors: starting dosage—100 mg twice a day. Maintenance dosage—100–200 mg twice a day.

Child: not recommended.

Overdosage

Overdose slows heart rate and causes an excessive drop in blood pressure. The possible consequences of these effects can be treated only in a hospital emergency room. ALWAYS bring the prescription bottle or container.

Special Information

You may experience scalp tingling, especially when you first start taking labetalol.

Labetalol is meant to be taken on a continuing basis. Do not stop this drug unless instructed to do so by your doctor.

Weakness; swelling of your ankles, feet, or legs; breathing difficulties; or other side effects should be reported to your doctor as soon as possible. Most side effects are not serious, but about 7% of people have to switch to another drug because of them.

If you forget a dose, take it as soon as possible. If it is within 8 hours of your next dose, skip the dose you forgot and go back to your regular schedule. Do not take a double dose.

Special Populations

Pregnancy/Breast-feeding: Labetalol enters the fetal circulation. Women who are or might be pregnant should not take this drug without their doctor's approval. When the drug is considered crucial by your doctor, its possible benefits must be carefully weighed against its risks.

This drug passes into breast milk. Nursing mothers who must take labetalol should consider using infant formula.

Seniors: Seniors may be more sensitive to the effects of labetalol. Your dosage must be individually adjusted by your doctor, especially if you have liver disease. Seniors may be more likely to suffer from cold hands and feet, reduced body temperature, chest pain, feeling unwell, sudden breathing difficulties, sweating, or changes in heartbeat.

Lamictal   *see Lamotrigine, below*

Generic Name

Lamotrigine   (lam-OE-trih-jene)

Brand Names
Lamictal   Lamictal CD

Type of Drug
Anticonvulsant.

Prescribed For
Adult epilepsy and partial seizure; tonic-clonic, temporal lobe, absence, and myoclonic seizures; bipolar disorder; and for infants and children with Lennox-Gastaut syndrome.

General Information
Much like phenytoin and carbamazepine, lamotrigine stabilizes voltage-dependent channels in the brain. This prevents the release

of chemicals that would stimulate the nervous system and lead to seizure. It reaches maximum blood concentration in 1½–5 hours. Lamotrigine is eliminated from the body by the liver.

Cautions and Warnings

Do not take lamotrigine if you are **allergic** or **sensitive** to any of its ingredients.

Lamotrigine may cause severe and possibly life-threatening rashes, nearly always within 2–8 weeks of use. Minor rashes also occur, but it is not possible to tell which ones may become life threatening. If you develop a rash or swollen glands while taking this drug, call your doctor at once.

Twenty sudden and unexplained deaths occurred among 4700 people taking lamotrigine before it was approved for general use. These deaths are thought to be unrelated to lamotrigine.

Five people taking lamotrigine died from acute liver failure or multi-organ failure before the drug was approved for general use. It is not known if the drug played a role in these deaths.

Lamotrigine is not recommended for general use in **children under age 18**.

Lamotrigine binds to melanin, a body hormone found in the skin and eyes. The long-term effects of lamotrigine on the eyes are not known.

When you stop taking lamotrigine, the dose should be reduced gradually over a period of 2 weeks or more to prevent withdrawal seizures.

Status epilepticus, a severe seizure disorder, and **worsening of existing seizure disorders** may develop in a small number of people taking lamotrigine.

People with **heart disease** or severe **kidney or liver disease** should use this drug with caution.

Lamotrigine may cause unusual sensitivity to the sun. Wear protective clothing and use sunscreen.

Possible Side Effects

▼ Most common: headache, dizziness, nausea, vomiting, weakness, tiredness, loss of coordination, double vision, and blurred vision.

▼ Common: accidental injury, flu-like symptoms, abdominal pain, infection, neck pain, feeling unwell, worsening of seizure, diarrhea, upset stomach, constipation, dental problems,

Possible Side Effects (continued)

sleeplessness, tremors, depression, anxiety, convulsions, irritability, itching, visual difficulties, painful menstruation, and vaginal irritation.

▼ Less common: chills, hot flashes, heart palpitations, appetite loss, dry mouth, joint ache, muscle weakness, speech disorders, sore throat, coughing, memory loss, confusion, loss of concentration, emotional upset, fainting, racing thoughts, rolling of the eyes, muscle spasm, breathing difficulties, hair loss, acne, ear pain, ringing or buzzing in the ears, and missed periods.

▼ Rare: Rare side effects can occur in almost any part of the body. Contact your doctor if you experience any side effect not listed above.

Drug Interactions

- Combining lamotrigine and sodium valproate doubles lamotrigine concentrations in the blood and reduces those of valproate by ¼. Dosage adjustments are necessary. Combining these drugs may also increase the risk of rash.

- Combining carbamazepine and lamotrigine increases carbamazepine blood levels, possibly leading to side effects, and reduces the amount of lamotrigine in the blood by 40%.

- Combining acetaminophen and lamotrigine can slightly increase the rate at which lamotrigine is broken down, but occasional use of the 2 drugs together is not likely to be a problem. Regular acetaminophen users may require more lamotrigine.

- Anti-folate drugs—often used in cancer treatment—can increase the effects of lamotrigine.

- Phenobarbital and primidone may reduce the effects of lamotrigine.

- Phenytoin reduces the amount of lamotrigine in the blood by about ½.

- Rifamycins, succinimides, contraceptive drugs, progestins, and oxcarbazepine may reduce the effectiveness of lamotrigine.

Food Interactions

None known.

Usual Dose

Adult and Child (age 12 and over): starting dosage—25 mg every other day or 25–50 mg every day depending on other medications being taken concurrently for seizure control. Increase gradually to a maximum daily dosage of 500 mg. Lamotrigine is usually taken twice a day; be sure to take your doses 12 hours apart. The chewable tablets can be swallowed whole, chewed, or dissolved in water or fruit juice.

Child (under age 12): Consult your doctor.

Overdosage

Symptoms include dizziness, headache, sleepiness, and coma. Take the victim to a hospital emergency room at once. ALWAYS bring the prescription bottle or container.

Special Information

Dosage increases may be required if your liver starts breaking down the drug faster over time. Periodic monitoring of lamotrigine blood levels is necessary to determine this.

People with impaired kidney or liver function may require smaller dosages.

Call your doctor at once if you develop a rash or swollen glands, but do not change your lamotrigine dosage or stop taking it until your doctor tells you to do so. If you stop taking lamotrigine on your own, do not restart it without telling your doctor.

Lamotrigine may cause drowsiness, dizziness, or blurred vision, effects that are increased by alcohol. Be careful while driving or engaging in any activity requiring concentration, alertness, and coordination.

If you take acetaminophen while you are taking lamotrigine, especially for a lamotrigine headache, do not take more acetaminophen than is recommended on the package.

If you take lamotrigine once a day and forget a dose, take it as soon as you remember. If it is within 8 hours of your next dose, skip the one you forgot and continue with your regular schedule. Do not take a double dose.

After the first 2 weeks of treatment, most people take lamotrigine twice a day. If you take it twice a day, be sure to take your medication every 12 hours. If you forget a dose, take it as soon as you remember. If it is within 4 hours of your next dose, take 1 dose as soon as you remember and another in 5 or 6 hours, then go back to your regular schedule.

Special Populations

Pregnancy/Breast-feeding: Animal studies suggest that lamotrigine causes fetal injury. It reduces the amount of folate in the fetus, an effect that is associated with birth defects. Seizure disorder itself also increases the risk of birth defects. Pregnant women should take lamotrigine only after discussing with their doctors its potential benefits and risks.

Lamotrigine passes into breast milk. Nursing mothers who must take it should use infant formula.

Seniors: Seniors may take lamotrigine without special restriction.

Lantus   see *Insulin,* page 585

Generic Name

Leflunomide   (leh-FLUE-noe-mide)

Brand Name

Arava

Type of Drug

Anti-inflammatory and antiproliferative (cell growth slower).

Prescribed For

Rheumatoid arthritis.

General Information

Leflunomide can help relieve symptoms of rheumatoid arthritis and slow the structural damage and erosion of tissues in affected joints. In studies, it was found to be as effective as methotrexate and sulfasalazine. It takes about a month for leflunomide to begin working and it reaches maximum effect in 3–6 months. The maximum effect is retained for as long as you take this medicine. Leflunomide is broken down in the liver.

Cautions and Warnings

Do not take leflunomide if you are **allergic** or **sensitive** to any of its ingredients.

Leflunomide causes birth defects and should not be taken during **pregnancy**.

Leflunomide causes liver irritation and an increase in certain liver enzymes. Your dosage may have to be reduced or the drug discontinued if the effect is severe. People with **liver disease** or **hepatitis B or C** should not take this drug. People with **kidney problems** should use it with caution.

New or worsening cough and difficulty breathing with or without fever may be a sign of an important drug side effect. Call your doctor at once if this happens.

Leflunomide is not recommended for people with severely **depressed immune systems, abnormal bone marrow,** or severe and uncontrolled **infection**.

Use of **live-virus vaccines** is not recommended while taking leflunomide.

Rare, serious skin reactions can occur with this drug. Call your doctor if you develop a skin rash or lesion in your mouth, nose, or rectum.

Possible Side Effects

▼ Most common: diarrhea, high blood pressure, nausea, hair loss, rash, and respiratory infection.

▼ Common: headache, upset stomach, stomach or abdominal pain, abnormal liver function, bronchitis, generalized pain, back pain, urinary infection, and accidents or injuries.

▼ Less common: chest pain, dizziness, tingling in the hands or feet, eczema, mouth ulcer, tooth disorder, itching, dry skin, appetite loss, vomiting, low blood potassium, weight loss, muscle pain, leg cramps, inflamed tendons, arthritis, cough, sore throat, pneumonia, runny nose, sinus irritation, allergic reaction, weakness, flu-like symptoms, and infections.

▼ Rare: Rare side effects can occur in almost any part of the body. Contact your doctor if you experience any side effect not listed above.

Drug Interactions

● Cholestyramine and charcoal rapidly reduce leflunomide blood levels.

- Rifampin increases the amount of leflunomide in the blood by 40%. These drugs should be mixed with caution.
- Leflunomide can increase the liver toxicity of other drugs that are toxic to the liver, such as methotrexate.
- Leflunomide increases blood levels of nonsteroidal anti-inflammatory drugs (NSAIDs). The importance of this effect is unclear.
- Leflunomide increases the amount of tolbutamide (an anti-diabetes drug) in the blood by up to 50%. The importance of this effect is unclear.
- Leflunomide, in rare cases, can increase the effects of warfarin.

Food Interactions

Leflunomide may be taken without regard to food or meals.

Usual Dose

Adult: 100 mg once a day for 3 days, then 20 mg once a day. If the side effects are intolerable, the dose may be lowered to 10 mg a day.

Child: not recommended.

When you stop taking leflunomide, it is recommended that you follow a drug elimination procedure: Take 8 g of cholestyramine (ordinarily used to help lower blood cholesterol) 3 times a day for 11 days. Without this procedure, it may take up to 2 years to eliminate the drug and its breakdown products from your body.

Overdosage

Symptoms are likely to include drug side effects. Take the victim to a hospital emergency room at once. ALWAYS bring the prescription bottle or container.

Special Information

Your liver function must be monitored regularly while you take this drug.

If you forget a dose, take it as soon as you remember. If it is almost time for your next dose, skip the one you forgot and continue with your regular schedule.

Special Populations

Pregnancy/Breast-feeding: Leflunomide causes birth defects and should not be used during pregnancy. Women of childbearing age must be tested for pregnancy before taking leflunomide and use effective contraception during treatment and until the drug is completely eliminated from the body. Women who plan to become pregnant after discontinuing the drug must follow the drug elimination procedure (see "Usual Dose").

Leflunomide may pass into breast milk. Nursing mothers who must take it should use infant formula.

Seniors: Seniors may take this drug without special precaution.

Generic Name

Lenalidomide (len-ah-LID-oh-mide)

Brand Name

Revlimid

Type of Drug

Immune system modulator.

Prescribed For

Multiple myeloma and transfusion-dependent anemia.

General Information

Lenalidomide has a number of known actions, including antineoplastic, immune system modulating and stopping cancerous tumors from growing new blood vessels that feed them so they can continue to grow, and acting as an anti-inflammatory agent by decreasing inflammatory and increasing anti-inflammatory proteins in the body. Its exact mechanism of action in multiple myeloma and anemia is not known. When prescribed for multiple myeloma, it is accompanied by dexamethasone, a corticosteroid drug. It is rapidly absorbed into the bloodstream and probably passes out of the body in the urine. Lenalidomide is available only through doctors and pharmacies that have registered with a special distribution program called RevAssist designed to prevent pregnant women from taking it.

Cautions and Warnings

Do not take lenalidomide if you are **allergic** or **sensitive** to any of its ingredients.

Lenalidomide can cause birth defects and fetal death. Do not take it if you are **pregnant**. Women of child-bearing potential must have 2 negative pregnancy tests and use an effective form of birth control for 4 weeks prior to starting treatment with lenalidomide.

Men taking this drug—even those who have had a vasectomy—must wear a condom to protect female partners from exposure to semen containing lenalidomide and continue this practice for 4 weeks after stopping the medicine. For more information, see "Pregnancy/Breast Feeding."

Lenalidomide is associated with significant reductions in white-blood-cell and platelet counts, so people taking it should have blood counts every week for the first 8 weeks of therapy.

Lenalidomide increases the risk of blood clots in the lungs and deep veins in the legs. Shortness of breath, chest pain, and arm or leg swelling can be signs a clot has formed.

The safety of lenalidomide in people with **kidney disease** is not known.

Possible Side Effects

▼ Most common: reduced white-blood-cell count without fever and reduced platelet count, itching, rash, dry skin, diarrhea, constipation, nausea, abdominal pains, vomiting, sore throat, nose and throat irritation, cough, difficulty breathing, nose bleeds, fatigue, fever, arm or leg swelling, generalized pain, joint pain, muscle cramps, leg pain, dizziness, and headache.

▼ Common: reduced white-blood-cell count with fever, dry mouth, bruising, night sweats, increase in overall sweating, nosebleeds, swelling, loose stools, shortness of breath after exercise, runny nose, bronchitis, shaking chills, muscle pain, reduced sense of touch, taste changes, tingling or pain in the hands or feet, low blood potassium or magnesium, appetite loss, sleeplessness, depression, high blood pressure, pain on urination, heart palpitations, and low thyroid activity.

▼ Less common: fainting, respiratory and other infections, fluid in the lungs, multi-organ failure, weakness, and confusion.

▼ Rare: Rare side effects can affect almost any part of the body. Contact your doctor if you experience any side effect not listed above.

Drug Interactions

● Lenalidomide can increase blood levels of digoxin by 14%. Periodic testing of digoxin blood levels with possible dose adjustment is recommended.

Food Interactions

This medicine can be taken without regard to food or meals.

Usual Dose

Adult (age 18 and over): 5–25 mg a day with water. Starting dose varies according to the condition being treated and is adjusted according to response and side effects.

Child (under age 18): not recommended.

Overdosage

There is no information on lenalidomide overdose. Take the overdose victim to a hospital emergency room at once for treatment. ALWAYS bring the prescription bottle or container.

Special Information

Do not break, chew, or open these capsules.

Call your doctor at once if you develop difficulty breathing, chest pain, or arm or leg swelling.

If you forget a dose of lenalidomide, take it as soon as you remember. If you do not remember until it is almost time for your next dose, skip the one you forgot and continue with your regular schedule. Do not take a double dose of this medicine.

Special Populations

Pregnancy/Breast-feeding: Lenalidomide is related to thalidomide, a drug known to damage or kill a developing fetus. Pregnant woman should not take lenalidomide. If you miss a period or have irregular bleeding, you may be pregnant. Women who suspect that they are pregnant must call their doctor at once and stop taking lenalidomide immediately.

Women of childbearing age must have a negative pregnancy test within 10–14 days before treatment and again within a day before starting the drug, weekly for the first month and then once a month in women with regular cycles or every 2 weeks in women with irregular cycles. Women of childbearing age with no alternative to lenalidomide must use 2 contraceptive methods; a highly effective one such as a hormonal contraceptive, an IUD, a surgical method such as a tubal ligation (tubes tied) or vasectomy for the male partner, and a less reliable one such as a condom, diaphragm, or cervical cap. These protective measures should begin 4 weeks before starting on lenalidomide and continue until at least 4 weeks after treatment has been completed.

It is not known whether this drug passes into breast milk. Nursing mothers who must take lenalidomide should use infant formula.

Seniors: Seniors are likely to have more drug side effects with the same drug effectiveness as younger adults, due to age-related reductions in kidney function.

Type of Drug

Leukotriene Antagonists/ Inhibitors (LUE-koe-treen)

Brand Names

Generic Ingredient: Montelukast Sodium
Singulair   Singulair Granules

Generic Ingredient: Zafirlukast
Accolate

Generic Ingredient: Zileuton
Zileuton CR   Zyflo CR
Zyflo

Prescribed For

Asthma; also seasonal allergic rhinitis (montelukast), chronic uticaria (montelukast and zafirlukast), and atopic dermatitis (montelukast).

General Information

Leukotrienes play an important role in the body's allergic response. They are associated with the swelling of tissues and tightening of muscles in the throat that cause the throat to close during an asthma attack. Leukotriene receptor antagonists (montelukast and zafirlukast) help to prevent attacks by blocking leukotrienes from binding to special tissue receptors. Zileuton interferes with the formation of leukotrienes and has no effect on the receptors. When taken on a regular basis, they can reduce the number of asthma attacks you experience, but do not treat them once they occur; other drugs must be used to treat acute attacks.

Cautions and Warnings

Do not take leukotriene antagonists or inhibitors if you are **allergic** or **sensitive** to any of their ingredients. It may be possible to be sensitive to one drug and tolerate another.

Do not use these drugs to treat an **acute asthma attack**.

Avoid aspirin and other nonsteroidal anti-inflammatory drugs (NSAIDs) if they have triggered an asthma attack in the past. These drugs may not offer protection against **NSAID-related asthma attacks.**

Keep your regular inhalants and other asthma drugs handy at all times in case you have an asthma attack. These drugs do not prevent all attacks.

People **age 55 and older** taking zafirlukast reported more mild to moderate respiratory infections than those taking a placebo (sugar pill). Infections were more common in people taking larger dosages of zafirlukast and among those who took zafirlukast with an inhaled corticosteroid.

People with **cirrhosis of the liver** may require lower dosages of zafirlukast and montelukast. People taking these drugs should have their liver enzymes measured periodically by their doctor. Life-threatening liver failure and unexplained liver injury have developed in people taking zafirlukast.

Possible Side Effects

Montelukast

▼ Most common: headache.
▼ Less common: flu, dizziness, upset stomach, gastroenteritis (inflammation of the mucous lining of the stomach and intestine), cough, stuffy nose, abdominal pain, hypersensitivity reactions, tingling in the hands and feet, reduced sense of touch, dream abnormalities, drowsiness, irritability, and restlessness.
▼ Rare: dental pain, rash, fever, injuries, liver damage, weakness, and tiredness. Contact your doctor if you experience any side effect not listed above.

Zafirlukast

▼ Most common: headache.
▼ Less common: nausea, diarrhea, infections, dizziness, abdominal pain, vomiting, generalized pain, weakness, accidental injury, muscle aches, fever, back pain, and upset stomach.
▼ Rare: liver inflammation or damage, low white-blood-cell count, rash, worsening asthma, heart problems, nerve damage, bleeding, bruising, swelling, joint or muscle pain,

---

Possible Side Effects *(continued)*

---

sleeplessness, itching, and not feeling well. Contact your doctor if you experience any side effect not listed above.

Zileuton

▼ Most common: headache.

▼ Common: general pains, upset stomach, nausea, and liver inflammation.

▼ Less common: abdominal pain, weakness, accidental injury, and muscle aches.

▼ Rare: joint pain, chest pain, eye redness, constipation, dizziness, fever, gas, muscle stiffness, sleeplessness, swollen lymph glands, feeling unwell, neck pain or rigidity, nervousness, itching, tiredness, urinary infections, vaginal inflammation, vomiting, and jaundice. Contact your doctor if you experience any side effect not listed above.

Drug Interactions

Montelukast

- Phenobarbital and rifampin can reduce blood levels of montelukast, but dosage adjustment is not needed.
- The adverse effects of prednisone may be increased when combined with montelukast.

Zafirlukast

- Aspirin increases the amount of zafirlukast in the blood by 45%.
- Zafirlukast may increase the effects of other drugs broken down in the liver.
- Erythromycin, terfenadine, and theophylline may reduce zafirlukast's effectiveness.
- Zafirlukast increases the effects of astemizole, carbamazepine, cisapride, cyclosporine, felodipine, isradipine, nicardipine, nifedipine, nimodipine, phenytoin, tolbutamide, and warfarin.

Zileuton

- Alcohol use and liver disease may increase the risk of serious side effects.
- Zileuton increases the effects of astemizole, beta blockers, cisapride, cyclosporine, felodipine, isradipine, ketoconazole,

methergine, nicardipine, nifedipine, nimodipine, theophylline, tizanidine, and warfarin. Dosage adjustments are necessary.

Food Interactions

Zileuton and montelukast may be taken with or without food. Zileuton CR tablets should be taken within an hour after breakfast and dinner. For optimal effectiveness, take each dose of zafirlukast at least 1 hour before or 2 hours after meals.

Usual Dose

Montelukast

Those with asthma doses should take this medicine every evening. Allergy patients may take this medicine at any time according to individual need.

Adult and Child (age 15 and over): 10 mg every evening.

Child (age 6–14): 5-mg chewable tablet every evening.

Child (age 2–5): 4-mg chewable tablet or one 4-mg packet of oral granules daily.

Child (age 6 to 23 months): 4-mg packet of oral granules a day.

Zafirlukast

Adult and Child (age 12 and over): 20 mg twice a day. Take this medication on an empty stomach, at least 1 hour before or 2 hours after meals.

Child (age 5–11): 10 mg twice a day.

Child (under age 5): not recommended.

Zileuton

Adult and Child (age 12 and over): 600 mg 4 times a day.

Child (under age 12): not recommended.

Zileuton CR

Adult and Child (age 12 and over): Two 600-mg tablets within an hour after breakfast and dinner.

Child (under age 12): not recommended.

Overdosage

The most common symptoms of montelukast overdose include thirst, tiredness, dilation of the pupils of the eyes, excessive movement, and abdominal pain. Symptoms of zafirlukast overdose include rash and upset stomach. Call your local poison control center or a hospital emergency room for more information. If you seek treatment, ALWAYS bring the prescription bottle or container.

Special Information

These drugs must be taken on a regular basis to prevent asthma attacks. You should continue taking them even if you are having an asthma attack, unless instructed by your doctor to stop.

Your dosage of inhaled corticosteroids, commonly used for asthma prevention, may be gradually reduced if you take these drugs. This reduction should be gradual and occur only under your doctor's supervision. Do not stop using your corticosteroid inhaler without your doctor's knowledge.

Call your doctor if you develop pain in the upper right portion of your abdomen, nausea, fatigue, lethargy, severe itching, yellowing of the skin or whites of the eyes, flu-like symptoms, and loss of appetite. They may be signs of liver damage.

Call your doctor if, after starting on leukotriene antagonist/inhibitor, your need for your regular asthma drug increases.

If you are using montelukast oral granules, the packet should not be opened until you are ready to use it. After opening the packet, the full dose must be administered within 15 minutes. The granules can be swallowed directly, dissolved in a teaspoonful of cold or room temperature baby formula or breast milk, or mixed with a spoonful of certain foods at either cold or room temperature. Only applesauce, carrots, rice, or ice cream should be used. If mixed with baby formula, breast milk, or food, montelukast oral granules must not be stored for future use. Throw away any unused portion.

If you forget a dose, take it as soon as you remember. If it is almost time for your next dose, skip the one you forgot and continue with your regular schedule. Do not take a double dose.

Special Populations

Pregnancy/Breast-feeding: Montelukast passes into fetal circulation. Zafirlukast and zileuton have harmed the fetus in animal studies using more than 400 times the human dose. When your doctor considers one of these drugs crucial, its potential benefits must be carefully weighed against its risks.

These drugs pass into breast milk. Nursing mothers who must take any of these drugs should use infant formula.

Seniors: In studies, people age 55 and older who took zafirlukast reported more infections (see "Cautions and Warnings"). Seniors taking this drug may require reduced dosage.

Levaquin *see Fluoroquinolone Anti-Infectives,*
page 495

Generic Name

Levetiracetam (leh-veh-tir-AS-eh-tam)

Brand Name
Keppra

Type of Drug
Antiepileptic.

Prescribed For
Partial onset seizures.

General Information
Levetiracetam works differently than other antiepileptic drugs. While it does not affect any pathway known to either block or stimulate nerve transmissions, research shows that it can help prevent seizures in adults with epilepsy. Levetiracetam is always prescribed in combination with other antiepileptic medicines.

Cautions and Warnings
Do not take this drug if you are **allergic** or **sensitive** to any of its ingredients.

People with **kidney problems** require reduced dosage.

Levetiracetam is a nervous system depressant and can cause fatigue, sleepiness, poor coordination, and behavioral changes (including aggression, agitation, anger, anxiety, apathy, depression, emotional instability, and psychosis) in adults, most commonly during the first 4 weeks of treatment. Almost 40% of **children** taking this drug will become sleepy, fatigued, and develop unusual behaviors including agitation, anxiety, apathy, depersonalization, depression, emotional instability, hostility, nervousness, neurosis, hyperactivity, and personality disorders.

Levetiracetam can cause reductions in white- and red-blood-cell counts in children and adults. Your doctor will evaluate your blood components periodically.

People with **impaired kidney function** should use levetiracetam with caution.

Possible Side Effects

Adult

▼ Most common: tiredness, headache, weakness, and infection.

▼ Common: dizziness, pain, and sore throat.

▼ Less common: appetite loss, memory loss, anxiety, poor muscle coordination, depression, emotional upset, hostility, nervousness, tingling in the hands or feet, fainting, cough, runny nose, sinus irritation, and double vision.

▼ Rare: muscle aches, diarrhea, constipation, stomach problems, chest pain, black-and-blue marks, fever, flu-like symptoms, convulsions, sleeplessness, rash, middle ear infection, tremors, swollen gums, weight gain, reduced platelet and white-blood-cell counts, inflammation of the pancreas, bone marrow suppression, and hair loss. Contact your doctor if you experience any side effect not listed above.

Child (4–16 years)

▼ Most common: hostility, sleepiness, nervousness, accidental injury, vomiting, appetite loss, runny nose, sore throat, and coughing.

▼ Common: weakness, pain, diarrhea, personality changes, dizziness, emotional instability, and agitation.

▼ Less common: itching, skin discoloration, flu-like symptoms and viral infections, facial swelling, neck pain, constipation, stomach pain, black-and-blue marks, depression, confusion, increased reflexes, conjunctivitis (pinkeye), reduced vision in one eye, ear pain, dehydration, and urine abnormalities.

▼ Rare: abdominal pain, allergic reaction, loss of muscle coordination, rash, sinus irritation, abnormal thinking, tremors, poor urinary control, convulsions, nosebleeds, fever, headache, hyperactivity, infection, insomnia, and nausea. Contact your doctor if your child experiences any side effect not listed above.

Drug Interactions

Levetiracetam has been studied in adults with a number of other commonly used medicines, including valproate, phenytoin, contraceptive drugs, digoxin, warfarin, and probenecid. No important interactions have been found.

In children, levetiracetam had no effect on blood levels of carbamazepine, valproate, topiramate, or lamotrigine. Some other seizure control medicines caused an apparent increase in the rate at which this drug is released from the body, but no dose adjustment is needed to account for this effect.

Food Interactions

None known.

Usual Dose

Adult (age 16 and over): starting dosage—500 mg twice a day. Dosage should be increased by 1000 mg a day every 2 weeks to a maximum of 3000 mg a day. Maintenance dosage—1500 mg twice a day.

Child (age 4–15, less than 44 lbs.): 4.5–27.35 mg per lb. of body weight twice a day.

Child (age 4–15, 44 lbs. or more): 250–1500 mg twice a day, depending on body weight.

Child (under age 4): not recommended.

Overdosage

The largest known individual dose taken was 6000 mg of levetiracetam. Symptoms may include drowsiness, agitation, aggression, loss of consciousness, difficulty breathing, and coma. Take the overdose victim to a hospital emergency room for treatment. ALWAYS bring the prescription bottle or container.

Special Information

Levetiracetam must be discontinued gradually. Stopping the drug too suddenly can lead to withdrawal seizures.

Levetiracetam causes dizziness and tiredness. Be careful when driving or performing any task that requires concentration.

Call your doctor if you become pregnant or are planning on becoming pregnant while taking this medication.

If you forget a dose, take it as soon as you remember. If it is almost time for your next dose, skip the one you forgot and continue with your regular schedule. Do not take a double dose.

Special Populations

Pregnancy/Breast-feeding: Animal studies show that levetiracetam can cause birth defects. When your doctor considers this drug crucial, its potential benefits must be carefully weighed against its risks. The manufacturer of this drug sponsors a registry to keep track of women who take levetiracetam during pregnancy and their outcomes.

This drug passes into breast milk. Nursing mothers who must take it should use infant formula.

Seniors: Seniors may need less of this medicine than younger adults because of normal declines in kidney function.

Levothroid *see Thyroid Hormone Replacements,*
page 1118

Levoxyl *see Thyroid Hormone Replacements,*
page 1118

Lexapro *see Selective Serotonin Reuptake Inhibitors, page 1020*

Brand Name

Lexxel

Generic Ingredients
Enalapril + Felodipine

Type of Drug
Antihypertensive combination.

Prescribed For
Hypertension (high blood pressure).

General Information

Lexxel contains 5 mg of felodipine, a calcium channel blocker, and 5 mg of enalapril, an angiotensin-converting enzyme (ACE) inhibitor. The 2 drugs in this combination belong to widely prescribed groups of hypertension medication. Lexxel is not meant for the initial treatment of hypertension. Most people taking this product have taken 1 of the ingredients as an individual pill and need more medication to control their blood pressure.

Felodipine works by blocking the passage of calcium into heart and smooth-muscle tissue, especially the smooth muscle found in arteries. Since calcium is an essential factor in muscle contraction, any drug that affects calcium in this way will interfere with the contraction of these muscles. This causes the veins to dilate (widen), reducing blood pressure. Also, the amount of oxygen used by these muscles is reduced.

ACE inhibitors such as enalapril work by preventing the conversion of a hormone called angiotensin I to another hormone called angiotensin II, a potent blood-vessel constrictor. Preventing this conversion relaxes blood vessels and helps to reduce blood pressure and relieve the symptoms of heart failure. Enalapril's effect on other hormones may also help to promote blood-vessel dilation. It begins working about 1 hour after you take it and continues to work for 24 hours. (See Enalapril, page 407, and Felodipine, page 471 for more information.)

Cautions and Warnings

Do not take Lexxel if you are **allergic** or **sensitive** to any of its ingredients. Rarely, it causes very low blood pressure. It may also affect your kidneys, especially if you have **congestive heart failure (CHF).** Your doctor should check your urine for protein content during the first few months of treatment. Lexxel should be used with caution by people with **kidney disease**.

Enalapril may affect white-blood-cell counts, possibly increasing your susceptibility to infection. Your doctor should monitor your blood counts periodically.

ACE inhibitors can cause injury or death to a developing fetus in the last 2 trimesters. **Pregnant women** should not take Lexxel or any ACE inhibitor.

People taking a **beta-blocking drug** who begin taking felodipine may develop heart failure or increased angina pain. Angina pain may also increase if your felodipine dosage is increased. People with severe **liver disease** break down felodipine much more slowly than those with less severe disease or normal livers.

A sudden, painless swelling in the hands, face, feet, lips, tongue, or throat may develop while you are taking any ACE inhibitor. If this happens, you must call your doctor and stop taking the medication at once. This condition usually goes away on its own, though antihistamines may also prove helpful. **Black patients** experience this condition more often than other patients.

Possible Side Effects

Calcium-channel-blocker side effects are generally mild. Side effects are more common with higher dosages and increasing age.

▼ Most common: swelling in the ankles, feet, and legs; dizziness; lightheadedness; muscle weakness or cramps; facial flushing; headache; fatigue; nausea; and chronic (long-term) cough. The cough usually goes away a few days after you stop taking the medication.

▼ Less common: respiratory infection, cough, tingling in the hands or feet, upset stomach, abdominal pain, chest pain, constipation, diarrhea, heart palpitations, sore throat, runny nose, back pain, rash, angina (condition characterized by brief attacks of chest pain), dizziness when rising from a sitting or lying position, fainting, vomiting, bronchitis, urinary tract infection, breathing difficulties, and weakness.

▼ Rare: Rare side effects can affect your heart, muscles and joints, stomach and intestines, sexual function, kidney or liver, and other body parts. Contact your doctor if you experience any side effect not listed above.

Drug Interactions

- The blood-pressure-lowering effect of Lexxel adds to that of diuretic (agent that increases urination) drugs or beta blockers. Any other drug that causes a rapid blood-pressure drop should be used with caution if you are taking Lexxel.
- Lexxel may raise blood-potassium levels, especially when taken with Dyazide or other potassium-sparing diuretics.
- Lexxel may increase the effects of lithium; this combination should be used with caution.
- Capsaicin may cause or aggravate the cough associated with Lexxel therapy.

- Nonsteroidal anti-inflammatory drugs (NSAIDs) may interfere with the blood-pressure-lowering effect of Lexxel.
- Phenothiazine sedatives and antiemetics may increase the effects of Lexxel.
- Rifampin may reduce the effects of Lexxel.
- Combining allopurinol with Lexxel increases the risk of an adverse drug reaction.
- Cimetidine, indinavir, nelfinavir, ritonavir, saquinavir, clarithromycin, nefazodone, ketoconazole, itraconazole, erythromycin, telithromycin, aprepitant, fluconazole, and verapamil increase the amount of felodipine in the blood, causing a slight increase in the drug's effect and possible side effects.
- Phenytoin and other hydantoin anti-seizure drugs, carbamazepine, and barbiturate sleeping pills and sedatives may decrease the amount of felodipine in the blood, reducing its effect.
- Felodipine may increase the effects of theophylline (a drug used to treat asthma and other respiratory problems) and oral anticoagulant (blood-thinning) drugs.
- Felodipine may increase blood levels of tacrolimus. Tacrolimus dose adjustment may be needed.
- Felodipine may interact with quinidine (an antiarrhythmic) to produce low blood pressure, very slow heart rate, abnormal heart rhythms, and swelling in the arms or legs.

Food Interactions

Lexxel may be taken without regard to food or meals; you may take it with food if it upsets your stomach. Avoid grapefruit juice while you are on Lexxel.

Usual Dose

Adult: 1 tablet a day. May be increased to 2 tablets if further blood pressure reduction is necessary after 1–2 weeks of treatment.
Child: not recommended.

Overdosage

Overdose may cause low blood pressure. In case of overdose, call your doctor or go to a hospital emergency room. ALWAYS bring the prescription bottle or container.

Special Information

Call your doctor if you develop a sore throat, mouth sores, abnormal heartbeat, chest pain, a persistent rash, loss of taste perception, constipation, nausea, very low blood pressure, breathing difficulties, increased heart pain, dizziness, lightheadedness, or any bothersome or persistent side effect.

Continue taking your medication and follow any instructions for diet restriction or other treatments to help maintain lower blood pressure, even if you feel well. Hypertension may be present without symptoms.

Do not break, crush, or chew Lexxel tablets.

Maintain good dental hygiene while taking Lexxel and use extra care when brushing or flossing because of the increased risk of oral infection associated with Lexxel.

Avoid over-the-counter diet pills, decongestants, and stimulants while taking Lexxel; they may raise blood pressure.

If you forget a dose, take it as soon as you remember. If it is almost time for your next dose, skip the dose you forgot and continue with your regular schedule. Do not take a double dose.

Special Populations

Pregnancy/Breast-feeding: Women who are or might be pregnant should not take Lexxel. ACE inhibitors have caused low blood pressure, kidney failure, slow skull formation, and death in the fetus when taken during the last 6 months of pregnancy. Women of childbearing age who must take Lexxel must use an effective contraceptive method. If you become pregnant, stop taking the medication and call your doctor immediately.

Small amounts of enalapril + felodipine pass into breast milk. Nursing mothers who must take Lexxel should use infant formula.

Seniors: Seniors, especially those with liver disease, may be more sensitive to the drug's effects.

Generic Name

Lidocaine (lie-DOE-cane) Ⓖ

Brand Name
Lidoderm

Combination Product
Generic Ingredients: Lidocaine + Prilocaine
EMLA

Type of Drug

Topical anesthetic.

Prescribed For

Skin pain.

General Information

The anesthetic ingredients in these products penetrate all layers of skin, dulling nerve endings and providing a local anesthetic effect comparable with that produced by injectable drugs. Lidocaine transdermal patch is approved for chronic nerve pain experienced after shingles, but is used for other types of skin pain as well. It alleviates pain specifically associated with postherpetic neuralgia (PHN), an extremely painful complication of the herpes virus. PHN can be severe and debilitating, and over 50% of shingles patients over age 60 and 75% of patients over age 70 experience long-term pain associated with PHN.

EMLA—which stands for Eutectic Mixture of Local Anesthetics —is a mixture of anesthetics that turns to liquid on contact with the skin. EMLA can prevent or treat virtually any kind of skin pain and may be used by people of almost any age. It has been used to relieve the pain of intravenous catheter placement, minor plastic and skin surgery, shingles, and injections. EMLA is also available in patch form.

Cautions and Warnings

Do not use these products if you are **allergic** or **sensitive** to any of their ingredients or to amide anesthetics.

People with **methemoglobinemia** (a rare blood condition) should not use these products (see "Drug Interactions").

People with a history of **drug sensitivities** should use these products with caution.

People with severe **liver disease** are more prone to developing toxic blood concentrations of anesthetics because of their impaired ability to metabolize these drugs.

Do not apply EMLA cream beyond the area prescribed by your doctor—otherwise, too much anesthetic may enter your blood and cause systemic side effects. Do not put EMLA cream in your eyes, ears, or mouth. EMLA may, however, be used on genital mucous membranes as an anesthetic for minor surgery. Do not apply either patches or cream to **open wounds, burns,** or **broken or inflamed**

skin. Do not apply the patch for longer than the recommended wearing time, as it could lead to serious adverse reactions.

Keep out of the reach of children at all times, and dispose of used patches immediately.

Possible Side Effects

▼ Most common: blisters, bruising, irritation, redness, burning, and swelling of the area to which it is applied.

▼ Common: skin pallor, patches of white skin, itching, rash, and changes in how skin temperature is sensed.

▼ Rare: In rare cases when these topical anesthetic products are applied in excess, are used too often, or when too much anesthetic is absorbed, the following reactions may occur: nervous system excitation; nervousness; apprehension; lightheadedness; euphoria (feeling "high"); confusion; dizziness; drowsiness; ringing or buzzing in the ears; blurred or double vision; vomiting; feelings of warmth, coldness, or numbness; twitching; tremors; convulsions; unconsciousness; or a very slow breathing rate or cessation of breathing. Contact your doctor if you experience any side effect not listed above.

Drug Interactions

● Combining lidocaine with antiarrhythmic drugs such as quinidine, procainamide, tocainide, and mexiletine may increase the risk of serious side effects.

● Do not use more than 1 topical anesthetic at a time because of the risk of absorbing too much of these drugs.

● Drugs that can cause methemoglobinemia—including acetaminophen, sulfa drugs, oral antidiabetes drugs, thiazide diuretics, phenacetin, phenobarbital, phenytoin, primaquine, quinine, benzocaine, chloroquine, and nitrites (preservatives used in meats)—should not be taken with lidocaine products. This interaction is generally limited to children under age 1.

Usual Dose

EMLA Cream

Adult and Child (age 1 month and over): Apply a thick layer—2.5 g or ½ tsp.—and cover with the dressing provided in the package or some other occlusive bandage. Leave in place for at least

1–2 hours. The cream should be wiped away immediately before any surgical procedure or injection.

EMLA Patch: Apply to designated area and leave in place for at least 1–2 hours before removing.

Lidoderm Patch: Use this product to cover the most painful area. Apply up to 3 patches once every 12 hours within a 24-hour period.

Overdosage
Accidental ingestion of these medicines may affect the heart by making it less efficient. Call your local poison control center or a hospital emergency room for more information. If you seek treatment, ALWAYS bring the prescription container.

Special Information
Apply the patch immediately after removing from its protective envelope. Patches may be cut into smaller pieces with scissors while lining is still attached.

If irritation or burning occurs during application, remove the patch(es) and do not reapply until symptoms subside.

When you apply EMLA cream, place the entire dose in the center of the designated area. Then cover it with the occlusive dressing and allow the pressure of the dressing to spread the cream. Since the cream numbs the skin, be careful not to accidentally scratch or burn yourself after the product has been applied.

Wash hands after handling the lidocaine patch or cream. Be sure to properly dispose of the patch immediately after use, as leftover amounts of lidocaine remain and can be accidentally ingested by children or pets.

Do not apply these products near the eyes or to open wounds.

Call your doctor if you develop severe, persistent, or bothersome side effects.

Special Populations
Pregnancy/Breast-feeding: The safety of using the lidocaine patch or cream during pregnancy is not known, though animal studies have revealed no harm to the fetus. When this drug is considered crucial by your doctor, its potential benefits must be carefully weighed against its risks.

The anesthetics in these products pass into breast milk. Nursing mothers who must use these drugs should consider using infant formula.

Seniors: Seniors may be more sensitive to the side effects of lidocaine, and may require a smaller dose.

Lidoderm   see *Lidocaine,* page 638

Generic Name

Linezolid (lie-NEZ-oh-lid)

Brand Name
Zyvox

Type of Drug
Antibiotic.

Prescribed For
Staphylococcus, streptococcus, and enterococcus infections.

General Information
Linezolid is the first of a new group of antibiotics for infections that cannot be treated by other antibiotics. It does not kill bacteria, but rather interferes with their reproduction. The oral form of this antibiotic can be directly substituted for the intravenous form. This is helpful for people who may have been started on linezolid in a hospital or emergency room with an intravenous dose and who can then continue taking linezolid at home.

Cautions and Warnings
Do not use linezolid if you are **allergic** or **sensitive** to any of its ingredients.

Colitis has been associated with nearly all antibiotic drugs, including linezolid. Mild colitis usually abates when the drug is stopped, but it is possible for drug-associated colitis to be fatal.

Linezolid can cause tingling or pain in the hands or feet and visual problems. Blurred vision has occurred in some people who took this medicine for 28 days or less. Blindness has occurred in some people who took this medicine for more than 28 days. Call your doctor immediately if you experience any changes in the quality of your vision or the color of your vision, blurred vision, or tunnel vision.

Low levels of different blood cell types have developed in people taking linezolid, which can lead to anemia and a higher risk of bleeding. This effect usually reverses after the drug is stopped. Your doctor may do blood tests.

Lactic acidosis, which causes nausea and vomiting, has been reported with the use of linezolid.

Possible Side Effects

▼ Common: diarrhea, headache, and nausea.
▼ Less common: bleeding due to low blood-platelet counts, and vaginal fungus infection.
▼ Rare: dizziness, vomiting, abdominal or stomach pain, taste changes, tongue discoloration, and oral fungus infection. Contact your doctor if you experience any side effect not listed above.

Drug Interactions

- Linezolid inhibits the enzyme monamine oxidase (MAO). MAO is a key component of the nervous system and linezolid may interact with any stimulant or agent that activates the nervous system, such as dopamine or noradrenaline.
- People taking any antidepressant drugs should be extremely cautious about taking this medicine because of the risk of serious and even fatal reactions. This applies to both the selective serotonin reuptake inhibitors (SSRIs) antidepressants and the tricyclic antidepressants. Two weeks should elapse between stopping the antidepressant and starting linezolid.
- Mixing linezolid with anesthetics, barbiturates, antidiabetes drugs, beta blockers, bupropion, buspirone, carbamazepine, cyclobenzaprine, methyldopa, meperidine, rauwolfia drugs, sulfa drugs, sumatriptan, and diuretics can lead to severely exaggerated drug side effects.
- Mixing linezolid with dextromethorphan may lead to severe reactions including high fever, abnormal muscle movement, psychosis, coma, and low blood pressure.
- The stimulant and blood pressure effects of levodopa + carbidopa, pseudoephedrine, phenylephrine, and similar agents may be enhanced by linezolid.

Food Interactions

Avoid foods that have been fermented, pickled, aged, or smoked. These include pickles, tap beer, fava beans, cheddar cheese, red wine, soy sauce, sauerkraut, and smoked meats or fish. These foods contain tyramine and can cause very high blood pressure if mixed with linezolid.

Usual Dose

Adult: 800–1200 mg a day for 10–28 days.
Child: Consult your doctor.

Overdosage

Overdose symptoms may include vomiting, tremors, poor muscle coordination, and reduced activity. Overdose victims should be taken to a hospital emergency room. ALWAYS bring the prescription bottle or container.

Special Information

Be sure to tell your doctor if you have or have had high blood pressure, and if you are taking or plan to take any cold remedies or decongestants.

Avoid foods that have been pickled, smoked, aged, or fermented.

Linezolid oral suspension contains phenylalanine. The intravenous and oral forms do not.

If you forget a dose of linezolid, take it as soon as you remember. If it is almost time for your next dose, skip the dose you forgot and continue with your regular schedule. Do not take a double dose.

Special Populations

Pregnancy/Breast-feeding: There is no information on the effect of linezolid during pregnancy. When it is considered crucial by your doctor, its potential benefits must be weighed against its risks.

Linezolid passes into the breast milk of laboratory animals but it is not known if the drug passes into human breast milk. Nursing mothers should consider using infant formula.

Seniors: Seniors may take this medication without special restriction.

Lipitor   *see Statin Cholesterol-Lowering Agents,*
page 1052

Generic Name

Lisinopril (lih-SIN-oe-pril) Ⓖ

Brand Names

Prinivil   Zestril

Combination Products

Generic Ingredients: Lisinopril + Hydrochlorothiazide Ⓖ
Prinzide   Zestoretic

Type of Drug

Angiotensin-converting enzyme (ACE) inhibitor.

Prescribed For

Hypertension (high blood pressure), heart failure, and improving survival after a heart attack. Also prescribed for migraine prevention, kidney failure, kidney hypertension, post–heart attack management, management of people with a high risk of heart disease, kidney protection in people with diabetes, chronic kidney disease, and preventing a second stroke.

General Information

Lisinopril and other ACE inhibitors work by preventing the conversion of a hormone called angiotensin I to another hormone called angiotensin II, a potent blood-vessel constrictor. Preventing this conversion relaxes blood vessels, thus reducing blood pressure and relieving the symptoms of heart failure. Lisinopril also affects the production of other hormones and enzymes that participate in the regulation of blood vessel dilation. Lisinopril begins working about 1 hour after you take it and lasts for 24 hours.

Cautions and Warnings

Do not take lisinopril if you are **allergic** or **sensitive** to any of its ingredients. Occasionally, severe allergic reactions have occurred in people undergoing **desensitization treatments** such as **venom immunizations** or certain kinds of **kidney dialysis**.

Swelling of the face, extremeties, or throat has been known to occur with lisinopril, which can be dangerous (see "Special Information").

Lisinopril occasionally causes very low blood pressure.

Lisinopril can affect your kidneys, especially if you have **congestive heart failure**. Your doctor should check your urine for changes during the first few months of treatment. Dosage adjustment is required if you have **reduced kidney function**.

ACE inhibitors can affect white-blood-cell counts, possibly increasing your susceptibility to infection. Blood counts should be monitored periodically.

Lisinopril can cause serious injury or death to the fetus if taken during **pregnancy**. Pregnant women should not take lisinopril.

ACE inhibitors may be less effective in some **black patients** with high blood pressure, especially when dietary salt intake is high. Nevertheless, they should still be considered useful blood pressure treatments. Swelling beneath the skin to form welts is more common among black patients.

Possible Side Effects

▼ Most common: headache, dizziness, fatigue, low blood pressure, nausea, diarrhea, and chronic cough. The cough is more common in women and usually goes away a few days after the medication is stopped.

▼ Less common: chest pain, vomiting, upset stomach, breathing difficulties, rash, and muscle weakness.

▼ Rare: Rare side effects can affect your muscles and joints, sex drive, liver, mental status, and respiratory tract. Contact your doctor if you experience any side effect not listed above.

Drug Interactions

- The blood-pressure-lowering effect of lisinopril is additive with diuretic drugs and beta blockers. Any other drug that can reduce blood pressure should be used with caution if you are taking an ACE inhibitor.
- Lisinopril may increase the effects of lithium; this combination should be used with caution.
- Aspirin and other nonsteroidal anti-inflammatory drugs (NSAIDs) reduce the blood pressure-lowering effects of lisinopril and other ACE inhibitors. The combination can cause reductions in kidney function.
- Lisinopril may increase your blood potassium levels, especially when taken with dyazide or other potassium-sparing diuretics.

- Antacids and lisinopril should be taken at least 2 hours apart.
- Capsaicin may trigger or aggravate lisinopril cough.
- Indomethacin and other NSAIDs may reduce the blood-pressure-lowering effect of lisinopril.
- Phenothiazine sedatives and antiemetics may increase the effects of lisinopril.
- Lisinopril may affect blood levels of digoxin. More digoxin in the blood increases the chance of digoxin-related side effects while less digoxin in the blood can compromise its effectiveness.
- Combining lisinopril with antidiabetes drugs or insulin may increase the risk of hypoglycemia.
- Severe sensitivity reactions can occur in those taking allopurinol.

Food Interactions
None known.

Usual Dose
Adult: 5–40 mg a day. People with severe kidney disease should start treatment with 2.5 mg a day; dosage may then be increased up to 5–20 mg a day.

Overdosage
The principal effect of lisinopril overdose is a rapid drop in blood pressure, as evidenced by dizziness or fainting. Take the overdose victim to a hospital emergency room immediately. ALWAYS remember to bring the prescription bottle or container.

Special Information
Call your doctor if you develop swelling of the face or throat, if you have sudden difficulty in breathing, a sore throat, mouth sores, abnormal heartbeat, chest pain, a persistent rash, or loss of taste perception.

Unexplained swelling of the face, lips, hands, and feet can also affect the larynx (throat) and tongue and interfere with breathing. If this happens, the victim should be taken to a hospital emergency room at once for treatment. You may require a longer period of hospital/emergency room observation, even if your reaction is only swelling of the tongue, because antihistamines and corticosteroids may not be sufficient treatment.

Some people who start taking an ACE inhibitor after they are already on a diuretic (an agent that increases urination) experience a rapid drop in blood pressure after their first doses or when the dosage is increased. To prevent this from happening, you may be told to stop taking the diuretic 2 or 3 days before starting the ACE inhibitor or to increase your salt intake during that time. The diuretic may then be restarted gradually.

You may get dizzy if you rise quickly from a sitting or lying position when taking lisinopril.

Avoid strenuous exercise and very hot weather because heavy sweating or dehydration can cause a rapid drop in blood pressure.

Avoid over-the-counter diet pills, decongestants, and other stimulants that can raise blood pressure. Also, do not take potassium supplements or salt substitutes containing potassium without consulting your doctor.

If you forget to take a dose of lisinopril, take it as soon as you remember. If it is within 8 hours of your next dose, skip the one you forgot and continue with your regular schedule. Do not take a double dose.

Special Populations

Pregnancy/Breast-feeding: ACE inhibitors can cause fetal injury or death. Women who are or might be pregnant should not take lisinopril. Stop taking the medication and contact your doctor if you become pregnant.

It is not known if lisinopril passes into breast milk. Nursing mothers who must take this drug should use infant formula.

Seniors: Seniors may be more sensitive to the effects of lisinopril due to age-related kidney impairment.

Generic Name

Lithium Carbonate
(LITH-ee-um CAR-buh-nate) Ⓖ

Brand Names

Cibalith-S	Lithobid
Eskalith	Lithonate
Eskalith CR	Lithotabs
Lithane	

The information in this profile also applies to the following drug:

Generic Ingredient: Lithium Citrate Ⓖ

Type of Drug

Antipsychotic and antimanic.

Prescribed For

Bipolar (manic-depressive) disorder, especially suppression of manic attacks or reduction in their number and intensity; also prescribed to improve white-blood-cell count in those with cancer undergoing chemotherapy and in those with human immunodeficiency virus (HIV), and for premenstrual tension, bulimia, postpartum psychosis, overactive thyroid, and alcoholism, especially in people who are also depressed. Lithium lotion has been used for genital herpes and dandruff.

General Information

Lithium carbonate and lithium citrate are the only effective antimanic drugs. They reduce the levels of manic episodes and may produce normal activity within the first 3 weeks of treatment. Typical manic symptoms include rapid speech, elation, hyperactive movements, little need for sleep, grandiose ideas, poor judgment, aggressiveness, and hostility.

Cautions and Warnings

Do not take lithium if you are **allergic** or **sensitive** to any of its ingredients.

Lithium should not be taken by people with **heart or kidney disease, dehydration, low blood sodium,** or those taking **diuretic drugs** or **angiotensin converting enzyme (ACE) inhibitors**. If such people require lithium carbonate, they must be very carefully monitored by their doctors, and hospitalization may be needed until the lithium carbonate dose is stabilized.

A few people treated with both lithium carbonate and haloperidol or another antipsychotic have developed encephalopathic syndrome (symptoms include weakness, tiredness, fever, confusion, tremulousness, and uncontrollable muscle spasms). In addition, your doctor may find laboratory indicators of liver or kidney disease. Rarely, this combination of symptoms is followed by irreversible brain damage.

Up to 20% of people on long-term lithium carbonate treatment develop structural changes in their kidneys and reduced kidney function.

Long-term use of this drug may lead to reduced thyroid activity, enlargement of the thyroid gland, and increased blood levels of thyroid-stimulating hormone. All of these conditions may be treated with thyroid hormone replacement therapy. Overactive thyroid has occasionally occurred.

Frequent urination and thirst associated with lithium carbonate may be a sign of a condition known as diabetes insipidus, in which the kidney stops responding to a hormone called vasopressin. This causes the kidney to reabsorb water and make concentrated urine. Lithium carbonate may reverse the kidneys' ability to perform this function, but things usually go back to normal when lithium carbonate treatment is stopped, dosage is reduced, or small doses of a thiazide diuretic are taken.

Your lithium carbonate dosage may have to be temporarily reduced if you develop an infection or fever.

Some lithium carbonate products contain tartrazine dyes for coloring purposes. Tartrazine can stimulate allergic responses in some people, including asthma.

Possible Side Effects

Side effects of lithium carbonate are directly related to the amount of drug in the bloodstream.

▼ Most common: fine hand tremor, thirst, and excessive urination, especially when treatment is first started; mild nausea and discomfort during the first few days of treatment.

▼ Less common: diarrhea, vomiting, drowsiness, muscle weakness, poor coordination, giddiness, ringing or buzzing in the ears, and blurred vision.

▼ Rare: Rare side effects can affect muscles and nerves (blackouts, seizures, and dizziness), stomach and intestines, kidneys and urinary tract, skin, and thyroid function. Contact your doctor if you experience any side effect not listed above. Lithium carbonate can also affect tests used to monitor heart and brain function. Contact your doctor if you experience any side effect not listed above.

Drug Interactions

• When lithium carbonate is combined with haloperidol, weakness, tiredness, fever, or confusion may result. In some people, these symptoms have been followed by permanent brain damage. Also, haloperidol may increase the effect of lithium carbonate.

- Lithium may interfere with the effectiveness of phenothiazine drugs. Combining these drugs can have serious side effects.
- Lithium carbonate is counteracted by acetazolamide, urea, mannitol, urinary alkalinizers such as sodium bicarbonate, and theophylline drugs. Verapamil can raise or lower blood levels of lithium carbonate.
- Lithium's effect may be increased by methyldopa, fluoxetine and other selective serotonin reuptake inhibitors (SSRIs), carbamazepine, thiazide and loop diuretics, ACE inhibitors, and nonsteroidal anti-inflammatory drugs (NSAIDs).
- Lithium carbonate may increase the effects of tricyclic antidepressant medications.
- Lithium may interfere with the effectiveness of stimulant drugs.
- Lithium may increase the effects of neuromuscular blocking agents, which can lead to severe respiratory side effects.
- Use of metronidazole with lithium can cause lithium toxicity. Careful monitoring is required with this combination.

Food Interactions

Lithium carbonate should be taken immediately after meals or with food or milk.

Usual Dose

Adult: Dosage must be individualized. Most people respond to 1800 mg a day at first in 2 or 3 divided doses. Once the person has responded, daily lithium dosage is reduced to the lowest effective level, usually 300 mg 3–4 times a day.

Child: not recommended.

Overdosage

Toxic blood levels of lithium carbonate are only slightly above the levels required for treatment. Signs of drug toxicity may be diarrhea, vomiting, nausea, tremors, drowsiness, poor coordination, giddiness, weakness, blurred vision, ringing or buzzing in the ears, dizziness, fainting, confusion, muscle twitching, uncontrollable muscle movements, loss of bladder control, worsening of manic symptoms, overactive reflexes, and painful muscles or joints. If any of these symptoms occur, stop taking the medication and call your doctor immediately. ALWAYS bring the prescription bottle or container with you when you go to an emergency room.

Special Information

Lithium carbonate may cause drowsiness. Be cautious while driving or operating hazardous machinery.

Lithium carbonate causes your body to lose sodium (salt). You must maintain a well-balanced diet and drink 8–12 glasses of water a day while taking this drug. Excessive sweating or diarrhea may make you more sensitive to side effects.

Call your doctor if you develop diarrhea, vomiting, unsteady walking, tremors, drowsiness, or muscle weakness.

To avoid side effects, your doctor may need to reduce your dosage once manic symptoms decline.

If you forget to take a dose of lithium carbonate, take it as soon as possible. However, if it is within 2 hours of your next dose, or 6 hours if you take the long-acting form, skip the missed dose and go back to your regular schedule. Do not take a double dose. Call your doctor if you miss more than 1 dose.

Special Populations

Pregnancy/Breast-feeding: Lithium can cause heart and thyroid birth defects, especially if taken during the first 3 months of pregnancy. Talk with your doctor about the risks of taking lithium during pregnancy.

Lithium carbonate passes into breast milk. It may cause weak muscle tone, low body temperature, bluish discoloration of the skin, and abnormal heart rhythm in an infant. Nursing mothers who must take this drug should use infant formula.

Seniors: Seniors are more sensitive to the effects of lithium carbonate. Because seniors have a higher frequency of heart, liver, and kidney problems, they should be monitored carefully and started on the low end of the dosage range.

Type of Drug

Loop Diuretics

Brand Names

Generic Ingredient: Bumetanide Ⓖ
Bumex

Generic Ingredient: Ethacrynic Acid
Edecrin

Generic Ingredient: Furosemide Ⓖ
Lasix

Generic Ingredient: Torsemide
Demadex

Prescribed For

Congestive heart failure (CHF), cirrhosis of the liver, fluid accumulation in the lungs, kidney dysfunction, high blood pressure, and other conditions where it may be desirable to rid the body of excess fluid. Bumetanide can be used to treat people who urinate frequently at night.

General Information

Stronger than thiazide diuretics, loop diuretics work in a similar fashion. Not only do they affect the same part of the kidney as thiazide diuretics, they also act in another portion called the "loop of Henle." This dual action is what makes loop diuretics so potent. All 4 loop diuretics can be used for the same purposes, but their dosages vary.

Cautions and Warnings

Do not take loop diuretics if you are **allergic** or **sensitive** to any of their ingredients. People allergic to sulfa drugs may also be allergic to furosemide, torsemide, or bumetanide.

Loop diuretics can cause depletion of water and electrolytes. They should not be taken without constant medical supervision. Frequent lab evaluations of electrolytes should be performed during therapy and periodically thereafter. You should not take these drugs if your urine production has been decreased abnormally by **kidney disease**.

Excessive use of loop diuretics results in dehydration or reduction in blood volume, and may cause circulatory collapse or other related problems, particularly in **older adults**.

Ringing or buzzing in the ears, hearing loss, deafness, fainting, and a sensation of fullness in the ears can occur with these drugs. Hearing usually returns within 24 hours, but some loss may be permanent.

These drugs may worsen systemic **lupus erythematosus**. Diarrhea may occur with ethacrynic acid or furosemide solution. Rarely, people taking bumetanide develop thrombocytopenia (low blood-platelet count).

People taking a loop diuretic may develop increased levels of total cholesterol, low-density lipoprotein (LDL) cholesterol, and triglycerides.

If you have **diabetes mellitus**, you may develop high blood sugar or sugar in the urine. To treat this problem, the dosage of your antidiabetes drugs must be increased.

Possible Side Effects

▼ Common: Changes may occur in blood levels of potassium or other electrolytes. Hypokalemia (low blood potassium), may cause dry mouth, excessive thirst, weakness, lethargy, drowsiness, restlessness, muscle pain or cramps, muscular tiredness, low blood pressure, decreased frequency of urination and urine volume, abnormal heart rate, and upset stomach, including nausea and vomiting. Loop diuretics may alter sugar metabolism.

▼ Less common: abdominal discomfort, nausea, vomiting, diarrhea, rash, dizziness, lightheadedness, headache, blurred vision, fatigue, weakness, jaundice (symptoms include yellowing of the skin or whites of the eyes), acute gout attacks, dermatitis and other skin reactions, tingling in the extremities, dizziness upon rising quickly from a sitting or lying position, and anemia.

▼ Rare: a sweet taste in the mouth, a burning sensation in the stomach or mouth, excessive thirst, increased perspiration, and frequent urination. Contact your doctor if you experience any side effect not listed above.

Drug Interactions

- Loop diuretics increase the effects of other blood-pressure-lowering drugs. This is beneficial and is frequently used to help lower blood pressure in people with hypertension.
- Combining a loop diuretic and digitalis drugs or adrenal corticosteroids increases the risk of developing electrolyte imbalances. Potassium loss caused by loop diuretics significantly increases the toxicity of digitalis.
- Loop diuretics may increase the effect of oral anticoagulants (blood thinners); a dosage adjustment may be needed.
- The dosage of an oral antidiabetes drug—except metformin —may need to be altered if you start taking a loop diuretic.

- The effect of theophylline may be altered by any loop diuretic. Your doctor should check your theophylline levels after you have started on a loop diuretic.
- If you are taking lithium carbonate, you should probably not take a diuretic, which greatly increases the risk of lithium side effects.
- People taking chloral hydrate as a nighttime sedative may, in rare cases, experience hot flashes, high blood pressure, sweating, abnormal heart rhythms, weakness, and nausea when they also take a loop diuretic.
- Periodic hearing loss or ringing or buzzing in the ears may occur if a loop diuretic is taken with cisplatin (an anticancer drug) or an aminoglycoside antibiotic. Make sure your doctor knows you are taking a loop diuretic before giving you an injection of either of these.
- Clofibrate and thiazide diuretics increase the effect of loop diuretics.
- Charcoal tablets, phenytoin, probenecid, aspirin and other salicylate drugs, and nonsteroidal anti-inflammatory drugs (NSAIDs) may decrease the effectiveness of loop diuretics.
- If you are taking a loop diuretic for high blood pressure or CHF, avoid over-the-counter (OTC) cough, cold, and allergy products, which often contain stimulant drugs that can raise your blood pressure. Check with your pharmacist before taking any OTC drug if you are taking a loop diuretic.

Food Interactions

Furosemide should be taken on an empty stomach at least 1 hour before or 2 hours after meals. The other loop diuretics may be taken with food if they upset your stomach.

Usual Dose
Bumetanide
Adult: 0.5–2 mg a day, up to 10 mg a day. It may also be taken every other day for 3–4 consecutive days followed by 1–2 days off the drug.

Child (under age 18): not recommended.

Ethacrynic Acid
Adult: 50–200 mg taken every day or every other day.

Child: starting dose—25 mg; increase slowly.

Furosemide

Adult: 20–80 mg a day. Dosages of 600 mg or more a day have been prescribed.

Child: 0.9 mg per lb. of body weight in a single daily dose. If therapy is not successful, the dosage may be increased in small steps up to 2.7 mg per lb. a day.

Torsemide

Adult: 5–20 mg once a day. Dosages up to 40 mg may be prescribed.

Child: not recommended.

Maintenance dosages for all of the loop diuretics are adjusted to individual needs.

Overdosage

Symptoms include dehydration, reduced blood volume, high urine volume, weakness, dizziness, confusion, appetite loss, tiredness, vomiting, circulatory collapse, and cramps. Take the victim to a hospital emergency room. ALWAYS bring the prescription bottle or container.

Special Information

If the amount of urine you produce each day is dropping, or if you suffer from cramps, significant appetite loss, muscle weakness, tiredness, or nausea, contact your doctor immediately.

Loop diuretics are usually taken once a day after breakfast. If a second dose is needed, it should be taken no later than 2 p.m. to avoid nighttime urination.

To avoid the dizziness associated with these drugs, rise slowly and carefully from a sitting or lying position.

Loop diuretics rob your body of potassium. To counteract this effect, be sure to eat high-potassium foods such as bananas, citrus fruits, melons, and tomatoes.

Loop diuretics can increase your sensitivity to the sun. Use sunscreen and wear protective clothing.

If you forget a dose, take it as soon as you remember. If it is almost time for your next dose, skip the one you forgot and continue with your regular schedule. Do not take a double dose.

Special Populations

Pregnancy/Breast-feeding: Loop diuretics have been used to treat specific conditions in pregnancy, but they should be used only when absolutely necessary.

Furosemide passes into breast milk, and the other loop diuretics may pass into breast milk. Nursing mothers who must take any of these drugs should use infant formula.

Seniors: Seniors are more sensitive to the effects of these drugs.

Generic Name

Loperamide (loe-PER-uh-mide) Ⓖ

Brand Names

Diar-Aid	K-Pek II
Imodium	Neo-Diaral
Imodium A-D	Pepto Diarrhea Control

Type of Drug
Antidiarrheal.

Prescribed For
Acute and chronic diarrhea; also prescribed to reduce the amount of discharge in an ileostomy (surgical procedure in which a hole is made in the small intestine, usually through the abdominal wall).

General Information
Loperamide hydrochloride, which relieves diarrhea but does not address the underlying cause, should be used only for short periods. It works by slowing intestinal movement and affecting the movement of water and salts in the intestines. In some cases antidiarrheals should not be used at all; these drugs may harm people with bowel, stomach, or other diseases. Loperamide is available over-the-counter (OTC) under a variety of brand names. OTC loperamide products are used to treat acute diarrhea and traveler's diarrhea.

Cautions and Warnings
Do not use loperamide if you are **allergic** or **sensitive** to any of its ingredients. Drug allergy to loperamide is rare.

Do not take loperamide if you suffer from diarrhea associated with **colitis** or you have an **intestinal infection** of *Escherichia coli, Salmonella,* or *Shigella,* or abdominal pain without diarrhea.

If you have **ulcerative colitis** and start taking loperamide, stop the drug at once and call your doctor if you develop abdominal problems of any kind.

Do not use loperamide to treat infants younger than 2 years old.

Stop taking loperamide if you develop constipation, abdominal distention, or intestinal blockage.

Use this drug with caution if you have **liver disease.**

Possible Side Effects

Incidence of side effects is low. They are most likely to occur when loperamide is taken over longer periods to treat chronic diarrhea.

▼ Most common: stomach and abdominal pain, bloating or other discomfort, constipation, dry mouth, dizziness, tiredness, nausea and vomiting, and drug-sensitivity reactions, including rash.

Other side effects that have occurred with loperamide are itching; hives; swelling of the tongue, lips, or face; rare but serious skin reactions; gas; severe bowel reactions; and urinary difficulty.

Drug Interactions

- Loperamide increases the effects of sleeping pills, sedatives, and alcohol. Avoid these combinations.
- Loperamide should not be taken with clindamycin or lincomycin, agents that can cause severe and possibly fatal colitis.
- Quinidine and ritonavir can increase the effects of loperamide. These drugs should be mixed with caution.
- Loperamide reduces saquinavir levels by more than 50%, interfering with the effects of that drug. Saquinavir dose adjustment may be necessary.

Food Interactions

Loperamide should be taken on an empty stomach.

Usual Dose

Acute Diarrhea

Adult and Child (age 12 and over): 4 mg to start, followed by 2 mg after each loose stool, up to 16 mg a day maximum. Improvement should be seen in 2 days.

Child (age 9–12): 2 mg 3 times a day to start, followed by 1 mg per 22 lbs. of body weight after each loose stool, up to 6 mg a day maximum.

Child (age 6–8): 2 mg twice a day to start, followed by 1 mg per 22 lbs. of body weight after each loose stool, up to 4 mg a day maximum.

Child (age 2–5): 1 mg 3 times a day to start, followed by 1 mg per 22 lbs. of body weight after each loose stool, up to 3 mg a day maximum.

Child (under age 2): not recommended.

Chronic Diarrhea

Adult and Child (age 12 and over): 4 mg to start, followed by 2 mg after each loose stool, until symptoms are controlled. Then dosage should be tailored to individual needs—usually 4–8 mg a day. Loperamide is usually effective within 10 days or not at all.

Child (under age 12): not recommended.

OTC (acute diarrhea, including traveler's diarrhea)

Adult: 4 mg to start, followed by 2 mg after each loose stool. No more than 8 mg a day, for no more than 2 days.

Child (age 9–11): 2 mg to start, followed by 1 mg after each loose stool. No more than 6 mg a day for no more than 2 days.

Child (age 6–8): 1 mg to start, followed by 1 mg after each loose stool. No more than 4 mg a day for no more than 2 days.

Child (under 6): Consult your doctor.

Overdosage

Symptoms include constipation, difficulty urinating, irritation of the stomach, tiredness, and CNS depression. Children may be more sensitive to loperamide overdose than adults. Large doses usually cause vomiting. Take the victim to a hospital emergency room immediately. ALWAYS bring the prescription bottle or container.

Special Information

Loperamide depresses the central nervous system (CNS), which may cause drowsiness: Be careful when driving or performing any task that requires concentration.

Loperamide may cause dry mouth. Drink plenty of water or other clear fluids to prevent dehydration due to diarrhea. It is important to maintain a proper diet and drink plenty of fluids to restore normal bowel function.

Call your doctor if diarrhea persists after a few days of loperamide treatment or if you develop abdominal discomfort or pain, fever, or any bothersome or persistent side effect.

If you forget a dose, skip it and go back to your regular schedule. Do not take a double dose.

Special Populations

Pregnancy/Breast-feeding: Loperamide has not been found to cause birth defects; however, women who are or might be pregnant should not take this drug without their doctor's approval. When loperamide is considered crucial by your doctor, its potential benefits must be carefully weighed against its risks.

It is not known if loperamide passes into breast milk. Nursing mothers who must take this drug should consider using infant formula.

Seniors: Seniors may be more sensitive to the constipating effects of loperamide but no dosage adjustment is necessary.

Generic Name

Loratadine (lor-AH-tuh-dene) Ⓖ

Brand Names

Alavert	Claritin Reditabs
Alavert Children's	Clear-Atadine
Claritin	Dimetapp Children's ND
Claritin 24-Hour Allergy	Allergy
Claritin Children's Allergy	Tavist ND
Claritin Hives	Triaminic Allerchews

The information in this profile also applies to the following drug:

Generic Ingredient: Desloratadine

Clarinex   Clarinex RediTabs

Type of Drug

Antihistamine.

Prescribed For

Stuffy and runny nose, itchy eyes, and scratchy throat caused by seasonal allergy and for other symptoms of allergy such as rash, itching, and hives; also prescribed for asthma.

General Information

Antihistamines generally work by blocking the release of histamine (chemical released by body tissue during an allergic reaction) from cells at the H_1 histamine receptor site, drying up secretions of the nose, throat, and eyes. Loratadine causes less sedation than most antihistamines and appears to be just as effective.

Cautions and Warnings

Do not take loratadine if you are **allergic** or **sensitive** to any of its ingredients.

People with **liver disease** and **kidney disease** require reduced dosage.

Possible Side Effects

▼ Less common: sore throat, headache, dry mouth, muscle aches, drowsiness, fatigue, and painful menstruation. Other side effects include heart palpitations, drug sensitivity reactions (rash, itching, hives, swelling, and difficulty breathing), hyperactivity, seizures, liver irritation, and hepatitis.

▼ Rare: Rare side effects can occur in almost any part of the body. Contact your doctor if you experience any side effect not listed above.

Drug Interactions

- Loratadine may interact with ketoconazole, erythromycin, and theophylline, but the evidence for this interaction is inconclusive.
- Cimetidine can substantially increase the amount of loratadine in the bloodstream.
- Combine loratadine with monoamine oxidase inhibitor antidepressants with caution, as it can increase side effects.
- Combining loratadine with alcohol or nervous system depressants can cause increased nervous system depression.

Food Interactions

Loratadine is best taken on an empty stomach 1 hour before or 2 hours after eating; it may be taken with food or milk if it upsets your stomach. Desloratadine may be taken with or without food.

Usual Dose

Loratadine

Adult and Child (over age 6): 10 mg once a day. People with liver disease should take 10 mg every other day.

Child (age 2–5): 5 mg a day of loratadine syrup. Children with liver disease should take 5 mg every other day.

Child (under age 2): not recommended.

Desloratadine
   Adult and Child (age 12 and over): 5 mg once a day. People with liver disease should take one 5-mg tablet every other day.
   Child (age 6–11): 2.5 mg once a day.
   Child (age 12 months–5 years): 1.25 mg once a day.
   Child (age 6 months–11 months): 1 mg once a day.

Overdosage

Overdose is likely to cause drowsiness, headache, rapid heartbeat, or severe side effects. Overdose victims should be given ipecac syrup—available at any pharmacy—to make them vomit and should be taken to a hospital emergency room for treatment. Call your local poison control center or hospital emergency room for instructions. ALWAYS bring the prescription bottle or container.

Special Information

Dizziness or fainting may be the first sign of a serious side effect. Call your doctor at once if this happens to you. Also report sore throat, trouble swallowing or speaking, swelling of the tongue, wheezing, dizziness or fainting, swelling around the mouth, drooling, or any other unusual side effect.

   If you forget to take a dose of loratadine, take it as soon as you remember. If it is almost time for your next dose, skip the one you forgot and continue with your regular schedule. Do not take a double dose.

   Rapidly disintegrating loratadine tablets must be used as soon as they are removed from their foil package. Place on your tongue and allow to dissolve. You may drink water or another liquid with it but it is not necessary.

Special Populations

Pregnancy/Breast-feeding: Do not take any antihistamine without your doctor's knowledge if you are or might be pregnant—especially during the last 3 months of pregnancy—because newborns may have severe reactions to antihistamines.

   Loratadine passes into breast milk. Nursing mothers who must take loratadine should use infant formula.

Seniors: Seniors are unlikely to experience nervous system effects with loratadine as opposed to the older, more sedating antihistamines. However, seniors, especially those with liver disease, are more likely to experience side effects than are younger adults. Seniors should take the smallest effective dose.

Brand Name

Lotrel

Generic Ingredients

Amlodipine + Benazepril Hydrochloride

Type of Drug

Antihypertensive combination.

Prescribed For

High blood pressure.

General Information

Lotrel combines the calcium channel blocker amlodipine with the angiotensin-converting enzyme (ACE) inhibitor benazepril. Both drugs are often prescribed individually for hypertension. Lotrel is not intended as a first treatment for hypertension. You should take Lotrel only after you have tried an ACE inhibitor or calcium channel blocker alone and your doctor feels you need an additional drug to control your blood pressure. (See Amlodipine, page 65, and Benazepril, page 145, for more information.)

Cautions and Warnings

Do not take Lotrel if you are **allergic** or **sensitive** to any of its ingredients or to any other ACE inhibitor. People taking any ACE inhibitor may experience severe drug reactions, including swelling of the face, throat, lips, tongue, hands, and feet—this reaction occurs in about 5 in 1000 people.

Lotrel or any ACE inhibitor should not be taken by **pregnant women.**

In rare instances, people taking a calcium channel blocker who have severe **heart disease** develop increased angina pain or a heart attack.

In people with **heart failure,** ACE inhibitors may cause very low blood pressure, kidney failure, and death. People with heart failure who start Lotrel must be under a doctor's care.

This medication may cause high blood potassium, especially in people with **diabetes** or **kidney disease**, which can lead to abnormal heart rhythms.

Another ACE inhibitor has caused depression of bone marrow and reduced white-blood-cell counts, especially in people with **kidney failure.** Fever and chills can be a sign of this problem.

Lotrel should be used with caution by people with **kidney** or **liver disease.**

In rare instances, people taking ACE inhibitors have developed liver failure.

All ACE inhibitors may cause a persistent cough.

ACE inhibitors may be less effective in some **black patients** with high blood pressure, especially when dietary salt intake is high. Nevertheless, they should still be considered useful blood pressure treatments. Swelling beneath the skin to form welts is more common among black patients.

Possible Side Effects

Side effects are generally mild and temporary.
▼ Most common: cough, headache, dizziness, and swelling.
▼ Less common: allergic reactions, weakness, fatigue, dry mouth, nausea, abdominal pain, constipation, diarrhea, upset stomach, throat irritation, low blood-potassium levels, back pain, muscle cramps and pain, sleeplessness, nervousness, anxiety, tremors, reduced sex drive, impotence, flushing, hot flashes, rash, and frequent urination.
▼ Rare: inflammation of the pancreas, hemolytic anemia, chest pain, abnormal heart rhythms, gout, neuritis, ringing or buzzing in the ears, and hair loss. Contact your doctor if you experience any side effect not listed above.

Drug Interactions
- Combining a diuretic and Lotrel lowers blood pressure, possibly excessively.
- Combining potassium supplements or a potassium-sparing diuretic such as spironolactone, amiloride, or triamterene and benazepril increases the risk of high blood potassium. High blood-potassium levels may lead to abnormal heart rhythms.
- Combining lithium with benazepril may increase blood-lithium levels and lithium side effects.
- Use alcohol cautiously with Lotrel.

Food Interactions
Food does not affect individual tablets of amlodipine and benazepril, but the effects of food on Lotrel have not been studied.

Until more information is available, take Lotrel on an empty stomach at least 1 hour before or 2 hours after meals.

Usual Dose

Adult: Daily doses range from 2.5 mg of amlodipine and 10 mg of benazepril to 10 mg of amlodipine and 20 mg of benazepril. Dosage depends on your need for each of the 2 ingredients. Small or frail people or those with liver failure should follow dosage recommendations for seniors.

Senior: Start with 2.5 mg of amlodipine and 10 mg of benazepril a day and increase gradually. You may need to take amlodipine and benazepril in separate pills until your daily needs are established.

Child: not recommended.

Overdosage

Little is known about the effects of Lotrel overdose. Call your local poison control center for more information. Overdose victims should be taken to a hospital emergency room for treatment. ALWAYS bring the prescription bottle or container.

Special Information

Continue taking your medication and follow all instructions including diet restriction and other treatments, even if you feel well. Hypertension may be present without symptoms.

Lotrel may increase the risk of dangerous allergic reactions. Call your doctor if you develop swelling in the hands, feet, face, or throat; sudden breathing difficulties; a sore throat; mouth sores; abnormal heartbeat; increased chest pain; persistent rash; constipation; nausea; weakness; dizziness; loss of the sense of taste; or any bothersome or persistent side effect.

You may get dizzy if you rise to your feet quickly from a sitting or lying position. If you experience any dizziness or drowsiness, avoid driving or performing hazardous activities.

Avoid strenuous exercise and very hot weather because heavy sweating or dehydration may lead to a rapid drop in blood pressure.

Avoid over-the-counter stimulants that can raise blood pressure, including diet pills and decongestants.

Maintain good dental hygiene while taking Lotrel and use extra care when brushing or flossing because of the increased risk of oral infection associated with Lotrel.

If you forget a dose, take it as soon as you remember. If it is within 8 hours of your next dose, skip the one you forgot and continue with your regular schedule. Do not take a double dose.

Special Populations

Pregnancy/Breast-feeding: ACE inhibitors may cause fetal damage or death. Lotrel should not be taken by pregnant women. If you are taking Lotrel and become pregnant, see your doctor at once about changing drugs. Women of childbearing age who must take Lotrel must use an effective contraceptive method.

Small amounts of both active ingredients pass into breast milk. Nursing mothers who must take Lotrel should use infant formula.

Seniors: Seniors should begin with the lowest strength of Lotrel available—2.5 mg of amlodipine and 10 mg of benazepril.

Brand Name

Lotrisone

Generic Ingredients

Betamethasone Dipropionate + Clotrimazole [G]

Type of Drug

Corticosteroid and antifungal combination.

Prescribed For

Severe fungal infection such as athlete's foot, jock itch, and ringworm.

General Information

The corticosteroid in Lotrisone is betamethasone dipropionate; the antifungal is clotrimazole. Lotrisone is used to relieve the symptoms of itching, rash, or skin inflammation associated with a severe fungal infection. It may also treat the underlying cause of the skin problem by killing the fungus. Improvement usually occurs within the first week of treatment. Creams that contain only clotrimazole or only betamethasone—as betamethasone diproprionate or in a slightly different form called betamethasone valerate—may be more effective than a combination product such as Lotrisone for certain skin conditions.

Cautions and Warnings

Do not use Lotrisone if you are **allergic** or **sensitive** to any of its ingredients.

Do not apply Lotrisone near or in your eyes, nose, or mouth. Avoid using this product on the ear if the eardrum is perforated, unless specifically directed to do so by your doctor.

Do not use an old tube of Lotrisone for a new skin problem without your doctor's knowledge.

Lotrisone may cause viral skin infections such as **chickenpox** and **herpes** to spread. It may also worsen **tuberculosis (TB) of the skin, bacterial skin infections, skin diseases** that affect circulation, and **diaper rash**. Do not use this medication on **children under the age of 2** without your doctor's approval.

Lotrisone may increase glucose levels in the blood or urine, especially in people with severe **diabetes**.

Do not use Lotrisone to treat **eye infections.**

Possible Side Effects

▼ Most common: itching, stinging, burning, peeling skin, redness, and swelling.

Food and Drug Interactions
None known.

Usual Dose
Adult and Child (age 17 and over): Gently rub a thin film onto the affected area and surrounding skin 2 times a day for 2–4 weeks, washing hands before and after application.

Child (under age 17): not recommended.

Overdosage
Accidental ingestion of Lotrisone may cause nausea and vomiting. Call your local poison control center or a hospital emergency room for more information. If you seek treatment, ALWAYS bring the prescription bottle or container.

Special Information
Washing or soaking the skin before applying the medication may increase the amount that penetrates into your skin.

Applying this drug to the face, underarms, groin, genitals or genital areas, abdomen, or between the toes for more than a few days may result in stretch marks.

Wear loose fitting clothing (preferably cotton) after applying Lotrisone, especially when applied to the genitals or genital areas.

Stop using the medication and call your doctor if Lotrisone causes itching, burning, or skin irritation.

Although prolonged treatment with Lotrisone is not recommended, it is important to take this drug for the entire period prescribed by your doctor, even if you are no longer experiencing symptoms.

Call your doctor if you develop acne or oily skin, bruising, white spots, increased hair growth, or inflammation of hair follicles.

If you do not see results after 1–2 weeks, your doctor may need to prescribe a different medication.

People with ringworm should wash their clothes separately from other household members' clothes.

If you forget a dose, apply it as soon as you remember. If it is almost time for your next application, skip the dose you forgot and continue with your regular schedule.

Special Populations

Pregnancy/Breast-feeding: Lotrisone can adversely affect fetal development. Pregnant women should not apply Lotrisone over large areas of skin or use it for a prolonged period. When this drug is considered crucial by your doctor, its potential benefits must be weighed against its risks.

The ingredients in Lotrisone may pass into breast milk when applied to the breast. Nursing mothers who must apply it there should use infant formula.

Seniors: Seniors may use Lotrisone without special restriction.

Generic Name

Lubiprostone (lew-bee-PROSS-tone)

Brand Name
Amitiza

Type of Drug
Local chloride channel activator.

Prescribed For
Chronic constipation.

General Information
One way to treat chronic constipation is to add fluid to the insides of the gut. Lubiprostone accomplishes this by acting inside the

gastrointestinal (GI) tract to increase intestinal fluid secretion. This increases intestinal movement and speeds stool passage through the GI tract, eliminating symptoms of chronic constipation. Lubiprostone improves intestinal fluid secretion without altering sodium and potassium concentrations in the serum. Other constipation treatments work in a similar way but can be associated with other potential problems.

Cautions and Warnings

Do not take lubiprostone if you are **allergic** or **sensitive** to any of its ingredients, or if you have or have had a **blockage in the stomach or intestinal area**.

This drug has not been studied in people with **liver or kidney problems** and it has not been studied in **children**.

People with **diarrhea** should not take this medication.

Drug Interactions

The chances of lubiprostone interacting with other medications after they have been absorbed is small because very little lubiprostone is absorbed into the blood. There is no information on the interaction of lubiprostone with other medications in the GI tract.

Food Interactions

This drug may be taken with food or meals.

Usual Dose

Adult: 24 mcg twice a day with food.
Child: not recommended.

Possible Side Effects
Side effects increase with higher doses.
▼ Most common: nausea, diarrhea, and headache.
▼ Common: stomach bloating and fullness, abdominal pain, headache, and gas.
▼ Less common: sinusitis, urinary tract infection, upper respiratory infections, irritation of the nose and throat, flu or other viral infections, vomiting, loose stools, stomach or abdominal discomfort, upset stomach, upper or lower abdominal pain, gastroesophageal reflux disease (GERD), dry mouth, constipation, dizziness, swelling in the arms and legs, fatigue, chest pain or discomforts, fever, joint pain,

Possible Side Effects (continued)

   back pain, leg or arm pain, difficulty breathing, cough, pain
   in the lower part of the throat (larynx or pharynx), depression, anxiety, and sleeplessness.
▼ Rare: loss of the sense of touch, muscle cramps, weight
   gain, and high blood pressure. Contact your doctor if you
   experience any side effect not listed above.

Overdosage

There have been 2 confirmed reports of overdosage with lubiprostone. The first report involved a 3-year-old child who accidentally ingested 7–8 capsules of 24 mcg of lubiprostone and fully
recovered. The second report was a study subject who self-
administered a total of 96 mcg lubiprostone a day for 8 days. This
person experienced no drug side effects during this time. High
doses of lubiprostone cause drug side effects or other reactions.
Call your local poison control center or a hospital emergency room
for more information. If you seek treatment, ALWAYS bring the prescription bottle or container.

Special Information

Taking lubiprostone with food may lessen symptoms of nausea if
they occur. If you experience severe diarrhea while taking lubiprostone, contact your doctor.
   Men and women respond similarly to this drug.
   If you forget a dose of lubiprostone, take it as soon as you remember. If it is almost time for the next dose, skip the one you forgot and continue with your regular schedule. Do not apply a double
dose.

Special Populations

Pregnancy/Breast-feeding: Animal studies have shown lubiprostone can damage a developing fetus. Pregnant women should
take this drug only if its potential benefits outweigh the possible
risks. Women who might become pregnant and who are starting
on this medicine must take a pregnancy test before starting treatment to be sure they are not pregnant. Women taking lubiprostone should use birth control while taking it.
   It is not known if lubiprostone passes into breast milk, however
nursing mothers should either not take lubiprostone if it is pre-

scribed or use infant formula while on this drug because of the possibility of side effects appearing in the nursing baby.

Seniors: Seniors may use this drug with no special precaution.

Lunesta   *see **Eszopiclone**, page 449*

Type of Drug

Luteinizing Hormone Inhibitors

Brand Names

Generic Ingredient: Cetrorelix
Cetrotide

Generic Ingredient: Ganirelix Acetate Ⓖ

Prescribed For

Infertility.

General Information

Luteinizing hormone inhibitors are prescribed as part of a treatment program offered by fertility specialists to help stimulate the development of follicles into mature eggs in women who have had difficulty becoming pregnant. These drugs block the release of gonadotropin-releasing hormones (GnRH), which stimulate the production and release of 2 other hormones: luteinizing hormone (LH) and follicle-stimulating hormone (FSH). LH and FSH levels return to normal within 48 hours after treatment is stopped.

A luteinizing hormone inhibitor may be taken once a day by subcutaneous (under the skin) injection during the several days after FSH is given, specifically on day 2 or 3 of the cycle. Treatment with an LH inhibitor continues until chorionic gonadotropin (hCG)—the final drug in the sequence—is given. Your doctor will determine when enough follicles have reached an adequate size by ultrasound. In some cases hCG is given to help the follicles develop into mature eggs.

Cautions and Warnings

Do not use luteinizing hormone inhibitors if you are **allergic** or **sensitive** to any of their ingredients.

People with a **latex allergy** may react adversely to ganirelix.

People who are allergic to **mannitol** should not use cetrorelix.

People who are allergic to **gonadotropin-releasing hormone** must be monitored carefully after the first injection. A severe reaction associated with cough, rash, and hypotension occurred in 1 patient after 7 months of treatment with cetrorelix, when taken at a dosage of 10 mg a day, in a study for a use unrelated to infertility.

People with severe **kidney impairment** should not use cetrorelix.

Possible Side Effects

▼ Less common: abdominal pain, headache, miscarriage, hyperstimulation of the ovary, vaginal bleeding, injection-site allergy (symptoms include redness, rash, bruising, itching, and swelling), and nausea.

Drug Interactions

Ganirelix can suppress the secretion of pituitary gonadotropins, and may require dose adjustments of exogenous gonadotropins.

Food Interactions

None known.

Usual Dose

Cetrorelix: single-dose regimen—one 3 mg subcutaneous dose, usually on stimulation day 7 (range: day 5–9). If hCG is not given within 4 days after injection of 3 mg cetrorelix, then cetrorelix 0.25 mg once daily is prescribed until the day of hCG administration.

Multiple-dose regimen—0.25 mg of cetrorelix, on either stimulation day 5 (morning or evening) or day 6 (morning). Continue every day until the day of hCG administration.

Ganirelix: 250 mcg once daily after starting FSH therapy on day 2 or 3 of the cycle. Treatment is continued until the day of hCG administration.

Overdosage

Very high doses of these medicines have been employed in clinical trials without serious side effects. Call your local poison center or a hospital emergency room for more information. If you seek treatment, ALWAYS bring the prescription bottle or container.

Special Information

This drug is given by injection under the skin. For more information on how to properly administer this drug, see page 1242.

If taking a multiple-dose regimen, change the injection site regularly to minimize irritation.

Cetrorelix powder for injection requires more manipulation than Cetrotide, which comes in pre-filled syringes. You must dissolve the powder with sterile water provided by the manufacturer before it is injected. Follow the directions for dilution in the package.

Special Populations

Pregnancy/Breast-feeding: Women who are pregnant should not take these drugs because they may harm a developing fetus.

It is not known if these drugs pass into breast milk. Nursing mothers who must use luteinizing hormone inhibitors should use infant formula.

Seniors: These medicines are not intended for use by seniors.

Lyrica   see **_Pregabalin,_** page 914

Generic Name

Malathion   (MAL-uh-thye-on)

Brand Name

Ovide

Type of Drug

Scabicide.

Prescribed For

Head lice.

General Information

Originally used as an agricultural insecticide, malathion is effective against common lice and the eggs they leave behind in the scalp. Malathion works by interfering with the breakdown of acetylcholine, a neurohormone that carries nervous-system impulses. The excess acetylcholine produced by malathion kills lice and their eggs.

Once applied to the hair, malathion binds with the hair shaft within 6–12 hours, providing some protection against future infestations.

Cautions and Warnings

Do not use malathion if you are **allergic** or **sensitive** to any of its ingredients.

Malathion is extremely toxic if swallowed (see "Overdosage").

Normally, about 89% of the malathion applied to the skin is absorbed into the bloodstream; more may be absorbed if it is applied to **broken skin or open sores**—this may cause a toxic reaction.

Malathion lotion is flammable. Do not expose the lotion or hair that is still wet with the lotion to an open flame or an electric dryer because of the risk of fire. Allow hair to dry naturally after application.

Malathion can damage the eyes and cause conjunctivitis (pinkeye). If it gets into your eyes, flush them with water immediately.

People who have had a recent **heart attack** or who have any of the following conditions should be cautious when using malathion because it can precipitate an attack or worsen your condition: **asthma,** very **slow heartbeat, low blood pressure, stomach spasms or ulcer,** or **Parkinson's disease**.

Do not use malathion in **children under age 2,** as they may absorb too much of it through the scalp.

Malathion can worsen the following conditions: **severe anemia, dehydration, insecticide exposure effects, liver disease** or **cirrhosis, malnutrition, myasthenia or other neuromuscular diseases,** and **seizure** disorders.

People with recent **brain surgery** should be cautious about using this product because it can initiate toxic nervous system effects, including seizures.

Possible Side Effects

▼ Common: scalp irritation.
▼ Rare: Convulsions and other side effects can occur if too much of the drug is absorbed into the blood through the scalp (see "Overdosage"). Contact your doctor if you experience any side effect not listed above.

Drug Interactions

- Large dosages of malathion may interact with aminoglycosides (injectable antibiotics) to cause breathing problems, with local anesthetics to cause systemic side effects, and with glaucoma eyedrops—physostigmine, echothiophate, demecarium, and isoflurophate—to cause side effects.

- Combining malathion and anticholinesterase muscle stimulants used to treat myasthenia gravis may lead to increased side effects.

Usual Dose

Adult and Child (age 6 and over): Sprinkle the lotion onto dry hair and rub it in until the hair and scalp are wet. Pay special attention to the back of your head and neck. Avoid contact with the eyes. Immediately after applying the lotion, wash your hands. Allow the treated hair to dry naturally; do not cover it or use an electric dryer or other heat source. After 8–12 hours, wash your hair with a plain shampoo. Remove dead lice and eggs from the scalp with a fine-toothed comb. Repeat after 7–9 days if necessary.

Child (age 2–6): Consult your doctor.

Child (under age 2): not recommended.

Overdosage

Accidental ingestion or absorbing too much drug through the skin is serious and potentially fatal. Symptoms of malathion toxicity include abdominal cramps; anxiety; restlessness; clumsiness or unsteadiness; confusion; depression; diarrhea; dizziness; drowsiness; increased sweating; watery eyes or mouth; loss of bowel or bladder control; muscle twitching in the eyelids, face, or neck; pinpointed pupils; difficulty breathing; seizures; slow heartbeat; trembling; and weakness. People who swallow this drug may not experience toxic effects for up to 12 hours. In case of accidental ingestion induce vomiting with ipecac syrup—available at any pharmacy. Take the victim to a hospital emergency room. ALWAYS bring the prescription bottle or container.

Special Information

Follow your prescription exactly, paying careful attention to dosage, duration of exposure, and frequency of application. Do not increase the chance of absorption through the skin as it may lead to overtoxicity.

Malathion should only be used on scalp hair.

Pregnant women should not handle this medication or apply it to others.

Avoid exposure to other insecticides while being treated with malathion.

Head lice can be easily transferred to people in close contact. Be sure to examine and treat other family members if necessary.

Special Populations

Pregnancy/Breast-feeding: Animal studies of malathion have revealed no drug-related birth defects. Since animal studies may not predict human results and up to 8% of malathion applied to the skin may be absorbed, pregnant women should not use it or apply it to others.

It is not known if this drug passes into breast milk. Nursing mothers who must use it should use infant formula.

Seniors: Seniors may use this drug without special restriction.

Generic Name

Maraviroc (muh-RAH-vih-roc)

Brand Name

Selzentry

Type of Drug

CCR5 co-receptor antagonist.

Prescribed For

Human immunodeficiency virus (HIV) infection in people whose virus is resistant to multiple-drug treatment, in combination with other HIV antiviral drugs.

General Information

Maraviroc is the first of a new class of HIV antiviral drugs called CCR5 blockers. These drugs are prescribed together with other antiviral medications. Maraviroc is used to treat HIV virus that utilizes the CCR5 receptor on the surface of the white blood cell to get inside the cell and take it over. Other HIV antivirals work inside white blood cells, but maraviroc prevents the virus from entering uninfected cells by blocking the virus' major route of entry, the CCR5 co-receptor. CCR5 is a protein found on the surface of some types of immune cells. Half or more of people who have previously been treated for HIV have CCR5-tropic HIV virus in their blood. Maraviroc has not been tested in adults or children who have not already been treated with another HIV antiviral.

Cautions and Warnings

Do not take maraviroc if you are **allergic** or **sensitive** to it. Drug allergy may appear before maraviroc affects the liver. Maraviroc should be used with caution if you have **liver disease, heart disease** or **hepatitis B.** It should be used with caution by people with **kidney disease** because about 25% of the drug passes out of the body through the kidneys.

About 20% of people on combination antiretroviral therapies develop Immune Reconstitution Syndrome within a month or 2 after starting treatment. If this happens, people start feeling worse even though their HIV is better because infections, hepatitis, or other conditions that may have been dormant now begin to express themselves. Maraviroc can increase the risk of infection.

Possible Side Effects

▼ Most common: fever, cough, upper respiratory infection, rash, dizziness, muscle and joint pain, and stomach and abdominal pain.

▼ Common: herpes infections, constipation, fainting when rising quickly from a sitting or lying position, sinusitis, bronchitis, appetite changes, sensory changes, changes in consciousness, and nerve pain.

▼ Less common: high blood pressure, upset stomach, ulcers of the stomach or mouth, pain and discomfort, flu, pneumonia, genital warts, infection of hair follicles, benign skin tumors, kidney problems, breathing difficulty, sinus disorders, respiratory disorders, bronchial spasm, itching, sweat gland disorders, eczema, and dermatitis, and body fat redistribution.

▼ Rare: Other side effects can involve almost any body part, including the brain (stroke) heart (angina, heart failure, heart attack, and coronary artery occlusion), liver and bile system. Contact your doctor if you experience any side effect not listed above.

Drug Interactions

- The daily dosage of maraviroc is doubled to 600 mg in people taking other drugs that speed its breakdown in the liver, including efavirenz, rifampin, carbamazepine, phenobarbital, and phenytoin. Other drugs that can interact in the same way are barbiturates, glitazone antidiabetes drugs, modafinil, oxcarbazine, and rifabutin.

- Do not take maraviroc with St. John's wort because it will unpredictably reduce maraviroc blood levels.
- The daily dosage of maraviroc is reduced to ½ or 150 mg a day in people also taking other drugs that slow its breakdown in the liver such as delavirdine, indinavir, or nelfinavir. Other drugs that inhibit the enzyme that breaks down maraviroc are amiodarone, aprepitant, chloramphenicol, cimetidine, clarithromycin, diltiazem, erythromycin, fluconazole, fluvoxamine, gestodene, imatinib, itraconazole, ketoconazole, mifepristone, nefazodone, norfloxacin, norfluoxetine, mibefradil, verapamil, and voriconazole.
- HIV antiviral drugs that do not dictate maraviroc dose adjustment include the protease inhibitors tipranavir and ritonavir, enfurvitide, the reverse transcriptase inhibitors zidovudine (AZT), azidothymidine, didanosine, stavudine, lamivudine, abacavir, emtricitabine, nevirapine, tenofovir, and adefovir.

Food Interactions

This drug may be taken without regard to food or meals. Do not drink grapefruit juice or eat any grapefruit-containing product while taking this medicine. Grapefruit and star fruit (carambola) slow the breakdown of maraviroc in the liver.

Usual Dose

Adult (age 16 and over): 150–600 mg twice a day depending on specific drug combinations.

Child (under age 16): not recommended.

Overdosage

Overdose symptoms can be expected to include drug side effects, especially dizziness or fainting. Overdose victims should be taken to a hospital emergency room for treatment because of the possibility of an impact on the heart. ALWAYS bring the prescription bottle or container.

Special Information

Maraviroc is not a cure for HIV. It will not prevent you from transmitting the HIV virus to another person; you must still practice safe sex. People taking maraviroc may still develop opportunistic infections and other complications associated with HIV infection. It is very important that you take this drug exactly as prescribed.

Call your doctor at once if you have an allergic reaction to maraviroc.

Your doctor should test your liver function regularly while you are taking maraviroc, and should monitor you for signs of any infection.

Maraviroc can make you dizzy or lightheaded. Take extreme care while driving or operating any complex equipment or machinery.

If you forget a dose, take it as soon as you remember. If it is almost time for the next dose, skip the one you forgot and continue with your regular schedule. Do not take a double dose.

Special Populations

Pregnancy/Breast-feeding: Animal studies of maraviroc have not shown it to be toxic to a developing fetus. Pregnant women should take maraviroc only if its potential benefits outweigh its risks. Pregnant women who decide to take maraviroc can be included in a company-sponsored registry by their doctor to help track the drug's effect.

It is not known if maraviroc passes into breast milk, however mothers with HIV should always use infant formula, regardless of whether they take this drug, to avoid transmitting the virus to their child.

Seniors: Seniors may experience more drug side effects than younger adults. Caution should be used when seniors take maraviroc.

Generic Name

Medroxyprogesterone
(med-rok-see-proe-JES-ter-one) [G]

Brand Names

Depo-Provera   Provera

The information in this profile also applies to the following drugs:

Generic Ingredient: Megestrol
Megace

Generic Ingredient: Norethindrone [G]
Aygestin

Generic Ingredient: Progesterone

Crinone   Prometrium
Endometrin Vaginal Insert

Type of Drug

Progestin.

Prescribed For

Absence of menstruation, abnormal uterine bleeding caused by fibroids or uterine cancer, and menopausal changes in the lining of the uterus—in conjunction with estrogen replacement therapy (ERT); also prescribed to stimulate breathing in people who suffer from sleep apnea and for other conditions in which breathing rate is abnormally slow or stops completely for short periods of time. Norethindrone may be used for endometriosis. Progesterone has been used to treat premenstrual syndrome (PMS), prevent spontaneous abortion or premature labor, and support embryo implantation and help maintain pregnancy in some assisted reproductive technology (ART) procedures.

General Information

Progesterone is the principal hormone involved in the process of pregnancy. It helps to prepare the womb to accept the fertilized egg and maintain the growth and development of the fetus. The decision to take medroxyprogesterone on a regular basis should be made carefully by you and your doctor because of this drug's risks.

Megestrol is used in advanced breast and endometrial cancer to reduce symptoms of the disease, and for weight loss and decreased appetite in people living with HIV.

Cautions and Warnings

Do not take medroxyprogesterone if you are **allergic** or **sensitive** to any of its ingredients or to any progestin.

If you have a history of **stroke, blood clots or similar disorders, varicose veins, liver or gallbladder disease,** known or suspected **breast or genital cancer,** undiagnosed **vaginal bleeding,** or **miscarriage**, do not take medroxyprogesterone. Medroxyprogesterone and other progestins should not be used regularly to treat weight loss.

Smoking may increase the risk of a stroke or blood clot.

Although progestins have been used to prevent spontaneous abortion, such treatment can harm a fetus if given during the first 4 months of pregnancy.

Medroxyprogesterone use should be carefully considered if you have had **asthma, cardiac insufficiency, epilepsy, HIV infection, migraine, kidney problems, ectopic pregnancy, high blood cholesterol,** or **depression**. People with **diabetes** may experience a decrease in glucose tolerance, worsening their condition.

Possible Side Effects

There is a strong relationship between the use of progestin drugs and the development of blood clots in the veins, lungs, or brain.

Medroxyprogesterone, Megestrol, and Norethindrone

▼ Most common: breakthrough bleeding, spotting, changes in or loss of menstrual flow, water retention, weight change, breast tenderness, jaundice, acne, rash with or without itching, and depression.

▼ Common: changes in sex drive, changes in appetite and mood, headache, nervousness, dizziness, tiredness, backache, loss of scalp hair, hair growth in unusual quantities or places, itching, symptoms similar to those of a urinary infection, and unusual rashes.

▼ Rare: allergy, fatigue, fever, flu-like symptoms, bloating, asthma, back or leg pain, sinus inflammation, respiratory infection, upset stomach, stomach gas or noise, emotional instability, sleeplessness, acne, itching, painful urination, and urinary infections. Contact your doctor if you experience any side effect not listed above.

Progesterone Gel

Side effects are less common if you use this drug once a day.

▼ Most common: pelvic or abdominal pain or cramps, sleepiness, tiredness, headache, nervousness, depression, reduced sex drive, constipation, nausea, breast enlargement, and nighttime urination.

▼ Common: bloating, dizziness, diarrhea, vomiting, painful intercourse, joint pain, itching, and vaginal infection or discharge.

Drug Interactions

- Rifampin and aminoglutethimide may reduce medroxyprogesterone acetate's effectiveness.

Food Interactions

You may take this drug with food if it upsets your stomach.

Usual Dose

Medroxyprogesterone: 5–10 mg a day for 5–10 days.

Megestrol: breast cancer—40 mg 4 times a day; endometrial carcinoma—40–320 mg a day in divided doses; weight or appetite loss—400–800 mg a day.

Norethindrone: endometriosis—5 mg a day for 14 days, then increased gradually up to 15 mg a day; treatment may continue for 6–9 months. Abnormal periodic bleeding or no period—2.5–10 mg a day for 5–10 days during the second half of the menstrual cycle.

Progesterone Capsules: 5–10 mg a day for 6–8 days.

Progesterone Gel: Apply a single-use disposable unit once or twice a day.

Progesterone Insert: 100 mg 2 or 3 times a day.

Overdosage

Symptoms may include severe side effects, though small overdoses generally do not cause unusual symptoms. Call your local poison control center or a hospital emergency room for more information. If you seek treatment, ALWAYS bring the prescription bottle or container.

Special Information

Your need for this medication should be evaluated at least every 6 months.

This drug may make you drowsy. Be careful when driving or performing any tasks that require concentration.

Stop taking this drug immediately and call your doctor if you experience sudden, partial, or complete loss of vision; double vision; sudden falling; calf pain, swelling, and redness; numbness in an arm or leg; leg cramp; water retention; unusual vaginal bleeding; migraine or a sudden and severe headache; depression; or if you think you have become pregnant.

Medroxyprogesterone may increase your sensitivity to the sun. Use sunscreen and wear protective clothing.

Avoid excessive salt intake while taking medroxyprogesterone.

Medroxyprogesterone may mask symptoms of menopause.

If you forget a dose, take it as soon as you remember. If it is almost time for your next dose, skip the one you forgot and continue with your regular schedule. Do not take a double dose.

Special Populations

Pregnancy/Breast-feeding: Medroxyprogesterone, megestrol, and norethindrone may cause birth defects or interfere with fetal development; they can double the rate of certain birth defects if used during the first 4 months of pregnancy. They are not considered safe for use during pregnancy, except under very specific circumstances. Progesterone gel is used to support embryo implantation and help maintain pregnancies in some ART procedures.

Medroxyprogesterone passes into breast milk. It may also increase the amount of milk produced and the duration of milk production when taken after childbirth. Nursing mothers who must use this drug should consider using infant formula.

Seniors: Seniors with severe liver disease are more sensitive to the effects of this drug.

Generic Name

Memantine (meh-MAN-teen)

Brand Name

Namenda

Type of Drug

N-methyl-D-aspartate (NMDA) receptor inhibitor.

Prescribed For

Moderate to severe Alzheimer's disease (AD). It is also used to treat vascular dementia.

General Information

Overstimulation of nerve cells in the brain by a chemical called glutamate, which causes nerve degeneration, is thought to be a cause of AD symptoms. Memantine hydrochloride blocks NMDA receptors in the brain, which decreases the effects of glutamate, but it does not stop the nerve degeneration that is a normal part of AD. Thus, the drug is not a cure for AD, but can be expected to improve symptoms and delay a patient's mental decline. Other available AD treatments work differently and are only approved for mild to moderate AD, although they have been studied in people with severe AD.

Cautions and Warnings

Do not take this drug if you are **allergic** or **sensitive** to any of its ingredients.

People with **kidney disease** may retain more memantine in their bodies. People with severe kidney disease should not use this drug.

Some memantine is broken down by the liver. People with severe **liver disease** may require lower doses of this medication and should use it with caution. Those with mild or moderate disease may use it without dose adjustment.

Memantine has not been studied in people with **seizure disorders.** A very small number of people taking memantine in drug studies had seizures, but the number was similar to that which occurred in people taking a placebo (sugar pill).

Possible Side Effects

In most cases, memantine side effects reported in clinical studies were similar to those reported by people who took a placebo.

▼ Common: dizziness, headache, confusion, and constipation.
▼ Less common: fatigue, hallucinations, vomiting, difficulty breathing, high blood pressure, and back pain.
▼ Rare: Other side effects, including chest pain, stroke, convulsions, liver failure, low blood sugar, high blood lipids, impotence, and severe allergic reactions, can affect almost any part of the body. Contact your doctor if you experience any side effect not listed above.

Drug Interactions

- Carbonic anhydrase inhibitors (such as acetazolamide) and bicarbonate of soda (or "baking soda")—drugs that reduce the acidity of urine—can cause the body to eliminate about 80% less memantine through the kidneys.
- Memantine does not interfere with the ability of donepezil and other cholinesterase inhibitors to function.
- Dextromethorphan, a common ingredient in over-the-counter cough medicines, should be avoided when you are taking memantine.

Food Interactions

This drug can be taken without regard to food or meals.

Usual Dose

Adult: starting dose—5 mg a day. Dose is increased weekly in 5 mg increments up to 20 mg a day.

Child: not recommended.

Overdosage

Symptoms include restlessness, psychosis, hallucinations, sleepiness, stupor, and loss of consciousness. Take the victim to a hospital emergency room. ALWAYS bring the prescription bottle or container.

Special Information

Patient caregivers who are responsible for ensuring that medicines are taken correctly must understand how memantine is taken and its dosage regimen.

Special Populations

Pregnancy/Breast-feeding: Animal studies with memantine revealed no danger to a developing fetus, even at the highest dosage. When this drug is considered crucial by your doctor, its potential benefits must be carefully weighed against its risks.

It is not known if memantine passes into breast milk. Nursing mothers who must take it should use infant formula.

Seniors: Seniors may use this drug without special precaution. Those with kidney disease may require lower doses.

Generic Name

Meperidine (muh-PER-ih-dine) Ⓖ

Brand Name

Demerol

Type of Drug

Narcotic analgesic (pain reliever).

Prescribed For

Moderate to severe pain.

General Information

Meperidine hydrochloride is a potent narcotic analgesic and cough suppressant. It is also used before surgery to reduce anxiety and help bring the patient into early stages of anesthesia. Meperidine is probably the most widely used narcotic in American hospitals. It compares favorably with morphine sulfate, the standard for narcotic analgesics.

It is useful for mild to moderate pain; 25–50 mg of meperidine are approximately equal in pain-relieving effect to two 325-mg aspirin tablets. Meperidine may be less effective than aspirin for pain associated with inflammation because aspirin reduces inflammation, but meperidine does not. Meperidine suppresses the cough reflex but does not cure the underlying cause of the cough.

Cautions and Warnings

Do not take meperidine if you are **allergic** or **sensitive** to any of its ingredients.

Use this drug with extreme caution if you suffer from **asthma or other breathing problems** or if you have a **head injury** or other condition causing **increased pressure to the brain**.

Meperidine should be used with caution if you have **kidney, heart, or liver disease,** a history of **seizures, sickle cell anemia, hypothyroidism** (underactive thyroid gland), **Addison's disease, pheochromocytoma, inflammatory bowel disease, gallstones** or **gallbladder disease, enlarged prostate,** or **urinary difficulties**.

Meperidine may cause postural low blood pressure (symptoms include dizziness or fainting when rising from a sitting or lying position). High blood pressure has also been reported with meperidine use.

Chronic (long-term) use of meperidine may cause drug dependence or addiction.

Meperidine is a respiratory depressant and affects the central nervous system (CNS), producing sleepiness, tiredness, and an inability to concentrate. Alcohol may increase the CNS depression caused by this drug.

Possible Side Effects

▼ Most common: lightheadedness, dizziness, sleepiness, nausea, vomiting, appetite loss, and increased sweating. These side effects usually disappear if you lie down. More serious side effects of meperidine are shallow breathing or breathing difficulties.

▼ Less common: euphoria (feeling "high"), weakness, headache, agitation, uncoordinated muscle movement, minor

Possible Side Effects *(continued)*

hallucinations, disorientation, visual disturbances, dry mouth, constipation, flushing of the face, rapid heartbeat, palpitations, faintness, urinary difficulties or hesitancy, reduced sex drive or potency, itching, rash, anemia, lowered blood sugar, and yellowing of the skin or whites of the eyes. Narcotic analgesics may aggravate convulsions in those who have had them.

Drug Interactions

- Because of its depressant effect and potential effect on breathing, meperidine should be taken with extreme caution in combination with alcohol, sleeping medications, antihistamines, sedatives, or other depressant drugs.
- Meperidine should not be taken with ritonavir.
- Caution should be used when combining meperidine with isoniazid. Frequent blood pressure monitoring at initiation of therapy is necessary.
- Mixing cimetidine and a narcotic analgesic may cause confusion, disorientation, depression, seizure, or breathing difficulties. Cimetidine slows the clearance of meperidine from the body.
- Combining meperidine and a monoamine oxidase inhibitor (MAOI) antidepressant may lead to breathing difficulties; blood pressure changes; bluish discoloration of the lips, fingernails, or skin; coma; or death. Do not take meperidine within 2 weeks of your last dose of an MAOI.
- Meperidine should not be combined with sibutramine (Meridia).
- Combining meperidine and the antipsychotic drug chlorpromazine (Thorazine) or thioridazine may lead to serious side effects.
- Hydantoin anticonvulsant drugs (phenytoin) may decrease the effectiveness of meperidine, while enhancing its side effects. Anticonvulsant drugs like phenytoin increase the breakdown of meperidine in the liver.
- Combining meperidine and a protease inhibitor may increase the risk of CNS depressant and breathing difficulties. These medications should not be used together.
- Acyclovir increases blood levels of meperidine. Use this combination with caution.

Food Interactions

Meperidine may be taken with food to reduce upset stomach.

Usual Dose

Adult: 50–150 mg every 3–4 hours as needed.

Child: 0.5–0.8 mg per lb. of body weight every 3–4 hours as needed, up to the adult dosage.

Overdosage

Symptoms include slow breathing, extreme tiredness progressing to stupor and then coma, pinpointed pupils, no response to pain stimulation, cold or clammy skin, slow heartbeat, low blood pressure, convulsions, and cardiac arrest. The victim should be taken to a hospital emergency room immediately. ALWAYS bring the prescription bottle or container.

Special Information

Be extremely careful when driving or doing any task that requires concentration. Avoid alcohol.

Call your doctor if you develop nausea, vomiting, constipation, breathing difficulties, or any bothersome or persistent side effect.

Ask your doctor to consider lowering your meperidine dosage if you experience lightheadedness, dizziness, sleepiness, nausea, vomiting, appetite loss, or increased sweating.

If you have been taking meperidine for more than a few weeks, do not stop taking it without your doctor's instruction. Suddenly stopping this drug may lead to withdrawal symptoms.

If you forget a dose, take it as soon as you remember. If it is almost time for your next dose, skip the one you forgot and continue with your regular schedule. Do not take a double dose.

Special Populations

Pregnancy/Breast-feeding: Meperidine should not be used in pregnancy prior to the labor period. When this drug is considered crucial by your doctor, its potential benefits must be carefully weighed against its risks.

Meperidine passes into breast milk. Nursing mothers who must take this drug should use infant formula.

Seniors: Seniors are more likely to experience side effects and should take the smallest effective dosage.

Generic Name

Meprobamate (meh-proe-BUH-mate) Ⓖ

Type of Drug

Antianxiety agent.

Prescribed For

Short-term anxiety and tension.

General Information

Meprobamate works by directly affecting several areas of the brain. It can relax you, relieve anxiety, and act as a muscle relaxant, anti-convulsant, or sleeping pill. This drug should be used for less than 4 months.

Cautions and Warnings

Do not take meprobamate if you are **allergic** or **sensitive** to any of its ingredients or to a related drug such as carbromal, cariso-prodol, felbamate, or mebutamate.

Do not use meprobamate if you have **intermittent porphyria**.

People with **epilepsy** should use this drug with caution because it may cause seizures in these people.

Meprobamate should be used with caution by people with **kidney disease,** who may need to take lower dosages.

Some people taking meprobamate have developed severe physical and psychological drug dependence. This drug can produce chronic intoxication after prolonged use or if used in greater than recommended doses. Symptoms include slurred speech, dizziness, general sleepiness, and depression. Suddenly stopping meprobamate after prolonged and excessive use may result in drug withdrawal symptoms, including severe anxiety, vomiting, appetite loss, sleeplessness, tremors, muscle twitching, confusion, hallucinations, and convulsions. Withdrawal symptoms usually begin 12–48 hours after meprobamate has been stopped and may last 1–4 days. When stopping treatment with meprobamate, the drug should be reduced gradually over 1 or 2 weeks.

Possible Side Effects

▼ Most common: drowsiness, sleepiness, dizziness, slurred speech, poor muscle coordination, headache, weakness, tingling in the arms and legs, and euphoria (feeling "high").

Possible Side Effects *(continued)*

▼ Less common: nausea, vomiting, diarrhea, abnormal heart rhythm, excitement or overstimulation, low blood pressure, itching, rash, and changes in blood components.

▼ Rare: allergic reactions, including high fever, chills, bronchospasm (closing of the throat), and reduced urinary function. Contact your doctor if you experience any side effect not listed above.

Drug Interactions

● Combining meprobamate with central-nervous-system (CNS) depressants, including alcohol, other sedatives, narcotics, sleeping pills, or antihistamines, can cause excess sedation, depression, sleepiness, or fatigue.

Food Interactions

Take this drug with food if it upsets your stomach.

Usual Dose

Adult and Child (age 13 and over): 1200–1600 mg a day in 3–4 doses; maximum daily dose, 2400 mg.

Child (age 6–12): 100–200 mg 2–3 times a day.

Child (under age 6): not recommended.

Overdosage

Overdose symptoms include extreme drowsiness, lethargy, stupor, and coma, with possible shock and respiratory collapse. If alcohol or another depressant has also been taken, small overdoses can be fatal. After a large overdose, the victim will go to sleep very quickly, and blood pressure, pulse, and breathing levels will drop rapidly. The overdose victim must immediately be taken to a hospital emergency room. ALWAYS bring the prescription bottle or container.

Special Information

Take this drug according to your doctor's direction. Do not change your dose without your doctor's approval. Do not crush or chew meprobamate tablets.

This drug causes drowsiness and poor concentration. Be careful when driving or performing complex activities. Avoid alcohol and other CNS depressants because they increase these effects.

Call your doctor if you develop fever, sore throat, rash, mouth sores, nosebleeds, unexplained black-and-blue marks, or easy bruising or bleeding, or if you become pregnant.

If you forget a dose and remember within about 1 hour of your regular time, take it right away. If you do not remember until later, skip the dose you forgot and go back to your regular schedule. Do not take a double dose.

Special Populations

Pregnancy/Breast-feeding: Meprobamate increases the risk of birth defects, particularly during the first 3 months of pregnancy. Inform your doctor immediately if you are taking this drug and are pregnant. When this drug is considered crucial by your doctor, its potential benefits must be carefully weighed against its risks.

Large amounts of meprobamate pass into breast milk. Nursing mothers who must take this drug should use infant formula.

Seniors: Seniors are more sensitive to the sedative and other effects of this drug and should take the lowest effective dosage.

Generic Name

Metaproterenol (meh-tuh-proe-TER-uh-nol) Ⓖ

Brand Name
Alupent

Type of Drug
Bronchodilator.

Prescribed For
Asthma, bronchospasm, and emphysema.

General Information
Metaproterenol sulfate can be taken both by mouth as a tablet or syrup and by inhalation. This drug may be used with other drugs to produce relief from asthma symptoms. Oral metaproterenol begins working 15–30 minutes after a dose; its effects may last for up to 4 hours. Metaproterenol inhalation begins working in 5–30 minutes and lasts for 2–6 hours.

Cautions and Warnings
Do not take metaproterenol if you are **allergic** or **sensitive** to any of its ingredients, or if you have **cardiac arrhythmia** (irregular heartbeat).

This drug should be used with caution by people with a history of **angina pectoris, heart disease, high blood pressure, stroke, seizures, diabetes, thyroid disease, prostate disease,** or **glaucoma**. Excessive use of metaproterenol could lead to worsening of your condition. Using excessive amounts of metaproterenol can lead to increased breathing difficulties rather than relief. In the most extreme cases, people have had heart attacks after using excessive amounts of inhalant.

Possible Side Effects

▼ Common: heart palpitations, rapid heartbeat, tremors, convulsions, shakiness, nervous tension, dizziness, fainting, headache, heartburn, upset stomach, nausea and vomiting, cough, dry or sore and irritated throat, muscle cramps, and urinary difficulties.

▼ Less common: high blood pressure, abnormal heart rhythms, and angina. Metaproterenol inhalation is less likely to cause these effects than some of the older asthma drugs. It can also cause diarrhea, unusual tastes or smells, dry mouth, drowsiness, hoarseness, stuffy nose, worsening of asthma, backache, fatigue, and rash.

Drug Interactions

- The effect of this drug may be increased by antidepressant drugs, such as monoamine oxidase inhibitors, some antihistamines, and levothyroxine.
- The risk of cardiac toxicity may be increased in people combining metaproterenol and theophylline.
- Beta-blocking drugs such as propanolol reduce the effect of metaproterenol. Metaproterenol may reduce the effects of blood-pressure-lowering drugs, especially reserpine, methyldopa, and guanethidine.

Food Interactions

If the tablets upset your stomach, they may be taken with food.

Usual Dose

Tablets or Syrup

    Adult and Child (age 10 or 60 lbs. and over): 60–80 mg a day.

    Child (age 6–9 or under 60 lbs.): 30–40 mg a day.

Child (under age 6): 0.6–1.2 mg per lb. of body weight a day. Children this age should be treated only with metaproterenol syrup.

Inhalation

Adult and Child (age 12 and over): 2–3 puffs every 3–4 hours. Each canister contains about 300 inhalations. Do not use more than 12 puffs a day.

Child (under age 12): not recommended.

Overdosage

Symptoms include palpitations, abnormal heart rhythm, rapid or slow heartbeat, chest pain, high blood pressure, fever, chills, cold sweat, blanching of the skin, nausea, vomiting, sleeplessness, delirium, tremor, pinpoint pupils, convulsions, coma, and collapse. The victim should see a doctor or be taken to a hospital emergency room. ALWAYS bring the prescription bottle or container.

Special Information

Be sure to follow your doctor's instructions for using metaproterenol. Using more than the amount prescribed can lead to drug tolerance and actually worsen your symptoms. If your condition worsens rather than improves after taking metaproterenol, stop taking it and call your doctor.

Metaproterenol inhalation should be breathed in during the second half of your inward breath, since this allows it to reach more deeply into your lungs.

Call your doctor immediately if you develop chest pain, palpitations, rapid heartbeat, muscle tremors, dizziness, headache, facial flushing, or urinary difficulty, or if you still have trouble breathing after using this medication.

If you miss a dose of metaproterenol, take it as soon as possible. Take the rest of that day's dose at regularly spaced time intervals. Go back to your regular schedule the next day.

Special Populations

Pregnancy/Breast-feeding: Metaproterenol has caused birth defects when given in large amounts to pregnant animals. When this drug is considered crucial by your doctor, its potential benefits must be carefully weighed against its risks.

It is not known if metaproterenol passes into breast milk. Nursing mothers who must use it should use infant formula.

Seniors: Seniors are more sensitive to the effects of this drug.

Generic Name

Metaxalone (meh-TAX-uh-lone)

Brand Name

Skelaxin

Type of Drug

Skeletal muscle relaxant.

Prescribed For

Muscle spasms.

General Information

Metaxalone is prescribed as part of a coordinated program of rest, physical therapy, and other measures for the relief of acute, painful spasm conditions. Exactly how metaxalone works is unknown.

Cautions and Warnings

Do not take metaxalone if you are **allergic** or **sensitive** to any of its ingredients.

Do not take metaxalone if you have a tendency toward **anemia,** or have serious **kidney or liver disease.**

Possible Side Effects

▼ Most common: nausea, vomiting, upset stomach, stomach cramps, drowsiness, dizziness, headache, nervousness, and irritability.

▼ Less common: rash, itching, low white-blood-cell count, low red-blood-cell count (symptoms include chills, fatigue, pale skin color, shortness of breath, rapid or pounding heartbeat, and dark urine), liver inflammation, and yellowing of the skin or whites of the eyes.

▼ Rare: drug sensitivity reactions (symptoms include hives, changes in facial color, and breathing difficulties). Contact your doctor if you experience any side effect not listed above.

Drug Interactions

● Sedatives, alcohol, and other nervous system depressants may increase the depressant effects of metaxalone.

Food Interactions

Metaxalone may be taken with food or meals if it upsets your stomach. Avoid high fat-content meals.

Usual Dose

Adult and Child (age 12 and over): 800 mg 3 or 4 times a day.
Child (under age 12): not recommended.

Overdosage

Symptoms are likely to be severe side effects but may include some less common reactions as well. Overdose victims should be taken to a hospital emergency room. ALWAYS bring the prescription bottle or container.

Special Information

Long-term metaxalone treatment may cause liver toxicity or damage. If you are using this medicine for an extended period, your doctor should check your liver function about every 1–2 months.

Metaxalone may cause tiredness, dizziness, and lightheadedness. Be careful when driving or performing tasks that require concentration and coordination.

Call your doctor if you develop breathing difficulties, unusual tiredness or weakness, fever, chills, cough or hoarseness, lower back or side pain, painful urination, yellowing of the skin or whites of the eyes, rash, hives, itching, redness, or any other bothersome or persistent symptom.

If you miss a dose of metaxalone, take it as soon as you remember. If it is almost time for your next dose, take 1 dose as soon as you remember, another in 3 or 4 hours, and then go back to your regular schedule. Do not take a double dose.

Special Populations

Pregnancy/Breast-feeding: The safety of metaxalone in pregnant women is unknown. Pregnant women should not use metaxalone unless its benefits have been carefully weighed against its risks.

It is not known if metaxalone passes into breast milk. Nursing mothers who must take it should use infant formula.

Seniors: Seniors with reduced kidney or liver function may require less metaxalone.

Generic Name

Metformin (met-FOR-min) Ⓖ

Brand Names

Fortamet   Glumetza
Glucophage   Riomet
Glucophage XR

Type of Drug

Biguanide antihyperglycemic.

Prescribed For

Type 2 diabetes; insulin-resistant and prediabetic conditions including impaired glucose tolerance, obesity, polycystic ovary syndrome, and metabolic abnormalities associated with HIV disease.

General Information

Metformin hydrochloride lowers the amount of glucose (sugar) produced by the liver, reduces the amount of glucose you absorb from food, and helps cells use glucose. If metformin fails to control your blood sugar, combining it with another antidiabetic drug may control your diabetes. Metformin can also moderately lower blood fats.

Metformin is available in either tablet form or as an oral solution.

Cautions and Warnings

Do not take metformin if you are **allergic** or **sensitive** to any of its ingredients or have **heart failure**. Metformin should not be taken by people with **kidney disease**. If you are having surgery or an x-ray that requires the injection of an iodine-based contrast material, you should temporarily stop taking metformin because the combination could result in acute kidney problems.

Metformin is related to an older antidiabetes drug that was removed from the market because of the risk of a very rare but serious complication known as lactic acidosis. Lactic acidosis is fatal about ½ of the time. It may also occur in association with a number of conditions, including diabetes mellitus. The risk of lactic acidosis increases with age, the presence of heart failure, and worsening kidney function. Regular monitoring of kidney function minimizes the risk of developing lactic acidosis, as does using the minimum effective dosage of metformin. Metformin should not be taken by people with acidosis, including those with diabetic ketoacidosis. Diabetic ketoacidosis should be treated with insulin.

People with **liver disease** should not take metformin because of the increased risk of lactic acidosis.

Possible Side Effects

People who have been stabilized on metformin should not consider gastrointestinal (GI) symptoms to be related to the drug unless other causes or lactic acidosis have been excluded.

▼ Most common: diarrhea, nausea, vomiting, abdominal bloating, gas, and appetite loss. These symptoms tend to occur when you first start taking metformin but are generally transient and resolve on their own. Occasionally, temporary dosage reduction is useful.

▼ Less common: weakness, stomach pain, and headache.

▼ Rare: an unpleasant or metallic taste in the mouth (this usually resolves on its own) and low blood levels of vitamin B_{12}. Blood levels of vitamin B_{12} should be periodically checked, or you may take a B_{12} supplement. Contact your doctor if you experience any side effect not listed above.

Drug Interactions

- Metformin may reduce the effect of glyburide (a sulfonylurea) but this interaction is highly variable from 1 person to another.
- Alcohol increases the risk of developing lactic acidosis while taking metformin.
- Metformin may interfere with amiloride, digoxin, morphine, procainamide, quinidine, quinine, ranitidine, triamterene, trimethoprim, and vancomycin. Careful monitoring is necessary.
- Cimetidine, nifedipine, and furosemide can cause a large increase in metformin blood levels and possible side effects. Furosemide levels are reduced by metformin.

Food Interactions

Metformin may be taken with food to reduce upset stomach.

Usual Dose

Adult: 500 mg twice daily or 850 mg once daily, increased gradually to a maximum daily dosage of 2550 mg. Older adults should start with the regular dosage but generally are not given the maximum.

Child (age 10 and over): same as adult dosage, but with a maximum of 2000 mg. Extended-release tablets should not be taken by those under age 17.

Overdosage

Lactic acidosis has occurred in some cases. Take the victim to a hospital emergency room at once. ALWAYS bring the prescription bottle or container.

Special Information

Diet and exercise are the mainstays of diabetes treatment. Be sure to follow your doctor's directions in these areas while taking your medication.

Alcohol increases the risk of developing lactic acidosis while taking metformin.

Lactic acidosis is a medical emergency. Metformin treatment must be stopped immediately if you develop it. This disease is often subtle and is accompanied only by nonspecific symptoms such as feeling unwell, muscle aches, breathing difficulties, tiredness, and nonspecific upset stomach. Low body temperature, low blood pressure, and slow heartbeat can develop with more severe acidosis. Call your doctor at once if you develop these symptoms.

Stomach and intestinal side effects may be reduced by gradually increasing your dosage and by taking metformin with meals.

Metformin should be temporarily stopped if you have severe diarrhea or vomiting. However, do not stop taking your medication without first consulting your doctor.

If you forget a dose, take it as soon as you remember. If it is almost time for your next dose, skip the dose you forgot and continue with your regular schedule. Do not take a double dose.

Special Populations

Pregnancy/Breast-feeding: The safety of using metformin during pregnancy is not known. Pregnant women with diabetes should take insulin.

Metformin passes into breast milk. Nursing mothers who must take it should consider using infant formula.

Seniors: Seniors may require reduced dosage.

Generic Name

Methotrexate (meth-oe-TREK-sate) [G]

Brand Name

Rheumatrex

Type of Drug

Antimetabolite, antiarthritic, and anti-inflammatory agent.

Prescribed For

Cancer chemotherapy; psoriasis; and adult and juvenile rheumatoid arthritis. Also used for Reiter's disease and severe asthma.

General Information

Used effectively in cancer treatment since the late 1940s, methotrexate is also prescribed for other conditions that respond to immune-system suppressants. Dosage varies widely depending on the disease being treated. Even relatively low dosages, such as those prescribed for rheumatoid arthritis, can be extremely toxic. Because of the risks associated with methotrexate, it should be used in noncancerous conditions only when the disease is severe and other treatments have failed. Only doctors who are familiar with methotrexate and its risks should prescribe it.

Cautions and Warnings

Do not take methotrexate if you are **allergic** or **sensitive** to any of its ingredients.

Methotrexate should not be used in pregnant women to treat psoriasis or rheumatoid arthritis. It should only be used in pregnant women for cancer treatment when the potential benefits outweigh the risks.

People with **alcoholism** should not take methotrexate.

Methotrexate can trigger a unique and dangerous form of lung disease at any time during your course of therapy. It can occur at dosages as low as 7.5 mg per week—the antiarthritis dosage. Symptoms of this condition are cough, respiratory infection, difficulty breathing, abnormal chest X-ray, and low blood-oxygen levels. Report any changes in breathing or lung status to your doctor.

Methotrexate can cause severe liver damage; this usually occurs only after taking it over a long period. Changes in liver enzymes, as measured by a blood test, are common. People with chronic **liver disease** should not take methotrexate.

People with **kidney disease** should use this drug with caution and receive a reduced dosage.

Methotrexate can severely lower red- and white-blood-cell and blood-platelet counts. Your doctor should periodically evaluate your kidney and liver function and blood components.

Methotrexate suppresses the immune system and can make you more likely to develop an opportunistic infection such as pneumocystis, especially if your **immune system is already weakened** by disease or another medication.

Methotrexate can cause severe diarrhea, stomach irritation, and mouth or gum sores. Death can result from intestinal perforation caused by methotrexate.

Methotrexate has been studied as an abortion drug in combination with misoprostol (see "Misoprostol").

Possible Side Effects

▼ Most common: liver irritation, loss of kidney function, reduced blood-platelet count, nausea, vomiting, diarrhea, stomach upset and irritation, itching, rash, hair loss, dizziness, and risk of infection.

▼ Less common: reduced red-blood-cell count, unusual sensitivity to the sun, acne, headache, drowsiness, blurred vision, respiratory infection and breathing problems, appetite loss, muscle aches, chest pain, coughing, painful urination, eye discomfort, nosebleeds, fever, infection, blood in the urine, sweating, ringing or buzzing in the ears, defective sperm production, reduced sperm count, menstrual dysfunction, vaginal discharge, convulsions, and slight paralysis.

Drug Interactions

• Aspirin and other nonsteroidal anti-inflammatory drugs (NSAIDs), as well as low-dose corticosteroid treatment, may be continued in most cases while you are taking methotrexate for rheumatoid arthritis, although an increase in drug toxicity is possible. However, fatal reactions have developed in 4 people taking methotrexate and an NSAID—3 with ketoprofen, 1 with naproxen. Do not take methotrexate and an anti-inflammatory or antiarthritic drug—even over-the-counter drugs such as ibuprofen or naproxen sodium—without your doctor's knowledge.

- Aspirin and other salicylates, anticancer drugs, etretinate, phenytoin, penicillins, probenecid, and sulfa drugs can increase the therapeutic and toxic effects of methotrexate.
- Combining phenylbutazone and methotrexate increases the risk of severe white-blood-cell count reductions, but may be medically necessary. In these cases, your doctor should monitor your health for signs of drug toxicity (see "Cautions and Warnings").
- Oral antibiotics may counteract the effects of methotrexate.
- Methotrexate may raise theophylline blood levels. Theophylline levels should be monitored when it is used with methotrexate.

Food Interactions

For optimal effectiveness, take this drug on an empty stomach, at least 1 hour before or 2 hours after meals. It may be taken with food if it upsets your stomach.

Usual Dose

Cancer: Dosage varies. Some cancers are treated with 10–30 mg a day, while others require 100s or 1000s of mg given intravenously.

Rheumatoid Arthritis: starting dosage—7.5 mg a week by mouth, either as a single dose or in 3 separate doses of 2.5 mg taken every 12 hours. Weekly dosage may be increased gradually up to 20 mg. Dosages above 20 mg a week are more likely to cause severe side effects.

Psoriasis: 2.5–6.5 mg a day by mouth, not to exceed 30 mg a week.

Overdosage

Methotrexate overdose can be serious and life threatening. Victims should be taken to a hospital emergency room immediately. A specific antidote to the effects of methotrexate, calcium leucovorin, is available in every hospital. ALWAYS bring the prescription bottle or container.

Special Information

If you vomit after taking a dose of methotrexate, do not take a replacement dose unless instructed to do so by your doctor.

Women taking this drug must use effective birth control.

People at risk of liver or kidney damage must be regularly monitored by their doctor for possible damage caused by methotrexate.

To avoid birth defects, men should not conceive during treatment or for 3 months after treatment has been completed.

Call your doctor immediately if you develop diarrhea, fever or chills, skin reddening, mouth or lip sores, stomach pain, unusual bleeding or bruising, blurred vision, seizures, cough, or breathing difficulties.

The following symptoms are less severe but should still be reported to your doctor: back pain, darkened urine, dizziness, drowsiness, headache, unusual tiredness or sickness, and yellowing of the skin or whites of the eyes.

If you forget a dose, skip it and continue with your regular schedule. Call your doctor at once. Do not take a double dose.

Special Populations

Pregnancy/Breast-feeding: Methotrexate can cause spontaneous abortion, stillbirth, and severe birth defects. Pregnant women should take methotrexate only after discussing the potential benefits versus risks with their doctor. Methotrexate should not be given to pregnant women to treat psoriasis or rheumatoid arthritis. Do not attempt to achieve pregnancy during methotrexate treatment or for at least 1 menstrual cycle after the treatment is completed. Use effective birth control while taking this drug. To avoid birth defects, men should not conceive during treatment or for 3 months after treatment has been completed. Methotrexate reduces sperm counts and may compromise sperm health.

This drug passes into breast milk. Nursing mothers should not take methotrexate.

Seniors: Seniors may be more susceptible to side effects and may obtain maximum benefit with smaller dosages.

Generic Name

Methyldopa (meth-ul-DOPE-uh) Ⓖ

The information in this profile also applies to the following drug:

Generic Ingredients: Methyldopa + Hydrochlorothiazide Ⓖ

Type of Drug

Antihypertensive.

Prescribed For

High blood pressure.

General Information

How methyldopa works is not well understood. It may lower blood pressure by stimulating receptors in the central nervous system (CNS), and by inhibiting or reducing levels of important pressure-regulating hormones such as norepinephrine and serotonin. It takes about 2 days for methyldopa to reach its maximal antihypertensive (blood-pressure-lowering) effect. It is usually prescribed with one or more other antihypertensive drugs or a diuretic.

Cautions and Warnings

Do not take methyldopa if you are **allergic** or **sensitive** to any of its ingredients or any other ingredient in the formulation, including sulfites.

Do not take this drug if you have had a previous **liver-related reaction** to it, or if you have liver disease such as **hepatitis** or **cirrhosis**. People taking this drug may develop a fever with changes in liver function within the first 3 weeks of treatment. Some people develop jaundice (symptoms include yellowing of the skin or whites of the eyes) during the first 2 or 3 months of treatment. Your doctor should periodically evaluate your liver function during the first 3 months of methyldopa treatment, or if you develop an unexplained fever.

Methyldopa should be used with caution in people with severe **kidney disease,** who may need reduced dosage.

Methyldopa may increase the risk of hemolytic anemia.

Some people taking methyldopa experience swelling or weight gain. This can usually be controlled when this drug is combined with a diuretic. Do not continue taking methyldopa if swelling progresses or you experience signs of heart failure.

Possible Side Effects

Most people have little trouble with methyldopa, but it can cause temporary sedation in the first few weeks of treatment or when the dose is increased. Passing headache and weakness are other possible early side effects.

▼ Less common: headache; dizziness; lightheadedness; tingling in the extremities; muscle spasms or weakness; decreased mental acuity; psychological disturbances including nightmares, mild psychosis, and depression; rash; changes in heart rate; increased angina pain; water retention, resulting in weight gain; nausea; vomiting; constipation;

Possible Side Effects (*continued*)

---

diarrhea; mild dry mouth; sore or black tongue; stuffy nose; male breast enlargement or pain; lactation in females; impotence or decreased sex drive in males; mild arthritis symptoms; and skin reactions.

▼ Rare: Methyldopa may affect white blood cells or blood platelets. It may also cause involuntary jerky movements, twitching, restlessness, and slow, continuous, wormlike movements of the fingers, toes, hands, or other body parts. Contact your doctor if you experience any side effect not listed above.

Drug Interactions

- Do not combine methyldopa and a monoamine oxidase inhibitor antidepressant. This combination can cause excessive stimulation.
- Methyldopa increases the effect of other blood-pressure-lowering drugs. This is a desirable interaction for people with hypertension. However, the combination of methyldopa and propranolol or nadolol—2 beta blockers often prescribed for hypertension—has, rarely, caused an increase in blood pressure.
- Avoid over-the-counter cough medicines, cold and allergy remedies, and appetite suppressants. These products contain stimulant ingredients that can increase blood pressure.
- Methyldopa may increase the blood-sugar-lowering effect of tolbutamide or other sulfonylurea-type oral antidiabetic drugs.
- If methyldopa is combined with phenoxybenzamine, urinary incontinence (inability to control the bladder) may result.
- The effect of methyldopa may be reduced by barbiturates, tricyclic antidepressants, and iron.
- The combination of methyldopa and lithium may cause symptoms of lithium overdose—upset stomach, frequent urination, muscle weakness, tiredness, and tremors—even though blood levels of lithium have not changed.
- Methyldopa in combination with haloperidol may produce irritability, aggressiveness, assaultive behavior, or other psychiatric symptoms.
- Combining methyldopa with levodopa + carbidopa may increase all their effects.

- Combining methyldopa with stimulants or a phenothiazine-type drug may lead to a serious increase in blood pressure.
- Reduced doses of anesthetics may be required while taking methyldopa.

Food Interactions

Methyldopa is best taken on an empty stomach, but you may take it with food if it upsets your stomach.

Usual Dose

Adult: starting dosage—250-mg tablet 2–3 times a day for the first 2 days. Dosage may then be increased until lower blood pressure is achieved. Maintenance dose—500–2000 mg a day in 2–4 divided doses, depending on individual need.

Child: 4.5 mg per lb. of body weight a day in 2–4 divided doses, depending on individual need. Do not exceed 30 mg per lb. of body weight or 3 g a day, whichever is less.

Overdosage

Symptoms include sedation, very low blood pressure, weakness, dizziness, lightheadedness, fainting, slow heartbeat, constipation, abdominal gas or bulging, nausea, vomiting, and coma. Overdose victims should be made to vomit if they are still conscious by using ipecac syrup—available at any pharmacy—and then taken to a hospital emergency room. If some time has passed since the overdose was taken, take the victim directly to an emergency room. ALWAYS bring the prescription bottle or container.

Special Information

Take methyldopa exactly as prescribed to maintain maximum control of your hypertension. Do not stop taking this drug unless you are told to do so by your doctor.

A mild sedative effect is to be expected from methyldopa and will resolve within several days. Be careful when driving, operating hazardous machinery, or performing any task that requires concentration.

Your urine may darken if left exposed to air. This is normal and not a cause for alarm.

You may experience dizziness when rising suddenly from a sitting or lying position. However, call your doctor if you develop fever, prolonged general tiredness, or general dizziness. If you develop involuntary muscle movements, fever, or jaundice, stop taking the drug and contact your doctor immediately. If these reactions are due to methyldopa, your temperature or liver abnormalities will begin to normalize as soon as you stop taking it.

If you forget a dose, take it as soon as you remember. If it is almost time for your next dose, skip the one you forgot and continue with your regular schedule. Do not take a double dose.

Special Populations

Pregnancy/Breast-feeding: Methyldopa crosses into the fetal circulation. When this drug is considered crucial by your doctor, its potential benefits must be carefully weighed against its risks.

Small amounts of methyldopa pass into breast milk. Nursing mothers who must take this drug should use infant formula.

Seniors: Seniors are more sensitive to the sedating and blood-pressure-lowering effects of methyldopa and may experience dizziness or fainting. Older adults should receive reduced dosage.

Generic Name

Methylphenidate (meth-ul-FEN-ih-date) G

Brand Names

Concerta	Methylin
Daytrana Patch	Methylin ER
Metadate	Ritalin
Metadate CD	Ritalin LA
Metadate ER	Ritalin-SR

The information in this profile also applies to the following drug:

Generic Ingredient: Dexmethylphenidate
Focalin   Focalin XR

Type of Drug

Mild central-nervous-system stimulant.

Prescribed for

Attention-deficit hyperactivity disorder (ADHD); also prescribed for psychological, educational, or social disorders; narcolepsy; and mild depression in the elderly. Methylphenidate is also used in cancer treatment and stroke recovery and for treating hiccups after anesthesia.

General Information

Methylphenidate hydrochloride is prescribed for the treatment of ADHD in children. It should be used only after conducting a complete evaluation of the child. Frequency and severity of symptoms and their appropriateness for the age of the child—not solely the presence of certain behavioral characteristics—determine whether drug therapy is required. Many experts believe that methylphenidate offers only a temporary solution because it does not permanently change behavioral patterns. Psychological measures must also be taken to ensure successful treatment in the long term.

Cautions and Warnings

Do not take methylphenidate if you are **allergic** or **sensitive** to any of its ingredients.

Do not take methylphenidate if you have **glaucoma or other visual problems,** a **seizure** disorder, severe **depression, tics** or **Tourette's syndrome,** or if you are extremely **tense or agitated**.

People with a history of **drug dependence** or **alcoholism** should use methylphenidate with caution. Chronic or abusive use of methylphenidate can lead to drug dependence or addiction. This drug can also cause severe psychotic episodes. Do not use methylphenidate for the prevention or treatment of normal fatigue.

Methylphenidate should be used with caution if you have **high blood pressure**, and your doctor should monitor your blood pressure frequently while you take this drug.

Stimulants like methylphenidate are not effective in children whose symptoms are related to environmental factors or to primary psychiatric conditions, including psychosis. Methylphenidate should not be used to treat a primary stress reaction.

Possible Side Effects

Adult

▼ Most common: nervousness and inability to sleep, which doctors generally control by reducing or eliminating the afternoon or evening dose.

▼ Rare: rash, itching, fever, symptoms resembling those of arthritis, appetite loss, nausea, dizziness, abnormal heart rhythm, headache, drowsiness, changes in blood pressure or pulse, chest pain, stomach pain, psychotic reactions, changes in blood components, and loss of some scalp hair.

Possible Side Effects (continued)

Contact your doctor if you experience any side effect not listed above.

Child
▼ Most common: headache, appetite loss; stomach pain; weight loss, especially during prolonged therapy; sleeping difficulties; and abnormal heart rhythm.

Drug Interactions

- Methylphenidate reduces the effectiveness of guanethidine (an antihypertensive drug) and of coumarin anticoagulants (blood thinners).
- Monoamine oxidase inhibitor (MAOI) antidepressants may significantly increase the effect of methylphenidate, which may lead to extreme high blood pressure. Do not take these drugs together, or take methylphenidate for 14 days after you stop taking an MAOI.
- Methylphenidate may increase tricyclic and selective serotonin reuptake inhibitors (SSRI) antidepressant blood levels and the risk of side effects.
- Methylphenidate may increase anticonvulsant blood levels.
- If you take methylphenidate regularly, avoid alcohol. This combination increases drowsiness.

Food Interactions

This medication is best taken 30–45 minutes before meals.

Usual Dose

Oral Tablets

Adult: Doses range from 10–30 mg a day but can be as high as 60 mg. The immediate-release drug is taken 2–3 times a day.

Child (age 6 and over): starting dosage—5 mg before breakfast and lunch. Increase by 5–10 mg each week as required, not to exceed 60 mg a day.

Child (under age 6): not recommended.

SR tablets and ER tablets are designed to last for 8 hours, and Concerta, Ritalin LA, and Metadate CD last 8–12 hours. These medications may be used in place of more frequent doses during the same period of time.

Skin Patch: The methylphenidate patch should be applied to the hip area about 2 hours before an effect is needed and should be removed 9 hours after application. Apply the patch as close to the same time every day as possible to obtain consistent daily dosing.

Overdosage

Symptoms include vomiting, agitation, uncontrollable twitching of the muscles, convulsions followed by coma, euphoria (feeling "high"), confusion, hallucinations, delirium, sweating, flushing, headache, high fever, abnormal heart rate, high blood pressure, and dryness of the mouth and nose. Take the victim to a hospital emergency room immediately. ALWAYS bring the prescription bottle or container.

Special Information

Methylphenidate can mask the signs of temporary drowsiness or fatigue: Be careful when driving or doing any task that requires concentration. Take your last daily dose no later than 6 p.m. to avoid sleeping difficulties.

Call your doctor if you develop any persistent or bothersome side effect. Do not increase your dosage without your doctor's knowledge.

If improvement is not seen after 1 month of adequate dosage, discontinue use of this drug.

Suppression of growth in children has been reported with long-term use of this drug. Contact your doctor if your child does not grow or gain weight as expected.

ER and SR tablets must be swallowed whole, never crushed or chewed.

Use of the methylphenidate skin patch should be stopped if an intense local reaction (redness, plus small solid rounded bumps and pustules) that does not get much better within 48 hours or spreads beyond the patch site. Redness is common and, by itself, not a severe reaction. Call your doctor if a skin reaction develops; you may need to take the oral form in this case.

If you miss a dose, take it as soon as possible. Space the remaining daily dosage evenly throughout the day. Go back to your regular schedule the next day.

Special Populations

Pregnancy/Breast-feeding: Methylphenidate crosses into the fetal circulation. When this drug is considered crucial by your doctor, its potential benefits must be carefully weighed against its risks.

It is not known whether this drug passes into breast milk. Nursing mothers who must take this drug should consider using infant formula.

Seniors: Seniors may take this drug without special restriction.

Generic Name

Metoclopramide (met-oe-KLOE-pruh-mide) Ⓖ

Brand Names

Octamide   Reglan*
Reclomide

Some products in this brand-name group are alcohol- or sugar-free. Consult your pharmacist.

Type of Drug

Antiemetic and gastrointestinal (GI) stimulant.

Prescribed For

Diabetic gastropareisis (stomach paralysis associated with diabetes; symptoms include nausea, vomiting, heartburn, persistent feeling of fullness, and appetite loss), gastroesophageal reflux disease (GERD), stomach ulcer, anorexia nervosa, and bleeding from blood vessels in the esophagus—often associated with severe liver disease. It also facilitates diagnostic x-ray procedures and improves the absorption of anti-migraine medication and narcotic pain relievers. Nursing mothers are occasionally given metoclopramide to increase milk production.

General Information

Metoclopramide stimulates movement of the upper GI tract without producing excess stomach acids or other secretions. Doctors believe that it prevents nausea and vomiting primarily by affecting dopamine receptors in the brain. Metoclopramide also affects the secretion of a variety of hormones and may improve the absorption of other drugs into the bloodstream.

Cautions and Warnings

Do not take metoclopramide if you are **allergic** or **sensitive** to any of its ingredients.

People with **high blood pressure, Parkinson's disease, asthma,** or **liver or kidney failure** should use metoclopramide with caution. Do not take this drug if you have a **seizure disorder.** Metoclopramide should not be used if you have a **bleeding ulcer** or any condition that makes stimulation of the GI tract dangerous.

Mild to severe depression has occurred with metoclopramide.

Uncontrollable motions similar to those associated with Parkinson's disease have developed as a side effect of this drug. These generally occur within 6 months after starting metoclopramide and subside within 2–3 months.

This drug may cause extrapyramidal side effects similar to those associated with phenothiazine drugs. These effects, which occur in 0.2–1% of the people taking the drug, include restlessness and involuntary movements of the arms and legs, face, tongue, lips, and other parts of the body. Do not combine metoclopramide with a phenothiazine drug because this may increase the risk of extrapyramidal effects.

Women taking this drug develop chronic elevations of the hormone prolactin. About 33% of breast tumors are prolactin-dependent, a factor that you should consider before taking metoclopramide.

Metoclopramide is only prescribed for short-term relief of symptoms. Treatment with metoclopramide lasting longer than 12 weeks has not been studied and is not recommended.

Possible Side Effects

Mild side effects occur in 20–30% of people. Side effects increase with dosage or prolonged use.

▼ Most common: restlessness, drowsiness, fatigue, sleeplessness, dizziness, anxiety, loss of muscle control, nausea, diarrhea, headache, muscle spasm, confusion, and severe depression.

▼ Less common: rash, diarrhea, blood-pressure changes, abnormal heart rhythms, slow heartbeat, oozing from the nipples, tender nipples, loss of regular menstrual periods, breast swelling and tenderness, impotence, reduced white-blood-cell counts, frequent urination, loss of urinary control, visual disturbances, worsening of bronchial spasm, convulsions, and hallucinations.

▼ Rare: People taking this drug may develop a group of possibly fatal symptoms collectively called neuroleptic malignant syndrome. These symptoms include very high fever,

Possible Side Effects *(continued)*

semi-consciousness, and rigid muscles. Flushing of the face and upper body as well as liver toxicity after high doses have also occurred. Contact your doctor if you experience any side effect not listed above.

Drug Interactions

- Narcotics and anticholinergic drugs interfere with metoclopramide's effect on stomach acid.
- Due to metoclopramide's effect on food absorption, injected insulin doses may need adjustment.
- Metoclopramide may increase the sedative effects of nervous system depressants, including sedatives and sleeping pills.
- Metoclopramide may increase blood levels of acetaminophen, tetracycline, ethanol, and cyclosporine.
- Metoclopramide and levodopa + carbidopa interfere with each other.
- Metoclopramide may reduce the effects of digoxin and cimetidine.
- Combining metoclopramide and a monoamine oxidase inhibitor antidepressant may cause very high blood pressure.

Food Interactions

Take this drug 30 minutes before meals and at bedtime.

Usual Dose

Adult and Child (age 15 and over): 5–15 mg before meals and at bedtime. Single doses of 10–20 mg are used before x-ray diagnostic procedures.

Senior: starting dosage—5 mg.

Child (age 6–14): ¼–½ the adult dosage.

Child (under age 6): 0.05 mg per lb. of body weight per dose.

Overdosage

Symptoms of overdose include drowsiness, disorientation, restlessness, or uncontrollable muscle movement. These usually disappear within 24 hours after the drug has been stopped. Anticholinergic drugs help control overdose symptoms. Call your local poison control center or a hospital emergency room for more information.

Special Information

Call your doctor if you develop chills; fever; sore throat; dizziness; severe or persistent headache; feeling unwell; rapid or irregular heartbeat; difficulty speaking or swallowing; loss of balance; stiffness of the arms or legs; a shuffling walk; a mask-like face; lip-smacking or puckering; puffing of the cheeks; rapid, worm-like tongue movement; uncontrollable chewing movement; uncontrolled arm and leg movement; or any persistent or intolerable side effect.

Metoclopramide may cause dizziness, confusion, and drowsiness. Be careful when driving or doing any task that requires concentration. Avoid alcohol and be cautious about taking sedatives or sleeping pills.

If you forget a dose, take it as soon as you remember. If it is almost time for your next dose, skip the dose you forgot and continue with your regular schedule. Do not take a double dose.

Special Populations

Pregnancy/Breast-feeding: Metoclopramide enters the fetal circulation. When this drug is considered crucial by your doctor, its potential benefits must be carefully weighed against its risks.

This drug passes into breast milk. Nursing mothers occasionally receive metoclopramide to increase milk production. There appears to be no risk for the infant whose nursing mother takes 45 mg or less a day. Always consider possible effects on the nursing infant if breast-feeding while taking this drug.

Seniors: Seniors, especially women, are more sensitive to side effects (see "Cautions and Warnings"). Shuffling walk and shaking hands may be likely to occur in seniors after a prolonged use of metoclopramide. Dose adjustments may be necessary.

Generic Name

Metoprolol (meh-TOPE-roe-lol) Ⓖ

Brand Names

Lopressor   Toprol-XL

Combination Product
Generic Ingredients: Metoprolol + Hydrochlorthiazide
Dutoprol   Lopressor-HCT

The information in this profile also applies to the following drug:

Generic Ingredient: Penbutolol
Levatol

Type of Drug

Beta-adrenergic blocking agent.

Prescribed For

High blood pressure, angina pectoris, abnormal heart rhythms, prevention of second heart attack, migraine, tremors, side effects of antipsychotic drugs, congestive heart failure, and bleeding from the esophagus.

General Information

Metoprolol is one of many beta-adrenergic blocking drugs, or beta blockers, that interfere with the action of a specific part of the nervous system. Beta receptors are found all over the body and affect many body functions. Each beta blocker has particular characteristics that make it more suitable for certain conditions or people. Metoprolol is available in a sustained-release formulation, taken only once a day, that maintains a steady blood level of the drug for a full 24 hours.

Cautions and Warnings

Do not take metoprolol if you are **allergic** or **sensitive** to any of its ingredients or to beta blockers.

You should not take metoprolol if you have **asthma, a very slow heart rate,** or **heart block** (disruption of the electrical impulses that control heart rate) because the drug may aggravate these conditions.

People with **angina** who take metoprolol for high blood pressure risk aggravating their angina if they suddenly stop taking the drug. These people should have their drug dosage reduced gradually over 1–2 weeks.

Metoprolol should be used with caution if you have **liver or kidney disease** because your ability to eliminate the drug from your body may be impaired.

People with **pheochromocytoma** (adrenal gland tumor) need treatment with an alpha blocker before starting on a beta blocker drug.

Metoprolol reduces the amount of blood pumped by the heart with each beat. This reduction in blood flow may aggravate the condition of people with **heart failure, poor circulation,** or **circulatory disease**.

If you are undergoing **major surgery,** your doctor may want you to stop taking metoprolol at least 2 days before.

People with a history of **severe anaphylactic reaction** to allergens may be unresponsive to usual doses of epinephrine while taking beta blockers.

Possible Side Effects

Metoprolol side effects are relatively uncommon and usually mild.

▼ Less common: impotence, unusual tiredness or weakness, slow heartbeat, heart failure, dizziness, breathing difficulties, bronchospasm, depression, confusion, anxiety, nervousness, sleeplessness, disorientation, short-term memory loss, emotional instability, cold hands and feet, constipation, diarrhea, nausea, vomiting, upset stomach, increased sweating, urinary difficulties, cramps, blurred vision, rash, itching, hives, hair loss, stuffy nose, facial swelling, aggravation of lupus erythematosus, chest pain, back or joint pain, colitis, drug allergy (symptoms include fever and sore throat), and liver toxicity.

For side effects for Hydrochlorothiazide, see page 1113.

Drug Interactions

- Metoprolol may interact with surgical anesthetics to increase the risk of heart problems during surgery. Some anesthesiologists recommend gradually stopping the drug by 2 days before surgery.
- Metoprolol may interfere with the normal signs of low blood sugar and with the action of oral antidiabetes medications.
- Metoprolol increases the blood-pressure-lowering effect of other blood-pressure-reducing agents, including clonidine, guanabenz, and reserpine, as well as calcium-channel blockers such as nifedipine.
- Aspirin-containing drugs, indomethacin, sulfinpyrazone, and estrogen drugs may interfere with the blood-pressure-lowering effect of metoprolol.

- Cocaine may reduce the effectiveness of all beta blockers.
- Metoprolol may worsen the problem of cold hands and feet associated with taking ergot alkaloids, which are used to treat migraine. Gangrene is a possibility in people taking both an ergot and metoprolol.
- The effect of benzodiazepine antianxiety drugs may be increased by metoprolol.
- Thyroid hormone replacement will interfere with the effects of metoprolol.
- Combining metoprolol and prazosin may increase the risk of postural hypotension.
- Selective serotonin reuptake inhibitor antidepressants (SSRIs) may increase the side effects of metoprolol.
- Calcium channel blockers, flecainide, hydralazine, contraceptive drugs, propafenone, haloperidol, phenothiazine sedatives (molindone and others), quinolone antibacterials, and quinidine may increase the amount of metoprolol in the bloodstream and lead to increased metoprolol effects.
- Metoprolol should not be taken within 2 weeks of taking a monoamine oxidase inhibitor antidepressant.
- Aluminum salts, barbiturates, calcium salts, cholestyramine, colestipol, ampicillin, and rifampin may reduce the effectiveness of metoprolol.
- Cimetidine increases the amount of metoprolol absorbed into the bloodstream from oral tablets.
- Metoprolol may interfere with the effectiveness of some asthma medications, including theophylline and aminophylline, and especially ephedrine and isoproterenol.
- Combining metoprolol with phenytoin or digitalis drugs may result in excessive slowing of the heart, possibly causing heart block.
- Beta blockers may block the effects of epinephrine.
- If you stop smoking while taking metoprolol, your dose may have to be reduced because your liver will break down the drug more slowly afterward.

Food Interactions

Sustained-release metoprolol—Toprol-XL—may be taken with food if it upsets your stomach. Because food increases the amount of short-acting metoprolol—Lopressor—absorbed into the blood, take the short-acting form without food.

Usual Dose

Adult

Metoprolol: 100–450 mg a day; dosage must be tailored to your specific needs.

Metoprolol + Hydrochlorthiazide: 1 tablet daily. This is available in a number of dosage strengths for individualized treatment options.

Penbutolol: 20 mg once a day. Seniors may require more or less medication and must be carefully monitored by their doctors. People with liver problems may require lower dosage.

Child: not recommended.

Overdosage

Symptoms include changes in heartbeat—unusually slow, unusually fast, or irregular—severe dizziness or fainting, breathing difficulties, bluish-colored fingernails or palms, and seizures. The victim should be taken to a hospital emergency room. ALWAYS bring the prescription bottle or container.

Special Information

Metoprolol should be taken continuously. When ending metoprolol treatments, dosage should be lowered gradually over a period of about 2 weeks. Do not stop taking this drug unless directed to do so by your doctor; abrupt withdrawal may cause chest pain, breathing difficulties, increased sweating, and unusually fast or irregular heartbeat.

Call your doctor at once if you develop back or joint pain, breathing difficulties, cold hands or feet, depression, rash, or changes in heartbeat. This drug may produce an undesirable lowering of blood pressure, leading to dizziness or fainting; call your doctor if this happens to you. Call your doctor if you experience persistent or bothersome nausea or vomiting, upset stomach, diarrhea, constipation, impotence, headache, itching, anxiety, nightmares or vivid dreams, trouble sleeping, stuffy nose, frequent urination, unusual tiredness, or weakness.

Metoprolol can cause drowsiness, lightheadedness, dizziness, or blurred vision. Be careful when driving or performing complex tasks.

Do not crush or chew the sustained-release form of metoprolol.

It is best to take metoprolol at the same time each day. If you forget a dose, take it as soon as you remember. If you take metoprolol once a day and it is within 8 hours of your next dose, skip the dose you forgot and continue with your regular schedule. If you take it twice a day and it is within 4 hours of your next dose, skip the dose you forgot and continue with your regular schedule. Never take a double dose.

Special Populations

Pregnancy/Breast-feeding: Infants born to women who took a beta blocker while pregnant had lower birth weights, low blood pressure, and reduced heart rates. Metoprolol should be avoided by women who are or might be pregnant.

Small amounts of metoprolol pass into breast milk. Nursing mothers taking metoprolol should use infant formula.

Seniors: Seniors require less of the drug to achieve results. Seniors taking metoprolol may be more likely to suffer from cold hands and feet, reduced body temperature, chest pain, general feelings of ill health, sudden breathing difficulties, increased sweating, or changes in heartbeat.

Generic Name

Metronidazole (meh-troe-NYE-duh-zole) Ⓖ

Brand Names

Flagyl	MetroLotion
Flagyl ER	Noritate
MetroCream	Vandazole
MetroGel	

The information in this profile also applies to the following drug:

Generic Ingredient: Tinidazole
Tindamax

Type of Drug

Amoebicide and antibiotic.

Prescribed For

Metronidazole is prescribed for acute amoebic dysentery and infections of the vagina, bone, joint, brain, nervous system, urinary tract, abdomen, and skin; also prescribed for pneumonia, ulcers caused by *Helicobacter pylori,* inflammatory bowel disease, rosacea, colitis caused by other antibiotics, periodontal (gum) infection, and complications of severe liver disease. The gel may be used to treat acne, severe skin ulcers, and inflammation of the skin around the mouth.

Tinidazole is prescribed for bacterial vaginosis, vaginal infections with trichomonas, giardia infections in adults and children, and intestinal and liver infections caused by amoeba infection.

General Information

Metronidazole is an effective treatment for infections caused by a variety of fungi and some bacteria. Metronidazole kills these microorganisms by disrupting their DNA after they enter body cells. Tinidazole is a drug chemically related to metronidazole that has been proven to work on bacterial vaginosis, vaginal trichomonas, giardia, and amoeba infections of the bowel or liver. These drugs may be prescribed for symptomless diseases when the doctor feels that an underlying infection may be involved. For example, asymptomatic women may be treated with one of these drugs when vaginal examination shows evidence of trichomonas.

Cautions and Warnings

Do not take metronidazole if you are **allergic** or **sensitive** to any of its ingredients or if you have a history of **blood disease**.

Metronidazole has been found to cause cancer in lab animals. Unnecessary use of this drug should be avoided.

People taking metronidazole have experienced seizures and numbness or tingling in the hands or feet. This effect is rare with low dosages but may be more common in people taking larger dosages for long periods, as in Crohn's disease. If this occurs, stop taking the drug and call your doctor at once.

Metronidazole should be taken with caution if you have active **nervous system disease,** including **epilepsy,** or severe **liver problems.**

Metronidazole may cause *Candida* vaginitis in women.

Possible Side Effects

Metronidazole

▼ Most common: gastrointestinal symptoms (including nausea that is sometimes accompanied by headache), dizziness, appetite loss, vomiting, diarrhea, vaginitis, upset stomach, abdominal cramping, metallic taste, and constipation.

Possible Side Effects *(continued)*

▼ Less common: numbness or tingling in the extremities, joint pain, confusion, irritability, depression, difficulty sleeping, itching, pelvic pressure, and weakness.

▼ Rare: clumsiness or poor coordination, fever, increased urination, seizure, incontinence, and reduced sex drive. Contact your doctor if you experience any side effect not listed above.

Skin creams containing metronidazole may cause redness, itching, irritation, or worsening of rosacea.

Tinidazole

The chance of side effects increases with the amount of medication taken.

▼ Less common: metallic or bitter taste, nausea, loss of appetite, upset stomach, cramps, vomiting, constipation, weakness, fatigue, not feeling well, dizziness, and headache.

▼ Rare: drug sensitivity (itching, rash, flushing, sweating, dry mouth, fever, burning sensation, thirst, salivation, and swelling around the eyes or lips), which may also affect the nervous system, kidneys, heart, blood, and other systems. Contact your doctor if you experience any side effect not listed above.

Drug Interactions

- Do not use alcohol or take disulfiram with metronidazole because of the risk of serious interactions.
- Metronidazole may increase the side effects of 5-fluorouracil. Do not combine these treatments.
- Dosages of oral anticoagulants (blood thinners) such as warfarin must be reduced because metronidazole increases their effect.
- Metronidazole may increase lithium blood levels, effects, and side effects. Lithium levels should be monitored.
- Delaviridine, indinavir, nelfinavir, ritonavir, amiodarone, aprepitant, chloramphenicol, cimetidine, ciprofloxacin, clarithromycin, diltiazem, erythromycin, fluconazole, fluvoxamine, gestodene, itraconazole, ketoconazole, mifepristone, nefazodone, norfloxacin, norfluoxetine, mibefradil, and verapamil may increase blood levels of metronidazole by interfering

with their breakdown in the liver. Your metronidazole dosage may have to be reduced.

- Carbamazepine, rifabutin, rifampin, St. John's wort, phenytoin, fosphenytoin, as well as phenobarbital and other barbiturates may reduce the effectiveness of metronidazole by increasing the rate at which it is cleared from the body.
- The antibiotic oxytetracycline may antagonize the effects of metronidazole.
- Medications that cause nervous system toxicity—such as mexiletine, ethambutol, isoniazid, lindane, lincomycin, lithium, pemoline, quinacrine, and long-term, high-dose pyridoxine (vitamin B_6) should not be taken with metronidazole because nervous system side effects may be increased.
- Cholestyramine reduces the amount of metronidazole absorbed into the blood. Separate these medicines by at least 2 hours to avoid this interaction.

Food Interactions

Do not drink grapefruit juice while taking these medicines because it can interfere with the liver's ability to break them down. Metronidazole and tinidazole (when they must be taken for more than 1 day) should be taken with food to avoid upset stomach.

Usual Dose

Metronidazole

Adult: amoebic dysentery—750 mg 3 times a day for 5–10 days. Bacterial vaginosis—750 mg a day for 7 days. *H. pylori*—250 mg 4 times a day. Trichomonal infection—250 mg 3 times a day for 7 days; or 2 g in 1 dose. Reduced dosage may be necessary for seniors.

Child (age 3 and over): amoebic dysentery—16–23 mg per lb. of body weight daily, divided in 3 equal doses for 10 days. Trichomonal infection—2.25 mg per lb. of body weight 3 times a day for 7 days.

Skin creams should be applied 1–2 times a day. Vaginal creams should be used 1–2 times a day for 5 days.

Tinidazole

Adult: bacterial vaginosis—2 g a day for 2 days or 1 g a day for 5 days. Amoebic dysentery—2 g a day for 3 days. Amoebic liver abscesses: 2 g per day for 3–5 days taken with food. Trichomonal infection—1 dose of 2 g taken with food. Giardiasis—1 dose of 2 g taken with food. Reduced dosage may be necessary for seniors.

Child (age 3 and older): giardiasis or intestinal amebiasis—1 dose of 22.7 mg per lb. of body weight, up to 2 g, taken with food. Amoebic liver abscesses—1 dose of 22.7 mg per lb. of body weight, up to 2 g, taken with food, for 3–5 days.

Overdosage

Symptoms may include nausea, vomiting, clumsiness, unsteadiness, seizures, and pain or tingling in the hands or feet. Call your local poison control center or a hospital emergency room for more information. If you seek treatment, ALWAYS bring the prescription bottle or container.

Special Information

Call your doctor if you become dizzy or lightheaded while taking metronidazole, or if you develop numbness, tingling, pain, or weakness in your hands or feet; seizures; clumsiness or unsteadiness; mood changes; unusual vaginal irritation, discharge, or dryness; frequent or painful urination; rash, hives, or itching; severe pain in the back or abdomen accompanied by vomiting, appetite loss, or nausea; or any bothersome or persistent side effect.

Avoid drinking alcohol while taking metronidazole.

These medicines may cause darkening of your urine; this is probably not an important side effect, but inform your doctor if it happens.

Follow your doctor's dosage instructions exactly. Complete the full course of drug therapy.

Metronidazole may cause dry mouth, which usually can be relieved with ice, hard candy, or gum. Call your doctor or dentist if dry mouth persists for more than 2 weeks.

If you are taking these drugs for more than 1 day and forget a dose, take it as soon as you remember. If it is almost time for your next dose, skip the dose you forgot and continue with your regular schedule. Do not take a double dose.

Special Populations

Pregnancy/Breast-feeding: Metronidazole passes into the fetal circulation and should not be taken during the first 3 months of pregnancy and should be used with caution during the last 6 months of pregnancy.

Metronidazole passes into breast milk. Nursing mothers who must take this drug should use infant formula.

Seniors: Seniors, particularly those with advanced liver disease, are more sensitive to the effects of metronidazole and may require lower dosages.

Generic Name

Miconazole (mye-KON-uh-zole) Ⓖ

Brand Names

Monistat   Monistat-Derm

The information in this profile also applies to the following drugs:

Generic Ingredient: Butoconazole Nitrate
Femstat   Gynazole

Generic Ingredient: Oxiconazole
Oxistat

Generic Ingredient: Terconazole Ⓖ
Terazol

Generic Ingredient: Tioconazole
Vagistat

Type of Drug
Antifungal.

Prescribed For
Fungal infections of the vagina, skin, and blood.

General Information
Miconazole nitrate is used to treat a variety of fungal infections. Monistat-Derm cream and related products are applied directly to the skin to treat common fungal infections of the skin, including ringworm, athlete's foot, and jock itch. Monistat and similar products are used to treat vaginal yeast infections. Terconazole is prescribed exclusively for vaginal or skin infections. Oxiconazole is prescribed for fungal infections of the skin, including athlete's foot and jock itch. Little of the drug applied to the skin is absorbed into the bloodstream.

Cautions and Warnings

Do not use any of these drugs if you are **allergic** or **sensitive** to any of their ingredients. If a reaction (such as a sensitivity reaction or a chemical irritation) occurs while taking miconazole, discontinue use and consult your doctor.

Proper diagnosis is essential for effective treatment. Do not use this product without first consulting your doctor.

Possible Side Effects

Vaginal Administration

▼ Common: itching, burning, and irritation.

▼ Less common: pelvic cramps, hives, rash, and headache.

Topical Application

▼ Less common: headache (affects 1 in 4 people taking terconazole) and skin irritation, burning, rash, and redness.

▼ Rare: painful menstruation; genital pain; body pain; abdominal pain; fever; chills; and vaginal burning, itching, or irritation. Application of terconazole cream to the skin can cause unusual sensitivity to the sun. Contact your doctor if you experience any side effect not listed above.

Drug Interactions

These interactions do not apply to drugs applied to the skin.

- Miconazole may increase the effect of warfarin (an anticoagulant drug) which may cause bleeding problems, including nosebleeds, bleeding gums, and bruising.
- The use of miconazole and related drugs with some anticonvulsants may cause serious side effects.
- Miconazole may interact with oral antidiabetes drugs to produce very low blood sugar levels.

Food Interactions

None known.

Usual Dose

Vaginal Suppositories and Cream: 1 applicatorful or suppository into the vagina at bedtime for 1–7 days, depending on the product and how it is manufactured.

Topical Cream, Lotions, and Powder: Apply to affected areas twice a day, morning and evening, for up to 1 month, or as directed by your doctor.

Overdosage
Accidental ingestion may cause upset stomach. Call your local poison control center or hospital emergency room for more information. If you seek treatment, ALWAYS bring the prescription bottle or container.

Special Information
When using the vaginal cream, insert the whole applicator of cream high into the vagina and be sure to complete the full course of treatment. Call your doctor if you develop burning or itching.

Refrain from sexual intercourse or use a condom to avoid reinfection while using this product. Using sanitary napkins even if you do not have your period may prevent the product from staining your clothing.

If you forget to administer a dose of one of these drugs, do so as soon as you remember. If it is almost time for your next dose, skip the dose you forgot and continue with your regular schedule. Do not take a double dose.

Oxiconazole is meant only for application to the skin. Do not apply to your eyes or mouth.

Continue using these medicines for the prescribed time of treatment, even if symptoms improve.

Do not use a covered dressing unless instructed by your doctor.

Special Populations
Pregnancy/Breast-feeding: Pregnant women should not use the vaginal suppositories or tablets during the first trimester. Use during the following 6 months only if absolutely necessary and without an applicator (insert by hand). Creams applied to the skin are unlikely to be absorbed to the extent they would affect a pregnancy.

Miconazole has not been shown to cause problems in breast-fed infants. Nursing mothers taking oxiconazole or terconazole should consider using infant formula.

Seniors: Seniors may take these medications without special restriction.

Generic Name

Midodrine (MYE-doe-dreen) Ⓖ

Brand Names
Orvaten   ProAmatine

Type of Drug
Alpha stimulant.

Prescribed For
Dizziness or fainting when rising from a sitting position. Midodrine is also used for poor urinary control and retrograde ejaculation.

General Information
Midodrine is recommended only if other treatments for dizziness or fainting have failed and symptoms are severely interfering with your daily routine. It stimulates nerve endings in small veins and arteries, "tightening" them slightly to raise blood pressure. This helps control dizziness and fainting caused by poor blood flow to the brain. Systolic blood pressure increases by 15–30 points 1 hour after taking 10 mg of midodrine. The effect lasts about 2–3 hours.

Cautions and Warnings
Do not take midodrine if you are **allergic** or **sensitive** to any of its ingredients.

Do not take this drug if you **retain urine** or have severe **heart disease, kidney disease, pheochromocytoma** (adrenal gland tumor), a severely **overactive thyroid gland,** or excessive and persistent **high blood pressure** when lying down. If you have **diabetes** or **visual problems**, use this drug with caution.

High blood pressure—especially when lying down—can be the most serious side effect of midodrine. This problem may be prevented by not completely reclining, or by raising the head of your bed when you sleep.

People with **kidney disease** require reduced dosage. People with **liver disease** should be cautious about using midodrine because it may be partially broken down in the liver. Your doctor should evaluate your kidney and liver function periodically.

Heart rate may decrease while taking midodrine.

Possible Side Effects

▼ Most common: tingling in the hands or feet, pain, itching, goosebumps, painful urination, high blood pressure when lying down, and chills.

▼ Less common: headache, sensation of pressure in the head, facial flushing, confusion, abnormal thinking, dry mouth, nervousness, anxiety, and rash.

Possible Side Effects *(continued)*

▼ Rare: visual problems, dizziness, sensitive skin, sleeplessness, tiredness, canker sores, dry skin, urinary difficulties,
weakness, backache, nausea, upset stomach, gas, heartburn, and leg cramps. Contact your doctor if you experience any side effect not listed above.

Drug Interactions

- Midodrine increases the effects of digoxin and similar drugs,
  psychoactive medications, beta blockers, and other stimulants. Be very cautious when combining any of these drugs
  and midodrine.
- People taking fludrocortisone must have their dosage reduced or salt intake lowered before starting midodrine.
- Alpha blockers such as prazosin, terazosin, and doxazosin
  can block midodrine's effects.

Food Interactions

None known.

Usual Dose

Dizziness or Fainting

Adult: 10 mg 3 times a day. People with kidney failure should
start with 2.5 mg.

Child: not recommended.

Urinary Incontinence

Adult: 2.5–5 mg 2–3 times a day.

Child: not recommended.

Overdosage

Symptoms include high blood pressure, goosebumps, feeling cold,
and difficulty urinating. Take the victim to a hospital emergency
room. ALWAYS bring the prescription bottle or container.

Special Information

Your doctor may suggest that you take the medication about every
4 hours: when you get up, around noon, and in the late afternoon—
no later than 6 p.m. The drug may also be taken every 3 hours to
control symptoms. Do not take midodrine after dinner or less than
4 hours before you go to bed.

If you experience symptoms of high blood pressure when lying down, such as headache, pounding in the ears, blurred vision, and an acute awareness of your heartbeat, contact your doctor immediately.

Continue taking midodrine only if it works for you. If you forget a dose, take it as soon as you remember. If it is almost time for your next dose, skip the dose you forgot and continue with your regular schedule. Call your doctor if you miss 2 or more doses in a row.

Special Populations

Pregnancy/Breast-feeding: Midodrine may pass into fetal circulation. When this drug is considered crucial by your doctor, its potential benefits must be carefully weighed against its risks.

It is not known if midodrine passes into breast milk. Nursing mothers who must take it should consider using infant formula.

Seniors: Seniors may take midodrine without special precaution.

Generic Name

Mifepristone (mif-ih-PRIS-tone)

Brand Name

Mifeprex

Type of Drug

Abortifacient.

Prescribed For

Termination of pregnancies of less than 7 weeks. Also used as a "morning after" contraceptive and for uterine fibroids, fetal deaths or fetuses that are not viable in the early stages of pregnancy, meningioma that cannot be treated surgically, endometriosis, and Cushing's syndrome.

General Information

Formerly known as RU-486, mifepristone is a prostaglandin that works by interrupting the supply of hormones that maintain the interior of the uterus where the fetus attaches to obtain nourishment and grow. Without these hormones, the uterus cannot support the pregnancy and the contents of the uterus are expelled. It is related to misoprostol, a drug used to prevent gastrointestinal tract ulcers from aspirin and other nonsteroidal anti-inflammatory (NSAID)-

type drugs. Misoprostol is usually given 2 full days after mifepristone to complete the medical abortion.

Cautions and Warnings

Do not take mifepristone if you are **allergic** or **sensitive** to any of its ingredients.

Surgery may be needed if mifepristone treatment does not produce a complete termination. The same pre-surgical precautions should be taken with mifepristone as are taken with a surgical termination.

Death due to blood infection has occurred following a mifepristone-induced termination. Nausea, vomiting, or diarrhea and weakness, with or without abdominal pain or fever, developing more than 24 hours after taking mifepristone can be signs of infection. Go to your doctor or a hospital emergency room immediately.

Vaginal bleeding or spotting should be expected for 9–16 days. Up to 8% of women who use mifepristone can bleed for 30 days or more, which may lead to anemia.

There is no information on the effect of this drug in liver or kidney disease. You should not take this drug if you have problems with your **adrenal glands** or if you have an **IUD, ectopic pregnancy,** or a **bleeding disorder**.

Possible Side Effects

This drug is designed to produce the vaginal bleeding and cramping necessary to produce pregnancy termination. Nearly all women who use mifepristone can be expected to have at least 1 side effect.

▼ Most common: headache, abdominal cramps, uterine cramps, vaginal bleeding, nausea, vomiting, diarrhea, fatigue, and back pain.

▼ Common: uterine hemorrhage.

▼ Less common: upset stomach, vaginitis, pelvic pain, fever, viral infection, shaking chills, weakness, leg pain, anemia (reduced red-blood-cell count), sinus irritation, and fainting.

▼ Rare: liver irritation and increased white-blood-cell count. Contact your doctor if you experience any side effect not listed above.

Drug Interactions

- Mifepristone may be less effective if given less than 2 days after taking mifepristol.
- Do not take this drug if you are also taking a blood-thinning drug (e.g., warfarin) or a corticosteroid.
- Ketoconazole, itraconazole, and erythromycin may increase blood levels of mifepristone.
- Carbamazepine, dexamethasone, phenytoin, phenobarbital, rifampin, and St. John's wort may reduce the amount of mifepristone in the blood.
- Mifepristone stays in the body for a week or more and stimulates a particular liver enzyme involved in drug metabolism. This may lead to increases in blood levels of such drugs as benzodiazepine sedatives, statins, caffeine, cocaine, codeine and other narcotics, calcium channel blockers, some antibiotics and antiviral medications, cortisone drugs, hormone supplements, and other drugs broken down by this enzyme.

Food Interactions

Grapefruit juice may slow the breakdown of mifepristone in the liver, increasing drug levels in the blood.

Usual Dose

600 mcg of mifepristone on the first office visit. 400 mcg of misoprostol 2 days later.

Overdosage

No serious symptoms were reported in men and non-pregnant women who took up to 3 times the recommended dose of mifepristone. Massive overdose may lead to adrenal gland failure.

Special Information

Be sure to read all written information given to you by your doctor and that all your questions are answered before proceeding.

Tell your doctor if you have any clotting or bleeding problems, or if you are anemic.

You should have a follow-up visit with your doctor 2 weeks after treatment to make sure that a complete termination has occurred. Surgery may be needed if mifepristone results in an incomplete termination. When using this drug, be sure you know exactly what to do and where to go if something goes wrong.

Contact your doctor right away if you develop any symptoms of a serious infection (see "Cautions and Warnings").

You may become pregnant again after your pregnancy has been terminated and before your next period. Contraception may be started as soon as your doctor has confirmed the pregnancy termination.

Special Populations

Pregnancy/Breast-feeding: Pregnant women who are not interested in pregnancy termination may not take this drug for any reason. Failed mifepristone treatment may lead to birth defects.

Mifepristone may pass into breast milk. Nursing mothers who must take this drug should use infant formula for several days after taking mifepristone.

Generic Name

Miglitol (mig-LIH-tol)

Brand Name

Glyset

The information in this profile also applies to the following drug:

Generic Ingredient: Acarbose
Precose

Type of Drug

Antidiabetic.

Prescribed For

Type 2 diabetes.

General Information

Miglitol works differently from other oral antidiabetes drugs, which control blood sugar levels by increasing the production of insulin or helping the body to use the hormone more efficiently. Miglitol delays the digestion of carbohydrates (sugars) by acting in the cells that line the small intestine, where sugar is absorbed. This results in less sugar being absorbed into the blood and, therefore, a lower blood-sugar level. Miglitol also has some effect against the enzyme lactase, but usually does not cause lactose intolerance. Hypoglycemia (very low blood sugar) is unlikely with miglitol because of the way the drug works in diabetes.

People taking miglitol should have their blood sugar checked periodically to see how well the drug is working. (Home glucose monitors are available.) Miglitol may be prescribed with another antidiabetic drug if single-drug therapy is not enough to adequately control blood sugar levels.

Cautions and Warnings

Do not take miglitol if you are **sensitive** or **allergic** to any of its ingredients, or if you have **diabetic ketoacidosis, cirrhosis of the liver, inflammatory bowel disease, ulcers in the colon, intestinal obstruction, absorption or digestion diseases,** or if **intestinal gas** will be a severe problem.

People with kidney disease retain higher levels of miglitol in the blood, but this does not affect the drug's action because it acts locally in cells lining the small intestine. Those with **severe kidney disease** should not take this drug because of drug retention in the blood.

Acarbose may lead to liver inflammation.

Possible Side Effects

Acarbose

Intestinal side effects of acarbose tend to improve or go away after a few weeks.

▼ Most common: stomach gas (in 75% of people who take it), abdominal pain, and diarrhea. These side effects may be worse if you don't restrict the amount of carbohydrate in your diet.

▼ Less common: skin rashes, swelling and itching, hepatitis or yellowing of the skin or whites of the eyes, abdominal distress, or abdominal obstruction.

▼ Rare: liver irritation and minor abnormalities in blood tests. Contact your doctor if you experience any side effect not listed above.

Miglitol

Most side effects of miglitol go away with continued use of the drug.

▼ Most common: gas, diarrhea, and abdominal pain.

▼ Less common: rash and low blood iron.

Drug Interactions

• Thiazides and other diuretics, corticosteroid anti-inflammatory drugs, phenothiazines, thyroid drugs, estrogens, contraceptive drugs, phenytoin, nicotinic acid, stimulants, calcium channel blockers, and isoniazid may increase blood sugar levels. Your blood glucose should be carefully monitored if you add or withdraw any of these drugs while taking miglitol or acarbose.

- Miglitol and acarbose add to the blood-sugar-lowering effect of sulfonylureas, insulin, and other antidiabetes drugs and may increase the risk of hypoglycemia (low blood sugar) associated with these drugs.

- Miglitol may interfere with the absorption of several drugs into the blood, including propranolol, ranitidine, digoxin, glyburide, and metformin. Your doctor may need to adjust your dose of these drugs.

- Digestive enzyme preparations, charcoal, kaolin (an ingredient in Kaopectate), and antacids—as well as other drugs intended to absorb stomach contents—reduce the effects of miglitol and acarbose. Separate dosing of these drugs by at least 2 hours.

- Combining acarbose and digoxin may increase the effects of digoxin.

Food Interactions

Miglitol must be taken with the first bite of each main meal.

Usual Dose

Acarbose

Adult: 25–100 mg with breakfast, lunch, and dinner.
Child: not recommended.

Miglitol

Adult: 25–100 mg with breakfast, lunch, and dinner.
Child: not recommended.

Overdosage

Unlike other antidiabetic medicines, a miglitol overdose does not cause hypoglycemia. Overdose symptoms are likely to include gas, diarrhea, and pain. Call your local poison control center or hospital emergency room for more information. If you seek treatment, ALWAYS bring the prescription bottle or container.

Special Information

Follow your doctor's instructions for diet, exercise, and blood-sugar testing.

Miglitol prevents the breakdown of table sugar. If you take this drug in combination with insulin or a sulfonylurea drug, be sure to have a quick source of glucose (dextrose) with you to treat hypoglycemia (symptoms include tiredness, increased hunger, increased heart rate, sweating, and numbness in the arms and legs).

Read product labels carefully or check with your pharmacist before buying any nonprescription drug to be sure it is safe for diabetics to take with acarbose.

Take your dose with the first bite of each meal. The drug has to be present in your intestine to prevent the absorption of sugar into your blood.

If you forget to take a dose of miglitol with your meal, skip the dose you forgot, since it cannot work unless there is food in your stomach. Continue with your regular dose at the beginning of your next meal.

Special Populations

Pregnancy/Breast-feeding: The safety of using miglitol during pregnancy is not known. When this drug is considered crucial by your doctor, its potential benefits must be carefully weighed against its risks. Diabetes during pregnancy is usually treated with insulin.

Small amounts of miglitol pass into breast milk. Nursing mothers who must take this drug should use infant formula.

Seniors: Blood levels of acarbose are higher in older adults, but this is not considered important. Seniors with severe kidney disease should avoid this medication. Seniors may take this drug without special precaution.

Generic Name

Minoxidil (mih-NOX-ih-dil) G

Brand Names

Loniten   Rogaine

Type of Drug

Antihypertensive and hair-growth stimulant.

Prescribed For

Hypertension (high blood pressure), male-pattern baldness, and alopecia areata.

General Information

Oral minoxidil is prescribed for severe hypertension that has not responded to other drugs. It reduces blood pressure by dilating (widening) peripheral blood vessels, allowing more blood to flow through the arms and legs. This increased blood flow reduces resistance levels in central blood vessels—for example, in the heart, lungs, and kidneys—and therefore reduces blood pressure. Minoxidil's effect on blood pressure is seen 30 minutes after a dose is taken and lasts up to 3 days. Minoxidil, which is usually taken once or twice a day, reaches maximum effect in as little as 3 days if the dose is large enough—40 mg a day.

Topical minoxidil stimulates hair growth in men and women with hereditary hair loss. It is also used to treat alopecia areata, a condition in which patches of hair fall out all over the body. No one knows exactly how minoxidil produces this effect and it does not work for everyone. The ideal candidate is a man who has just started to lose hair. The drug is not effective unless hair in the balding area is at least ½ in. long, and it takes 4–6 months of applications before any effect can be expected. The application regimen must be followed carefully; stopping the drug will nullify its effects and new growth will be lost. In some men who used minoxidil for a year, hair loss was only slowed.

Cautions and Warnings

Do not take minoxidil if you are **allergic** or **sensitive** to any of its ingredients.

Oral minoxidil may cause severe adverse effects on the heart, including angina pain and fluid around the heart, which affects cardiac function. This drug is only indicated for extremely high blood pressure and should not be used for **mild hypertension** or **pulmonary hypertension.** It is usually prescribed with a beta-blocking drug to prevent rapid heartbeat and a diuretic to prevent fluid accumulation. Hospitalization may be recommended for some people when they start minoxidil to avoid an overly rapid drop in blood pressure.

People with **pheochromocytoma** (adrenal gland tumor) should not use this drug.

This drug has not been carefully studied in people who have suffered a **heart attack** within a month of beginning minoxidil; cardiac side effects may be particularly serious in people with a history of **heart disease.** People who use minoxidil for hair growth must have a healthy scalp and no heart disease.

Possible Side Effects

Tablets

Water and sodium retention may develop (which can worsen heart failure) as well as fluid in the sacs surrounding the heart.

▼ Most common: 80% of people experience thickening, elongation, and darkening of body hair within 3–6 weeks, first noticed on the temples, between the eyebrows, on the forehead, or on the upper cheek. Later it may extend to the back, arms, legs, and scalp. This effect stops when the drug is stopped, and symptoms usually disappear in 1–6 months. Heart rhythm changes occur in 60% of people, but cause no symptoms. Some laboratory tests, such as blood, liver, and kidney tests, may be affected by minoxidil.

▼ Less common: severe rash, nausea, vomiting, chest pain, edema, breast tenderness, and changes in blood composition and heart function.

Lotion

Not enough minoxidil is usually absorbed into the blood to affect blood pressure or cause serious side effects.

▼ Most common: People using 2% minoxidil lotion may experience irritation or itching.

▼ Less common: bronchitis or other respiratory infections, rash, eczema, fungal infection, itching, redness, dry skin or scalp, flaking, worsening of hair loss, diarrhea, nausea, headache, dizziness, fainting, back pain, broken bones, tendonitis, swelling of the arms or legs, chest pain, blood-pressure changes, heart palpitations, allergic reactions (symptoms include breathing difficulties, rash, and itching), hives, runny nose, facial swelling, conjunctivitis (pinkeye), ear infection, visual disturbances, urinary infection, inflammation of the prostate or urethra, vaginal discharge, pain during sex, anxiety, depression, menstrual changes, nonspecific breast symptoms, and pain, inflammation, or redness of the testes, vagina, or vulva.

Drug Interactions

- Minoxidil may interact with guanethidine to produce severe dizziness when rising from a sitting or lying position. These drugs should not be taken together.
- Do not use the lotion in conjunction with other topical drugs.

Food Interactions

None known.

Usual Dose

Tablets

   Adult and Child (age 12 and over): 5 mg a day to start; effective range is usually 10–40 mg a day. Do not exceed 100 mg a day.

   Child (under age 12): 0.1 mg per lb. of body weight a day to start; may be increased to 0.5 mg per lb. of body weight a day. Do not exceed 50 mg a day. Children should be monitored closely, as pediatric experience of this drug's effects is limited.

Minoxidil is usually taken with a diuretic, such as 100 mg of hydrochlorothiazide, 50–100 mg of chlorthalidone, or 80 mg of furosemide daily; and a beta blocker, such as 80–160 mg a day of propranolol. People who cannot take beta blockers may take 250–750 mg of methyldopa or 0.1–0.2 mg of clonidine daily.

Lotion: Apply to scalp twice a day.

Overdosage

Symptoms include dizziness, fainting, and rapid heartbeat. Call your local poison control center or a hospital emergency room for instructions. ALWAYS bring the prescription bottle or container if you seek treatment.

Special Information

Oral minoxidil is usually prescribed with 2 other drugs—a beta blocker and a diuretic; do not discontinue any of these drugs unless told to do so by your doctor. Take all medication exactly as prescribed.

   The effect of oral minoxidil on body hair (see "Possible Side Effects") is more of a nuisance than a risk and is not a reason to stop taking it.

   Call your doctor if you experience an increase in your pulse of 20 or more beats per minute; weight gain of more than 5 lbs.; swelling of your arms, legs, face, or stomach; chest pain; breathing difficulties; dizziness; or fainting spells.

   Minoxidil lotion has an alcohol base that may cause burning and irritation of the eyes. In case of accidental contact with eyes or other sensitive areas, flush with large amounts of cool tap water. Accidental ingestion of the lotion may lead to whole-body adverse effects.

If you forget a dose of oral minoxidil or an application of the lotion, take it as soon as you remember. If it is almost time for your next dose, skip the dose you forgot and continue with your regular schedule. Do not take a double dose.

Special Populations

Pregnancy/Breast-feeding: Oral minoxidil crosses into the fetal circulation. Women should avoid either form of minoxidil during pregnancy. When this drug is considered crucial by your doctor, its potential benefits must be carefully weighed against its risks.

Oral minoxidil passes into breast milk, as may the lotion. Nursing mothers who must take either form of minoxidil should use infant formula.

Seniors: Seniors may be more sensitive to the blood-pressure-lowering effect of the drug due to loss of kidney function.

Generic Name

Mirtazapine (mur-TAZ-uh-pene) Ⓖ

Brand Names

Remeron	Remeron SolTab

The information in this profile also applies to the following drug:

Generic Ingredient: Maprotiline Ⓖ

Type of Drug

Antidepressant.

Prescribed For

Major depressive disorder.

General Information

Mirtazapine blocks the passage of stimulant chemicals (serotonin and noradrenaline) in and out of nerve endings and has a sedative effect. It also moderately counteracts the effects of the neurohormone acetylcholine. Mirtazapine can elevate mood, increase physical activity and mental alertness, and improve appetite and sleep patterns 2–4 weeks after you start taking it. Mirtazapine is useful in treating mild forms of depression associated with anxiety. It can also significantly reduce tremors associated with Parkinson's disease and other causes, though the effect is lost soon after drug treatment is stopped. Mirtazapine is broken down in the liver. Women clear the drug more slowly than men.

Cautions and Warnings

Do not take mirtazapine if you are **allergic** or **sensitive** to any of its ingredients.

Antidepressants have been associated with an increased risk of suicide, especially in **teenagers**. Suicide is always a risk in severely depressed people, who should only be allowed to have minimal quantities of medication in their possession.

Mirtazapine should be taken with care if you have **heart disease.**

Antidepressants may aggravate the condition of people who are **schizophrenic** or **paranoid** and may cause people with **bipolar (manic-depressive) disorder** to switch phase. These reactions are also possible when changing or stopping antidepressants.

Care should be used when initiating mirtazapine in people with **epilepsy** or a history of **seizures**.

People taking mirtazapine may develop very low white-blood-cell counts, leading to infections, fever, and related problems. Call your doctor at once if you develop a sore throat, fever, infection, or mouth sores while taking this drug.

Mirtazapine should be taken with care if you have **kidney or liver disease.**

Mirtazapine may cause dizziness and sleepiness with potentially serious effects on performance.

Possible Side Effects

▼ Most common: tiredness, dizziness, dry mouth, constipation, abnormal dreams, increased appetite, weight gain, large increases in blood cholesterol or triglyceride levels, weakness, and flu-like symptoms.

▼ Less common: back pain, nausea, vomiting, muscle ache, abnormal thinking, anxiety, agitation, confusion, tremors, itching, rash, breathing difficulties, and frequent urination.

▼ Rare: blood-pressure changes, weakness, hair loss, uncontrollable muscle spasms or movements, hallucinations, manic reactions, and liver function changes. Other rare side effects can occur in almost any part of the body. Contact your doctor if you experience any side effect not listed above.

Drug Interactions
Mirtazapine and Maprotiline
- Combining mirtazapine or maprotiline with a monoamine oxidase inhibitor (MAOI) antidepressant may cause high fevers, convulsions, or death. Do not take an MAOI until at least 2 weeks after mirtazapine or maprotiline has been stopped.
- Mirtazapine and maprotiline increase the effects of alcohol and other sedative drugs.

Maprotiline
- Maprotiline interacts with guanethidine and clonidine (drugs used to treat high blood pressure). Tell your doctor if you are taking any drug for high blood pressure.
- Combining maprotiline and thyroid medication enhances the effects of both drugs and may cause abnormal heart rhythms.
- Combining mirtazapine and phenothiazide or benzodiazepine sedatives (when doses are rapidly tapered off) may increase the risk of seizures.
- Contraceptive drugs may reduce the effect of maprotiline, as may smoking. Charcoal tablets may block the absorption of maprotiline. Estrogen may increase or decrease the effect of maprotiline.
- Cimetidine and fluoxetine may increase the effects of maprotiline, while barbiturates and phenytoin may decrease effects. Dosage adjustments of maprotiline may be necessary.

Food Interactions
You may take mirtazapine with food if it upsets your stomach.

Usual Dose
Maprotiline
Adult: 75–150 mg a day. Severely depressed patients may need up to 225 mg a day.
Senior: usually 50–75 mg a day.

Mirtazapine
Adult: 15 mg at bedtime to start. After the first 1–2 weeks of taking the drug, dosage may be increased up to 45 mg a day. Dosage must be tailored to your needs.

Overdosage
Symptoms of mirtazapine overdose include disorientation, drowsiness, memory loss, and rapid heartbeat. Symptoms of maprotiline overdose include confusion, inability to concentrate, hallucinations, drowsiness, lowered body temperature, abnormal heart rate,

heart failure, enlarged pupils, seizures, convulsions, very low blood pressure, stupor, and coma; agitation, stiffening of muscles, vomiting, and high fever may also develop. The victim should be taken to a hospital emergency room immediately. ALWAYS bring the prescription bottle or container.

Special Information

Do not stop taking this drug without your doctor's knowledge. Abruptly stopping mirtazapine may cause nausea, headache, and feelings of ill health.

The following symptoms may occur early in treatment or when drug dosage is adjusted up or down: anxiety, agitation, panic attacks, sleeplessness, irritability, restlessness, hostility, aggressiveness, acting impulsively, a manic reaction, deepening of depression, other unusual changes in behavior, and suicidal thinking. Report any changes to your doctor at once.

Mirtazapine may cause drowsiness and dizziness. Be careful when driving or doing any task that requires concentration. Avoid alcohol and other depressant drugs. Avoid prolonged exposure to the sun.

Be careful when taking over-the-counter (OTC) medications because mirtazapine may interact with sedative ingredients in OTC products.

Call your doctor at once if you develop chills, difficult or rapid breathing, fever, sweating, blood-pressure changes, muscle stiffness, loss of bladder control, or unusual tiredness or weakness.

If your symptoms are unchanged after 6–8 weeks of treatment with an antidepressant, contact your doctor.

If you forget a dose, skip it and go back to your regular schedule. Do not take a double dose.

Special Populations

Pregnancy/Breast-feeding: Mirtazapine crosses into the fetal circulation and may cause birth defects. When this drug is considered crucial by your doctor, its potential benefits must be carefully weighed against its risks.

It is not known if mirtazapine passes into breast milk. Maprotiline is excreted in breast milk. Nursing mothers who must take these drugs should consider using infant formula.

Seniors: Seniors are more sensitive to side effects and may require reduced dosage. Older men may need less of the drug than women of the same age.

Generic Name

Misoprostol (mye-soe-PROS-tol) G

Brand Name
Cytotec

Type of Drug
Anti-ulcer.

Prescribed For
Stomach ulcer and prevention of kidney rejection after transplant. It may also be used to soften the cervix, inducing contractions to begin labor, and as part of a medical abortion drug regimen.

General Information
Like most anti-ulcer drugs, misoprostol suppresses stomach acid. It has a demonstrated ability to protect the stomach lining from damage, though the exact way misoprostol works is not known. It may increase production of stomach lining and the thickness of the protective gel layer lining the stomach. Misoprostol may also increase blood flow in and subsequent healing of the stomach lining in addition to increasing production of bicarbonate, a natural antacid found in the stomach.

Misoprostol is intended to prevent severe stomach irritation and ulcers in people taking a nonsteroidal anti-inflammatory drug (NSAID). It is helpful for seniors and others with a history of ulcer or stomach disease who require NSAID treatment for arthritis. It is often an effective ulcer treatment for people who do not respond to or cannot tolerate cimetidine, ranitidine, famotidine, or nizatidine.

Misoprostol is also used as a medical abortion drug along with mifepristone. It has additionally been used for labor induction, post-partum hemorrhaging, and chronic constipation.

Cautions and Warnings
Do not take misoprostol if you are **allergic** or **sensitive** to any of its ingredients or to any prostaglandin agent, or if you are **pregnant**. It has been shown to cause abortion, premature birth, and birth defects.

People with **kidney disease** may require reduced dosages.

People with **epilepsy** or **blood-vessel disease** in the heart or brain should be cautious about taking misoprostol, as should those with **heart disease**.

Possible Side Effects

▼ Most common: diarrhea and abdominal pain. Most cases of diarrhea are mild and last no more than 2–3 days.
▼ Less common: headache, nausea, vomiting, and stomach upset or gas.
▼ Rare: spotting, cramps, excessive menstrual bleeding, painful menstruation or other menstrual disorders, and vaginal bleeding. Rare side effects can occur in almost any part of the body. Contact your doctor if you experience any side effect not listed above.

Drug Interactions

- Misoprostol may interfere with the absorption of diazepam and theophylline.
- Rarely, antacids interfere with misoprostol's effectiveness. Magnesium-containing antacids may worsen misoprostol-induced diarrhea.

Food Interactions

Though food interferes with the absorption of this drug, it should be taken with or after meals (and at bedtime) to minimize gastrointestinal side effects.

Usual Dose

Adult: 100–200 mcg 4 times a day.
Child: not recommended.

Overdosage

Symptoms include sedation, tremors, convulsions, breathing difficulties, stomach pain, diarrhea, fever, changes in heart rate—either very fast or very slow, gastrointestinal lesions, testicular atrophy, liver damage, central-nervous-system depression, and low blood pressure. Take the victim to a hospital emergency room. ALWAYS bring the prescription bottle or container.

Special Information

Do not stop taking misoprostol, or take it for more than 4 weeks, without your doctor's knowledge.

Call your doctor if side effects, especially diarrhea or abdominal or stomach pain, become severe or intolerable. Women who experience menstrual problems and postmenopausal women who experience vaginal bleeding should discuss these side effects with their doctors.

If you forget a dose, take it as soon as you remember. If it is almost time for your next dose, skip the dose you forgot and continue with your regular schedule. Do not take a double dose.

Special Populations

Pregnancy/Breast-feeding: Pregnant women should not take this drug. Women of childbearing age should take misoprostol only if they absolutely must take an NSAID and already have, or are at high risk of developing, stomach ulcers. Misoprostol causes spontaneous miscarriage. Within 2 weeks of starting treatment, you must receive a negative blood test result for pregnancy—an over-the-counter urine test is not sufficient. Start taking misoprostol on day 2 or 3 of your period and use effective contraception throughout drug therapy.

It is not known if misoprostol passes into breast milk, although it is unlikely. Nursing mothers who must take this drug should use infant formula.

Seniors: Seniors should receive lower dosages if intolerable side effects develop.

Mobic *see Nonsteroidal Anti-inflammatory Drugs,*
page 821

see Nonsteroidal Anti-inflammatory Drugs, page 821

Generic Name

Modafinil (moe-DAF-ih-nil)

Brand Names
Provigil   Sparlon

The information in this profile also applies to the following drug:

Generic Ingredient: Armodafinil
Nuvigil

Type of Drug

Stimulant.

Prescribed For

Narcolepsy (uncontrollable desire to sleep); obstructive sleep apnea; ADHD (attention-deficit/hyperactivity disorder) in children and adolescents ages 6–17; shift-work sleep disorder.

General Information

Modafinil promotes wakefulness. Armodafinil is the active form of modafinil. While some of these actions are similar to those of amphetamine and methylphenidate, it may have more to do with the fact that these medications increase the amount of free dopamine, a major neurotransmitter, in the brain by reducing the amount reabsorbed into nerve endings. People taking these medications who continue to experience excessive sleepiness may not be able to recover their normal sleep patterns. People being treated with these drugs may experience euphoria (feeling "high"), anxiety, and changes in mood, mental state, and behavior. They are classified as Schedule IV controlled substances.

Cautions and Warnings

Do not take modafinil if you are **allergic** or **sensitive** to any of its ingredients. Serious reactions including rash and difficulty breathing and/or swallowing have been reported with armodafinil. Rarely, serious rash requiring hospitalization has occurred in both adults and children taking modafinil.

People with a history of **heart failure,** an **enlarged heart ventricle, angina, chest pain, abnormal heart rhythms,** or **mitral valve prolapse** should not take modafinil.

Modafinil has not been studied in people with **high blood pressure**. People with high blood pressure who take this drug must be closely monitored. Prazosin, a drug normally prescribed for high blood pressure, can counteract the wakefulness produced by these drugs.

People taking these medication may develop mania, delusions, hallucinations, and suicidal thoughts.

People with **cirrhosis of the liver** or **liver failure** may require reduced dosages.

People who regularly take large dosages (more than 400 mg a day) of modafinil may develop some resistance to its effects.

Possible Side Effects

▼ Most common: headache, nausea, and runny nose.
▼ Common: back pain, nervousness, dizziness, diarrhea, dry mouth, appetite loss, and sore throat.
▼ Less common: depression, anxiety, cataplexy (extreme muscle weakness, often precipitated by laughter, a surprised feeling, or emotions of fear or anger), sleeplessness, anxiety, tingling in the hands or feet, unusual facial or mouth movements, muscle stiffness, blood pressure changes, liver function problems, vomiting, lung problems, breathing difficulties, vision problems, chest pain, neck pain, chills, and high white-blood-cell counts.
▼ Rare: confusion, memory loss, emotional instability, euphoria (feeling "high"), changes in mood, manic behavior, delusions, hallucinations, suicidal thinking, flushing, fainting, dry skin, herpes infections, mouth sores, gum sores, thirst, difficulty urinating, abnormal urination, abnormal ejaculation, high blood sugar, nosebleeds, asthma, rigid neck, fever with chills, and joint problems. Contact your doctor if you experience any side effect not listed above.

Drug Interactions

- Combining these drugs with a monoamine oxidase inhibitor antidepressant may increase the effects of both drugs. Use this combination with caution and only under your doctor's supervision.
- Methylphenidate can delay these drugs' effects.
- Carbamazepine, phenobarbital, rifampin, ketoconazole, and itraconazole may reduce these drugs' effects.
- These drugs may reduce the effects of contraceptive drugs, theophylline, and cyclosporine.
- These drugs may elevate blood levels of clomipramine, clozapine, omeprazole, phenytoin, diazepam, propranolol, tricyclic antidepressants, and warfarin, increasing the risk of side effects—some of these can be very serious.
- Stimulants in some over-the-counter (OTC) decongestants, diet pills, and asthma drugs may cause excessive stimulation when combined with these medications.

Food Interactions

Food can slow the rate at which these drugs are absorbed into the blood but is unlikely to change the effect of modafinil. The action of armodafinil is more likely to be delayed and extended if it is taken with food.

Usual Dose

Armodafinil

Adult (age 18 and over): 150–250 mg every morning.
Child (under age 18): not recommended.

Modafinil

Adult (age 18 and over): 200 mg every morning; 100 mg daily for people with cirrhosis or liver failure.
Child (under age 18): not recommended.

Overdosage

Symptoms include excitation, sleeplessness, sleep disturbances, anxiety, irritability, aggressiveness, confusion, nervousness, tremors, heart palpitations, nausea, diarrhea, and bleeding. Take the victim to a hospital emergency room. ALWAYS bring the prescription bottle or container.

Special Information

Call your doctor at once if you develop a fever; rash; hives; swelling of the face, eyes, lips, tongue, or larynx; hoarseness; or other signs of a drug reaction or allergy.

Modafinil's beneficial effects on mood, thought, and perception may produce psychological dependence, though drug withdrawal symptoms have not been reported.

Be careful when driving or doing any task that requires concentration. Avoid alcohol.

Special Populations

Pregnancy/Breast-feeding: These drugs cause fetal malformation in animal studies. When these drugs are considered crucial by your doctor, their potential benefits must be carefully weighed against their risks.

These drugs may pass into breast milk. Nursing mothers who must take them should consider using infant formula.

Seniors: Seniors with kidney or liver problems may require reduced dosage.

Generic Name

Moexipril (moe-EX-uh-pril) Ⓖ

Brand Name

Univasc

Combination Product

Generic Ingredients: Moexipril + Hydrochlorothiazide Ⓖ
Uniretic

Type of Drug

Angiotensin-converting enzyme (ACE) inhibitor.

Prescribed For

Hypertension (high blood pressure). Also prescribed for kidney failure, kidney hypertension, heart failure, post–heart attack management, management of people with a high risk of heart disease, diabetes, chronic kidney disease, and preventing a second stroke.

General Information

Moexipril hydrochloride and other ACE inhibitors work by preventing the conversion of a hormone called angiotensin I to another hormone called angiotensin II, a potent blood-vessel constrictor. Preventing this conversion relaxes blood vessels, thus reducing blood pressure and relieving the symptoms of heart failure. Moexipril also affects production of other hormones and enzymes that participate in the regulation of blood vessel dilation. Moexipril begins working about 1 hour after you take it and continues to work for 24 hours.

Cautions and Warnings

Do not take moexipril if you are **allergic** or **sensitive** to any of its ingredients.

Swelling of the face, extremities, or throat has been known to occur with moexipril, which can be dangerous (see "Special Information").

Moexipril occasionally causes very low blood pressure.

Moexipril may cause a decline in kidney function, especially if you have **congestive heart failure**. Your doctor should check your urine for changes during the first few months of treatment. Dosage adjustment may be necessary.

Moexipril can occasionally affect white-blood-cell count, possibly increasing your susceptibility to infection. Blood counts should be monitored periodically.

The risk of severe sensitivity reactions is greater in **hemodialysis** patients and those undergoing **venom immunization**.

Moexipril can cause injury and death to the fetus during pregnancy. **Pregnant women** should not take moexipril.

ACE inhibitors may be less effective in some **black patients** with high blood pressure, especially when dietary salt intake is high. Nevertheless, they should still be considered useful blood pressure treatments. Swelling beneath the skin to form welts is more common among black patients.

Possible Side Effects

▼ Most common: dizziness, tiredness, diarrhea, headache, nausea, low blood pressure, chest pain, and chronic cough. The cough usually goes away a few days after you stop taking the medicine.

▼ Less common: angina, dizziness when rising from a sitting or lying position, fainting, abdominal pain, vomiting, breathing difficulties, weakness, and rash.

▼ Rare: Rare side effects can occur in almost any part of the body. Contact your doctor if you experience any side effect not listed above.

Drug Interactions

- The blood-pressure-lowering effect of moexipril is increased by taking diuretic drugs and beta blockers. Any other drug that causes a rapid drop in blood pressure should be used with caution if you are taking an ACE inhibitor.
- Moexipril may increase the effects of lithium; this combination should be used with caution.
- Aspirin and other nonsteroidal anti-inflammatory drugs (NSAIDs) reduce the blood-pressure-lowering effects of moexipril and other ACE inhibitors. The combination may cause reductions in kidney function.
- Moexipril may increase potassium levels in your blood, especially when taken with dyazide or other potassium-sparing diuretics.
- Antacids and moexipril should be taken at least 2 hours apart.

- Capsaicin may trigger or aggravate the cough associated with moexipril therapy.
- Indomethacin may reduce the blood-pressure-lowering effect of moexipril.
- Phenothiazine sedatives and antiemetics may increase the effects of moexipril.
- Allopurinol increases the risk of severe sensitivity reactions.
- Moexipril may affect blood levels of digoxin. More digoxin in the blood increases the chance of digoxin-related side effects, while less digoxin in the blood can compromise its effectiveness.

Food Interactions

Moexipril should be taken 1 hour before meals.

Usual Dose

Adult: 7.5–30 mg once a day. Some people may divide their daily dosage into 2 doses. People with poor kidney function should take ½ the usual dose.

Overdosage

The principal effect of moexipril overdose is a rapid drop in blood pressure, as evidenced by dizziness or fainting. Take the victim to a hospital emergency room immediately. ALWAYS bring the prescription bottle or container.

Special Information

Call your doctor if you develop swelling of the face or throat, if you have sudden difficulty in breathing, a sore throat, mouth sores, abnormal heartbeat, chest pain, a persistent rash, or loss of taste perception. Unexplained swelling of the face, lips, hands, and feet can also affect the larynx (throat) and tongue and interfere with breathing. If this happens, the victim should be taken to a hospital emergency room at once for treatment.

Some people who start taking an ACE inhibitor after they are already on a diuretic (an agent that increases urination) experience a rapid drop in blood pressure after their first doses or when the dosage is increased. To prevent this from happening, you may be told to stop taking the diuretic 2 or 3 days before starting the ACE inhibitor, or to increase your salt intake during that time. The diuretic may then be restarted gradually.

You may get dizzy if you rise to your feet quickly from a sitting or lying position when taking moexipril.

Avoid strenuous exercise and very hot weather because heavy sweating or dehydration can cause a rapid blood pressure drop.

Avoid over-the-counter diet pills, decongestants, and other stimulants that can raise blood pressure. Also, do not take potassium supplements or salt substitutes containing potassium without consulting your doctor.

If you take moexipril on a regular schedule and forget a dose, take it as soon as you remember. If you take it once a day and it is within 8 hours of your next dose, skip the one you forgot and continue with your regular schedule. If you take moexipril twice a day and it is within 4 hours of your next dose, take 1 dose as soon as you remember and another in 5 or 6 hours, then go back to your regular schedule. Never take a double dose.

Special Populations
Pregnancy/Breast-feeding: ACE inhibitors can cause fetal injury or death. Women who are or might be pregnant should not take moexipril. Stop taking the medication and contact your doctor if you become pregnant.

Small amounts of moexipril pass into breast milk. Nursing mothers who must take this drug should use infant formula.

Seniors: Seniors may be more sensitive to the effects of moexipril due to possible kidney impairment.

Brand Name

Motofen

Generic Ingredients
Difenoxin Hydrochloride + Atropine Sulfate Ⓖ

Type of Drug
Antidiarrheal.

Prescribed For
Acute and chronic diarrhea.

General Information
Difenoxin is an antidiarrheal agent related to meperidine, a narcotic analgesic (pain reliever) used in Demerol. Difenoxin, which can be addictive, works by slowing the contractions of intestinal-wall muscles. The atropine sulfate ingredient in Motofen guards against drug overdose or abuse by producing undesirable effects

at small dosages, thus deterring users from taking larger amounts of Motofen, as this drug is a Schedule IV controlled substance. This drug, which relieves diarrhea but does not address the underlying cause, should only be used for short periods and in cases that do not respond to other treatment.

Cautions and Warnings

Do not take Motofen if you are **allergic** or **sensitive** to any of its ingredients or to Lomotil. Some people should not use this drug even if diarrhea is present. Antidiarrheal drugs may harm people with **stomach, bowel, or other conditions.**

Avoid Motofen if you have advanced **liver disease** or have **jaundice** (symptoms include yellowing of the skin or whites of the eyes), or if your diarrhea was caused by taking clindamycin or another antibiotic.

People with **ulcerative colitis** or a history of **drug addiction** should use Motofen with caution.

Possible Side Effects

▼ Most common: nausea, vomiting, dry mouth, dizziness, lightheadedness, drowsiness, and headache.

▼ Less common: constipation, upset stomach, bloating, confusion, nervousness, tiredness, and sleeplessness.

▼ Rare: a burning sensation in the eyes, blurred vision, dry skin, rapid heartbeat, elevated temperature, and urinary difficulties. Contact your doctor if you experience any side effect not listed above.

Drug Interactions

- Motofen may increase the effects of alcohol, barbiturates, sedatives, pain relievers, and other nervous system depressants. Avoid these combinations.
- Monoamine oxidase inhibitor (MAOI) antidepressants may, in theory, produce a high-blood-pressure crisis in combination with Motofen. Do not use Motofen if you are taking an MAOI unless you are under a doctor's care.

Food Interactions

None known.

Usual Dose

Adult and Child (age 12 and over): 2 tablets to start, then 1 after each loose stool or every 3–4 hours, as needed; up to 8 tablets a day. Treatment for more than 2 consecutive days is usually not needed.

Child (under age 12): not recommended.

Overdosage

It is crucial to keep this medication out of reach from children at all times because of the risk of accidental overdosage. Symptoms include dry skin, mouth, and nose; flushing; fever; and rapid heartbeat. These symptoms may be followed by loss of reflexes, pinpointed pupils, droopy eyelids, breathing difficulty, and lethargy or coma, which in extreme cases can lead to brain damage or death. Take the victim to a hospital emergency room immediately. ALWAYS bring the prescription bottle or container.

Special Information

Motofen can make you tired, dizzy, or lightheaded. Be careful when driving or doing any task that requires concentration. Alcohol, sedatives, and other nervous system depressants increase the depressant effects of this drug.

Your doctor may prescribe fluid and salt mixtures to replace the body fluids you lose while taking Motofen.

Call your doctor if you develop heart palpitations or your symptoms do not clear up in 2 days. You may need a different dosage or drug.

If you forget a dose, take it as soon as you remember. If it is almost time for your next dose, skip the one you forgot and continue with your regular schedule. Do not take a double dose.

Special Populations

Pregnancy/Breast-feeding: Animal studies with very large dosages of Motofen showed an increase in stillbirths. When this drug is considered crucial by your doctor, its potential benefits must be carefully weighed against its risks.

The ingredients in Motofen may pass into breast milk. Nursing mothers taking Motofen should use infant formula.

Seniors: Seniors with severe kidney or liver disease require reduced dosage.

Type of Drug

Multiple Kinase Inhibitors

Generic Ingredient: Dasatinib
Sprycel

Generic Ingredient: Gefitinib
Iressa

Generic Ingredient: Imatinib
Gleevec

Generic Ingredient: Lapitinib
Tykerb

Generic Ingredient: Nilotinib
Tasigna

Generic Ingredient: Sorafenib
Nexavar

Generic Ingredient: Sunitinib
Sutent

Prescribed For

Dasatinib is prescribed for adults with leukemias that have not responded to other therapies. Gefitinib may be prescribed for non-small-cell lung cancer in people who have not responded to other treatments. Imatinib is prescribed for chronic myeloid leukemia (CML), gastrointestinal (GI) tumors, and other cancers. Lapitinib is prescribed together with capecitabine for HER2-positive advanced or metastatic breast cancer and is being studied for lung cancer. Nilotinib is prescribed for chronic and accelerated Philadelphia chromosome positive CML in adults resistant or intolerant to prior therapy that included imatinib. Sorafenib is prescribed for advanced kidney cancer. Sunitinib is prescribed for advanced kidney cancer and a rare cancer of the stomach, bowel, or esophagus.

General Information

These drugs are members of a new class of anti-cancer drugs. The kinase enzymes they inhibit are central switches to many processes within the cancer cell. They can overcome drug resistance that involves a family of kinase proteins responsible for the uncontrolled growth of some cancer cells, several of which are known to drive tumor growth and progression. Dasatinib is intended for people with specific leukemias who have been treated with but not responded to imatinib and those who are no longer able to take imatinib because of tolerance issues or a drug side effect. It is being studied in the treatment of solid tumors. Gefitinib inhibits the stimulation of the "epidermal growth receptor" found on the surface of many cancer cells. When stimulated, the receptor triggers processes inside the cell to make it grow and divide. Gefitinib interferes with this process. It is also used for breast, colorectal, and prostate cancers. Imatinib can be prescribed for CML and other blood cancers, breast cancer, GI tumors, and other cancer types. Lapitinib, in combination with capecitabine, is effective for some advanced or metastatic solid breast tumors that have failed treatment with traditional chemotherapy treatments. Sorafenib decreases the spread of tumor cells. In some studies, it was found to reduce the growth of new blood vessels that are necessary to feed the growth of a cancerous tumor. Sunitinib is recommended for a gastrointestinal cancer that does not respond to imatinib. These drugs are rapidly absorbed into the bloodstream, are broken down by enzymes in the liver, and eliminated primarily in the stool. The assessment of dasatinib's effectiveness was based on improvement in lab tests. No studies of either dasatinib or sunitinib have proven that people taking them live longer, though the drugs can extend the time until the cancer gets worse.

Cautions and Warnings

Do not take these drugs if you are **allergic** or **sensitive** to any of their ingredients.

Dasatinib should only be prescribed if you have already been **treated with imatinib**.

People with **liver disease** should use these drugs with caution, and dosage reduction may be needed. Sorafenib may be used in mild to moderate liver disease, but not in **severe liver or kidney disease**. One in 100 gefitinib patients can develop severe and sometimes fatal lung disease. People with **pre-existing lung disease** are more likely to experience a decline in health while taking gefitinib than those without pre-existing lung conditions.

Sunitinib should not be used if you have **liver or pancreatic failure**.

Dasatinib may affect **male and female fertility** and the developing fetus. Sexually active men and women taking this drug should use effective birth control while they are taking this drug.

Imatinib and dasatinib can severely reduce the numbers of blood platelets and white and red cells. Internal bleeding can be associated with platelet reductions induced by these drugs. Bleeding can occur while you are taking sorafenib, which may affect wound healing. Interrupt treatment if you are undergoing **major surgery**. Your doctor will check blood counts every week for the first 2 months and then once a month to monitor for changes. These effects are generally reversible by reducing drug dosage or temporarily stopping treatment.

Severe fluid retention can occur in people taking dasatinib and imatinib. This includes fluid in the lungs, around the heart, and in the abdomen.

These drugs can affect the heart by interfering with the conduction of electrical signals, which changes the heart's rhythm. Inform your doctor if you have **heart problems, low blood potassium or magnesium levels,** or are taking drugs for **abnormal heart rhythms.** Be sure your cardiologist knows you are starting on this medication. People taking nilotinib have died suddenly, possibly because of cardiac complications. Imatinib, lapitinib, and sunitinib can worsen **heart failure.** There are more heart attacks and other cardiac problems in people taking sorafenib. People with **high blood pressure** should use caution while taking sorafenib, because high blood pressure is a common side effect of this drug. Blood pressure should be checked during the first 6 weeks of treatment.

Sunitinib has also been associated with reduced thyroid and adrenal gland function, and high blood pressure.

Lapitinib can cause diarrhea. Call your doctor if this happens to you because it should be treated aggressively to avoid significant fluid and electrolyte loss.

Possible Side Effects

Dasatinib

▼ Most common: abdominal pain; pain; difficulty breathing; cough; fever; chills; pneumonia; infections, including herpes virus and blood infection; fluid retention; nausea; vomiting; diarrhea; constipation; appetite loss; weight loss; abdominal enlargement; headache; muscle and joint pain; fatigue; skin rashes; itching; weakness; inflammation and ulcers in the mouth, GI tract, or anus; chest pain; tingling

Possible Side Effects *(continued)*

in the hands or feet; nerve inflammation; and abnormal heart rhythms.

▼ Common: fluid in the lungs, fever with very low white-blood-cell count, GI bleeding, reduced blood-platelet count, upset stomach, dental disorders, colitis, stomach pain, anal fissure, not feeling well, sweating, hair loss, dry skin, acne, unusual sun sensitivity, nail disorders, skin color changes, asthma, taste changes, tiredness, fainting, tremors, convulsions, muscle inflammation, muscle stiffness, elevated blood uric acid level, heart palpitations, angina pain, heart enlargement, heart attack, conjunctivitis (pinkeye), dry eye, flushing, blood pressure changes, sleeplessness, depression, anxiety, confusion, affect changes, male breast enlargement, bruising, dizziness, ringing or buzzing in the ears, frequent urination, and kidney failure.

▼ Less common: anemia, heart failure, bleeding in the brain, and reduced sex drive.

▼ Rare: Rare side effects can occur in almost any part of the body. Contact your doctor if you experience any side effect not listed above.

Gefitinib

The risk of drug side effects increases when taking high doses of gefitinib.

▼ Most common: rash, acne, dry skin, nausea, and diarrhea.

▼ Common: vomiting, dry mouth, itching, appetite loss, and weakness.

▼ Less common: weight loss, swelling in the arms or legs, poor vision in one eye, conjunctivitis (pinkeye), mild rash, mouth ulcers, and difficulty breathing, with or without cough and fever, that may become severe in a very short period of time.

▼ Rare: eye pain, erosion of the cornea, eye ulcer, unusual eyelash growth, bleeding in the eye, severe skin reaction, and allergic reaction. Contact your doctor if you experience any side effect not listed above.

Imatinib

Most side effects are mild to moderate, but are very common in patients experiencing a myeloid blast crisis. As many as 5%

Possible Side Effects (continued)

of people taking the drug in clinical studies stopped because of side effects. Women taking imatinib are likely to develop more swelling around the eyes, headache, and fatigue.

▼ Most common: nausea, diarrhea, vomiting, swelling around the eyes, leg swelling and muscle cramps, and upset stomach.

▼ Common: muscle pain, fever, cough, rash, and difficulty breathing.

▼ Less common: headache, fatigue, severe joint pain, weight gain, abdominal pain, appetite loss, constipation, irritation of the nose or nasal cavity, night sweats, and weakness.

▼ Rare: severe fluid retention, bleeding, easy bruising, and pneumonia. Contact your doctor if you experience any side effect not listed above.

Lapitinib

▼ Most common: Diarrhea, nausea, vomiting, stomach irritation and pain, upset stomach, dry skin, rash, skin peeling on your palms and soles of your feet, inflamed mucosal tissue, pain in the hands or feet, back pain, difficulty breathing, and sleeplessness.

Nilotinib

▼ Most common: rash, itching, nausea, constipation, diarrhea, vomiting, fatigue, headache, fever, swelling in the arms or legs, bone and joint pain, arm or leg pain, back pain, muscle spasms, cough, difficulty breathing, and nose and throat infections.

▼ Rare: Rare side effects can occur in almost any part of the body. Contact your doctor if you experience any side effect not listed above.

Sorafenib

▼ Most common: high blood pressure; fatigue; swelling; blisters; rash and other skin reactions, especially on the soles of the feet and palms; hair loss; itching; diarrhea; nausea; appetite loss; vomiting; constipation; bleeding; cough; and difficulty breathing.

▼ Common: weight loss, numbness, tingling in the hands or feet, sensitivity to bright light, joint pain, abdominal pain, headache, hoarseness, erectile dysfunction, depression,

Possible Side Effects *(continued)*

anemia, low levels of white blood cells, increased liver enzyme levels, flu-like symptoms, and fever.

▼ Less common: GI tract perforation.

▼ Rare: Rare side effects can occur in almost any part of the body. Contact your doctor if you experience any side effect not listed above.

Sunitinib

▼ Most common: fatigue; fever; weakness; diarrhea; nausea; vomiting; constipation; abdominal pain; upset stomach; inflammation and ulceration in the mouth and GI tract; dry mouth; cough; difficulty breathing; high blood pressure; rash; dry skin; pain, redness, tenderness, and peeling of the palms of the hands and soles of the feet; skin discoloration; taste changes; appetite loss; sleeplessness; and bleeding.

▼ Common: oral pain, hair color changes, hair loss, gastroesophageal reflux disease (GERD) with or without irritation and swelling of the esophagus, gas, tongue pain, swelling in the arms or legs, dizziness, and depression.

Drug Interactions

- Ketoconazole, itraconazole, erythromycin, clarithromycin, atazanavir, indinavir, nefazodone, nelfinavir, ritonavir, saquinavir, simvastatin, telithromycin, and voriconazole will increase blood levels of these drugs. They should be avoided if possible. If they must be taken together, dose modification is necessary.

- Carbamazepine, dexamethasone, phenytoin, phenobarbital and rifampin, rifabutin, and rifapentin will substantially reduce blood levels of all these drugs. They should be avoided if possible. Dose adjustment may be needed.

- Imatinib stimulates enzymes in the liver that break down phenytoin. Patients taking this combination may need to increase their phenytoin dosage to maintain seizure control.

- St. John's wort also reduces blood levels of these drugs, but the effect is unpredictable. Do not mix these medications.

- Long term use of antacids or drugs that reduce stomach acid production (esomeprazole, lansoprozole, omeprazole, pantoprazole, rabeprazole, ranitidine, famotidine and cimetidine) can make dasatinib and gefitinib less soluble in the GI tract, cutting blood levels in half. Avoid taking any product aimed at reducing stomach acid for 2 hours before or after a dose of dasatinib.

- People taking warfarin or another anticoagulant should be cautious when imatinib, dasatinib, or sorafenib is started because of the increased chance of bleeding. You may be switched to a heparin (injectable) blood thinner to avoid this interaction.
- Imatinib and dasatinib may increase blood levels of alfentanil, astemizole, cisapride, cyclosporine, fentanyl, pimozide, quinidine, sirolimus, tacrolimus, terfenidine, some calcium channel blockers, and ergot-based migraine medicines. These drugs should be mixed with caution.
- Imatinib increases the amount of simvastatin in the blood by 3½ times. Other statin drugs may be similarly affected.
- Gefitinib can increase the effect of warfarin, causing bleeding episodes. Your doctor must check your blood regularly and may have to adjust your warfarin dose while you are taking gefitinib.
- Sorafenib may increase blood levels of the following drugs by interfering with the breakdown in the liver: bupropion, cyclophosphamide, efavirenz, ifosfamide, methadone, paclitaxel, torsemide, amodiaquine, cerivastatin and repaglinide.
- Sorafenib also inhibits the liver's ability to break down toxic chemicals and drugs including acetaminophen. The importance of this effect is not yet known.
- Sorafenib causes a 21% increase in blood levels of the anticancer drug doxorubicin and a 26–42% increase in blood levels of the drug irinotecan. The clinical importance of these interactions is not known but these combinations should be used with caution. Sorafenib has been used safely together with a variety of other anticancer drugs.

Food Interactions

Imatinib can cause stomach and intestinal irritation. Take each dose with food and a glass of water to minimize this side effect. Dasatinib, gefitinib, and sunitinib may be taken without regard to meals. Lapitinib, nilotinib, and sorafenib should be taken on an empty stomach, at least 1 hour before or 2 hours after a meal. Do not drink or eat any grapefruit product with imatinib, nilotinib, or sunitinib. Grapefruit stimulates liver enzymes that remove these drugs from the bloodstream.

Usual Dose

Dasatinib

Adult (age 18 and over): 100–140 mg a day in 1 or 2 doses. Always take this medication at the same time every day. Modifications of 20 mg/day may be based on response or toxicity assessments. To deal with drug interactions, other medications with the same effect may be substituted for the interacting drugs or the dasatinib dose may be altered.

Child (under age 18): not recommended.

Gefitinib

Adult: 250 mg once a day.

Child: not recommended.

Imatinib

Adult and Child (age 3 and over): 400–800 mg a day. Treatment should be continued for as long as the patient continues to benefit. Drug dosage should be reduced or stopped if severe liver or other problems develop until they resolve. Children 3 years of age and older can take imatinib in either 1 or 2 daily doses.

Child (under age 3): not recommended.

Lapitinib

Adult (age 18 and over): 5 tablets once a day for 3 weeks plus capecitabine twice a day for 2 weeks.

Child (under age 18): not recommended.

Nilotinib

Adult: two 200-mg capsules every 12 hours. This dose may be modified based on certain lab tests and your heart function.

Child: not recommended.

Sorafenib

Adult: two 200-mg tablets twice a day at least 1 hour before or 2 hours after a meal. Drug dosage may be reduced if you experience a serious side effect.

Child: not recommended.

Sunitinib

Adult: 50 mg once a day for 4 weeks. Then stop for 2 weeks and repeat the 4-week treatment as prescribed. Daily dose may be adjusted in 12.5 mg steps.

Child: not recommended.

Overdosage

Animal overdose studies of dasatinib showed cardiac toxicity, bleeding, and high blood pressure. Likely gefitinib and sorafenib overdose symptoms include diarrhea and skin rash. Symptoms should be treated individually but it is particularly important to pay attention to severe diarrhea. There is little experience with imatinib doses larger than 800 mg a day, the maximum human dose. Some overdose effects are muscle cramps and elevated liver enzymes. Lapitinib overdose can cause diarrhea, vomiting, and other drug side effects. Take the overdose victim to your doctor or emergency room. Nilotinib overdose has not been reported. Sunitinib overdose can cause loss of muscle coordination; head shakes; slowing of thought, speech, and movement; eye discharge; upset stomach; and standing of small hairs on the arm or back of the neck. If you seek treatment, ALWAYS bring the prescription bottle or container with you.

Special Information

You must report any severe side effect or anything unusual to your doctor, especially shortness of breath, fatigue, or heart palpitations. These may be signs of heart failure. Treatment may have to be stopped until the side effect improves or resolves. Then, treatment may be resumed.

These drugs can cause liver toxicity. Symptoms of liver toxicity may include yellowing of the skin or whites of the eyes.

Dasatinib contains lactose and may cause GI distress in people who are lactose intolerant.

Crushing dasatinib tablets is not recommended. However, if this is necessary, women who are or who may be pregnant must avoid contact with the crushed tablets because of risk to the developing fetus. The medication is coated to protect people from unecessary exposure to dasatinib.

Sorafenib can pass into male ejaculate. Men must use a condom while taking this drug and for 2 weeks after stopping it.

If you are taking gefitinib, call your doctor at once if you develop cough, wheezing, or difficulty breathing and fever. You may have to stop taking gefitinib until the reason for your symptoms is discovered. These symptoms are fatal in 1/3 of people who develop them. Other reasons to call your doctor right away are severe or persistent diarrhea, nausea, appetite loss, vomiting, eye irritation, or any other new symptom. If your diarrhea is severe, your doctor may have you discontinue the drug for 2 weeks to rest your GI system.

Do not stop or change the dose of these medications unless instructed to do so by your doctor. You should make a special effort to take these medications at the same time every day. Do not take a double dose of dasatinib. If you take dasatinib twice a day and forget a dose, take it if you remember within an hour of your regular time, and then continue with your regular schedule. Otherwise, skip the forgotten dose. If you take dasatinib once a day and forget a dose, take it if you remember within 12 hours of your regular time. Otherwise, skip the forgotten dose and continue with your regular schedule.

If you forget a dose of imatinib or sorafenib, take it as soon as you remember. If it is almost time for your next dose, space out the remaining doses for the day to allow you to take your total prescribed dosage for the day. Contact your doctor if you forget more than 1 dose in a row or if you take too much medication.

If you forget your daily dose of gefitinib, lapitinib, nilotinib, or sunitinib, skip the forgotten dose and continue with your regular schedule. Tell your doctor if you forget to take any doses of these drugs. Do not take a double dose.

Special Populations

Pregnancy/Breast-feeding: These drugs are not recommended during pregnancy, as they are known to enter the blood circulation of the developing fetus and may cause birth defects. Women who are pregnant or may become pregnant should discuss these drugs with their doctor. When these drugs are considered crucial by your doctor, their potential benefits must be carefully weighed against their risks. If you become pregnant while taking one of these drugs, call your doctor at once.

It is estimated that about 1.5% of each dose of imatinib passes into breast milk. It is not known if dasatinib, gefitinib, or sunitinib pass into breast milk. Nursing mothers taking one of these medicines should always use infant formula because of the risk of drug side effects to the nursing infant.

Seniors: Seniors have been able to take dasatinib without special precaution, though they may be more sensitive to some side effects, especially fluid retention. No differences in side effect sensitivity have been noted with gefitinib, lapitinib, or sunitinib.

Generic Name

Mupirocin (mue-PYE-roe-sin) Ⓖ

Brand Names

Bactroban   Centany

Type of Drug

Topical antibiotic.

Prescribed For

Impetigo (streptococcal skin infections), eczema, inflammation of the hair follicles, and minor bacterial skin infections. Mupirocin nasal is used to prevent resistant *Staphylococcus aureus* infections from spreading during outbreaks of the infection. Mupirocin can also be used to treat diaper rash.

General Information

Mupirocin is a unique, non-penicillin drug that works against the common microorganisms that cause impetigo in children. It is used to supplement other treatments for impetigo, although many doctors prefer oral medication. Mupirocin works by interfering with bacteria's ability to make the proteins it needs for survival. Large amounts of mupirocin kill bacteria and smaller amounts stop the bacteria from growing. It may be effective against antibiotic-resistant bacteria.

Cautions and Warnings

Do not use a mupirocin product if you are **allergic** or **sensitive** to any of its ingredients. Mupirocin ointment is not for use in the eye.

Mupirocin nasal should be used only to treat *Staphylococcus aureus* infections, not to prevent them.

Large quantities of mupirocin ointment should not be applied to an open wound because polyethylene glycol—used as a base in mupirocin ointment—may be absorbed through the wound and damage the kidneys.

Long-term or chronic use of mupirocin may lead to secondary infection caused by drug-resistant bacteria or fungi.

Possible Side Effects

Ointment

▼ Less common: burning, pain, and itching.

Possible Side Effects *(continued)*

▼ Rare: rash, stinging, or pain where the ointment is applied; nausea, skin redness, dry skin, tenderness, swelling, and increased oozing from impetigo lesions. Contact your doctor if you experience any side effect not listed above.

Cream
▼ Less common: headache, rash, and nausea.
▼ Rare: abdominal pain, burning, irritation, inflammation, dizziness, itching, secondary infection, and mouth ulcer. Contact your doctor if you experience any side effect not listed above.

Nasal Ointment
▼ Most common: headache and runny nose.
▼ Less common: respiratory congestion, sore throat, changes in sense of taste, burning or stinging, cough, and itching.
▼ Rare: eyelid inflammation, diarrhea, dry mouth, ear pain, nosebleeds, nausea, and rash. Contact your doctor if you experience any side effect not listed above.

Drug Interactions
- Do not use mupirocin nasal at the same time as any other prescription or over-the-counter nasal drug product.
- Taking other antibiotics while using mupirocin can lead to the development of resistant bacteria.

Usual Dose
Ointment and Cream: Apply a small amount to the affected area 3 times a day. Cover with gauze if desired.

Nasal Ointment: Put half the ointment from a single-use tube in each nostril morning and evening for 5 days. After the ointment is applied, gently squeeze your nostrils closed and allow them to open again. Repeat this continuously for about 1 minute.

Overdosage
Little is known about the effects of accidental ingestion. Call your local poison control center or a hospital emergency room for more information. If you seek treatment, ALWAYS bring the prescription bottle or container.

Special Information

Call your doctor if this medication does not work within 3–5 days or if any of the following symptoms develop: dry skin or redness, rash, itching, stinging, pain, or other possible drug reactions.

If you forget a dose, apply it as you remember. If it is almost time for your next dose, skip the one you forgot and continue with your regular schedule. Do not apply a double dose.

Special Populations

Pregnancy/Breast-feeding: The safety of using mupirocin during pregnancy is not known. When this drug is considered crucial by your doctor, its potential benefits must be carefully weighed against its risks.

It is not known if mupirocin passes into breast milk. Nursing mothers who must take this drug should use infant formula.

Seniors: Seniors may use mupirocin without special restriction.

Generic Name

Muromonab-CD3 (muh-ROE-moe-nab)

Brand Name

Orthoclone OKT3 Sterile Solution

Type of Drug

Immunosuppressant.

Prescribed For

Kidney, heart, and liver transplantation.

General Information

Muromonab-CD3 is an important alternative to cyclosporine in treating acute organ transplant rejection. By blocking the activity of T-cells, which protect the body against invading microorganisms or foreign substances, this drug suppresses the immune system and reverses organ rejection. The drug starts working in minutes and continues working for as long as it is used. T-cells rapidly return to normal within 1 week after the medication is stopped.

Cautions and Warnings

Muromonab-CD3 should only be prescribed by physicians experienced in immunosuppressive therapy and the care of organ-transplant patients.

Do not use muromonab if you are **allergic** or **sensitive** to any of its ingredients.

This drug should not be used by people with uncontrolled **hypertension,** untreated **heart failure, fluid overload,** or a history of **seizures**. Severe allergic reactions can occur, including arthritis, serum sickness, treatment failure, angioedema (a life-threatening syndrome involving swelling of the lips, eyelids, and throat), and anaphylactic shock.

Muromonab-CD3 is made in cells from mouse tissue and causes the development of anti-mouse antibodies in humans. People who have received other drugs made in this way may already have high levels of this kind of antibody in their blood and, if they do, should not be treated with muromonab-CD3. Your doctor will test for antibody levels.

People who receive this drug usually develop cytokine release syndrome (CRS) from 30 minutes to 2 days after the first dose is given. CRS symptoms range from mild, flu-like symptoms such as fever, chills, joint aches, weakness, and headaches, to a less common, life-threatening shock-like reaction that involves the heart and nervous system. Some of the more severe symptoms of CRS are shortness of breath, high fever—up to 107°F, wheezing, rapid heartbeat, chest pain, respiratory collapse or failure, heart attack, severe drug reactions, seizures, confusion, hallucinations, stiff neck, brain swelling, headache, tremor, confusion, altered thinking or mood, lethargy, weakness, and involuntary movements. People who are at risk for more severe forms of CRS include those with a **recent heart attack** or uncontrolled **angina pectoris, heart failure, fluid in the lungs, serious lung disease**, and a history of **seizure or shock.** CRS may be prevented or minimized by giving methylprednisolone 1–4 hours before the first dose of muromonab-CD3. CRS symptoms usually become less severe with repeated doses of muromonab-CD3.

People receiving this drug are more likely to develop infection. Preventive antibiotic therapy is sometimes used to reduce the risk of infection.

Possible Side Effects

More than 90% of people receiving muromonab-CD3 experience some form of CRS, though it is usually mild (see "Cautions and Warnings" for symptoms list).

Possible Side Effects *(continued)*

▼ Common: infections, lymphoma, and allergic reactions.
▼ Rare: Rare side effects can occur in almost any part of the body. Contact your doctor if you experience any bothersome or persistent side effect, or any side effect not listed above.

Drug Interactions

- Other immunosuppressants (corticosteroids, cyclosporine, and azathioprine) and indomethacin increase the effect of muromonab-CD3, in turn increasing the risk of CRS.

Food Interactions

Muromonab-CD3 may be taken without regard to food.

Usual Dose

Adult and Child (age 12 and over): 5 mg intravenously a day for 10–14 days.

Child (under age 12): 2.5 mg intravenously a day for 10–14 days.

Overdosage

Little is known about the effects of muromonab-CD3 overdose. Call your local poison control center or a hospital emergency room for information.

Special Information

Call your doctor at the first sign of rash, itching, rapid heartbeat, difficulty swallowing, breathing difficulties, unusual swelling, allergic reaction, or if you experience any bothersome or persistent side effect. It is essential to maintain close contact with your doctor while taking muromonab-CD3.

Mild reactions due to CRS may be treated by taking acetaminophen or antihistamines. Your body temperature should be no higher than 100°F when each dose is given.

Avoid exposure to bacterial infection and immunizations while you are taking this drug. If an infection develops, your doctor will have to stop muromonab-CD3 therapy and treat the infection.

Maintain good dental hygiene while taking muromonab-CD3 and use extra care when brushing and flossing because this drug increases your risk of oral infection. See your dentist regularly.

This drug may cause confusion or interfere with your alertness, dexterity, or coordination. Be careful when driving or doing any task that requires concentration.

It is essential to complete the full course of treatment. This medication should not be stopped unless an infection or other severe side effect develops. If you miss a dose, take it as soon as you remember and call your doctor.

Special Populations

Pregnancy/Breast-feeding: Muromonab-CD3 may cross into the fetal circulation. When this drug is considered crucial by your doctor, its potential benefits must be carefully weighed against its risks.

It is not known if muromonab-CD3 passes into breast milk. Nursing mothers who must take this drug should use infant formula.

Seniors: Seniors may use this drug without special restriction.

Generic Name

Mycophenolate (mye-coe-FEN-oe-late)

Brand Name
CellCept

Type of Drug
Immunosuppressant.

Prescribed For
Kidney, liver, and heart transplantation.

General Information
Mycophenolate mofetil is used with corticosteroids and cyclosporine to prevent the rejection of transplanted kidneys and other organs. In the body, the drug is metabolized into MPA, the active form of mycophenolate. MPA blocks the activity of T and B lymphocytes, which protect the body against invading microorganisms or foreign substances. MPA also suppresses antibody formation and may act directly on inflammation and organ rejection sites to prevent tissue rejection.

Cautions and Warnings

Mycophenolate should only be prescribed by physicians experienced in immunosuppressive therapy and the care of organ-transplant patients.

Do not take mycophenolate if you are **allergic** or **sensitive** to any of its ingredients or to mycophenolic acid or polisorbate 80. As with other immunosuppressants, people taking mycophenolate are at increased risk of infections or developing a lymphoma or other malignancy. The risk increases with the degree of immune suppression and the length of time that the drug is taken.

About 2 in 100 people receiving mycophenolate develop a severe reduction in white-blood-cell count. Call your doctor if you develop symptoms of viral infection or other unusual symptoms.

Mycophenolate increases your sensitivity to the sun and susceptibility to skin cancer. Always exercise caution outdoors and wear protective clothing.

About 3 in 100 people who take this drug develop stomach or intestinal bleeding, though many of these people are also taking other drugs that may affect the gastrointestinal (GI) tract. People with **stomach or intestinal disease** should take this drug with caution.

People with **kidney disease** should receive lower dosages. People who experience post-transplant reduction in liver function may develop kidney damage.

Mild to moderate hypertension (high blood pressure) is a common side effect of mycophenolate and may be a sign of kidney damage. People taking this drug should measure their blood pressure regularly.

Possible Side Effects

▼ Most common: general pain, abdominal pain, fever, headache, infection, blood infection, weakness, chest pain, back pain, hypertension, anemia, reduced white-blood-cell and platelet counts, urinary infection, blood in the urine, swelling of the arms or legs, diarrhea, anxiety, numbness or tingling, constipation, nausea, vomiting, upset stomach, oral fungus infection, respiratory infection, cough, increased incidence of other opportunistic infections, breathing difficulties, and tremors.

Possible Side Effects *(continued)*

▼ Common: kidney damage, urinary tract problems, high blood cholesterol, low blood-phosphate levels, fluid retention, changes in blood-potassium levels, high blood sugar, sore throat, pneumonia, bronchitis, acne, rash, sleeplessness, and dizziness.

▼ Less common: painful urination, impotence, frequent urination, pyelonephritis, urinary disorder, angina pain, heart palpitations, low blood pressure, dizziness when rising from a sitting or lying position, cardiovascular disorders, appetite loss, gas, stomach irritation or bleeding, gum irritation or enlargement, liver irritation, mouth ulcer, asthma, lung disorder, stuffy or runny nose, sinus irritation, hair loss, itching, sweating, skin ulcer, anxiety, depression, stiff muscles, tingling in the hands or feet, joint or muscle pain, leg cramps, double vision, cataracts, conjunctivitis (pinkeye), chills and fever, abdominal enlargement, facial swelling, cysts, flu-like symptoms, bleeding, hernia, feeling sick, pelvic pain, and black-and-blue marks.

▼ Rare: lymphoma, skin cancer—not melanomas—and other malignancies, herpes, chickenpox or shingles, fungus infection, and pneumocystis and other opportunistic infections that usually only develop in people with suppressed immune systems. Contact your doctor if you experience any side effect not listed above.

Children receiving mycophenalate experience similar side effects as adults, as well as fever, infection, pain, blood infection, diarrhea, vomiting, sore throat, respiratory tract infection, high blood pressure, low white-blood-cell count, and anemia.

Drug Interactions

- Combining mycophenolate and acyclovir or ganciclovir (antiviral drugs) increases blood levels of both drugs.
- Cholestyramine and aluminum/magnesium antacids decrease mycophenolate blood levels. Aluminum/magnesium antacids should be separated from mycophenolate by at least 1 hour and cholestyramine and myophenolate should not be taken together.

- Azathioprine (an immune-system suppressant) should not be combined with mycophenolate because of the risk of excess immune-system suppression.
- Probenecid may double or triple mycophenolate blood levels. Aspirin also increases mycophenolate blood levels.
- Mycophenolate may moderately increase phenytoin and theophylline blood levels.
- Mycophenolate may reduce the effectiveness of some contraceptive drugs.
- Mycophenolate should not be combined with iron supplements, as iron decreases blood levels of mycophenolate.
- Mycophenolate can make vaccines less effective, although a flu vaccine may be recommended.
- Salicylates increase mycophenolate levels.
- Trimethoprim and sulfamethoxazole may lower mycophenolate levels slightly.

Food Interactions

Mycophenolate should be taken at least 1 hour before or 2 hours after meals.

Usual Dose

Adult: 2–3 g a day divided into 2 doses.

Child (age 3 months and over): capsules—1.5–2 g a day divided into 2 doses. Oral suspension—600 mg/m^2 twice daily up to a maximum daily dose of 2 g/10 mL oral suspension.

Overdosage

Overdose is likely to cause side effects—especially those relating to the stomach and intestines—and blood abnormalities. Take the victim to a hospital emergency room. ALWAYS bring the prescription bottle or container.

Special Information

It is extremely important to take this drug exactly as prescribed. If you forget a dose, take it as soon as you remember. If it is almost time for your next dose, skip the dose you forgot and continue with your regular schedule. Do not take a double dose. Call your doctor if you forget 2 or more doses in a row.

Because this drug causes birth defects in animals, take extra caution when handling the capsules. Do not open or crush them. Avoid inhaling the powder or allowing it to touch your skin or the inside of your mouth or nose. If such contact does occur, wash thoroughly with soap and water. If the powder gets into your eyes, rinse them thoroughly with plain water.

People taking mycophenolate require regular testing to monitor their progress.

Call your doctor at the first sign of fever; sore throat; tiredness; weakness; nervousness; unusual bleeding or bruising; tender or swollen gums; convulsions; irregular heartbeat; confusion; numbness or tingling of your hands, feet, or lips; breathing difficulties; severe stomach pain with nausea; or blood in the urine. Other side effects are less serious but should be brought to your doctor's attention, particularly if they are bothersome or persistent.

Maintain good dental hygiene while taking mycophenolate and use extra care when brushing or flossing because this drug increases your risk of oral infection. See your dentist regularly.

This drug should be continued for as long as prescribed by your doctor. Do not stop taking it because of side effects or other problems without your doctor's knowledge.

Special Populations

Pregnancy/Breast-feeding: Pregnant women should not take this drug. Women of childbearing age should have a negative pregnancy test at least 1 week before treatment is started. They should either use 2 effective contraceptive methods before treatment is started and continue until 6 weeks after mycophenolate is discontinued, or they should practice abstinence during this period. Should you accidentally become pregnant during mycophenolate treatment, discuss with your doctor the advisability of continuing the pregnancy. When this drug is considered crucial by your doctor, its potential benefits must be carefully weighed against its risks.

Mycophenolate passes into breast milk. Nursing mothers who must take this drug should use infant formula.

Seniors: Seniors may require reduced dosage due to loss of kidney and cardiac function.

Generic Name

Naltrexone (nal-TRECK-sohn) Ⓖ

Brand Names

Depade	ReVia

The information in this profile also applies to the following drugs:

Generic Ingredient: Buprenorphine
Subutex

Generic Ingredients: Buprenorphine + Naloxone
Suboxone

Type of Drug

Opioid receptor antagonist.

Prescribed For

Narcotic or alcohol addiction.

General Information

Naltrexone is a pure antagonist of opioid receptors in the brain that are stimulated by narcotic drugs. Buprenorphine is a pure antagonist of one of the opioid receptors and a partial stimulator of another. Buprenorphine satisfies narcotic cravings but seems to have a limit to its effect. Naloxone is an opioid receptor antagonist, added to prevent product abuse. When taken on a regular basis, these drugs block the actions of and physical dependence to narcotic drugs including methadone, morphine, and heroin. Naltrexone is also beneficial in the treatment of alcoholism and helps reduce alcohol cravings and number of drinking days. How naltrexone blocks alcohol craving is not known, but it may involve the same brain receptors as narcotic dependence. Naltrexone is a long-acting drug, with effects lasting for 2–3 days.

Cautions and Warnings

Do not take these medications if you are **allergic** or **sensitive** to any of their ingredients.

Do not take naltrexone if you have taken any narcotic drug within the previous 7–10 days or are **dependent on narcotic drugs**. Taking naltrexone may produce severe drug withdrawal symptoms. People who attempt to overcome the blocking effects of naltrexone by taking large doses of a narcotic drug are at risk for drug overdose. People who had been taking naltrexone are likely to be more sensitive to narcotic drugs.

Naltrexone should be used with caution if you have **active liver disease**, **hepatitis**, or **liver failure**.

Naltrexone passes out of the body through the urine. People with **kidney disease** should use it with caution.

Buprenorphine should be used with caution by people with **severe kidney disease**. The effect of **kidney failure** on naloxone is not known. These 2 drugs are broken down in the liver. Hepatitis and jaundice have developed in people taking buprenorphine. People with **liver disease** should receive lower doses of buprenorphine.

Buprenorphine should be used with caution by people who have a **lung or breathing disorder**. It can cause nervous system depression and interfere with your ability to breathe especially when it is accompanied by a benzodiazepine drug or other depressant. Caution should also be exercised by people with a **thyroid disorder, Addison's disease, nervous system depression, toxic psychosis, prostate enlargement, acute alcoholism,** or **delirium tremens (DTs).**

Buprenorphine produces **drug dependence** and will lead to withdrawal symptoms if it is suddenly stopped or the dose is not tapered over a long enough time. Buprenorphine and naloxone will cause more intense withdrawal symptoms.

These drugs should be used with caution by people with **head injuries** or **brain lesions.**

It is not known if naltrexone is safe for use in **rapid detoxification** programs.

The **risk of suicide**, which always accompanies drug abuse, is not reduced by these medications.

Possible Side Effects

Buprenorphine

Side effects increase with drug dosage.

▼ Most common: weakness, headache, infections, pain, back pain, drug withdrawal symptoms, constipation, nausea, anxiety, depression, sleeplessness, and sweating.

▼ Common: chills, flu-like symptoms, diarrhea, vomiting, dizziness, nervousness, runny eyes, and tiredness.

▼ Less common: abscesses, fever, accidental injury, and upset stomach.

Buprenorphine + Naloxone

▼ Most common: headache, pain, abdominal pain, drug withdrawal symptoms, flushing, low blood pressure, nausea, sleeplessness, and sweating.

▼ Common: weakness, chills, infections, constipation, vomiting, and runny nose.

▼ Less common: back pain and diarrhea.

Possible Side Effects (continued)

Naltrexone

Most naltrexone side effects appear early in treatment and then improve with time.

▼ Common: headache, nausea, sleeplessness, nervousness, abdominal cramps, and nausea or vomiting.

▼ Less common: dizziness, fatigue, anxiety, tiredness, and weight changes.

▼ Rare: Rare side effects can occur in the gastrointestinal tract, heart and blood vessels, respiratory tract, eyes, and ears. Contact your doctor if you experience any side effect not listed above.

Drug Interactions

Buprenorphine and Buprenorphine + Naloxone

- Ketoconazole, itraconazole, erythromycin, clarithromycin, atazanavir, indinavir, nefazodone, nelfinavir, ritonavir, simvastatin, and telithromycin may increase buprenorphine blood levels. Dose reduction may be necessary.
- Carbamazepine, dexamethasone, phenytoin, phenobarbital, and rifampin may reduce buprenorphine blood levels. Dose adjustment may be needed.

Naltrexone

- Mixing naltrexone and thioridazine can cause lethargy and tiredness.
- People taking naltrexone will not benefit from narcotic cough suppressants and pain relievers.
- The consequences of mixing naltrexone and disulfiram (for alcohol abuse) are not known.

Food Interactions

None known.

Usual Dose

Buprenorphine and Buprenorphine + Naloxone

Adult (age 16 and over): 8 mg to start, then 12–16 mg a day. These drugs are interchangeable.

Child (under age 16): not recommended.

Naltrexone

Adult (age 18 and over): 25–50 mg once a day to start. Individualization of drug dosage may be needed.

Child: not recommended.

Overdosage

Buprenorphine

Overdose symptoms are those associated with a narcotic overdose: pinpoint pupils, sedation, low blood pressure, and difficulty breathing. Take the victim to a hospital emergency room at once. ALWAYS bring the prescription bottle or container.

Naltrexone

There is little experience with naltrexone overdose in humans. However, doses of 50 mg or more can cause liver damage. Take the victim to a hospital emergency room. ALWAYS bring the prescription bottle or container.

Special Information

Naltrexone can cause narcotic withdrawal symptoms. Do not take this drug if you have used any narcotic within the past 7–10 days.

Wear a special identification bracelet or carry an ID card saying you are taking this drug. This may be important if you require emergency medical care.

If you are using heroin, wait at least 4 hours or when early withdrawal signs start to appear before taking buprenorphine. Withdrawal symptoms are possible if you are using methadone, especially if you take more than 30 mg a day.

Buprenorphine and buprenorphine + naloxone sublingual tablets should be placed under the tongue and allowed to dissolve there. If you take more than 2 tablets at a time, either place all the tablets under the tongue at once or 2 at a time.

Take these drugs as directed. If you skip a dose, take it as soon as you remember. If it is almost time for your next dose, skip the forgotten dose and continue with your regular schedule.

Call your doctor at once and stop taking naltrexone if you develop abdominal pain lasting more than a few days, white bowel movements, dark urine, or yellowing of your eyes.

Call your doctor if you are taking buprenorphine and develop a rash, hives, or itching. Do not stop taking buprenorphine without your doctor's permission. Stopping suddenly or too quickly can lead to drug withdrawal symptoms.

Special Populations

Pregnancy/Breast-feeding: These drugs have been found to damage a developing animal fetus but there is no information on how these drugs will affect pregnant women. They should be used during pregnancy only after carefully weighing their potential benefits against their risks. Babies born to mothers taking buprenorphine may go through drug withdrawal.

Buprenorphine passes into breast milk.

It is not known if naltrexone passes into human breast milk. Nursing mothers who must take these medications should consider using infant formula.

Seniors: Seniors may be more sensitive to the effects of naltrexone, but dosage adjustments are not needed. Seniors should use buprenorphine with caution.

Namenda   *see Memantine, page 683*

Nasacort AQ   *see Corticosteroids, Nasal, page 309*

Nasonex   *see Corticosteroids, Nasal, page 309*

Generic Name

Nefazodone   (neh-FAZ-oe-don) Ⓖ

Type of Drug

Antidepressant.

Prescribed For

Depression.

General Information

A unique compound, nefazodone is chemically unrelated to other antidepressants. It interferes with the ability of nerve endings in the brain to absorb serotonin and norepinephrine, two key neuro-hormones. Nefazodone is broken down in the liver; severe liver disease may increase nefazodone blood levels by 25%. Very little of the drug is released through the kidneys.

Cautions and Warnings

Do not take nefazodone if you are **allergic** or **sensitive** to any of its ingredients.

Antidepressants have been associated with an increased risk of suicide, especially in **teenagers** and **children**. Suicide is always a risk in severely depressed people, who should only be allowed to have minimal quantities of medication in their possession.

Nefazodone may precipitate a manic phase in those with pre-viously undiagnosed bipolar (manic-depressive disorder. Nefa-zodone is not used to treat this disorder.

Nefazodone has been associated with potentially fatal liver fail-ure. People with **liver disease** should use nefazodone with caution.

People with a history of **seizure disorders** may experience seizures while taking nefazodone.

People who have recently had a **heart attack** should use this drug with caution because it can substantially reduce heart rate.

Possible Side Effects

▼ Most common: weakness, dry mouth, nausea, headache, constipation, blurred or abnormal vision, tiredness, dizzi-ness, insomnia, agitation, lightheadedness, and confusion.

▼ Common: upset stomach, increased appetite, cough, memory loss, tingling in the hands or feet, flushing or feel-ings of warmth, poor muscle coordination, and dizziness when rising from a lying or sitting position.

▼ Less common: low blood pressure, fever, chills, flu-like symptoms, joint pain, stiff neck, itching, rash, diarrhea, nau-sea, vomiting, thirst, sore throat, changes in sense of taste, ringing or buzzing in the ear, unusual dreams, poor coordi-nation, tremors, muscle stiffness, reduced sex drive, uri-nary difficulties including infection, vaginitis, and breast pain.

Possible Side Effects (continued)

▼ Rare: Rare side effects can affect your liver, gastrointestinal tract, joints, sexual function, and skin. Severe nefazodone allergy is rare. Contact your doctor if you experience any side effect not listed above.

Drug Interactions

- People who take nefazodone within 2 weeks of taking a monoamine oxidase inhibitor (MAOI) antidepressant may experience severe reactions including high fever, muscle rigidity or spasm, changes in mental state, and fluctuations in pulse, temperature, and breathing rate. People stopping nefazodone should wait at least 1 week before starting an MAOI.
- Nefazodone should not be taken with terfenadine, astemizole, cisapride, pimozide, or carbamazepine.
- Combining nefazodone and sumatriptan or sibutramine may cause "serotonin syndrome"; avoid these combinations if possible.
- Combining buspirone and nefazodone may lead to increased side effects.
- Nefazodone may increase blood levels of alprazolam and triazolam (benzodiazepine anti-anxiety drugs). Do not combine these drugs with nefazodone.
- Blood levels of digoxin may be substantially increased by nefazodone. People taking these drugs together should have their digoxin blood levels checked periodically.
- The clearance of haloperidol (an antipsychotic drug) may be drastically reduced by nefazodone; dosage adjustments for haloperidol may be necessary.
- Combining nefazodone and propranolol may cause substantial reductions in propranolol blood levels and substantial increases in blood levels of nefazodone. Do not take these drugs together.
- Avoid drinking alcohol or taking St. John's wort while taking nefazodone.

Food Interactions

Take this drug on an empty stomach at least 1 hour before or 2 hours after meals.

Usual Dose

Adult: 100 mg twice a day to start. Dosage may be increased by 100–200 mg a week to a maximum daily dose of approximately 600 mg.

Senior: Start at ½ the regular adult dose and increase as needed up to 600 mg a day.

Child (under age 18): Consult your physician.

Overdosage

Symptoms of overdose include nausea, vomiting, and sleepiness. Overdose victims should be taken to a hospital emergency room. ALWAYS bring the prescription bottle or container.

Special Information

Several weeks of nefazodone treatment may be necessary before you notice any effect. Continue taking the medication during this period. The following symptoms may occur early in treatment or when the dosage is adjusted: anxiety, agitation, panic attacks, sleeplessness, irritability, restlessness, hostility, aggressiveness, acting impulsively, manic reaction, deepening of depression, other unusual changes in behavior, and suicidal thinking. Report any changes to your doctor.

Call your doctor at once if you develop hives, rash, or other allergic side effects while taking nefazodone.

Nefazodone may make you drowsy. Be careful when driving or doing any task that requires concentration. Avoid alcohol.

Check with your pharmacist or doctor before taking any over-the-counter medication because of the risk of drug interactions.

Special Populations

Pregnancy/Breast-feeding: Animal studies of nefazodone suggest decreased fertility and a risk of fetal damage. When this drug is considered crucial by your doctor, its potential benefits must be carefully weighed against its risks.

It is not known if nefazodone passes into breast milk. Nursing mothers who must take this drug should consider using infant formula.

Seniors: Seniors, especially women, should start treatment at ½ the usual dose. Dosage may be gradually increased as needed, up to the maximum recommended dosage.

Generic Name

Nelfinavir (nel-FIN-uh-vere)

Brand Name

Viracept

Type of Drug

Protease inhibitor.

Prescribed For

Human immunodeficiency virus (HIV) infection.

General Information

Part of the triple-drug "cocktail" responsible for the most important gains in the fight against acquired immunodeficiency syndrome (AIDS), nelfinavir belongs to a group of anti-HIV drugs called protease inhibitors. Triple-drug cocktails are considered responsible for the first overall reduction in the AIDS death rate, recorded in 1996. When the HIV virus attacks a cell, it must be converted into viral DNA. Older drugs known as reverse transcriptase inhibitors interfered with this step but are inferior to protease inhibitors. Protease inhibitors work at the end of the process of HIV reproduction, at the point when proteins are "cut" into strands of exactly the right size to duplicate HIV; these proteins are cut by protease enzymes. Protease inhibitors prevent the mature HIV virus from being formed by interfering with this cutting process. Proteins that are cut to the wrong length or remain uncut are inactive. Protease inhibitors are not a cure for HIV infection or AIDS.

Protease inhibitors are always taken with 1 or 2 nucleoside antiviral drugs such as efavirenz, emtricitabine, lamivudine, tenofovir, or zidovudine (AZT). Protease inhibitors revolutionized HIV treatment because, when taken in combination with other drugs, they reduce the amount of HIV virus in the bloodstream to levels that are often undetectable by current methods such as CD4 cell counts of immune system cells and viral load (amount of virus in the blood) measurements. Multiple-drug therapy has changed the current view of HIV disease from a fatal disease to a manageable chronic illness.

People taking a protease inhibitor may still develop infection or other conditions normally associated with HIV disease. Because of this, it is very important for you to remain under the care of a doctor or other health care provider. The long-term effects of nelfinavir are not known. You may be able to spread the HIV virus to others even if you are on triple-drug therapy.

Cautions and Warnings

Do not take nelfinavir if you are **allergic** or **sensitve** to any of its ingredients. People with **liver disease** or **cirrhosis** break down nelfinavir more slowly than do those with normal liver function.

Nelfinavir may raise blood sugar, worsen **diabetes**, or cause new cases of diabetes to develop. It can also increase risks of bleeding for patients with **hemophilia**. It may produce changes in body fat as well. The long-term effects of these changes are not known.

Immune reconstitution syndrome has occurred in people treated with combination HIV therapy, including nelfinavir. In this syndrome, people develop an immune response to opportunistic infections living in the body, including *Mycobacterium,* cytomegalovirus, *Pneumocystis carinii* pneumonia, or tuberculosis. As the immune system is revived, it sees these organisms and starts responding to them. Additional treatment may be needed.

Excess levels of a potential cancer-causing substance called ethyl methanesulfonate (EMS) were discovered in Viracept in mid-2007. The manufacturer is currently working to reduce the amount of EMS contained in Viracept. The decision to continue individual treatment must be made on a case-by-case basis to determine if this drug's benefits outweigh its possible risks.

Possible Side Effects

▼ Most common: diarrhea.
▼ Common: liver inflammation and nausea.
▼ Less common: abdominal pain, gas, weakness, night-mares, agitation, gallstones, and rash.
▼ Rare: Rare side effects can occur in almost any part of the body including your blood, muscles and joints, gastro-intestinal tract, kidneys, and eyes, and can affect your men-tal state and sexual function. Contact your doctor if you experience any side effect not listed above.

Drug Interactions

● Anticonvulsant medication such as carbamazepine, pheny-toin, or phenobarbital may reduce the amount of nelfinavir in the blood.

- Nelfinavir interferes with the liver's ability to break down triazolam, midazolam, statin drugs (except pravastatin), sildenafil, ergot derivatives, amiodarone, inhaled fluticasone, immunosuppressants, trazodone, azithromycin, and quinidine. These drugs should be mixed with caution.
- Combining nelfinavir with indinavir or saquinavir, other protease inhibitors, results in large increases in the amounts of both drugs in the blood. Other drugs that increase the amount of nelfinavir in the blood are ketoconazole and ritonavir.
- Combining rifabutin with nelfinavir lowers the amount of nelfinavir in the blood and raises the amount of rifabutin. Rifabutin dosage should be cut in half when this combination is used.
- Do not combine rifampin or pimozide and nelfinavir. Combine nelfinavir and sildenafil or vardenafil with extreme caution.
- Nelfinavir reduces the amount of hormonal contraceptive in your bloodstream (see "Special Information").
- If you combine nelfinavir, lamivudine, and zidovudine (an HIV drug—also known as AZT), your AZT dosage may have to be increased.
- St. John's wort may decrease the effectiveness of nelfinavir. Avoid this combination.

Food Interactions

Take nelfinavir with food. If taking the oral powder form, it may be mixed with a small amount of water, milk, soy milk, or dairy foods such as pudding or ice cream. If the entire dose is not consumed, it may be refrigerated for up to 6 hours. Do not heat the mixed dose after refrigeration.

Usual Dose

Adult and Child (age 14 and over): 1250 mg twice daily or 750 mg 3 times a day.

Child (age 2–13): 9–13 mg per lb. of body weight, 3 times a day.

Child (under age 2): not recommended.

Overdosage

Little is known about the effects of nelfinavir overdose except that it may cause severe side effects. Take overdose victims to a hospital emergency room for treatment. ALWAYS bring the prescription bottle or container.

Special Information

Nelfinavir does not cure AIDS. It will not prevent you from transmitting the HIV virus to another person; you must still practice safe sex. You may still develop opportunistic infections or other complications associated with HIV infection.

It is imperative for you to take your HIV medication exactly as prescribed. Missing or skipping doses of nelfinavir increases your risk of becoming resistant to the drug and losing the benefits of nelfinavir therapy.

Diarrhea associated with nelfinavir may be controlled by using loperamide, an over-the-counter remedy.

Do not depend on contraceptive drugs while taking nelfinavir. Use another contraceptive method.

Report anything unusual to your doctor.

If you forget a dose, take it as soon as you remember. If it is almost time for your next dose, skip the dose you forgot and continue with your regular schedule. Do not take a double dose.

Special Populations

Pregnancy/Breast-feeding: Nelfinavir should not be used by pregnant woment. In rare cases when this drug is considered crucial by your doctor, its potential benefits must be carefully weighed against its risks.

Mothers with HIV should always use infant formula, regardless of whether they take this drug, to avoid transmitting the virus to their child.

Seniors: Seniors may take nelfinavir without special restriction.

Brand Name

Neosporin Ophthalmic

Generic Ingredients

Gramicidin + Neomycin Sulfate + Polymyxin B Sulfate Ⓖ

Other Brand Names

AK-Spore

Type of Drug

Ophthalmic and antibiotic combination.

Prescribed For

Superficial eye infection.

General Information

Neosporin Ophthalmic is a combination of antibiotics that is effective against the most common types of eye infection. It is most useful when the infecting organism is known to be sensitive to any of the 3 antibiotics contained in Neosporin Ophthalmic. It may also be useful when the infecting organism is not known because of the drug's broad range of coverage. This product is also available as an eye ointment with a minor formula change—bacitracin is substituted for gramicidin. Both the eyedrops and eye ointment are used for the same kinds of eye infection.

Cautions and Warnings

Do not use Neosporin Ophthalmic if you are **allergic** or **sensitive** to any of its ingredients.

Prolonged use of any antibiotic product in the eye should be avoided because of the risk of becoming sensitive to it and because other organisms such as fungi may grow. If the infection does not clear up within a few days, call your doctor.

Possible Side Effects

▼ Less common: occasional eye irritation, itching, swelling, or burning.

Drug Interactions

None known.

Usual Dose

1 or 2 drops in the affected eye every 4 hours for 7–10 days. For severe infections, dosage may be increased to as much as 2 drops every hour.

Overdosage

There is not enough medicine in this product to cause serious problems. Call your local poison control center or a hospital emergency room for more information. If you seek treatment, ALWAYS bring the prescription bottle or container.

Special Information

To avoid infection, always wash hands first; do not touch the eyedropper tip to your finger, eyelid, or any other surface. Wait at least 5 minutes before using another eyedrop or eye ointment.

Call your doctor if the itching or burning does not go away after a few minutes, or if redness, irritation, swelling, visual disturbance, loss of vision, or eye pain persists.

In general, you should not wear contact lenses if you have an eye infection but your doctor may determine that the use of lenses is acceptable in your situation.

If you forget to administer a dose, do so as soon as you remember. If it is almost time for your next dose, skip the forgotten dose and continue with your regular schedule. Do not take a double dose.

Special Populations

Pregnancy/Breast-feeding: This drug has been found to be safe for use during pregnancy and breast-feeding, but should only be taken by pregnant women if clearly needed. Check with your doctor before taking Neosporin Opthalmic if you are pregnant.

Seniors: Seniors may take this drug without special restriction.

Nexium see *Proton-Pump Inhibitors,* page 939

Generic Name

Niacin (NYE-uh-sin) Ⓖ

Brand Names

Niacor	Nicotinex
Niaspan	Slo-Niacin

Type of Drug

Vitamin.

Prescribed For

Pellagra (niacin deficiency); also prescribed for high blood levels of cholesterol and triglycerides and to dilate (widen) blood vessels.

General Information

Niacin, also known as vitamin B_3 and nicotinic acid, is essential in maintaining health because of the role it plays in enzyme activity. It is effective in lowering blood fat levels as part of a comprehensive program including diet and exercise, and helps to dilate blood vessels, but it is not known exactly how it works. The effect of niacin on blood fats is seen as early as 1 week after treatment is started.

Cautions and Warnings

Do not take niacin if you are **allergic** or **sensitive** to any of its ingredients or to niacin-related drugs. Those who have **liver disease, stomach ulcer,** or a history of **arterial bleeding** should not take niacin. Niacin should be used with caution by people with **kidney disease, heart disease, glaucoma, gallbladder disease,** severely **low blood pressure,** or **alcoholism**.

When you are taking niacin in therapeutic dosages, your doctor should periodically check your liver function and blood-sugar level. People with **diabetes** may experience an increase in blood sugar. Blood levels of uric acid may rise; people who are prone to **gout** may experience an attack.

Niacin may cause postural low blood pressure (symptoms include dizziness or fainting when rising from a sitting or lying position).

Possible Side Effects

Most side effects are experienced by people taking niacin in higher doses. Taking a sustained-release form of niacin may reduce the risk of side effects.

▼ Most common: flushing, which may occur within 2 hours of taking the first dose of niacin. Flushing may be accompanied by dizziness, rapid heartbeat, heart palpitations, shortness of breath, sweating, chills, and/or swelling, and, rarely, fainting.

▼ Common: headache, itching, skin rash, and gastrointestinal problems.

▼ Less common: decreased sugar tolerance in people with diabetes, nausea, vomiting, abdominal pain, diarrhea, upset stomach, yellowing of the skin or whites of the eyes, oily or dry skin, aggravation of skin conditions such as acne, itching, high blood levels of uric acid, low blood pressure, runny nose, tingling in the hands or feet, rash, abnormal heartbeats, and dizziness.

▼ Rare: Rare side effects can occur in almost any part of the body. Contact your doctor if you experience any side effect not listed above.

Drug Interactions

- Niacin may increase the effect of blood-pressure-lowering drugs, causing dizziness when rising quickly from a sitting or lying position.
- Niacin may interfere with sulfinpyrazone (a gout medication).
- Combining niacin and a statin-type drug such as lovastatin may lead to the destruction of skeletal muscle.
- Aspirin may slow the removal of niacin from the body, but the importance of this interaction is not known.
- Separate any niacin product from cholestyramine or colestipol by at least 4–6 hours to avoid most of the niacin from being tied up by the other medication.
- Niacin extended-release tablets should be taken with caution with anticoagulants (blood thinners). Blood-platelet counts should be monitored closely.

Food Interactions

Take niacin with or after meals to reduce the risk of upset stomach. Sustained-release niacin products should be taken at bedtime with a low-fat snack. Avoid drinking grapefruit juice while taking niacin.

Usual Dose

Vitamin Supplement
Adult and Child (age 16 and over)
Men: 15–20 mg a day.
Women: 13–15 mg a day.

Child (under age 16): not recommended.

Pellegra
Adult and Child (age 16 and over): up to 500 mg a day.
Child (under age 16): not recommended.

High Blood-Fat Levels
Immediate-Release
Adult and Child (age 16 and over): 250 mg after the evening meal to start; increase dosage slowly, to 1500–3000 mg a day. Do not take more than 6000 mg a day.
Child (under age 16): not recommended.

Sustained-Release
Adult (age 21 and over): 500 mg at bedtime for 1–4 weeks, then 1000 mg for weeks 5–8. Can increase dose slowly if

needed (no more than 500 mg increase in a 4-week period). Do not exceed 2000 mg a day.

Child (under age 21): not recommended.

Overdosage

Symptoms may include drug side effects. Take the victim to a hospital emergency room. ALWAYS bring the prescription bottle or container.

Special Information

Skin reactions may occur within 2 hours of the first dose and include flushing and warmth, especially in the face, ears, or neck; tingling; itching; and headache. Call your doctor if these effects do not disappear as you continue taking niacin.

You can minimize flushing by taking aspirin or a nonsteroidal anti-inflammatory drug (NSAID) such as ibuprofen 30 minutes before your sustained-release niacin tablets. Avoid alcohol or hot drinks around the time you take sustained-release niacin to minimize flushing. Sustained-release niacin tablets should be swallowed whole, not broken, crushed, or chewed.

Stop taking this drug and call your doctor immediately if you experience irregular heartbeat, blurred vision, loss of appetite, flu-like symptoms, nausea, vomiting, dark-colored urine, or reduced urination.

Call your doctor if you have diabetes and notice your blood sugars changing.

If you forget a dose, take it as soon as you remember. If it is almost time for your next dose, skip the missed dose and continue with your regular schedule. Do not take a double dose.

Special Populations

Pregnancy/Breast-feeding

When used in normal dosages, niacin may and should be taken during pregnancy as part of a prenatal vitamin formulation. Dosages larger than 20 mg a day are not recommended during pregnancy because their effect on the fetus is unknown.

Niacin passes into human breast milk. Usual doses (up to 20 mg a day) will not affect a nursing infant. Larger doses used for lowering blood fats may affect a nursing infant and should be avoided if you are nursing.

Seniors: Seniors may be more sensitive to drug side effects than younger adults.

Niaspan *see Niacin, page 787*

see Niacin, page 787

Generic Name

Nicardipine (nye-KAR-dih-pene) Ⓖ

Brand Names

Cardene   Cardene SR

Type of Drug

Calcium channel blocker.

Prescribed For

Angina pectoris, high blood pressure, and congestive heart failure.

General Information

Nicardipine hydrochloride is one of many calcium channel blockers available in the U.S. These drugs block the passage of calcium, an essential factor in muscle contraction, into the heart and smooth muscles. Such blockage of calcium interferes with the contraction of these muscles, which in turn dilates (widens) the veins and vessels that supply blood to them. This dilating effect reduces blood pressure, the amount of oxygen used by the heart muscle, and the risk of blood vessel spasm. Nicardipine is therefore useful in treating not only high blood pressure but also angina pectoris (brief attacks of chest pain), a condition related to poor oxygen supply to the heart muscle.

Nicardipine affects the movement of calcium only into muscle cells; it has no effect on calcium in the blood.

Cautions and Warnings

Do not take nicardipine if you are **allergic** or **sensitive** to any of its ingredients.

Nicardipine can slow your heart rate and interfere with normal electrical conduction in heart muscle. For some people, this action can result in temporary heart stoppage, but such a reaction will not occur in people whose hearts are otherwise healthy.

You should not use nicardipine if you have had a **stroke** or **bleeding in the brain** or if you have advanced **hardening of the arteries**—particularly the aorta—because the drug can cause heart failure.

People who take nicardipine for congestive **heart failure** should be aware that the drug may aggravate the condition.

If you are also taking a **beta blocker,** its dosage should be reduced gradually rather than stopped abruptly when starting on nicardipine. Nicardipine may increase the risk of developing low blood pressure, especially if you are also taking beta blockers.

Nicardipine dosage should be adjusted in the presence of **kidney or liver disease**.

Nicardipine may cause angina when treatment is first started, when dosage is increased, or if the drug is rapidly withdrawn. This can be avoided by reducing dosage gradually.

Studies of calcium channel blockers—usually those taken several times a day, not those taken only once daily—have shown that people taking them are more likely to have a heart attack than are people taking beta blockers or other medication for the same purposes. Discuss this with your doctor to be sure you are receiving the best possible treatment.

Calcium channel blockers may interfere with blood clot formation, especially if taken with aspirin. Call your doctor if you develop unusual bruises or bleeding.

Possible Side Effects

▼ Most common: dizziness or lightheadedness; fluid accumulation in the hands, legs, or feet; headache; weakness or fatigue; heart palpitations; angina; and facial flushing.

▼ Less common: low blood pressure; abnormal heart rhythms; fainting; increase or decrease in heart rate; heart failure; nausea; rash; nervousness; tingling in the hands or feet; hallucinations; temporary memory loss; difficulty sleeping; weakness; diarrhea; vomiting; constipation; upset stomach; itching; unusual sensitivity to the sun; painful or stiff joints; liver inflammation; increased urination, especially at night; infection; allergic reactions; sore throat; and hyperactivity.

Drug Interactions

• Combining nicardipine with a beta-blocking drug in order to treat high blood pressure is usually well tolerated but may lead to heart failure in susceptible people.

- Blood levels of cyclosporine may be increased by nicardipine, increasing the chance for cyclosporine-related kidney damage.
- The effect of quinidine (an antiarrhythmic) may be altered by nicardipine.
- Cimetidine and ranitidine may increase the amount of nicardipine in the bloodstream.
- Combining nicardipine with fentanyl or other anesthetics may cause very low blood pressure.
- Rifampin may decrease nicardipine's effectiveness.
- Calcium channel blockers may cause bleeding when taken alone or combined with aspirin.

Food Interactions

Nicardipine is best taken on an empty stomach at least 1 hour before or 2 hours after meals, but it may be taken with food or milk if it upsets your stomach. Avoid high-fat meals and grapefruit juice while on this drug.

Usual Dose

Immediate-Release: 20–40 mg 3 times a day. People with kidney disease should take 20 mg 3 times a day. People with liver disease should take 20 mg twice a day. Seniors should start with 20 mg 2–3 times a day and increase dosage gradually.

Sustained-Release: 30–60 mg twice a day. People with kidney disease should take 30 mg twice a day.

Overdosage

Symptoms of nicardipine overdose are very low blood pressure and reduced heart rate. Nicardipine can be removed from the victim's stomach by inducing vomiting with ipecac syrup—available at any pharmacy. This must be done within 30 minutes of the actual overdose, before the drug can be absorbed into the blood. Once symptoms develop or if more than 30 minutes have passed since the overdose, the victim must be taken to an emergency room. ALWAYS bring the prescription bottle or container.

Special Information

Call your doctor if you develop any of the following symptoms: worsening angina pain; swelling of the hands, legs, or feet; severe dizziness; fainting; rash; constipation or nausea; or very low blood pressure.

Some people may experience a slight increase in blood pressure just before their next dose is due. You will be able to see this effect only if you use a home blood-pressure-monitoring device. If this happens, contact your doctor.

Use alcohol with caution while taking nicardipine. Alcohol may further lower blood pressure and could increase drowsiness or dizziness.

If you take nicardipine 3 times a day and forget a dose, take it as soon as you remember. If it is almost time for your next dose, take it and space the remaining doses evenly throughout the rest of the day. If you take nicardipine 2 times a day and forget a dose, take it as soon as you remember. If it is almost time for your next dose, skip the dose you forgot and continue with your regular schedule. Never take a double dose.

Do not crush, chew, or break the sustained-release capsules.

Special Populations

Pregnancy/Breast-feeding: In animal studies, large doses of nicardipine have been shown to harm the fetus. Nicardipine should be avoided by women who are or might be pregnant. When your doctor considers this drug crucial, its potential benefits must be carefully weighed against its risks.

Nicardipine passes into breast milk; nursing mothers who must take this drug should use infant formula.

Seniors: Seniors may be more sensitive to the side effects of nicardipine and require reduced dosage.

Generic Name

Nicotine (NIK-uh-teen) Ⓖ

Brand Names

Commit	Nicorette DS
Habitrol	Nicotrol
Nicoderm	Nicotrol Inhaler
Nicoderm CQ	Nicotrol NS
Nicorelief	ProStep
Nicorette	Thrive

Type of Drug

Smoking deterrent.

Prescribed For

Addiction to cigarettes. Nicotine gum has also been prescribed with haloperidol for children with Tourette's syndrome.

General Information

Nicotine replacement products are prescribed for short-term treatment and make cigarette withdrawal easier for many people. Because nicotine addiction also has a psychological component, counseling or other psychological support is necessary in order for a smoking cessation program to be successful. Patches, inhalers, chewing gum, lozenges, and nasal sprays are available.

Cautions and Warnings

Do not use nicotine if you are **allergic** or **sensitive** to any of its ingredients.

Nicotine should be used only by people addicted to nicotine. It should not be used during the period immediately following a **heart attack** or if you have severe **abnormal heart rhythms** or **angina pain**.

People with **heart conditions** must be evaluated by a cardiologist before starting treatment.

People with severe **temporomandibular joint (TMJ) disease** should not chew nicotine gum.

Nicotine should be used with caution by people with **diabetes** who take insulin and by people with an **overactive thyroid, kidney or liver disease, pheochromocytoma** (adrenal gland tumor), **hypertension** (high blood pressure), stomach **ulcer,** or chronic **dental problems** that might be worsened by nicotine chewing gum.

The nasal spray should not be used by people with **asthma, bronchospasm, allergic rhinitis, sinusitis,** or **nasal polyps**.

The inhaler should not be used by people with **asthma** or **chronic pulmonary disease.** It should be used with caution in people with **lung problems** or **bronchospasm.**

It is possible to become addicted to nicotine replacement products. Your nicotine addiction may worsen while using this product.

Possible Side Effects

Chewing Gum and Lozenges

▼ Most common: injury to the gums, jaw, or teeth; sore mouth or throat; and stomach growling due to swallowing air while chewing.

Possible Side Effects (continued)

▼ Common: nausea, vomiting, upset stomach, and hiccups.
▼ Less common: excessive salivation, dizziness, lightheadedness, irritability, headache, more frequent bowel movements, diarrhea, constipation, gas pain, dry mouth, hoarseness, flushing, sneezing, coughing, sleeplessness, swelling of the arms or legs, high blood pressure, heart palpitations, rapid and abnormal heartbeat, confusion, convulsions, depression, euphoria (feeling "high"), numbness, tingling in the hands or feet, ringing or buzzing in the ears, fainting, weakness, redness, itching, and rash.

Transdermal Patch

▼ Most common: feeling tired and irritation at the patch site. Transdermal systems may be more irritating to people with eczema or other skin conditions.
▼ Common: weakness, back pain, body ache, diarrhea, upset stomach, headache, sleeplessness, dizziness, nervousness, unusual dreams, increased cough or sore throat, muscle and joint pain, changes in sense of taste, and painful menstruation.
▼ Less common: chest pain, allergic reaction (symptoms include hives, breathing difficulties, and peeling skin), dry mouth, abdominal pain, vomiting, poor concentration, tingling in the hands or feet, sinus irritation or inflammation, increased sweating, and high blood pressure.

Nasal Spray

▼ Most common: headache, chest tightness, tingling in the hands or feet, constipation, inflammation of the mucous membranes of the mouth, and irritation of the nose, throat, or eye.
▼ Common: back pain, difficulty breathing, nausea, and joint pain.
▼ Less common: menstrual disorder, heart palpitations, gas, tooth and gum problems, muscle aches, abdominal pains, confusion, acne, and itching.

Inhaler

▼ Most common: irritation of the mouth or throat, cough, runny nose, upset stomach, and headache.

Possible Side Effects *(continued)*

▼ Common: changes in taste, flu-like symptoms, nausea, and diarrhea.

▼ Less common: pain in the neck or jaw, dental problems, sinus inflammation, back pain, numbness or tingling, gas, and fever.

Drug Interactions

● Nicotine—and cigarette smoking—reduces the effects of alcohol, benzodiazepine sedatives, sleeping pills, beta blockers, caffeine, clozapine, fluvoxamine, olanzapine, tacrine, theophylline, clorazepate, oral lidocaine, estradiol, imipramine, flecainide, heparin, insulin, mexiletine, opioids, propanolol, and pentazocine.

Food Interactions

Do not eat or drink anything while or immediately after you chew nicotine gum. Caffeine, juice, wine, and soft drinks may interfere with its effects.

Usual Dose

Chewing Gum: 1 piece of gum whenever you feel the urge for a cigarette; do not use more than 24 pieces a day. Gradually reduce the number of pieces you chew and the time you chew each piece every 4–7 days. Substituting sugarless gum for nicotine gum may help in the process of gradual dosage reduction. Each piece contains 2–4 mg of nicotine.

Lozenge: 1 lozenge every 1–2 hours for the first 6 weeks, gradually reduced over 12 weeks to 1 lozenge every 4–8 hours. Do not use more than 20 lozenges a day. Each lozenge contains 2 or 4 mg of nicotine.

Transdermal Patch: Apply the patch to the skin as soon as you remove it from the package. Nicotrol patches should be applied when you get up in the morning and removed at bedtime. Prescription nicotine patches should be left on for 16–24 hours, depending on the brand. The dosage of the patch will be gradually reduced by your doctor. Use a different skin site when applying a new patch.

Nasal Spray: 1–2 sprays in each nostril up to 5 times an hour. The spray should be used at least 8 times a day to ease symptoms of nicotine withdrawal. Do not use more than 40 doses a day.

Inhaler: Use as needed, generally 3–6 cartridges a day for the first 3–6 weeks; some people use up to 16 cartridges a day. Dosage should be gradually reduced after 12 weeks until you are able to stop.

Overdosage

Nicotine overdose may be deadly. Symptoms include excessive salivation, nausea, vomiting, diarrhea, abdominal pain, headache, cold sweats, dizziness, hearing and visual disturbances, weakness, and confusion. These symptoms may be followed by fainting; very low blood pressure; a pulse that is weak, rapid, and irregular; convulsions; and death by paralysis of the muscles that control breathing.

Nicotine stimulates the brain's vomiting center, making this reaction common but not automatic; spontaneous vomiting may be sufficient to remove the poison from the victim's system. In case of overdose, call your local poison control center or a hospital emergency room. If the victim has not already vomited, you may be told to induce vomiting with ipecac syrup—available at any pharmacy—before taking the victim to an emergency room. If you seek treatment, ALWAYS bring the nicotine package.

Special Information

When using the gum, follow the product instructions. Chew each piece slowly and intermittently for about 30 minutes. Rapid chewing releases the nicotine too quickly and may lead to side effects including nausea, hiccups, and throat irritation. Do not chew more than 24 pieces a day. The amount of gum chewed should be gradually reduced and stopped after 3 months of successful treatment.

When using lozenges, place the lozenge in your mouth and let it dissolve, moving it back and forth from time to time. Each lozenge will last 20–30 minutes. Since lozenges come in the form of hard candy, be sure to keep them away from children.

When administering the nasal spray, tilt your head back slightly and do not sniff or inhale through your nose. A dose consists of 1 spray in each nostril. Administering fewer than 8 doses a day may not be effective. Do not exceed 40 doses a day. The spray should not be used for longer than 6 months.

Do not store nicotine patches in an area that is warmer than 86°F. Slight discoloration is not a sign of loss of potency, but do not store a patch after you have removed it from its pouch. Nicotine patches should not be used for more than 3 consecutive months.

Stop smoking completely when using the nicotine inhaler. When using the inhaler, inhale deeply into the back of your throat or puff in short breaths. Use often and longer at first to control cravings. Nicotine in cartridges is used up after about 20 minutes of active puffing. Do not use more than 16 cartridges a day.

Keep nicotine patches, inhalers, and nasal spray containers—used or unused—out of the reach of children and pets to avoid accidental poisoning.

Consult with your doctor if you continue to smoke while using nicotine products, as you may experience potentially dangerous adverse effects. You dosage may need to be adjusted.

Special Populations

Pregnancy/Breast-feeding: Nicotine is not safe for use during pregnancy. It is known to cause fetal harm when used during the last 3 months of pregnancy and is associated with breathing difficulties in newborns and miscarriage.

Nicotine passes into breast milk. Nursing mothers who use it should use infant formula.

Seniors: Seniors may be more sensitive to side effects, including weakness, dizziness, and body aches.

Generic Name

Nifedipine (nih-FED-ih-pene) Ⓖ

Brand Names

Adalat CC	Procardia
Afeditab CR	Procardia XL
Nifedical XL	

The information in this profile also applies to the following drugs:

Generic Ingredient: Isradipine Ⓖ
DynaCirc CR

Generic Ingredient: Nisoldipine

Sular	Sular CD

Type of Drug

Calcium channel blocker.

Prescribed For

Angina pectoris, Prinzmetal's angina, and high blood pressure; also prescribed for migraine headache prevention, asthma, heart failure, Raynaud's disease, disorders of the esophagus, gallbladder and kidney stone attacks, severe high blood pressure triggered by pregnancy, and premature labor.

General Information

Nifedipine is one of many calcium channel blockers available in the U.S. These drugs block the passage of calcium, an essential factor in muscle contractions, into the heart and smooth muscles. Such blockage of calcium interferes with the contraction of these muscles, which in turn dilates (widens) the veins and vessels that supply blood to them. This dilating effect reduces blood pressure, the amount of oxygen used by the heart muscle, and the risk of blood vessel spasm. Nifedipine is therefore useful in treating not only high blood pressure but also angina pectoris (brief attacks of chest pain), a condition related to poor oxygen supply to the heart muscle.

Nifedipine affects the movement of calcium only into muscle cells; it has no effect on calcium in the blood.

Nifedipine capsules contain liquid medication. In cases in which the drug is needed in the blood immediately, the capsules may be punctured and their content squeezed under the tongue; the medication is rapidly absorbed into the blood when taken in this manner. Thus nifedipine capsules are particularly useful when extremely high blood pressure must be lowered as quickly as possible. Some researchers assert that biting the capsule and swallowing the contents is an even faster way of absorbing the drug.

Cautions and Warnings

Do not take nifedipine if you are **allergic** or **sensitive** to any of its ingredients.

These drugs may cause unwanted low blood pressure in some people who take it for reasons other than hypertension.

Patients taking a beta-blocking drug who begin taking these drugs may develop an increase in episodes of **angina** pain. Angina may also intensify when these drugs are first started, when they are increased, or if they are stopped abruptly.

Calcium channel blockers may cause low blood pressure, particularly if taken with beta blockers.

Studies have shown that people taking calcium channel blockers—usually those taken several times a day, not those that are taken only once daily—have a greater chance of having a heart attack than people taking beta blockers or other medications for the same purposes. Discuss this with your doctor to be sure you are receiving the best possible treatment.

Congestive heart failure has, on rare occasions, developed in people taking nifedipine.

Nifedipine may interfere with one of the mechanisms by which blood clots form, especially if you are also taking aspirin. Call your doctor if you develop unusual bruises, bleeding, or black-and-blue marks.

People with **kidney disease** or **severe liver disease** may require dosage adjustments.

Possible Side Effects

Nifedipine

Nifedipine side effects are generally mild and rarely cause people to stop taking the drug.

▼ Most common: swelling of the ankles, feet, and legs; dizziness or lightheadedness; flushing; a feeling of warmth; and headache.

▼ Less common: nausea; weakness, shakiness, or jitteriness; giddiness; muscle cramps, inflammation, and pain; nervousness; mood changes; heart palpitations; heart failure; heart attack; breathing difficulties; coughing; fluid in the lungs; wheezing; stuffy nose; fever and chills; and sore throat.

▼ Rare: Rare side effects can occur in your heart, stomach or intestines, urinary tract, and joints and muscles and can affect your mental and sexual function, hearing, and balance. Contact your doctor if you experience any side effect not listed above.

Isradipine

Isradipine side effects are generally mild and self-limiting.

▼ Most common: headache.

▼ Less common: low blood pressure, chest pain, abdominal pain, rapid heartbeat, dizziness, diarrhea, a feeling of warmth, nausea, lightheadedness, fatigue and lethargy, itching, rash, flushing, changes in certain blood-cell components, and swelling of the legs, ankles, or feet.

Possible Side Effects *(continued)*

Nisoldipine

▼ Most common: headache and swelling in the arms or legs.

▼ Common: sore throat, sinus irritation, heart palpitations, and dizziness.

▼ Less common: chest pain, nausea, and rash.

Drug Interactions

- These drugs may interact with beta-blocking drugs to cause heart failure, very low blood pressure, or an increased incidence of angina pain. However, in many cases these drugs have been taken together with no problem. Regular monitoring is necessary.
- Mixing nifedipine with another calcium channel blocker can increase the amount of nifedipine in the blood. Dosage reduction may be needed.
- Taking doxazosin (for high blood pressure) with nifedipine may reduce blood pressure. Regular blood pressure monitoring is necessary with this combination.
- Nifedipine may cause unexpected blood pressure reduction in patients who also take other drugs to control their high blood pressure. Low blood pressure can also result from taking nifedipine with fentanyl and other anesthetics.
- Cimetidine, erythromycin, amprenavir, atanazavir, delavirdine, fosamprenavir, indinavir, nelfinavir, nefazodone, ritonavir, and valproic acid can increase the amount of these drugs in the blood and may account for an increase in their effect. A reduction in the dose of nifedipine may be needed.
- St. John's wort, rifampin, nafcillin, phenytoin, phenobarbital, and carbamazepine increase the rate at which nifedipine is broken down in the body. An increase in the dose of nifedipine may be required.
- The combination of quinidine (an antiarrhythmic) and nifedipine must be used with caution because it can produce low blood pressure, very slow heart rate, abnormal heart rhythm, and swelling in the arms or legs. Flecainide, another drug for abnormal heart rhythms, may also interact with nifedipine.
- On rare occasions, nifedipine may increase the effects of warfarin and similar oral anticoagulant (blood-thinning) drugs.

There is no interaction with drugs that affect platelets such as clopidogrel.

- Calcium channel blockers may cause bleeding when taken alone or combined with aspirin.
- Ketoconazole, itraconazole, and fluconazole can slow the breakdown of nifedipine, further reducing blood pressure. Blood pressure should be monitored if you are taking this combination. A reduction in the dose of nifedipine may be needed.
- Nifedipine may intensify the effects of cyclosporine, digoxin, and theophylline products, increasing the chances of side effects from those drugs. Regular drug monitoring may be required.
- Nifedipine slows the breakdown of tacrolimus (immune system suppressant). Dosage reduction of tacrolimus may be needed. Sirolimus is not affected by this interaction.
- Nifedipine tends to raise blood sugar. Diabetics taking this medicine should check their blood sugar regularly. Some dosage adjustments of diabetes medication may be needed.
- Drugs that may increase blood levels of isradipine include itraconazole, and cimetidine; dosage adjustments may be necessary.
- Rifampin may decrease the effects of isradipine, which may also require dosage adjustment.
- Isradipine may lower blood levels of lovastatin, requiring dosage adjustment.
- When nisoldipine is combined with cimetidine, blood levels of nisoldipine increase substantially.
- Quinidine reduces the amount of nisoldipine in the blood, but maximum levels remain unaffected.

Food Interactions

Avoid drinking grapefruit juice if you are taking these drugs and be sure to stop drinking or eating grapefruit at least 3 days before you start taking nifedipine. Avoid fatty foods when taking nisoldipine.

Usual Dose

Nifedipine

Immediate-Release: 10–30 mg 3 times a day. Do not take more than 180 mg a day.

Sustained-Release: 30–60 mg once a day.

Do not stop taking nifedipine abruptly. The dosage should be reduced gradually.

Isradipine: 5–20 mg a day in 2 doses. Do not stop taking the drug abruptly. The dosage should be reduced gradually over a period of time.

Nisoldipine
Sular
Adult: starting dosage—20 mg a day. Maintenance dosage—20–40 mg, as needed, up to a maximum of 60 mg.

Seniors and People with Liver Disease: starting dosage—10 mg a day. Maintenance dosage—20–40 mg, as needed and tolerated, up to a maximum of 60 mg.

Child: not recommended.

Sular CR
Adult: starting dosage—17 mg a day. Maintenance dosage—17–34 mg, as needed, up to a maximum of 51 mg.

Seniors and People with Liver Disease: starting dosage—8.5 mg a day. Maintenance dosage—17–34 mg, as needed and tolerated, up to a maximum of 51 mg.

Child: not recommended.

Overdosage
Overdose of these drugs can cause low blood pressure, nausea, weakness, dizziness, drowsiness, confusion, and slurred speech. If you think you have taken an overdose of nifedipine, call your doctor or go to a hospital emergency room. ALWAYS bring the prescription bottle or container.

Special Information
Call your doctor if you develop constipation, nausea, very low blood pressure, swelling in the arms or legs, worsening angina, swelling in the hands or feet, breathing difficulties, increased heart pain, or dizziness or lightheadedness, or if other side effects are particularly bothersome or persistent.

If you are taking nifedipine for high blood pressure, be sure to continue taking your medication and follow any instructions for diet restriction or other treatments.

If you take Procardia XL, be sure not to break or crush the tablets. You may notice an empty tablet in your stool. This is not a cause for alarm, because the drug is normally released without actually destroying the tablet.

It is important to maintain good dental hygiene while taking nifedipine and to use extra care when using your toothbrush or dental floss: The drug may make you more susceptible to some infections.

If you forget a dose of nifedipine and you take it 3 or more times a day, take it as soon as you remember. If it is almost time for your next dose, take the dose you forgot and space the rest evenly throughout the remainder of the day. If you take nifedipine twice a day and forget a dose, take it as soon as you remember. If it is almost time for your next dose, skip the dose you forgot and continue with your regular schedule. Never take a double dose.

Special Populations

Pregnancy/Breast-feeding: Nifedipine crosses into the fetal blood circulation. It has been used to treat severe high blood pressure associated with pregnancy without causing any unusual effect on the fetus. Nevertheless, women who are or might be pregnant should not take nifedipine without their doctor's approval. When this drug is considered crucial by your doctor, its potential benefits must be carefully weighed against its risks.

Small amounts of nifedipine may pass into breast milk. Nursing mothers who must take this drug should use infant formula.

Seniors: Seniors are more sensitive to the effects of nifedipine and may require dosage adjustments.

Generic Name

Nimodipine (nih-MOE-dih-pene) Ⓖ

Brand Name

Nimotop

Type of Drug

Calcium channel blocker.

Prescribed For

Functional losses following a hemorrhagic stroke; also used for the prevention of migraine and cluster headaches.

General Information

Unlike other calcium channel blockers, nimodipine has a negligible effect on the heart. It is the only calcium channel blocker proven to improve neurological function after a stroke. Nimodipine has a greater effect on blood vessels in the brain than on those in other parts of the body.

Cautions and Warnings

Do not take nimodipine if you are **allergic** or **sensitive** to any of its ingredients or to other calcium channel blockers.

People with **liver disease,** including cirrhosis, may require reduced dosage.

Nimodipine should not be administered intravenously. Serious adverse reactions, including death, have been reported due to parenteral infection of this drug.

Possible Side Effects

▼ Most common: diarrhea, low blood pressure, rash, and headache.

▼ Less common: swelling of the arms or legs, high blood pressure, heart failure, rapid heartbeat, changes in the electrocardiogram, depression, memory loss, psychosis, paranoid feelings, hallucinations, nausea, itching, acne, anemia, bleeding or bruising, abnormal blood clotting, flushing, breathing difficulties, stomach bleeding, and muscle cramps.

▼ Rare: dizziness, heart attack, liver inflammation or jaundice, vomiting, intestinal blockage, and sexual difficulties. Contact your doctor if you experience any side effect not listed above.

Drug Interactions

- Calcium channel blockers may cause bleeding when taken alone or combined with aspirin.
- Combining nimodipine with a beta-blocking drug is usually tolerated well but may lead to heart failure in susceptible people.
- Calcium channel blockers, including nimodipine, may add to the effects of digoxin.
- Cimetidine may increase blood levels of nimodipine.

Food Interactions

Nimodipine is best taken at least 1 hour before or 2 hours after meals, but may be taken with food or milk if it upsets your stomach. Avoid drinking grapefruit juice if you are taking this drug.

Usual Dose

Stroke: 60 mg 4 times a day, beginning within 96 hours after the stroke and continuing for 21 days.

Migraine Headache: 40 mg 3 times a day.

Overdosage

Symptoms of nimodipine overdose are nausea, weakness, dizziness, drowsiness, confusion, and slurred speech. Blood pressure and heart rate may also be affected. Nimodipine can be removed from a victim's stomach by giving ipecac syrup—available at any pharmacy—to induce vomiting, but this should be done only under a doctor's supervision or direction. Once symptoms develop, the victim must be taken to a hospital emergency room for treatment. ALWAYS bring the prescription bottle or container.

Special Information

Call your doctor if you develop any of the following symptoms: swelling of the arms or legs, breathing difficulties, severe dizziness, constipation, or nausea.

Patients who are unable to swallow nimodipine capsules because of their condition may have the liquid withdrawn from the capsule with a syringe, mixed with other liquids, and given orally or through a feeding tube. Do not administer this drug intravenously.

If you forget a dose of nimodipine, take it as soon as you remember. If it is almost time for your next dose, skip the dose you forgot and continue with your regular schedule. Call your doctor if you miss more than 2 consecutive doses.

Special Populations

Pregnancy/Breast-feeding: Animal studies have shown that nimodipine may cause fetal malformation. Nimodipine should be avoided by women who are or might be pregnant. When your doctor considers this drug crucial, its potential benefits must be carefully weighed against its risks.

Nimodipine passes into breast milk. Nursing mothers who must take nimodipine should use infant formula.

Seniors: Seniors, especially those with severe liver disease, may be more sensitive to side effects.

Generic Name

Nitazoxanide (neye-tan-OX-ah-nyde)

Brand Name

Alinia

Type of Drug

Antiprotozoal.

Prescribed for

Diarrhea caused by the parasites *Giardia lamblia* and *Cryptosporidium parvum*.

General Information

Specific enzyme reactions that occur in the body are used by the *Giardia lamblia* and *Cryptosporidium parvum* microorganisms for energy production, allowing them to thrive inside the body. Nitazoxanide works by blocking these specific enzyme reactions, preventing them from thriving inside humans. It is broken down in the liver.

Cautions and Warnings

Do not take nitazoxanide if you are **allergic** or **sensitive** to any of its ingredients.

People with **liver or kidney disease** should take this drug with caution since it has not been studied in people with these conditions.

This drug may not be effective in people whose **immune system** is compromised.

The safety of nitazoxanide in people with **AIDS** and those who are **HIV positive** has not been established.

Possible Side Effects

Most side effects are mild and pass with time.

▼ Most common: abdominal pain.

▼ Less common: headache, diarrhea, nausea, and vomiting.

▼ Rare: Other side effects of nitazoxanide can affect almost any body system. Contact your doctor if you experience any side effect not listed above.

Drug Interactions

- Nitazoxanide is highly bound to proteins in the bloodstream and may interact with warfarin, digoxin, and other highly bound drugs; however, no specific interactions have been reported.

Food Interactions

Take this drug with food or meals for maximum effect.

Usual Dose

Adult and Child (over age 11): one 500-mg tablet or 5 tsp. every 12 hours with food.

Child (age 4–11): 2 tsp. every 12 hours for 3 days.

Child (age 1–4): 1 tsp. every 12 hours for 3 days.

Child (under 1 year): not recommended.

Overdosage

Single doses of nitazoxanide up to 4000 mg have been taken by adults without significant side effects. Overdose victims should be taken to a hospital emergency room for evaluation. ALWAYS bring the prescription bottle or container.

Special Information

This product contains 1.48 g of sugar in each teaspoonful of the suspension. This information may be of importance for people with diabetes and others who must manage their sugar intake.

Special Populations

Pregnancy/Breast-feeding: Animal studies using doses about 48 times the usual dose have revealed no adverse reproductive effects. The safety of nitazoxanide during pregnancy is not known. While animal studies reveal no damage to the fetus, this drug should only be used during pregnancy after carefully weighing its potential benefits against its risks.

It is not known if nitazoxanide passes into breast milk. Nursing mothers who must take it should use infant formula.

Seniors: This drug has been studied in too few seniors to draw definite conclusions about its safety. However, seniors with reduced kidney, liver, or heart function; other diseases; and those taking other medications may respond differently to this medication.

Generic Name

Nitrofurantoin (NYE-troe-few-RAN-toe-in) Ⓖ

Brand Names

Furadantin   Macrodantin
Macrobid

Type of Drug

Urinary anti-infective.

Prescribed For

Treatment or prevention of acute, uncomplicated urinary tract infections (UTIs), also known as acute cystitis.

General Information

Nitrofurantoin is helpful in treating UTIs because large amounts of it pass into the urine. It works by interfering with the metabolism of carbohydrates, or sugars, in the infecting bacteria. It may also interfere with the formation of the bacterial cell wall.

Cautions and Warnings

Do not take nitrofurantoin if you are **allergic** or **sensitive** to any of its ingredients or if you have **kidney disease**.

Rarely, severe chest pain, breathing difficulties, cough, fever, and chills may develop within a few hours to 3 weeks after taking nitrofurantoin. These symptoms usually go away within 1–2 days after you stop taking it. Nitrofurantoin therapy may cause cough, breathing difficulties, and feelings of ill health after 1–6 months. Respiratory failure and death have occurred in a few cases. Chronic respiratory reactions generally occur in patients receiving continuous treatment for 6 months or longer. These chronic reactions due to longer-term therapy may remain even after treatment has stopped.

Diarrhea caused by antibiotics is a common problem that is usually mild and ends when the antibiotic is discontinued, but it can be serious or even fatal. People can develop watery and bloody stools without stomach cramps and fever as long as 2 months or more after taking the last antibiotic dose. If this happens, contact your doctor right away.

Rarely, nitrofurantoin causes hemolytic anemia. People with a **deficiency of the enzyme G-6-PD** are most susceptible to this reaction and should not take nitrofurantoin.

Rarely, nitrofurantoin causes hepatitis, which may lead to death. It is most likely to develop during long-term treatment.

This drug may cause serious or irreversible peripheral neuropathy (damage to the nerves in the arms and legs). People with **kidney disease, anemia, diabetes, electrolyte imbalance,** or **vitamin B deficiency** are at increased risk.

This drug is only used to treat UTIs caused by organisms susceptible to nitrofurantoin. It should not be used to treat **infections in other parts of the body.** Long-term or chronic use of nitrofurantoin may lead to secondary infection caused by drug-resistant bacteria or fungi.

This drug may cause a false positive result in urine tests for glucose.

Possible Side Effects

Side effects are less prominent with Macrodantin than with Furadantin.

▼ Most common: loss of appetite, nausea, vomiting, stomach pain, gas, and diarrhea. Some people develop hepatitis-like symptoms.

▼ Less common: fever, chills, cough, chest pain, breathing difficulties, and development of fluid in the lungs. If these reactions occur in the first week of therapy, they can generally be resolved by stopping the medication. If they develop after taking nitrofurantoin for a longer period, they are considered chronic and may be more serious.

▼ Rare: rash, itching, asthmatic attacks in people with a history of asthma, drug fever, symptoms similar to arthritis, jaundice (yellowing of the skin or whites of the eyes), effects on components of the blood, headache, dizziness, drowsiness, and temporary hair loss. Contact your doctor if you experience any side effect not listed above.

This drug is known to cause changes in white and red blood cells. It should be used only under the strict supervision of your doctor.

Drug Interactions

- Nitrofurantoin may increase other drugs' toxic effects on the liver and the risk of hemolytic anemia if you are taking another drug associated with that condition. These drugs include oral antidiabetes drugs, methyldopa, primaquine, procainamide, quinidine, quinine, and sulfa drugs.

- Nitrofurantoin may interfere with nalidixic acid, norfloxacin, and other fluoroquinolones. Do not combine these drugs.
- Sulfinpyrazone and probenecid may reduce this drug's effectiveness and increase side effects.
- Anticholinergic drugs, including propantheline, may increase the risk of nitrofurantoin side effects.
- Magnesium, found most commonly in antacids, delays the absorption of nitrofurantoin or reduces the amount absorbed.
- Combining nitrofurantoin and metronidazole, mexiletine, ethambutol, isoniazid, lindane, lincomycin, lithium, pemoline, quinacrine, or long-term high-dose pyridoxine (vitamin B_6), may increase the risk of nervous system effects. Do not combine nitrofurantoin and any of these drugs.

Food Interactions

Nitrofurantoin should be taken with food to minimize upset stomach, loss of appetite, nausea, or other gastrointestinal symptoms. For optimal effectiveness, avoid citrus fruits while taking nitrofurantoin.

Usual Dose

Adult: 50–100 mg 4 times a day, with meals and at bedtime.

Child (over age 1 month): 2–3 mg per lb. of body weight in 4 doses.

Child (under age 1 month): not recommended.

People with chronic urinary infections may require lower-dosage, longer-term therapy for up to 6 months. Therapy for longer than 6 months should only be continued when the benefits outweigh the risks.

Overdosage

Induce vomiting with ipecac syrup—available at any pharmacy— and take the victim to a hospital emergency room for treatment. If you seek treatment, ALWAYS bring the prescription bottle or container.

Special Information

Call your doctor if you develop chest pain or breathing difficulties; cough; sore throat; pale skin; unusual tiredness or weakness; dizziness; drowsiness; headache; rash and itching; yellow skin; achy joints; fever and chills; numbness, tingling, or burning of the fingers or toes; severe diarrhea; abdominal pain; bloody stool; or any persistent or bothersome side effect.

Continue taking this drug until your prescription is finished even if you stop experiencing symptoms of a UTI.

Nitrofurantoin may give your urine a brownish color. This is not a cause for concern.

The liquid form can stain your teeth if you do not swallow it rapidly.

If you miss a dose, take it as soon as possible. If it is almost time for your next dose and you take it 3 or more times a day, space the missed dose and your next dose by 2–4 hours.

Special Populations

Pregnancy/Breast-feeding: Nitrofurantoin should never be taken by pregnant women with G-6-PD deficiency or those who are near term because it can interfere with the immature enzyme systems of the fetus and cause hemolytic anemia. When this drug is considered crucial by your doctor, its potential benefits must be carefully weighed against its risks.

This drug passes into breast milk. Nursing mothers who must take nitrofurantoin should use infant formula, especially if the baby is G-6-PD deficient.

Seniors: Seniors with kidney disease may be more sensitive to nervous-system and lung effects. Seniors may also require reduced dosage due to reduction of kidney function.

Generic Name

Nitroglycerin (nye-troe-GLIH-ser-in) Ⓖ

Brand Names

Minitran	Nitrolingual
Nitrek	Nitromist
Nitrocine	Nitrong
Nitro-Derm	NitroQuick
Nitrodisc	Nitrostat
Nitro-Dur	NitroTab
Nitrogard	Nitro-Time
Nitroglyn	

Type of Drug

Antianginal agent.

Prescribed For

Chest pain associated with angina pectoris; prevention and management of angina; nitroglycerin injection is also used as a treatment after a heart attack, for congestive heart failure (CHF), and for high blood pressure.

General Information

Nitroglycerin and other nitrates are used to treat pain associated with heart problems. While the exact nature of their action is not fully understood, they relax vascular smooth muscle. Nitroglycerin is available in several forms: sublingual tablets, which are taken under the tongue and allowed to dissolve; capsules, which are swallowed; transmucosal tablets, which are placed between the lip or cheek and gum and allowed to dissolve; oral sprays, which are sprayed directly onto or under the tongue; transdermal patches, which deliver nitroglycerin for absorption through the skin over a 24-hour period; and ointment, which is usually spread over the chest or another area of the body. One or more forms of nitroglycerin are often used to prevent or alleviate chest pain associated with angina.

Cautions and Warnings

Do not take nitroglycerin if you are **allergic** or **sensitive** to any of its ingredients or to another nitrate product, such as isosorbide. Do not use the patch form if you are allergic to adhesives.

Nitroglycerin should be taken with great caution if **head trauma** or **bleeding in the head** is present.

This drug may be inappropriate for you if you have had a recent **heart attack** or **stroke,** or have severe **anemia, glaucoma,** severe **liver or kidney disease, overactive thyroid, cardiomyopathy** (loss of blood-pumping ability due to damaged heart muscle), or **low blood pressure,** especially postural low blood pressure (symptoms include dizziness or fainting when rising from a sitting or lying position).

Possible Side Effects

▼ Most common: flushing and headache, which may be severe or persistent.

▼ Less common: lightheadedness, dizziness, and weakness. Blurred vision and dry mouth may occur; if they do, stop

---

Possible Side Effects *(continued)*

taking the drug and call your doctor. In some people, the blood-pressure-lowering effect of nitroglycerin causes severe responses, including nausea, vomiting, weakness, restlessness, pallor (loss of facial color), increased perspiration, and collapse. Rash may also occur.

Drug Interactions

- Avoid over-the-counter drugs containing stimulants, such as cough, cold, and allergy remedies and appetite suppressants; they may aggravate heart disease.
- Do not take sildenafil, vardenafil, or taldenafil if you are taking nitroglycerin or another nitrate product. The combination can result in a rapid and potentially fatal drop in blood pressure.
- Interaction with large amounts of alcohol may rapidly lower blood pressure, resulting in weakness, dizziness, and fainting.
- Aspirin and calcium channel blockers may increase nitrate blood levels and the risk of side effects.
- Nitroglycerin may interfere with heparin (an injectable anticoagulant drug).
- Nitrates increase dihydroergotamine blood levels, which may raise blood pressure or block the effects of nitroglycerin.
- Use nitroglycerin with caution with antihypertensives such as beta blockers, phenothiazines, or other nitrates.

Food Interactions

Do not use any oral form of nitroglycerin with food or gum in your mouth. Nitroglycerin pills intended for swallowing are best taken on an empty stomach.

Usual Dose

Use only as much as is necessary to control chest pain. Nitroglycerin is not recommended for pediatric use.

Sublingual Tablets: Since this form acts within 10–15 seconds, it should be taken only when necessary. Dissolve 1 tablet under the tongue, or between the cheek and gum at first sign of attack. Do not swallow sublingual tablets. Repeat about every 5 minutes until you get relief; take no more than 3 tablets in 15 minutes. You may also take sublingual tablets as a preventative measure 5–10 minutes before an activity which might precipitate an attack.

Transmucosal Tablets: The tablets are placed between the upper lip and gum or between the cheek and gum and allowed to dissolve over a 3- to 5-hour period. The tablet releases the drug faster when touched with the tongue or when you drink a hot liquid. Insert another tablet after the previous one is dissolved. Do not sleep with a tablet in your mouth.

Sustained-Release Capsules and Tablets: Starting dose: 2.5–6.5 mg 2–4 times a day. Increase gradually, if needed, to a maximum of 26 mg 4 times a day. Swallow capsules or tablets whole.

Ointment: 1–2″ squeezed from the tube onto a specially marked piece of paper—some people may require as much as 4–5″. The ointment is spread on the skin every 4–8 hours as needed to control chest pain. The medication is absorbed through the skin. The application sites should be rotated to prevent skin inflammation and rash.

Transdermal Patch: The patch is placed on a hairless site on the body that is not associated with excess movement. It is applied once a day and removed after 12–14 hours. Dosages start at 0.2–0.4 mg per hour and may increase to 0.8 mg. Higher dosages are preferable for once-daily patch applications.

Aerosol: 1–2 sprays (0.4–0.8 mg) under or on your tongue; repeat as needed to relieve an angina attack, but use no more than 3 doses in a 15-minute period.

Overdosage

Overdose can result in low blood pressure; very rapid heartbeat; flushing; increased perspiration followed by cold, bluish, and clammy skin; headache; heart palpitations; blurred vision and other visual disturbances; dizziness; nausea; vomiting; slow and difficult breathing; slow pulse; confusion; moderate fever; and paralysis. Take the victim to a hospital emergency room immediately. ALWAYS bring the prescription bottle or container.

Special Information

Do not change brands of nitroglycerin without your doctor's and pharmacist's knowledge—they may not be equivalent.

Sublingual nitroglycerin should be acquired from your pharmacist only in the original, unopened bottle; the tablets must not be transferred to another bottle or container because they may lose potency. Close the bottle tightly after each use or the drug may evaporate from the tablets. Sublingual nitroglycerin should be taken while you are sitting down. Sublingual tablets should not be chewed, crushed, or swallowed. This form of nitroglycerin frequently produces a burning sensation under the tongue, but this sensation does not necessarily indicate that the drug is working for you. If 1 tablet does not relieve your symptoms in 5 minutes, take another. If the second one does not work, take a third. If the pain continues or worsens, call your doctor or go to an emergency room at once.

When applying nitroglycerin ointment, do not rub or massage it into the skin. Any excess ointment should be washed from the hands after application.

People who use transdermal patches for more than 12 hours a day for an extended period can build up a tolerance to the patch and may have to use another form of nitroglycerin.

Nitroglycerin patches contain a significant amount of medication even after they have been used. They can be a hazard to children and small pets; be certain to dispose of them properly.

Orthostatic hypotension may become a problem if you take nitroglycerin over a long period of time. More blood stays in the extremities and less becomes available to the brain, resulting in lightheadedness or faintness if you stand up suddenly. Avoid prolonged standing and always stand up slowly.

If you take nitroglycerin on a regular schedule and forget a dose, take it as soon as you remember. If you use immediate-release tablets and it is within 2 hours of your next dose, skip the dose you forgot and continue with your regular schedule. If you take sustained-release tablets or capsules and it is within 6 hours of your next dose, skip the dose you forgot and continue with your regular schedule. Do not take a double dose.

Special Populations

Pregnancy/Breast-feeding: Nitroglycerin crosses into the fetal circulation. When this drug is considered crucial by your doctor, its potential benefits must be carefully weighed against its risks.

Nitroglycerin passes into breast milk. Nursing mothers who must take it should consider using infant formula.

Seniors: Seniors may take nitroglycerin without special restriction. Because saliva is necessary for the absorption of sublingual nitroglycerin, seniors with reduced saliva secretion may need to use another form of nitroglycerin or add a saliva substitute; this also applies to younger people with dry mouth.

Generic Name

Nizatidine (nih-ZAY-tih-dene) Ⓖ

Brand Names

Axid   Axid Pulvules
Axid AR

Type of Drug

Histamine H_2 antagonist.

Prescribed For

Treatment and maintenance of ulcers of the stomach and duodenum (upper intestine); also used to treat gastroesophageal reflux disease (GERD) and associated heartburn.

General Information

H_2 antagonists work by turning off the system that produces stomach acid and other secretions. Nizatidine is effective in treating the symptoms of ulcer and preventing complications of the disease, although an ulcer that does not respond to another histamine H_2 antagonist will probably not respond to nizatidine. Histamine H_2 antagonists differ only in their potency. Cimetidine is the least potent; 1000 mg are roughly equal to 300 mg of either nizatidine or ranitidine, or 40 mg of famotidine. All these drugs have roughly equivalent success rates in treating ulcer disease and comparable risk of side effects.

Cautions and Warnings

Do not take nizatidine if you are **allergic** or **sensitive** to any of its ingredients or to any histamine H_2 antagonist.

People with **kidney or liver disease** should take nizatidine with caution because 1/3 of each dose is broken down in the liver and the rest passes out of the body through the kidneys.

Do not self-treat with over-the-counter (OTC) forms of nizatidine without the advice and supervision of your doctor.

Possible Side Effects

Side effects are infrequent.

▼ Most common: tiredness and increased sweating.

▼ Rare: Rare side effects can affect the heart, liver, kidneys, stomach and intestines, blood, joints and muscles, mental status, and sexual function. Contact your doctor if you experience any side effect not listed above.

Drug Interactions

- Antacids, anticholinergics, and metoclopramide may slightly reduce the amount of nizatidine absorbed into the blood, but no precaution is needed.
- Enteric-coated tablets should not be taken with nizatidine. The change in stomach acidity produced by nizatidine causes the tablets to disintegrate prematurely in the stomach.
- Nizatidine may increase blood levels of aspirin in people taking very large doses of aspirin.

Food Interactions

Take nizatidine up to 1 hour before eating to prevent heartburn, acid indigestion, or sour stomach. Otherwise you may take it without regard to food or meals.

Usual Dose

Adult

Ulcer: 300 mg at bedtime or 150 mg twice a day. Maintenance dose is 150 mg at bedtime. Dosage is reduced in people with kidney disease.

GERD: 150 mg twice a day.

Child: not recommended.

OTC forms of nizatidine should only be used for the temporary relief of heartburn, and are not recommended for children under 12 years of age. Do not take more than 2 capsules or chewable tablets in 24 hours.

Overdosage

Little is known about the effects of nizatidine overdose, but victims may experience exaggerated side effects. Your local poison control center may advise giving ipecac syrup—available at any pharmacy—to induce vomiting and remove any drug remaining in the stomach. Victims who have definite symptoms should be taken to a hospital emergency room. ALWAYS bring the prescription bottle or container.

Special Information

Take nizatidine exactly as directed and follow your doctor's instructions regarding diet and other treatments to get the maximum benefit from the drug. Antacids may be taken together with nizatidine, if needed.

Do not take the maximum dose continuously for more than 2 weeks without the consent and supervision of your doctor.

Cigarette smoking is associated with stomach ulcer and may reduce nizatidine's effectiveness.

Call your doctor at once if you develop any unusual side effects such as bleeding or bruising, tiredness, diarrhea, dizziness, or rash. Black or tarry stools or vomiting material that resembles coffee grounds may indicate that your ulcer is bleeding.

If you empty the nizatidine capsule and mix it with juice before taking it, you may keep it in the refrigerator. Do not store it for more than 2 days because the drug may lose potency.

If you forget a dose of nizatidine, take it as soon as you remember. If it is almost time for your next dose, skip the one you forgot and continue with your regular schedule. Do not take a double dose.

Special Populations

Pregnancy/Breast-feeding: Although animal studies revealed no damage to the fetus, nizatidine should be avoided by women who are or might be pregnant. When the drug is considered crucial by your doctor, its potential benefits must be carefully weighed against its risks.

Very small amounts of nizatidine may pass into breast milk. Nursing mothers who must take this drug should use infant formula.

Seniors: Seniors may need lower doses due to loss of kidney function and may be more susceptible to side effects.

Type of Drug

Nonsteroidal Anti-inflammatory Drugs

Brand Names

Generic Ingredient: Diclofenac Potassium Ⓖ
Cataflam

Generic Ingredient: Diclofenac Sodium Ⓖ

Flector	Voltaren
Solaraze	Voltaren-XR

Generic Ingredient: Diflunisal Ⓖ

Generic Ingredient: Etodolac Ⓖ
Lodine   Lodine XL

Generic Ingredient: Fenoprofen Calcium Ⓖ
Nalfon

Generic Ingredient: Flurbiprofen Ⓖ
Ansaid

Generic Ingredient: Ibuprofen Ⓖ

Advil*	Medipren
Bayer Select Pain Relief	Menadol
Formula	Motrin*
Cap-Profen	Motrin IB
Children's Advil*	Motrin Migraine Pain
Children's Motrin*	Pediacare Fever
Ibuprohm	Profen
Ibu-Tab	Tab-Profen
Infants' Motrin*	

Generic Ingredient: Ketoprofen Ⓖ

Generic Ingredient: Meclofenamate Sodium Ⓖ

Generic Ingredient: Mefenamic Acid
Ponstel

Generic Ingredient: Meloxicam Ⓖ
Mobic

Generic Ingredient: Nabumetone Ⓖ

Generic Ingredient: Naproxen/Naproxen Sodium Ⓖ

Aleve	Midol Extended Relief
Anaprox	Naprelan
Anaprox DS	Naprosyn
EC-Naprosyn	

Generic Ingredient: Oxaprozin Ⓖ
Daypro

Generic Ingredient: Piroxicam Ⓖ
Feldene

Generic Ingredient: Sulindac Ⓖ
Clinoril

Generic Ingredient: Tolmetin Sodium Ⓖ

Tolectin	Tolectin DS
Tolectin 600	

*Some products in this brand-name group are alcohol- or sugar-free. Consult your pharmacist.

Combination Products
Generic Ingredients: Hydrocodone Bitartrate + Ibuprofen

Reprexain	Vicoprofen

Generic Ingredients: Ibuprofen + Oxycodone
Combunox

Generic Ingredients: Diclofenac Sodium + Misoprostol
Arthrotec

Prescribed For

Rheumatoid arthritis, osteoarthritis, fever, mild to moderate pain, migraine, juvenile rheumatoid arthritis, sunburn, menstrual pain, acute shoulder pain, ankylosing spondylitis, tendinitis, bursitis, acute gout, and other inflammatory conditions.

General Information

NSAIDs are used to relieve pain and inflammation. We do not know exactly how NSAIDs work, but they may achieve their effects by blocking the body's production of a hormone called prostaglandin and the action of other body chemicals known as COX-1 and COX-2 enzymes. Pain relief comes within 1 hour after taking the first dose of these medicines, but their anti-inflammatory effects take several days to 2 weeks to become apparent and may take a month or more to reach their maximum effect.

Cataflam, a newer version of diclofenac, has no sodium and is preferred for menstrual pain and cramps. Voltaren, the older version of diclofenac, has sodium. Women taking Cataflam for menstrual problems should not switch to Voltaren. The combination of diclofenac and misoprostol is used to protect against stomach and intestinal irritation and ulcer.

Cautions and Warnings

Do not take ibuprofen or any other NSAID if you are **allergic** or **sensitive** to any of their ingredients. Those with a history of **asthma** attacks brought on by an NSAID, iodides, or aspirin should not take these medicines.

These drugs may cause gastrointestinal (GI) tract bleeding, ulcers, and perforation. This can occur at any time, with or without warning, in people who take ibuprofen regularly. People with a **history of active GI bleeding** should be cautious about taking any NSAID. **Alcoholism** may increase the risk of bleeding. People who develop these symptoms and continue NSAID treatment should be aware of the possibility of developing more serious side effects.

Anemia can develop in people taking an NSAID.

Children taking these medicines may be more likely to vomit blood, suffer acute kidney failure, and develop rashes.

Ibuprofen can affect platelets and blood clotting at high doses and should be avoided by **people with clotting problems** and those taking **warfarin**.

People with **heart failure** who use ibuprofen may experience swelling in their arms, legs, or feet.

Ibuprofen and other NSAIDs may increase the risk of high blood pressure, heart attacks, and stroke. This risk increases with the length of time you are taking the drug. People taking ibuprofen, especially those with a collagen disease such as **systemic lupus erythematosus,** may experience an unusually severe drug-sensitivity reaction. Report any unusual symptoms to your doctor at once.

Long-term use of ibuprofen may lead to severe kidney toxicity. Report any unusual side effects to your doctor, who might need to periodically test your kidney function. People with advanced **kidney disease** should avoid these medicines.

Diflunisal is a chemical similar to aspirin and should not be given to **children** or **teens**. It may cause a serious complication called Reye's syndrome.

Ibuprofen may make you unusually sensitive to the effects of the sun.

Ibuprofen may affect your liver, in rare cases with serious or fatal results.

Ibuprofen can cause blurred or impaired vision, including changes in color vision. People experiencing these symptoms should stop using the drug and get a vision test, including a test of color vision.

Possible Side Effects

▼ Common: diarrhea, nausea, vomiting, constipation, dizziness, rash, and minor stomach upset, distress, or gas, especially during the first few days of treatment.

▼ Less common: stomach ulcers, gastrointestinal bleeding, appetite loss, hepatitis, gallbladder attacks, painful urination, poor kidney function, kidney inflammation, blood and protein in the urine, fainting, nervousness, depression, confusion, disorientation, tingling in the hands or feet, lightheadedness, itching, sweating, dry nose and mouth, heart palpitations, chest pain, breathing difficulties, and muscle cramps.

▼ Rare: severe allergic reactions including closing of the throat, fever and chills, changes in liver function, hallucinations, jaundice (yellowing of the skin and whites of the eyes), and kidney failure. These must be treated in a hospital emergency room or doctor's office. NSAIDs have caused severe skin reactions; see your doctor immediately if this happens to you. Contact your doctor if you experience any side effect not listed above.

Drug Interactions

- These drugs may increase the effects of oral anticoagulant (blood-thinning) drugs such as warfarin. Your anticoagulant dose may need to be reduced.

- These drugs may reduce the blood-pressure-lowering effect of beta blockers, ACE inhibitors, and diuretics.
- Combining these drugs with cyclosporine may increase the kidney-related side effects of both drugs.
- Ibuprofen may increase digoxin blood levels and toxicity.
- Ibuprofen may increase phenytoin side effects.
- Lithium blood levels and side effects may be increased by ibuprofen.
- Methotrexate side effects may be increased in people also taking ibuprofen.
- Blood levels of these drugs may be affected by cimetidine.
- Probenecid may increase the risk of NSAID side effects.
- Aspirin and other salicylates should never be combined with an NSAID in the treatment of arthritis.

Food Interactions
Take these drugs with food or a magnesium/aluminum antacid if they upset your stomach.

Usual Dose
Diclofenac Tablets
Adult: 100–200 mg a day.
Senior: starting dose—⅓–½ the usual dosage.

Diclofenac + Misoprostol
Adult: one 50/200 tablet 3 or 4 times a day or one 75/200 tablet 3 times a day. For seniors, taking the combination product 4 times a day provides better ulcer protection, but arthritis relief does not improve.

Diflunisal: starting dosage—500–1000 mg. Maintenance dosage—250–500 mg every 8–12 hours. Do not take more than 1500 mg a day. Do not crush or chew diflunisal tablets.

Etodolac
Adult (age 18 and over): 200–400 mg every 6–12 hours, not to exceed 1200 mg a day. People weighing 132 lbs. or less should not take more than 20 mg for every 2.2 lbs. of body weight.

Fenoprofen
Adult: mild to moderate pain—200 mg every 4–6 hours. Arthritis—300–600 mg 3–4 times a day to start, individualized to your needs. Total daily dose should not exceed 3200 mg.
Child: not recommended.

Flurbiprofen: 200–300 mg a day in divided doses.

Ibuprofen
   Adult and Child (age 12 and over): 200–800 mg 4 times a day depending on the condition being treated; follow your doctor's directions. 200 mg every 4–6 hours is appropriate for mild to moderate pain.
   Child (6 months–12 years): juvenile arthritis—9–18 mg per lb. of body weight a day, divided into several doses.

Ketoprofen: 50–75 mg 3–4 times a day. Do not exceed 300 mg a day. Seniors and people with kidney problems should start with ⅓–½ of the usual dose.

Ketoprofen ER: 150–200 mg once a day.

Meclofenamate
   Adult and Child (age 14 and over): 200–400 mg a day in divided doses.
   Child (under age 14): not recommended.

Mefenamic Acid
   Adult and Child (age 14 and over): 500 mg to start, then 250 mg every 6 hours in divided doses.
   Child (under age 14): not recommended.

Meloxicam: 7.5–15 mg once a day.

Nabumetone: 1000–2000 mg a day, taken in 1 or 2 doses.

Naproxen
   Adult: starting dose—250–500 mg morning and evening; up to 1500 mg a day if needed. Mild to moderate pain—take 250–275 mg every 6–8 hours.
   Child (age 2 and over): 4.5 mg per lb. of body weight divided into 2 doses a day.
   Child (under age 2): not recommended.

Oxaprozin: 600–1200 mg once a day. May be increased to up to 1800 mg a day in divided doses. Do not exceed 12 mg per lb. of body weight daily.

Piroxicam
   Adult (age 18 and over): 20 mg a day.
   Child: not recommended.

Sulindac
Adult (age 18 and over): 150–200 mg twice a day.
Child: not recommended.

Tolmetin
Adult (age 18 and over): 400 mg 3 times a day.
Child (age 2 and over): 9 mg per lb. of body weight divided into 3 or 4 doses a day.
Child (under age 2): not recommended.

Overdosage
People have died from NSAID overdoses. Common signs of overdose are drowsiness, nausea, vomiting, diarrhea, abdominal pain, rapid breathing, rapid heartbeat, sweating, ringing or buzzing in the ears, confusion, disorientation, stupor, and coma. Take the victim to a hospital emergency room at once for treatment. ALWAYS bring the prescription bottle or container.

Special Information
Take each dose with a full glass of water and do not lie down for 15–30 minutes afterward.

NSAIDs may make you drowsy or tired: Be careful when driving or operating hazardous equipment. Do not take over-the-counter products containing aspirin while taking ibuprofen. Avoid alcohol.

Contact your doctor if you develop rash, itching, visual disturbances, weight gain, breathing difficulties, fluid retention, hallucinations, black stools, persistent headache, or any unusual or intolerable side effect.

If you forget a dose of any of these drugs, take it as soon as you remember. If you take several doses a day and it is within 4 hours of your next dose, skip the dose you forgot and continue with your regular schedule. Do not take a double dose.

Special Populations
Pregnancy/Breast-feeding: NSAIDs may affect the developing fetal heart during the last half of pregnancy. Women who are or might become pregnant should not take ibuprofen without their doctor's approval. When the drug is considered crucial by your doctor, its potential benefits must be carefully weighed against its risks.

Arthrotec, a combination product, contains an ingredient called misoprostol that can induce labor. Pregnant women should never take this product.

NSAIDs may pass into breast milk. There is a possibility that a nursing mother taking ibuprofen could affect her baby's heart or cardiovascular system. Nursing mothers who must take this drug should use infant formula.

Seniors: Seniors, especially those with poor kidney or liver function, may be more susceptible to side effects.

Type of Drug

Nonsteroidal Anti-inflammatory Drug Eyedrops

Brand Names

Generic Ingredient: Bromfenac
Xibrom

Generic Ingredient: Diclofenac
Voltaren

Generic Ingredient: Ketorolac
Acular

Generic Ingredient: Flurbiprofen Sodium Ⓖ
Ocufen

Generic Ingredient: Nepafenac
Nevanac

Prescribed For

Eye redness and inflammation caused by seasonal allergies; inflammation during and after eye surgery.

General Information

Nonsteroidal anti-inflammatory drug (NSAID) eyedrops are used during eye surgery to prevent movement of the eye muscles and are used after surgery to relieve inflammation, pain, and aversion to light. They are also used to treat itching and redness due to seasonal allergies. After cataract surgery, they are used to prevent inflammation.

Cautions and Warnings

Do not take NSAID eyedrops if you are **allergic** or **sensitive** to any of their ingredients. Those with a history of **asthma** attacks brought on by an NSAID, iodides, or aspirin should not take these medicines.

Small amounts of these eyedrops are absorbed into the bloodstream. NSAIDs may cause gastrointestinal (GI) tract bleeding, ulcers, or stomach perforation. They should be used with caution in people with known **bleeding disorders** or those taking other medications that prolong bleeding time.

NSAIDs may increase the risk of high blood pressure, heart disease, and stroke.

They can cause severe toxic effects to the kidney. Report anything to your doctor, who might need to periodically test your kidney function. People taking NSAIDs on a regular basis should also have their liver function tested regularly.

NSAIDs may make make you unusually sensitive to the effects of the sun.

Possible Side Effects

▼ Most common: temporary burning, stinging, or other minor eye irritation.

▼ Less common: nausea, vomiting, viral infections, and eye reactions including persistent redness, burning, itching, or tearing. The risk of developing bleeding problems or other systemic (whole-body) side effects with NSAID eyedrops is low because only a small amount of the drug is absorbed into the blood.

Drug Interactions

None known.

Food Interactions

None.

Usual Dose

Bromfenac: 1 drop twice a day, beginning 24 hours after cataract surgery and continuing for 2 weeks.

Diclofenac: 1 drop 4 times a day for 2 weeks, beginning 24 hours after cataract surgery.

Flurbiprofen: 1 drop every 30 minutes, beginning 2 hours before surgery (total of 4 drops).

Ketorolac: 1 drop 4 times a day for itching and irritation due to seasonal allergies.

Nepafenac: 1 drop 3 times a day for 2 weeks, beginning 1 day before cataract surgery. Shake this product before using it.

Overdosage

People have died from overdoses of NSAID pills but there is not enough medicine in a bottle of eyedrops to cause a severe effect. Call a hospital emergency room or local poison center for more information. ALWAYS bring the prescription bottle or container.

Special Information

To prevent possible infection, do not allow the dropper to touch your fingers, eyelids, or any surface. Wait at least 5 minutes before using any other eyedrops.

Take out contact lenses before using these eyedrops.

These medicines may cause blurred vision. Use caution while driving or performing other tasks requiring alertness, coordination, or physical dexterity.

If you forget to administer a dose of NSAID eyedrops, do so as soon as you remember. If it is almost time for your next dose, skip the dose you forgot and continue with your regular schedule. Do not take a double dose.

Special Populations

Pregnancy/Breast-feeding: NSAID eyedrops should not be taken by pregnant women because they may affect fetal blood circulation and prevent normal labor.

NSAID eyedrops may pass into breast milk. There is a possibility that a nursing mother taking NSAIDs could affect her baby's heart or cardiovascular system. Nursing mothers who must take these drugs should use infant formula.

Seniors: Seniors may be more susceptible to side effects, especially ulcer disease.

Norvasc   *see **Amlodipine**, page 65*

Nuvaring   *see **Contraceptives**, page 287*

Generic Name

Nystatin (nye-STAH-tin)

Brand Names

Mycostatin   Nilstat

The information in this profile also applies to the following drug:

Generic Ingredients: Nystatin + Triamcinoline Acetonide [G]
Mykacet

Type of Drug

Antifungal.

Prescribed For

Fungal infections of the skin, mouth, vagina, and gastrointestinal tract.

General Information

Nystatin comes in a number of dosage forms and can be prescribed when fungal infection is a possible complication of a disease or treatment. Very little nystatin is absorbed into the blood when the product is swallowed. In most cases, nystatin relieves symptoms in 1–3 days. Nystatin vaginal tablets effectively control symptoms such as itching, inflammation, and discharge. Generally, 2 weeks of therapy is sufficient, but prolonged treatment may be necessary. It is important that you continue using this drug during menstruation. This drug has been used to prevent thrush or *Candida* in newborns by treating the mother for 3–6 weeks before her due date. Triamcinoline acetonide is a corticosteroid added to nystatin to relieve the discomfort and inflammation associated with a fungal skin infection.

Cautions and Warnings

Do not take this drug if you are **sensitive** or **allergic** to any of its ingredients.

Proper diagnosis is essential for effective treatment. Do not use nystatin without first consulting your doctor.

If large amounts of nystatin + triamcinoline acetonide are applied for prolonged periods, the corticosteroid may enter the bloodstream and in rare cases may cause serious side effects, especially in children.

Possible Side Effects

Nystatin is generally well tolerated.

Oral Form
▼ Less common: nausea, upset stomach, and diarrhea may occur with large doses.

Topical Form
Nystatin
▼ Less common: skin irritation.

Nystatin + Triamcinoline Acetonide
▼ Less common: skin irritation, burning, and dryness.

Vaginal Form
▼ Less common: vaginal irritation; if this occurs, discontinue the drug and contact your doctor.

Drug Interactions

None known.

Food Interactions

None known.

Usual Dose

Lozenges
   Adult and Child: 200,000–400,000 units 4–5 times a day for as long as 14 days if necessary. Allow the lozenges to dissolve slowly on your tongue.

Oral Suspension
   Adult and Child: 200,000–600,000 units 4 or 5 times a day. Shake the bottle well before using.

Oral Tablets
   Adult and Child: 500,000–1,000,000 units 3 times a day.

Topical Form
   Adult and Child: Apply twice a day for as long as your doctor recommends.

Vaginal Tablets
   Adult: 1 tablet inserted high in the vagina daily for 2 weeks, or 3–6 weeks before delivery in pregnant women.
   Child: not recommended.

Overdosage

Nystatin overdose may cause stomach irritation or upset. Call your local poison control center for more information. If you seek treatment, ALWAYS bring the prescription bottle or container.

Special Information

If you are taking nystatin + triamcinoline acetonide and you notice stretch marks, skin thinning or discoloration, acne, hair growth, or signs of an allergic reaction (which include rash, swelling, dizziness, and trouble breathing), contact your doctor immediately.

Call your doctor if you develop diarrhea, upset stomach, stomach pain, or skin rash.

Do not stop taking nystatin just because you begin to feel better. You must continue taking the medication as prescribed for at least 2 days after the relief of symptoms.

Insert the vaginal tablets or cream high into the vagina. They each come with a special applicator and directions. Be sure to unwrap the vaginal tablets just before inserting them. Read the directions provided with the tablets or cream and follow these steps:

—Fill the special applicator to the level indicated.

—Lie on your back with your knees drawn upward and spread apart.

—Gently insert the applicator into your vagina and push the plunger to release the medication.

—Withdraw the applicator and wash it with soap and warm water.

—Wash your hands promptly to avoid spreading the infection.

You may want to wear a sanitary pad while using the vaginal cream to protect your clothing against stains. Do not use a tampon because it will absorb the drug. Do not douche unless your doctor tells you to do so. Continue using nystatin vaginal cream or tablets even if you get your period during treatment.

Some nystatin brands require storage in the refrigerator. Ask your pharmacist for specific instructions.

If you forget to administer a dose, do so as soon as you remember. If it is almost time for your next dose, skip the one you forgot and continue with your regular schedule. Do not take a double dose.

Special Populations

Pregnancy/Breast-feeding: Pregnant and breast-feeding women may use nystatin with no restrictions. Pregnant women should use nystatin + triamcinoline acetonide only when absolutely necessary. Women who are using nystatin + triamcinoline acetonide and breast-feeding should consider using infant formula.

Seniors: Seniors may use nystatin without special precaution.

Generic Name

Olanzapine (oeh-LAN-zuh-pene)

Brand Names
Zyprexa   Zyprexa Zydis

Combination Product
Generic Ingredients: Olanzapine + Fluoxetine
Symbyax

Type of Drug
Antipsychotic.

Prescribed For
Schizophrenia and bipolar disorder; agitation associated with schizophrenia and bipolar disorder; and depression or mania associated with bipolar disorder. Olanzapine may be prescribed both for acute and chronic conditions.

General Information
Olanzapine is a potent antipsychotic that blocks several different chemical receptors in the brain. The exact way in which olanzapine works is not known, but its antipsychotic effect may be produced by its effect on dopamine and serotonin receptors. A small portion of each dose of olanzapine is eliminated through the kidneys, but most of it is broken down in the liver. The combination of olanzapine and fluoxetine is thought to be more effective in severe depression than either drug alone because of the combination of nervous system receptors it blocks. See "Fluoxetine," page 1020, for more information.

Cautions and Warnings
Do not take olanzapine if you are **allergic** or **sensitive** to any of its ingredients.

Olanzapine has been associated with increased mortality in seniors with **dementia** or **Alzheimer's disease**. The specific causes of death related to olanzapine and other atypical antipsychotic drugs were either due to a heart-related event or infection, mostly pneumonia. Olanzapine and olanzapine + fluoxetine are not approved for use in treatment of dementia-related psychosis.

Suicide is a danger with all psychotics and antidepressants. People taking this drug should be limited to a 30-day supply of medication at any time to reduce the chances of possible overdose.

Olanzapine has been associated with obesity, high cholesterol, high blood sugar, and diabetes. Olanzapine alone often causes significant weight gain over time, but this has not been seen in the combination product. People with **diabetes** or **risk factors for diabetes** such as elevated blood glucose levels or a family history of diabetes should have their blood glucose levels monitored regularly and be vigilant for the symptoms of hyperglycemia including increased thirst, frequent urination, and fatigue.

Women eliminate olanzapine about 30% more slowly than men, but this effect is not considered a problem. Women may respond to lower olanzapine doses than men.

Smokers eliminate olanzapine from their bodies about 40% faster than non-smokers, but most people do not require dose adjustments.

People with **liver disease** may require dosage adjustments.

A serious set of side effects known as neuroleptic malignant syndrome (NMS) includes a high fever, convulsions, difficult or fast breathing, rapid heartbeat, and rapid pulse. This condition has been associated with antipsychotic medicines. Other symptoms of NMS include muscle rigidity, mental changes, irregular pulse or blood pressure, and increased sweating. NMS can be fatal and requires immediate medical attention.

Tardive dyskinesia (symptoms include lip smacking or puckering, puffing of the cheeks, rapid or worm-like movements of the tongue, uncontrolled chewing motions, and uncontrolled arm or leg movements) can occur and is often considered a reason to stop taking this drug. Report any of these side effects to your doctor.

People with **heart disease** and those **taking medications that reduce blood pressure** should use olanzapine with caution.

Olanzapine can cause dizziness or fainting when rising from a sitting or standing position, especially when people first start taking the drug.

Antipsychotics can upset the body's temperature-regulating mechanism, creating the risk for heat stroke and dehydration.

Swallowing problems and inhaling food have been experienced by people taking antipsychotics, including olanzapine.

Seizures occur in a small number of people taking olanzapine. Olanzapine should be taken with care if you have had **seizures** or are at increased risk.

Possible Side Effects

▼ Most common: headache, tiredness, agitation, sleepless-ness, nervousness, hostility, dizziness, and runny nose.

▼ Less common: fever; abdominal, back, or chest pains; a rigid neck; dizziness or fainting when rising from a sitting or standing position; rapid heartbeat; low blood pressure; constipation; dry mouth; increased appetite; weight gain; swelling in the arms or legs; joint pain; arm or leg pain; twitching; anxiety; personality changes; restlessness or a feeling that you need to keep moving; muscle stiffness; tremors; memory loss; difficulty speaking or expressing thoughts; euphoria (feeling "high"); stuttering; cough; sore throat; double vision or other eye problems; and symptoms of premenstrual syndrome (PMS).

▼ Rare: Other side effects can occur in almost any part of the body. Contact your doctor if you experience any side effect not listed above.

Drug Interactions

- Alcohol should be avoided when taking olanzapine.
- The dosage of olanzapine must be adjusted when the drug is combined with carbamazepine.
- Olanzapine increases the effects of blood-pressure-lowering drugs and nervous system depressants. Dosage adjustments may be needed if you add olanzapine to another medicine.
- Do not take the combination of olanzapine and fluoxetine if you are taking a monoamine oxidase inhibitor (MAOI) anti-depressant, or have taken one of these drugs in the past 2 weeks. Do not start taking a MAOI until at least 5 weeks after you stop taking the olanzapine + fluoxetine combination.
- Do not take the combination of olanzapine + fluoxetine if you are taking thioridazine for mental problems. Mixing these drugs increases your chances of having a serious or life-threatening heart problem. Do not start taking thioridazine

until at least 5 weeks after you stop taking olanzapine + fluoxetine.

- Combining olanzapine with fluvoxamine may cause elevations in olanzapine blood levels and added side effects.
- Mixing olanzapine + fluoxetine with aspirin or a nonsteroidal anti-inflammatory drug (NSAID) may increase your risk of bleeding.
- Combining olanzapine with ritonavir may decrease the effectiveness of olanzapine.
- The combination of olanzapine and a tricyclic antidepressant may cause increased side effects, such as seizures. This combination should be used with caution.

Food Interactions

Take olanzapine without regard to food or meals; it can be taken with food if it upsets your stomach.

Usual Dose

Olanzapine

Adult: starting dosage—5–10 mg a day. Maintenance dosage increases gradually up to 20 mg a day if needed. Seniors should start with lower doses and increase gradually until maximum benefit is achieved.

Child (under age 18): not recommended.

Olanzapine + Fluoxetine

Adult: one 6/25 capsule every evening to start. Dosage may be increased gradually to one 12/50 capsule in the evening. Higher doses have not been studied. Lower doses may be needed by women, seniors, people with liver disease, and those with low blood pressure or those who are inclined to dizziness or fainting.

Overdosage

Overdose symptoms are drowsiness and slurred speech. Overdose victims should be taken to a hospital emergency room for treatment. ALWAYS bring the prescription bottle or container.

Special Information

Sleepiness occurs in about 25% of people who take olanzapine; this effect may increase with larger doses. Take care when engaging in activities, such as driving, that require concentration or coordination.

Avoid alcohol and other nervous system depressants while taking olanzapine.

Avoid being exposed to extreme heat while taking olanzapine.

Olanzapine can cause dry mouth. See your dentist regularly while you are taking this medication, since dental problems are more likely.

Be sure your doctor knows all the medication you are taking, including over-the-counter products.

If you forget to take a dose of olanzapine, take it as soon as you remember. If it is almost time for your next dose, skip the dose you forgot and continue with your regular schedule. Do not take a double dose.

To use olanzapine orally disintegrating tablets, remove the tablet from its blister pack by peeling back the foil; do not push the tablet through the foil. Handle the tablet with clean dry hands and place it in your mouth. The tablet will dissolve with or without water or another liquid. Orally disintegrating tablets must be used as soon as they are removed from their packaging.

Special Populations

Pregnancy/Breast-feeding: Pregnant women should only take olanzapine if the potential benefits outweigh the risks. Birth defects and other problems have occurred in women taking olanzapine but there is no definite link between the drug and these effects.

It is not known if olanzapine passes into breast milk. Nursing mothers who must take this medication should use infant formula.

Seniors: Seniors taking olanzapine are more likely to suffer a stroke. Seniors usually need less olanzapine than younger adults.

Generic Name

Olopatadine (oe-loe-PAT-uh-dene) Ⓖ

Brand Name

Patanol

The information in this profile also applies to the following drugs:

Generic Ingredient: Azelastine
Optivar

Generic Ingredient: Levocabastine
Livostin

Type of Drug

Antihistamine and mast-cell stabilizer.

Prescribed For

Eye itching due to allergy.

General Information

Olopatadine hydrochloride is an antihistamine eyedrop that alleviates irritation caused by conjunctivitis (pinkeye). It prevents the release of chemicals from mast cells in the eye that cause allergic symptoms and minimizes the response of nerve endings to these chemicals. Levocabastine only affects the nerve endings to minimize the allergic response.

Cautions and Warnings

Do not use olopatadine if you are **allergic** or **sensitive** to any of its ingredients.

Possible Side Effects

Side effects are generally mild and subside as your body gets used to the drug.

Azelastine

▼ Common: eye stinging or burning, headache, and bitter taste in the mouth.

▼ Less common: asthma, difficulty breathing, eye pain or blurriness, fatigue, flu-like symptoms, itching, and sinus inflammation.

Levocabastine

▼ Most common: mild stinging or burning.

▼ Common: headache.

▼ Less common: dry mouth, visual disturbances, tiredness, sore throat, eye redness, eye tearing or discharge, eye pain or dryness, cough, nausea, skin rash or redness, eyelid swelling, and difficulty breathing.

Olopatadine

▼ Common: headache.

▼ Less common: burning or stinging in the eye, dry eye, sensation that something is in your eye, eye redness, inflammation of the cornea, eyelid swelling, itching, weakness, sore throat, runny nose, common cold symptoms, sinus inflammation, and changes in sense of taste.

Drug Interactions

If you use several different eyedrops, separate them by 5 minutes.

Usual Dose

Azelastine
Adult (age 3 and over): 1 drop in the affected eye twice a day.
Child (under age 3): not recommended.

Levocabastine
Adult and Child (age 12 and over): 1 drop in the affected eye 4 times a day for up to 2 weeks; be sure to shake the bottle well before using.
Child (under age 12): not recommended.

Olopatadine
Adult and Child (age 3 and over): 1–2 drops in each affected eye 2 times a day, 6–8 hours apart.
Child (under age 3): not recommended.

Overdosage

Little is known about the effects of olopatadine overdose, but it is likely to increase side effects. Accidental ingestion of olopatadine is not likely to be associated with side effects because each bottle contains only small amounts of the active drug. Call your local poison control center or hospital emergency room for more information. If you seek treatment, ALWAYS bring the prescription bottle.

Special Information

Do not wear contact lenses if your affected eye is red. If you wear soft contact lenses and your eye is not red, wait at least 15 minutes after using olopatadine before putting in your lenses.

To avoid infection, do not touch the dropper tip to your finger, eyelid, or any other surface. Wait at least 5 minutes before using another eyedrop or eye ointment.

If you forget a dose of olopatadine, administer it as soon as you remember. If it is almost time for your next dose, skip the one you forgot and continue with your regular schedule. Do not take a double dose.

Special Populations

Pregnancy/Breast-feeding: Olopatadine can cause birth defects when given to laboratory animals in extremely high doses (nearly 100,000 times the maximum recommended dosage equivalency for humans). There is no information on its effect in women during pregnancy. When your doctor considers this drug crucial, the potential benefits must be carefully weighed against its risks.

Olopatadine may pass into breast milk. Nursing mothers using olopatadine should use infant formula.

Seniors: Seniors may take olopatadine without special precaution.

Omnicef   see **Cephalosporin Antibiotics,** page 210

Generic Name

Orlistat (OR-lih-stat)

Brand Names

Alli   Xenical

Type of Drug

Fat blocker.

Prescribed For

Weight reduction and maintenance.

General Information

Orlistat is the first "fat blocker" to be approved by the Food and Drug Administration (FDA). It works in the stomach and intestine by interfering with an enzyme that is key to the breakdown and absorption of one kind of fat. The unabsorbed fat, about 30% of that in your diet, passes out of the body in the stool. Since fat is the most concentrated form of calories, blocking fat absorption also reduces the number of calories you take in. People taking orlistat usually begin losing weight in a few weeks and continue to lose it for 6 months to a year. After that, weight loss is maintained. If you increase your exercise level or further reduce your caloric intake, you may lose more weight. More than 50% of people taking orlistat in clinical studies lost at least 5% of their body weight after a year of continuous treatment. About 18% lost more than 10% of body weight.

By losing weight, people taking orlistat achieved improved blood-fat profiles and lower blood pressure and blood sugar. They also reduced their waist and hip measurements—2″ and 2.5″, respectively—more than people taking a placebo (sugar pill) and following a weight-loss diet.

Cautions and Warnings

Do not take orlistat if you are **allergic** or **sensitive** to any of its ingredients.

Orlistat should not be used by those with **gastrointestinal absorption disorders** or **cholestasis** (bile duct obstruction).

Some people may develop **kidney stones** while taking this drug, especially those prone to kidney stones.

Orlistat, like any weight-loss drug, may be abused or misused. Orlistat should never be used by those with eating disorders such as **anorexia** or **bulimia.**

The cause of obesity must be determined before taking orlistat; it is not recommended for people who have **hyperthyroidism** or other organic causes of **obesity**.

A reduction in oral hypoglycemic medication or insulin may be necessary for **diabetic patients taking orlistat.**

Possible Side Effects

Most side effects are mild and temporary and tend to decrease during the second year of treatment.

▼ Most common: oily underwear spotting, gas with discharge, the feeling that you have to move your bowels, an oily or fat-laden stool, releasing an oily liquid during a bowel movement, more frequent bowel movements, abdominal pain or discomfort, flu, respiratory infections, back pain, and headache.

▼ Common: an inability to control bowel movements, nausea, infectious diarrhea, rectal pain or discomfort, arthritis, dizziness, fatigue, rash, menstrual problems, and urinary infection.

▼ Less common: tooth or gum problems; vomiting; ear, nose, or throat problems; muscle pain; joint problems; tendonitis; sleep disturbances; dry skin; vaginal irritation; anxiety; depression; and swollen feet.

▼ Rare: Rare side effects can occur in almost any part of the body. Contact your doctor if you experience any side effect not listed above.

Drug Interactions

- Orlistat causes blood levels of cyclosporine to decrease when they are taken together. Orlistat and cyclosporine doses should be separated by at least 2 hours.
- Orlistat interferes with the absorption of fat-soluble vitamins and drugs.
- The blood-fat-lowering effect of statin cholesterol-lowering drugs is increased by orlistat.
- Orlistat may increase the effect of warfarin by interfering with the absorption of vitamin K. Warfarin dosage reduction may be needed.

Food Interactions

Take a dose with, or within an hour of, a fat-containing meal.

Usual Dose

Alli

   Adult (age 18 and over): 60 mg taken 3 times a day with, or within an hour of, each main meal containing fat.

   Child (under age 18): not recommended.

Xenical

   Adult: 120 mg taken 3 times a day with, or within an hour of, each main meal containing fat.

   Child: not recommended.

Overdosage

Symptoms are likely to include side effects, especially those related to the stomach and intestines. Take the victim to a hospital emergency room. ALWAYS bring the prescription bottle or container.

Special Information

Orlistat should be taken as part of a program of diet and exercise. Taking more than 1 capsule with each meal does not provide extra benefit.

   Daily fat intake should be distributed over 3 meals to reduce the risk of developing a stomach or gastrointestinal (GI) problem.

   Orlistat can interfere with the absorption of the fat-soluble vitamins A, D, and E. Take a multivitamin supplement while using this drug, separated by at least 2 hours.

   If you forget to take an orlistat capsule within an hour of any meal, skip the forgotten dose and take a capsule with your next meal. Do not take a double dose.

Special Populations

Pregnancy/Breast-feeding: While animal studies of orlistat reveal no damage to the fetus, this drug is not recommended during pregnancy and should only be used after carefully weighing its potential benefits against its risks.

It is not known if orlistat passes into breast milk. Nursing mothers who must take this drug should use infant formula.

Seniors: Orlistat has not been studied in older adults, who should use caution.

Ortho-Evra *see Contraceptives, page 287*

Ortho-Tri-Cyclen Lo *see Contraceptives, page 287*

Generic Name

Oseltamivir (oe-sel-TAM-ih-veer)

Brand Name
Tamiflu

Type of Drug
Antiviral.

Prescribed For
Influenza type A and B and for prevention of influenza following exposure.

General Information
Oseltamivir is the first pill approved to treat both type A and B influenza. It may also lessen the effects of other types of flu. It is thought to work by interfering with a virus enzyme called neuraminidase; this interference limits the spread of virus particles through the respiratory tract. In studies, people taking the drug for 5 days

got better 1.3 days sooner than those taking a placebo (sugar pill). Oseltamivir is only prescribed for adults and children over 1 year who have had flu symptoms for no more than 2 days. It may also be used to prevent the flu in children and adults. Studies have shown that it reduces the chances of catching the flu from 17% down to 3%. This drug is broken down in the liver.

Cautions and Warnings

Do not take oseltamivir if you are **allergic** or **sensitive** to any of its ingredients.

The effect of oseltamivir in people with **chronic heart disease, lung disease,** or any condition requiring hospitalization is not known. The safety and effectiveness of repeated oseltamivir use is not known.

Flu viruses can become resistant to oseltamivir, especially those already resistant to zanamivir (another flu medication).

People with moderate **kidney disease** require reduced dosage. People with severe kidney disease should be cautious about using oseltamivir because it has not been studied in this group.

Possible Side Effects

▼ Most common: nausea and vomiting.

▼ Common: diarrhea.

▼ Less common: bronchitis, abdominal pain, dizziness or fainting, headache, cough, sleeplessness, abnormal behavior or confusion leading to possible self-injury, fatigue, nosebleeds (occurs mainly in children), and ear disorder (occurs mainly in children).

▼ Rare: chest pain, anemia, colitis, bone fracture, pneumonia, fever, and abscesses around the tonsils. Contact your doctor if you experience any side effect not listed above.

Drug Interactions

• There is a possible interference between oseltamivir and live attenuated influenza vaccine (LAIV). For this reason, LAIV should not be administered within 2 weeks before or 48 hours after use of oseltamivir.

Food Interactions

Oseltamivir may be taken with food it it upsets your stomach.

Usual Dose

Treatment of Influenza

Adult and Child (age 13 and over): 75 mg twice a day for 5 days. Daily dosage may be reduced to a single 75-mg capsule in people with kidney disease.

Child (age 1 and over and more than 88 lbs.): 75 mg (1¼ tsp.) twice a day.

Child (age 1 and over and 52–88 lbs.): 60 mg (1 tsp.) twice a day.

Child (age 1 and over and 34–51 lbs.): 45 mg (¾ tsp.) twice a day.

Child (age 1 and over and less than 34 lbs.): 30 mg (½ tsp.) twice a day.

Child (under 1 year): not recommended.

Prevention of Influenza

Adult and Child (age 13 and over): 75 mg once a day for 10 days. Therapy should begin within 2 days of exposure.

Child (age 1 and over and more than 88 lbs.): 75 mg (1¼ tsp.) once a day.

Child (age 1 and over and 52–88 lbs.): 60 mg (1 tsp.) once a day.

Child (age 1 and over and 34–51 lbs.): 45 mg (¾ tsp.) once a day.

Child (age 1 and over and less than 34 lbs.): 30 mg (½ tsp.) once a day.

Child (under 1 year): not recommended.

Overdosage

Little is known about the effects of oseltamivir overdose, though symptoms may include nausea and vomiting. Call your local poison control center or a hospital emergency room for more information. If you seek treatment, ALWAYS bring the prescription bottle or container.

Special Information

Oseltamivir should be taken from the first appearance of flu symptoms. Taking oseltamivir is not a substitute for an annual flu shot.

If you forget a dose, take it as soon as you remember. If it is almost time for your next dose, skip the one you forgot and continue with your regular schedule. Do not take a double dose.

Special Populations

Pregnancy/Breast-feeding: Animal studies indicate that oseltamivir may cause fetal abnormalities. When this drug is considered crucial by your doctor, its potential benefits must be carefully weighed against its risks.

This drug may pass into breast milk. Nursing mothers who must take it should use infant formula.

Seniors: Oseltamivir may be less effective in seniors.

Generic Name

Oxcarbazepine (oks-kar-BAZ-e-peen)

Brand Name
Trileptal

Type of Drug
Anticonvulsant.

Prescribed For
Partial seizures in adults, and children age 2–16 with epilepsy.

General Information
The exact way that oxcarbazepine works is unknown. It may stabilize sodium and calcium channels in the brain, thereby preventing the spread of seizure in the brain.

Cautions and Warnings
Do not take oxcarbazepine if you are **allergic** or **sensitive** to any of its ingredients. About ¼ of those who have had a reaction to **carbamazepine** will also react to oxcarbazepine.

A small number of hypersensitivity reactions involving multiple organs have occurred close to starting oxcarbazepine in adults and children. Many of these people were hospitalized and some had life-threatening circumstances. Typical signs and symptoms of this reaction are fever and rash associated with swollen lymph glands, hepatitis, abnormal liver and blood tests, itching, kidney inflammation, inability to urinate, joint pains, and weakness.

People taking this drug occasionally develop very low blood sodium levels (symptoms include nausea, feeling sick, headache, tiredness, confusion, and reduced pain sensitivity) during the first 3 months of treatment. Your doctor will check your blood periodically and may stop the drug or lower the dose to eliminate this problem.

Serious, possibly life-threatening skin reactions, including Stevens-Johnson syndrome, have occurred in children and adults taking this medicine. Tell your doctor at once if you develop any type of skin reaction to the drug.

Possible Side Effects

▼ Most common: nausea, vomiting, abdominal pain, upset stomach, fatigue, headache, dizziness, tiredness, tremor, and double vision or abnormal vision.

▼ Common: poor muscle coordination, unusual eye movements, abnormal walking, memory loss, worsened convulsions, and fainting.

▼ Less common: emotional upset, reduced sensitivity to stimulation, nervousness, taste changes, earache, fever, allergy, weakness, swollen legs, weight gain, low blood pressure, speech or language problems, confusion, abnormal thinking, acne, hot flushes, rash, appetite loss, dry mouth, rectal bleeding, toothache, diarrhea, constipation, stomach irritation, thirst, runny nose, coughing, bronchitis, sore throat, nosebleed, and back pain.

▼ Rare: Rare side effects can occur in almost any part of the body. Contact your doctor if you experience any side effect not listed above.

Drug Interactions

● Carbamazepine (400–2000 mg a day), phenobarbital, and phenytoin reduce the amount of a metabolite of oxcarbazepine in the blood.

● Oxcarbazepine reduces the amount of felodipine, cyclosporine, and contraceptive drugs in the blood, possibly interfering with their effectiveness. Other drugs that may be reduced in the blood by oxcarbazepine are clarithromycin, erythromycin, quinidine, benzodiazepine sedatives, tacrolimus, indinavir, nelfinavir, ritonavir, saquinavir, astemizole, chlorpheniramine, terfenidine, calcium channel blocker drugs, statin-type cholesterol-lowering drugs (except pravastatin), hydrocortisone, testosterone, buspirone, codeine, dextromethorphan, finasteride, haloperidol, methadone, ondansetron, pimozide, quinine, salmeterol, sildenafil, tamoxifen, paclitaxel, terfenadine, trazodone, vincristine, zaleplon, and zolpidem.

● Oxcarbazepine may increase the amount of phenobarbital and phenytoin in the blood. It may also increase levels of amitriptyline and other tricyclic antidepressants, clomipramine, cyclophosphamide, hexobarbital, indomethacin, nilu-

tamide, progesterone, tenoposide, lansoprozole, omeprazole, pantoprozole, and warfarin.
- Valproic acid and verapamil reduce oxcarbazepine levels in
the blood.

Food Interactions

Oxcarbazepine can be taken with or without food.

Usual Dose

Adult and Child (age 16 and over): 600–2400 mg a day. People
with poor kidney function should start at ½ the dosage and increase slowly until the desired response is reached.

Child (age 4–15): 3.75–4.5 mg per lb. up to 600 mg a day to start.
Increase gradually to 900–1800 mg a day, according to body
weight.

Overdosage

All overdose patients have recovered with treatment. Symptoms
are likely to be exaggerated drug side effects. Overdose victims
should be taken to a hospital emergency room. ALWAYS bring the
prescription bottle or container.

Special Information

This drug may reduce the effectiveness of contraceptive drugs.
Use an alternate contraceptive method while taking oxcarbazepine.

Like all anticonvulsant medicines, oxcarbazepine must be gradually stopped to avoid experiencing sudden seizures.

Alcohol can enhance the depressive effects of this drug.

Oxcarbazepine can cause tiredness and confusion, especially
when the drug is started. Driving or performing any tasks that require intense concentration should be delayed until you have taken
oxcarbazepine for a while and have become used to its effects.

If you forget to take a dose of oxcarbazepine, take it as soon
as you remember. If it is almost time for your next dose, skip the
dose you forgot and continue with your regular schedule. Do not
take a double dose. Contact your doctor if you forget 2 or more
doses in a row.

Special Populations

Pregnancy/Breast-feeding: Oxcarbazepine passes into the fetus
and fetal damage has been seen in animals given the drug. There
is no experience with oxcarbazepine in women, but it is likely
to cause fetal damage in humans. When this drug is considered

crucial by your doctor, its potential benefits must be weighed against its risks.

Oxcarbazepine passes into breast milk. Nursing mothers who must take it should consider using infant formula.

Seniors: Older adults are likely to have 30–60% more oxcarbazepine in their blood than younger people because of age-related differences in kidney function. Lower doses may be as effective as higher ones.

Generic Name

Oxybutynin (ox-ee-BYUE-tih-nin) Ⓖ

Brand Names
Ditropan   Oxytrol
Ditropan XL

Type of Drug
Antispasmodic and anticholinergic.

Prescribed For
Bladder instability including an urgent need to urinate, frequent urination, urinary leakage, and painful urination.

General Information
Oxybutynin directly affects the smooth muscle that controls the opening and closing of the bladder. It is 4–10 times more potent than atropine but much less likely to cause side effects.

Cautions and Warnings
Do not take oxybutynin if you are **allergic** or **sensitive** to any of its ingredients.

Oxybutynin should be used with caution if you have **glaucoma, urinary retention, intestinal obstruction or poor intestinal function, gastroesophageal reflux disease (GERD), megacolon,** severe or ulcerative **colitis, myasthenia gravis,** or unstable **heart disease** including abnormal heart rhythms, heart failure, or recent heart attack.

Oxybutynin should be used with caution if you have **liver or kidney disease.** It may worsen symptoms of an **overactive thyroid gland, coronary heart disease, abnormal heart rhythms, rapid heartbeat, high blood pressure, prostate disease,** or hiatal hernia.

Heat prostration may develop more easily while you are taking this drug because it makes you more sensitive to high temperatures. Oxybutynin should not be started in people with **diarrhea.**

Possible Side Effects

▼ Most common: dry mouth, drowsiness, decreased sweating, and constipation. Transdermal patch—itching where the patch is placed.

▼ Less common: diarrhea, upset stomach, headache, difficulty urinating, blurred vision, enlarging of the pupils, worsening of glaucoma, palpitations, sleeplessness, weakness, nausea, bloating, impotence, reduced production of breast milk, rash, and itching.

Drug Interactions

- Oxybutynin should be used with caution when combined with alcohol or other sedative medications.
- Combining oxybutynin and atenolol may increase the effect of atenolol.
- The use of oxybutynin with other anticholinergic agents may produce increased side effects and affect the absorption of other medications.
- Oxybutynin may affect haloperidol blood levels, which in turn may worsen schizophrenic symptoms.
- Oxybutynin may increase blood levels of digoxin, increasing the risk of side effects.
- Oxybutynin may interfere with levodopa + carbidopa.
- Oxybutynin may increase the effects of beta-blocking medications.
- Amantadine may increase oxybutynin side effects.
- Combining oxybutynin with a phenothiazine antipsychotic drug may decrease phenothiazine blood levels.

Food Interactions

Take oxybutynin with food or milk if it upsets your stomach.

Usual Dose

Ditropan

    Adult: 5–20 mg a day in divided doses.

    Child (age 6 and over): 5–15 mg a day in divided doses.

    Child (age 5 and under): not recommended.

Ditropan XL

Adult (age 18 and over): 5–30 mg once a day.
Child (age 6 and over): 5–20 mg once a day.
Child (age 5 and under): not recommended.

Transdermal System (Oxytrol)

Adult: Apply to dry, intact skin on the abdomen or buttock twice a week.

Overdosage

Symptoms may include restlessness, tremors, irritability, convulsions, hallucinations, flushing, fever, nausea, vomiting, rapid heartbeat, blood-pressure changes, respiratory failure, paralysis, delirium, urinary retention, and coma. Take the victim to a hospital emergency room at once. ALWAYS bring the prescription bottle or container.

Special Information

Contact your doctor if you develop severe or persistent diarrhea.

Oxybutynin can make you dizzy, blur your vision, and interfere with your ability to concentrate. Be careful while driving or doing any task that requires concentration or clear vision. Your eyes may also become more sensitive to bright light; wearing sunglasses should help to alleviate this problem.

In warm weather, people taking oxybutynin may be at an increased risk for heatstroke due to decreased sweating.

Dry mouth may be relieved with sugarless gum, candy, or ice chips. Excessive mouth dryness may lead to tooth decay and should be brought to your dentist's attention if it lasts for more than 2 weeks.

If you forget a dose, take it as soon as you remember. If it is almost time for your next dose, skip the dose you forgot and continue with your regular schedule. Do not take a double dose.

Special Populations

Pregnancy/Breast-feeding: The safety of using oxybutynin during pregnancy is not known. When this drug is considered crucial by your doctor, its potential benefits must be carefully weighed against its risks.

It is not known if oxybutynin passes into breast milk. Nursing mothers who must take this drug should consider using infant formula.

Seniors: Seniors may be more susceptible to side effects and should take this drug with caution.

Patanol   see *Olopatadine, page 838*

Paxil   see *Selective Serotonin Reuptake Inhibitors (SSRIs), page 1020*

Generic Name

Pemirolast   (pe-MEER-oh-last)

Brand Name
Alamast

Type of Drug
Ophthalmic mast cell stabilizer.

Prescribed For
Eye allergies and redness.

General Information
Pemirolast helps relieve allergy-related itchy, red eyes by stabilizing cells in eye tissue that are responsible for releasing a number of different chemicals that cause inflammation when in the presence of an allergen.

Cautions and Warnings
Do not use pemirolast if you are **allergic** or **sensitive** to any of its ingredients.

Do not wear **contact lenses** if your eyes are red or use pemirolast for irritation caused by contact lenses because the preservative in this drug may be absorbed by soft contacts.

Do not use this drug if you have an **eye infection,** unless you are also being treated for it.

Possible Side Effects

Serious side effects are not expected with pemirolast.
▼ Most common: burning, irritation, or dryness of the eyes or a feeling of having something in the eye.
▼ Common: headache, inflammation of the mucous membranes of the nose, and flu-like symptoms.

Food and Drug Interactions
None known.

Usual Dose
Adult and Child (age 3 and over): 1–2 drops in each affected eye 4 times a day.
Child (under age 3): not recommended.

Overdosage
The amount absorbed into the blood from a dose is very small but overdose might be expected to produce ordinary drug side effects. Call your local poison control center for more information.

Special Information
To avoid infection, do not touch the dropper tip to your finger, eyelid or any other surface. Keep the bottle cap tightly closed when it is not being used.

Do not wear contact lenses if your eyes are red. If you wear soft contact lenses, and your eyes are not red, remove them before each dose and wait at least 10 minutes after using pemirolast before putting in your lenses.

If you forget a dose of pemirolast, administer it as soon as you remember. If it is almost time for your next dose, skip the dose you forgot and continue with your regular schedule. Do not take a double dose.

Special Populations
Pregnancy/Breast-feeding: Pemirolast, given orally, causes birth defects and miscarriage in animals. Pregnant women should only use this drug if its potential benefits outweigh the possible risks.

Pemirolast passes into the breast milk of animals but no information is available for humans. Nursing mothers should consider using infant formula.

Seniors: Seniors may use pemirolast without special restriction.

Generic Name

Penciclovir (pen-SYE-kloe-veer)

Brand Name

Denavir

Type of Drug

Antiviral.

Prescribed For

Cold sores.

General Information

Penciclovir works against the different types of herpes viruses responsible for common cold sores. Cold sores treated with penciclovir cream go away sooner and are less painful than those that are not treated. Once applied to the skin, penciclovir is converted to its active form and interferes with DNA production inside the viral particle; this inhibits the reproduction process of the herpes virus.

Cautions and Warnings

Do not use penciclovir if you are **allergic** or **sensitive** to any of its ingredients.

Penciclovir should be applied only to the face or lips. Avoid applying it near your eyes because it may be irritating. The effectiveness of penciclovir in people with **compromised immune systems** is not known.

Male animals given massive doses of penciclovir intravenously suffered damage to the testicles. This effect appears to be related to the dose of penciclovir. Men using famciclovir—the oral form of penciclovir—for 8–13 weeks experienced no changes in sperm count.

Drug resistance may develop with repeated use.

Possible Side Effects

Side effects are generally mild and infrequent. In studies, side effects were similar in type and frequency among people who used penciclovir and those who used an inactive cream.

▼ Common: headache, redness, and swelling.

▼ Less common: skin reactions to the cream.

Possible Side Effects (continued)

▼ Rare: loss of skin sensation where the cream has been applied, changes in the sense of taste, and rash. Contact your doctor if you experience any side effect not listed above.

Drug and Food Interactions

None known.

Usual Dose

Adult and Child (age 12 and over): Apply to affected areas every 2 hours, during waking hours, for 4 days.

Child (under age 12): not recommended.

Overdosage

Little is known about the effects of penciclovir overdose or accidental ingestion. Call your poison control center or a hospital emergency room for more information. ALWAYS bring the prescription bottle or container.

Special Information

Begin cold sore treatment as early as possible. Early application of penciclovir cream will help prevent cold sores from appearing and reduce accompanying pain.

It is very important to apply penciclovir cream every 2 hours during the day for the drug to work. If you forget to apply a dose of penciclovir, apply it as soon as you remember. If you realize you forgot a dose within 30–45 minutes of your next dose, skip the dose you forgot and continue with your regular schedule.

Special Populations

Pregnancy/Breast-feeding: In animal studies, penciclovir had no effect on the fetus. There is no information on the effect of penciclovir in pregnant women. This drug should be used during pregnancy only if its possible benefits outweigh its risks.

It is not known if penciclovir passes into breast milk, though famciclovir—the oral form of penciclovir—passes into breast milk in concentrations larger than those found in the mother's blood. Nursing mothers who must use penciclovir should use infant formula.

Seniors: Seniors may use this drug without special precaution.

Type of Drug

Penicillin Antibiotics (pen-ih-SIL-in)

Brand Names

Generic Ingredient: Amoxicillin G
Amoxil   Larotid
DisperMox   Trimox

Generic Ingredients: Amoxicillin + Potassium Clavulanate G
Augmentin   Augmentin XR
Augmentin ES-600

Generic Ingredient: Carbenicillin Indanyl Sodium
Geocillin

Generic Ingredient: Cloxacillin Sodium G
Cloxapen

Generic Ingredient: Dicloxacillin Sodium G

Generic Ingredient: Oxacillin G
Bactocill

Generic Ingredient: Penicillin V Potassium G
Penicillin VK   Veetids

Prescribed For
Bacterial and other infections.

General Information
Penicillin antibiotics kill bacteria and other microorganisms by destroying the cell wall of the invading organisms. Many infections respond to almost any kind of penicillin; some respond only to a specific penicillin antibiotic. Penicillin cannot cure a cold, the flu, or any other viral infection and should never be taken unless prescribed by a doctor for a specific condition. Always take penicillin exactly as prescribed, including the number of pills to take every day and number of days to take the drug, otherwise you will not get the drug's full effect.

Cautions and Warnings
Do not take penicillin antibiotics if you are **allergic** or **sensitive** to any of their ingredients. Some of these medications contain

tartrazine dyes or sulfites, which may cause allergic reactions in certain people.

Serious and sometimes fatal allergic reactions have occurred with penicillin. Though more common following penicillin injections, these reactions have also occurred with oral penicillin. Reactions are more common among people who have had a previous penicillin reaction and those who have had asthma, hay fever, or other allergies. Allergic symptoms include itching, rash, swelling, breathing difficulties, very low blood pressure, blood vessel collapse, peeling skin, chills, fever, muscle aches, arthritis-like pains, and feeling unwell. Sometimes, when an infection is life-threatening and can only be treated with penicillin, minor reactions may be treated with another drug while the penicillin is continued. About 1 in 20 people allergic to a penicillin antibiotic are also allergic to the cephalosporin antibiotics.

Cystic fibrosis patients are more likely to suffer from side effects of certain penicillins.

People with **kidney disease** should not take carbenicillin.

Prolonged or repeated use of penicillin may lead to a secondary infection that cannot be treated by the penicillin being used.

Colitis is possible with any broad-spectrum antibiotic; contact your doctor if you have severe cramps or bloody diarrhea while taking penicillin.

Possible Side Effects

The most common penicillin side effect, seen in up to 10% of people, is allergy. About 9% of ampicillin users develop an itchy rash, which is not a true allergic reaction.

▼ Common: upset stomach, abdominal pain, nausea, vomiting, diarrhea, colitis (symptoms include severe abdominal cramps and severe, persistent, and possibly bloody diarrhea), sore mouth, coated tongue, anemia, bleeding abnormalities, low platelet and white-blood-cell counts, and oral or rectal fungal infections.

▼ Less common: vaginal irritation, appetite loss, itchy eyes, and feelings of body warmth.

▼ Rare: yellowing of the skin or whites of the eyes. Contact your doctor if you experience any side effect not listed above.

Drug Interactions

- Penicillin should not be combined with a bacteriostatic antibiotic such as chloramphenicol, erythromycin, tetracycline, or neomycin. These drugs can interfere with each other.
- Penicillin can interfere with contraceptive drugs. Use additional contraception while taking a penicillin drug. Breakthrough bleeding may occur.
- Penicillin allergies may be intensified by beta-blocking drugs.
- Combining some penicillins and allopurinol may increase the risk of rash and itching.
- Ampicillin may reduce the effect of atenolol.
- Combining penicillins and probenecid may increase blood levels of penicillin.
- Dicloxacillin may interfere with the effects of anticoagulant (blood-thinning) drugs such as warfarin.

Food Interactions

Do not take penicillin with fruit juice or carbonated beverages. The acid in these beverages may destroy the drug.

Drink a full glass of water with each glass of cloxacillin.

Most penicillins are best absorbed on an empty stomach. These medications may be taken 1 hour before or 2 hours after meals, or first thing in the morning and last thing at night with the other doses spaced evenly throughout the day.

Amoxicillin and penicillin V may be taken without regard to food.

Augmentin (amoxicillin + potassium clavulanate) is best taken right before a meal for optimum effectiveness and minimum stomach upset.

Usual Dose

Amoxicillin

Adult: 250–500 mg every 8 hours. Severe infections may require 875 mg every 12 hours.

Child (age 12 weeks and over): 10–20 mg per lb. a day divided into 3 doses.

Amoxicillin and Potassium Clavulanate

Adult: one 250-mg tablet every 8 hours; one 500-mg or 875-mg tablet every 12 hours. Different strengths of this product are not interchangeable. Take only the exact strength and product your doctor has prescribed.

Child (age 12 weeks and over): 10–20 mg per lb. a day divided into 2–3 doses.

Carbenicillin Indanyl Sodium
Adult: 1–2 tablets 4 times a day.
Child: not recommended.

Cloxacillin Sodium
Adult and Child (45 lbs. and over): 250–500 mg every 6 hours.
Child (under 45 lbs.): 11–23 mg per lb. a day divided into 4 doses.

Dicloxacillin Sodium
Adult and Child (90 lbs. and over): 125–250 mg every 6 hours.
Child (under 90 lbs.): 6–12 mg per lb. a day divided into 4 doses.

Oxacillin
Adult and Child (90 lbs. and over): 500–1000 mg every 4–6 hours.
Child (under 90 lbs.): 25–50 mg per lb. a day divided into 4 or 6 doses.

Penicillin V Potassium
Adult (age 12 and over): 125–500 mg every 6–8 hours. People with severe kidney disease should not take more than 250 mg every 6 hours.
Child (under age 12): 12–25 mg per lb. a day divided into 3 or 4 doses.

Overdosage

Overdose is unlikely, but diarrhea or upset stomach is the primary symptom. Massive overdose may result in seizure or excitability. Call your local poison control center or a hospital emergency room for more information. ALWAYS bring the prescription bottle or container.

Special Information

Liquid penicillin should be refrigerated and must be thrown out after 14 days in the refrigerator or 7 days at room temperature.

Call your doctor if you develop black tongue, rash, itching, hives, diarrhea, breathing difficulties, sore throat, nausea, vomiting, fever, swollen joints, unusual bleeding or bruising, or if you are feeling unwell.

Penicillin eradicates most susceptible organisms in 7–10 days; be sure to take all the medication prescribed for the full period of the prescription. It is best taken at evenly spaced intervals throughout the day.

Prolonged use of antibiotics may lead to a vaginal yeast infection. Contact your doctor if you develop symptoms such as vaginal itching, irritation, or discharge.

If you miss a dose, take it as soon as possible. If it is almost time for your next dose, space the missed dose and your next dose by 2–4 hours and then continue with your regular schedule.

Special Populations

Pregnancy/Breast-feeding: Penicillin crosses into the fetal circulation but has not been known to cause birth defects and is often prescribed for pregnant women. When this drug is considered crucial by your doctor, its potential benefits must be carefully weighed against its risks.

Penicillin is generally safe during breastfeeding; however, small amounts may pass into breast milk and cause upset stomach, diarrhea, allergic reaction, or other problems in the nursing infant. Women who are breastfeeding may want to consider using infant formula.

Seniors: Seniors may take penicillin without special precaution.

Generic Name

Pentosan Polysulfate Sodium
(PEN-toe-san pol-ee-SUL-fate)

Brand Name
Elmiron

Type of Drug
Kidney analgesic (pain reliever).

Prescribed For
Bladder pain or discomfort due to cystitis.

General Information
Interstitial cystitis is a painful, long-term infection of the bladder. Pentosan does not affect the infectious process, but it may stick to the membranes of the bladder wall, preventing irritating substances from reaching bladder cells. About ⅓ of people who take this drug for 3 months or more have less cystitis pain.

Cautions and Warnings

Do not take pentosan polysulfate sodium if you are **allergic** or **sensitive** to any of its ingredients.

Pentosan is a weak anticoagulant and can cause black-and-blue marks, nosebleeds, and bleeding gums. People with **aneurysms, thrombocytopenia, hemophilia,** or **gastrointestinal ulcerations, polyps, or diverticula** should be carefully evaluated before beginning therapy. People taking this drug who are also **taking another anticoagulant drug** or having **surgery** must be screened for internal bleeding by their doctor.

People with **liver disease** should use this drug with caution because its breakdown can be reduced in people with liver problems. Pentosan may also cause mild liver toxicity.

Possible Side Effects

▼ Most common: patchy hair loss beginning within 4 weeks of treatment, diarrhea, and nausea.

▼ Common: headache, emotional upset or depression, dizziness, abdominal pain, upset stomach, and rash.

▼ Rare: Rare side effects can include sleeplessness, bleeding, and effects on your blood, eyes, breathing, stomach and intestines, ears, and liver. Contact your doctor if you experience any side effect not listed above.

Drug Interactions

- Aspirin, clopidogrel, warfarin, and other blood-thinning drugs should be taken with caution if you are already taking pentosan. Pentosan may increase the anticoagulant effect of these drugs.

Food Interactions

Take this drug with water on an empty stomach, at least 1 hour before or 2 hours after a meal.

Usual Dose

Adult: 100 mg 3 times a day.
Child (under age 16): not recommended.

Overdosage

Symptoms may include bleeding, liver problems, and upset stomach. Overdose victims should be taken to a hospital emergency room at once. ALWAYS bring the prescription bottle or container.

Special Information

Pentosan has a mild anticoagulant effect. Make sure that your pharmacist, dentist, and all of your doctors know you are taking pentosan. Check with your doctor before combining aspirin or other drugs with pentosan.

Patchy hair loss, usually starting within the first 4 weeks of taking pentosan, occurs in about 4% of people who take this medication.

Pentosan should be taken exactly as directed. If you forget to take a dose of pentosan, take it as soon as you remember. If it is almost time for your next dose, skip the dose you forgot and continue with your regular schedule. Do not take a double dose.

Special Populations

Pregnancy/Breast-feeding: While animal studies of pentosan reveal no damage to the fetus, this drug should only be used during pregnancy after carefully weighing its potential benefits against its risks.

It is not known if pentosan passes into breast milk. Nursing mothers who must take it should consider using infant formula.

Seniors: Seniors may use this medication without special precaution.

Brand Name

Percocet

Generic Ingredients

Acetaminophen + Oxycodone Hydrochloride Ⓖ

Other Brand Names

Endocet	Roxicet 5/500
Magnacet	Roxilox
Perloxx	Tylox
Roxicet	

The information in this profile also applies to the following drugs:

Generic Ingredients: Acetaminophen + Codeine Phosphate Ⓖ

Aceta with Codeine	Tylenol with Codeine No. 2
Capital with Codeine	Tylenol with Codeine No. 3
Fioricet with Codeine	Tylenol with Codeine No. 4
Tylenol with Codeine	Vopac

Generic Ingredients: Acetaminophen + Hydrocodone Bitartrate G

Allay	Lorcet 10/650
Anexsia	Lortab
Anexsia 5/500	Lortab 2.5/500
Anexsia 7.5/650	Lortab 5/500
Anexsia 10/660	Lortab 7.5/500
Bancap HC	Lortab 10/500
Ceta-Plus	Margesic H
Co-Gesic	Maxidone
Dolacet	Norco
Duocet	Norco 5/325
Duradyne DHE	Panacet 5/500
Hycet	Stagesic
Hydrocet	T-Gesic
Hydrogesic	Vicodin
Hy-Phen	Vicodin-ES
Liquicet	Vicodin-HP
Lorcet-HD	Xodol
Lorcet Plus	Zydone

Generic Ingredients: Acetaminophen + Pentazocine G
Talacen

Generic Ingredient: Oxycodone Hydrochloride G

ETH-Oxydose	OxyIR
M-Oxy	Percolone
OxyContin	Roxicodone
OxyFast	

Type of Drug

Narcotic and analgesic (pain reliever) combination.

Prescribed For

Mild to moderate pain.

General Information

Percocet is generally prescribed for those who require a greater analgesic effect than acetaminophen alone can deliver or for those who cannot take aspirin. This medication is intended for those who need continuous pain management for an extended period of time; it is not used on an as-needed basis. Percocet is not considered effective for arthritis or other pain caused by inflammation because it does not reduce inflammation.

Cautions and Warnings

Do not take Percocet if you are **allergic** or **sensitive** to any of its ingredients.

Use this drug with extreme caution if you suffer from **asthma** or **other breathing problems** or have **kidney or liver disease** or **viral infection of the liver**. This drug should be used with caution if you have **head injuries, brain disease,** a history of **seizures, hypothyroidism** (underactive thyroid gland), **inflammatory bowel disease, gallstones or gallbladder disease, enlarged prostate,** or **urinary difficulties**.

Chronic (long-term) use of Percocet may cause drug dependence or addiction.

Percocet may cause postural low blood pressure (symptoms include dizziness or fainting when rising from a sitting or lying position).

Oxycodone is a respiratory depressant and affects the central nervous system (CNS), producing sleepiness, tiredness, and an inability to concentrate. **Alcohol** may increase the risk of oxycodone-related drowsiness.

For additional information see "Cautions and Warnings" in Acetaminophen, page 7.

Possible Side Effects

▼ Most common: lightheadedness, dizziness, sleepiness, nausea, vomiting, appetite loss, and increased sweating. If any of these effects occur, ask your doctor to consider lowering your dosage. Most of these side effects disappear if you lie down. More serious side effects, including shallow breathing or breathing difficulties, may occur at higher dosages.

▼ Less common: euphoria (feeling "high"), weakness, headache, agitation, uncoordinated muscle movements, minor hallucinations, disorientation, visual disturbances, dry mouth, constipation, facial flushing, rapid heartbeat, palpitations, feeling faint, urinary difficulties, reduced sex drive, impotence, rash, itching, depression, abdominal pain,

---

Possible Side Effects *(continued)*

anemia, low blood sugar, and yellowing of the skin or whites of the eyes. Narcotic pain relievers may aggravate convulsions in those who have had them.

For additional information see "Possible Side Effects" in Acetaminophen, page 7.

Drug Interactions

- Because of its depressant effect and potential effect on breathing, Percocet should be taken with extreme care in combination with alcohol, sleeping medications, sedatives, antihistamines, or other drugs producing sedation.
- The use of Percocet with anticholinergic medications may cause intestinal obstruction (severe constipation).

For additional information see "Drug Interactions" in Acetaminophen, page 7.

Food Interactions

Percocet is best taken with food or at least half a glass of water to prevent upset stomach.

Usual Dose

Acetaminophen + Codeine

Tablets

Adult and Child (age 12 and over): equivalent of 15–60 mg of codeine every 4 hours; do not exceed 360 mg a day.

Child (age 12 and under): equivalent of 0.22–0.45 mg of codeine per lb. every 4–6 hours; do not exceed 260 mg a day.

Child (under age 3): not recommended.

Elixir

Child (age 12 and over): 15mL every 4 hours.

Child (age 7–12 years): 10mL 3–4 times a day.

Child (age 3–6 years): 5mL 3–4 times a day.

Child (under age 3): not recommended.

Acetaminophen + Hydrocodone

Adult: 1 tablet every 4–6 hours; do not exceed 5 tablets a day.

Child: not recommended.

Acetaminophen + Oxycodone

Adult: 1–2 tablets every 4–6 hours. The daily dose should not exceed 8–12 tablets a day depending on the formulation.

Child: not recommended.

Acetaminophen + Pentazocine

Adult: 1 tablet every 4 hours; do not exceed 6 tablets a day.

Child: not recommended.

Oxycodone

Adult: starting dose—5–15 mg every 4–6 hours. Maintenance doses should be based on the lowest effective dosage given often enough to prevent severe pain from reoccurring.

Child: not recommended.

Overdosage

Symptoms include depressed respiration, extreme tiredness progressing to stupor and then coma, pinpointed pupils, no response to pain stimulation, cold and clammy skin, slowing of heart rate, lowering of blood pressure, yellowing of the skin or whites of the eyes, bluish discoloration of the hands or feet, fever, excitement, delirium, convulsions, cardiac arrest, and liver toxicity (symptoms include nausea, vomiting, abdominal pain, and diarrhea). Induce vomiting with ipecac syrup—available at any pharmacy—and take the victim to a hospital emergency room immediately. ALWAYS bring the prescription bottle or container.

Special Information

Percocet is a respiratory depressant that affects the CNS, producing sleepiness, tiredness, and inability to concentrate. Be careful when driving or performing any task that requires concentration.

Take Percocet before pain becomes too severe.

If you have been taking this medication for more than a few weeks, do not stop taking it without your doctor's instruction. Suddenly stopping this drug may lead to withdrawal symptoms.

Call you doctor if you experience breathing difficulties; persistent nausea, vomiting, or constipation; blurred vision; rash; or yellowing of the skin or eyes.

Take these medications whole; do not crush or chew tablets.

If you forget a dose, take it as soon as you remember. If it is almost time for your next dose, skip the dose you forgot and continue with your regular schedule. Do not take a double dose.

For additional information see "Special Information" in Acetaminophen, page 7.

Special Populations

Pregnancy/Breast-feeding: High doses of acetaminophen, one of the ingredients in Percocet, have caused problems when taken during pregnancy. Regular use of oxycodone, the other active ingredient in Percocet, during pregnancy may cause addiction in newborns. If used during labor, it may cause breathing problems in the infant. When this drug is considered crucial by your doctor, its potential benefits must be weighed against its risks.

The ingredients in Percocet may pass into breast milk. Nursing mothers who must take this drug should wait 4–6 hours after their last dose before nursing or they should consider using infant formula.

Seniors: Seniors may be sensitive to the depressant effects of this drug and may experience dizziness, lightheadedness, and fainting, particularly upon rising from a sitting or lying position.

Brand Name

Percodan

Generic Ingredients

Aspirin + Oxycodone Hydrochloride + Oxycodone Terephthalate G

Other Brand Names
Percodan-Demi   Roxiprin

The information in this profile also applies to the following drugs:

Generic Ingredients: Aspirin + Codeine Phosphate G
Ascomp with Codeine   Empirin with Codeine No. 4
Empirin with Codeine No. 3   Fiorinal with Codeine

Generic Ingredients: Aspirin + Caffeine + Dihydrocodeine Bitartrate G
Synalgos-DC

Generic Ingredients: Ibuprofen + Hydrocodone Bitartrate G
Reprexain   Vicoprofen

Generic Ingredients: Pentazocine + Aspirin
Talwin Compound

Generic Ingredients: Pentazocine + Naloxone Ⓖ
Talwin Nx

Type of Drug

Narcotic and aspirin combination.

Prescribed For

Moderate to moderately severe pain.

General Information

Percodan is one of many combination products containing a narcotic and a non-narcotic analgesic (pain reliever). It is prescribed to relieve pain and reduce inflammation.

Cautions and Warnings

Do not take Percodan if you are **allergic** or **sensitive** to any of its ingredients.

Use this medication with extreme caution if you suffer from **asthma** or **other breathing problems**. Percodan should also be used with caution if you have **kidney or liver disease, head injuries, brain disease,** a history of **seizures, hypothyroidism** (underactive thyroid gland), **inflammatory bowel disease, gallstones or gallbladder disease, peptic ulcer, enlarged prostate,** or **urinary difficulties**.

Percodan may cause postural low blood pressure (symptoms include dizziness or fainting when rising from a sitting or lying position).

Chronic (long-term) use of this drug may cause drug dependence or addiction.

Percodan is a respiratory depressant and affects the central nervous system (CNS), producing sleepiness, tiredness, and an inability to concentrate. **Alcohol** may increase the CNS depression caused by this drug.

For additional information, see "Cautions and Warnings" in Aspirin, page 110, and Ibuprofen, page 821.

Possible Side Effects

▼ Most common: lightheadedness, dizziness, sleepiness, nausea, vomiting, appetite loss, and increased sweating.

Possible Side Effects (continued)

If these occur, ask your doctor to consider lowering your dosage. Usually they go away if you lie down. More serious side effects, including shallow breathing or other breathing difficulties, may occur at higher dosages.

▼ Less common: euphoria (feeling "high"), depression, constipation, itching, low blood sugar, and yellowing of the skin or whites of the eyes. These drugs may aggravate convulsions in those who have had them.

For additional information, see "Possible Side Effects" in Aspirin, page 110, and Ibuprofen, page 821.

Drug Interactions

- Combining Percodan and alcohol, sedatives, barbiturates, sleeping medications, antihistamines, or other drugs producing sedation increases sleepiness or an inability to concentrate and significantly increases Percodan's depressive effect.

For additional information, see "Drug Interactions" in Aspirin, page 110, and Ibuprofen, page 821.

Food Interactions

Take with food or half a glass of water to prevent upset stomach.

Usual Dose

Percodan

Adult: 1 tablet every 6 hours as needed for pain; the maximum daily dose of aspirin should not exceed 4 g or 12 tablets.

Child: not recommended.

Empirin with Codeine, Ascomp with Codeine, and Fiorinal with Codeine

Adult: 1–2 tablets every 4 hours; not to exceed 6 tablets a day.

Child: not recommended.

Synalgos-DC

Adult: 2 capsules every 4 hours.

Child: not recommended.

Talwin Compound

Adult: 2 tablets 3–4 times a day.

Child: not recommended.

Talwin NX
Adult: 50 mg every 3–4 hours; increase to 100 mg if necessary. Daily dose should not exceed 600 mg.
Child: not recommended.

Vicoprofen
Adult: 1 tablet every 4–6 hours, up to 5 tablets a day.
Child: not recommended.

Overdosage

Symptoms include breathing difficulties, extreme tiredness progressing to stupor and then coma, pinpointed pupils, no response to pain stimulation, cold and clammy skin, slowing of heartbeat, dizziness or fainting, convulsions, cardiac arrest, fever, excitement, confusion, liver or kidney failure, and bleeding. Symptoms of mild overdose include nausea, vomiting, dizziness, ringing or buzzing in the ears, flushing, increased sweating, thirst, headache, drowsiness, diarrhea, and rapid heartbeat. Take the victim to a hospital emergency room immediately. ALWAYS bring the prescription bottle or container.

Special Information

Percodan may produce sleepiness, tiredness, or an inability to concentrate. Be careful when driving or performing any tasks that require concentration.

If you have been taking this medication for more than a few weeks, do not stop taking it without your doctor's instructions. Suddenly stopping this drug may lead to withdrawal symptoms.

Call your doctor if you experience breathing difficulties or persistent nausea, vomiting, or constipation.

If you forget a dose, take it as soon as you remember. If it is almost time for your next dose, skip the one you forgot and continue with your regular schedule. Do not take a double dose.

For additional information, see "Special Information" in Aspirin, page 110, and Ibuprofen, page 821.

Special Populations

Pregnancy/Breast-feeding: Aspirin, one of the ingredients in Percodan, may cause bleeding problems in the fetus, particularly during the last 2 weeks of pregnancy. Taking aspirin during the last 3 months of pregnancy may produce a low-birth-weight infant, prolong labor, and extend the duration of pregnancy; it may also cause bleeding in the mother before, during, or after delivery. Large amounts of oxycodone, the other ingredient in Percodan, may cause addiction in newborns. It may also cause breathing problems in newborns if taken just before delivery. When Percodan is considered crucial by your doctor, its potential benefits must be carefully weighed against its risks.

The ingredients in Percodan may pass into breast milk. Nursing mothers who must take this drug should consider using infant formula.

Seniors: Seniors may be more sensitive to the depressant effects of this drug as well as dizziness, lightheadedness, and fainting, particularly upon rising suddenly from a sitting or lying position.

Generic Name

Permethrin (per-MEE-thrin) Ⓖ

Brand Names

Acticin   Elimite

Type of Drug

Scabicide.

Prescribed For

Scabies and head lice.

General Information

Permethrin is a synthetic chemical that kills lice, ticks, mites, and fleas. It paralyzes the parasite by interfering with its nervous system. Less than 1% of people who use permethrin for head lice need to be retreated because it kills both the parasite and its eggs. Permethrin, which remains on hair shafts after application, prevents reinfection for up to 2 weeks. Less than 2% of permethrin is absorbed through the skin into the bloodstream.

Cautions and Warnings

Do not use permethrin if you are **allergic** or **sensitive** to any of its ingredients or to chrysanthemums. Stop using permethrin if you develop a reaction to it.

Permethrin may cause breathing difficulties, especially in those with **asthma**.

<hr>

Possible Side Effects

Cream

▼ Most common: burning and stinging.

▼ Common: mild, temporary itching.

▼ Rare: tingling, numbness, mild swelling, and rash. Contact your doctor if you experience any side effect not listed above.

Liquid

▼ Common: mild, temporary itching.

▼ Less common: mild, temporary burning or stinging; tingling; numbness; discomfort; mild swelling; and rash.

<hr>

Drug Interactions

● Do not apply this product with any other topical medication.

Usual Dose

Adult and Child (age 2 months and over)

Cream (for scabies): Thoroughly massage the cream into the skin from the head to the soles of the feet; 1 oz. (30 g) is usually enough for a single treatment of an adult. Infants should be treated at the hairline, neck, scalp, and forehead. Leave the cream on for 8–14 hours and then remove it by washing.

Liquid (for head lice): Wash your hair with regular shampoo, rinse, and towel dry. Then, apply enough permethrin liquid to saturate the hair and scalp; leave it in for 10 minutes. Rinse off with water. Repeat if lice reoccur within 7 days.

Child (under age 2 months): not recommended.

Overdosage

In case of accidental ingestion, call your local poison control center or a hospital emergency room. You may be told to induce vomiting with ipecac syrup—available at any pharmacy—before taking the victim to an emergency room. If you seek treatment, ALWAYS bring the prescription bottle or container.

Special Information

This drug should be applied only to the skin. It should never be swallowed.

Do not apply permethrin to areas around the eyes, nose, or mouth. Call your doctor if anything unusual develops or if irritation continues after you have stopped using the drug.

Use the comb provided to remove any remaining nits.

Be sure to wash any personal articles that may be infected such as clothing, sheets, pillows, combs, and brushes in hot water.

Special Populations

Pregnancy/Breast-feeding: The safety of using permethrin during pregnancy is not known. When this drug is considered crucial by your doctor, its potential benefits must be carefully weighed against its risks.

It is not known if permethrin passes into breast milk. Nursing mothers who must use it should use infant formula.

Seniors: This drug may be used without special precaution.

Generic Name

Phenelzine (FEH-nel-zeen) Ⓖ

Brand Name

Nardil

The information in this profile also applies to the following drug:

Generic Ingredient: Tranylcypromine Sulfate Ⓖ
Parnate

Type of Drug

Monoamine oxidase inhibitor (MAOI).

Prescribed For

Atypical depression and depression that does not respond to other drugs; also prescribed for a variety of conditions including bulimia, night terrors, bipolar depression, panic disorder, post-traumatic stress disorder, chronic migraine, and social anxiety disorder.

General Information

Monoamine oxidase (MAO) is a complex enzyme system found throughout the body. MAO is responsible for breaking down hormones that make the nervous system work. MAO inhibitors (MAOIs) such as phenelzine interfere with MAO action, causing an increase in the amount of serotonin, dopamine, and norepinephrine stored throughout the nervous system. This increase is what gives phenelzine its therapeutic effect, which is long-lasting and may continue for up to 2 weeks after you stop taking it.

Cautions and Warnings

Do not take phenelzine if you are **allergic** or **sensitive** to any of its ingredients or to any MAOI.

Do not take phenelzine if you have **pheochromocytoma** (adrenal gland tumor), **heart failure, liver disease** or **abnormal liver function,** severe **kidney-function loss, heart disease,** or a history of **headaches, stroke, transient ischemic attack** (TIA)— "mini-stroke"—or **high blood pressure**.

The most severe reactions to phenelzine, which can be deadly, involve very high blood pressure. Bleeding in the brain has occurred in people with very high blood pressure. Serious, potentially fatal reactions may occur if phenelzine and another antidepressant, especially a **selective serotonin reuptake inhibitor (SSRI),** are taken together (see "Drug Interactions").

Suicidal thoughts and actions have occurred in **children** and **teens** taking phenelzine. Warning signs to look for include agitation, irritability, and unusual behavior changes, especially during the first few months of drug therapy or when drug dosage is increased or decreased. Phenelzine is not approved for use in children under age 16.

Possible Side Effects

Phenelzine
▼ Common: dizziness, especially when rising from a sitting or lying position, drowsiness, fatigue, sleep disturbances, twitching, constipation, weight gain, dry mouth, and sexual disturbances.
▼ Less common: jitteriness, euphoria (feeling "high"), rash, sweating, blurred vision, and electric-shock sensations.

Tranylcypromine
▼ Common: dizziness, restlessness, jitteriness, dry mouth, diarrhea, insomnia, headache, weight loss, and nausea.
▼ Less common: fast heartbeat, drowsiness, constipation, blurred vision, electric-shock sensations, and jerkiness.

Drug Interactions

- Do not ever combine phenelzine with meperidine, as fatal effects may occur.
- Bupropion, buspirone, sibutramine, atomoxetine, or carbamazepine should not be combined with phenelzine.

- Phenelzine interferes with the blood-pressure-lowering effect of guanethidine. Do not combine these drugs.
- Taking an SSRI antidepressant and phenelzine at the same time or too close together may result in a serious, sometimes fatal reaction characterized by very high fever, rigidity, muscle spasms, and changes in mental state, blood pressure, pulse, and breathing rate. Two weeks should elapse between stopping an MAOI and starting an SSRI. At least 2 weeks should usually elapse between stopping an SSRI and starting an MAOI; for fluoxetine, the wait is 5 weeks.
- A tricyclic antidepressant and phenelzine may be combined only under your doctor's direct supervision. If dosages are not strictly controlled, this combination can lead to seizures, sweating, coma, hyperexcitability, high fever, rapid heartbeat, rapid breathing, headache, dilated pupils, flushing, confusion, and low blood pressure. When severe, this reaction can be fatal. Generally, 2 weeks must pass between stopping phenelzine and taking a tricyclic antidepressant.
- Phenelzine increases the effects of sulfonylurea-type antidiabetic drugs, barbiturates, beta blockers, levodopa + carbidopa, methyldopa, rauwolfia drugs, sulfa drugs, sumatriptan, stimulants, thiazide-type diuretics, and L-tryptophan. The combination of any of these drugs and phenelzine can result in severe reactions.
- Combining dextromethorphan (a cough suppressant found in many over-the-counter products) and phenelzine may lead to a high fever and low blood pressure. Avoid this combination.
- Combining phenelzine with another MAOI, methylphenidate, or dexmethylphenidate may lead to excessively high blood pressure.
- Combining tranylcypromine sulfate and disulfiram may lead to delirium, agitation, disorientation, and hallucinations.
- Do not combine phenelzine with ginseng.

Food Interactions

Avoid foods with a high dopamine, tyramine, or tryptophan level such as the following while taking phenelzine and for at least 2 weeks after stopping phenelzine as they may lead to severe high blood pressure:

Alcohol: imported beer and ale; red wine, especially Chianti; sherry; vermouth; and distilled spirits.

Cheese and Dairy: processed American cheese, blue cheese, Boursault, natural brick cheese, Brie, Camembert, cheddar, Emmenthaler, Gruyere, mozzarella, Parmesan, Romano, Roquefort, sour cream, Stilton, Swiss cheese, and yogurt.

Fruits and Vegetables: avocados, especially when overripe; yeast extracts, including Marmite; canned figs; raisins; sauerkraut; soy sauce; miso soup; and bean curd.

Meat and Fish: beef or chicken liver, meats prepared with a tenderizer, summer sausage, bologna, pepperoni, salami, game, meat extracts, caviar, dried fish, anchovies, salted herring, pickled and spoiled herring, and shrimp paste.

Other: fava beans, ginseng, caffeine, and some chocolate.

Many other foods are contraindicated as well. Consult your doctor for a list of these foods.

Usual Dose
Phenelzine
Adult and Child (age 16 and over): 15 mg 3 times a day to start, increased gradually to 60–90 mg a day.

Senior: 15 mg in the morning. Dosage is increased very gradually.

Child (under age 16): not recommended.

Tranylcypromine Sulfate
Adult and Child (age 16 and over): 10–60 mg a day. Usual dosage is 30 mg a day.

Senior: starting dosage—2.5–5 mg a day.

Child (under age 16): not recommended.

Overdosage
Early symptoms may include excitement; irritability; hyperactivity; anxiety; low blood pressure; vascular system collapse; sleeplessness; restlessness; dizziness; fainting; weakness; drowsiness; hallucinations; jaw-muscle spasms; flushing; sweating; rapid breathing; rapid heartbeat; movement disorders, including grimacing, rigidity, muscle tremors, and large-muscle spasms; and severe headache. Death may occur. Take the victim to a hospital emergency room at once. ALWAYS bring the prescription bottle or container.

Special Information
Serious side effects include intense headache; heart palpitations; stiff or sore neck; nausea; vomiting; sweating, sometimes accompanied by fever or cold, clammy skin; dilated pupils; and

sensitivity to bright light. Report these or any bothersome or persistent side effect to your doctor.

Vivid nightmares, agitation, psychosis, and convulsions occasionally occur 1–3 days after phenelzine is abruptly stopped. Gradually stopping phenelzine should prevent these problems.

Phenelzine may cause drowsiness and blurred vision. Be careful when driving or performing any task that requires concentration. Avoid alcohol.

People with diabetes should be cautious because this drug may lower blood-sugar readings.

Be sure your surgeon or dentist knows that you are taking phenelzine before administering any anesthetic drug.

Do not take any other prescription or over-the-counter drug without first checking with your pharmacist or the doctor who prescribed phenelzine. Specific drugs to avoid include cough and cold medicines, decongestants, hay fever and asthma medicines, sinus medicines, weight-loss medications, energy pills and drinks, and products containing l-tryptophan.

If you forget a dose, take it as soon as possible. If it is less than 2 hours until your next dose, skip the dose you forgot and continue with your regular schedule. Do not take a double dose.

Special Populations

Pregnancy/Breast-feeding: Phenelzine may pass into the fetal circulation. When this drug is considered crucial by your doctor, its potential benefits must be carefully weighed against its risks.

This drug may pass into breast milk. Nursing mothers who must take it should use infant formula.

Seniors: Seniors are more susceptible to side effects and must use caution.

Generic Name

Phenobarbital (FEEN-oe-BAR-bih-tol) Ⓖ

Brand Name
Solfoton

Type of Drug
Hypnotic, sedative, and anticonvulsant.

Prescribed For

Epileptic and other seizures, convulsions, daytime sedation, and sleeplessness in the short term.

General Information

Phenobarbital is a sustained-release barbiturate. It takes 30–60 minutes to start working and its effect lasts for 10–16 hours. Like other barbiturates, phenobarbital appears to act by interfering with nerve impulses to the brain. When used as an anticonvulsant, phenobarbital is not very effective by itself; when used with anticonvulsant agents such as phenytoin, the combined action is dramatic. This combination has been used very successfully to control epileptic seizures. When used to treat insomnia, phenobarbital loses its effectiveness after 2 weeks.

Cautions and Warnings

Do not take phenobarbital if you are **allergic** or **sensitive** to any of its ingredients or to any barbiturate, have been **addicted to sedatives or hypnotics**, or have a **respiratory condition**.

Phenobarbital may dull your physical and mental reflexes. Be extremely careful when driving or performing any task that requires concentration.

Phenobarbital is a Schedule IV drug and is considered a controlled substance. It may be addictive if taken for an extended period of time. It may also cause signs of intoxication including slurred speech, a wobbly walk, rolling of the eyes, confusion, poor judgment, irritability, and sleeplessness. Combining this drug with alcohol or any other central-nervous-system (CNS) depressant worsens the situation. Barbiturates should be used with caution by people who have **depression** or **suicidal tendencies.**

Barbiturates are broken down in the liver and eliminated through the kidneys; people with **liver or kidney disease** should be cautious about taking phenobarbital.

People with **chronic pain** should be careful about taking this drug because it may mask symptoms or cause stimulation, though using phenobarbital after surgery and in people with cancer has proven effective.

People abruptly stopping this drug may develop seizures. Dosage should be reduced gradually. The symptoms of barbiturate withdrawal may be severe and can be fatal.

Barbiturates may increase your need for vitamin D; take a vitamin supplement while using this drug.

Possible Side Effects

▼ Most common: drowsiness, lethargy, headache, dizziness, drug "hangover," breathing difficulties, rash, and general allergic reaction (symptoms include runny nose, watery eyes, sneezing, scratchy throat, and cough).

▼ Less common: nausea, vomiting, constipation, diarrhea, slow heartbeat, low blood pressure, and fainting. Severe adverse reactions may include anemia and yellowing of the skin or whites of the eyes.

Drug Interactions

- Alcohol and other CNS depressants, monoamine oxidase inhibitor antidepressants, and valproic acid increase the effects of phenobarbital.
- Charcoal, chloramphenicol, and rifampin may counteract the effects of phenobarbital.
- Amphetamines can delay the absorption of phenobarbital into the bloodstream.
- Phenobarbital interferes with the effects of anticoagulant (blood-thinning) drugs, beta-blocking drugs, carbamazepine, chloramphenicol, contraceptive drugs, corticosteroids, clonazepam, digitoxin, doxorubicin, doxycycline, felodipine, fenoprofen, griseofulvin, metronidazole, phenylbutazone, quinidine, theophylline, and verapamil.
- Phenobarbital enhances the toxic effects of acetaminophen and methoxyflurane (an anesthetic).
- Phenobarbital has a variable effect on phenytoin and other antiseizure medication and on narcotic drugs. Dosage adjustments are necessary.

Food Interactions

Phenobarbital is best taken on an empty stomach but may be taken with food if it upsets your stomach.

Usual Dose

Anticonvulsant

    Adult: 60–100 mg a day.

    Child: 1.3–2.25 mg per lb. of body weight divided into 2 or 3 doses a day.

Sleeplessness: 100–200 mg at bedtime.

Daytime Sedation
    Adult: 30–120 mg in 2–3 divided doses.
    Child: 8–32 mg a day.

Overdosage

Severe barbiturate overdose may be fatal. Overdose symptoms include breathing difficulties, moderate reduction in pupil size, lowered body temperature progressing to fever, fluid in the lungs, and eventually coma. Take the victim to a hospital emergency room immediately. ALWAYS bring the prescription bottle or container.

Special Information

Avoid alcohol and other drugs that depress the nervous system such as other sedatives, hypnotics, or antihistamines.

Take this medication exactly as prescribed.

This drug causes drowsiness. Be careful when driving or doing any task that requires concentration.

Call your doctor at once if you develop fever, sore throat, nosebleeds, mouth sores, unexplainable black-and-blue marks, or easy bruising or bleeding.

If you forget a dose, take it as soon as you remember. If it is almost time for your next dose, skip the one you forgot and continue with your regular schedule. Do not take a double dose.

Special Populations

Pregnancy/Breast-feeding: Barbiturate use during pregnancy may increase the risk of birth defects and cause bleeding problems, brain tumors, and breathing difficulties in newborns. Regular use of a barbiturate during the last 3 months of pregnancy may cause drug dependency in newborns. However, phenobarbital may be necessary to control major episodes of seizure during pregnancy. Talk to your doctor about the potential benefits and risks of using phenobarbital.

Barbiturates pass into breast milk. They may cause drowsiness, slow heartbeat, and breathing difficulties in infants. Nursing mothers who must take phenobarbital should use infant formula.

Seniors: Seniors are more sensitive to the effects of barbiturates and often need less medication.

Generic Name

Phenytoin (FEN-ih-toin) Ⓖ

Brand Names

Dilantin	Dilantin Kapseals
Dilantin-125	Phenytek
Dilantin Infatab	

The information in this profile also applies to the following drugs:

Generic Ingredient: Ethotoin
Peganone

Generic Ingredient: Fosphenytoin
Cerebyx

Type of Drug

Hydantoin anticonvulsant.

Prescribed For

Epileptic seizure; also prescribed for prevention of seizure following neurosurgery in nonepileptics and for abnormal heart rhythm.

General Information

Phenytoin is the most widely prescribed of several hydantoin antiseizure drugs. These drugs all inhibit activity in that area of the brain responsible for grand mal seizures. People may respond to some hydantoins and not others.

Immediate-release phenytoin must be taken several times a day, while the sustained-release form can be taken either once or several times a day. Many people find the latter more convenient, but the immediate-release form allows your doctor more flexibility in designing an effective dosage schedule. Phenytoin may be used together with other anticonvulsants, such as phenobarbital.

Drugs that control grand mal seizures do not affect petit mal seizures. Combined drug therapy is needed if both conditions are to be treated.

Cautions and Warnings

Do not take phenytoin if you are **allergic** or **sensitive** to any of its ingredients or to any hydantoin anticonvulsant.

When discontinuing phenytoin, dosage should be gradually reduced over a period of about a week—otherwise, severe seizures may occur.

Phenytoin should not be used if you have **low blood pressure, myocardial insufficiency,** a very **slow heart rate,** or certain other **heart conditions**.

People with **liver disease** are more likely to experience phenytoin side effects.

Periodic blood tests are necessary to monitor red- and white-blood-cell counts. Sore throat, feeling unwell, fever, mucous-membrane bleeding, swollen glands, nosebleeds, black-and-blue marks, and easy bruising may be signs of blood disorders.

Rash may be a sign of a serious reaction and cause for stopping this medication. Tell your doctor at once if this happens.

If lymph node enlargement occurs, contact your doctor; you may be advised to substitute another anticonvulsant drug or drug combination.

Possible Side Effects

▼ Most common: drowsiness, rapid or unusual growth of the gums, slurred speech, mental confusion, nystagmus (rhythmic, uncontrolled movement of the eye), dizziness, insomnia, nervousness, uncontrollable twitching, double vision, tiredness, irritability, depression, tremors, and headache. These side effects generally disappear as therapy continues and dosage is reduced.

▼ Less common: nausea, vomiting, diarrhea, constipation, fever, rash, balding, weight gain, numbness in the hands or feet, chest pain, bronchitis, cough, water retention, sensitivity to bright light (especially sunlight), conjunctivitis (pink-eye), joint pain and inflammation, and high blood sugar. Phenytoin may cause coarse facial features, lip enlargement, and Peyronie's disease (in which the penis is permanently deformed or misshapen). Phenytoin rash may be accompanied by fever and may be serious or fatal. Some fatal blood-system side effects have occurred with phenytoin.

▼ Rare: liver damage (including hepatitis and jaundice) and unusual body-hair growth. Contact your doctor if you experience any side effect not listed above.

Drug Interactions

- The following drugs may increase the effects of phenytoin, possibly necessitating a decrease in phenytoin dosage: alcohol in small amounts, allopurinol, amiodarone, aspirin and other salicylate drugs, benzodiazepine drugs, chloramphenicol, chlorpheniramine, cimetidine, disulfiram, fluconazole, ibuprofen, isoniazid, metronidazole, miconazole, omeprazole, phenacemide, phenothiazine antipsychotic drugs, phenylbutazone, succinimide antiseizure drugs, sulfa drugs, tricyclic antidepressants, trimethoprim, and valproic acid.
- The following drugs may interfere with the effects of phenytoin, possibly necessitating an increase in phenytoin dosage: large amounts of alcohol, antacids, anticancer drugs, barbiturates, carbamazepine, charcoal tablets, diazoxide, folic acid, influenza virus vaccine, loxapine succinate, nitrofurantoin, pyridoxine, rifampin, sucralfate, and theophylline drugs.
- Calcium supplements may slow the absorption of phenytoin.
- Phenytoin may reduce the effectiveness of acetaminophen, amiodarone, carbamazepine, corticosteroids, dicumarol, digitalis drugs, disopyramide, doxycycline, estrogen drugs, haloperidol, methadone, metyrapone, mexiletine, contraceptive drugs, quinidine, theophylline drugs, and valproic acid. Dosage increases may be necessary.
- Phenytoin may increase the risk of liver toxicity caused by acetaminophen, especially if phenytoin is taken regularly.
- Phenytoin may affect certain other drugs in an unpredictable manner. If you take phenytoin and one or more of these drugs, your doctor will have to determine if dosage adjustment is needed: cyclosporine, dopamine, furosemide, levodopa + carbidopa, levonorgestrel, mebendazole, phenothiazine antipsychotic drugs, and oral antidiabetes drugs.
- Combining clonazepam and phenytoin yields unpredictable results: The effect of either drug may be reduced or phenytoin side effects may occur.
- Corticosteroid drugs may mask the effects of phenytoin sensitivity reactions.
- Lithium toxicity may be increased if lithium is taken with phenytoin.
- Phenytoin may decrease meperidine's pain-relieving effects and increase the risk of meperidine side effects. This combination is not recommended.

- Long-term phenytoin therapy may result in extreme folic acid deficiency, or megaloblastic anemia. This imbalance may be corrected with folic acid supplements.
- Warfarin's effects may be increased by phenytoin; warfarin dosage must be adjusted.

Food Interactions

Take phenytoin with food to avoid stomach upset. Calcium can slow phenytoin absorption. Separate your phenytoin dose from high-calcium foods, such as milk, cheese, almonds, hazelnuts, and sesame seeds and calcium supplements, by 1–2 hours.

Usual Dose

Adult: starting dosage—300 mg a day. Maintenance dosage—300–400 mg a day. Dosage can be raised gradually to 600 mg a day. Sustained-release phenytoin is taken once a day; the immediate-release form must be taken throughout the day.

Child: starting dosage—2.5 mg per lb. of body weight a day, divided into 2 or 3 equal doses. Maintenance dosage—2–4 mg per lb. of body weight a day. Dosage should be adjusted according to the child's needs. Children age 6 and over may take the adult dosage, but no child should take more than 300 mg a day.

Overdosage

Initial symptoms include drug side effects. At lethal doses, victim may become comatose with unresponsive pupils. Take the victim to a hospital emergency room at once. ALWAYS bring the prescription bottle or container.

Special Information

Call your doctor at once if you feel unwell or develop a rash, severe nausea or vomiting, swollen glands, swollen or tender gums, yellowing of the skin or whites of the eyes, joint pain, sore throat, fever, unusual bleeding or bruising, persistent headache, infection, slurred speech, or poor coordination.

Always carry a medic alert identification that indicates your medication usage and epilepsy status.

Do not stop taking phenytoin or change dosage without your doctor's knowledge.

Phenytoin may cause drowsiness, dizziness, or blurred vision, effects which are increased by alcoholic beverages. Be careful when driving or doing any task that requires concentration.

Phenytoin sometimes produces a pink-brown color in the urine, which is normal and not a cause for concern.

People with diabetes who take phenytoin must monitor their urine regularly and report any changes to their doctors.

Good oral hygiene—including gum massage, frequent brushing, and flossing—is very important because phenytoin can cause abnormal growth of your gums.

Do not switch phenytoin brands without notifying your doctor. Different brands may not be equivalent.

If you use phenytoin suspension, be sure to shake the bottle vigorously just before a dose.

Do not use phenytoin capsules that have become discolored. Throw them away.

If you forget a dose, take it as soon as you remember. If you take phenytoin once a day and it is almost time for your next dose, skip the one you forgot and continue with your regular schedule. If you take phenytoin several times a day and do not remember it within 4 hours of your regular time, skip the forgotten dose and go back to your regular schedule. Never take a double dose.

Special Populations

Pregnancy/Breast-feeding: Phenytoin crosses into the fetal circulation. The great majority of mothers who take phenytoin deliver healthy babies, but some are born with cleft lip, cleft palate, or heart malformations. There is a recognized group of deformities, fetal hydantoin syndrome, which affects children of women taking phenytoin, though the drug has not been definitively established as the cause. This syndrome consists of skull and face abnormalities, reduced brain size, growth deficiency, deformed fingernails, and mental deficiency. Phenytoin increases the risk of vitamin K deficiency in newborns, which can lead to serious, life-threatening bleeding during the first 24 hours of life. Also, mothers taking phenytoin may be deficient in vitamin K, increasing the risk of bleeding during delivery.

Phenytoin passes into breast milk. Nursing mothers who must take it should use infant formula.

Seniors: Seniors are more sensitive to side effects.

Generic Name

Pimecrolimus (pih-meh-CRO-lim-us)

Brand Name

Elidel Cream

Type of Drug

Immune system modulator.

Prescribed For

Mild to moderate eczema.

General Information

The exact way that pimecrolimus works in the management of mild to moderate dermatitis is unknown. However, it is related to drugs that are used to prevent organ rejection in transplant patients. Extremely small amounts of pimecrolimus are absorbed into the blood after application to the skin. Even after long-term use on more than half of the body, blood levels of pimecrolimus cannot be detected.

Cautions and Warnings

Do not take pimecrolimus if you are **allergic** or **sensitive** to any of its ingredients or to other related drugs.

Do not apply pimecrolimus cream to infected skin.

Pimecrolimus may cause a mild warmth or burning sensation. Contact your doctor if this reaction persists for more than 1 week.

Pimecrolimus has been linked to an increased risk of cancer. Use for the shortest amount of time possible and only after other treatments have failed.

Pimecrolimus should not be used on children under age 2.

Possible Side Effects

▼ Most common: skin burning, headache, sore throat (with or without nasal pain), infections, fever, and cough.

▼ Less common: tonsillitis, sore throat, chickenpox, runny nose, worsening asthma, wheezing, nosebleeds, painful menstruation, conjunctivitis (pinkeye), eye irritation after application near eyes or lids, skin irritation, back pain, joint pain, and earache.

Possible Side Effects *(continued)*

▼ Rare: herpes infection; itching; allergic reations; swelling of the face, lips, or other application site; toothache; constipation or loose stool; and abdominal pain. Contact your doctor if you experience any side effect not listed above.

Drug Interactions

Potential interactions between pimecrolimus and other drugs, including immunizations, have not been studied. Interactions are not expected but may still occur.

- Patients with widespread skin disease should avoid combining pimecrolimus with drugs that inhibit the liver enzyme CYP3A, including calcium channel blockers, cimetidine, erythromycin, fluconazole, itraconazole, and ketoconazole.

Food Interactions

None known.

Usual Dose

Adult and Child (age 2 and over): apply a thin layer of pimecrolimus to the affected skin twice a day. Rub in gently and completely.

Child (under age 2): not recommended.

Overdosage

There have been no cases of pimecrolimus accidental ingestion. Call your local poison control center or emergency room for more information. If you seek treatment, ALWAYS bring the prescription bottle or container.

Special Information

Call your doctor if your condition does not improve after 6 weeks of using pimecrolimus cream.

Notify your doctor if you develop swollen lymph glands, or if warts, blemishes, or any other side effect worsen while using pimecrolimus.

Drinking alcohol while using pimecrolimus may cause adverse effects such as skin flushing or redness.

Avoid exposure to the sun or to artificial sun lamps while using pimecrolimus.

Use pimecrolimus cream only as directed by your doctor. It is only for external application to the skin.

Wash your hands after applying pimecrolimus cream, unless your hands are the area being treated.

Do not bathe, shower, or swim immediately after applying pimecrolimus cream. This could wash off the cream.

Stop using pimecrolimus after your eczema has healed. You can begin using pimecrolimus cream again if the condition recurs.

Do not cover the skin being treated with bandages, dressings, or wraps.

Special Populations

Pregnancy/Breast-feeding: While animal studies of pimecrolimus reveal no damage to the fetus, this drug should only be used during pregnancy after carefully weighing its potential benefits against its risks.

It is not known if pimecrolimus passes into breast milk. Nursing mothers who must take it should use infant formula.

Seniors: The effects of pimecrolimus on seniors is not known.

Generic Name

Pindolol (PIN-doe-lol) G

Brand Name

Visken

Type of Drug

Beta-adrenergic blocking agent.

Prescribed For

High blood pressure, abnormal heart rhythms, side effects of antipsychotic drugs, and stage fright and other anxieties.

General Information

Pindolol is one of many beta-adrenergic blocking drugs, or beta blockers, that interfere with the action of a specific part of the nervous system. Beta receptors are found all over the body and affect many body functions. Each beta blocker has particular characteristics that make it more suitable for certain conditions or people. Pindolol is a mild heart stimulant, which is an advantage for some. When prescribed to treat high blood pressure, pindolol may be taken alone or in combination with other antihypertensive drugs.

Cautions and Warnings

Do not take pindolol if you are **allergic** or **sensitive** to any ingredients or to beta blockers.

You should be cautious about taking pindolol if you have **asthma, severe heart failure,** a **very slow heart rate,** or **heart block** (disruption of the electrical impulses that control heart rate) because the drug may aggravate these conditions.

Pindolol should be used with caution if you have **chronic bronchitis** or **emphysema**, as it may block bronchodilation.

Do not stop taking pindolol without consulting your doctor, as the result may be chest pain or heart attack.

People with **angina** who take pindolol for high blood pressure risk aggravating their angina if they suddenly stop taking the drug. These people should have their drug dosage reduced gradually over 1–2 weeks.

Pindolol should be used with caution if you have **liver or kidney disease** because your ability to eliminate the drug from your body may be impaired.

Pindolol reduces the amount of blood pumped by the heart with each beat. This reduction in blood flow may aggravate the condition of people with **poor circulation** or **circulatory disease**.

Pindolol should be used with caution in people with **diabetes,** as it may affect glycemic response.

If you are undergoing **major surgery,** your doctor may want you to stop taking pindolol at least 2 days before surgery (see "Drug Interactions"). This is a controversial practice and may not be recommended for all surgeries.

People with a history of **severe anaphylactic reaction** to allergens may be unresponsive to usual doses of epinephrine while taking beta blockers.

Possible Side Effects

Side effects are relatively uncommon and usually mild.
▼ Most common: impotence.
▼ Less common: unusual tiredness or weakness, slow heartbeat, heart failure, dizziness, breathing difficulties, bronchospasm, depression, confusion, anxiety, nervousness, sleeplessness, disorientation, short-term memory loss, emotional instability, cold hands and feet, constipation, diarrhea,

Possible Side Effects (continued)

nausea, vomiting, upset stomach, increased sweating, urinary difficulties, cramps, blurred vision, rash, hair loss, stuffy nose, facial swelling, aggravation of lupus erythematosus, itching, chest pain, back or joint pain, colitis, drug allergy (symptoms include fever and sore throat), and liver toxicity.

Drug Interactions

- Pindolol may interact with surgical anesthetics to increase the risk of heart problems during surgery. Some anesthesiologists recommend gradually stopping the drug by 2 days before surgery.
- Pindolol may interfere with the normal signs of low blood sugar and with the action of oral antidiabetes drugs.
- Pindolol increases the blood-pressure-lowering effect of other blood-pressure-reducing agents, including clonidine, guanabenz, and reserpine as well as calcium channel blockers such as nifedipine.
- Aspirin, indomethacin, sulfinpyrazone, and estrogen drugs may interfere with the blood-pressure-lowering effect of pindolol.
- Cocaine may reduce the effectiveness of all beta blockers.
- Pindolol may worsen the cold hands and feet associated with taking ergot alkaloids for migraine. Gangrene is possible in people taking both ergot alkaloids and pindolol.
- Pindolol counteracts thyroid hormone replacements.
- Calcium channel blockers, flecainide, hydralazine, contraceptive drugs, propafenone, haloperidol, phenothiazine sedatives—molindone and others—quinolone antibacterials, and quinidine may increase the amount of pindolol in the bloodstream and lead to increased pindolol effects.
- Pindolol should not be taken within 2 weeks of taking a monoamine oxidase inhibitor antidepressant.
- Cimetidine increases the amount of pindolol absorbed into the bloodstream from oral tablets.
- Pindolol may interfere with the effectiveness of some anti-asthma drugs, including theophylline and aminophylline, and especially ephedrine and isoproterenol.

- Combining pindolol and phenytoin or digitalis drugs may result in excessive slowing of the heart, possibly causing heart block.
- If you stop smoking while taking pindolol, your dose may have to be reduced because your liver will break down the drug more slowly afterward.
- Aluminum salts, barbiturates, calcium salts, cholestyranine, colestipol, ampicillin, and rifampin may reduce the effectiveness of pindolol.
- Beta blockers may block the effects of epinephrine.

Food Interactions

None known.

Usual Dose

    Adult: 5–60 mg a day.
    Child: not recommended.

Overdosage

Symptoms include changes in heartbeat—unusually slow, unusually fast, or irregular; severe dizziness or fainting; breathing difficulties; bluish-colored fingernails or palms; and seizures. The victim should be taken to a hospital emergency room. ALWAYS bring the prescription bottle or container.

Special Information

Pindolol is taken continuously. When ending pindolol treatment, dosage should be reduced gradually over about 2 weeks. Do not stop taking this drug unless directed to do so by your doctor: Abrupt withdrawal may cause chest pain, breathing difficulties, increased sweating, and unusually fast or irregular heartbeat.

    Call your doctor at once if you develop back or joint pain, breathing difficulties, cold hands or feet, depression, rash, or changes in heartbeat. Pindolol may produce an undesirable lowering of blood pressure, leading to dizziness or fainting; call your doctor if this happens to you. Call your doctor if you experience persistent or bothersome anxiety, diarrhea, constipation, impotence, headache, itching, nausea or vomiting, nightmares or vivid dreams, upset stomach, trouble sleeping, stuffy nose, frequent urination, unusual tiredness, or weakness.

    Pindolol may cause drowsiness, blurred vision, dizziness, and lightheadedness. Be careful when driving or performing complex tasks.

Consult your pharmacist or doctor before using nasal decongestants or over-the-counter cold medications while taking pindolol.

It is best to take pindolol at the same time each day. If you forget a dose, take it as soon as you remember. If you take pindolol once a day and it is within 8 hours of your next dose, skip the dose you forgot and continue with your regular schedule. If you take it twice a day and it is within 4 hours of your next dose, skip the one you forgot and continue with your regular schedule. Never take a double dose.

Special Populations

Pregnancy/Breast-feeding: In studies, infants born to women who took a beta blocker while pregnant had lower birth weights, low blood pressure, and reduced heart rate. Pindolol should be avoided by women who are pregnant.

Pindolol passes into breast milk. Nursing mothers who must take it should use infant formula.

Seniors: Seniors may require less of the drug to achieve results. Seniors taking pindolol may be more likely to suffer from cold hands and feet, reduced body temperature, chest pain, general feelings of ill health, sudden breathing difficulties, increased sweating, or changes in heartbeat.

Plavix   see *Clopidogrel, page 265*

see *Clopidogrel, page 265*

Generic Name

Podofilox (poe-DUH-fil-ox) Ⓖ

Brand Name
Condylox

Type of Drug
Antimitotic drug.

Prescribed For
External genital and perianal warts.

General Information

Podofilox, which can be either manufactured from chemicals or purified from natural sources, kills visible wart tissues. Exactly how it works is not known. Condylomas or genital warts are caused by the human papillomavirus and can appear in various places including the sex organs, anus, and abdomen. Podofilox is not recommended for treatment of mucous membrane warts. The risk of developing warts increases if your immune system is suppressed.

Cautions and Warnings

Do not use podofilox if you are **allergic** or **sensitive** to any of its ingredients.

Proper diagnosis of genital warts is necessary before you use this product. See your doctor before you start using podofilox. Podofilox is for external use only. Do not use podofilox for any other purpose.

If you get podofilox in your eyes, wash it out at once with cool water and seek medical attention.

Podofilox is flammable. Keep away from any open flame.

Possible Side Effects

▼ Most common: burning, pain, inflammation, skin erosion, itching, and bleeding.

▼ Common: pain during intercourse, sleeplessness, tingling, tenderness, chafing, bad odor, dizziness, scarring, small sores or ulcers, dryness, difficulty retracting the foreskin, blood in the urine, vomiting, headache, stinging, and redness.

▼ Less common: skin peeling, scabbing, skin discoloration, tenderness, crusting, skin cracks, soreness, swelling, rash, and blisters.

Drug Interactions

None known.

Usual Dose

Adult

Podofilox can be applied as a solution or as a gel.

Apply morning and night—every 12 hours—for 3 consecutive days, and then apply nothing for 4 days. Repeat this cycle for up to 4 weeks in a row. Use the cotton-tipped applicator supplied with the solution, or your finger if you are using the gel. Try to limit the amount of podofilox that gets on intact skin. Thoroughly wash your hands before and after each application.

Child: not recommended.

Overdosage

Swallowing podofilox may lead to nausea, vomiting, fever, diarrhea, mouth sores, tingling in the hands or feet, changes in mental state, lethargy, coma, rapid breathing, respiratory failure, blood in the urine, kidney failure, and seizures. Excess podofilox should be washed off the skin as soon as possible. In case of overdose or accidental ingestion, take the victim to a hospital emergency room. ALWAYS bring the prescription bottle or container.

Special Information

Call your doctor if you develop any bothersome or persistent side effect. If you do not see any improvement in 4 weeks, stop using the drug and call your doctor.

Data is not available on the use of podofilox solution for the treatment of warts in the perianal area. Consult with your doctor if this treatment is necessary.

If you forget a dose, apply it as soon as you remember. If it is within 4 hours of your next dose, skip the dose you forgot and continue with your regular schedule.

Special Populations

Pregnancy/Breast-feeding: Podofilox is toxic to animal fetuses at very high dosages. When this drug is considered crucial by your doctor, its potential benefits must be carefully weighed against its risks.

It is not known if podofilox passes into breast milk. Nursing mothers who must use it should use infant formula.

Seniors: Seniors may use podofilox without special precaution.

Generic Name

Polyethylene Glycol 3350

(pah-lee-ETH-ih-leen GLYE-cohl) Ⓖ

Brand Names

Glycolax   Miralax

Type of Drug

Osmotic laxative.

Prescribed For

Occasional constipation.

General Information

Polyethylene glycol (PEG) laxatives work by preventing water in the stool from being reabsorbed into the body. Other osmotic laxatives such as lactulose, phosphates, citrate of magnesia, and milk of magnesia work by this same mechanism. However, they are not always interchangeable. PEG laxatives soften the stool and help it to pass out of the body. PEG laxatives usually take 2–4 days to produce a bowel movement. Regularity may take a week or more. PEG is also an ingredient in other laxative products, which can contain a stimulant laxative, vitamin C, sodium, and potassium.

Cautions and Warnings

Do not use a PEG laxative if you are **sensitive** or **allergic** to any of its ingredients. The chances of having a PEG allergy are very rare.

Excess use of a PEG laxative can lead to diarrhea and dehydration.

PEG laxatives should be used with caution if you have appendicitis or signs of **appendicitis** (**rectal bleeding**, **colostomy**, **ileostomy**) or signs of **intestinal blockage** (**nausea**, **vomiting**, **abdominal pain**, or **distention**).

PEG laxatives may be preferable over other laxative types for people with **high blood pressure**, **heart or kidney disease**, or some **gastrointestinal** (**GI**) **diseases**.

People with **eating disorders** should not use these products without consulting a doctor.

Overuse of this or any other laxative product can lead to laxative dependence and chronic constipation.

Possible Side Effects

▼ Common: nausea, cramps, and stomach gas.
▼ Less common: confusion, dizziness or lightheadedness, bloating, thirst, and diarrhea.
▼ Rare: sweating, irregular heartbeat, unusual tiredness or weakness, and blood in the stool. Contact your doctor if you experience any side effect not listed above.

Drug Interactions

- Laxatives can interfere with the absorption of drugs in the GI tract. Other oral medicines must be taken at least 1 hour before or 2 hours after your laxative dose.

Food Interactions

These products can be taken without regard to food or meals.

Usual Dose

Adult and Child (age 6 and over): 17 g (about 1 heaping tbsp.) once a day for up to 14 days.

Child (age 6 and under): 1 mg per lb. of body weight once a day; up to a maximum dose of 17 g.

Overdosage

Overdose of PEG laxatives can lead to dehydration and sodium and potassium imbalance, which can cause abnormal heart rhythms and other heart problems. Overdose victims may be taken to a hospital emergency room for treatment. ALWAYS bring the prescription bottle or container.

Special Information

Call your doctor if you have had no bowel movement or are still irregular after taking a PEG laxative for 7 days in a row, or if you develop bloody diarrhea, blood in the stool, severe cramping, or signs of a drug reaction or allergy (rash, itching, swelling, or dizziness).

Tell your doctor if you have nausea, vomiting, severe stomach pain, ulcerative colitis, irritable bowel syndrome, kidney disease, or if you have had a sudden change in bowel habits that has lasted 2 weeks or longer.

Mix the powder with a full glass of water, juice, soda, coffee, or tea. Stir well until the powder is completely dissolved before swallowing the mixture.

If you forget a dose of your PEG laxative, take it as soon as you remember. If you do not remember until it is almost time for your next dose, skip the one you forgot and continue with your regular schedule. Do not take a double dose of this medicine.

Special Populations

Pregnancy/Breast-feeding: PEG laxatives may be used during pregnancy if needed but can be harmful to the developing fetus if they are overused. Other laxative types, such as stool softeners or bulk-forming laxatives, are used more commonly. Tell your doctor if you are pregnant or become pregnant while using a PEG laxative. It is unlikely that this drug will directly affect a nursing infant. Nursing mothers may occasionally use PEG laxative products if needed.

Seniors: Seniors may be more sensitive to the laxative effects of PEG laxatives; diarrhea is more likely.

Brand Name

Poly-Vi-Flor

Generic Ingredients

Folic Acid + Sodium Fluoride + Vitamin A + Vitamin B_1 (Thiamine) + Vitamin B_2 (Riboflavin) + Vitamin B_3 (Niacin) + Vitamin B_6 (Pyridoxine) + Vitamin B_{12} (Cyanocobalamin) + Vitamin C + Vitamin D + Vitamin E Ⓖ

Other Brand Names

Florvite*	Soluvite*
Polytabs-F	Tri-Vi-Flor
Poly-Vi-Flor with Iron	Vi-Daylin/F*

*Some products in this brand-name group are alcohol- or sugar-free. Consult your pharmacist.

Type of Drug

Multivitamin supplement with fluoride.

Prescribed For

Vitamin deficiencies and prevention of dental cavities in infants and children.

General Information

Fluoride taken in small daily dosages has been effective in preventing cavities in children by strengthening the teeth. Multivitamins with fluoride are also available in preparations with iron.

Cautions and Warnings

Do not use Poly-Vi-Flor if you are **allergic** or **sensitive** to any of its ingredients.

Too much fluoride can damage teeth. Because of this, Poly-Vi-Flor should not be used where the fluoride content of the water supply exceeds 0.7 parts per million (ppm)—consult your pediatrician or local water company.

Possible Side Effects

▼ Common: occasional rash, itching, upset stomach, constipation, nausea, headache, and weakness.

Food and Drug Interactions

Avoid foods containing calcium such as milk or yogurt for at least 2 hours before or after taking Poly-Vi-Flor, as they may decrease its effectiveness.

Usual Dose

1 tablet or 1 mL-dropperful a day. Tablets and drops come in a range of 0.25 mg–1 mg. Consult your pediatrician for the correct dosage.

Overdosage

Symptoms include tarry stools, bloody vomit, diarrhea, drowsiness, faintness, increased watering of the mouth or eyes, shallow breathing, stomach cramps, aching bones, rash, mouth or lip sores, or discoloration of the teeth. Check with your doctor immediately or take the victim to a hospital emergency room. ALWAYS bring the prescription bottle or container.

Special Information

If you forget to give your child a dose of Poly-Vi-Flor, do so as soon as you remember. If it is almost time for the next dose, skip the dose you forgot and continue with the regular schedule. Do not give a double dose.

Type of Drug

Potassium Replacements

Brand Names

Generic Ingredient: Potassium Chloride (Liquid) Ⓖ

Cena-K Ⓢ	Klorvess
Kaon-Cl 20% Ⓢ	Potasalan Ⓢ
Kay Ciel Ⓢ	

Generic Ingredient: Potassium Gluconate (Liquid) Ⓖ

Kaon Ⓢ	K-G Elixir
Kaylixir Ⓢ	

Generic Ingredient: Potassium Salt Combination (Liquid) G

Kolyum [$]	Twin-K [$]
Tri-K	

Generic Ingredient: Potassium Chloride (Powder) G

Kay Ciel [$]	K+Care [$]
K-Lor [$]	K-Lyte/Cl
Klor-Con [$]	K-Lyte/Cl 50
Klor-Con/25 [$]	Micro-K LS

Generic Ingredient: Potassium Salt Combination (Powder) G

Klorvess [$]	Kolyum [$]

Generic Ingredient: Potassium (Effervescent Tablets) G

Effer-K	Klorvess [$]
K+Care ET	K-Lyte
Klor-Con/EF [$]	K-Lyte DS

Generic Ingredient: Potassium Chloride (Controlled-Release) G

K+8	Klor-Con M15
K+10	Klor-Con M20
Kaon-Cl-10	Klotrix
K-Dur 10	K-Tab
K-Dur 20	Micro-K Extencaps
Klor-Con 8	Micro-K 10 Extencaps
Klor-Con 10	Ten-K
Klor-Con M10	

Generic Ingredient: Potassium Gluconate (Tablets) G
Only available in generic form.

Prescribed For

Hypokalemia (low blood-potassium levels) and mild hypertension (high blood pressure).

General Information

A major component of body fluids, potassium helps to maintain electrolyte balance, kidney function, and blood pressure. Low potassium levels, which can affect the central nervous system (CNS) and heart functions, are usually caused by extended diuretic treatment, severe diarrhea, vomiting, complications of diabetes, or other medical conditions.

Potassium supplements are available in different types and forms. Potassium chloride is most often prescribed because it contains the most potassium per unit weight. Another advantage of potassium chloride is that it provides chloride ion, an important body-fluid component. Potassium gluconate provides about ⅓ as much potassium as the chloride, so you have to take 3 times as much to get an equal dose of potassium. However, it is preferable to potassium chloride in circumstances where chloride is undesirable.

Cautions and Warnings

Potassium replacement therapy should always be monitored and controlled by your doctor.

Potassium tablets have caused ulcers of the esophagus in some people with compression of the esophagus, who should use the liquid form. Potassium tablets have been reported to cause small bowel ulcer, leading to obstruction or perforation (formation of a hole through the bowel into the abdomen). Symptoms of bowel obstruction or perforation are severe vomiting, abdominal pain or distention, and gastrointestinal (GI) bleeding (indicated by black or tarry stools). **Seniors,** people with **diabetes** or **scleroderma,** and people who have had **mitral valve replacement** may be at higher risk for ulcers.

People who take potassium may develop hyperkalemia (high blood-potassium levels). Hyperkalemia can develop rapidly, without warning or symptoms, and is potentially fatal. It is often discovered through an EKG, but the following symptoms may also occur: tingling in the hands and feet, a feeling of heaviness or weakness in the muscles, listlessness, confusion, low blood pressure, extreme difficulty moving the arms and legs, abnormal heart rhythms, weak pulse, loss of consciousness, pallor, restlessness, and low urine output.

Do not take potassium if you are **dehydrated** or experiencing **muscle cramps** due to excessive sun or heat exposure. Potassium should be used with caution in people with **kidney or heart disease** or untreated **Addison's disease.**

Possible Side Effects

▼ Most common: nausea, vomiting, diarrhea, gas, and abdominal discomfort.

Possible Side Effects *(continued)*

▼ Rare: skin rash. Contact your doctor immediately if you experience tingling in the hands or feet, weakness and heaviness in the legs, listlessness, mental confusion, decreased blood pressure, and heart-rhythm changes.

Drug Interactions

- Potassium supplements should not be taken with the potassium-sparing diuretics spironolactone, triamterene, or amiloride. Severe hyperkalemia may occur.
- Combining supplements with an angiotensin-converting enzyme (ACE) inhibitor may result in hyperkalemia.
- People taking digitalis drugs must keep their blood-potassium levels within acceptable limits. Too little potassium in the blood may increase digitalis side effects and toxic reactions.

Food Interactions

Eating excess salt contributes to the problem of potassium depletion. Salt substitutes contain large amounts of potassium; do not use them while taking a potassium supplement unless directed by your doctor. If stomach upset occurs, take potassium supplements after meals or with food.

Usual Dose

Hypokalemia: 16–24 milliequivalents (mEq) a day.

Potassium Depletion: 40–100 milliequivalents (mEq) a day.

Overdosage

Symptoms include muscle weakness, tingling in the hands or feet, a feeling of heaviness in the legs, listlessness, confusion, breathing difficulties, low blood pressure, shock, abnormal heart rhythms, and heart attack. Call your local poison control center or a hospital emergency room for more information. If you seek treatment, ALWAYS bring the prescription bottle or container.

Special Information

Directions for taking and using any potassium supplement must be followed closely. Effervescent tablets, powders, and liquids should be properly and completely dissolved, or diluted in 3–8 oz. of cold water or juice and drunk slowly. Noneffervescent tablets or capsules should never be chewed or crushed; they must be swallowed whole, preferably after a meal and with a full glass of water.

Many of the controlled-release potassium supplements contain potassium distributed throughout an indigestible wax core or matrix; you may notice the depleted wax matrix in your stool several hours after swallowing a tablet. This is normal and not a cause for alarm.

Call your doctor at once if you experience tingling in your hands or feet, a feeling of heaviness in the legs, unusual tiredness or weakness, nausea, vomiting, continued abdominal pain, black stool, if you have trouble swallowing the tablets, or if the tablets seem to stick in your throat.

If you forget a dose, take it right away if you remember within 2 hours of your regular time. If you do not remember until later, skip the dose you forgot and go back to your regular schedule. Do not take a double dose.

Special Populations

Pregnancy/Breast-feeding: The safety of using potassium salts is not known. When this medication is considered crucial by your doctor, its potential benefits must be carefully weighed against its risks.

Normal doses of potassium supplements add little to the potassium already in breast milk. Exercise caution and do not take higher dosages without consulting your doctor.

Seniors: Seniors may be at higher risk for ulcers caused by potassium supplements.

Generic Name

Pramipexole (pram-ih-PEX-ole)

Brand Name
Mirapex

Type of Drug
Antiparkinsonian.

Prescribed For
Parkinson's disease and moderate-to-severe restless legs syndrome.

General Information

Pramipexole is thought to relieve symptoms of Parkinson's disease and restless legs syndrome by stimulating dopamine receptors in the brain. Studies of pramipexole in people with early Parkinson's disease showed improvement after 4 weeks of treatment. People with advanced Parkinson's disease showed improvement after 6 months.

Restless legs syndrome is a condition that affects about 1 out of every 10 people. Symptoms include an urge to move the legs, usually accompanied by, or caused by, uncomfortable leg sensations. Symptoms begin or worsen during periods of rest or inactivity for most people and are partly or totally relieved by movement. Symptoms usually worsen or occur only in the evening or at night, and can disturb sleep. People with restless legs syndrome taking pramipexole may show improvement in symptoms as early as 3 weeks.

Cautions and Warnings

Do not take pramipexole if you are **allergic** or **sensitive** to any of its ingredients.

Pramipexole may cause low blood pressure and make you dizzy or faint when rising from a sitting or lying position, especially during the early stages of treatment.

About 1 in 10–15 people who take pramipexole experience hallucinations that may be serious enough to require stopping drug therapy.

Pramipexole may make you fall asleep, sometimes suddenly, during the day. Use extreme caution when driving or engaging in a potentially hazardous activity.

One person taking pramipexole developed a disease in which skeletal muscle is destroyed.

People who stop taking other antiparkinsonians may develop high fever and confusion. Breathing difficulties caused by lung changes have also occurred with other antiparkinsonians. These symptoms have not been associated with pramipexole, but there is a risk that you may experience similar problems if you stop taking pramipexole.

Pramipexole, like other dopaminergic drugs, may cause pathological gambling, hypersexuality, or overeating, or other impulsive/compulsive behaviors, which are generally reversible if the dose is reduced or the drug stopped.

Twenty percent of people taking pramipexole for restless legs syndrome experienced their symptoms 2 hours earlier than usual; the reason is unknown.

Possible Side Effects

Early Parkinson's Disease
▼ Most common: sleepiness or tiredness and nausea.
▼ Common: insomnia, hallucinations, and constipation.
▼ Less common: dizziness, confusion, memory loss, reduced touch sensation, loss of muscle tone, a tendency to frequently change positions or pace the floor, odd thoughts, loss of sex drive, impotence, unusual muscle spasms, swelling in the arms or legs, generalized swelling, appetite loss, difficulty swallowing, weight loss, weakness, feeling unwell, fever, and abnormal vision.

Advanced Parkinson's Disease
▼ Most common: dizziness or fainting when rising from a sitting or lying position, abnormal movements, tremors, muscle rigidity, and hallucinations.
▼ Common: insomnia.
▼ Less common: accidental injury, weakness, generalized swelling, chest pain, feeling unwell, abnormal dreaming, confusion, sleepiness, unusual muscle spasms, unusual walking, muscle stiffness, memory loss, a tendency to frequently change positions or pace the floor, odd thoughts, paranoid reactions, delusions, sleeping problems, urinary problems, swelling in the arms or legs, arthritis, twitching, bursitis, muscle weakness, breathing difficulties, runny nose, pneumonia, visual difficulties, constipation, dry mouth, and rash.

Restless Legs Syndrome
▼ Most common: nausea, tiredness, and sleepiness.
▼ Common: constipation.
▼ Less common: diarrhea, dry mouth, fatigue, insomnia, and abnormal dreaming.

Drug Interactions
• Pramipexole increases levodopa + carbidopa blood levels and may worsen the uncontrolled muscle spasms that occur

with levodopa + carbidopa. Your doctor may reduce your dosage of levodopa + carbidopa.

- Cimetidine increases the amount of pramipexole absorbed by 50% and lengthens the time it takes for pramipexole to leave your body by 40%. Dose adjustment may be required if you take both drugs.
- Drugs that are eliminated through the kidneys—including amantadine, cimetidine, ranitidine, diltiazem, triamterene, verapamil, quinidine, and quinine—reduce the ability to clear pramipexole from the body. Dosage adjustment may be required.
- Phenothiazine sedatives, haloperidol and other antipsychotics, thioxanthene sedatives, metoclopramide, and other drugs that antagonize the effects of dopamine can reduce the effect of pramipexole.
- Pramipexole increases the sedative effect of benzodiazepines, sleeping pills, and other nervous system depressants.

Food Interactions

You may take this drug with food to prevent nausea.

Usual Dose

Parkinson's Disease

Adult: 0.125 mg 3 times a day to start, gradually increasing to a maximum of 4.5 mg a day. Dosage is reduced for people with kidney disease.

Child: not recommended.

Restless Legs Syndrome

Adult: 0.125 mg 3 times a day 2–3 hours before bedtime to start, gradually increasing to a maximum of 0.5 a day.

Child: not recommended.

Overdosage

Little is known about the effects of pramipexole overdose. Symptoms are likely to include the most common side effects. Take the victim to a hospital emergency room. ALWAYS bring the prescription bottle or container.

Special Information

Take this drug exactly as prescribed.

Pramipexole causes sedation. Be careful when driving or performing any task that requires concentration. Avoid alcohol and other nervous system depressants.

Call your doctor if you develop hallucinations or any bothersome or persistent side effect.

If you forget a dose, take it as soon as you remember. For Parkinson's disease, space the remaining daily dosage evenly throughout the day. Continue with your regular schedule on the next day. Do not take a double dose.

Special Populations

Pregnancy/Breast-feeding: The safety of using pramipexole during pregnancy is not known. When this drug is considered crucial by your doctor, its potential benefits must be carefully weighed against its risks.

It is not known if pramipexole passes into breast milk but this drug can interfere with milk production. Nursing mothers who must take this drug should use infant formula.

Seniors: Seniors are more likely to experience side effects.

Generic Name

Pramlintide (PRAM-lin-tide)

Brand Name

Symlin

Type of Drug

Amylinomimetic.

Prescribed For

Type 1 and 2 diabetics who use mealtime insulin therapy without satisfactory control.

General Information

Pramlintide acetate is a synthetic form of amylin, a natural hormone that helps control blood sugar. Natural amylin is found in the same part of the pancreas as insulin and it is released into the blood at the same time as insulin. Amylin is also deficient when inadequate amounts of insulin are released by the pancreas. Amylin affects blood sugar levels in 3 ways. First, it slows the movement of food from the stomach to the small intestine without reducing the overall type and amount of nutrient absorbed from the food. Slowing the movement of food helps because it spreads out the absorption of sugar from food, avoiding dangerous sugar spikes. Second, amylin also reduces the amount of glucagon released into the bloodstream. Glucagon is a hormone that raises blood sugar released from storage sites in the liver. Third, amylin helps to control your appetite, reducing overall food intake. Pramlintide exerts all the same effects as natural amylin.

Cautions and Warnings

Do not take pramlintide if you are **allergic** or **sensitive** to it or any of its ingredients, including metacresol.

Do not take this drug if you have **gastroparesis**, a diabetes-related condition in which stomach emptying is delayed.

The combination of insulin and pramlintide has been associated with an increased risk of very low blood sugar, especially in people with type 1 diabetes. People who have difficulty detecting if or when they have low blood sugar should not use pramlintide. If very low blood sugar is going to occur, it will be within 3 hours after pramlintide injection. Pramlintide injections must be given separately from insulin. They cannot be mixed.

Do not take pramlintide if you have trouble following your current insulin regimen; have trouble doing regular blood-sugar testing; have a **hemoglobin A1C level above 9%**; have had several bouts of low blood sugar requiring a doctor's assistance in the past 6 months; or if you use **medicines that stimulate gastrointestinal motility**.

This drug should not be used by **children**.

Antibodies to pramlintide may develop, but antibody levels generally go down with time. Most patients who develop antibodies still have good sugar control and similar types of side effects as people who do not develop pramlintide antibodies.

Possible Side Effects

▼ Most common: nausea (usually clears up on its own), appetite loss, headache, vomiting, and very low blood sugar (type 1 diabetics).

▼ Common: abdominal pain, dizziness, coughing, sore throat, joint pain, fatigue, allergic reaction, and dizziness.

Possible Side Effects (continued)

▼ Less common: very low blood sugar (type 2 diabetics).
▼ Rare: Rare side effects can occur in almost any part of the body. Contact your doctor if you experience any side effect not listed above.

Drug Interactions

- Pramlintide will slow the rate, but not the total amount, at which some drugs are absorbed into the bloodstream. Take all your pills at least 1 hour before or 2 hours after you inject pramlintide to avoid this interaction.
- Beta blockers, clonidine, guanethidine, and reserpine can mask signs of low blood sugar.
- Doses of oral blood-sugar-lowering drugs may have to be modified when you start taking pramlintide. Other drugs that can increase the blood-sugar-lowering effect of this drug include ACE inhibitors, disopyramide, fibrates, fluoxetine, monoamine oxidase inhibitor antidepressants, pentoxifylline, propoxyphene, salicylates, and sulfa antibiotics.
- Do not take pramlintide if you take drugs that affect stomach emptying, including atropine.
- Drugs prescribed for overactive bladder (tolterodine and others) should not be taken with pramlintide.

Food Interactions

None known.

Usual Dose

Adult: 15–60 mcg (type 1 diabetes) or 60–120 mcg (type 2 diabetes) by subcutaneous injection immediately before all major meals (250 or more calories; 30 or more grams of carbohydrate).
Child: not recommended.

Overdosage

The effects of pramlintide overdose are severe nausea, vomiting, diarrhea, dizziness, flushing, and drops in blood pressure. Blood sugar is not affected. Overdose victims should be taken to a hospital emergency room for evaluation and treatment. ALWAYS bring the prescription bottle or container.

Special Information

Pramlintide injections must be given separately from insulin. These drugs cannot be mixed.

Each dose of pramlintide must be given as an injection under the skin of the thigh or abdomen immediately before all your meals. Do not inject pramlintide into the arm. For information on how to administer injections, see page 1242.

If you forget a dose of pramlintide, skip the forgotten dose and continue with your regular injection just before your next meal. Do not take a double dose.

Always use a new needle and syringe for each insulin and pramlintide injection.

Unopened pramlintide should be kept in a refrigerator. Never freeze it. Opened vials of pramlintide may be stored for 28 days in a refrigerator or at room temperature no greater than 77 degrees. Frozen, overheated, or opened vials older than 28 days must be thrown away.

Pramlintide injection is a clear solution. Do not use it if there is any discoloration, cloudiness, or if there are any particles floating in it.

Make sure you know the signs and symptoms of low blood sugar (hunger, headache, sweating, tremor, or irritability; severe symptoms include difficulty concentrating, loss of consciousness, coma, or seizure) and are aware of how your body reacts. Serious injuries can occur if very low blood sugar develops while you are driving, operating heavy machinery, or engaging in other high-risk activities. Your doctor may cut your pre-meal short-acting insulin dose in half when you start taking pramlintide.

Do frequent pre- and post-meal blood sugar testing, and keep a source of sugar on hand.

This drug can cause appetite loss and weight reduction. Do not change your regular dosage if this happens to you.

Tell your doctor if you are pregnant, planning on becoming pregnant, or nursing your baby.

Special Populations

Pregnancy/Breast-feeding: In animal studies of up to 47 times the usual human dose, pramlintide was associated with some birth defects. If you are or might be pregnant and your doctor considers this drug crucial, its potential benefits must be weighed against its risks.

It is not known if this drug passes into breast milk. Nursing mothers taking pramlintide should consider using infant formula.

Seniors: Seniors may take this drug without special restriction. Careful monitoring and management to avoid very low blood sugar is important.

Pravachol *see Statin Cholesterol-Lowering Agents,* page 1052

Generic Name

Prazosin (PRAY-zoe-sin) G

Brand Names
Minipress   Minipress XL

Type of Drug
Antihypertensive.

Prescribed For
High blood pressure, benign prostatic hyperplasia (BPH), congestive heart failure (CHF), and Raynaud's disease. Prasozin combined with the diuretic polythiazide is used to treat high blood pressure.

General Information
Prazosin hydrochloride and other alpha-adrenergic blocking agents, or alpha blockers, reduce blood pressure by dilating (widening) blood vessels. They achieve this effect by blocking nerve endings known as alpha$_1$ receptors. The maximum blood-pressure-lowering effect of prazosin is seen between 2 and 6 hours after taking a dose. Prazosin's effect in CHF is seen within 1 hour of taking the drug. In BPH treatment, prazosin works by relaxing smooth muscles in the prostate and neck of the bladder. Despite the fact that prazosin reduces the symptoms of BPH, the drug's long-term effect on complications of BPH or the need for urinary

surgery is not known. Prazosin's effect lasts between 6 and 10 hours. It is broken down in the liver.

Prazosin may slightly reduce cholesterol levels and improve the ratio of high-density lipoprotein (HDL)—"good" cholesterol—and low-density lipoprotein (LDL), a positive step for people with a blood-cholesterol problem.

Cautions and Warnings

Do not take prazosin if you are **allergic** or **sensitive** to any of its ingredients or to any alpha blocker.

Prazosin may cause dizziness and fainting, especially with the first few doses. This is known as the first-dose effect, which can be minimized by limiting the first dose to 1 mg at bedtime. First-dose effects occur in about 1% of people taking an alpha blocker and may recur if the drug is stopped for a few days and then restarted.

Possible Side Effects

Side effects occur less often with prazosin than with other alpha blockers.

▼ Most common: dizziness, drowsiness, weakness, nausea, headache, and heart palpitations.

▼ Less common: low blood pressure, dizziness when rising from a sitting or lying position, rapid heartbeat, vomiting, dry mouth, diarrhea, constipation, abdominal pain or discomfort, breathing difficulties, stuffy nose, nosebleed, joint or muscle pain, blurred vision, conjunctivitis (pinkeye), ringing or buzzing in the ears, depression, nervousness, tingling in the hands or feet, frequent urination, impotence, poor urinary control, painful erection, itching, sweating, rash, hair loss, fluid retention, and fever. Contact your doctor if you experience any side effect not listed above.

Drug Interactions

- Prazosin may interact with beta blockers to increase the risk of dizziness or fainting after the first dose of prazosin. Prazosin dosage may need to be reduced.
- The blood-pressure-lowering effect of prazosin may be reduced by indomethacin.

- When taken with verapamil, prazosin produces an exaggerated reduction of blood pressure.
- The blood-pressure-lowering effect of clonidine may be reduced by prazosin.
- People taking this drug for high blood pressure should avoid over-the-counter cough medicine, cold and allergy remedies, and appetite suppressants. These products often contain stimulant ingredients that can increase blood pressure.
- People taking prazosin should avoid alcohol, which may increase the risk of low blood pressure.

Food Interactions

None known.

Usual Dose

Adult: 1 mg 2–3 times a day to start; may be increased to a total daily dose of 20 mg, although 40 mg a day (in divided doses) has been used in some cases.

Child: not recommended.

Overdosage

Overdose may produce drowsiness, poor reflexes, and very low blood pressure. Overdose victims should be taken to a hospital emergency room immediately. ALWAYS bring the prescription bottle or container.

Special Information

Take prazosin exactly as prescribed. Do not stop taking prazosin unless directed to do so by your doctor.

Prazosin may cause dizziness, headache, and drowsiness, especially 2–6 hours after you take your first dose, although these effects can persist after the first few doses. Use caution when getting up from a sitting or lying position.

Call your doctor if you develop severe dizziness, heart palpitations, or any bothersome or persistent side effect.

Wait 12–24 hours after taking your first dose of prazosin before driving or doing anything that requires intense concentration. Take your dose at bedtime to minimize this problem.

If you forget a dose, take it as soon as you remember. If it is almost time for your next dose, skip the dose you forgot and continue with your regular schedule. Do not take a double dose.

Special Populations

Pregnancy/Breast-feeding: The safety of using prazosin during pregnancy is not known, although animal studies have shown that alpha blockers may affect fetal development. When this drug is considered crucial by your doctor, its potential benefits must be carefully weighed against its risks.

Small amounts of prazosin pass into breast milk. Nursing mothers who must take this drug should use infant formula.

Seniors: Seniors, especially those with CHF or kidney disease, may be more sensitive to the side effects of prazosin.

Generic Name

Pregabalin (Pre-GAB-ah-lin)

Brand Name

Lyrica

Type of Drug

Anticonvulsant, pain reliever.

Prescribed For

Fibromyalgia, nerve pain associated with diabetes, pain after herpes zoster (shingles) infection, and partial onset seizures.

General Information

The exact mechanism of pregabalin is not known, but it does bind to tissues in the central nervous system where there is a high flow of calcium. Limiting calcium flow may be the key to its pain-relieving and antiseizure effects. For fibromyalgia, it relieves pain and helps improve daily functioning, but it may not work for everyone. This drug is unique because, unlike others prescribed for partial onset seizures, it does not bind to or affect GABA receptors or GABA itself in the brain. It does not affect the flow of sodium in the brain or stimulate opiate receptors. It also does not affect dopamine, serotonin, or norepinephrine, common areas of action for other central-nervous-system drugs.

Cautions and Warnings

Do not take this drug if you are **allergic** or **sensitive** to any of its ingredients. Potentially serious reactions include swelling of the face, mouth, lips, gums, tongue, or neck and trouble breathing. Other reactions included rash, hives, and blisters.

People with a **history of drug abuse** may be more likely to become dependent on this medicine.

Pregabalin passes out of the body through the kidneys. People with **kidney disease** require lower doses or an extended time between doses.

Pregabalin may make you dizzy or tired, or interfere with your concentration. Pregabalin may also cause blurred vision.

People taking this drug may gain weight. In one study of more than 325 people, they gained an average of more than 11 lbs. over 2 years.

People taking pregabalin may accumulate fluid in their legs or arms. This, and weight gain, are more common in people taking both pregabalin for diabetic nerve pain and rosiglitazone or pioglitazone.

People with **liver or heart disease**, including **heart failure**, should take this drug with caution.

In animal studies, pregabalin reduced sperm counts, increased the numbers of abnormal sperm, and interfered with the ability to father a child. There were also birth defects. These effects have been studied in humans but are not confirmed.

Possible Side Effects

▼ Common: dizziness, tiredness, dry mouth, loss of muscular coordination, swelling in the arms or legs, blurred or double vision, weight gain, and loss of concentration.

▼ Less common: accidental injury, increased appetite, constipation, tremors, headache, memory loss, speech disorders, walking abnormally, and urinary problems.

▼ Rare: Rare side effects can occur in almost any part of the body, but may not depend on the amount of pregabalin you are taking. Contact your doctor if you experience any side effect not listed above.

Drug Interactions

- Alcohol, sedatives, lorazepam, opiates, and other nervous system depressants may increase the depressant effects of pregabalin.

Food Interactions

This drug may be taken with or without food.

Usual Dose

Adult (age 19 and over): 50–200 mg 3 times a day, depending on the condition being treated. People with reduced kidney function must receive lower doses of pregabalin.

Child (under age 18): not recommended.

Overdosage

Accidental overdoses as high as 8000 mg have been taken with no symptoms other than side effects. Take the victim to a hospital emergency room for treatment and evaluation. ALWAYS bring the prescription bottle or container.

Special Information

Pregabalin can make you dizzy or tired, or interfere with your concentration. Be extremely careful when driving or performing any task that requires concentration. Sedatives, alcohol, and other nervous system depressants will worsen these effects.

Take this medicine exactly as prescribed by your doctor. Suddenly stopping it may lead to seizures, sleeplessness, nausea, headache, and diarrhea. The dose of pregabalin should be reduced gradually over at least one week rather than discontinued abruptly.

Tell your doctor if you experience unexplained muscle pain, changes in vision, weight gain, swollen feet or hands, or any bothersome or persistent side effect.

Diabetic patients may develop skin lesions while taking pregabalin.

If you forget a dose, take it as soon as you remember. If it is almost time for your next dose, take the dose you forgot and space the remaining daily dosage evenly throughout the rest of the day. Do not take a double dose.

Special Populations

Pregnancy/Breast-feeding: This medication causes birth defects in laboratory animals given 5 or more times the usual human dose. Also, seizure disorders have been associated with an increased risk of birth defects. Women who are or may become pregnant should take this medicine only if the potential benefits outweigh its risks.

Pregabalin passes into the breast milk of test animals but it is not known if this also happens in humans. Nursing mothers who must take pregabalin should use infant formula.

Seniors: Seniors may take pregabalin without special precaution, but may require reduced drug dosage because of declining kidney function with advanced age.

Premarin *see Estrogens, page 441*

Prempro *see Estrogens, page 441*

Prevacid *see Proton-Pump Inhibitors, page 939*

Generic Name

Procainamide (proe-KAY-nuh-mide) Ⓖ

Brand Name

Pronestyl

Type of Drug

Antiarrhythmic.

Prescribed For

Abnormal heart rhythms.

General Information

Procainamide hydrochloride works by slowing the response of heart muscle to nervous system stimulation. It also slows the rate at which nervous system impulses are carried through the heart. Procainamide begins working 30 minutes after you take it and continues working for 3 or more hours. As with other antiarrhythmic drugs, studies have not proven that people who take procainamide live longer than people who do not take it.

Procainamide should only be used to treat life-threatening irregular heartbeat. It has been associated with an increased risk of death when used to treat non-life-threatening irregular heartbeat.

Cautions and Warnings

Do not take procainamide if you are **allergic** or **sensitive** to any of its ingredients. Tell your doctor if you are allergic to anesthetics (particularly **procaine**) or aspirin.

About 1 in 200 people taking procainamide in the usual dosage range develop bone marrow depression, a drastic drop in white-blood-cell count, low platelet count, or other abnormalities of blood components. Because these abnormalities happen most often during the first 3 months of taking procainamide, you should be checked with weekly blood counts during your first 3 months on this drug.

Procainamide and other antiarrhythmic agents should be taken only by patients with **life-threatening ventricular arrhythmias.**

Procainamide should not be taken by people who have complete **heart block** or the arrhythmia called **"torsade de pointes."** Long-term use may cause up to 30% of people taking procainamide to test positive for **lupus erythematosus** (long-term condition affecting the body's connective tissues). If you already have this condition, you should not take procainamide.

If you have **myasthenia gravis,** tell your doctor when procainamide is first prescribed; you should be taking a drug other than procainamide.

Procainamide may aggravate **congestive heart failure**.

This drug is eliminated from the body through the kidney and liver. If you have either **kidney or liver disease,** your dosage of procainamide may have to be adjusted.

Possible Side Effects

▼ Common: appetite loss; nausea; itching; symptoms resembling the disease lupus erythematosus (fever and chills, nausea, vomiting, muscle aches, skin lesions, arthritis, and abdominal pains); enlargement of the liver or changes in blood tests that indicate a change in the liver; soreness of the mouth or throat; unusual bleeding; rash; and fever. If any of these symptoms occur while you are taking procainamide, tell your doctor immediately.

▼ Less common: bitter taste in the mouth, vomiting, diarrhea, weakness, dizziness, mental depression, giddiness, hallucinations, and drug allergy (symptoms include rash, itching, and fever).

Drug Interactions

- Procainamide blood levels and the risk of side effects are increased by propranolol and other beta blockers; cimetidine, ranitidine, and other H_2 antagonists; ketolide, macrolide, or quinolone antibiotics; terfenadine; trimethoprim; and ziprasidone.
- Procainamide may increase the action of lidocaine, producing dangerous side effects. Procainamide may also increase the effects of succinylcholine.
- Do not take procainamide with other antiarrhythmic drugs such as amiodarone or quinidine unless specifically instructed by your doctor. These combinations can depress heart function.
- The interaction between alcohol and procainamide is variable and may alter the effects of procainamide.
- Avoid over-the-counter (OTC) cough, cold, or allergy remedies containing drugs that have a stimulating effect on the heart. Ask your pharmacist about the ingredients in OTC remedies.

Food Interactions

This medication is best taken on an empty stomach, but you may take it with food if it upsets your stomach.

Usual Dose

Starting dosage—1000 mg in divided doses. Maintenance dosage—23 mg a day per lb. of body weight, in doses every 3 hours around the clock, adjusted according to individual needs. Seniors and people with kidney or liver disease are treated with lower dosages or given the medication less often.

Overdosage

Symptoms include abnormal heart rhythms, slow heart rate, low blood pressure, tremors, and nervous system depression. Overdose victims should be taken to an emergency room immediately. ALWAYS bring the prescription bottle or container.

Special Information

Call your doctor at once if you develop any sign of infection, including fever, chills, sore throat, or mouth sores, or if you develop any of the following: joint or muscle pain, dark urine, wheezing, weakness, chest or abdominal pains, heart palpitations, nausea, vomiting, diarrhea, appetite loss, dizziness, depression, hallucinations, or unusual bruising or bleeding.

Be sure you discuss with your doctor any drug sensitivity or reaction, especially to procaine, other local anesthetics, or aspirin. Also, be sure your doctor knows if you have heart failure, lupus erythematosus, liver or kidney disease, or myasthenia gravis.

Because procainamide is taken so frequently during the day, it is essential that you follow your doctor's directions about taking your medicine. Taking more medicine will not necessarily help you, and skipping doses or taking them less often than directed may lead to a loss of control over your heart problem.

Procainamide may make you drowsy. Do not drive a car or operate machinery until you know how this drug affects you.

If you forget to take a dose of procainamide and remember within 2 hours, take it right away. If it is almost time for your next dose, skip the one you forgot and continue with your regular schedule. Do not take a double dose.

Special Populations

Pregnancy/Breast-feeding: Procainamide passes into fetal circulation. When this drug is considered crucial by your doctor, its potential benefits must be carefully weighed against its risks.

This drug passes into breast milk. Nursing mothers who must take it should use infant formula.

Seniors: Seniors are more sensitive to procainamide.

Generic Name

Prochlorperazine (proe-klor-PER-uh-zeen) Ⓖ

Brand Names

Compazine   Compro
Compazine Spansule

Type of Drug

Antinauseant and phenothiazine antipsychotic.

Prescribed For

Severe nausea and vomiting; also prescribed for psychotic disorders such as schizophrenia, excessive anxiety, tension, and agitation.

General Information

Prochlorperazine and other phenothiazine drugs act on a portion of the brain called the hypothalamus. They affect areas of the hypothalamus that control metabolism, body temperature, alertness, muscle tone, hormone balance, and vomiting. How phenothiazines work is not completely understood.

Cautions and Warnings

Do not take prochlorperazine if you are **allergic** or **sensitive** to any of its ingredients or to any phenothiazine drug.

Do not take prochlorperazine if you have **very high or low blood pressure**; **Parkinson's disease**; or **blood**, **lung**, **liver**, **kidney**, **or heart disease**.

If you have **glaucoma**, **epilepsy**, **ulcers**, **intestinal obstruction**, or **difficulty passing urine**, prochlorperazine should be used with caution and under the strict supervision of your doctor.

Prochlorperazine may depress the gag (cough) reflex. Some people who have taken this drug have accidentally choked to death because the gag reflex failed to respond. Because it can prevent vomiting, prochlorperazine may obscure symptoms of disease or drug toxicity.

Because this drug may both increase the risk of **Reye's syndrome** and mask its symptoms, it should not be used to treat vomiting in children when the underlying cause is unknown. It should be used with caution in children with acute illnesses such as **chickenpox, measles, central-nervous-system (CNS) infections, gastroenteritis,** or any illness that causes **dehydration**.

Some people taking prochlorperazine develop tardive dyskinesia (symptoms include lip smacking or puckering, puffing of the cheeks, rapid or worm-like tongue movements, uncontrolled chewing motions, and uncontrolled arm and leg movements). This risk increases with long-term use of the medication.

A potentially fatal condition called Neuroleptic Malignant Syndrome (NMS) has been linked to the use of phenothiazine drugs. Symptoms include elevated body temperature, muscle stiffness, altered mental states, and irregularities in pulse or blood pressure.

Avoid extreme heat because prochlorperazine can upset your body's temperature-control mechanism.

Possible Side Effects

▼ Most common: drowsiness, especially during the first or second week of therapy. If the drowsiness becomes troublesome, call your doctor. Prochlorperazine can cause jaundice (symptoms include yellowing of the skin or whites of the eyes), typically within the first 4 weeks of treatment. It usually goes away when the drug is discontinued. If you notice this effect or feel feverish or unwell, call your doctor immediately.

▼ Less common: changes in blood components including anemia (condition characterized by a reduction in the number of red blood cells, amount of hemoglobin, or blood), raised or lowered blood pressure, abnormal heart rate, heart attack, feeling faint, and dizziness. Phenothiazines may produce extrapyramidal effects such as spasm of the neck muscles, rolling back of the eyes, convulsions, difficulty swallowing, and symptoms associated with Parkinson's disease. These effects look very serious but disappear after the drug is withdrawn; however, face, tongue, and jaw symptoms may persist for several years, especially in seniors with a history of brain damage. If you experience extrapyramidal effects, contact your doctor immediately.

▼ Rare: Prochlorperazine may cause an increase in psychotic symptoms or cause paranoid reactions. Other rare side effects can occur in almost any part of the body. Contact your doctor if you experience any side effect not listed above.

Drug Interactions

- Be cautious about combining prochlorperazine and barbiturates, sleeping pills, narcotics, sedatives, other phenothiazines, or other drugs that produce a depressive effect. Avoid alcohol.

- Aluminum antacids may reduce the effectiveness of prochlorperazine. Anticholinergic drugs may reduce the effectiveness of prochlorperazine and increase the risk of side effects.

- Prochlorperazine may reduce the effects of bromocriptine and appetite suppressants. The blood-pressure-lowering effect of guanethidine may be counteracted by this drug.
- Combining lithium and prochlorperazine may lead to disorientation, loss of consciousness, and uncontrolled muscle movements.
- Combining propranolol and prochlorperazine may lead to unusually low blood pressure.
- Combining phenytoin and prochlorperazine may either increase or decrease phenytoin levels in the blood.
- Prochlorperazine may increase blood levels of tricyclic antidepressants and the risk of their side effects.

Food Interactions

Prochlorperazine's effectiveness as an antipsychotic may be counteracted by beverages or foods containing caffeine.

Usual Dose

Adult: by mouth for nausea and vomiting—15–40 mg a day; rectal suppositories—25 mg twice a day; psychosis—15–150 mg a day.

Child (40–85 lbs.): 2.5 mg 3 times a day or 5 mg twice a day. The syrup form contains 5 mg of prochlorperazine per tsp.

Child (30–39 lbs.): 2.5 mg 2–3 times a day.

Child (20–29 lbs.): 2.5 mg 1–2 times a day.

Child (under age 2 or 20 lbs.): not recommended unless considered to be life-saving. Usually only 1–2 days of therapy are needed to relieve nausea and vomiting.

Overdosage

Symptoms include depression, extreme weakness, tiredness or a desire to sleep, lowered blood pressure, uncontrolled muscle spasms, agitation, restlessness, convulsions, fever, dry mouth, abnormal heart rhythms, deep sleep, and coma. Take the victim to a hospital emergency room immediately. ALWAYS bring the prescription bottle or container.

Special Information

Prochlorperazine is a sedative and may have a depressive effect, especially during the first few days of therapy. Be careful when driving or performing any task that requires concentration.

Call your doctor if you develop symptoms of tardive dyskinesia or NMS (see "Cautions and Warnings") or sore throat, fever, rash, weakness, tremors, visual disturbances, or yellowing of the skin or whites of the eyes.

Do not take any over-the-counter medications without first consulting your doctor.

Prochlorperazine may cause increased sensitivity to the sun. It may also turn your urine reddish-brown to pink; this is not a cause for concern.

If dizziness occurs, avoid sudden changes in posture and climbing stairs. Use caution in hot weather because this medication may make you more prone to heatstroke.

The liquid form of prochlorperazine may cause skin irritation or rash; do not get it on your skin. Liquid prochlorperazine must be protected from light. Do not remove it from its opaque bottle.

If you miss a dose, take it as soon as you remember. If it is almost time for your next dose, skip the dose you forgot and go back to your regular schedule. Do not take a double dose.

Special Populations

Pregnancy/Breast-feeding: Taking prochlorperazine during pregnancy may cause jaundice and CNS effects in newborns. When this drug is considered crucial by your doctor, its potential benefits must be carefully weighed against its risks.

Prochlorperazine may pass into breast milk. Nursing mothers who must take it should consider using infant formula.

Seniors: Seniors are more sensitive to prochlorperazine's effects and usually require lower dosages to achieve desired results. Some experts feel that they should be treated with 25–50% of the usual adult dosage.

Generic Name

Promethazine (proe-METH-uh-zeen) Ⓖ

Brand Names

Phenergan	Promethegen
Promethacon	Prometh Plain

Combination Products

Generic Ingredients: Promethazine + Codeine Phosphate Ⓖ
Phenergan with Codeine Syrup

Pherazine with Codeine Syrup
Prometh with Codeine Syrup

Generic Ingredients: Promethazine + Dextromethorphan Hydrobromide **[G]**
Phenergan with Dextromethorphan Syrup
Pherazine DM Syrup
Prometh with Dextromethorphan Syrup

Generic Ingredients: Promethazine + Phenylephrine Hydrochloride **[G]**
Phenergan VC Syrup
Promethazine VC Plain Syrup
Prometh VC Plain Liquid **[A]**

Generic Ingredients: Promethazine + Codeine Phosphate + Phenylephrine Hydrochloride **[G]**
Phenergan VC with Codeine Syrup
Pherazine VC with Codeine Syrup
Prometh VC with Codeine Liquid **[A]**

Type of Drug
Antihistamine.

Prescribed For
Allergy, motion sickness, nausea, vomiting, nighttime sedation, and pain relief following surgery. Combination products are used to treat cough and stuffy/runny nose due to allergy or cold.

General Information
Promethazine hydrochloride, one of the older members of the phenothiazine antihistamine group, is used alone and in combination with cough suppressants and decongestants.

Cautions and Warnings
Do not use promethazine if you are **allergic** or **sensitive** to any of its ingredients or if you cannot tolerate any other phenothiazine drug such as chlorpromazine and prochlorperazine.

This medication is not to be used in any **child under age 2** because of potentially fatal slowing of breathing. Use caution when using this drug in a child age 2 and older. The lowest effective dose should be used.

Promethazine should be used with caution if you have **very low blood pressure; sleep apnea; Parkinson's disease; intestinal**

obstruction; or **heart, blood, respiratory, liver, or kidney disease.** This drug should be used under your doctor's strict supervision if you have an **ulcer,** a **seizure disorder, bone-marrow depression, glaucoma,** or **urinary difficulties,** including an enlarged prostate.

A potentially fatal condition called Neuroleptic Malignant Syndrome (NMS) has been linked to the use of phenothiazine drugs. Symptoms include elevated body temperature, muscle stiffness, altered mental states, and irregularities in pulse or blood pressure.

Children with **liver disease,** any illness that causes **dehydration,** a history of **sleep apnea,** a family history of **sudden infant death syndrome** (SIDS), or **Reye's syndrome** should not take promethazine.

Possible Side Effects

The suppositories can cause rectal burning or stinging.

▼ Most common: drowsiness, thick mucous, and sedation.

▼ Less common: sore throat and fever; unusual bleeding or bruising; tiredness; weakness; dizziness; feeling faint; clumsiness; unsteadiness; dry mouth, nose, or throat; facial redness; breathing difficulties; hallucinations; confusion; seizure; muscle spasm, especially in the back and neck; restlessness; a shuffling walk; jerky movements of the head and face; shaking and trembling of the hands; blurred vision or other changes in vision; urinary difficulties; rapid heartbeat; sensitivity to the sun; increased sweating; and appetite loss. Children and older adults are more likely to develop difficulty sleeping, excitability, nervousness, restlessness, or irritability.

Drug Interactions

- This drug should not be taken with a monoamine oxidase inhibitor antidepressant.
- The sedating effects of promethazine are increased by central nervous system (CNS) depressants including alcohol, hypnotics, sedatives, antianxiety drugs, and narcotics. These combinations should be used with extreme caution.
- Promethazine will antagonize the effects of amphetamines and other appetite suppressants such as diet pills.

- The combination of promethazine and an oral anti-thyroid drug may increase the risk of agranulocytosis (condition characterized by a reduction in the number of white blood cells).
- The combination of quinidine and promethazine may increase the cardiac effects of both drugs.
- Increasing the dosage of anticonvulsant medication, bromocriptine, guanadrel, guanethidine, or levodopa + carbidopa may be necessary when any of these drugs are taken with promethazine.
- Riboflavin requirements are increased in people taking promethazine.
- Promethazine may interfere with blood-sugar tests and home pregnancy tests.

Food Interactions

Take promethazine with food if it upsets your stomach.

Usual Dose
Allergy
Adult: 12.5 mg before meals and 12.5–25 mg at bedtime.

Child (age 2 and over): 6.25–12.5 mg 3 times a day or 25 mg at bedtime.

Motion Sickness
Adult: 12.5–25 mg ½ hour before travel; repeat in 8–12 hours if needed. Then take 1 dose upon arising and another before dinner.

Child (age 2 and over): 12.5–25 mg twice a day.

Nausea and Vomiting
Adult: 12.5–25 mg when needed, up to 6 times a day if necessary.

Child (age 2 and over): 10–25 mg when needed, or 0.5 mg per lb. of body weight; 10–25 mg every 4–6 hours if necessary.

Nighttime Sedation
Adult: 25–50 mg at bedtime.

Child (age 2 and over): 12.5–25 mg at bedtime.

Overdosage

Symptoms include drowsiness; confusion; clumsiness; dry mouth, nose, or throat; hallucinations; seizure; and other promethazine side effects. Overdose victims should be taken to a hospital emergency room for treatment. ALWAYS bring the prescription bottle or container.

Special Information

Be careful when performing tasks requiring concentration and co-ordination, such as driving, because promethazine may cause tiredness, dizziness, or lightheadedness. Avoid alcohol.

Call your doctor if you develop sore throat; dry mouth, nose, or throat; fever; chills; unusual bleeding or bruising; tiredness; weakness; clumsiness; unsteadiness; hallucinations; seizure; sleeping problems; feeling faint; flushing; breathing difficulties; or any bothersome or persistent side effect.

Maintain good dental hygiene while taking promethazine because dry mouth may cause you to be more susceptible to oral infections. If the dry mouth caused by promethazine is not eased by gum or hard candy or lasts more than 2 weeks, call your doctor or dentist. Any dental work should be completed prior to starting on this drug.

If you forget a dose of promethazine, take it as soon as you remember. If you take it twice a day and it is almost time for your next dose, take 1 dose right away and another in 5 or 6 hours, then continue with your regular schedule. If you take promethazine 3 or more times a day and forget a dose, take it as soon as you remember. If it is almost time for your next dose, take 1 dose right away and another in 3 or 4 hours, then continue with your regular schedule. Never take a double dose.

Special Populations

Pregnancy/Breast-feeding: Babies born to women who took phenothiazines have suffered side effects at birth such as yellowing of the skin and whites of the eyes, CNS effects, and blood-clotting problems. Do not take any antihistamine without your doctor's knowledge if you are or might be pregnant—especially during the last 3 months of pregnancy—because newborns may have severe reactions to antihistamines.

Nursing mothers who must take promethazine should use infant formula.

Seniors: Seniors are more sensitive to side effects and may require lower dosages.

Generic Name

Propoxyphene Hydrochloride
(proe-POK-sih-fene hye-droe-KLOR-ide) G

Brand Names
Darvon Compound-65   Darvon Pulvules

Combination Products
Generic Ingredients: Propoxyphene Hydrochloride + Aspirin + Caffeine G
Darvon Compound

Generic Ingredients: Propoxyphene Hydrochloride + Acetaminophen G
Wygesic

The information in this profile also applies to the following drugs:

Generic Ingredient: Propoxyphene Napsylate
Darvon-N

Generic Ingredients: Propoxyphene Napsylate + Acetaminophen G
Darvocet A500   Darvocet-N 100
Darvocet-N 50

Type of Drug
Analgesic (pain reliever).

Prescribed For
Mild to moderate pain.

General Information
A chemical derivative of methadone (a narcotic pain reliever), propoxyphene hydrochloride is widely used for mild pain. It is estimated that propoxyphene hydrochloride is about ½–⅔ as strong a pain reliever as codeine and about as equally effective as aspirin. Propoxyphene hydrochloride is more effective when combined with aspirin or acetaminophen than when used alone. Propoxyphene hydrochloride is about 30% more potent than propoxyphene napsylate.

Cautions and Warnings

Do not take propoxyphene hydrochloride if you are **allergic** or **sensitive** to any of its ingredients or to similar drugs. This medication should be used with caution if you have **liver or kidney disease**.

Psychological or physical drug dependence (addiction) may result when propoxyphene hydrochloride is taken in doses larger than those needed for pain relief for long periods of time. The major sign of psychological dependence is anxiety when the drug is suddenly stopped. People may also become physically addicted to propoxyphene hydrochloride; it can be abused to the same degree as codeine.

Never take more of this medication than is prescribed by your doctor. Use this medication with extreme caution if you also take **sedatives** or **antidepressants**.

Propoxyphene hydrochloride should be considered a potentially dangerous drug, especially in the hands of anyone with a history of addiction or severe depression. Excessive doses of propoxyphene hydrochloride, either by itself or together with alcohol or other central-nervous-system (CNS) depressants, are a major cause of drug-related deaths. Many of these deaths have occurred in people with a **history of emotional disturbances**, **suicidal ideas or suicide attempts**, and **misuse of sedatives**, **alcohol**, and other **CNS depressants**.

Propoxyphene hydrochloride should not be taken by **children**.

For more information about combination products, see Acetaminophen, page 7.

Possible Side Effects

▼ Common: dizziness, sedation, nausea, and vomiting. These effects usually disappear if you lie down and relax for a few moments.

▼ Less common: constipation, stomach pain, rash, light-headedness, headache, weakness, euphoria (feeling "high"), dysphoria (feeling sad), hallucinations, insomnia, and minor visual disturbances.

▼ Rare: jaundice. Contact your doctor if you experience any side effect not listed above.

Taking propoxyphene hydrochloride over long periods of time and in high doses may cause physical or psychological dependence.

Possible Side Effects *(continued)*

For more information about combination products, see Acetaminophen, page 7.

Drug Interactions

- Propoxyphene hydrochloride may cause drowsiness when taken with other drugs that cause drowsiness, such as sedatives, hypnotics, narcotics, alcohol, and possibly antihistamines.
- Carbamazepine levels may be increased by propoxyphene hydrochloride, resulting in dizziness, nausea, and poor coordination.
- Charcoal tablets decrease the absorption of propoxyphene hydrochloride into the bloodstream.
- Cigarette smoking increases the rate at which this drug is broken down in the liver. Heavy smokers may need more propoxyphene hydrochloride to obtain pain relief but will have to take less of the drug if they stop smoking.
- Propoxyphene hydrochloride may increase the anticoagulant (blood-thinning) effect of warfarin.
- Combining propoxyphene hydrochloride and protease inhibitors is not recommended.

For more information about combination products, see Acetaminophen, page 7.

Food Interactions

Take propoxyphene hydrochloride with a full glass of water or with food if it upsets your stomach.

Usual Dose

Propoxyphene Hydrochloride: 65 mg every 4 hours as needed. Do not exceed 390 mg per day.

Propoxyphene Napsylate: 100 mg every 4 hours as needed. Seniors and people with poor liver or kidney function may need to take the medication less often.

Overdosage

Symptoms include a decrease in respiratory rate, changes in breathing pattern, pinpointed pupils, convulsions, extreme sleepiness leading to stupor or coma, and abnormal heart rhythms. The overdose victim should be taken to a hospital emergency room immediately. ALWAYS bring the prescription bottle or container.

Special Information

Use caution while driving or performing any tasks that require you to be awake and alert. Avoid alcohol and other CNS depressants.

Call your doctor if you develop nausea or vomiting while taking this drug, or if you develop breathing difficulties.

If you forget a dose, take it as soon as you remember. If it is almost time for your next dose, skip the one you forgot and continue with your regular schedule. Do not take a double dose.

For more information about combination products, see Acetaminophen, page 7.

Special Populations

Pregnancy/Breast-feeding: No clinical studies of this medication have been conducted in pregnant women, but a survey of almost 3000 pregnant women who took propoxyphene hydrochloride found that 46—1.6%—had infants with birth defects. Animal studies show that high doses of the drug can cause problems in a fetus. Pregnant women who must take propoxyphene hydrochloride should talk to their doctor about the risks of this drug.

Small amounts of propoxyphene hydrochloride pass into breast milk. Nursing mothers who must take this drug should consider using infant formula.

Seniors: Seniors, especially those with reduced kidney or liver function, are more likely to be sensitive to the effects of this drug and should be treated with smaller dosages.

Generic Name

Propranolol (proe-PRAN-oe-lol) G

Brand Names

Inderal

Inderal LA

Innopran XL

Combination Products

Generic Ingredients: Propranolol + Hydrochlorothiazide G

Inderide

Inderide LA

Type of Drug

Beta-adrenergic blocking agent.

Prescribed For

High blood pressure, angina pectoris, abnormal heart rhythm, prevention of second heart attack or migraine, tremors, aggressive behavior, side effects of antipsychotic drugs, acute panic, stage fright and other anxieties, and schizophrenia; also used to treat bleeding from the stomach or esophagus, and symptoms of hyperthyroidism (overactive thyroid gland).

General Information

Propranolol hydrochloride is one of many beta-adrenergic blocking drugs, or beta blockers, that interfere with the action of a specific part of the nervous system. Beta receptors are found all over the body and affect many body functions. Each beta blocker has particular characteristics that make it more suitable for certain conditions or people.

Cautions and Warnings

Do not take propanolol if you are **allergic** or **sensitive** to any of its ingredients or to beta blockers.

You should be cautious about taking propranolol if you have **asthma, severe heart failure,** a very **slow heart rate,** or **heart block** (disruption of the electrical impulses that control heart rate) because the drug may aggravate these conditions.

People with **angina** who take propranolol for high blood pressure risk aggravating their angina if they suddenly stop taking the drug. These people should have their drug dosage reduced gradually over 1–2 weeks.

Propranolol should be used with caution if you have **liver or kidney disease** because your ability to eliminate this drug from your body may be impaired.

Propranolol reduces the amount of blood pumped by the heart with each beat. This reduction in blood flow may aggravate the condition of people with **poor circulation** or **circulatory disease**.

If you are undergoing major **surgery**, your doctor may want you to stop taking propranolol at least 2 days before surgery.

People with a history of **severe anaphylactic reaction** to allergens may be unresponsive to usual doses of epinephrine while taking beta blockers.

Possible Side Effects

Side effects are relatively uncommon and usually mild.
▼ Most common: impotence.

Possible Side Effects *(continued)*

▼ Less common: tiredness or weakness, slow heartbeat, heart failure, dizziness, breathing difficulties, bronchospasm, depression, confusion, anxiety, nervousness, sleeplessness, disorientation, short-term memory loss, emotional instability, cold hands and feet, constipation, diarrhea, nausea, vomiting, upset stomach, increased sweating, urinary difficulties, cramps, blurred vision, rash, hair loss, stuffy nose, facial swelling, aggravation of lupus erythematosus, itching, chest pain, back or joint pain, colitis, drug allergy (symptoms include fever and sore throat), and liver toxicity.

Drug Interactions

- Propranolol may interact with surgical anesthetics to increase the risk of heart problems during surgery. Some anesthesiologists recommend gradually stopping the drug by 2 days before surgery.
- Propranolol may interfere with the normal signs of low blood sugar and with the action of oral antidiabetes medications.
- Propranolol increases the blood-pressure-lowering effect of other blood-pressure-reducing agents including clonidine, guanabenz, and reserpine, as well as calcium channel blockers such as nifedipine.
- Aspirin-containing drugs, indomethacin, sulfinpyrazone, and estrogen drugs may interfere with the blood-pressure-lowering effect of propranolol.
- Cocaine may reduce the effectiveness of all beta blockers.
- Propranolol may worsen the problem of cold hands and feet associated with ergot alkaloids, used to treat migraine. Gangrene is a possibility in people taking both ergot and propranolol.
- The effect of benzodiazepine antianxiety drugs may be increased by propranolol.
- Propranolol will counteract thyroid hormone replacements.
- Calcium channel blockers, flecainide, hydralazine, contraceptive drugs, propafenone, haloperidol, phenothiazine sedatives—molindone and others—quinolone antibacterials, and quinidine may increase the amount of propranolol in the bloodstream and lead to increased propranolol effects.
- Propranolol should not be taken within 2 weeks of taking a monoamine oxidase inhibitor antidepressant.

- Cimetidine increases the amount of propranolol absorbed into the bloodstream from oral tablets.
- Propranolol may interfere with the effectiveness of some anti-asthma medications, including theophylline and amino-phylline, and especially ephedrine and isoproterenol.
- Combining propranolol and phenytoin or digitalis drugs may result in excessive slowing of the heart, possibly causing heart block.
- Your propranolol dose may have to be reduced if you stop smoking because your liver will break down the drug more slowly after you stop.
- Aluminum salts, barbiturates, calcium salts, cholestyramine, colestipol, ampicillin, and rifampin may reduce the effectiveness of propranolol.
- Propanolol may increase the anticoagulant effect of warfarin.
- Beta blockers may block the effects of epinephrine.
- Alcohol may increase blood plasma levels of propranolol.

Food Interactions

Although it is best to take propranolol without food or on an empty stomach, it is more important to be consistent about taking it with or without food in order to maintain consistent effects.

Usual Dose

Adult: 30–700 mg a day. Take once daily at bedtime.
Child: not recommended.

Overdosage

Symptoms include changes in heartbeat—unusually slow, fast, or irregular; severe dizziness or fainting; breathing difficulties; bluish-colored fingernails or palms; and seizures. The victim should be taken to a hospital emergency room. ALWAYS bring the prescription bottle or container.

Special Information

Propranolol is for continuous use. Do not stop taking this drug unless directed to do so by your doctor. Abrupt withdrawal may cause chest pain, breathing difficulties, increased sweating, and unusually fast or irregular heartbeat. When ending propranolol treatment, dosage should be reduced gradually over a period of about 2 weeks.

Call your doctor at once if you develop back or joint pain, breathing difficulties, cold hands or feet, depression, rash, or changes in heartbeat. Propranolol may produce an undesirable lowering of blood pressure, leading to dizziness or fainting; call your doctor if this happens to you. Call your doctor if you experience persistent or bothersome anxiety, diarrhea, constipation, impotence, headache, itching, nausea or vomiting, nightmares or vivid dreams, upset stomach, trouble sleeping, stuffy nose, frequent urination, unusual tiredness, or weakness.

Propranolol may cause drowsiness, lightheadedness, dizziness, or blurred vision. Be careful when driving or performing complex tasks.

It is best to take propranolol at the same time each day. If you forget a dose, take it as soon as you remember. If you take propranolol once a day and it is within 8 hours of your next dose, skip the dose you forgot and continue with your regular schedule. If you take it twice a day and it is within 4 hours of your next dose, skip the dose you forgot and continue with your regular schedule. Never take a double dose.

Special Populations

Pregnancy/Breast-feeding: In studies, infants born to women who took a beta blocker while pregnant had lower birth weights, low blood pressure, low blood sugar, difficulty breathing, and reduced heart rates. Propranolol should be avoided by pregnant women.

Propranolol passes into breast milk in concentrations too small to have any effect.

Seniors: Seniors may require less of the drug to achieve results. Seniors taking propranolol may be more likely to suffer from cold hands and feet, reduced body temperature, chest pain, general feelings of ill health, sudden breathing difficulties, increased sweating, or changes in heartbeat.

Type of Drug

Prostaglandin Agonists

Brand Names

Generic Ingredient: Bimatoprost
Lumigan

Generic Ingredient: Travoprost
Travatan Z

Generic Ingredient: Latanoprost
Xalatan

Prescribed For

Open-angle glaucoma and ocular hypertension (high pressure inside the eye). May also be prescribed for angle closure, inflammatory, or neovascular glaucoma.

General Information

Prostaglandin agonists are believed to reduce pressure inside the eye by combining with prostaglandin receptors to increase the outflow of eye fluid. They are absorbed through the cornea, where all but bimatoprost are transformed into their active forms. Pressure is lowered within 2 hours and lasts up to 12 hours.

Cautions and Warnings

Do not use prostaglandin agonists if you are **allergic** or **sensitive** to any of their ingredients. Sensitivity to one member of this group may not indicate sensitivity to all.

Prostaglandin agonists may change your eye color because they increase the number of pigment granules in the cornea, which in turn increases brown pigment in the iris. This color change occurs gradually over a period of months or years. Typically, the brown color around the pupil spreads slowly to the outer part of the iris. This change is more noticeable in people with green-brown, blue/gray-brown or yellow-brown eye color. The long-term effect of these medicines on eye pigment granules is not known; your doctor may tell you to stop using these eyedrops if the color change persists or is especially noticeable. They can also darken eyelid color and increase eyelash color and length, as well as the number of eyelashes.

The effect of prostaglandin agonists on the cornea is not known.

Possible Side Effects

▼ Most common: blurred vision; stinging, burning, itching, and redness of the eyes; and brownish eye coloration.
▼ Common: abnormal vision, eyelid problems, excessive tearing, and a sensation of something in the eye.

Possible Side Effects *(continued)*

▼ Less common: dry eye; swelling or redness of the eyelid; eyelid discomfort, inflammation, or pain; and increased sensitivity to bright light.

▼ Rare: blood clot in the artery supplying the retina, bleeding inside the eye, detachment of the retina, increased eye pressure, color blindness, corneal deposits, corneal swelling, droopy eyelid, and irritation of the iris. Contact your doctor if you experience any side effect not listed above.

Systemic side effects from traces of these drugs passing into the blood

▼ Common: cold, flu, or other respiratory infections.

▼ Less common: muscle, joint or back pain, accidental injury, chest pain, angina pain, bronchitis, cough, diabetes, dizziness, headache, high blood pressure, sleeplessness, sore throat, runny nose, sinus irritation, and rash or allergic reactions.

Drug Interactions

• If you use other eyedrops that contain a thimerosal preservative, separate the administration of each eyedrop by at least 5 minutes.

Usual Dose

Bimatoprost, Latanoprost, and Travoprost

   Adult: 1 drop in the affected eye every evening.
   Child: not recommended.

Overdosage

Overdose symptoms include eye irritation and redness. Severe overdosage may also cause abdominal pain, dizziness, fatigue, flushing, nausea, and sweating. Call your doctor, local poison control center, or a hospital emergency room for more information. If you go to a hospital emergency room ALWAYS bring the prescription bottle or container.

Special Information

Call your doctor if you develop eye irritation or any other side effect.

   If you use any other eye medication, wait 5 minutes between each application.

To prevent infection, keep the eyedropper from touching your fingers, eyelids, or any surface.

Contact your doctor immediately if you are having eye surgery, experience an eye injury, develop an eye infection such as conjunctivitis (pinkeye), or develop an eyelid reaction to determine if you should continue to use the eyedrops.

If you wear contact lenses, take them out before using these eyedrops and wait 15 minutes before reinserting them. They contain a benzalkonium preservative that can be absorbed by the contacts.

Store unopened bottles of latanoprost in the refrigerator. Once opened, the eyedrops can be kept at room temperature—up to 77°F—for 6 weeks. All other products can be stored at room temperature and should be discarded 6–8 weeks after opening.

Do not take more medication than your doctor has prescribed. Taking it more often may actually reduce its effectiveness. If you forget to administer a dose, do so as soon as you remember. If it is almost time for your next dose, skip the one you forgot and continue with your regular schedule. Do not take a double dose.

Special Populations

Pregnancy/Breast-feeding: Animal studies have shown that prostaglandin agonists may be harmful to the fetus at extremely high dosages. When your doctor considers this drug crucial, its potential benefits must be carefully weighed against its risks.

It is not known if these medications pass into breast milk. Nursing mothers who must use a prostaglandin agonist should consider using infant formula.

Seniors: Seniors may use these medicines without special precaution.

Protonix *see Proton-Pump Inhibitors, below*

Type of Drug

Proton-Pump Inhibitors

Brand Names

Generic Ingredient: Esomeprazole Magnesium
Nexium

Generic Ingredient: Lansoprazole
Prevacid

Generic Ingredients: Lansoprazole + Amoxicillin + Clarithromycin
Prevpac

Generic Ingredients: Lansoprazole + Naproxen
NapraPAC

Generic Ingredient: Omeprazole Ⓖ
Prilosec

Generic Ingredients: Omeprazole + Sodium Bicarbonate
Zegerid

Generic Ingredient: Pantoprazole Sodium Ⓖ
Protonix

Generic Ingredient: Rabeprazole Sodium
Aciphex

Prescribed For

Stomach or duodenal (upper intestinal) ulcers, gastroesophageal reflux disease (GERD), and conditions in which there is an excess of stomach acid; also used to treat and maintain healing of ulcers of the esophagus.

General Information

Proton-pump inhibitors (PPIs) stop the production of stomach acid by interfering with the "proton pump" in the mucous lining of the stomach at the last stage of acid production. PPIs can turn off stomach acid production within 1 hour. These drugs are useful in treating conditions in which stomach acid plays a key role, as with ulcers and GERD. It is prescribed together with amoxicillin and clarithromycin for people with ulcers caused by *Heliobacter pylori* infections.

Cautions and Warnings

Do not take PPIs if you are **allergic** or **sensitive** to any of their ingredients.

PPIs should not be taken as maintenance treatment for **duodenal ulcers** and are not recommended for treatment of **GERD** beyond 8–16 weeks.

People with **liver disease** may need to take a lower dose of PPIs.

Possible Side Effects

Generally, PPIs cause few side effects.

▼ Common: headache, diarrhea, nausea, gas, abdominal pain, constipation, and dry mouth.

▼ Less common: sore throat, upper respiratory infection, fever, vomiting, dizziness, rash, constipation, muscle pain, unusual tiredness, cough, and back pain.

▼ Rare: Drug sensitivity reactions, including severe skin reactions, may occur. Other rare side effects can affect almost any part of the body. Contact your doctor if you experience any side effect not listed above.

Drug Interactions

- PPIs may increase the effects of benzodiazapines, phenytoin, and warfarin. They may also interact with other drugs broken down by the liver.
- Combining PPIs and clarithromycin may increase blood levels of both drugs.
- Sucralfate may interfere with the absorption of PPIs into the blood.
- PPIs may interfere with the absorption of iron, ampicillin, ketoconazole, itraconazole, and digoxin.
- PPIs may increase the effects of drugs that reduce the production of blood cells by bone marrow.
- Combining PPIs and aspirin may increase gastric side effects.
- PPIs may reduce the effectiveness of protease inhibitors (HIV drugs). Do not combine PPIs with atazanavir in particular.
- Lansoprazole may reduce the amount of theophylline drugs in the blood.
- Omeprazole may increase the effects of cilostazol.

Food Interactions

PPIs should be taken immediately before a meal, preferably breakfast. Esomeprazole and Zegerid must taken at least 1 hour before a meal.

Usual Dose

Esomeprazole

Adult: 20–40 mg a day, 1 hour before a meal. Capsules may be opened and mixed with a tablespoon of cool applesauce for people having difficulty swallowing. Eat the mixture right away, and do not chew the pellets.

Child (under age 18): not recommended.

Lansoprazole

Adult: 15–30 mg a day. Capsules may be opened and mixed with 1 tbsp. of cool applesauce for people having difficulty swallowing. People with liver disease need a lower dosage.

Child: (age 1–11): 15–30 mg a day.

NapraPAC

Adult: 15 mg lansoprazole/375–500 mg naproxen a day.

Omeprazole

Adult: 20–40 mg a day. Antacids may be taken with omeprazole.

Child (age 2 and over): 10–20 mg a day.

Pantoprazole

Adult: 40 mg once a day, preferably in the morning.

Prevpac: 2 amoxicillin (Trimox) capsules, 1 clarithromycin (Biaxin) tablet, and 1 lansoprazole (Prevacid) capsule before breakfast and dinner.

Rabeprazole

Adult: 20 mg a day.

Child (under age 18): not recommended.

Zegerid

Adult: 1 capsule (20 or 40 mg) or 1 powder packet (20 or 40 mg) a day with water. Do not use other liquids or foods. Take at least 1 hour before a meal, on an empty stomach.

Child (under age 18): not recommended.

Overdosage

Little is known about the effects of PPI overdose. Symptoms are likely to resemble side effects. Call your local poison control center or a hospital emergency room for more information. If you seek treatment, ALWAYS bring the prescription bottle or container.

Special Information

Call your doctor if you are unusually tired or weak, or if you develop a sore throat, fever, sores in the mouth that do not heal, unusual bleeding or bruising, bloody or cloudy urine, urinary difficulties, or any persistent or bothersome side effect.

Take the full course of treatment prescribed, even if your symptoms improve after 1 or 2 weeks.

If you forget a dose, take it as soon as you remember. If it is almost time for your next dose, skip the one you forgot and continue with your regular schedule. Do not take a double dose.

Special Populations

Pregnancy/Breast-feeding: PPIs may be toxic to pregnant animals. When your doctor considers this drug crucial, its potential benefits must be carefully weighed against its risks.

It is not known if PPIs pass into breast milk. Nursing mothers who use this drug should consider using infant formula.

Seniors: Seniors report the same side effects as younger adults.

Generic Name

Quetiapine (kwe-TYE-uh-pene)

Brand Names

Seroquel   Seroquel XR

Type of Drug

Antipsychotic.

Prescribed For

Psychotic disorders, bipolar disorder, and schizophrenia.

General Information

Quetiapine fumarate is effective against a wide variety of symptoms. It may work by antagonizing a number of different types of brain receptors. This means that the drug decreases levels of certain neurotransmitters including serotonin, dopamine, and histamine, by preventing them from binding to cell receptors. Quetiapine is broken down by the liver.

Cautions and Warnings

Do not take quetiapine if you are **allergic** or **sensitive** to any of its ingredients. Severe reactions include swelling of the lips, tongue, face, arms, or legs; closing of the throat; and intestinal reactions.

Quetiapine has been associated with increased mortality in seniors with **dementia** or **Alzheimer's disease**. The causes of death were due to a heart-related event or infection, mainly pneumonia.

Quetiapine should not be used in people with dementia-related psychosis.

Antidepressants have been linked to an increase in suicidal behavior amongst **teens** and **adolescents**. All patients started on quetiapine should be closely monitored, especially in the first few months of treatment, for changes in behavior, worsening of symptoms, or suicidal tendencies.

A potentially fatal condition called **neuroleptic malignant syndrome** (symptoms include convulsions, breathing difficulties, and back, neck, or leg pain) may occur with some antipsychotic drugs. People who have experienced this syndrome with another antipsychotic drug should be cautious when taking quetiapine.

Antipsychotic drugs are often associated with involuntary, uncoordinated, and uncontrolled movements. This reaction is most common among older adults, especially women. Contact your doctor if you develop any unusual movements while taking quetiapine.

Quetiapine should be used with caution if you have had a **seizure,** or have a seizure disorder or other condition that may make you more susceptible to seizures.

Quetiapine may make you dizzy or cause you to faint if you rise suddenly from a sitting or lying position. It should be used with caution if you have a **history of heart disease** including **heart attack, angina pains,** and **abnormal heart rhythms**. Take this drug with caution if you have a condition or take any drug that can cause **low blood pressure**.

People taking this drug for a long period have developed cataracts, but they have not been directly related to the drug. People taking quetiapine should have an eye exam when they start the drug and every 6 months thereafter to detect any cataract formation.

Quetiapine treatment has been associated with low levels of thyroid hormone in the blood. This is usually not a problem, although a small percentage of people taking this drug may need a thyroid supplement.

Quetiapine may cause increases in blood cholesterol and triglyceride levels.

Quetiapine has caused liver inflammation without any symptoms, as measured by increases in enzymes produced by the liver. These enzymes generally return to normal with continued treatment.

Antipsychotics can upset the body's temperature-regulating mechanism creating the risk for heat stroke or dehydration.

Swallowing problems and inhaling food have been experienced by people taking other antipsychotics and may present problems for those taking quetiapine.

Quetiapine has been associated with obesity, high cholesterol, high blood sugar, and diabetes. Very severe high blood sugar that is not treated can be fatal. People with **diabetes** or those who are at **risk for diabetes** should have their blood glucose levels monitored while taking quetiapine.

Possible Side Effects

▼ Most common: dizziness, headache, agitation, upset stomach, tiredness, sleepiness, dizziness or fainting when rising from a sitting or lying position, abdominal pain, weight gain, and dry mouth.

▼ Common: swelling in the arms or legs, heart palpitations, spastic movements, difficulty talking, sore throat, runny nose, increased coughing, breathing difficulties, flu-like symptoms, appetite loss, sweating, and low white-blood-cell counts.

▼ Less common: Other side effects can occur in almost any part of the body. Contact your doctor if you experience any side effect not listed above.

Drug Interactions

- Drinking alcohol while taking quetiapine can cause drowsiness.
- Quetiapine may antagonize the effects of drugs used to treat Parkinson's disease.
- Combining quetiapine with phenytoin increases the rate at which quetiapine is released from the body by 5 times. You may require an increase in quetiapine dosage to achieve the same effect. Once dosage has been adjusted, special caution should be taken if phenytoin is replaced by another anti-seizure drug that does not stimulate the body's breakdown of quetiapine. Other drugs that have a similar effect on quetiapine are thioridazine, carbamazepine, barbiturates, rifampin, and oral corticosteroids.

- Ketoconazole, itraconazole, fluconazole, and erythromycin may affect quetiapine. Caution should be exercised when combining these drugs with quetiapine.
- Quetiapine may reduce the rate at which the body clears lorazepam.
- Quetiapine may enhance the effects of blood-pressure-lowering drugs.

Food Interactions

Taking quetiapine with food increases the amount of drug absorbed by a small amount. This is not likely to change its effect on your body.

Usual Dose

Quetiapine
Adult: 150–750 mg a day. Seniors may obtain maximum benefit with smaller doses.

Quetiapine XR
Adult: 400–800 mg a day.

Overdosage

Overdose victims should be taken to a hospital emergency room at once. ALWAYS bring the prescription bottle or container.

Special Information

Quetiapine may make you drowsy. Take care while driving or performing any task that requires concentration.

Antipsychotic drugs may increase your sensitivity to hot weather and your susceptibility to dehydration by interfering with temperature-control mechanisms.

Special Populations

Pregnancy/Breast-feeding: Quetiapine should only be taken during pregnancy if the possible benefits outweigh the risks. Talk to your doctor if you become pregnant or are trying to become pregnant while taking this drug.

Quetiapine passes into breast milk. Nursing mothers who must take quetiapine should use infant formula.

Seniors: Seniors may be more sensitive to side effects, especially dizziness, fainting, and tiredness.

Generic Name

Quinapril (QUIN-uh-pril) Ⓖ

Brand Name
Accupril

Combination Products
Generic Ingredients: Quinapril + Hydrochlorothiazide Ⓖ
Accuretic   Quinaretic

The information in this profile also applies to the following drugs:

Generic Ingredient: Perindopril
Aceon

Generic Ingredient: Ramipril
Altace

Type of Drug
Angiotensin-converting enzyme (ACE) inhibitor.

Prescribed For
High blood pressure and congestive heart failure. Also prescribed for kidney failure, kidney hypertension, post–heart attack management, management of people with a high risk of heart disease, diabetes, chronic kidney disease, and preventing a second stroke.

General Information
Quinapril hydrochloride and other ACE inhibitors work by preventing the conversion of a hormone called angiotensin I to another hormone called angiotensin II, a potent blood-vessel constrictor. Preventing this conversion relaxes blood vessels, thus reducing blood pressure and relieving the symptoms of heart failure. Quinapril also affects the production of other hormones and enzymes that participate in the regulation of blood-vessel dilation. Quinapril begins working about 1 hour after you take it and lasts for 24 hours.

Cautions and Warnings
Do not take quinapril if you are **allergic** or **sensitive** to any of its ingredients. Severe sensitivity reactions can occur in people taking an ACE inhibitor while on **hemodialysis** or undergoing **venom immunization**.

    Quinapril occasionally causes very low blood pressure. Quinapril can affect your kidneys, especially if you have **congestive heart**

failure. It is advisable for your doctor to check your urine for changes during the first few months of treatment. Dosage adjustment is necessary if you have **reduced kidney function**.

Rarely, quinapril affects white-blood-cell count, possibly increasing your susceptibility to infection. Blood counts should be monitored periodically.

Quinapril can cause fetal injury or death; do not take quinapril if you are **pregnant.**

ACE inhibitors may be less effective in some **black patients** with high blood pressure, especially when dietary salt intake is high. Nevertheless, they should still be considered useful blood pressure treatments. Swelling beneath the skin to form welts is more common among black patients.

Possible Side Effects

▼ Most common: dizziness, tiredness, headache, and chronic cough. The cough usually goes away a few days after you stop taking the medication.

▼ Less common: nausea, vomiting, and abdominal pain.

▼ Rare: Rare side effects can occur in almost any part of the body. Contact your doctor if you experience any side effect not listed above.

Drug Interactions

- The blood-pressure-lowering effect of quinapril is additive with diuretic drugs and beta blockers. Any other drug that causes a rapid drop in blood pressure should be used with caution if you are taking an ACE inhibitor.
- Quinapril may increase the effects of lithium; this combination should be used with caution.
- Aspirin and other nonsteroidal anti-inflammatory drugs (NSAIDs) reduce the blood-pressure-lowering effects of quinapril and other ACE inhibitors. The combination may cause reductions in kidney function.
- Quinapril may increase potassium levels in your blood, especially when taken with dyazide or other potassium-sparing diuretics.
- Antacids and quinapril should be taken at least 2 hours apart.
- Quinapril decreases the absorption of tetracycline by about $1/3$, possibly because of the high magnesium content of quinapril tablets.

- Quinapril may affect blood levels of digoxin. More digoxin in the blood increases the chance of digoxin-related side effects while less digoxin in the blood can compromise its effectiveness.
- Capsaicin may trigger or aggravate the cough associated with quinapril therapy.
- Indomethacin may reduce the blood-pressure-lowering effect of quinapril.
- Phenothiazine sedatives and antiemetics may increase the effects of quinapril.
- Combining allopurinol and quinapril can produce a severe sensitivity reaction.
- The combination of perindopril and gentamicin should be used with caution.

Food Interactions

Quinapril can be taken with food if it upsets your stomach.

Usual Dose

Quinapril: Adult dosage is 10–80 mg a day in 1 or 2 doses. Seniors and people with kidney disease may require a lower dosage.

Accuretic: 1 tablet a day.

Perindopril: Adult dosage is 4–8 mg a day. Seniors and people with kidney disease may require a lower dosage.

Ramipril: Adult dosage is 2.5–20 mg a day. Seniors and people with moderate to severe kidney disease should begin with 1.25 mg a day; dosage may then be increased up to 5 mg a day.

Overdosage

The principal effect of quinapril overdose is a rapid drop in blood pressure, as evidenced by dizziness and fainting. Take the overdose victim to a hospital emergency room at once. ALWAYS bring the prescription bottle or container.

Special Information

ACE inhibitors may cause unexplained swelling of the face, lips, hands, and feet. This swelling can also affect the larynx (throat) and tongue and interfere with breathing. If this happens, go to a hospital emergency room for treatment immediately. Call your doctor if you develop a sore throat, mouth sores, abnormal heartbeat, chest pain, a persistent rash, or loss of taste perception.

Some people who start taking an ACE inhibitor after they are already on a diuretic (an agent that increases urination) experience a rapid blood-pressure drop after their first doses or when the dosage is increased. To prevent this from happening, you may be told to stop taking the diuretic 2 or 3 days before starting the ACE inhibitor or to increase your salt intake during that time. The diuretic may then be restarted gradually.

You may get dizzy if you rise too quickly from a sitting or lying position when taking quinapril.

Avoid strenuous exercise and very hot weather because heavy sweating or dehydration can cause a rapid drop in blood pressure.

Avoid over-the-counter diet pills, decongestants, and other stimulants that can raise blood pressure. Also do not take potassium supplements or salt substitutes containing potassium without consulting your doctor.

If you forget a dose, take it as soon as you remember. If it is within 8 hours of your next dose, skip the one you forgot and continue with your regular schedule. Do not take a double dose.

Special Populations

Pregnancy/Breast-feeding: ACE inhibitors can cause fetal injury or death. Women who are or might be pregnant should not take quinapril. Stop taking the medication and contact your doctor if you become pregnant.

Small amounts of quinapril pass into breast milk. Nursing mothers who must take this drug should use infant formula.

Seniors: Seniors may be more sensitive to the effects of quinapril due to age-related kidney impairment. The dosage for seniors is often lower.

Generic Name

Quinidine (QUIN-ih-dene) Ⓖ

Brand Names

Cardioquin
Quinaglute Dura-Tabs

Quinidex Extentabs
Quin-Release

Type of Drug

Antiarrhythmic.

Prescribed For

Abnormal heart rhythms.

General Information

Derived from the bark of the cinchona tree, which also gives us quinine, quinidine works by affecting the flow of potassium into and out of heart muscle cells. This helps quinidine slow the flow of nerve impulses throughout the heart muscle, which allows control mechanisms in the heart to take over and keep the heart beating at a normal, even rate. The 3 kinds of quinidine—gluconate, polygalacturonate, and sulfate—provide different amounts of active drug and cannot be interchanged without dosage adjustments.

Cautions and Warnings

Do not take quinidine if you are **allergic** or **sensitive** to any of its ingredients or to quinine or a related drug. Quinidine sensitivity may be masked if you have **asthma, muscle weakness,** or an **infection** when you start taking the drug.

Liver toxicity related to quinidine sensitivity occurs rarely. Unexplained fever or liver inflammation may indicate this effect. Your doctor should monitor your liver function during the first 4–8 weeks of therapy. People with **kidney or liver disease** may require lower dosages.

Quinidine can also cause abnormal heart rhythms.

People taking quinidine for long periods may experience sudden fainting or an abnormal heart rhythm. Occasionally, these episodes may be fatal.

Possible Side Effects

▼ Most common: nausea, vomiting, abdominal pain, diarrhea, and appetite loss. These may be accompanied by fever.

▼ Less common: unusual heart rhythms, altering of blood components, irritation of the esophagus, headache, dizziness, feelings of apprehension or excitement, confusion, delirium, muscle ache or joint pain, ringing or buzzing in the ears, mild hearing loss, blurred vision, changes in color perception, sensitivity to bright light, double vision, difficulty seeing at night, flushing of the skin, itching, sensitivity to the

---

Possible Side Effects (continued)

sun, cramps, an unusual urge to defecate or urinate, and cold sweat.

▼ Rare: collapse of blood vessels; asthma; swelling of the face, hands, and feet; respiratory collapse; and liver problems.

High dosages of quinidine may cause rash, hearing loss, dizziness, ringing in the ears, headache, nausea, or disturbed vision. This group of symptoms, called cinchonism, is usually related to taking a large amount of quinidine but may appear after a single dose of the medication. Cinchonism is not necessarily a toxic reaction, but you should immediately report any sign of it to your doctor. Do not stop taking this drug unless instructed to do so by your doctor. Contact your doctor if you experience any side effect not listed above.

Drug Interactions

- Quinidine increases the effect of warfarin and other oral anticoagulants (blood thinners).
- Quinidine may increase the effects of metoprolol, procainamide, propafenone, propranolol, and other beta blockers; succinylcholine; benztropine, oxybutynin, atropine, trihexyphenidyl, and other anticholinergic drugs; and tricyclic antidepressants.
- The effect of quinidine may be decreased by the following medicines: phenobarbital and other barbiturates, phenytoin and other hydantoins, nifedipine, rifampin, sucralfate, and cholinergic drugs such as bethanechol.
- The effectiveness and side effects of quinidine may be increased by taking amiodarone, some antacids, cimetidine, clarithromycin, diltiazem, erythromycin, fluvoxamine, itraconazole, ketoconazole, indinavir, mibefradil, nefazodone, nelfinavir, ritonavir, troleandomycin, verapamil, or anything that decreases urine acid levels.
- Quinidine may dramatically increase the amount of digoxin in the blood, causing possible digoxin toxicity. This combination should be monitored closely by your doctor.
- The combination of disopyramide and quinidine may result in increased disopyramide levels and possible side effects; reduced quinidine activity may also result.

- Avoid over-the-counter cough, cold, allergy, and diet preparations. These medications may contain drugs that stimulate the heart and may be dangerous in combination with quinidine.
- St. John's wort may decrease quinidine levels.
- Avoid taking megadoses of vitamin C while taking this drug.

Food Interactions

You may take quinidine with food if it upsets your stomach. Some forms of quinidine may be less irritating to the stomach. Avoid drinking grapefruit juice.

Usual Dose

Immediate-Release
Adult: extremely variable; generally, 600–1200 mg a day.
Child: not recommended.

Sustained-Release
Adult: generally, 600–1800 mg a day.
Child: not recommended.

Overdosage

Overdose produces depressed mental function, including lethargy, decreased breathing, seizures, and coma. Other symptoms are abdominal pain and diarrhea, abnormal heart rhythms, and symptoms of cinchonism (see "Possible Side Effects"). The victim should be taken to a hospital emergency room. ALWAYS bring the prescription bottle or container.

Special Information

Call your doctor if you develop ringing or buzzing in the ears, hearing or visual disturbances, dizziness, headache, nausea, rash, breathing difficulties, or any intolerable side effect.

Do not crush or chew the sustained-release products.

Some side effects of quinidine may lead to oral discomfort including dry mouth, cavities, periodontal disease, and oral Candida infections. See your dentist regularly while taking this drug.

If you forget to take a dose of quinidine and you remember within 2 hours of your regular time, take it right away. If you do not remember until later, skip the dose you forgot and continue your regular schedule. Do not take a double dose.

Special Populations

Pregnancy/Breast-feeding: Quinidine may cause birth defects. When this drug is considered crucial by your doctor, its potential benefits must be carefully weighed against its risks.

Quinidine passes into breast milk but is considered acceptable for use while breast-feeding. Consult your doctor.

Seniors: Seniors may be more sensitive to the effects of this medication due to decreased kidney function.

Generic Name

Raloxifene (rah-LOX-ih-feen)

Brand Name

Evista

Type of Drug

Selective Estrogen Receptor Modulator (SERM).

Prescribed For

Osteoporosis prevention and treatment. Also used for breast cancer prevention.

General Information

The female hormone estrogen plays an important role in maintaining bone strength in women by regulating the body's use of calcium. When the ovaries stop producing estrogen after menopause, a woman's risk of developing osteoporosis increases significantly. Raloxifene hydrochloride, which belongs to the SERM class of drugs, is used to increase bone density and prevent broken bones in postmenopausal women by mimicking the protective effect that estrogen has on bone. This drug also lowers cholesterol levels by acting like estrogen therapy in the cardiovascular system. Raloxifene has a potential advantage over estrogen therapy in the treatment of osteoporosis because it does not appear to have an estrogen-like effect in the breast or uterus, where the hormone may increase cancer risk. Raloxifene is broken down in the liver.

Cautions and Warnings

Do not take raloxifene if you are **allergic** or **sensitive** to any of its ingredients; are **pregnant;** or have had **blood-clotting problems** or clots in the lung, leg, eye, or another part of the body.

Only **postmenopausal women** should use raloxifene.

People with moderate to severe **kidney or liver disease** should use this drug with caution.

Raloxifene should not be used to prevent **heart disease**. **Women** taking raloxifene have a greater risk of dying of a stroke, though the overall risk of a stroke is small—1.2%. Triglycerides should be closely monitored in women with **high blood triglyceride levels** as this drug can further increase triglycerides, a risk factor for heart disease.

There is an increased risk of **venous thromboembolism** with raloxifene; women with a history of this disorder should not take this drug.

There is no information on the use of this drug by **men**.

Possible Side Effects

▼ Most common: infections, flu-like symptoms, hot flashes, joint pain, and sinus irritation.

▼ Common: depression, sleeplessness, headaches, rash, nausea, diarrhea, upset stomach, weight gain, muscle aches, leg cramps, sore throat, and cough.

▼ Less common: chest pain, fever, migraine, sweating, vomiting, gas, stomach and intestinal problems, vaginal irritation, vaginal discharge, urinary infection, cystitis, endometrial problems, swelling in the arms or legs, arthritis, pneumonia, and laryngitis.

▼ Rare: coughing up of blood; loss of or changes in speech, coordination, or vision; pain or numbness in the chest, arm, or leg; and shortness of breath. Rare side effects can occur in almost any part of the body. Contact your doctor if you experience any side effect not listed above.

Raloxifene is more likely to cause hot flashes, infection, and chest pain than estrogen therapy but is much less likely to cause abdominal pain, vaginal bleeding, breast pain, and gas.

Drug Interactions

• Taking raloxifene and estrogen therapy is not recommended because the effects of this combination are unknown.

• Raloxifene can increase blood levels of clofibrate, indomethacin, naproxen, ibuprofen, diazepam, and diazoxide.

• Ampicillin can reduce the absorption of raloxifene, but this interaction is not considered important.

- Cholestyramine can reduce the amount of raloxifene absorbed by 60%. Separate doses of these drugs by 2 hours or more.
- Raloxifene can reduce the effect of warfarin (a blood thinner). Your warfarin dosage may need adjustment.
- Raloxifene interferes with the absorption and effectiveness of levothyroxine. Separate these two medicines by 12 hours.

Food Interactions

Raloxifene can be taken with or without food.

Usual Dose

Adult: 60 mg once a day.
Child: not recommended.

Overdosage

Little is known about the effects of raloxifene overdose. Call your local poison control center or a hospital emergency room for information. If you seek treatment, ALWAYS bring the prescription bottle or container.

Special Information

Raloxifene can increase your risk of developing a blood clot in the lung, leg, or another part of the body during any extended period of inactivity. Stop taking raloxifene 3 days before surgery, a long period of bed rest, or lengthy plane or car trips.

It is very important for all postmenopausal women and women age 51 and over to get 1200 mg of calcium and 10 mcg (400 IU) of vitamin D every day, either from food or a dietary supplement. Women age 70 and over require 1200 mg of calcium and 15 mcg (600 IU) of vitamin D daily.

Regular exercise is recommended for all postmenopausal women because it helps build strong bones.

Raloxifene does not reduce the hot flashes or flushes associated with menopause. Call your doctor if you experience hot flashes or flushes, uterine bleeding, or breast changes while taking raloxifene.

If you forget a dose, take it as soon as you remember. If a whole day has passed without taking your medication, skip the forgotten dose and continue with your regular schedule. Do not take a double dose.

Special Populations

Pregnancy/Breast-feeding: Raloxifene can harm the fetus. It is not considered safe for use during pregnancy.

It is not known if raloxifene passes into breast milk. Nursing mothers who must take it should use infant formula.

Seniors: Seniors can use raloxifene without special precaution.

Generic Name

Raltegravir (rahl-TEG-rah-veer)

Brand Name
Isentress

Type of Drug
HIV integrase inhibitor.

Prescribed For
Human immunodeficiency virus (HIV).

General Information
Raltegravir is the first HIV integrase strand transfer inhibitor. HIV integrase is an enzyme required for the HIV virus to reproduce. It is responsible for the integration of HIV-1 DNA into an infected cell. Once introduced into a cell, the DNA forms the provirus that is required to create new HIV virus. Raltegravir's unique mechanism of action makes it a valuable addition to other HIV drug treatments that attack different aspects of HIV reproduction. It is recommended only for adults who have been unsuccessfully treated with other HIV antiviral medicines. It is broken down in the liver. Resistance to the effects of raltegravir can develop in a number of different ways.

Cautions and Warnings
Do not take raltegravir if you are **allergic** or **sensitive** to any of its ingredients.

When beginning treatment with raltegravir, some patients who respond to therapy sometimes develop an inflammatory response to infectious organisms already in the body but in an inactive state such as *Mycobacterium,* cytomegalovirus, *pneumocystis* pneumonia, or tuberculosis, or they may experience a reactivation of varicella zoster virus, which may necessitate further evaluation and treatment.

Raltegravir can cause muscle aches and destruction of muscle tissue.

Possible Side Effects

▼ Most common: diarrhea.
▼ Common: nausea, headache, and fever.
▼ Less common: abdominal pain, vomiting, weakness, fatigue, dizziness, selective loss of body fat, anemia, heart attack, reduced white-blood-cell count, hepatitis, herpes simplex infection, gastritis (a burning pain in your upper abdomen, bloating, belching, nausea, or vomiting), and kidney disease.
▼ Rare: Cancers have been reported in people taking this drug. The type and frequency is consistent with those found in people with poorly functioning immune systems. Contact your doctor if you experience any side effect not listed above.

Drug Interactions

- Rifampin, phenytoin, and phenobarbital reduce the amount of raltegravir in the blood; dose adjustment may be needed.
- Efavirenz, nevirapine, rifabutin, St. John's wort, and tipranavir + ritonavir may reduce raltegravir blood concentrations, but dose adjustment is not needed.
- Atazanavir and atazanavir + ritonavir increase the amount of raltegravir in the blood, but dose adjustment is not needed.

Food Interactions

Raltegravir can be taken without regard to food or meals.

Usual Dose

Adult (age 16 and over): 400 mg twice a day. Dosage range is 100–1600 mg a day.

Child: not recommended.

Overdosage

No specific information is available on raltegravir overdose. Take the victim to a hospital emergency room at once for treatment. ALWAYS bring the prescription bottle or container.

Special Information

This drug is not a cure for HIV. It will not prevent you from transmitting the HIV virus to another person; you must still practice safe sex. People taking this drug may still develop opportunistic infections and other complications of advanced HIV infection. It is very important to take these drugs exactly as prescribed. Every dose of HIV medication you forget or skip can make it more difficult for the drugs to do their job and can lead to the development of HIV resistance.

People infected with HIV must take especially good care of their teeth and gums to minimize the risk of developing oral infections.

If you forget a dose of raltegravir, take it as soon as you remember. If you do not remember until it is almost time for your next dose, skip the one you forgot and continue with your regular schedule. Do not take a double dose of this medicine. Call you doctor if you forget 2 or more doses in a row.

Special Populations

Pregnancy/Breast-feeding: Animal studies of raltegravir have not shown it to be toxic to the developing fetus. However, pregnant women should only use raltegravir if its potential benefits outweigh its risks.

It is not known if raltegravir passes into breast milk. Mothers with HIV should always use infant formula, regardless of whether they take this drug, to avoid transmitting the virus to their child.

Seniors: Studies have not revealed any differences in response between seniors and younger adults. Caution is recommended because of the likelihood of other concurrent diseases and drug therapy, and reduced liver, kidney, and heart function in seniors.

Generic Name

Ramelteon (RAM-el-tee-on)

Brand Name

Rozerem

Type of Drug

Hypnotic.

Prescribed For

Insomnia characterized by difficulty falling asleep.

General Information

Ramelteon is a unique hypnotic that activates the same nerve endings in the brain that are acted on by melatonin, the hormone that is essential to natural sleep and our normal circadian rhythms that dictate sleep-wake patterns. Some have called this drug "super-melatonin." It does not act on brain receptors targeted by other widely used sedatives and hypnotics.

Ramelteon studies have shown it has no potential for abuse and it is not considered a controlled substance under federal laws. Studies of up to 20 times the recommended dosage showed no indication of abuse potential with this drug. There was also no evidence of memory loss or hangover after 2 days of taking ramelteon. But in a study where adults with chronic trouble sleeping took ramelteon for 35 consecutive nights, there was some morning-after fatigue and sluggishness as well as short-term memory difficulties. Information from this study also showed no risk for drug withdrawal symptoms or sleeplessness after stopping ramelteon.

Ramelteon passes rapidly into the blood and starts working in a few minutes. It is broken down in the liver and mostly passes out of the body in the urine.

Cautions and Warnings

Do not take ramelteon if you are **allergic** or **sensitive** to any of its ingredients.

Complex sleep-related behaviors including driving, eating, and walking while asleep, with no memory of the event afterward, can occur with ramelteon and other sleep medications. These activities happen after taking a sedative-hypnotic product while you are not fully awake.

People with **severe liver disease** should not take this drug. Even those with mild liver disease can have as much as 4 times as much ramelteon in their blood as those with normal liver function.

Studies of ramelteon show it does not cause difficulty breathing. However, people with **chronic obstructive pulmonary disease** and other respiratory conditions have not yet been studied with this drug.

Difficulty sleeping may be a sign of another physical or psychiatric problem. If ramelteon does not help you, ask your doctor to look for other issues that might be interfering with your sleep and have not yet been discovered.

People with **severe sleep apnea** should use ramelteon with caution because it has not been studied in this group. Ramelteon does not worsen mild to moderate sleep apnea.

In **depressed** patients taking any hypnotic drug, worsening depression, including suicidal thoughts, is possible.

Ramelteon can affect hormone levels in adults, decreasing testosterone and increasing prolactin.

The effects of ramelteon on reproductive system development in growing **children** are not known.

Possible Side Effects

▼ Common: headache, tiredness, and dizziness.
▼ Less common: fatigue, nausea, diarrhea, worsening sleeplessness, upper respiratory infections, muscle aches, depression, taste changes, joint pains, and flu infections.

Report any other side effects, particularly changes in behavior, to your doctor.

Drug Interactions

- Fluvoxamine can dramatically increase the amount of ramelteon in the blood by interfering with enzymes in the liver that break it down. Do not take ramelteon if you are also taking fluvoxamine.
- Ketoconazole and fluconazole increase the amount of ramelteon in the blood by affecting its breakdown in the liver. This combination should be used with caution.
- Rifampin increases the rate at which the liver breaks down ramelteon and can reduce its effectiveness.
- Alcohol can increase ramelteon's effects. Avoid alcoholic beverages before you take ramelteon or during the 30 minutes between taking ramelteon and going to sleep.

Food Interactions

This drug is best taken on an empty stomach. Taking it with or immediately after a high-fat meal will delay the absorption of ramelteon into the bloodstream.

Usual Dose

Adult: 8 mg taken 30 minutes before sleep.
Child: not recommended.

Overdosage

There have been no reports of ramelteon overdose, although symptoms are likely to be sleepiness and some of its side effects. Overdose victims should be taken to a hospital emergency room at once. ALWAYS bring the prescription bottle or container.

Special Information

Avoid alcohol.

Avoid engaging in activities that require concentration (such as operating a motor vehicle or heavy machinery) after taking ramelteon.

Take ramelteon within 30 minutes of going to bed. After taking this drug, you should restrict your activities, since you are likely to become sleepy within a few minutes.

Call your doctor if your insomnia gets worse while taking ramelteon or if you develop any behavioral changes, reduced sex drive (men or women), skipped periods, release of breast milk (women), or fertility problems (men or women).

Do not take more than 1 dose a day.

Special Populations

Pregnancy/Breast-feeding: In animal studies, ramelteon affected the development of a growing fetus, but its effects on the human fetus are unknown. This drug should be taken during pregnancy only if its potential benefits outweigh its possible risks.

In animal studies, ramelteon passed into the breast milk of nursing animals, but it is not known if this drug passes into human milk. Nursing mothers who must take it should consider using infant formula.

Seniors: Seniors retain almost twice as much ramelteon as younger adults and should use the lowest effective dose.

Generic Name

Ranitidine (rah-NIT-ih-deen) Ⓖ

Brand Name

Zantac

Type of Drug

Antiulcer and histamine H_2 antagonist.

Prescribed For

Duodenal (intestinal) and gastric (stomach) ulcers, gastroesophageal reflux disease (GERD), and erosive esophagitis; also prescribed for other conditions characterized by the secretion of large amounts of gastric fluids, and to prevent bleeding in the stomach and upper intestines, stress ulcers, stomach damage caused by nonsteroidal anti-inflammatory drugs (NSAIDs), and the production of stomach acid during surgery.

General Information

Ranitidine hydrochloride and other H_2 antagonists work by turning off the system that produces stomach acid and other secretions. Ranitidine starts working within 1 hour and reaches its peak effect in 1–3 hours. Its effect lasts for up to 15 hours. Ranitidine is effective in treating ulcer symptoms and preventing complications of the disease. It is prescribed for short-term and maintenance therapy. Since all H_2 antagonists work in the same way, ulcers that do not respond to one will probably not respond to another. The only difference among H_2 antagonists is their potency. Cimetidine is the least potent, with 1000 mg roughly equal to 300 mg of ranitidine and nizatidine or 40 mg of famotidine. The ulcer-healing rates of all of these drugs are roughly equivalent, as is the risk of side effects.

Cautions and Warnings

Do not take ranitidine if you are **allergic** or **sensitive** to any of its ingredients or to another H_2 antagonist.

Caution must be exercised by people with **kidney or liver disease** who take ranitidine because the drug is partly broken down in the liver and passes out of the body through the kidneys. Occasionally, reversible hepatitis or other liver abnormality may occur, with or without jaundice (symptoms include yellowing of the skin or whites of the eyes).

Reducing stomach acid levels in a person with **compromised immune function** may increase the risk of intestinal worm infection.

Ranitidine should not be used in people with **acute porphyria.**

Possible Side Effects

Side effects with ranitidine are rare.

▼ Most common: dizziness, confusion, hallucinations, depression, sleeplessness, hair loss, inflammation of the pancreas, joint pain, and drug reactions.

▼ Less common: headache, blurred vision, agitation or anxiety, nausea, vomiting, constipation, diarrhea, abdominal discomfort, painful breast swelling, impotence, loss of sex drive, and rash.

▼ Rare: rapid or irregular heartbeat, reversible reduction in white-blood-cell or blood-platelet count, and hepatitis. Contact your doctor if you experience any side effect not listed above.

Drug Interactions

- Antacids slightly reduce the effects of ranitidine. To avoid this interaction, separate doses of these drugs by about 2–3 hours.
- Ranitidine may interfere with the absorption of diazepam tablets. This interaction is considered minor and is unlikely to affect most people.
- Ranitidine may increase blood concentrations of glipizide, glyburide, theophylline drugs, and procainamide, increasing the risk of side effects. Interactions between ranitidine and glyburide or a theophylline drug are rare.
- Ranitidine may interact with warfarin, an anticoagulant (blood thinner). Your warfarin dosage may need an adjustment.

Food Interactions

You may take ranitidine with or without food.

Usual Dose

Adult: 150–300 mg a day. People with severe conditions may require up to 600 mg a day. People with severe kidney disease need less medication.

Child (age 1 month–16 years): 0.42–0.9 mg per lb. every 12 hours up to the 150–300 mg a day maintenance dose.

Child (under 1 month): 0.9–1.8 mg per lb. divided into 2 or 3 doses a day.

Overdosage

Little is known about the effects of ranitidine overdose, although symptoms are likely to include severe side effects. Induce vomiting with ipecac syrup—available at any pharmacy. Call your doctor or a local poison control center before doing this. If you seek treatment, ALWAYS bring the prescription bottle or container.

Special Information

It may take several days for ranitidine to begin to relieve stomach pain. You must take this drug exactly as directed and follow your doctor's instructions for diet and other treatments to get the maximum benefit from it.

Call your doctor at once if any unusual side effects develop. Especially important are unusual bleeding or bruising, unusual tiredness, diarrhea, dizziness, rash, or hallucinations. Black, tarry stools or vomiting "coffee-ground"-like material may indicate that your ulcer is bleeding.

If you forget a dose, take it as soon as you remember. If it is almost time for your next dose, skip the one you forgot and continue with your regular schedule. Do not take a double dose.

Special Populations

Pregnancy/Breast-feeding: While animal studies of ranitidine reveal no damage to the fetus, this drug should only be used during pregnancy after carefully weighing its potential benefits against its risks.

Large amounts of ranitidine pass into breast milk. Nursing mothers who must take this drug should consider using infant formula.

Seniors: Seniors may obtain maximum benefit with smaller dosages. They also may be more susceptible to side effects, especially confusion.

Generic Name

Ranolazine (rah-NO-la-zeen)

Brand Name

Ranexa

Type of Drug

Antianginal agent.

Prescribed For

Treatment of chronic angina that has not responded to other treatments.

General Information

Ranolazine has been studied in people with angina who had not responded to maximum doses of other antianginal drugs. These studies showed significant reductions in the number of angina attacks in people taking ranolazine. It is intended to reduce the number of angina attacks, not to treat an acute attack. Its exact mechanism is unknown, but some common ways of relieving chest pain, such as reducing heart rate and blood pressure, are not part of how ranolazine works. It is broken down in the gut and the liver, so its absorption into the bloodstream can be very variable. It takes about 3 days of medicine to produce a steady blood level in your body. About ¾ of each dose passes out of the body via the urine. Ranolazine is prescribed in combination with other antianginal drugs including some calcium channel blockers, beta blockers, and nitrates. Men appear to benefit more from ranolazine than women.

Cautions and Warnings

Do not take ranolazine if you are **allergic** or **sensitive** to any of its ingredients.

Ranolazine should be used with caution if you have **liver disease.** People with **severe kidney disease** may experience significant blood pressure increases. Check your blood pressure regularly. People with an **abnormal electrocardiogram** should not take this medicine.

Possible Side Effects

▼ Common: headache, dizziness, constipation, and nausea.
▼ Less common: palpitations, ringing in the ears, fainting, dry mouth, abdominal pains, vomiting, swelling in the arms or legs, and difficulty breathing.
▼ Rare: slow heart beat, blood in the urine, reduced touch sensitivity, low blood pressure, dizziness when rising from a sitting or lying position, tingling in the hands or feet, tremors, and blurred vision. Contact your doctor if you experience any side effect not listed above.

Drug Interactions

- Ketoconazole, itraconazole, voriconazole, diltiazem, verapamil, erythromycin, clarithromycin, and protease inhibitors
  interfere with one of the enzymes that break down ranolazine.
  Do not take these drugs with ranolazine because they can
  raise the amount of ranolazine in the blood, leading to drug
  side effects.
- Caution should be exercised if you are taking ranolazine with
  cyclosporine or ritonavir.
- Blood levels of simvastatin can be doubled when taken with
  ranolazine. Simvastatin dosage adjustment is necessary.
- Ranolazine may increase blood levels of digoxin, tricyclic antidepressants, and antipsychotic drugs. Dosage adjustments
  may be needed.
- Many drugs can also affect the electrocardiogram in the same
  way as ranolazine, including amiodarone, bepridil, cisapride,
  dofetilide, dolasetron, droperidol, erythromycin, fluoxetine,
  halofantrine, haloperidol, mesoridazine, moexepril quinidine,
  sotalol, thioridazine, ziprasidone and others. These drugs
  should not be taken with ranolazine.

Food Interactions

This drug may be taken without regard to food or meals. Do not
drink grapefruit juice or eat any grapefruit-containing products
while taking this medicine.

Usual Dose

Adult (age 18 and over): 500–1000 mg twice a day. Do not chew,
crush, or break the tablets.

Child (under age 18): not recommended.

Overdosage

There are no cases of ranolazine overdose. Overdose symptoms
may include drug side effects. Overdose patients should be taken
to a hospital emergency room for treatment because of the possibility of an impact on the heart. ALWAYS bring the prescription
bottle or container.

Special Information

Ranolazine should only be taken when other antianginal drugs
have not worked.

Do not take more than 1000 mg twice a day. Larger doses are likely to affect your heart without producing a greater benefit.

Call your doctor at once if you faint or have heart palpitations.

Ranolazine can make you dizzy or lightheaded. Take extreme care while driving or operating any complex equipment or machinery.

If you forget a dose, take it as soon as you remember. If it is almost time for the next dose, skip the one you forgot and continue with your regular schedule. Do not take a double dose

Special Populations

Pregnancy/Breast-feeding: There are no studies of ranolazine in pregnant women or of its effect on the developing fetus. Pregnant women should take it only if its potential benefits outweigh the possible risks.

It is not known if ranolazine passes into breast milk, however nursing mothers should consider using infant formula while on this medicine because of the possibility of ranolazine side effects appearing in the nursing baby.

Seniors: Seniors age 75 and older may experience more ranolazine side effects than younger adults. Seniors should be started on the lowest effective dose of ranolazine.

Generic Name

Rasagiline (rah-SAY-jill-ene)

Brand Name
Azilect

Type of Drug
Monoamine oxidase inhibitor (MAOI).

Prescribed For
Parkinson's disease.

General Information
Rasagiline's exact mechanism of action is unknown, but it is believed to be related to the ability of rasagiline to inhibit one type of MAO, MAO-B, in the brain, which leads to an increase in levels of dopamine. The symptoms of Parkinson's disease are related to a deficiency of dopamine, so any treatment that increases dopamine will improve the symptoms of Parkinson's, but it does not cure the

disease. Over 90% of MAO inhibition is achieved after only 3 days of taking rasagiline, and the effect lasts 1 week after the medicine is stopped. Rasagiline is broken down by enzymes in the liver. It may be prescribed alone or together with another antiparkinsonian drug, such as the combination levodopa + carbidopa.

Cautions and Warnings

Do not take rasagiline if you are **sensitive** or **allergic** to any of its ingredients.

Rasagiline should be used with caution if you have mild **liver disease** because blood levels of the drug can be doubled. People with moderate or severe liver disease should not take this medication.

Rasagiline is a drug that has some very important and potentially deadly drug interactions (see "Drug Interactions" for details). It also has important food interactions (see "Food Interactions" for details).

Rasagiline should be stopped at least 14 days before **elective surgery.** People taking rasagiline should not undergo elective surgery requiring general anesthesia. Also, they should not be given cocaine or local anesthesia containing epinephrine or another blood-vessel-constricting medicine.

When taken with levodopa + carbidopa, rasagiline may worsen the difficulty or distortion experienced while performing voluntary muscle movements associated with levodopa and dizziness or fainting when rising from a sitting or lying position. Dizziness and fainting is most common during the first 2 months of treatment and then becomes less common.

Hallucinations may occur in a small number of people taking rasagiline by itself and a larger number of those taking it together with levodopa + carbidopa. Report any hallucinations to your doctor at once.

As with other MAOIs, rasagiline should not be taken by anyone with **pheochromocytoma**, a rare adrenal gland tumor.

Possible Side Effects

▼ Most common: headache.
▼ Common: joint pain, upset stomach, depression, falling, and flu-like symptoms.
▼ Less common: conjunctivitis (pinkeye), fever, inflammation of the stomach and/or intestines, runny nose, arthritis,

Possible Side Effects *(continued)*

black-and-blue marks, neck pain, not feeling well, tingling in the hands or feet, and dizziness.

▼ Rare: diarrhea, chest pain, protein in the urine, allergic reactions, hair loss, angina pains, appetite loss, asthma, hallucinations, erectile dysfunction, reduction in white-blood-cell count, reduced sex drive, abnormal liver function tests, skin cancer, fainting, rash, and vomiting. Contact your doctor if you experience any side effect not listed above.

Drug Interactions

- Serious reactions can occur if you combine rasagiline with meperidine, tramadol, methadone, or propoxyphene, including coma, severe changes in blood pressure, severe reduction in breathing rate, convulsions, very high fever, excitation, collapsed blood vessels, and death. Allow at least 2 weeks to elapse between taking meperidine and rasagiline.
- Do not combine any antidepressant medicine, including St. John's wort, with rasagiline. The combination may lead to high fever and death.
- Do not mix any MAOI, including rasagiline, with the cough suppressant dextromethorphan, found in many over-the-counter products. The combination has been reported to cause brief episodes of psychosis or bizarre behavior.
- Like other MAOIs, rasagiline should not be taken with stimulant drugs, including amphetamines or any over-the-counter or prescription medicine containing pseudoephedrine, phenylephrine, phenylpropanolamine, or ephedrine. Severe high blood pressure has followed the mixing of these medicines.
- Do not combine rasagiline with any other MAOI. This combination can lead to severe hypertension. Allow at least 2 weeks to elapse between taking rasagiline and any other MAOI.
- Ciprofloxacin and other fluoroquinolones, cimetidine, fluvoxamine, and ticlopidine inhibit the enzyme that breaks down rasagiline. Mixing these drugs with rasagiline can cause a substantial increase in the amount of rasagiline in the blood.

- Tobacco smoking stimulates the enzyme system responsible for breaking down rasagiline and may increase the speed at which rasagiline is broken down by the liver.

Food Interactions

This drug may be taken with or without food or meals. Avoid all of the following listed foods while you are taking rasagiline and for at least 2 weeks after you stop because they are rich in the amino acid tyramine. Eating these foods while taking this or any MAOI can lead to severe and dangerous high blood pressure: air-dried, aged, and fermented meats, sausages, and salamis; pickled herring; any spoiled or improperly stored meat, poultry, animal livers, or fish; broad bean pods (fava bean pods); aged cheeses; tap beers and beers that have not been pasteurized; red wines; concentrated yeast extract (eg, Marmite); sauerkraut; most soybean products (including soy sauce and tofu); and any supplements containing tyramine.

Usual Dose

Adult (age 18 and over): 1 mg a day. Adjunctive therapy—0.5– 1 mg a day.

People with mild liver disease: no more than 0.5 mg a day.

Child (age 17 and under): not recommended.

Overdosage

There have been no cases of rasagiline overdose. Overdose symptoms may be similar to other MAOIs: drowsiness, dizziness, faintness, irritability, hyperactivity, agitation, severe headache, hallucinations, contraction of muscles of your mouth, rigidity and severe arching of the back with the head thrown backward, convulsions, coma, rapid and irregular pulse, high or low blood pressure and blood vessel collapse, heart pain, respiratory depression or failure, high fever, sweating, and cool, clammy skin. Overdose patients should be taken to a hospital emergency room for treatment. ALWAYS bring the prescription bottle or container with you.

Special Information

Rasagiline can cause a marked increase in blood pressure if mixed with a variety of other drugs (see "Drug Interactions") or foods rich in tyramine (see "Food Interactions") that can be a hypertensive emergency requiring immediate treatment or hospitalization. Some symptoms of this reaction are severe headache, blurred vision or visual disturbances, difficulty thinking, stupor or coma, seizures, chest pain, unexplained nausea or vomiting, or the signs or symptoms of a stroke. If this happens, contact your doctor immediately and consider taking the person to a hospital emergency room for treatment. Always bring the medicine bottle with you.

If you forget a dose of rasagiline, take it as soon as you remember. If it is almost time for the next dose, skip the one you forgot and continue with your regular schedule. Do not take a double dose.

Special Populations

Pregnancy/Breast-feeding: Animal studies have shown this drug may damage a developing fetus. Pregnant women should take it only if its potential benefits outweigh the risks.

Rasagiline may reduce the volume of breast milk. It is not known if this drug passes into breast milk; however, nursing mothers should strongly consider using infant formula while taking rasagiline because of the possibility of rasagiline side effects appearing in the nursing baby.

Seniors: Seniors may take this drug with no special precaution.

Brand Name

Rebetron

Generic Ingredients
Interferon Alpha-2b + Ribavirin

Type of Drug
Antiviral combination.

Prescribed For
Hepatitis C virus (HCV) infection.

General Information
This combination should be used only when interferon alpha, the only other approved treatment for HCV, has failed. Ribavirin is not effective against HCV by itself. The way that this combination works against HCV is not known.

HCV infection can be especially serious in people with HIV. Interferon alpha or a long-acting (pegylated) interferon called Pegasys, taken either alone or in combination with the antiviral pill ribavirin, can be given to people coinfected with chronic HCV and HIV, who are at greatest risk for progression to serious disease. Treatment does not always work, but HIV-infected patients may benefit from treatment with this combination.

For more information on both of these drugs, see also their individual drug profiles, Interferon Alpha, page 590, and Ribavirin, page 981.

Cautions and Warnings

Do not take Rebetron if you are **allergic** or **sensitive** to any of its ingredients.

All people taking this combination must be closely monitored by their doctors, including having periodic blood, liver, and thyroid function tests.

People with **kidney disease**, **heart disease**, **sickle-cell anemia,** or **thalassemia** should use this medication with caution. If heart disease worsens during treatment, the drug should be discontinued.

Hearing disorders and fainting have occurred in people taking this medication.

Rebetron can affect both sperm and egg. Men and women taking Rebetron must **use effective contraception** during treatment and for 6 months after treatment is completed. Call your doctor if pregnancy occurs.

People with **autoimmune hepatitis** should not use Rebetron.

People who develop severe side effects or become depressed while taking this medication should have their interferon dosage temporarily lowered. The medication should be stopped if severe depression develops.

Children as young as age 1 have been treated with interferon alpha, but the combination product has not been studied in **children** of any age.

Possible Side Effects

Some people experience no side effects while taking Rebetron, and most feel well enough to work and travel during treatment.

▼ Most common: depression, fever, tiredness, headache, muscle aches, chills, flu-like symptoms, irritability, nausea, diarrhea, appetite loss, abdominal pain, weakness, joint and muscle pain, and feeling unwell.

Possible Side Effects (continued)

▼ Common: dry mouth, thirst, dizziness, tingling in the hands or feet, sleep disturbances, vomiting, upset stomach, weight loss, and hemolytic anemia (red-blood-cell destruction).

▼ Less common: loss of concentration, nervousness, constipation, loose stools, changes in sense of taste, sore throat, breathing difficulties, sinus irritation, inflamed injection site (interferon only), chest pain, and sweating.

▼ Rare: confusion, loss of sex drive, stuffy nose, coughing, facial swelling, and cold sores. Other rare side effects can occur in almost any part of the body. Contact your doctor if you experience any side effect not listed above.

Drug Interactions

- Antacids may reduce the amount of ribavirin absorbed.
- Interferon alpha-2b can significantly increase the level of theophyline in the blood.
- Combining interferon alpha-2b with zidovudine (AZT) may result in serious side effects. If taking this combination, your white-blood-cell count must be monitored carefully.

Food Interactions

High-fat meals can increase the amount of ribavirin absorbed, though the importance of this is not known. These drugs may be taken with or without food.

Usual Dose

Adult (under 166 lbs.): ribavirin—400 mg in the morning and 600 mg at night. Interferon alpha—3 million units 3 times a week by injection under the skin.

Adult (166 lbs. and over): ribavirin—600 mg morning and night. Interferon alpha—3 million units 3 times a week by injection under the skin.

Child (110–134 lbs.): ribavirin—400 mg morning and night. Interferon alpha—3 million units 3 times a week by injection under skin.

Child (81–109 lbs.): ribavirin—200 mg morning and 400 mg at night. Interferon alpha—3 million units 3 times a week by injection under skin.

Child (55–80 lbs.): ribavirin—200 mg morning and night. Interferon alpha—3 million units 3 times a week by injection under skin.

Child (under 55 lbs.): not recommended.

Overdosage

Little is known about the effects of Rebetron overdose. Take the victim to a hospital emergency room. ALWAYS bring the prescription bottle or container.

Special Information

Rebetron is administered in 2 forms—capsule (ribavirin) and injection (interferon alpha-2b). For information on how to properly administer injections, see page 1242.

This medication can make you drowsy. Be careful when driving or performing any task that requires concentration.

Drink lots of water while using Rebetron to make sure you are well hydrated.

Call your doctor at once if hives, itching, chest tightness, coughing, breathing difficulties, visual difficulties, wheezing, low blood pressure, or lightheadedness develop. These can be signs of drug allergy.

Rebetron can make you more sensitive to the sun. Avoid spending a lot of time in the sun while taking it.

If you forget to take a dose of interferon, take it as soon as you remember. If it is almost time for your next dose, space your remaining weekly doses throughout the rest of the week. If you forget a dose of ribavirin, take it as soon as you remember. If it is almost time for your next dose, skip the dose you forgot and continue with your regular schedule. Do not take a double dose. Call your doctor if you forget 2 or more doses in a row.

Do not change brands of interferon without your doctor's knowledge—they may not be equivalent.

Special Populations

Pregnancy/Breast-feeding: Rebetron should not be taken by pregnant women or their male partners because of its effect on the sperm, egg, and fetus. Women must be tested monthly to be sure they are not pregnant.

It is not known if the ingredients in Rebetron pass into breast milk. Nursing mothers who must take this medication should use infant formula.

Seniors: Rebetron is partially passed out of the body through the kidneys. Seniors should use this drug with caution because of the risk of kidney damage.

Generic Name

Repaglinide (reh-PAG-lih-nide)

Brand Name
Prandin

The information in this profile also applies to the following drug:

Generic Ingredient: Nateglinide
Starlix

Type of Drug
Antidiabetic.

Prescribed For
Type 2 diabetes.

General Information
In people with type 2 diabetes, the pancreas does not make
enough insulin, or the hormone fails to work. Because insulin reg-
ulates the amount of sugar in the blood, lack of this hormone
causes blood sugar to rise to unhealthy levels. Repaglinide is the
first in a group of drugs designed to control diabetes by increasing insulin production. When taken with meals, this drug temporarily stimulates the pancreas to release more insulin when it is
needed to help process dietary sugar. This helps to stabilize blood
sugar. Repaglinide may be used alone or combined with metformin
or other antidiabetes drugs. Repaglinide works only if beta cells
in the pancreas are functioning.

Cautions and Warnings
Do not use repaglinide if you are **allergic** or **sensitive** to its
ingredients.

Because repaglinide is broken down in the liver, people with
liver problems may require reduced dosage or more time between
doses.

People with severe **kidney disease** must start with the lowest
effective dose of repaglinide.

Any antidiabetes drug can excessively **lower blood sugar.** Do
not use **NPH insulin** while taking one of these drugs. Low blood
sugar can develop when you do not consume enough calories,
overexert yourself physically, drink alcohol, or combine blood-

sugar-lowering drugs (see "Overdosage" for low blood sugar symptoms).

You may need to temporarily switch to insulin therapy if you have **surgery** or experience **fever, infection,** or **trauma**.

Possible Side Effects

Nateglinide
▼ Most common: respiratory infection.
▼ Less common: bronchitis, cough, back pain, flu-like symptoms, dizziness, joint disease, diarrhea, accidents, and low blood sugar.

Repaglinide
▼ Most common: low blood sugar, headache, and respiratory infection.
▼ Common: sinus irritation, runny nose, bronchitis, nausea, diarrhea, and back or joint pain.
▼ Less common: constipation, vomiting, upset stomach, tingling in the hands or feet, chest pain, urinary infection, and tooth problems.
▼ Rare: allergy. Contact your doctor if you experience any side effect not listed above.

Drug Interactions

- Combining repaglinide with ketoconazole, miconazole, erythromycin, gemfibrozil, or clarithromycin may result in severely low blood sugar.
- Combining repaglinide and rifampin, barbiturates, gemfibrozil, or carbamazepine may result in high blood sugar.
- The blood sugar-lowering effect of all antidiabetes drugs may be increased by sulfa drugs; aspirin, ibuprofen, and other nonsteroidal anti-inflammatory drugs (NSAIDs); chloramphenicol; coumadin-type anticoagulants (blood thinners); probenecid; monoamine oxidase inhibitor antidepressants; and beta blockers.
- Thiazides and other diuretics, corticosteroid anti-inflammatory drugs, phenothiazines, thyroid drugs, estrogens, contraceptive drugs, phenytoin, nicotinic acid, stimulants, calcium channel blockers, and isoniazid may increase blood sugar levels. Your dosage of repaglinide may need to be increased if you combine it with any of these drugs.

Food Interactions

Repaglinide should be taken before meals because food interferes with its absorption in the blood.

Usual Dose

Nateglinide

   Adult: 60–120 mg 1–30 minutes before each meal, 3 times a day.

   Child: not recommended.

Repaglinide

   Adult: 0.5–4 mg 15–30 minutes before each meal, up to 4 times a day. Adults with severe kidney disease should start at 0.5mg before each meal.

   Child: not recommended.

Overdosage

People taking up to 80 mg a day of repaglinide for 2 weeks had few problems other than low blood sugar. Up to 720 mg a day of nateglinide has been taken for 7 days with no adverse effect, but low blood sugar may occur. Symptoms of low blood sugar are cold sweats, anxiety, cool and pale skin, difficulty concentrating, drowsiness, excessive hunger, headache, nausea, nervousness, rapid pulse, shakiness, unusual tiredness or weakness, and vision changes. Take the overdose victim to a hospital emergency room. ALWAYS bring the prescription bottle or container.

Special Information

Measurements of blood sugar and glycosylated hemoglobin (A1C) are essential to your doctor's evaluation of your progress. See your doctor regularly.

   Repaglinide must be taken before you eat. If you skip a meal, do not take this drug. If you have an extra meal, take an extra dose of repaglinide before that meal.

   The timing of each repaglinide dose is key to its effectiveness. If you forget to take repaglinide before a meal, take it during the meal. If you have already eaten and forgotten your medication, skip the forgotten dose. If you cannot remember to take repaglinide before each meal, talk to your doctor about changing drugs.

Special Populations

Pregnancy/Breast-feeding: Repaglinide should not be taken during pregnancy. Animal studies indicate that it may affect the skeletal development of the fetus. Most experts recommend that diabetes be controlled with insulin during pregnancy.

It is not known if repaglinide passes into breast milk. Nursing mothers who must take it should use infant formula.

Seniors: Some seniors may be more sensitive to the effects of this drug.

Generic Name

Retapamulin (reh-tah-PAM-u-lin)

Brand Name

Altabax

Type of Drug

Antibacterial.

Prescribed For

Impetigo.

General Information

Retapamulin is an antibiotic ointment that is applied directly to the impetigo blisters, especially those that have burst and are leaking pus. Impetigo is a skin infection caused by *Staphylococcus aureus* or *Streptococcus pyogenes*. The condition is most common in children between the ages of 2 and 6, but it can affect people of all ages. Impetigo usually begins when bacteria enter a break in the skin, such as a cut, scratch, or insect bite. Early symptoms include red or pimple-like sores surrounded by red skin. These sores can be anywhere, but usually they occur on the face, arms, and legs. The sores fill with pus, then break open after a few days and form a thick crust. They are often itchy, but scratching them can spread the sores. Impetigo can spread by contact with sores or nasal discharge from an infected person.

Cautions and Warnings

Do not use retapamulin if you are **sensitive** or **allergic** to any of its ingredients. Stop using retapamulin if it causes a severe skin irritation.

Do not swallow this ointment or apply it directly to the eye or to the inside of the mouth, nose, or vagina.

Possible Side Effects

Adult

▼ Less common: headache, skin irritation at the application site, diarrhea, nausea, and irritation of the nose and throat.

▼ Rare: pain at the application site, local swelling, and contact dermatitis. Contact your doctor if you experience any side effect not listed above.

Child

▼ Less common: itchy skin at the application site and general itchiness, diarrhea, irritation of the nose and throat, eczema, headache, and fever.

▼ Rare: pain at the application site, local swelling, and contact dermatitis. Contact your doctor if you experience any side effect not listed above.

Drug Interactions

None known.

Food Interactions

None known.

Usual Dose

Adult and Child (9 months and over): Apply a thin layer of ointment to the affected areas twice a day for 5 days. You should not cover an area of more than 4″ by 4″ on any day because of the possibility of absorbing too much antibiotic into the blood. Covering the ointment with sterile gauze helps prevent scratching of itchy sores and also prevents accidentally getting the ointment into your eye.

Overdosage

Little is known about retapamulin overdosage, but it can cause treatment-resistant bacteria. Call your local poison control center or a hospital emergency room for more information. If you seek treatment, ALWAYS bring the prescription container.

Special Information

Do not use this ointment more often than prescribed or for longer than 5 days. Excessive use can lead to the development of resistant bacteria, making this and other infections harder to treat.

Impetigo is highly contagious. You should try to avoid scratching the infected areas. Scratching or touching the infected skin and then touching another part of the body can spread the infection to that area. Impetigo can also spread from one person to another. Contact with an infected person's hands is the most common way that impetigo spreads.

If you forget a dose, apply it as soon as you remember. If it is almost time for the next dose, skip the one you forgot and continue with your regular schedule. Do not apply a double dose.

Special Populations

Pregnancy/Breast-feeding: Animal studies indicate no effects of retapamulin on a developing fetus. However, because there are no studies in pregnant women, its potential benefits should be weighed against its potential risks.

It is not known if retapamulin passes into breast milk. Nursing mothers should consider using infant formula.

Seniors: Seniors may use this drug with no special precaution.

Rhinocort Aqua *see **Corticosteroids, Nasal,***
page 309

Generic Name

Ribavirin (ry-bah-VY-rin) Ⓖ

Brand Names

Copegus   Ribasphere
Rebetol

Type of Drug

Antiviral.

Prescribed For

Hepatitis C virus (HCV) infection.

General Information

Ribavirin is part of a two-drug combination (with peginterferon injection) that has become a primary treatment for active HCV infection in adults with some liver disease. The exact way that it works against the hepatitis C virus is not known. Ribavirin is not effective for chronic HCV infections without interferon injections or for any other type of virus infection. It does not work against any other form of hepatitis.

HCV infection can be especially serious in people with HIV. Interferon alpha or a long-acting (pegylated) interferon called Pegasys, either alone or taken in combination with ribavirin, can be given to people coinfected with chronic HCV and HIV, who are at greatest risk for progression to serious disease. Treatment does not always work, but HIV-infected patients may benefit from treatment with this combination.

Because this drug is always taken in combination with injectable interferon alpha, see Interferon Alpha, page 590, for further information.

Cautions and Warnings

Do not take this drug if you are **allergic** or **sensitive** to any of its ingredients.

People with **kidney damage** and those with moderate to severe **liver disease** or liver disease caused by an autoimmune reaction (in which the liver is attacked by the body's own defense system) should not take this medicine.

People with **cancer** and those taking anti-rejection drugs because they have had an **organ transplant** should not take ribavirin.

Ribavirin may worsen **heart disease,** causing high blood pressure, increased heart rate, and chest pain.

People with **sickle-cell disease, thalassemia,** and other hemoglobin abnormalities should not take ribavirin.

Serious side effects of combination therapy include severe depression, hemolytic anemia, suppression of bone marrow function, autoimmune and infectious disorders, pulmonary dysfunction, pancreatitis, and diabetes. Ribavirin should not be used by **pregnant** women or by men whose female partners are pregnant.

Possible Side Effects

Virtually every person who takes ribavirin + interferon for HCV will develop a drug side effect.

▼ Most common: nausea and vomiting, diarrhea, depression, insomnia, irritability, anxiety, inability to concentrate, flu-like symptoms such as fatigue, fever and chills, joint pains and muscle aches, headache, bacterial infections, severe anemia (usually within the first 2 weeks of ribavirin therapy) and

Possible Side Effects *(continued)*

reductions in white-blood-cell counts, difficulty breathing, fluid in the lungs, pneumonia, inflammation of the pancreas, hair loss, itching, and rashes.

▼ Common: loss of appetite, diarrhea, abdominal pain, injection-site reactions, liver failure, dizziness, confusion, back pain, mood changes, tiredness or fatigue, dry mouth, coughing, unusual shortness of breath after exertion, upset stomach, reduced thyroid gland activity, reduced blood-platelet count, blurred vision, sweating, and eczema.

▼ Rare: Rare side effects can occur in almost any part of the body. Some rare side effects include suicidal thoughts, psychosis, aggression, anxiety, drug abuse and drug overdose, heart pain, liver damage, abnormal heart rhythms, worsening diabetes, overactive thyroid, systemic lupus erythematosus, rheumatoid arthritis, nerve damage, aplastic anemia, stomach ulcers, gastrointestinal bleeding, colitis, corneal ulcer, pulmonary embolism, coma, myositis, and stroke. Contact your doctor if you experience any side effect not listed above.

For further side effects for combination treatments, see Interferon Alpha, page 590.

Drug Interactions

- Ribavirin increases blood levels of didanosine and can increase the risk of drug side effects, including fatal liver failure, pancreas inflammation, and nervous system problems. This combination should be avoided.
- Ribavirin should be used with caution with nucleoside analogues.
- Ribavirin slows the metabolism of several HIV antivirals (lamivudine, stavudine, and zidovudine). This may increase the risk of drug side effects, including anemia.
- Treatment with interferon, typically prescribed with ribavirin, increases blood levels of theophylline by 25%, increasing the risk of drug side effects.

For further drug interactions for combination treatments, see Interferon Alpha, page 590.

Food Interactions

Take this medicine with food.

Usual Dose

Adult: 400–600 mg twice a day, depending on body weight and the type of hepatitis C infection. Dosage adjustments may be required if severe side effects occur.

Child (under age 18): not recommended.

Overdosage

Take the overdose victim to a hospital emergency room at once. ALWAYS bring the prescription bottle or container.

Special Information

Call your doctor at once if you begin to have trouble breathing or develop pneumonia or abdominal pains.

Call your doctor if you become severely depressed or suicidal or develop flu-like symptoms, fever, chills, muscle pain, headache, hives or swelling, severe stomach pain, lower back pain, bruising or unusual bleeding, worsening psoriasis, changes in your vision, tiredness or weakness, appetite loss, nausea, vomiting, sore throat, unusual bleeding or bruising, yellowing of the skin or whites of the eyes, rash, or itching.

This drug can cause dizziness, confusion, tiredness, or fatigue. Avoid driving or operating machinery until you know how this drug affects you.

Alcoholic beverages can worsen liver disease and should be avoided if you have any form of hepatitis.

If you forget a dose of ribavirin, take it as soon as you remember. If it is almost time for your next dose, skip the forgotten dose and continue with your regular schedule. Do not take a double dose. Regularly missing doses of this medicine will reduce the ability of this drug to fight HCV.

Special Populations

Pregnancy/Breast-feeding: Ribavirin is toxic to a developing fetus and causes birth defects, and it remains in the body for up to 6 months after a course of treatment is finished. Pregnant women and their male partners and women who may be pregnant must avoid this drug.

Use at least 2 reliable forms of contraception to avoid becoming pregnant during treatment and for at least 6 months after a course of ribavirin therapy has been completed. The female partners of men taking ribavirin should also practice this form of contraception.

This drug may pass into breast milk. Nursing mothers who take ribavirin should use infant formula.

Seniors: Seniors should use this drug with caution because of the risk of kidney damage.

Generic Name

Rifampin (rih-FAM-pin) Ⓖ

Brand Names
Rifadin   Rimactane

Combination Products
Generic Ingredients: Rifampin + Isoniazid Ⓖ
Rifamate

Generic Ingredients: Rifampin + Isoniazid + Pyrazinamide
Rifater

Type of Drug
Antitubercular.

Prescribed For
Tuberculosis, meningitis carriers, and other infections.

General Information
Rifampin, an important agent in the treatment of tuberculosis, is always used with at least one other tuberculosis drug. It is also prescribed to eradicate the organism that causes meningitis in carriers—people who are not infected themselves but carry the organism and can spread it to others. Rifampin can be used to treat strep throat; staphylococcal infections of the skin, bones, or prostate; cat scratch disease; legionnaires' disease; leprosy; and to prevent meningitis caused by *Haemophilus influenzae.*

Cautions and Warnings
Do not take rifampin if you are **allergic** or **sensitive** to any of its ingredients, or to rifabutin, prescribed for *Mycobacterium avium* complex (an infection associated with advanced cases of AIDS).

Liver damage and death have been reported in people taking rifabutin, a drug that is very similar to rifampin. It is also the principal side effect of pyrazinamide, an ingredient in Rifater. People taking other drugs that may cause liver damage should avoid rifampin.

If you have **liver disease,** your doctor should monitor your liver function.

Reduced white-blood-cell and platelet counts that may be severe can occur with high doses of rifampin.

Bacterial resistance develops very quickly if rifampin is used for active **meningococcus infection**. It should not be used for this purpose.

Rifampin should not be used in people with **porphyria**.

It is very important that you comply with the full course of therapy and not miss any doses; otherwise, the drug may not work and may cause increased side effects.

Possible Side Effects

▼ Most common: flu-like symptoms; heartburn; upset stomach; appetite loss; nausea; vomiting; gas; cramps; diarrhea; headache; drowsiness; tiredness; menstrual disturbances; dizziness; fever; pain in the joints, arms, and legs; confusion; visual disturbances; numbness; and hypersensitivity to the drug.

▼ Less common: effects on the blood, kidneys, or liver.

▼ Rare: Rare side effects can occur in almost any part of the body. Contact your doctor if you experience any side effect not listed above.

Drug Interactions

- Severe and sometimes fatal hepatitis has also occurred in people taking isoniazid, another antitubercular drug often combined with rifampin. This combination produces more liver damage than either drug taken alone. People with liver disease should be carefully monitored by their doctors and receive reduced dosage.

- Severe liver damage, including hepatitis, may develop when rifampin is combined with other drugs that may cause liver toxicity, such as the protease inhibitors saquinavir and ritonavir. Do not use rifampin with any protease inhibitor; their effectiveness may also be affected.

- Rifampin may increase your need for oral anticoagulant (blood-thinning) drugs and may also affect angiotensin-converting enzyme (ACE) inhibitors, especially enalapril.

- Rifampin may reduce the effectiveness of acetaminophen; anticonvulsants; oral antidiabetes drugs; barbiturates; benzodiazepines; beta blockers; buspirone; clarithromycin, erythromycin, and other macrolide antibiotics; chloramphenicol; corticosteroids; cyclosporine; digoxin; disopyramide; doxycycline; estrogens; fluroquinolone anti-infectives; haloperidol; inamrinone; itraconazole; ketoconazole; losartan; narcotics; ondansetron; phenytoin; methadone; mexiletine; quinine drugs; quinidine; sulfa drugs; tacrolimus; theophylline drugs; tocainide; tricyclic antidepressants; thyroid hormones; verapamil; zidovudine; and zolpidem.

- Drugs that can interfere with rifampin include aminosalicylic acid, itraconazole, and ketoconazole.
- Women taking contraceptive drugs should use another contraceptive method while taking rifampin.
- Liver toxicity has developed when people taking rifampin were given halothane, a general anesthetic, prior to surgery.

Food Interactions

Take rifampin and all rifampin combinations 1 hour before or 2 hours after a meal, at the same time every day.

Usual Dose

Rifampin
Adult: 4.5 mg per lb., up to 600 mg a day.
Child: 4.5–9 mg per lb., up to 600 mg a day.

Rifamate
Adult: 2 capsules once a day.

Rifater
Adult (age 15 and over): This drug is dosed according to body weight. The following dose should be taken once a day on an empty stomach, either 1 hour before or 2 hours after a meal, with a full glass of water.
   Weight
   97 lbs. or less—4 tablets
   100–120 lbs.—5 tablets
   120 lbs. or more—6 tablets
Child: not recommended.

Overdosage

Take the overdose victim to a hospital emergency room at once. ALWAYS bring the prescription bottle or container.

Symptoms of rifampin overdose include nausea, vomiting, and tiredness. Unconsciousness is possible in cases of severe liver damage. Brown-red or orange skin discoloration may also develop.

Overdose symptoms of isoniazid, an ingredient in Rifater, include nausea, vomiting, dizziness, slurring of speech, blurring of vision, and visual hallucinations, and are among the early manifestations. Respiratory distress and central-nervous-system depression, moving rapidly from stupor to profound coma, are to be expected with marked overdosage, along with severe, intractable seizures.

Pyrazinamide overdose is likely to cause liver problems.

Special Information

Rifampin may cause a red-brown or orange discoloration of the urine, stool, saliva, sweat, or tears; this is not harmful. Soft contact lenses and dentures may become permanently stained.

Call your doctor if you develop flu-like symptoms, fever, chills, muscle pain, headache, tiredness or weakness, appetite loss, nausea, vomiting, sore throat, unusual bleeding or bruising, yellowing of the skin or whites of the eyes, rash, or itching.

If you take rifampin once a day and miss a dose, take it as soon as you remember. If it is almost time for your next dose, skip the dose you forgot and continue with your regular schedule. Do not take a double dose. Regularly missing doses of rifampin increases the risk of side effects.

Special Populations

Pregnancy/Breast-feeding: Animal studies indicate that rifampin may cause cleft palate and spina bifida (birth defect in which bones of the lower spinal column do not form properly, leaving the spinal canal partially exposed) in the fetus. Pregnant women should use this drug only if absolutely necessary.

This drug may pass into breast milk. Nursing mothers who must take it should use infant formula.

Seniors: Seniors with liver disease may be more sensitive to the effects of this drug.

Generic Name

Rifaximin (rih-FAX-ih-min)

Brand Name

Xifaxan

Type of Drug
Antibiotic.

Prescribed For
Rifaximin is used to treat diarrhea caused by eating food or drinking water contaminated with *E. coli* bacteria.

General Information
Many people who travel outside of the United States develop "traveler's diarrhea" because their food and water is contaminated with the bacteria *E. coli*. This bacteria is also responsible for the majority of food poisoning cases in the United States, and some have said that the common "stomach flu" is really just a minor case of food poisoning. Other antibiotics have been successful in treating *E. coli* bacteria, but this product's advantage is that only a very small amount of it is absorbed into the blood. It stays in the intestines where the offending bacteria are located.

Cautions and Warnings
Do not take rifaximin if you are **allergic** or **sensitive** to any of its ingredients or to any of the group of antibiotics known as rifamycins. The best known member of the group is rifampin. Reported allergic reations include severe rash, swelling of the face and tongue, difficulty swallowing, hives, flushing, and itching. Some of these reactions have occurred as soon as 15 minutes after taking this medicine.

Do not take rifaximin if you have **fever** and/or **bloody stool** unless you consult your doctor.

Rifaximin should not be used to treat the form of diarrhea known as **dysentery**. Dysentery symptoms are often mild and vague. Usually there is persistent discomfort, nausea, and mild diarrhea with blood and mucous. Occasionally there is also tenderness over the area of the liver.

Treatment with antibiotics can cause diarrhea or, more seriously, colitis. Contact your doctor if you develop diarrhea while taking rifaximin.

Possible Side Effects
▼ Most common: intestinal gas, headache, abdominal pain, urgent bowel movements, nausea, and constipation.
▼ Common: fever and vomiting.
▼ Less common: dizziness, hives, and skin rash.

Possible Side Effects *(continued)*

▼ Rare: Rare side effects can occur in almost any part of the body. Contact your doctor if you experience any side effect not listed above.

Drug Interactions
None known.

Food Interactions
You can take this drug without regard to food or meals.

Usual Dose
Adult: 1 tablet (200 mg) 3 times a day for 3 days.
Child (under age 12): not recommended.

Overdosage
There is no experience with rifaximin overdose, although people in studies using doses larger than the usual dose of 600 mg per day have experienced the same side effects as those taking the usual dose. Call your poison center or local emergency room for more information. If you do take an overdose victim to an emergency room, ALWAYS bring the prescription bottle or container.

Special Information
You should contact your doctor if you think your condition is getting worse, if diarrhea develops, or if you are not improving after 24–48 hours (1–2 days) while taking rifaximin.

If you forget a dose, take it as soon as you remember. If it is almost time for your next dose, skip the dose you forgot and continue with your regular schedule. Do not take a double dose.

Special Populations
Pregnancy/Breast-feeding: Animal studies of rifaximin show that it causes birth defects. Pregnant women and those who may be pregnant should only take this drug if it is considered crucial by your doctor. The potential benefit of rifaximin must be carefully weighed against its risks.

It is not known if rifaximin passes into breast milk. Nursing mothers who must take this drug should consider using infant formula.

Seniors: There is not enough information on seniors and rifaximin to determine whether they react differently than younger adults to this medication.

Generic Name

Riluzole (RIL-ue-zole) Ⓖ

Brand Name

Rilutek

Type of Drug

Glutamate-release blocker.

Prescribed For

Amyotrophic lateral sclerosis (ALS), also known as Lou Gehrig's disease.

General Information

ALS is a chronic disease of the nervous system. Riluzole, the only drug proven to affect ALS, has a number of different actions, though nobody knows exactly how it works. The drug slows the release of glutamate, which is thought to damage important nerve centers in the brains of people with ALS, and protects other aspects of nerve function. Riluzole extended survival in people with ALS during 18 months of treatment, though muscle strength and nerve function did not improve. Overall, death rates at the end of the studies were the same whether people took riluzole or not. In one study, the average life extension for people taking riluzole was 60 days. Riluzole is broken down in the liver.

Cautions and Warnings

Do not take riluzole if you are **allergic** or **sensitive** to any of its ingredients.

Riluzole causes liver inflammation; people with **severe liver disease** should use this drug with caution. Liver function should be evaluated regularly. People with **kidney disease** should also use riluzole with caution.

Rarely, there have been cases of neutropenia (low white-blood-cell count) and anemia in people taking riluzole. Report any sign of fever to your doctor, who should check your levels of white blood cells.

Women and **people of Japanese descent** may eliminate riluzole from their bodies twice as slowly as do male Caucasians. The drug may be eliminated more slowly due to genetic factors or because of differences in diet such as decreased use of alcohol, nicotine, and caffeine.

Cigarette smoking is likely to increase the rate at which riluzole is broken down by the liver. The drug may break down more quickly in women than in men. There is no indication that either of these factors is important in determining riluzole dosage.

Taking more than 100 mg a day of riluzole increases side effects and is not more effective.

Possible Side Effects

About 14% of people stop taking riluzole because of side effects.

▼ Most common: weakness, nausea, dizziness (twice as common in women), diarrhea, a tingling sensation around the mouth, appetite loss, fainting, and tiredness. These effects increase with dosage.

▼ Common: poor lung function, abdominal pain, pneumonia, and vomiting.

▼ Less common: back pain, headache, upset stomach at high dosages, gas, stuffy nose, runny nose, cough, high blood pressure, joint aches, and swelling in the arms and legs. At high dosages—urinary infection and painful urination, and dizziness when rising from a lying or sitting position.

▼ Rare: aggravation, feeling unwell, mouth infection, eczema, rapid heartbeat, and vein irritation. Other rare side effects can occur in almost any part of the body. Contact your doctor if you experience any side effects not listed above.

Drug Interactions

• Allopurinol, methyldopa, sulfasalazine, and other drugs that are toxic to the liver may interact with riluzole. Combinations of liver-toxic drugs should be taken with caution.

• Caffeine, theophylline, phenacetin, amitriptyline, and quinolone antibacterials may slow the elimination of riluzole, increasing the risk of drug side effects.

• Rifampin and omeprazole may quicken the elimination of riluzole.

• Riluzole can accelerate the breakdown of caffeine, theophylline, and tacrine, but these effects have not actually been seen in people.

Food Interactions

Take riluzole on an empty stomach, at least 1 hour before or 2 hours after meals. Avoid charcoal-broiled foods, which may speed the elimination of riluzole. Avoid high-fat meals, which decrease the absorption of riluzole.

Usual Dose

Adult: 50 mg every 12 hours.
Child: not recommended.

Overdosage

Little is known about the effects of riluzole overdose. Take the victim to a hospital emergency room at once. ALWAYS bring the prescription bottle or container.

Special Information

Taking more than 50 mg twice a day will not improve your condition and may increase drug side effects.

Call your doctor at once if you become feverish or ill. This could be a sign of a very low white-blood-cell count.

Riluzole should be taken at the same time each day—morning and evening—to achieve maximum benefit.

Riluzole can make you dizzy, tired, or faint. Be careful when driving or doing any task that requires concentration.

People taking riluzole should not drink excessive amounts of alcohol.

Store riluzole tablets between 68°F and 77°F and protect them from bright light.

If you forget a dose, take it as soon as you remember. If it is almost time for your next dose, skip the dose you forgot and continue with your regular schedule.

Special Populations

Pregnancy/Breast-feeding: Riluzole is toxic to pregnant lab animals at high dosages. When this drug is considered crucial by your doctor, its potential benefits must be carefully weighed against its risks.

It is not known if riluzole passes into breast milk. Nursing mothers who must take it should use infant formula.

Seniors: Seniors with kidney or liver disease should use riluzole with caution.

Generic Name

Rimantadine (rih-MAN-tuh-dene) Ⓖ

Brand Name

Flumadine

Type of Drug

Antiviral.

Prescribed For

Influenza A viral infection (type A flu).

General Information

Rimantadine hydrochloride is a synthetic antiviral agent that appears to interfere with the reproduction of various strains of the influenza A virus, a common cause of viral infection. Rimantadine is used both to treat and to prevent type A flu; however, it is indicated only for infuenza A prevention in children. Annual vaccination against the virus is the best way of preventing the flu, but immunity takes 2–4 weeks to develop. In the meantime, rimantadine may be taken to prevent viral infection in high-risk people or people who may experience greater exposure to the virus.

Cautions and Warnings

Do not take rimantadine if you are **allergic** or **sensitive** to any of its ingredients or to amantadine.

People with severe **liver or kidney disease** clear this drug from their bodies only half as fast as those with normal organ function; they will need to have their dosage adjusted appropriately.

People with a history of **seizures** are likely to suffer another one while taking rimantadine. Call your doctor if this happens to you.

The influenza virus may become resistant to rimantadine in up to 30% of people taking the drug. When this happens, the resistant virus can infect people who are not protected by the vaccine.

Possible Side Effects

▼ Most common: sleeplessness, nervousness, loss of concentration, headache, fatigue, weakness, nausea, vomiting, appetite loss, dry mouth, and abdominal pains.

▼ Less common: diarrhea, upset stomach, dizziness, depression, euphoria (feeling "high"), changes in gait or walk,

---

Possible Side Effects *(continued)*

tremors, hallucinations, convulsions, fainting, ringing or buzzing in the ears, changes in or loss of the senses of taste or smell, breathing difficulties, pallor, rash, heart palpitations, rapid heartbeat, high blood pressure, heart failure, swelling of the ankles or feet, and heart block.

▼ Rare: constipation, swallowing difficulties, mouth sores, agitation, sweating, diminished sense of touch, eye pain or tearing, cough, bronchospasm, increased urination, fever, and fluid oozing from the nipples in women. Contact your doctor if you experience any side effect not listed above.

Drug Interactions

The importance of rimantadine's drug interactions is not known because there is no established relationship between the amount of drug in the blood and its antiviral effect.

- Aspirin and acetaminophen may reduce the amount of rimantadine in the blood by about 10%.
- Cimetidine decreases the rate at which rimantadine is broken down by the liver.
- Do not use rimantadine concurrently with live intranasal influenza virus vaccine, such as FluMist. Wait at least 48 hours between uses of either medicine.

Food Interactions

Rimantadine is best taken on an empty stomach, or at least 1 hour before or 2 hours after meals. You may take it with food if it upsets your stomach.

Usual Dose

Adult and Child (age 10 and over): 100 mg twice a day. People with severe liver or kidney disease—no more than 100 mg a day.

Child (age 1–10): 2.25 mg per lb. of body weight, up to 150 mg, taken once a day.

Child (under 1 year): not recommended.

Overdosage

Symptoms include agitation, hallucination, and abnormal heart rhythm. Overdose victims should be made to vomit with ipecac syrup—available at any pharmacy—as soon as possible. Call your local poison control center or a hospital emergency room before giving ipecac. Take overdose victims to a hospital emergency room. ALWAYS bring the prescription bottle or container.

Special Information

Rimantadine may be given to children to prevent influenza infection, but it is not recommended for treatment of their flu symptoms.

Call your doctor if you develop seizures, convulsions, or any other serious or unusual side effects.

If you forget a dose, take it as soon as you remember. If it is almost time for your next dose, skip the dose you forgot and continue with your regular schedule. Do not take a double dose.

Special Populations

Pregnancy/Breast-feeding: In animal studies, rimantadine is toxic to fetuses. When this drug is considered crucial by your doctor, its potential benefits must be carefully weighed against its risks.

Rimantadine passes into breast milk. Nursing mothers who must take it should use infant formula.

Seniors: Seniors are more likely to suffer from rimantadine side effects of the nervous system, stomach, and intestine and may require reduced dosage due to liver or kidney dysfunction.

Risperdal   *see **Risperidone**, below*

Generic Name

Risperidone (ris-PER-ih-done)

Brand Names

Risperdal
Risperdal M-Tab Orally Disintegrating Tablets

Type of Drug

Antipsychotic.

The information in this profile also applies to the following drug:

Generic Ingredient: Paliperidone
Invega

Prescribed For

Psychotic disorders and schizophrenia; risperidone is also prescribed for bipolar disorders, symptoms of Alzheimer's disease, and treatment-resistant depression.

General Information

Paliperidone is a major product of the breakdown of risperidone, so these medications work in exactly the same way and have the same safety profile. They affect brain receptors for serotonin and dopamine, two important neurohormones. They are broken down in the liver. Between 6–8% of Caucasians and a very small number of Asians have little of the liver enzyme that breaks down these medications and are considered to be "poor metabolizers" of the drug. Because these people break down these medications very slowly, it takes about 5 days for the drug to reach a steady level in their blood. People with normal amounts of the enzyme reach a steady level in about 1 day. People with kidney or liver disease require reduced dosage.

Cautions and Warnings

Do not take either of these medications if you are **allergic** or **sensitive** to any of their ingredients.

People taking them for longer than 6–8 weeks must be re-evaluated at least every 2 months.

Risperidone and paliperidone have been associated with increased mortality in seniors with **dementia** or **Alzheimer's disease**. The specific causes of death related to atypical antipsychotic drugs were either due to a heart-related event or infection, mostly pneumonia. The drugs should not be used to treat people with dementia-related psychosis.

A serious set of side effects known as neuroleptic malignant syndrome (NMS) has been associated with some antipsychotic drugs. The symptoms that constitute NMS include high fever, muscle rigidity, mental changes, irregular pulse or blood pressure, sweating, and abnormal heart rhythm. NMS is potentially fatal and requires immediate medical attention.

Risperidone and paliperidone can produce uncontrolled movements, including tremor, spasm of the neck muscles, rolling back of the eyes, convulsions, difficulty swallowing, and symptoms associated with Parkinson's disease. These effects usually disappear after the drug has been discontinued. Face, tongue, and jaw symptoms may persist, especially in **older women**. Contact your doctor immediately if you experience any of these symptoms.

Risperidone and paliperidone can cause a life-threatening abnormal heart rhythm called torsade de pointes. These drugs should therefore be used with caution in people with **heart disease. Slow heart rate**, **electrolyte imbalance**, and taking other drugs that carry a risk of torsade de pointes may increase the chances of developing this abnormality. Dizziness and fainting can also occur.

Risperidone and paliperidone raise levels of a hormone called prolactin. Increased prolactin has been associated with tumors of the pituitary gland, breast, and pancreas.

Risperidone and paliperidone have been associated with obesity, high cholesterol, and diabetes. People with **diabetes** and those who are at **risk for diabetes** should have their blood glucose levels checked regularly while taking these drugs.

Paliperidone should not be given to people with **severe narrowing of the gastrointestinal tract** (a result of some disorders of the esophagus), **small bowel inflammation**, **narrowing of the bowels**, **slowed gastrointestinal motility**, past history of **peritonitis**, or **cystic fibrosis**.

Possible Side Effects

Risperidone

▼ Most common: sleepiness, sleeplessness, agitation, anxiety, uncontrolled movements, headache, and nasal stuffiness and irritation.

▼ Less common: dizziness, constipation, nausea, vomiting, upset stomach, abdominal pain, weight gain, absence of menstrual periods, increased sleep duration, coughing, upper respiratory infection, sinus infection, sore throat, breathing difficulties, rapid heartbeat, joint or back pain, chest pain, fever, abnormal vision, rash, dry skin, and dandruff.

Paliperidone

▼ Most common: rapid heart beat, headache, and tiredness.

▼ Common: nausea, anxiety, inability to sit still or remain motionless, dizziness, extrapyrimidal syndrome (involuntary movements, muscle tremors, and rigidity, body restlessness, muscle contractions, and changes in breathing and heart rate), and weight gain.

▼ Less common: other heart disorders, cardiogram changes, blurred vision, upper abdominal pain, dry mouth, upset

Possible Side Effects *(continued)*

stomach, excess saliva, weakness, fatigue, fever, high blood pressure, back pain, pain in the arms or legs, twisting and repetitive movement or abnormal postures, muscle tightness that can lead to deformity and functional loss, Parkinson's-like symptoms, tremors, coughing, and dizziness or fainting when rising from a sitting or lying position.
Rare side effects of these medications can occur in almost any part of the body. Contact your doctor if you experience any side effect not listed above.

Drug Interactions

- Risperidone and paliperidone may decrease the effects of levodopa + carbidopa and other dopamine agonists.
- Clozapine, ritonavir, fluoxetine, and paroxetine may increase the effect of these drugs and their side effects.
- Carbamazepine and clozapine may reduce the effect of these drugs.
- Risperidone and paliperidone increase the effects of blood-pressure-lowering drugs and central-nervous-system depressants.
- Combining alcohol with these drugs may cause weakness and poor coordination.

Food Interactions

These drugs may be taken without regard to food or meals.

Usual Dose

Risperidone
Adult: starting dosage—1 mg twice a day. Daily dosage—may be increased gradually up to 8 mg a day if needed.
Senior: starting dosage—0.5 mg twice a day. Increase gradually if needed.
Child: not recommended.

Risperidone dosages should be reduced in patients with liver or kidney disease.

Paliperidone
Adult: 6 mg once a day to start. Daily dosage may be increased to 12 mg if needed.
Child (under age 17): not recommended.

No dose adjustment is required in people with mild to moderate liver disease. People with mild kidney disease need less medication.

Overdosage

Symptoms include drowsiness, rapid heartbeat, low blood pressure, and abnormal and uncontrolled muscle movements. Overdose victims should be taken to a hospital emergency room. ALWAYS bring the prescription bottle or container.

Special Information

These drugs can make you tired and affect your judgment, an effect that increases with dosage. Be careful when driving or performing any task that requires concentration. Avoid alcohol.

Some antipsychotic drugs can interfere with the body's temperature-regulating mechanism. Avoid extreme heat while you are taking risperidone or paliperidone.

Some people develop a rapid heartbeat and become dizzy or faint when first taking risperidone. This risk can be minimized by starting at a low dose.

These drugs can make you unusually sensitive to the sun. Wear protective clothes and use sunscreen.

Because of the controlled release design of the paliperidone tablet, it should only be taken by people who are able to swallow the tablet whole. It should not be cut or split.

If you forget a dose, take it as soon as you remember. If it is almost time for your next dose, skip the dose you forgot and continue with your regular schedule. Call your doctor if you forget 2 doses in a row.

Special Populations

Pregnancy/Breast-feeding: Studies of risperidone in animals show an increase in birth defects and stillbirth. There is also a report of an infant who was born with an abnormally developed brain after the mother took risperidone. Risperidone and paliperidone should not be taken by pregnant women unless the potential benefits are carefully weighed against the risks.

Both risperidone and paliperidone pass into breast milk. Nursing mothers who must take these medications should use infant formula.

Seniors: Seniors with reduced kidney function require lower dosages. Seniors may also be more sensitive to side effects.

Generic Name

Ritonavir (rih-TON-uh-vere)

Brand Name
Norvir

Combination Product
Generic Ingredients: Ritonavir + Lopinavir
Kaletra

Type of Drug
Protease inhibitor.

Prescribed For
Human immunodeficiency virus (HIV) infection.

General Information
Part of the multidrug "cocktail" responsible for the most important gains in the fight against acquired immunodeficiency syndrome (AIDS), ritonavir and lopinavir belong to a group of anti-HIV drugs called protease inhibitors. Triple-drug cocktails are considered responsible for the first overall reduction in the AIDS death rate, recorded in 1996. Protease inhibitors work in a unique way but are not a cure for HIV infection or AIDS. When the HIV virus attacks a cell, it must be converted into viral DNA. Older drugs, known as reverse-transcriptase inhibitors, interfere with this step, but they need help in fighting HIV. Protease inhibitors work at the end of the HIV reproduction process, when proteins are "cut" into strands of exactly the right size to duplicate HIV. The protein is cut by a protease enzyme. Protease inhibitors prevent the mature HIV virus from being formed by interfering with this cutting process. Proteins that are cut to the wrong length or that remain uncut are inactive.

Protease inhibitors are always taken with 1 or 2 nucleoside antiviral drugs such as efavirenz, emtricitabine, lamivudine, tenofovir, or zidovudine (AZT). Protease inhibitors revolutionized HIV treatment because when taken in combination, they reduce the amount of HIV virus in the bloodstream to levels that are often undetectable by current methods—CD_4 cell counts (immune system cells) and viral load (amount of virus in the blood) measurements. Multiple-drug therapy has changed the current view of HIV from a fatal disease to a manageable chronic illness.

People taking a protease inhibitor may still develop infections or other conditions associated with HIV disease. Because of this, it is very important for you to remain under the care of a doctor or other health care provider. You may be able to pass the HIV virus to others even if you are on triple-drug therapy.

Cautions and Warnings

Do not take ritonavir if you are **allergic** or **sensitive** to any of its ingredients. People with mild or moderate **liver disease** and **cirrhosis** break down ritonavir more slowly than those with normal liver function and may be more likely to develop side effects. People with cirrhosis should receive a reduced dose of ritonavir.

Ritonavir may raise your blood sugar, worsen your **diabetes,** or bring out latent diabetes. Diabetics who take ritonavir may have to have the dosage of their antidiabetes medication adjusted.

Ritonavir may cause pancreatitis, a dangerous condition. Symptoms include nausea, vomiting, and abdominal pain.

Some of ritonavir's drug interactions may be dangerous (see "Drug Interactions").

Ritonavir can affect a wide variety of blood tests, including those for triglycerides, liver function, and blood sugar.

Some patients experience changes in body fat. The long-term effects of these changes are not known.

Possible Side Effects

▼ Most common: weakness, tiredness, nausea, abnormal stools, diarrhea (more common with once-daily dosage), vomiting, appetite loss, abdominal pains, taste changes, and tingling around the mouth and in the hands or feet.

▼ Less common: increased levels of cholesterol and other blood fats, rash, diabetes, and high blood sugar, and increased fat deposits in some areas of the body, including the back of the neck.

▼ Rare: Rare side effects can occur in almost any part of the body, including muscles and joints, blood components, and the mouth, stomach and intestines, nervous system, skin, kidneys, liver, and urinary and respiratory tracts. Changes in mental state and sexual function may also occur. Contact your doctor if you experience any side effect not listed above.

Drug Interactions

- Combining ritonavir and lopinavir with statin-type cholesterol-lowering drugs can result in serious reactions.
- The following drugs should not be combined with ritonavir: amiodarone, astemizole, bepridil, bupropion, clozapine, encainide, flecainide, meperidine, piroxicam, propafenone, propoxyphene, quinidine, rifabutin, and sildenafil. Ritonavir can be expected to substantially raise the blood levels of all these drugs, which may cause serious abnormal heart rhythms, blood problems, seizures, and other serious side effects.
- Combining ritonavir with any of the following drugs may cause excessive sedation and breathing difficulties: alprazolam, clorazepate, diazepam, estazolam, flurazepam, midazolam, triazolam, and zolpidem. The effectiveness of other sedative-hypnotics is likely to be reduced by ritonavir. Ritonavir may interact with narcotic pain relievers, but the exact interaction is not predictable.
- Rifampin substantially decreases the amount of ritonavir and lopinavir absorbed into the blood and should be avoided.
- Ritonavir should not be used with the antimigraine drugs dihydroergotamine and ergotamine.
- Ritonavir and lopinavir should not be combined with pimozide.
- Combining ritonavir with clarithromycin raises the amount of clarithromycin in the blood.
- Mixing ritonavir with isoniazid increases the amount of isoniazid in the blood.
- Combining ritonavir with didanosine (ddI) may reduce the amount of ddI in the blood by about 15%. Take ddI 1 hour before or 2 hours after taking ritonavir.
- Combining fluconazole or fluoxetine with ritonavir increases the amount of ritonavir in the blood.
- Combining ritonavir with trazodone substantially increases the amount of these drugs in the blood. Dosage adjustment may be required.
- Do not combine ritonavir or ritonavir + lopinavir oral solutions with disulfiram or metronidazole. They contain alcohol, which may cause adverse reactions with these drugs.
- Combining ritonavir with methadone and with contraceptive drugs containing ethinyl estradiol can lower blood levels, possibly reducing their effectiveness.

- Combining ritonavir with saquinavir, another protease inhibitor, slows the breakdown of saquinavir and increases its blood levels.
- Ritonavir lowers the amount of sulfamethoxazole absorbed into the blood by about 20% and raises trimethoprim by about 20%.
- Combining ritonavir with theophylline reduces the amount of theophylline absorbed by about 40%.
- Taking ritonavir with AZT reduces the amount of AZT in the blood by about 10%.
- Ritonavir is likely to increase the absorption of these drugs into the blood: alpha blockers, antiarrhythmics, anticancer drugs, antidepressants, antiemetics, antifungals, antimalarials, beta blockers, blood-fat reducers, calcium entry blockers, cimetidine, desipramine, ergot alkaloids, erythromycin, immunosuppressants, indinavir, methylphenidate, pentoxifylline, phenothiazines, and warfarin.
- Ritonavir is likely to reduce the amount of these drugs absorbed into the blood: atovaquone, clofibrate, daunorubicin, diphenoxylate, theophylline, and metoclopramide. Dose adjustments may be needed.
- St. John's wort significantly reduces blood levels of ritonavir and they should not be used together.
- Ritonavir + lopinavir should not be taken with high doses (more than 200 mg a day) of ketoconazole or itraconazole. It should not be taken with voriconazole.
- Efavirenz and nevirapine reduce the amount of lopinavir in the blood. An increase in the ritonavir + lopinavir dose may be needed if you are taking either of those drugs. The ritonavir + lopinavir combination must be taken more than once daily if you are using either efavirenz or nevirapine.
- Delavirdine increases the amount of lopinavir in the blood. Proper dosing of this drug combination has not been established.
- Blood levels of tenofovir are increased by the ritonavir + lopinavir combination. The chance of tenofovir side effects is increased.
- Amprenavir blood levels are increased and lopinavir blood levels reduced when amprenavir is taken with ritonavir + lopinavir. Dosage adjustments are necessary. You will have to take ritonavir + lopinavir more than once a day. This same interaction exists if indinavir, nelfinavir, and saquinavir are substituted for amprenavir.

- Fosamprenavir reduces blood levels of both amprenavir and lopinavir. Do not mix these drugs.
- The anticonvulsant drugs carbamazepine, phenobarbital, and phenytoin reduce blood levels of ritonavir + lopinavir. If you take one of these drugs, your ritonavir + lopinavir dosage may have to be increased, and you will have to take it more than once a day.
- Ritonavir + lopinavir increases blood levels of felodipine, nifedipine, and nicardipine. Caution should be exercised when mixing these drugs because of the risk of an excessive blood-pressure drop.
- Dexamethasone reduces the amount of lopinavir in the blood, reducing its effectiveness.
- Ritonavir + lopinavir increases blood levels of erectile dysfunction drugs (sildenafil, tadalafil, and vardenafil). If you are taking one of these drugs, do not take more than 25 mg of sildenafil every 2 days, 10 mg of tadalafil once every 3 days, or 2.5 mg of vardenafil once every 3 days. Drug side effects may also increase.
- Atorvastatin blood levels are increased by the ritonavir + lopinavir combination. Use the lowest possible dose of atorvastatin. Pravastatin and fluvastatin are not subject to this interaction.
- Ritonavir + lopinavir increases blood levels of immune suppressants (cyclosporine, tacrolimus, and rapamycin).
- Blood levels of the inhaled corticosteroid fluticasone are increased when used with ritonavir or lopinavir. The combination is not recommended unless the potential benefit outweighs the risks.

Food Interactions

To increase the effectiveness of ritonavir capsules, take them with meals. Ritonavir oral solution should be taken on an empty stomach, 1 hour before or 2 hours after meals. The taste of the oral liquid may be improved by mixing it with chocolate milk, Ensure, or Advera. Do not mix earlier than 1 hour before you take your dose.

Usual Dose

Ritonavir

Adult: 600 mg twice a day. You may start with a lower dosage and increase gradually to avoid upset stomach.

Child (age 1 month and over): 250–400 mg per square meter of body surface area (BSA) twice a day. BSA is calculated by your doctor using height and weight.

Kaletra

Adult and Child (88 lbs. or more or age 12 and over): 2–4 capsules twice a day.

Child (age 6 months–11 years): Consult your doctor.

Overdosage

Little is known about the effects of ritonavir overdose. Take the victim to a hospital emergency room at once. ALWAYS bring the prescription bottle or container.

Special Information

Ritonavir is not a cure for HIV. It will not prevent you from transmitting the HIV virus to another person; you must still practice safe sex. People taking this drug may still develop opportunistic infections and other complications associated with HIV infection.

Take your HIV medication exactly as prescribed. Missing doses of ritonavir makes you more likely to become resistant to the drug and to lose the benefits of therapy.

Stay in close touch with your doctor while taking ritonavir and report unusual symptoms. Abdominal pain, nausea, and vomiting may be signs of pancreatitis (inflammation of the pancreas), which can be fatal.

Ritonavir and Kaletra capsules should be stored in the refrigerator. The ritonavir liquid may be kept at room temperature, but only for 30 days; Kaletra liquid may be kept at room temperature for 2 months.

If you forget a dose of these drugs, take it as soon as you remember. If it is almost time for your next dose, skip the dose you forgot and continue with your regular schedule. Do not take a double dose.

Special Populations

Pregnancy/Breast-feeding: Animal studies indicate that these drugs may affect the fetus. The effects of these drugs on pregnant women are not known. However, if your doctor considers them crucial, potential benefits must be carefully weighed against the risks.

It is not known if these drugs pass into breast milk. Mothers with HIV should always use infant formula, regardless of whether they take this drug, to avoid transmitting the virus to their child.

Seniors: Seniors may take ritonavir without special restriction.

Generic Name

Ropinirole (roe-PIN-ih-role)

Brand Name

Requip

Type of Drug

Antiparkinsonian.

Prescribed For

Parkinson's disease and moderate-to-severe restless legs syndrome (RLS).

General Information

Ropinirole relieves symptoms of Parkinson's disease and RLS by stimulating dopamine receptors in the brain. A study of people with early Parkinson's disease showed improvement in about 70% of people taking the drug for 10–12 weeks, compared to 40% of people taking a placebo (sugar pill). In another study, 28% of people with advanced Parkinson's disease who received ropinirole for 6 months showed improvement, compared to 11% of people in the placebo group. Ropinirole is broken down in the liver.

RLS is a condition that affects about 1 out of every 10 people. Symptoms include an urge to move the legs, usually accompanied by, or caused by, uncomfortable leg sensations. Symptoms begin or worsen during periods of rest or inactivity for most people and are partly or totally relieved by movement. Symptoms usually worsen or occur only in the evening or at night, and can disturb sleep.

Cautions and Warnings

Do not take ropinirole if you are **allergic** or **sensitive** to any of its ingredients.

Ropinirole may cause low blood pressure and make you dizzy or faint when rising from a sitting or lying position, especially during the early stages of treatment.

About 1 in 10–15 people who take ropinirole experience hallucinations that may be serious enough to require stopping drug therapy.

Ropinirole may make you fall asleep, sometimes suddenly, during the day. Use extreme caution when driving or engaging in a potentially hazardous activity.

People with **severe cardiovascular disease** should use ropinirole with caution.

Ropinirole, like other dopaminergic drugs, may cause pathological gambling, hypersexuality, or overeating, or other impulsive/compulsive behaviors, which are generally reversible if the dose is reduced or the drug is stopped.

People stopping other treatments for Parkinson's disease have developed high fever and confusion. Breathing difficulties caused by lung changes have occurred with the use of other antiparkinsonians. These problems have not been associated with ropinirole, but there is a risk that you may experience similar problems if you stop taking ropinirole.

Ropinirole may cause symptoms of RLS to occur earlier than usual or in other extremities; this has been seen with similar drugs, but has not been studied specifically in ropinirole.

Possible Side Effects

Early Parkinson's Disease
▼ Most common: sleepiness or tiredness, nausea, dizziness, fainting, upset stomach, vomiting, and virus infection.
▼ Common: general pain, sweating, weakness, fainting, abdominal pain, sore throat, and changes in vision.
▼ Less common: dry mouth, flushing, chest pain, feeling unwell, blood-pressure changes, heart palpitations, rapid heartbeat, hallucinations, confusion, memory loss, very sensitive reflexes, yawning, unusual movements, difficulty concentrating, appetite loss, gas, swollen arms or legs, runny nose, sinus irritation, bronchitis, breathing difficulties, eye problems, urinary infection, impotence, and poor blood supply to the hands, legs, and feet.

Advanced Parkinson's Disease
▼ Most common: abnormal movements, tremor, muscle rigidity, hallucinations, and urinary infection.
▼ Common: confusion, constipation, pneumonia, sweating, abdominal pain, and twitching.
▼ Less common: dizziness or fainting when rising from a sitting or lying position, unusual dreaming, changes in the way you walk, poor muscle coordination, memory loss, nervousness, tingling in the hands or feet, temporary paralysis, diarrhea, difficulty swallowing, gas, increased salivation,

Possible Side Effects *(continued)*

poor urinary control, pus in the urine, arthritis, breathing difficulties, dry mouth, anemia, and weight loss.

Restless Legs Syndrome
▼ Most common: nausea, tiredness, sleepiness, vomiting, dizziness, and fatigue.
▼ Common: sweating.
▼ Less common: dry mouth, diarrhea, nasal congestion, and swelling.

Drug Interactions

- Ropinirole increases levodopa + carbidopa blood levels and may worsen uncontrolled muscle spasm that occurs with levodopa + carbidopa. Your doctor may reduce your dosage.
- Ciprofloxacin, diltiazem, enoxacin, erythromycin, estrogen, fluvoxamine, mexilitene, norfloxacin, tacrine, cimetidine, and cigarette smoking increase ropinirole's effects.
- Phenothiazine sedatives, haloperidol and other antipsychotics, thioxanthene sedatives, and metoclopramide and other drugs that antagonize the effects of dopamine may reduce the effect of ropinirole.
- Ropinirole increases the sedative effect of benzodiazepines, sleeping pills, and other nervous system depressants.

Food Interactions

You may take this drug with food to prevent nausea.

Usual Dose

Parkinson's Disease

Adult: 0.25 mg 3 times a day to start, gradually increasing, if needed, in intervals of 0.75 mg a week, to a maximum of 24 mg a day. Dosage is reduced for people with kidney disease.

Child: not recommended.

Restless Legs Syndrome

Adult: 0.25–4 mg a day 1–3 hours before bedtime.

Child: not recommended.

Overdosage

Little is known about the effects of ropinirole overdose. Symptoms are likely to include the most common side effects. Take the victim to a hospital emergency room. ALWAYS bring the prescription bottle or container.

Special Information

Take this drug exactly as prescribed.

Ropinirole can cause sedation. Be careful when driving or performing any task that requires concentration. Avoid alcohol and other nervous system depressants.

Hallucinations may occur with this drug, especially among seniors. Call your doctor if you develop hallucinations or bothersome or persistent side effects.

If you forget a dose, take it as soon as you remember. For Parkinson's disease, space the remaining daily dosage evenly throughout the day. Go back to your regular schedule the next day. Do not take a double dose.

Special Populations

Pregnancy/Breast-feeding: In animal studies, ropinirole causes birth defects and damages the fetus. When this drug is considered crucial by your doctor, its potential benefits must be carefully weighed against its risks.

Animal studies show that ropinirole passes into breast milk, but it is not known if this occurs in humans. Ropinirole may interfere with milk production. Nursing mothers who must take this drug should use infant formula.

Seniors: Hallucinations are more likely to occur in seniors.

Generic Name

Rotigotine (row-TIH-go-tene)

Brand Name

Neupro

Type of Drug

Dopamine agonist.

Prescribed For

Early Parkinson's disease.

General Information

Rotigotine is thought to work by stimulating specific dopamine receptors in the brain. Almost half of the total content of the patch is released into the blood within 24 hours after it is applied to the skin. Maximum blood concentrations are usually achieved 15–18 hours after the patch is applied but can occur anywhere from 4–27 hours afterward. Rotigotine is broken down in the liver and is eliminated from the body within a day unless another patch is applied.

Cautions and Warnings

Do not use this drug is you are **allergic** or **sensitive** to any of its ingredients or to the patch. People with a **sulfite allergy** should avoid the rotigotine patch. Sulfite reactions can be mild to very severe and are more common in people with **asthma**.

Mild to moderate liver disease has no effect on rotigotine dosage but there is no information on the use of this drug by people with **severe liver disease**.

People with a **sleep disorder** should use this drug with caution. People using rotigotine may experience hallucinations.

Rotigotine may lower blood pressure, which can lead to dizziness or fainting. Rotigotine can also paradoxically increase blood pressure and heart rate. This effect increases with increasing dosage.

People using rotigotine may experience significant weight gain and swelling in the arms and legs.

Rotigotine may make you fall asleep, sometimes suddenly, during the day. Use extreme caution when driving or engaging in a potentially hazardous activity.

People who stop taking other antiparkinsonians may develop high fever and confusion. Breathing difficulties caused by lung changes have also occurred with other antiparkinsonians. These symptoms have not been associated with rotigotine, but there is a risk that you may experience similar problems if you stop taking rotigotine.

Rotigotine, like other dopaminergic drugs, may cause pathological gambling, hypersexuality, or overeating, or other impulsive/compulsive behaviors, which are generally reversible if the dose is reduced or the drug stopped.

The rotigotine patch contains aluminum. Remove the patch before undergoing an MRI scan or cardioversion to avoid skin burns.

Possible Side Effects

Most rotigotine side effects increase when the dose is increased.

▼ Most common: skin reactions where the patch is applied, drowsiness or fatigue, dizziness, nausea, headache, vomiting, and sleeplessness.

▼ Common: swelling in the arms or legs, constipation, and back pain.

▼ Less common: weight gain, sweating, dry mouth, high blood pressure, fainting, upset stomach, appetite loss, joint pain, unusual dreams, hallucinations, sinusitis, urinary infection, vision changes, and increased salivation.

▼ Rare: weakness, flu-like symptoms, diarrhea, depression, runny nose, frequent urination, upper respiratory infection, falling, tremors, cough, anxiety, and abdominal and chest pain. Contact your doctor if you experience any side effect not listed above.

Drug Interactions

- Rotigotine may increase the effects of sedatives and sleeping pills.
- Dopamine antagonists such as antipsychotics and metoclopramide can reduce rotigotine's effectiveness.

Food Interactions

Rotigotine may be taken with or without food.

Usual Dose

Adult (age 18 and over): Start with a 2 mg patch every 24 hours. Dosage may be increased as necessary, up to 6 mg a day.

Child (age 17 and under): not recommended.

Overdosage

There have been no cases of rotigotine overdose. Overdose is unlikely unless you forget to remove the previous day's patch after applying the current one. Overdose symptoms to be expected include nausea, vomiting, low blood pressure, involuntary movements, hallucinations, confusion, and convulsions. Call a hospital emergency room or your local poison control center for more information. If you take the victim to a hospital emergency room for treatment, ALWAYS bring the prescription bottle or container.

Special Information

Do not suddenly stop using this medicine. The dosage should be gradually reduced to avoid serious side effects.

Report fever, rigid muscles, muscle aches, perceptual changes, and any other unusual events to your doctor.

Avoid exposing the applied rotigotine patch to external sources of direct heat, including heating pads, electric blankets, heat lamps, saunas, hot tubs, heated water beds, and prolonged direct sunlight.

Apply one patch every day and be sure to always remove the old one. The adhesive side of the patch should be applied to clean, dry, intact skin on the front of the abdomen, thigh, hip, side, shoulder, or upper arm immediately after the patch is removed from its pouch. Do not place the patch onto skin that is oily, irritated, or damaged, or where it will be rubbed by tight clothes. If it is necessary to apply the patch to a hairy area, shave the area first so the patch can be placed on a hairless area. Do not use the same site more than once every 2 weeks.

If you forget a dose or if a patch falls off, apply a new one as soon as you remember. If it is almost time for the next dose, skip the one you forgot and continue with your regular schedule. Do not apply more than one rotigotine patch at a time.

Special Populations

Pregnancy/Breast-feeding: Animal studies have shown rotigotine may damage a developing fetus. Pregnant women should take it only if its potential benefits outweigh the risks.

Rotigotine may reduce the volume of breast milk and can pass into breast milk. Nursing mothers who use this medicine should consider using infant formula because of the possibility of causing drug-related side effects in the nursing infant.

Seniors: Seniors under age 80 may use this drug without special precaution. Those over 80 years of age may develop higher blood levels of rotigotine because the drug passes more easily through their skin.

Generic Name

Salmeterol (sal-METE-er-ol)

Brand Names

Serevent   Serevent Diskus

The information in this profile also applies to the following drugs:

Generic Ingredients: Salmeterol + Fluticasone
Advair Diskus   Advair HFA

Type of Drug

Bronchodilator.

Prescribed For

Asthma and bronchospasm.

General Information

Salmeterol xinafoate differs from other bronchodilators in that it does not provide immediate symptom relief, but is instead prescribed for long-term prevention. When you start salmeterol treatment, you may need to continue your other asthma inhalers for symptom relief. After a while, however, you should have less need for the other drugs. Salmeterol works like other bronchodilator drugs, such as albuterol, terbutaline, and metaproterenol, but it has a weaker effect on nerve receptors in the heart and blood vessels; for this reason, it is somewhat safer for people with heart conditions. Still, very large doses of salmeterol may lead to abnormal heart rhythms. Salmeterol begins working within 20 minutes after a dose and continues for 12 hours. Salmeterol and fluticasone, a corticosteriod, have been combined into a single product for inhalation because both drugs are prescribed in the long-term prevention of asthma.

Cautions and Warnings

Do not take salmeterol if you are **allergic** or **sensitive** to any of its ingredients.

Salmeterol should be used with caution by people with a history of **angina pectoris** (condition characterized by brief attacks of chest pain), **heart disease, high blood pressure, stroke** or **seizure, thyroid disease, prostate disease,** or **glaucoma.**

Used in excess, salmeterol can rarely lead to more severe asthma attacks, rather than asthma relief. In the most extreme cases, people have had heart attacks after using excessive amounts of inhalant bronchodilators such as salmeterol.

A large study comparing the safety of salmeterol to a placebo (sugar pill) showed a small but significant increase in asthma-related deaths among people taking salmeterol—13 deaths out of 13,174 patients treated for 28 weeks—versus only 3 deaths among

13,179 taking the placebo. The risk of asthma-related death might be greater in **black patients** than Caucasians.

Long-term use of salmeterol and related drugs can lead to increases in certain ovarian tumors.

Salmeterol should not be used by patients with **acutely deteriorating asthma**, which can lead to serious respiratory events.

Possible Side Effects

▼ Most common: heart palpitations, rapid heartbeat, tremors, cough, dizziness and fainting, shakiness, nervousness, tension, headache, diarrhea, heartburn or upset stomach, dry or sore or irritated throat, respiratory infections, and nasal or sinus conditions.

▼ Less common: nausea and vomiting, joint or back pain, muscle cramps, muscle soreness, muscle ache or pain, giddiness, viral stomach infections, itching, dental pain, not feeling well, rash, and menstrual irregularity.

Drug Interactions

- Monoamine oxidase inhibitor antidepressants, tricyclic antidepressants, thyroid drugs, other bronchodilator drugs, and some antihistamines may increase the effects of salmeterol.
- The risk of cardiotoxicity may be increased in people taking both salmeterol and theophylline.
- Beta-blocking drugs may reduce the effect of salmeterol, and may also produce severe bronchospasm in people with asthma.
- Salmeterol may exacerbate certain effects of non-potassium sparing (loop or thiazide) diuretics.
- Salmeterol may decrease the effects of blood-pressure-lowering drugs, especially reserpine, methyldopa, and guanethidine.

Food Interactions

None known.

Usual Dose

Salmeterol (aerosol)
> **Adult and Child (age 12 and over):** 2 inhalations every 12 hours.
> **Child (under age 12):** not recommended.

Salmeterol (powder)
    Adult and Child (age 4 and over): 1 inhalation every 12 hours.
    Child (under age 4): not recommended.

Salmeterol + Fluticasone
    Adult and Child (age 12 and over): 1 inhalation every 12 hours.
    Child (under age 12): not recommended.

Overdosage

Overdose of salmeterol inhalation usually results in exaggerated side effects, including chest pain and high blood pressure, although blood pressure may drop to a low level after a short period of elevation. People who inhale too much salmeterol should see a doctor. ALWAYS bring the prescription bottle or container.

Special Information

Be sure to follow the inhalation instructions that come with the product. Wait at least 1 minute between puffs. Do not inhale salmeterol if you have food or anything else in your mouth. Rinse mouth with water after each use.

Call your doctor immediately if you develop chest pain, palpitations, rapid heartbeat, muscle tremors, dizziness, headache, facial flushing, or urinary difficulty, or if you continue to experience difficulty in breathing after using salmeterol.

If you forget a dose of salmeterol, take it as soon as you remember. If it is almost time for your next dose, skip the one you forgot and go back to your regular schedule. Do not take a double dose.

If your doctor is switching you from an inhaled corticosteroid to the salmeterol + fluticasone combination, it is important for you to report any changes in symptoms as soon as they occur.

Special Populations

Pregnancy/Breast-feeding: When used during childbirth, salmeterol may slow or delay natural labor. It can cause rapid heartbeat and high blood sugar in the mother and rapid heartbeat and low blood sugar in the baby. It is not known whether salmeterol causes birth defects in humans, but it has caused defects in animals. When your doctor considers this drug crucial, its potential benefits must be carefully weighed against its risks.

Salmeterol may pass into breast milk. Nursing mothers who must take this drug should use infant formula.

Seniors: Seniors should use the same dosage of salmeterol as younger adults.

Generic Name

Saquinavir (suh-QUIN-uh-vere)

Brand Name

Invirase

Type of Drug

Protease inhibitor.

Prescribed For

Advanced human immunodeficiency virus (HIV) infection.

General Information

Part of the multidrug "cocktail" responsible for important gains in the fight against acquired immunodeficiency syndrome (AIDS), saquinavir is a member of a group of anti-HIV drugs called protease inhibitors. These drugs work at the end of the HIV reproduction process, when proteins are "cut" into strands of exactly the correct size to duplicate HIV. An enzyme known as protease cuts the protein. Protease inhibitors prevent the mature HIV virus from being formed by inhibiting this cutting process. Proteins that are cut to the wrong length or that remain uncut are inactive.

Protease inhibitors are always taken with 1 or 2 nucleoside antiviral drugs such as efavirenz, emtricitabine, lamivudine, tenofovir, or zidovudine (AZT). They revolutionized HIV treatment because, when taken in combination, they reduce the amount of HIV virus in the bloodstream to levels that are often undetectable by current methods—CD_4 cell (immune system cell) counts and viral load (amount of virus in the blood) measurements. Multiple-drug therapy has changed the current view of HIV from a fatal disease to a manageable chronic illness.

Cautions and Warnings

Do not take saquinavir if you are **allergic** or **sensitive** to any of its ingredients.

If a serious toxic reaction occurs while taking saquinavir, you should stop the drug until your doctor can determine the cause or until the reaction resolves itself. Then treatment can be resumed.

Use caution if you have moderate to severe **liver disease.**

Saquinavir may raise your blood sugar, worsen your **diabetes,** or bring out latent diabetes. People with diabetes who take saquinavir may need the dosage of their antidiabetes medication adjusted.

HIV virus may become resistant to saquinavir or other protease inhibitors. For this reason it is essential that you take saquinavir exactly according to your doctor's directions.

Possible Side Effects

Most side effects are mild. Other side effects become more prominent when saquinavir is taken together with antiretroviral drugs; these include weakness, muscle pain, and mouth ulcers.

▼ Most common: diarrhea, dyspepsia, nausea, and abdominal discomfort.

▼ Less common: upset stomach, abdominal pain, headache, tingling or numbness in the hands or feet, dizziness, nerve damage, changes in appetite, and rash.

▼ Rare: Rare side effects can occur in almost any part of the body. Contact your doctor if you experience any side effect not listed above.

Drug Interactions

- Rifampin and rifabutin reduce saquinavir blood levels by 80% and 40%, respectively. Rifabutin levels are increased. Another protease inhibitor may be added to compensate for the interaction's effect. Do not combine these drugs with saquinavir. Phenobarbital, phenytoin, dexamethasone, carbamazepine, garlic capsules, and nevirapine may also reduce blood levels of saquinavir.

- Blood levels of saquinavir may be elevated by terfenidine, astemizole, ketoconazole, and itraconazole. Other drugs that may lead to serious side effects when combined with saquinavir are amiodarone, bepridil, cisapride, calcium channel blockers, clarithomycin, clindamycin, delavirdine, ergot derivatives, flecainide, midazolam, propafenone, quinidine, rifampin, and triazolam. Do not combine these medications.

- Saquinavir increases blood levels of the benzodiazepines, cyclosporine, tacrolimus, rapamycin, tricylic antidepressants (amitripyline, imipramine), and pimozide. Dose reductions of these medicines may be needed.

- Saquinavir reduces blood levels of the narcotic analgesics and the estrogen part of contraceptive drugs. Talk to your doctor about additional or different contraceptive protection.
- Ritonavir increases blood levels of saquinavir and increases the risk of side effects. This combination is often used to boost the effects of saquinavir.
- Combining rifampin with ritonavir + saquinavir can lead to hepatitis and serious increases in liver enzymes.
- Do not mix lovastatin or simvastatin with saquinavir or ritonavir + saquinavir. The combination leads to muscle pain and damage and to kidney damage. Atorvastatin and other statin drugs may also produce this reaction and should be used with caution.
- St. John's wort decreases the effectiveness of saquinavir. Do not combine these medications.
- Protease inhibitors may drastically increase the blood levels of the erectile dysfunction (ED) drugs sildenafil, vardenafil, and tadalafil, increasing the risk of side effects including low blood pressure, visual changes, sudden hearing loss, and persistent, painful erection. Reduce ED drug dose by ½ and use with caution.
- People taking warfarin with saquinavir should have their blood tested periodically to be sure that their anticoagulant dose is correct.

Food Interactions

Take saquinavir within 2 hours after a full meal. The amount of saquinavir absorbed into the blood is vastly reduced when it is taken on an empty stomach, thus negating its antiviral effects.

Usual Dose

Adult (age 16 and over): 200 mg 5 times a day (usually administered with 100 mg of ritonavir twice a day), within 2 hours after a full meal.

Child (under age 16): Consult your doctor.

Overdosage

Little is known about the effects of saquinavir overdose. Take the victim to a hospital emergency room. ALWAYS bring the prescription bottle or container.

Special Information

Saquinavir is not a cure for HIV. It will not prevent you from transmitting the HIV virus to another person; you must still practice safe sex. People taking this drug may still develop opportunistic infections or other complications associated with HIV infection. The long-term effects of this drug are not known.

It is imperative for you to take this medication exactly according to your doctor's instructions. Missing doses of saquinavir increases the risk that you will become resistant to the drug. It should be taken after meals with your nucleoside antiviral drug. If you forget a dose of saquinavir, take it as soon as you remember. Do not take a double dose.

Special Populations

Pregnancy/Breast-feeding: While animal studies of saquinavir reveal no damage to the fetus, this drug should only be used during pregnancy after carefully weighing its potential benefits against its risks.

It is not known if saquinavir passes into breast milk. Mothers with HIV should always use infant formula, regardless of whether they take this drug, to avoid transmitting the virus to their child.

Seniors: Seniors should take this drug with caution because of the likelihood of heart, liver, or kidney issues with advancing age. The lowest effective dose should be used.

Type of Drug

Selective Serotonin Reuptake Inhibitors (SSRIs)

Brand Name

Generic Ingredient: Citalopram Hydrobromide G
Celexa

Generic Ingredient: Escitalopram Oxylate G
Lexapro

Generic Ingredient: Fluoxetine Hydrochloride G
Prozac   Sarafem
Prozac Weekly

Generic Ingredient: Fluvoxamine Maleate Ⓖ

Generic Ingredient: Paroxetine Hydrochloride Ⓖ
Paxil   Paxil CR

Generic Ingredient: Paroxetine Mesylate
Pexeva

Generic Ingredient: Sertraline Hydrochloride Ⓖ
Zoloft

Prescribed For

Depression, bulimic binge-eating and vomiting, obsessive-compulsive disorder (OCD), social anxiety disorder, generalized anxiety disorder, panic disorder, migraine, peripheral diabetic neuropathy, hot flashes, post-traumatic stress disorder (PTSD), premenstrual dysphoric disorder, Reynaud phenomenon, and borderline personality disorder. Also prescribed for alcoholism, anorexia, kleptomania, irritable bowel syndrome, dyskinetic side effects of levodopa + carbidopa, and Tourette's syndrome.

Fluoxetine is approved for treating major depressive disorder and OCD in children. Fluvoxamine is also approved for treating OCD in children. Other SSRIs are not approved for use in children for any indication.

General Information

SSRIs, which are chemically unrelated to other antidepressant drugs, prevent the movement of the neurotransmitter serotonin into nerve endings. This forces serotonin to remain in the spaces surrounding nerve endings, increasing its action. Abnormal serotonin function may be involved in depression, and the SSRIs are effective in treating the common symptoms of depression. For example, they can help improve mood and mental alertness, alleviate anxiety, and improve sleep patterns.

Cautions and Warnings

Do not take SSRIs if you are **allergic** or **sensitive** to any of their ingredients. Some people have experienced serious drug reactions to SSRIs.

SSRIs can increase the risk of suicidal thinking and behavior in adults, children, and teens. Patients who are started on therapy should be observed closely for clinical worsening of depression, suicidality, or unusual changes in behavior, especially at the beginning of therapy or when the dose is increased or decreased.

Serious, potentially fatal reactions may occur if SSRIs and a monoamine oxidase inhibitor (MAOI) antidepressant are taken within 2 weeks of one another (see "Drug Interactions").

The possibility of suicide exists especially in **severely depressed patients** and may be present until the condition is significantly improved. Severely depressed people should be allowed to carry only small quantities of SSRIs to limit the risk of overdose.

About 7% of people taking fluoxetine develop an itching rash, ⅓ of whom have to stop taking the medication.

As many as ⅓ of people taking an SSRI experience anxiety, sleeplessness, and nervousness.

Underweight depressed people who take fluoxetine may lose more weight. About 9% of people taking fluoxetine experience appetite loss, while 13% lose more than 5% of their body weight.

SSRIs may affect blood platelets, although their exact effect is not known. Some people have had abnormal bleeding while taking these drugs.

SSRIs are significantly broken down in the liver. People with **liver disease** should use these drugs with caution and may require lower doses than people without liver disease. People with severe **kidney disease** should begin with smaller doses of citalopram, escitalopram, paroxetine, and sertraline.

People taking SSRIs may experience a severe drop in their blood sodium level, especially if taking diuretics as well.

SSRIs should be used with caution by people with **seizure disorders** and in people with **glaucoma.**

People with **mania** or **hypomania** may experience an activation or worsening of their condition when taking SSRIs, especially if they are not also taking an antimanic medication.

Fluoxetine may alter blood sugar control in people with **diabetes**.

SSRIs should be discontinued gradually, as significant side effects from discontinuing too quickly may occur.

Rarely, people taking SSRIs develop a group of symptoms called serotonin syndrome, consisting of one or more of the following symptoms: excitement, a mild manic reaction, restlessness, loss of consciousness, confusion, disorientation, anxiety, agitation, muscle weakness, muscle spasms, tremors, involuntary muscle movements on one side of the body, shivering and dilated pupils, sweating, vomiting, and rapid heartbeat. Serotonin syndrome requires immediate medical treatment.

Possible Side Effects

▼ Common: headache, anxiety, nervousness, sleeplessness, drowsiness, tiredness, weakness, sexual dysfunction, tremors, sweating, dizziness, lightheadedness, dry mouth, upset or irritated stomach, appetite loss, appetite increase, nausea, vomiting, diarrhea, gas, rash, weight loss or gain, electric-shock sensations, increased sweating, increased yawning, tinnitus, abnormal dreams, difficulty concentrating, acne, hair loss, dry skin, dizziness or fainting when rising suddenly from a sitting or lying position, and itching.

▼ Less common: chest pain, allergy, runny nose, bronchitis, abnormal heart rhythms, blood pressure changes, bone pain, bursitis, twitching, breast pain, cystitis, urinary pain, double vision, eye or ear pain, conjunctivitis (pinkeye), anemia, swelling, low blood sugar, and low thyroid activity.

▼ Rare: Rare side effects can occur in almost any part of the body. Contact your doctor if you experience any side effect not listed above.

Drug Interactions

- Five weeks should elapse between stopping fluoxetine and starting an MAOI antidepressant. At least 2 weeks should elapse between stopping other SSRIs and starting an MAOI. Two weeks should elapse between stopping an MAOI and starting an SSRI. Taking these drugs too close together or at the same time may cause serious, life-threatening reactions.

- Combining an SSRI with metoclopramide, sibutramine, linezolid, tramadol, or St. John's wort may increase the risk of serotonin syndrome (see "Cautions and Warnings"). Avoid combining these medications.

- Fluvoxamine, fluoxetine, and paroxetine increase thioridazine levels. Do not combine these drugs.

- Combining sertraline or fluvoxamine with pimozide can significantly increase the amount of pimozide in the blood. Do not combine these drugs.

- Combining an SSRI and nonsteroidal anti-inflammatory drugs (NSAIDs) substantially increases the risk of gastrointestinal side effects. This combination should be avoided over the long term.

- Tricyclic antidepressant blood levels may increase if they are taken with SSRIs. Combine these drugs with caution.
- SSRIs affect lithium blood levels. Your lithium dosage may need to be adjusted.
- People taking warfarin and SSRIs may experience increased bleeding or increased warfarin side effects.
- Cyproheptadine (an antihistamine) may reverse the effects of SSRIs.
- SSRIs can increase blood levels of many drugs, including any other SSRI, amphetamines, carbamazepine, codeine, phenothiazines, and some antiarrhythmics (encainide, flecainide, propafenonol) leading to an increased risk of side effects.
- Hallucinations have occurred after combining fluoxetine with dextromethorphan (the most common cough suppressant in over-the-counter products).
- Combining fluoxetine, paroxetine, or sertraline with phenytoin can lead to increased phenytoin side effects and reduce blood levels of paroxetine.
- Fluoxetine, fluvoxamine, and sertraline can raise the blood level of the antipsychotic drugs clozapine, risperidone, and olanzapine.
- People who combine l-tryptophan and SSRIs may become agitated and restless, and may experience an upset stomach.
- Fluoxetine and fluvoxamine may reduce the effectiveness of buspirone, which can lead to a worsening of obsessive-compulsive disorder (OCD) in people taking this combination to treat OCD.
- Fluoxetine and fluvoxamine may increase the risk of carbamazepine side effects and increase haloperidol levels.
- Fluoxetine, fluvoxamine, and sertraline may increase the effect of benzodiazepine antianxiety drugs.
- Cimetidine can increase paroxetine, escitalopram, and citalopram levels in the blood.
- Alcohol may increase tiredness and other depressant effects of SSRIs.
- Paroxetine may increase risperidone blood levels and the combination may lead to serotonin syndrome (see "Cautions and Warnings").
- Fluoxetine may affect ritonavir, possibly leading to serotonin syndrome (see "Cautions and Warnings").
- Sertraline may increase the effects of zolpidem.

- Smoking increases the metabolism of fluvoxamine.
- Fluvoxamine, citalopram, and escitalopram may increase the effects of beta blockers.
- Paroxetine may affect the effectiveness of digoxin, and may increase phenothiazine levels and the effects of procyclidine.
- Fluvoxamine may increase methadone and tacrine blood levels, and may increase the effects of diltiazem.
- Paroxetine and fluvoxamine may increase the effects of sumatriptan and affect theophylline blood levels.
- Fluoxetine can raise the blood levels of pimozide and cyclosporine (an immune suppressant).

Food Interactions

These drugs may be taken without regard to food or meals.

Usual Dose

Citalopram

Adult: 20–40 mg a day. Seniors and people with liver disease should take no more than 20 mg a day. People with kidney disease may need a lower dose.
Child: not recommended.

Escitalopram

Adult: 10–20 mg once a day. Seniors and people with liver disease should take no more than 10 mg.
Child: not recommended.

Fluoxetine

Adult: 20–80 mg a day, taken in the morning, or a single 90 mg capsule weekly. Seniors, people with kidney or liver disease, and people taking several different drugs may need a lower dose.
Child (age 8–18): 10–60 mg a day.

Fluvoxamine

Adult: 50–300 mg a day at bedtime. Seniors and people with liver disease may need a lower dose.
Child (age 8–17): 25–200 mg a day. Doses larger than 50 mg should be divided in 2 and given morning and night. If the 2 divided doses are not equal, give the larger dose at bedtime.
Child (under age 8): not recommended.

Paroxetine

Adult: 20–60 mg a day, or 25–62.5 mg a day for the controlled-release form. Seniors and people with liver disease should start at

10 mg a day and take no more than 40 mg a day. People with kidney disease may need a lower dose.

Child: not recommended.

Prozac Weekly

Adult: 90 mg (1 capsule) every 7 days.

Child: not recommended.

Sertraline

Adult: 50–200 mg a day. Lower doses may be used to start, but most adults take at least 50 mg a day. Seniors and people with liver disease should take a lower dose.

Child: not recommended.

Overdosage

Overdose symptoms may include seizures, nausea, vomiting, agitation, restlessness, and nervous system excitation. Any person suspected of having taken an SSRI overdose should be taken to a hospital emergency room at once. ALWAYS bring the prescription bottle or container.

Special Information

SSRIs can make you dizzy or drowsy. Take care when driving or performing other tasks that require alertness and concentration, especially when you first start the drug or increase your dose. Avoid alcohol.

Be sure your doctor knows if you are pregnant, breast-feeding, or taking other drugs, including over-the-counter drugs, while taking an SSRI.

Call your doctor if you develop a rash or hives, become excessively nervous or anxious, lose your appetite—especially if you are already underweight—or experience any unusual side effects.

If you forget a dose, take it as soon as you remember. If it is almost time for your next dose, skip the dose you forgot and continue with your regular schedule. Do not take a double dose.

Discontinuing SSRIs suddenly may cause adverse effects including mood changes, irritability, agitation, dizziness, tingling in the hands or feet, anxiety, confusion, headache, tiredness, and insomnia. These effects can be serious but are usually temporary. A gradual reduction in dose is recommended.

Special Populations

Pregnancy/Breast-feeding: These drugs pass into the circulation of the developing fetus. Studies in animals and people have shown that SSRIs may cause birth defects and premature birth. Do not take an SSRI if you are or might be pregnant without first weighing the potential benefits and risks with your doctor.

These drugs pass into breast milk. Nursing mothers who must take an SSRI should consider using infant formula.

Seniors: Seniors generally start with lower doses and may need less of the drug to achieve the desired results.

Generic Name

Selegiline (seh-LEG-uh-leen) [G]

Brand Names

Eldepryl   Zelapar

Emsam

Type of Drug

Antiparkinsonian and selective monoamine oxidase inhibitor (MAOI).

Prescribed For

Parkinson's disease; also prescribed for depression.

General Information

Selegiline hydrochloride is usually combined with levodopa + carbidopa when used to control Parkinson's disease, particularly the symptoms that appear when there is a "wearing off" of the effects of levodopa + carbidopa. Selegiline blocks the effects of the enzyme monoamine oxidase; it interferes with a form of it (MAO-B, at the proper dosage) found almost exclusively in the brain, which in part increases dopamine. Selegiline also stimulates dopamine receptors. Enhancing dopamine in the brain is the effective method of treatment for Parkinson's disease. MAOIs are also used for depression, particularly atypical depression. Since selegiline inhibits only MAO-B, there is much less risk of serious food interactions with lower doses. With larger doses typically used for depression, this drug becomes non-selective and can cause a full blown MAOI reaction, just like the older MAOIs phenelzine and tranyleypromine.

Cautions and Warnings

Do not use selegiline if you are **allergic** or **sensitive** to any of its ingredients.

If you take **levodopa + carbidopa** and start taking selegiline, you may experience an increase in levodopa side effects. Your dosage of levodopa + carbidopa may need to be reduced.

Taking more than the prescribed dose of selegiline a day may cause severe reactions, including possibly fatal high blood pressure. There are no benefits to taking doses of this drug higher than the maximum dose recommended by your doctor and the manufacturer.

Selegiline should not be used with **meperidine or other narcotic drugs** because of the risk of severe, possibly fatal reactions.

Antidepressants, including selegiline, may increase suicidal thoughts or actions in **children, teens, and young adults,** especially within the first few weeks or months of treatment, or when the dose is increased or decreased. Warning signs may include agitation, irritability, and unusual behavior changes.

While taking selegiline you will need to watch your diet carefully. See "Food Interactions" for details.

Selegiline may cause dizziness or fainting when rising from a sitting or lying position.

People who cannot take **phenylalanine** should know that Zelapar contains phenylalanine.

Hallucinations may occur with selegiline. They should be reported immediately to your doctor.

Possible Side Effects

In Parkinson's disease, selegiline often increases the side effects of levodopa + carbidopa. Your doctor may reduce your dosage of levodopa + carbidopa.

▼ Most common: nausea, vomiting, dizziness, lightheadedness or fainting, headache, and insomnia.

▼ Common: constipation, agitation, anxiety, and muscle problems.

▼ Less common: dry mouth, abnormal movements, and hallucinations.

Drug Interactions

- Selegiline should not be used with meperidine or other narcotics because of the risk of severe, possibly fatal reactions (see "Cautions and Warnings").

- Do not combine selegiline with any SSRI/SNRI or tricyclic antidepressant. Serious, possibly fatal, reactions may occur.
- Do not combine selegiline with bupropion, mirtazapine, St. John's wort, carbamazepine, or oxcarbazepine.
- Do not combine selegiline with dextromethorphan due to the risk of a psychotic reaction.
- Contraceptive drugs may increase the effects of selegiline. Combine with caution.

Food Interactions

Do not eat or drink 5 minutes before or after taking Zelapar. While taking any form of selegiline, avoid the following: Chianti and red wine, vermouth, unpasteurized or imported beer, beef or chicken liver, fermented sausages, tenderized or prepared meats, caviar, dried fish, pickled herring, cheese (American, Brie, cheddar, Camembert, Emmentaler, Boursault, Stilton, and others), avocados, yeast extracts, bananas, figs, raisins, soy sauce, miso soup, bean curd, fava beans, caffeine, and some chocolate. Although reactions to these foods are unlikely, patients should be cautious, as possible effects include severe, sudden high blood pressure, which can be fatal. Reactions to the higher doses used for depression are much more likely and these foods should be avoided.

Usual Dose

Parkinson's Disease
Eldepryl
>Adult: 5 mg at breakfast and lunch.
>Child: not recommended.

Emsam
>Adult: 6–12 mg a day. Apply the patch to dry, clean skin once every 24 hours.
>Child: not recommended.

Zelapar (oral disintegrating tablets)
>Adult: 1.25–2.5 mg a day. Allow the tablet to dissolve on your tongue.
>Child: not recommended.

Depression
>Adult: 5 mg twice a day to start, increasing gradually as needed to 10–30 mg twice a day.
>Child: not recommended.

Overdosage

Symptoms may include excitement, irritability, anxiety, low blood pressure, sleeplessness, restlessness, dizziness, weakness, drowsiness, flushing, sweating, heart palpitations, and unusual movements, including grimacing and muscle twitching. Serious overdoses may lead to convulsions, incoherence or confusion, severe headache, high fever, heart attack, shock, and coma. Take the victim to a hospital emergency room. ALWAYS bring the prescription bottle or container.

Special Information

Any severe headache or unusual symptoms should be reported to your doctor immediately.

After you have taken selegiline for 2 or 3 days, your doctor will probably reduce your levodopa + carbidopa dosage by 10–30%. If the disease is still under control, your dosage may be reduced further.

Contact your doctor if you develop headache, unusual body movements or muscle spasms, mood changes, or any bothersome or persistent side effects. Do not stop taking selegiline or change your dosage without your doctor's knowledge.

Selegiline reduces saliva flow in the mouth and may increase the risk of cavities, gum disease, and oral infections. Use candy, ice, sugarless gum, or a saliva substitute to avoid dry mouth.

If you forget a dose, take it as soon as you remember. Do not take a double dose.

Special Populations

Pregnancy/Breast-feeding: The safety of using selegiline during pregnancy is not known. When this drug is considered crucial by your doctor, its potential benefits must be carefully weighed against its risks.

It is not known if selegiline passes into breast milk. Nursing mothers who must take it should consider using infant formula.

Seniors: Seniors should receive the lowest effective dosage to minimize side effects.

Brand Name

Septra

Generic Ingredients

Sulfamethoxazole + Trimethoprim G

Other Brand Names

Bactrim   Sulfamethoprim
Bactrim DS   Sulfatrim Pediatric
Septra DS

Type of Drug

Anti-infective.

Prescribed For

A wide variety of infections, including urinary tract infection, bronchitis, and ear infection in children; also prescribed for traveler's diarrhea, pneumocystis carinii pneumonia (PCP), acute exacerbations of chronic bronchitis in adults, prostate infection, cholera, nocardiosis (lung infection), and *Salmonella* infection.

General Information

Septra is effective in many situations where other drugs are not. It is unique because it interferes with the infecting microorganism's normal use of folic acid in two ways, making it more efficient than other antibacterial drugs.

Cautions and Warnings

Do not take Septra if you are **allergic** or **sensitive** to any of its ingredients or to any sulfa drug, antidiabetes drug, or thiazide-type diuretic.

Do not take Septra if you have a **folic acid deficiency**.

Septra should be used with caution by people with **liver or kidney disease** and those with a history of **alcoholism**.

Infants under 2 months of age should not be given this combination product.

Symptoms such as unusual bleeding or bruising, extreme tiredness, rash, sore throat, fever, pallor, or yellowing of the skin or eyes may be early indications of a serious blood disorder. If any of these effects occur, particularly a rash, contact your doctor immediately and stop taking the drug.

People taking Septra for **PCP** also have compromised immune function. They may not respond to Septra and are more likely to develop the less common side effects.

Those with **asthma** or **severe allergies** should alert their doctor.

Septra should not be used for **strep throat** because of a greater chance of treatment failure than with penicillin.

Colitis may occur with Septra. Contact your doctor if you experience diarrhea, especially if bloody.

Possible Side Effects

▼ Most common: nausea, vomiting, upset stomach, diarrhea, loss of appetite, fever, chills, cough, sensitivity to sunlight, and rash or itching.

▼ Less common: reduced levels of red and white blood cells and platelets, allergic reaction (symptoms include rash, itching, hives, and breathing difficulties), swelling around the eyes, arthritis-like pain, coating of the tongue, headache, tingling in the arms or legs, depression, convulsions, hallucinations, ringing in the ears, dizziness, difficulty sleeping, apathy, tiredness, weakness, and nervousness. Septra may also affect your kidneys and cause you to produce less urine.

Drug Interactions

- Septra may prolong the effects of anticoagulant (blood-thinning) agents—such as warfarin—and oral antidiabetes drugs.
- The trimethoprim in Septra may reduce the effectiveness of cyclosporine and increase its toxic effect on the kidney.
- The sulfamethoxazole in Septra can increase the amount of phenytoin and methotrexate in the bloodstream, increasing the chance of side effects. Dosage reduction of phenytoin or methotrexate may be needed to adjust for the presence of Septra.
- Older adults taking a thiazide diuretic with Septra are more likely to develop reduced levels of blood platelets and an increased chance of bleeding under the skin.
- Caution should be used when combining Septra with angiotensin converting enzyme inhibitors because your potassium levels may be affected. Seniors in particular are prone to dangerously high potassium levels.
- Taking Septra with leucovorin for AIDS-related pneumonia increases the risk of overall treatment failure.
- Septra can interfere with the elimination of zidovudine (AZT) through the kidneys, increasing the amount of AZT in the blood.

Food Interactions

Take each dose with a full glass of water. Continue to drink plenty of fluids throughout the day to decrease the risk of kidney-stone formation.

Usual Dose

Adult: 2 regular tablets or 1 Septra DS tablet every 12 hours for 5–14 days, depending on the condition being treated.

Child (67–88 lbs.): 4 tsp. (or 2 tablets) every 12 hours.

Child (45–66 lbs.): 3 tsp. (or 1½ tablets) every 12 hours.

Child (23–44 lbs.): 2 tsp. (or 1 tablet) every 12 hours.

Child (under 22 lbs.): 1 tsp. every 12 hours.

Child (under age 2 months): not recommended.

Overdosage

Large overdoses can cause exaggerated side effects. Call your local poison control center or emergency room for more information. If you go to the hospital for treatment, ALWAYS bring the prescription bottle or container.

Special Information

Take Septra exactly as prescribed for the full length of the prescription. Do not stop taking it just because you are beginning to feel better.

Call your doctor if you develop a sore throat, rash, unusual bleeding or bruising, or any other persistent or intolerable side effect.

You may develop unusual sensitivity to bright light, particularly sunlight. If you have a history of light sensitivity or if you have sensitive skin, avoid prolonged exposure to sunlight while using Septra.

If you miss a dose of Septra, take it as soon as possible. If you take it twice a day and it is almost time for your next dose, take 1 dose as soon as you remember and another in 5–6 hours, then go back to your regular schedule. If you take Septra 3 or more times a day and it is almost time for your next dose, take 1 dose as soon as you remember and another in 2–4 hours, then continue with your regular schedule. Never take a double dose.

Special Populations

Pregnancy/Breast-feeding: Septra may affect folic acid in the fetus throughout pregnancy and should be used with caution. It should never be taken near term because of the effects of sulfamethoxazole on the newborn, including yellowing of the skin or eyes. Talk to your doctor about Septra's risks versus its benefits if the drug is to be used during pregnancy.

Septra is not recommended for use if you are nursing because of possible effects on the newborn infant.

Seniors: Seniors are more likely to be sensitive to the effects of this drug, especially if they have liver or kidney problems; dosage adjustments may be required.

Seroquel *see **Quetiapine,** page 943*

Generic Name

Sevelamer (seh-VEL-ah-mer)

Brand Names

Renagel (sevelamer hydrochloride)
Renvela (sevelamer carbonate)

Type of Drug

Phosphate binder.

Prescribed For

High blood-phosphate levels in people with end-stage renal disease (ESRD).

General Information

People with ESRD, a form of kidney disease, tend to retain phosphorous. High phosphate levels, in turn, can affect calcium balance in the body and cause deposits of this mineral to build up in the wrong places. Sevelamer hydrochloride helps to reduce phosphate levels by limiting the amount of phosphorous absorbed from food. Sevelamer also lowers levels of total and low-density lipoprotein (LDL) cholesterol.

Cautions and Warnings

Do not take sevelamer if you are **allergic** or **sensitive** to any of its ingredients or you have a **low phosphate level** or a **bowel obstruction**.

Use this drug with caution if you have had **gastrointestinal (GI) surgery** or have **difficulty swallowing** or severe **stomach or intestinal problems**.

Possible Side Effects

▼ Most common: diarrhea, nausea, upset stomach, and vomiting.

▼ Common: abdominal pain, stomach gas, constipation, headache, infection, pain, blood pressure changes, and blood clotting problems.

▼ Less common: back pain, fever, and bowel impaction, obstruction, and perforation.

▼ Rare: Rare side effects can occur in almost any part of the body. Contact your doctor if you experience any side effect not listed above.

Drug Interactions

● Sevelamer may interfere with other drugs taken at the same time. Take sevelamer either 1 hour before or 3 hours after other medications.

● Sevelamer reduces the amount of ciprofloxacin in the blood by half.

● Sevelamer can interfere with the absorption of vitamins D, E, K, and folic acid in the blood.

Food Interactions

Sevelamer should be swallowed whole with meals.

Usual Dose

Renagel

Adult: starting dosage—1–4 capsules with each meal for people not taking a phosphate binder. For people switching from calcium acetate to sevelamer, consult your doctor for correct dosing.

Child: not recommended.

Renvela

Adult: starting dosage—1–2 800-mg tablets 3 times a day. Dose is adjusted every 2 weeks as needed to obtain target phosphorous level. The highest daily dose studied in trials was 17 tablets a day.

Child: not recommended.

Overdosage

Symptoms may include drug side effects. Call your local poison control center or a hospital emergency room for more information.

If you seek treatment, ALWAYS bring the prescription bottle or container.

Special Information

Sevelamer can interfere with the absorption of vitamins from food. Take a supplemental multivitamin while using this drug.

It is important to take sevelamer with each meal. If you forget a dose, skip it and continue to take the drug with subsequent meals.

Do not chew or dismantle the capsules before swallowing them.

Special Populations

Pregnancy/Breast-feeding: In animal studies, sevelamer interfered with fetal bone development. It also interferes with the absorption of vitamins and nutrients, which are essential for a healthy pregnancy. When this drug is considered crucial by your doctor, its potential benefits must be carefully weighed against its risks.

It is not known if sevelamer passes into breast milk. Nursing mothers who must take it should consider using infant formula.

Seniors: Seniors may take this drug without special precaution.

Generic Name

Sibutramine (sih-BYUE-trah-meen)

Brand Name

Meridia

Type of Drug

Appetite suppressant.

Prescribed For

Weight loss.

General Information

Sibutramine works by increasing levels of norepinephrine, serotonin, and dopamine in the brain. By preventing the re-uptake of these chemicals into nerve endings, sibutramine stimulates areas of the brain associated with appetite control. About 6 in 10 people who take sibutramine in conjunction with a diet and exercise program lose 4 lbs. or more during the first 4 weeks of treatment and are likely to lose about 5% of their total body weight in 6–12 months.

Cautions and Warnings

Do not take sibutramine if you are **allergic** or **sensitive** to any of its ingredients.

Sibutramine is a Schedule IV controlled substance. People taking sibutramine may develop drug dependency. As with other weight-loss drugs, sibutramine should not be used by people with eating disorders such as **anorexia** or **bulimia.**

People taking sibutramine may eventually become resistant to the drug, requiring increased dosage to achieve the same effect.

People who have had a **stroke** or who have **heart disease** should not take sibutramine.

People with **narrow-angle glaucoma** should take this drug with caution because it can dilate pupils.

Sibutramine should not be taken by people with severe **liver or kidney disease**.

Sibutramine can raise blood pressure and pulse rate, especially if you already have **high blood pressure**. Check your blood pressure and pulse regularly.

There have been reports of bleeding in people taking sibutramine. Use caution if you have a history of **bleeding disorders.**

Rarely, people taking sibutramine develop a group of symptoms called serotonin syndrome, consisting of one or more of the following symptoms: excitement, a mild manic reaction, restlessness, loss of consciousness, confusion, disorientation, anxiety, agitation, muscle weakness, muscle spasms, tremors, involuntary muscle movements on one side of the body, shivering and dilated pupils, sweating, vomiting, and rapid heartbeat. Serotonin syndrome requires immediate medical treatment.

Other weight loss drugs that act on the nervous system like sibutramine does can cause a rare condition called pulmonary hypertension. This has not been reported with sibutramine.

Rapid weight loss can cause or worsen **gallstones**.

People with a history of **seizures** should use caution when taking sibutramine.

Your doctor should rule out other causes of obesity such as untreated **hypothyroidism** before initiating treatment with sibutramine.

Possible Side Effects

▼ Most common: headache, dry mouth, sleeplessness, appetite loss, constipation, runny nose, and sore throat.

▼ Common: back pain, flu-like symptoms, injuries, weakness, dizziness, nervousness, increased appetite, nausea, joint pain, and sinus irritation.

▼ Less common: abdominal pain, chest pain, neck pain, allergy, rapid heartbeat, flushing, migraine, high blood pressure, heart palpitations, anxiety, depression, tingling in the hands or feet, tiredness, stimulation, emotional instability, rash, sweating, herpes infections, acne, upset stomach, stomach irritation, vomiting, rectal problems, painful menstruation, urinary or vaginal infections, excessive menstrual flow, thirst, swelling, muscle aches, tendon inflammation, joint problems, increased cough, laryngitis, changes in sense of taste, and ear problems.

▼ Rare: seizures, agitation, leg cramps, gas, tooth problems, abnormal thinking, bronchitis, asthma, breathing difficulties, bleeding problems, and kidney problems. Contact your doctor if you experience any side effect not listed above.

Drug Interactions

• Cimetidine, erythromycin, and ketoconazole can mildly increase sibutramine blood levels, but this effect is not considered important.

• Do not drink alcohol to excess while taking sibutramine.

• Do not combine a monoamine oxidase inhibitor (MAOI) or a selective serotonin reuptake inhibitor (SSRI) antidepressant with sibutramine. This combination could lead to serotonin syndrome (see "Cautions and Warnings"). Do not take MAOI drugs within 2 weeks of taking sibutramine.

• Do not combine sibutramine and other weight loss pills that act on the nervous system (usually these are prescription-only diet pills), triptan-type migraine drugs, dihydroergotamine, antidepressants, decongestants, cough medications, lithium, or l-tryptophan.

• Stimulants found in some over-the-counter medications—such as decongestants, weight loss pills, or cough, cold, or allergy drugs—can raise blood pressure or heart rate when combined with sibutramine.

Food Interactions

Sibutramine can be taken with or without food.

Usual Dose

Adult and Child (age 16 and over): 5–15 mg once a day.

Child (under age 16): not recommended.

Overdosage

Little is known about the effects of sibutramine overdose, though symptoms may include rapid heartbeat, high blood pressure, headache, and dizziness. Take the victim to a hospital emergency room. ALWAYS bring the prescription bottle or container.

Special Information

Call your doctor if you develop an allergic reaction such as rash or hives or experience any bothersome or persistent side effect.

This drug can cause an inability to concentrate. Be careful when driving or performing any task that requires concentration or good judgment.

If you forget a dose, take it as soon as you remember. If it is almost time for your next dose, skip the forgotten dose and continue with your regular schedule. Do not take a double dose.

Special Populations

Pregnancy/Breast-feeding: Pregnant women should not take sibutramine under any circumstances. Women of childbearing age should be sure to use effective contraception while taking this medication.

It is not known if sibutramine passes into breast milk. Nursing mothers who must take it should consider using infant formula.

Seniors: Seniors with reduced kidney or liver function should receive the lowest effective dosage.

Generic Name

Sinecatechins Ointment
(sin-eh-CAT-eh-kinz)

Brand Name

Veregen

Type of Drug

Botanical wart remover.

Prescribed For

External genital and perianal warts.

General Information

This drug is a botanical product which is a partially purified fraction of green tea leaves. It is 85–95% catechins and the rest consists of caffeine, theobromine, and undefined botanical ingredients found in green tea leaves. The exact way that sinecatechins ointment works is not known. It is an antioxidant but the importance of that action is not known. In clinical studies of this product, it improved wart clearance by about 20% over that produced by a placebo ointment. It is not known how often warts treated with sinecatechins recur after treatment is completed. If new warts develop during treatment, they should also be treated with the ointment. The effect of this product on spreading genital or perianal warts is not known.

Cautions and Warnings

Do not use sinecatechins ointment if you are **allergic** or **sensitive** to any of its ingredients. Stop using it if you develop an allergic reaction.

This medication has not been studied for use beyond 16 weeks in a row or for more than one treatment.

Do not apply this product inside the vagina, anus, or to the eye or inside the mouth. It may be applied only to the skin.

Avoid using this product on an open wound or upbraided skin.

Sinecatechins ointment has not been proven safe or effective in people whose immune system is not fully functional.

Avoid sun or UV light exposure to skin on which the ointment has been applied.

Possible Side Effects

▼ Most common: redness; raised blistery rash; skin erosion or ulceration; hardening of the skin to which the ointment is applied; swelling, itching, burning, pain, and discomfort at the site of application.

▼ Common: skin peeling.

▼ Less common: lymph node swelling, liquid discharge from the skin, bleeding, tightening of the foreskin (in uncircumcised men), allergic reaction, scarring, irritation, and rash.

Possible Side Effects *(continued)*

▼ Rare: severe pain and inflammation, irritation of the urinary tract, infection around the area of the anus, skin color changes, dryness, eczema, loss of feeling, and other side effects can also occur. Contact your doctor if you experience any side effect not listed above.

Drug Interactions

- Do not apply any other topical medication or skin product to the treatment area while using sinecatechins ointment.

Food Interactions

This drug may be taken without regard to food.

Usual Dose

Adult (age 18 and over): Apply 3 times a day to all warts as directed by your doctor. Do not bandage or wrap the area. Continue using the ointment until all warts have cleared, up to 16 weeks.

Child (under age 18): not recommended.

Overdosage

There have been no reports of sinecatechins overdose. In the event of an accidental overdose, call your local poison center for more information. If you seek treatment, ALWAYS bring the ointment container with you to the hospital emergency room.

Special Information

Wash your hands before and after applying the ointment. You must also wash and dry the skin before you apply the ointment; report severe skin reactions to your doctor. Should the reaction be very severe, you can remove the ointment by washing it off with mild soap and water.

Avoid sexual contact while the ointment is on the skin. If you choose to have sexual contact, wash the ointment off beforehand. Sinecatechins ointment can weaken condoms and diaphragms.

Women using tampons should insert the tampon before applying the ointment to avoid accidentally applying the ointment inside the vagina.

Uncircumcised men treating warts under their foreskin should pull back the foreskin and cleanse the area every day before applying the ointment directly to the warts.

Sinecatechins ointment can stain your clothing and bedding.

Special Populations

Pregnancy/Breast-feeding: This medication did affect some pregnant rabbits but was generally free of birth defects in animal studies. There is no information on how this drug will affect a pregnant woman. When sinecatechins ointment is considered crucial by your doctor, its potential benefits must be carefully weighed against its risks.

It is not known if sinecatechins ointment passes into breast milk. Nursing mothers who must take it should consider using infant formula.

Seniors: Only a small number of seniors have used this ointment. It is not known if there are any differences between seniors and younger adults.

Brand Name

Sinemet

Generic Ingredients

Carbidopa + Levodopa Ⓖ

Other Brand Names

Carbilev   Sinemet CR
Parcopa

The information in this profile also applies to the following drugs:

Generic Ingredient: Carbidopa
Lodosyn

Generic Ingredients: Carbidopa + Levodopa + Entacapone
Stalevo

Type of Drug

Antiparkinsonian.

Prescribed For

Parkinson's disease and Parkinsonism following nervous system damage.

General Information

In Sinemet, levodopa, which increases dopamine, is the active ingredient that affects Parkinson's disease; carbidopa slows the breakdown of levodopa, making more available to the brain, and reducing the side effects from levodopa. Carbidopa is sold under the brand name Lodosyn for people who need individual doses of carbidopa. Entacapone is added to levodopa + carbidopa to help alleviate periods when the levodopa stops working. Other anti-parkinsonian drugs are often prescribed with Sinemet.

Cautions and Warnings

Do not take Sinemet if you are **allergic** or **sensitive** to any of its ingredients.

The sustained-release form of Sinemet has a lesser incidence of nervous system side effects; the immediate-release version may produce such effects even at lower dosages.

Sinemet can make **narrow-angle glaucoma** worse, and can activate **melanoma**, a highly fatal kind of **skin cancer**; patients with suspected melanoma should not take Sinemet.

Patients should be monitored for depression and suicidal thinking.

For more information about Stalevo, see Entacapone, page 414.

Possible Side Effects

▼ Common: uncontrolled muscle movements, appetite loss, nausea, vomiting, stomach pain, dry mouth, difficulty swallowing, drooling, shaky hands, headache, dizziness, numbness, weakness, feeling faint, grinding of the teeth, confusion, sleeplessness, nightmares, hallucinations, anxiety, agitation, tiredness, feeling unwell, and euphoria (feeling "high").

▼ Less common: heart palpitations; chest pain; dizziness when rising quickly from a sitting or lying position; increased sex drive; sudden extreme slowness of movement ("on-off" phenomenon); changes in mental state, including paranoia, psychosis, depression, and a slowdown of mental functioning; difficulty urinating; muscle twitching; eyelid spasms; lockjaw; burning sensation on the tongue; bitter taste; diarrhea; constipation; gas; flushing; rash; sweating; drug allergy (including serious skin reactions); unusual breathing; blurred or double vision; pupil dilation; hot flashes; weight changes; and darkening of urine or sweat.

Possible Side Effects (*continued*)

▼ Rare: Rare side effects can occur in almost any part of the
   body. Contact your doctor if you experience any side effect not listed above.

For more information about Stalevo, see Entacapone, page
414.

Drug Interactions

- Combining Sinemet and a monoamine oxidase inhibitor
  (MAOI) antidepressant may cause a rapid increase in blood
  pressure. MAOIs should be stopped 2 weeks before starting
  on Sinemet. Do not combine these medications.
- Sinemet's effectiveness may be increased by anticholinergic
  drugs such as trihexyphenidyl.
- Methyldopa (an antihypertensive drug) may increase the
  amount of levodopa available in the central nervous system
  and may have a slight effect on Sinemet as well.
- People taking guanethidine or a diuretic to treat high blood
  pressure may need less of either if they start taking Sinemet.
- Reserpine, benzodiazepines, antipsychotic drugs, phenytoin,
  and papaverine may interfere with Sinemet.
- Sinemet may increase the effects of ephedrine, amphetamines, epinephrine, and isoproterenol. This interaction, which
  may also occur with antidepressant drugs, can result in adverse effects on the heart.
- Blood pressure medication, when taken with Sinemet, can
  cause postural problems.
- There are rare reports of high blood pressure and dyskinesia
  with a combination of Sinemet and tricyclic antidepressants.
- Metoclopromide may interfere with the effects of Sinemet.

For more information about Stalevo, see Entacapone, page 414.

Food Interactions

Immediate-release Sinemet may be taken with food to reduce
upset stomach. Sinemet CR, the sustained-release form, should
be taken on an empty stomach.

Usual Dose

Sinemet

Three Sinemet strengths are available: 10/100, 25/100, and 25/250.
The first number represents carbidopa content, the second the

levodopa content, in mg. Dosage must be individualized. Dosage adjustments are made by adding or omitting ½–1 tablet a day. Maximum daily dosage is 8 25/250-tablets. Sinemet CR is started at dosages roughly equal to 10% more levodopa a day than was being taken previously.

If extra carbidopa is needed, your doctor may prescribe Lodosyn to be taken together with Sinemet. Lodosyn is added in steps of no more than 25 mg a day until the desired effect is achieved.

Stalevo

Stalevo (12.5/50/200; 25/100/200; 37.5/150/200): 1 tablet every 3–8 hours, up to 8 tablets a day.

Stalevo (50/200/200): 1 tablet every 3–8 hours, up to 6 tablets a day.

Overdosage

Symptoms include exaggerated side effects. Take the victim to a hospital emergency room. ALWAYS bring the prescription bottle or container.

Special Information

Sinemet can cause tiredness or an inability to concentrate. Be careful when driving or doing any task that requires concentration.

Call your doctor if you experience dizziness; lightheadedness or fainting spells; changes in mood or mental state; abnormal heart rhythm or heart palpitations; difficulty urinating; persistent nausea, vomiting, or other stomach complaints; or uncontrollable movements of the face, eyelids, mouth, tongue, neck, arms, hands, or legs.

When stopping or reducing this drug, fever or hot flashes may be a symptom of a very dangerous condition similar to neuroleptic malignant syndrome. Contact your doctor immediately.

This drug may cause darkening of urine or sweat. This effect is not harmful, but may interfere with urine tests for diabetes. Make sure all your doctors know you are taking this medication.

Take Sinemet exactly as prescribed.

If you forget a dose, take it as soon as you remember. If it is within 2 hours of your next dose, skip the one you forgot and continue with your regular schedule. Do not take a double dose.

Do not cut, crush or chew Sinemet CR or Stalevo tablets.

Special Populations

Pregnancy/Breast-feeding: Both of the ingredients in Sinemet cause birth defects in animals. When this drug is considered crucial by your doctor, its potential benefits must be carefully weighed against its risks.

The ingredients in Sinemet may pass into breast milk and are considered unsafe for infants. Nursing mothers who must take this drug should use infant formula.

Seniors: Seniors may require reduced dosage. They are also more likely to develop abnormal heart rhythms or other cardiac side effects, especially if they have heart disease.

Singulair *see Leukotriene Antagonists/Inhibitors,* page 626

Generic Name

Sitagliptin (sit-ah-GLIP-tin)

Brand Name
Januvia

Type of Drug
DPP-4 inhibitor.

Prescribed For
Type 2 diabetes.

Combination Product
Generic Ingredients: Sitagliptin + Metformin Hydrochloride
Janumet

General Information
Sitagliptin is the first of a series of DPP-4 inhibitors to be approved in the US. These drugs prevent the breakdown of the incretin hormone GLP-1 by the enzyme DPP-4. GLP-1, a part of the body's blood sugar management system, is released in the intestine after a meal, which increases the secretion of insulin and also prevents the release of the hormone glucagon from the pancreas. Glucagon helps the liver maintain enough sugar in the blood to meet the

body's needs between meals. By stopping the breakdown of GLP-1, sitagliptin has clinical effects that are similar to the self-injected drug exenatide (page 457), which directly stimulates GLP-1 receptors in the pancreas to increase insulin and decrease glucagon production.

Sitagliptin has been studied by itself and in combination with metformin and glitazone medicines. It may also improve the efficiency of insulin by increasing insulin sensitivity in the body. Sitagliptin can be expected to reduce A1C levels between ½ and 1%. It is eliminated primarily through the kidneys. This medicine does not affect blood sugar in non-diabetic people. Sitagliptin increases the number of beta cells (that produce insulin) in animals and may have the same effect in humans. This could help reduce the need for other medicines and improve diabetes control.

Cautions and Warnings

Do not take this medicine if you are **sensitive or allergic** to it.

This drug should be used with caution in people with **kidney disease**, and a lower dosage may be prescribed. People with severe kidney disease should not take this drug. Sitagliptin should not be taken by people with **type 1 diabetes** because it will not help them.

Taking metformin can rarely lead to a condition known as lactic acidosis. Symptoms of lactic acidosis can include feeling ill, muscle aches, difficulty breathing, becoming increasingly tired, and pain or discomfort in your abdomen. Report any of these symptoms to your doctor at once.

Possible Side Effects

The overall risk of side effects with sitagliptin is very low.
▼ Most common: upper respiratory infection, common cold symptoms, and headache.
▼ Less common: abdominal pain, nausea, and diarrhea.
For more information about Janumet, see Metformin, page 696.

Drug Interactions

- If taken with the sulfonylurea drugs or insulin injections, sitagliptin may cause very low blood sugar.

- Sitagliptin causes a slight increase in the amount of digoxin absorbed into the system, but no dose adjustment is needed.

Food Interactions

This drug may be taken with or without food or meals.

Usual Dose

Januvia
> **Adult:** 100 mg once daily.
> **Child:** not recommended.

Janumet
> **Adult:** 50/500–50/1000 mg twice a day.
> **Child:** not recommended.

Overdosage

Clinical studies of sitagliptin used doses up to 800 mg. At these doses there were some effects on the cardiogram. Overdose victims should be taken to a hospital emergency room for treatment. ALWAYS bring the prescription bottle or container.

Special Information

If you forget a dose, take it as soon as you remember. If it is almost time for the next dose, skip the one you forgot and continue with your regular schedule. Do not take a double dose.

Call your doctor at once if you suddenly begin to feel ill, have muscle aches, difficulty breathing, become increasingly tired, or have pain or discomfort in your abdomen while taking Janumet. These could be signs of a condition called lactic acidosis.

Special Populations

Pregnancy/Breast-feeding: Animal studies using high doses of sitagliptin have shown it can cause some fetal malformations. Pregnant women should take this drug only if its potential benefits outweigh the possible risks.

It is not known if sitagliptin passes into breast milk. Because many drugs do pass into breast milk, nursing mothers should consider using infant formula.

Seniors: Seniors may require less sitagliptin to produce the desired effect because of reduced kidney function.

Skelaxin   see *Metaxalone, page 694*

Generic Name

Sodium Oxybate (so-DEE-um OX-ee-bate)

Brand Name
Xyrem

Type of Drug
Central-nervous-system (CNS) depressant.

Prescribed For
Narcolepsy, cataplexy, and fibromyalgia.

General Information
Sodium oxybate, also known as GHB, is a CNS depressant that reduces daytime sleepiness in people with narcolepsy, a condition in which people suddenly fall asleep without warning. People can stay asleep for anywhere from a few seconds to a few hours, and may continue to function as if they were completely awake and aware but later have no memory of the event. Some narcoleptic people also have attacks of cataplexy, in which they suddenly lose all muscle tone and strength. Cataplexy symptoms last for up to 30 minutes and can range from minor sagging of the facial muscles to dropping of the jaw or head, weak knees, or a total collapse. Speech is slurred, and double vision and inability to focus the eyes may occur, however hearing and awareness are unaffected. Cataplexy is often triggered by strong emotions including exhilaration, anger, fear, surprise, awe, embarrassment, laughter, or orgasm and is often confused with epilepsy. Sodium oxybate has also been used to treat fibromyalgia. This drug is available through a centralized pharmacy, and is distributed only to legitimate patients. Ninety five percent of this drug is broken down in the body to form carbon dioxide, which is then passed out through the lungs. The rest passes out of the body in the urine.

Cautions and Warnings
Do not take this drug if you are **allergic** or **sensitive** to it.

People with a rare genetic disease known as **SSD Deficiency** cannot take this drug.

Sodium oxybate (GHB) is a known drug of abuse and has been associated with important CNS side events. Prescribed sodium oxybate doses are much lower than those used by drug abusers.

Confusion, depression, breathing difficulty, and loss of consciousness can occur even at recommended doses.

People with **respiratory illnesses**, including **sleep apnea**, should use this drug with caution. Loss of consciousness in drug abusers taking GHB has lead to coma or death.

People with **liver disease** should take only ½ the usual dose of sodium oxybate. Some patients taking larger doses of sodium oxybate can experience nighttime urinary incontinence (bed wetting). Sleepwalking or confused nighttime behavior can occur.

This drug has large amounts of sodium. People with **heart failure, high blood pressure,** or **kidney disease** should avoid salt in their diet.

Possible Side Effects

Side effects increase noticeably as the drug dose increases.
▼ Most common: headache, nausea, and dizziness.
▼ Common: vomiting, tiredness, inflamed throat and nasal passages, throat pain, sleepiness, lethargy, weakness, loss of urinary control, ringing or buzzing in the ears, blurred vision, gastrointestinal (GI) pains, diarrhea, upset stomach, stomach virus, respiratory infections, increased blood pressure, back pain, reduced sense of touch, sleep paralysis, confusion, sleep disorders, and sleep walking.
▼ Less common: sweating, difficulty focusing or paying attention, depression, and nightmares.
▼ Rare: Other side effects can affect virtually every body system. Contact your doctor if you experience any side effect not listed above.

Drug Interactions

- Sodium oxybate should not be mixed with any other CNS depressant, including a sedative or hypnotic. Do not drink alcoholic beverages.
- Sodium oxybate may be mixed with other drugs often taken by people with narcolepsy, including zolpidem, protriptyline, and modafinil.

Food Interactions

Sodium oxybate must be taken on empty stomach, at least 2 hours after eating.

Usual Dose

Adult and Child (age 16 and over): 2.25 g at bedtime and again 2½–4 hours later to start. Your daily dose can be increased to 4.5 g in each of the doses. Most people require 6–9 g a day. People with liver disease should take half the regular dose.

Child (under age 16): not recommended.

Overdosage

Two overdoses were reported in clinical studies. Symptoms include drug side effects such as loss of consciousness, loss of urinary and stool control, blurred vision, seizures, and others. One patient died from an overdose of sodium oxybate with alcohol and other drugs. Sodium oxybate overdose victims are intoxicated and can injure themselves or pass out. In the past, people taking 18–250 g of GHB per day have become addicted to GHB. These people experienced withdrawal symptoms for several days to 2 weeks after abruptly stopping GHB. Overdose victims should be taken to a hospital emergency room at once for treatment. ALWAYS bring the prescription bottle or container with you.

Special Information

Sodium oxybate solution contains 2.5 g per 5ml. Each evening, measure both doses of sodium oxybate for the night using the oral syringe in the package and place them into the two dosing cups supplied in the package. Dilute each dose with 2 oz. of water. Set your alarm clock to wake up from 2½–4 hours after the first dose. Then, take your first dose while sitting in bed. When your alarm wakes you, take the second dose also while you are sitting in bed. Mixed solutions should be used on the same night.

Avoid any activity that requires coordination and alertness for at least 6 hours after you take this medication. Be aware that it can also affect your alertness and coordination during the day. Be careful until you know how it affects you.

Depression, psychosis, paranoia, hallucinations, agitation, or abnormal behavior or thinking should be reported to your doctor as soon as possible. They can be psychiatric side effects of sodium oxybate.

Do not allow children or pets access to your medication.

Special Populations

Pregnancy/Breast-feeding: Animal studies of sodium oxybate have found no effects on the developing fetus. However, there are no sodium oxybate studies in pregnant women. Pregnant women should discuss the risks and benefits of taking this drug with their doctor and only use it if absolutely necessary.

It is not known if this drug passes into breast milk. Nursing mothers should be cautious when taking sodium oxybate.

Seniors: This drug has not been studied in seniors.

Spiriva   *see Ipratropium, page 597*

Type of Drug

Statin Cholesterol-Lowering Agents

Brand Names

Generic Ingredient: Atorvastatin Calcium
Lipitor

Generic Ingredients: Atorvastatin Calcium + Amlodipine Besylate
Caduet

Generic Ingredient: Fluvastatin Sodium
Lescol   Lescol XL

Generic Ingredient: Lovastatin [G]
Altoprev   Mevacor

Generic Ingredients: Lovastatin + Niacin
Advicor

Generic Ingredient: Pravastatin Sodium [G]
Pravachol

Generic Ingredient: Rosuvastatin Calcium [G]
Crestor

Generic Ingredient: Simvastatin [G]
Zocor

Generic Ingredients: Simvastatin + Ezetimibe
Vytorin

Prescribed For

High blood levels of cholesterol, low-density lipoprotein (LDL) cholesterol, and triglycerides; also prescribed for atherosclerosis (hardening of the arteries), diabetes-related blood-fat problems, preventing heart attacks and strokes, and reducing the risk of cardiac bypass surgery. Some of these drugs may also be used for blood-fat disorders related to kidney disease and inherited blood-fat problems.

General Information

High blood-fat levels are believed to play a role in the development of cardiovascular disease. Statin drugs help to lower blood-fat levels by blocking the effects of the enzyme HMG-CoA reductase, which in turn interferes with the production of cholesterol in the body. They also increase levels of high-density lipoprotein (HDL) cholesterol, the "good" cholesterol considered to have a beneficial effect on heart health. Statin drugs are proven to slow the progression of atherosclerosis, help prevent heart attacks, and reduce the risk of dying from heart disease. Other related benefits have been discovered. Atorvastatin, for example, has been found to improve the ability of people with intermittent claudication (a blood-vessel disease) to walk. Advicor combines lovastatin with niacin, a nutrient that helps raise levels of "good" cholesterol. Vytorin combines 2 cholesterol drugs for further effectiveness. Caduet is another combination product used for heart attack prevention.

These drugs begin working quickly. Blood-fat levels are significantly improved after 1–2 weeks of treatment. Maximum effect occurs in 4–6 weeks, persists for the remainder of drug therapy, and continues for 4–6 weeks after you stop taking these drugs. These drugs are generally not recommended for people under age 30, although they may be prescribed for teenagers under certain circumstances. Only a small amount of these drugs enter the bloodstream. They are largely broken down in the liver.

Cautions and Warnings

Do not take statins if you are **allergic** or **sensitive** to any of their ingredients. It is possible to be allergic to one of these drugs and tolerate another.

People with a history of **liver disease** and those who drink large amounts of **alcohol** should avoid these drugs because they may aggravate or cause liver disease. About 1 in 100 people who take these drugs develops high liver-enzyme counts; the risk of this effect is highest with lovastatin and lowest with atorvastatin.

Your doctor should take a blood sample to test your liver function before you begin a statin drug and every month or so during the first year of treatment.

People taking these drugs may develop severe muscle aches or weakness, which can be a sign of a more serious condition. This is usually a rare problem but is more common at higher drug doses.

People with **kidney disease** who take pravastatin, rosuvastatin, or simvastatin must be closely monitored by their doctors.

People in early studies of lovastatin developed cloudy vision due to an effect on the lens of the eye, but this effect has not been seen in further studies. Statins have also been reported to cause degeneration of the optic nerve and cataracts at doses 30–60 times the average dose. Report any changes in vision to your doctor.

Possible Side Effects

Side effects are usually mild and temporary. Rare side effects associated with these drugs can occur in almost any part of the body. Contact your doctor if you experience any side effect not listed below.

Atorvastatin
▼ Most common: headache, diarrhea, joint pain, sinusitis, infection, and flu-like symptoms.
▼ Common: muscle aches and weakness.
▼ Less common: gas, upset stomach, itching, rash, and allergy.

Atorvastin + Amlodipine
See Amlodipine, page 65, for additional side effects.

Fluvastatin
▼ Most common: upper-respiratory infection, headache, upset stomach, and diarrhea.
▼ Common: muscle aches, abdominal pain or cramps, changes in sense of taste, flu-like symptoms, allergy, and back pain.
▼ Less common: dizziness, sleeplessness, nausea, vomiting, constipation, gas, tooth problems, arthritis, joint pain,

Possible Side Effects (continued)

runny nose, cough, sore throat, sinus irritation, itching, rash, and fatigue.

Lovastatin
▼ Common: stomach pain, cramps, gas, constipation, diarrhea, and headache.
▼ Less common: dizziness, heartburn, upset stomach, itching, rash, allergy, infection, nausea, vomiting, muscle aches or pain, joint pain, blurred vision, and eye irritation.

Lovastatin + Niacin
▼ Most common: flushing, which may occur within 2 hours of the first dose.
▼ Common: stomach pain, cramps, gas, and constipation.
▼ Less common: headache, dizziness, heartburn, upset stomach, itching, rash, allergy, infection, nausea, vomiting, diarrhea, muscle aches or pain, joint pain, blurred vision, eye irritation, decreased sugar tolerance in diabetics, stomach ulcer activation, jaundice (yellowing of the skin or eyes), oily or dry skin, aggravation of skin conditions such as acne, low blood pressure, tingling in the hands or feet, and abnormal heartbeat.

Pravastatin
▼ Most common: localized pain.
▼ Common: headache, nausea, vomiting, diarrhea, abdominal pain or cramps, and common cold symptoms.
▼ Less common: dizziness, constipation, heartburn, upset stomach, muscle aches, cough, runny nose, chest pain, itching, rash, flu-like symptoms, fatigue, and urinary difficulties.

Rosuvastatin
▼ Common: sore throat and headache.
▼ Less common: diarrhea, upset stomach, stomach pain, muscle aches, constipation, nausea, back pain, flu-like symptoms, weakness, accidental injury, chest pain, infection, pain, high blood pressure, swelling in the arms or legs, arthritis, joint pains, dizziness, sleeplessness, depression,

Possible Side Effects (*continued*)

tingling in the hands or feet, extreme muscle tension, coughing, bronchitis, and rash.

Simvastatin
▼ Less common: headache, weakness, nausea, vomiting, diarrhea, abdominal pain or cramps, constipation, gas, upset stomach, and respiratory infection.

Simvastatin and Ezetimibe
See Ezetimibe, page 460, for additional side effects.

Drug Interactions

- Antioxidant supplements, including vitamins E and C and beta carotene, may reverse the effects of statin drugs. These combinations should be avoided.
- Drinking alcohol regularly increases the amount of fluvastatin in the blood by 30%.
- Antacids reduce statin blood levels, although their actual cholesterol-lowering may not change. Separate doses of these drugs by at least 1 hour.
- Itraconazole, ketoconazole, clarithromycin, erythromycin, and protease inhibitors (indinavir, nelfinavir, ritonavir, saquinavir) can dramatically increase statin levels in the blood. Your doctor should reduce your statin dose while you are taking these drugs.
- Other drugs that interfere with the breakdown of statin drugs (except pravastatin) are danazol, delavirdine, amiodarone, cyclosporine, niacin, verapamil, gemfibrozil, fenofibrate, ciprofloxacin, diltiazem, fluconazole, fluvoxamine, mifepristone, nefazodone, norfloxacin, mibefradil, and telithromycin.
- Cimetidine, ranitidine, and omeprazole may increase the effects of fluvastatin.
- Adding glyburide to fluvastatin can affect the effects of both glyburide and fluvastatin.
- Carbamazepine, phenobarbital, phenytoin, pioglitazone, rosiglitazone, and rifampin may reduce statin drug blood levels by stimulating the liver to break it down faster than normal.
- The cholesterol-lowering effects of these drugs and cholestyramine are additive. Take a statin drug 1 hour before or 4 hours after cholestyramine. Colestipol reduces atorvastatin blood

levels, but this combination more effectively lowers blood-fat levels than either drug used alone.

- Digoxin can reduce fluvastatin blood levels. Statin drugs can increase the amount of digoxin in the blood by about 20%.
- Isradipine may speed the elimination of lovastatin from the body.
- Statins increase blood levels of estrogens and progestins in contraceptive drugs, which can lead to side effects. If you must take both drugs, talk to your doctor about switching to a lower dose hormonal contraceptive.
- These drugs may increase the effects of warfarin. People taking these drugs together should be periodically examined by their doctors. Warfarin dosage adjustment may be necessary.
- Propranolol can reduce the effectiveness of these drugs.
- St. John's wort may reduce the effectiveness of statins.

See Amlodipine, page 65, for further drug interactions for Caduet; see Ezetimibe, page 460, for further drug interactions for Vytorin.

Food Interactions

Grapefruit juice can slow the breakdown of statin drugs (except pravastatin) in the liver, increasing the risk of drug side effects. Lovastatin must be taken with meals. Other statin drugs may be taken with or without food.

Usual Dose

Atorvastatin
Adult: 10–80 mg a day.
Senior: 10–20 mg a day.
Child: not recommended.

Atorvastatin + Amlodipine
Adult: 2.5/10–10/80 mg a day.
Senior: Start on 2.5/10 mg a day.
Child (age 6–17): 2.5/10–5/20 mg a day.
Child (under age 6): not recommended.

Fluvastatin
Adult: 20–80 mg a day, taken in the evening.
Child: not recommended.

Lovastatin
Adult: 10–80 mg a day, usually taken with your evening meal.
Child: not recommended.

Lovastatin + Niacin
   Adult: 1 tablet, taken at bedtime.
   Child: not recommended.

Pravastatin
   Adult: 10–40 mg, taken at bedtime.
   Senior: 10–20 mg, taken at bedtime.
   Child: not recommended.

Rosuvastatin
   Adult: 5–20 mg a day. Dosage may be increased to a maximum of 40 mg a day.
   Child: not recommended.

Simvastatin
   Adults: 5–80 mg, taken in the evening.
   Senior: 5–20 mg, taken in the evening.
   Child: not recommended.

Simvastatin + Ezetimibe
   Adult: 10/10 mg–10/80 mg a day.
   Child: not recommended.

Overdosage

People taking overdoses of these drugs have experienced no specific symptoms and have recovered without a problem after the drug was removed by making them vomit. Overdose victims should be taken to a hospital emergency room for evaluation and treatment. ALWAYS bring the prescription bottle or container.

Special Information

Call your doctor if you develop blurred vision or muscle aches, pain, tenderness, or weakness, especially if you are also feverish or do not feel well.

Statin drugs are prescribed in combination with a low-fat diet. Following your doctor's dietary instructions will help reduce your blood fats and keep them low. Do not take more cholesterol-lowering medication than your doctor has prescribed. Do not stop taking it without your doctor's knowledge.

These drugs may cause increased sensitivity to the sun. Use sunscreen and wear protective clothing.

If you forget a dose, take it as soon as you remember. If it is almost time for your next dose, skip the one you forgot and continue with your regular schedule. Do not take a double dose.

Special Populations

Pregnancy/Breast-feeding: Pregnant women and those who might become pregnant must not take any of these drugs.

These drugs may pass into breast milk. Nursing mothers who must take them should use infant formula.

Seniors: Seniors are more sensitive to the effects of some statin drugs and may require reduced dosage.

Strattera *see **Atomexetine**, page 125*

Generic Name

Sucralfate (sue-KRAL-fate) Ⓖ

Brand Name
Carafate

Type of Drug
Antiulcer.

Prescribed For
Short-term (less than 8-week) treatment and maintenance therapy of duodenal (intestinal) ulcer. Also used for stomach ulcer, irritation, and bleeding; gastroesophageal reflux disease (GERD); irritation of the esophagus and mouth; throat ulcer; and prevention of stress ulcer and stomach bleeding.

General Information
Sucralfate works within the gastrointestinal (GI) tract by exerting a soothing local effect on ulcer tissue; very little of the drug is absorbed into the bloodstream. After the drug binds to proteins in the damaged mucous tissue within the ulcer, it forms a barrier to the normal acids and enzymes of the GI tract. This barrier protects ulcer tissue from further damage, allowing it to heal naturally. Sucralfate is not an antacid and works differently than cimetidine, omeprazole, and other antiulcer drugs, but it is as effective in treating duodenal ulcer disease as these drugs.

Cautions and Warnings

Do not take sucralfate if you are **allergic** or **sensitive** to any of its ingredients.

Small amounts of aluminum are absorbed while you take sucralfate. This can be a problem for people with chronic **kidney failure** and for those on **dialysis**.

Possible Side Effects

Side effects are usually minimal.
▼ Most common: constipation.
▼ Less common: diarrhea, nausea, upset stomach, indigestion, dry mouth, rash, itching, back pain, dizziness, and sleepiness.

Drug Interactions

- Sucralfate may interfere with the absorption of cimetidine, digoxin, diclofenac, levothyroxine, ketoconazole, phenytoin, quinidine, ranitidine, tetracycline, theophylline, warfarin, ciprofloxacin, norfloxacin, ofloxacin, and quinolone antibacterials. Separate these drugs and sucralfate by at least 2 hours to avoid this effect.
- Do not take antacids 30 minutes before or after taking sucralfate.
- Do not take aluminum-containing antacids at all while you are taking sucralfate. This combination increases aluminum absorption into the bloodstream and may lead to aluminum poisoning.

Food Interactions

Take each dose on an empty stomach, at least 1 hour before or 2 hours after meals.

Usual Dose

Adult: starting dosage—1 g 4 times a day for active ulcers. Maintenance dosage (tablets only)—1 tablet twice a day.
Child: not recommended.

Overdosage

Little is known about the effects of sucralfate overdose, although the risk associated with it is thought to be minimal. Call your local poison control center or a hospital emergency room for more information. If you seek treatment, ALWAYS bring the prescription bottle or container.

Special Information

Complete the full course of drug therapy.

Notify your doctor if you develop constipation, diarrhea, or other GI side effects.

If you forget a dose, take it as soon as you remember. If it is almost time for your next dose, skip the one you forgot and continue with your regular schedule. Do not take a double dose.

Special Populations

Pregnancy/Breast-feeding: While animal studies of sucralfate reveal no damage to the fetus, this drug should only be used during pregnancy after carefully weighing its potential benefits against its risks.

It is not known if sucralfate passes into breast milk. Nursing mothers who must take it should consider using infant formula.

Seniors: Seniors should take the lowest effective dose.

Type of Drug

Sulfa Drugs

Brand Names

Generic Ingredient: Sulfadiazine Ⓖ

Generic Ingredient: Sulfasalazine Ⓖ
Azulfidine   Azulfidine EN-Tabs

Generic Ingredient: Sulfisoxazole Ⓖ

Generic Ingredient: Sulfisoxazole Acetyl
Gantrisin Pediatric

Combination Product
Generic Ingredients: Sulfadoxine + Pyrimethamine
Fansidar

Prescribed For

Urinary and other infections; may also be prescribed for rheumatoid, juvenile, and psoriatic arthritis; ulcerative and other forms of colitis; Crohn's disease; ankylosing spondylitis; and psoriasis. Sulfisoxazole has also been used to prevent middle ear infection.

Fansidar (sufladoxine + pyrimethamine) is prescribed for the treatment and prevention of malaria.

General Information

In use for many years, sulfa drugs are prescribed for infections in various parts of the body but are particularly helpful for urinary tract infections. They kill bacteria and some fungi by interfering with the metabolic processes of these organisms. Some organisms may become resistant to the effects of sulfa drugs.

Sulfasalazine is different from the other sulfa drugs in that only about ⅓ of it is absorbed into the bloodstream; the rest remains in the intestines. Because of its specific anti-inflammatory and immune system effects, sulfasalazine is effective against colitis, intestinal irritation, and arthritis and other inflammatory conditions.

Cautions and Warnings

Do not take sulfa drugs if you are **allergic** or **sensitive** to any of their ingredients or to any drug chemically related to the sulfa drugs, including thiazide and loop diuretics, carbonic anhydrase inhibitors, and sulfonylurea-type oral antidiabetes drugs—which do not include metformin.

Do not use any sulfa drug if you are allergic to **aspirin, PABA-containing sunscreens, local anesthetics**, or if you have **porphyria**.

Fansidar has been associated with fatal rash and skin tissue decay. Stop taking this medication if you develop a skin rash or bacterial or fungal infection.

Sulfa drugs can cause increased sensitivity to the sun or bright light. Use sunscreen and wear protective clothing.

Sulfa drugs should be taken by people with severe **kidney or liver disease** only after a doctor has evaluated their condition and need for the drug.

Sulfasalazine should not be used by people with **intestinal or urinary obstruction** or by **children under age 2**.

Sulfa drugs should be used with caution in people with **severe allergies** or **bronchial asthma.**

Men taking sulfasalazine may have low sperm count or become infertile. This effect reverses when the drug is stopped.

Deaths in people taking sulfasalazine and sulfadiazine have been related to a variety of effects on the blood, liver damage, and nervous system changes. Deaths in people taking fansidar have occurred due to toxic skin reactions. Call your doctor if a rash or anything unusual develops while taking a sulfa drug.

Possible Side Effects

▼ Most common: headache, itching, rash, skin sensitivity to strong sunlight, nausea, vomiting, abdominal or stomach cramps or pain, feeling unwell, hallucinations, diarrhea, dizziness, ringing or buzzing in the ears, and chills.

▼ Less common: blood diseases or changes in blood composition, arthritic pain, appetite loss, drowsiness, hearing loss, itchy eyes, fever, hair loss, and yellowing of the skin or whites of the eyes. Sulfasalazine may reduce sperm count.

Drug Interactions

- Sulfa drugs may increase the effects of sulfonylurea-type oral antidiabetes drugs, methotrexate, warfarin and other anticoagulant drugs, and phenytoin and other hydantoin anti-seizure drugs. Dosages of these drugs may have to be reduced by your doctor.
- Cyclosporine blood levels may be reduced by sulfa drugs, possibly increasing kidney toxicity.
- Sulfa drugs may increase blood levels of indomethacin, probenecid, and aspirin and other salicylates, increasing the risks of side effects.
- When methenamine and a sulfa drug are taken together, an insoluble substance may form in acid urine. Avoid this combination.
- Erythromycin increases the effect of sulfa drugs against infections caused by *Haemophilus influenzae,* a common cause of middle ear infections.
- Do not take anti-folic drugs (eg, sulfonamides or trimethoprim-sulfamethoxazole) with Fansidar for malaria prevention.
- The effects of folic acid and digoxin may be diminished by sulfasalazine; dosage increases may be needed.
- Sulfa drugs may increase the effects of barbiturate anesthetics.
- Combining diuretics and sulfa drugs may lead to a decrease in blood platelets.

Food Interactions

Sulfa drugs should be taken on an empty stomach with a full glass of water. Sulfasalazine and Fansidar may be taken with food if they upset your stomach.

Usual Dose
Sulfadiazine
Adult: 2–4 g a day.

Child (age 2 months and over): 34–68 mg per lb. of body weight a day.

Child (under age 2 months): not recommended, except to treat certain infections present at birth. In these cases, dosage is 11.3 mg per lb. of body weight, 4 times a day.

Fansidar (Sulfadoxine + Pyrimethamine)
Adult: 2–3 tablets for an acute attack of malaria; for prevention, first dose prior to departure, then 1–2 tablets every week or every other week.

Child: ½–2 tablets for an acute attack of malaria; for prevention, first dose prior to departure, then ¼–1½ tablets every week or every other week.

Sulfasalazine
Adult: 1–4 g a day in evenly divided doses.

Child (age 2 and over): 18–27 mg per lb. of body weight a day, in evenly divided doses.

Child (under age 2): not recommended.

Sulfisoxazole
Adult: 4–8 g a day, in 4–6 divided doses.

Child (age 2 months and over): 34–68 mg per lb. of body weight a day, in 4–6 divided doses.

Overdosage
Symptoms include appetite loss, nausea, vomiting and colic, dizziness, headache, drowsiness, unconsciousness, high fever, severe bleeding or bruising, and irritation or soreness of the tongue. Take the victim to a hospital emergency room at once. ALWAYS take the prescription bottle or container.

Special Information
Sulfa drugs often cause increased sensitivity to the sun. Use sunscreen or wear protective clothing.

Sore throat, fever, chills, unusual bleeding or bruising, rash, and drowsiness are signs of serious blood disorders and should be reported to your doctor at once. Also contact your doctor if you experience ringing in the ears, blood in the urine, or breathing difficulties.

Be sure to take the full course of medication as prescribed, even if you notice an improvement in your symptoms.

Sulfasalazine may turn your urine orange-yellow. This is a harmless reaction. Skin discoloration has also occurred. This drug may permanently stain soft contact lenses.

Maintain adequate fluid intake to reduce the chance of kidney stone formation when taking sulfasalazine.

Sulfa drugs may interfere with some tests for sugar in the urine.

If you forget a dose, take it as soon as you remember. If you take the drug twice a day and it is almost time for your next dose, take 1 dose right away, another after 5–6 hours, and then go back to your regular schedule. If you take the drug 3 or more times a day and it is almost time for your next dose, take 1 dose right away, another after 2–4 hours, and then go back to your regular schedule. Never take a double dose.

Special Populations

Pregnancy/Breast-feeding: Sulfa drugs pass into the fetal circulation and may affect the fetus. Malformations have been seen in animal studies. Sulfa drugs are not recommended during pregnancy. When a sulfa drug is considered crucial by your doctor, its potential benefits must be carefully weighed against its risks.

Small amounts of sulfa drugs pass into breast milk. Nursing mothers who must take them should consider using infant formula, especially if their babies are premature, deficient in the enzyme G-6-PD, or have hyperbilirubinemia (condition in which there is too much bilirubin in the blood). Mothers taking sulfadoxine should not breast-feed.

Seniors: Seniors with kidney or liver problems should take sulfa drugs with caution.

Type of Drug

Sulfonylurea Antidiabetes Drugs

Brand Names

Generic Ingredient: Acetohexamide Ⓖ

Generic Ingredient: Chlorpropamide Ⓖ
Diabinese

Generic Ingredient: Glimepiride
Amaryl

Generic Ingredient: Glipizide Ⓖ

Glucotrol   Glucotrol XL

Generic Ingredient: Glyburide Ⓖ

DiaBeta   Micronase
Glynase

Generic Ingredient: Tolazamide Ⓖ

Tolinase

Generic Ingredient: Tolbutamide Ⓖ

Combination Products

Generic Ingredients: Glipizide + Metformin

Metaglip

Generic Ingredients: Glyburide + Metformin

Glucovance

Prescribed For

Type 2 diabetes mellitus. Chlorpropamide may also be used to treat diabetes insipidus (a hormonal condition unrelated to blood sugar).

General Information

The sulfonylureas stimulate the production and release of insulin from the pancreas. Some also help muscle and other cells to use glucose. They will not work in type 1 diabetes, as they do not lower blood sugar directly but require some functioning pancreas cells. These drugs differ from each other in how long they take to start working, the duration of their effectiveness, and the amount of each required to produce a roughly equivalent antidiabetic effect.

Glucovance and Metaglip consist of a sulfonylurea combined with metformin. Metformin lowers the amount of glucose produced by the liver, reduces the amount of glucose you absorb from food, and helps cells use glucose. Metformin can also moderately lower body fats.

These drugs may be used alone or in combination with other antidiabetes drugs to control your blood sugar.

Cautions and Warnings

Do not take a sulfonylurea if you are **allergic** or **sensitive** to any of its ingredients.

Infection, surgery, injury, or **emotional upset** reduce the effectiveness of these drugs. If you are having surgery or an X-ray that requires the injection of an iodine-based contract material, you should temporarily stop taking Glucovance or Metaglip because the combination could result in acute kidney problems. You must be under your doctor's continuous care while taking any of these drugs.

These drugs are not a form of oral insulin or a substitute for insulin. The pancreas must be functioning for them to work.

Studies conducted in the 1960s and the 1990s found that people taking sulfonylureas may be more likely to have fatal heart trouble than those whose diabetes is controlled with diet and/or other medications.

These drugs can cause low blood sugar (see "Overdosage") that may require medical attention.

These drugs should be used with caution if you have serious **liver, kidney, or endocrine disease;** monitor your blood sugar very closely.

Do not use Glucovance or Metaglip if you have **heart failure** or **liver or kidney disease**. These conditions increase the risk for lactic acidosis, a rare, potentially fatal condition that can occur with metformin treatment.

People with acidosis, including those with diabetic ketoacidosis, should not take Glucovance or Metaglip.

Possible Side Effects

▼ Most common: low blood sugar (see "Overdosage" for symptoms), loss of appetite, nausea, vomiting, stomach upset, and weakness or tingling in the hands and feet.

▼ Less common: sensitivity to sunlight, itching, dizziness, and headache.

▼ Rare: yellowing of the skin or whites of the eyes, itching, and rash. Usually these reactions will disappear in time. If they persist, contact your doctor. Contact your doctor if you experience any side effect not listed above.

For additional side effects of Glucovance and Metaglip, see Metformin, page 696.

Drug Interactions

● The following drugs may increase your need for sulfonylureas: beta blockers, calcium channel blockers, cholestyramine, contraceptive drugs, corticosteroids, diazoxide, estrogens, isoniazid, nicotinic acid, phenothiazines, phenytoin and other hydantoin drugs, rifampin, stimulants, thiazide diuretics, thyroid replacement drugs, charcoal tablets, and anything that makes your urine less acidic.

- The following drugs may decrease your need for sulfonylureas and some of these drugs can cause drastic drops in blood sugar levels: androgens (male hormones), anticoagulants, aspirin and other salicylates, bishydroxycoumarin, chloramphenicol, cimetidine, clarithromycin, clofibrate, dicumarol, famotidine, fenfluramine, fluconazole, gemfibrozil, itraconazole, ketoconazole, ranitidine, magnesium-containing products, methyldopa, miconazole, monoamine oxidase inhibitor antidepressants, nizatidine, oxyphenbutazone, phenylbutazone, probenecid, warfarin, phenyramidol, sulfa drugs, sulfinpyrazone, tricyclic antidepressants, large doses of vitamin C, and citrus fruits and other foods that make your urine more acidic.

- Mixing these drugs with alcohol can cause flushing and breathing difficulties. Other possible effects are throbbing pain in the head and neck, nausea, vomiting, increased sweating, excessive thirst, chest pains, palpitations, lowered blood pressure, weakness, dizziness, blurred vision, and confusion. Alcohol also increases the risk of lactic acidosis while taking Glucovance or Metaglip. If you experience any of these reactions, contact your doctor immediately.

- Combining a fluoroquinolone antibiotic, such as ciprofloxacin or gatifloxacin, with glyburide can increase its blood-sugar-lowering effect.

- Chlorpropamide may increase the effects of barbiturates.

- Glyburide may alter the effectiveness of oral anticoagulant (blood-thinning) drugs. Dosage may have to be adjusted by your doctor.

- These drugs may increase the effects of digitalis drugs.

- The stimulants in many over-the-counter cough, cold, and allergy remedies may affect your blood sugar; avoid them unless your doctor advises otherwise.

For additional drug interactions for Glucovance and Metaglip, see Metformin, page 696.

Food Interactions

All the sulfonylureas except glipizide may be taken with food. Glipizide should be taken 30 minutes before a meal for best results.

To minimize stomach problems, you should take Glucovance and Metaglip with food.

Usual Dose

Child: None of the sulfonylureas are recommended for children.

Acetohexamide
   Adult: 250–1500 mg a day.

Chlorpropamide
   Adult: starting dose—100–250 mg a day; maintenance dose—100–250 mg a day; rarely, 750 mg a day may be prescribed.

Glimepiride: 1–8 mg once a day.

Glipizide
   Adult: 5–20 mg once a day for extended release tablets; 5–40 mg a day in single or divided doses for immediate release tablets.
   Senior: start with 2.5 mg a day.

Glucovance
   Adult: 1.25/250 mg–20/2000 mg once or twice a day.

Glyburide
   DiaBeta/Micronase
      Adult: 2.5–20 mg a day, usually with a meal.
      Seniors: start with 1.25 mg a day.

   Glynase
      Adult: 1.5–12 mg a day, usually with breakfast or the first main meal.
      Seniors: start with 0.75 mg a day.
   Glynase is not equivalent to DiaBeta or Micronase and may not be substituted for either of them.

Metaglip: 2.5 mg/250 mg–10 mg/2000 mg once a day with a meal.

Tolazamide: 100–1000 mg a day.

Tolbutamide
   Adult: 1–3 g a day.

Overdosage

Sulfonylurea overdose will cause low blood sugar. Symptoms may occur suddenly and include weakness, fatigue, nervousness, confusion, headache, double vision, convulsions, dizziness, psychosis, unconsciousness, rapid and shallow breathing, numbness or tingling around the mouth, hunger, nausea, loss of skin color, dry skin, and pulse changes. Overdose victims should eat high-sugar, low-fat foods such as fruit juice or a glucose product for diabetics to raise blood-sugar levels. If victims are unable to eat or drink (due to a seizure, unconsciousness, or other debilitating condition), they should be immediately taken to a hospital emergency room. ALWAYS bring the prescription bottle or container.

Special Information

Managing diabetes is your responsibility. Follow your doctor's instructions about diet, exercise, hygiene, and measures to avoid infection. Take all your medicines as prescribed.

Call your doctor if you develop low blood sugar (see "Overdosage") or high blood sugar (symptoms include excessive thirst or urination and sugar or ketones in the urine), if you are not feeling well, or if you have symptoms such as itching, rash, yellowing of the whites of the eyes, abnormally light-colored stools, a low-grade fever, sore throat, diarrhea, or unusual bruising or bleeding.

Alcohol increases the risk of developing lactic acidosis while taking Glucovance or Metaglip. Lactic acidosis is a medical emergency. If you develop it, immediately call your doctor and stop taking these drugs. The symptoms of lactic acidosis (not feeling well, muscle aches, difficulty breathing, and slow heartbeat) can develop with more severe acidosis. Regular monitoring of kidney function minimizes the risk of developing lactic acidosis, as does using the smallest effective dosage of Glucovance or Metaglip.

Do not stop taking these drugs, except under your doctor's supervision. If you forget a dose, take it as soon as you remember. If it is almost time for your next dose, skip the one you forgot and continue with your regular schedule. Do not take a double dose.

Special Populations

Pregnancy/Breast-feeding: Animal studies have shown that all these drugs except glyburide cause birth defects or interfere with fetal development. Check with your doctor before taking a sulfonylurea if you are or might be pregnant. Pregnant women with diabetes should take insulin.

These drugs pass into breast milk. They may lower blood-sugar levels in an infant. Nursing mothers taking one of these medications should use infant formula.

Seniors: Seniors, especially those with reduced kidney function, are very sensitive to the blood-sugar-lowering effects and side ef-

fects of these drugs. Low blood sugar, the major sign of drug overdose, may be more difficult to identify in seniors and is more likely
to cause nervous system side effects. Seniors taking these drugs
must keep in close contact with their doctors and follow their directions. Doses should usually be lower, especially when first taking sulfonylureas.

Synthroid   see *Thyroid Hormone Replacements,*
page 1118

Generic Name

Tacrolimus   (tak-ROE-lim-us)

Brand Names

Prograf   Protopic Ointment

The information in this profile also applies to the following drug:

Generic Ingredient: Sirolimus
Rapamune

Type of Drug

Immunosuppressant.

Prescribed For

Organ transplant rejection, autoimmune disease, severe psoriasis, and atopic dermatitis.

General Information

Tacrolimus is derived from a bacterium and is used to prevent the
rejection of transplanted organs. The drug is used in liver transplants and has been studied in kidney, bone marrow, heart, pancreas, and small bowel transplants, among others. Tacrolimus
works by blocking the activity of T-cells, which protect the body
against invading microorganisms or foreign substances, producing immune-system suppression. Tacrolimus may be used with
corticosteroids and cyclosporine for further transplant protection.

Cautions and Warnings

Tacrolimus should only be prescribed by physicians experienced in immunosuppressive therapy and the care of organ-transplant patients.

Do not take tacrolimus if you are **allergic** or **sensitive** to any of its ingredients. Some people may be allergic to chemically modified castor oil, which is used in tacrolimus injection.

Between 10% and 20% of transplant patients treated with tacrolimus develop post-transplant diabetes mellitus (PTDM), though the condition is sometimes reversible.

Kidney toxicity has been found in more than 50% of kidney transplant patients and about 40% of liver transplant patients.

About 10–44% of liver transplant patients who take tacrolimus develop mild elevations of blood potassium.

Tremors, headaches, muscle function changes, changes in mental state and sense perception, or other nervous system problems occur in about ½ of the people receiving liver transplants. Seizure has also occurred. In some cases, these side effects may be associated with large amounts of tacrolimus in the blood.

As with other immune suppressants, people taking tacrolimus have an increased risk of developing a lymphoma or other malignancy. The risk increases with the degree of immune suppression and the length of time that the drug is taken. A disorder related to Epstein-Barr virus (EBV) infection has also been reported.

People with **kidney disease** should receive lower dosages. People who experience post-transplant reduction in liver function may develop kidney damage. Mild to moderate high blood pressure is a common side effect of tacrolimus and may be a sign of kidney damage. People taking this drug should measure their blood pressure regularly.

Sirolimus can cause increases in cholesterol and triglyceride levels that may require treatment with diet or lipid-lowering drugs.

Possible Side Effects

Sirolimus

Drug side effects increase as drug dosage increases.

▼ Most common: sore throat; difficulty breathing; upper respiratory infection; abdominal pain; weakness; back pain; chest pain; fever; headache; joint pain; urinary infection; high blood pressure; high blood lipids; tremors; acne; rash;

Possible Side Effects *(continued)*

constipation; diarrhea; nausea; vomiting; upset stomach; anemia; low blood-platelet levels; swollen legs, ankles, or arms; kidney damage; high blood potassium; low blood phosphate; and weight gain.

▼ Common: sleeplessness, low white-blood-cell counts, and nosebleeds.

▼ Rare: Rare side effects can occur in almost any part of the body. Contact your doctor if you experience any side effect not listed above.

Tacrolimus

▼ Most common: headache, tremors, sleeplessness, tingling in the hands or feet, diarrhea, nausea, constipation, appetite loss, vomiting, liver or kidney abnormalities, high blood pressure, urinary infection, infrequent urination, anemia, increased white-blood-cell counts, reduced blood-platelet counts, changes in blood-potassium level, reduced blood magnesium, high blood sugar, fluid in the lungs and other lung problems, breathing difficulties, itching, rash, abdominal pain, generalized pain, fever, weakness, back pain, abdominal-fluid buildup, and retention of fluid.

▼ Less common: abnormal dreaming, anxiety, confusion, depression, dizziness, instability, hallucination, poor coordination, muscle spasms, psychosis, tiredness, unusual thoughts, double vision or other visual disturbances, ringing or buzzing in the ears, upset stomach, yellowing of the skin or whites of the eyes, difficulty swallowing, gas, stomach bleeding, fungal infection of the mouth, blood in the urine, chest pain, rapid heartbeat, low blood pressure, diabetes, black-and-blue marks, muscle and joint aches, leg cramps, muscle weakness, asthma, bronchitis, coughing, sore throat, pneumonia, stuffy and runny nose, sinus irritation, voice changes, sweating, and herpes infection.

Protopic

▼ Most common: burning or itching skin, redness or infection of the skin, headache, and flu-like symptoms.

▼ Less common: herpes simplex, rash, acne, allergic reaction, asthma, sinusitis, sleeplessness, and painful menstruation.

Drug Interactions
Tacrolimus
- Tacrolimus should not be taken at the same time as other immune suppressants so as to avoid excessive suppression of the immune system.
- Combining tacrolimus with cyclosporine (another organ transplant drug) can worsen kidney disease. People switching from cyclosporine to tacrolimus should not begin tacrolimus therapy until at least 24 hours after the last cyclosporine dose.
- Tacrolimus may cause more kidney damage when combined with other drugs that also cause kidney problems, including aminoglycoside antibiotics, amphotericin B, and cisplatin.
- Antifungal drugs such as clotrimazole, fluconazole, itraconazole, ketoconazole, and voriconazole; bromocriptine; calcium channel blockers; cimetidine; clarithromycin; danazol; erythromycin; troleandomycin; methylprednisolone; protease inhibitors; omeprazole, cisapride; chloramphenicol; lansoprazole; nefazodone; and metoclopramide may increase tacrolimus blood levels and side effects.
- Carbamazepine, phenobarbital, phenytoin, rifampin, St. John's wort, rifabutin, caspofungin, and sirolimus may reduce tacrolimus blood levels.
- Vaccination may be less effective during tacrolimus use. Live virus vaccines such as those for measles, mumps, rubella, oral polio, BCG, yellow fever, and typhoid fever should be avoided.

Sirolimus
- Sirolimus should not be taken at the same time as other immune suppressants because of the risk of excessive immune system suppression.
- Cyclosporine can double the amount of sirolimus in the blood. Take sirolimus at least 4 hours after cyclosporine capsules or solution.
- Erythromycin and ketoconazole can increase the amount of sirolimus in the blood by up to 10 times. Do not mix these drugs with sirolimus.
- Other drugs that can increase sirolimus blood levels include bromocriptine, cimetidine, danazol, diltiazem, verapamil, fluconazole, clarithromycin, clotrimazole, itraconazole, metoclopramide, cisapride, nicardipine, protease inhibitors such as ritonavir and indinavir, rifabutin, erythromycin, telithromycin, troleandomycin, and voriconazole.

- Rifampin drastically reduces blood levels of sirolimus in the blood by increasing its metabolism. Do not mix these drugs.
- Other drugs that can reduce the amount of sirolimus in the blood include carbamazepine, phenobarbital, phenytoin, St. John's wort, and rifapentine.
- Sirolimus may be taken with acyclovir, digoxin, glyburide, nifedipine, ethinyl estradiol contraceptive (LoOvral), prednisolone, and Bactrim.

Food Interactions

Do not drink grapefruit juice while taking these drugs, since it can interfere with the breakdown of the drug. Take tacrolimus at least 1 hour before or 2 hours after meals. Sirolimus should be taken consistently before or after meals.

Usual Dose

Sirolimus

Adult and Child (age 13 and over): Dosage is individualized based on height and weight, and is usually in the range of 2–6 mg a day. Dosing is usually started at the high end of the recommended amount and then reduced to the lowest effective level. Mix the solution with only 2 or more oz. of water or orange juice.

Child (under age 13): A small number of younger children have been treated with sirolimus, but it is generally not recommended in this age group.

Tacrolimus

Adult and Child: 0.03–0.09 mg per lb. of body weight a day divided into 2 doses. Children may require more than adults. Dosing is usually started at the high end of the recommended amount and then reduced to the lowest effective level.

Protopic

Adult and Child: Rub ointment into affected areas twice a day and continue until symptoms go away. Call your doctor if your symptoms do not improve within 6 weeks of treatment.

Overdosage

Tacrolimus overdose produces expected drug side effects. Take the victim to a hospital emergency room. ALWAYS bring the prescription bottle or container.

Sirolimus overdose has produced abnormal heart rhythms.

Special Information

It is extremely important to take this drug exactly as prescribed. If you forget a dose, take it as soon as you remember. If it is almost time for your next dose, skip the forgotten dose and continue with your regular schedule. Do not take a double dose. Call your doctor if you forget 2 or more doses in a row.

Sirolimus solution must be stored in the refrigerator. If the solution becomes cloudy in the refrigerator, let it stand at room temperature until the cloudiness disappears. The cloudiness does not affect the quality of the drug.

If you are taking sirolimus oral solution, use the amber oral-dose syringe that comes in the package to withdraw the prescribed amount of medicine, and place that into a glass or plastic container with at least 2 oz. of water or orange juice. Do not use any other liquids, including grapefruit juice, for dilution. Stir the mixture and drink at once. Then pour another 4 oz. of water or orange juice into the same container, mix, and drink right away.

People taking these medicines require regular testing to monitor their progress.

Call your doctor at the first sign of fever; sore throat; tiredness; weakness; nervousness; unusual bleeding or bruising; tender or swollen gums; convulsions; irregular heartbeat; confusion; numbness or tingling of your hands, feet, or lips; breathing difficulties; severe stomach pain with nausea; or blood in the urine. Other side effects should be brought to your doctor's attention.

Maintain good dental hygiene while taking these drugs and use extra care when brushing and flossing because the drug increases your risk of oral infection. See your dentist regularly.

These drugs should be continued as long as prescribed by your doctor. Do not stop taking it because of side effects or other problems. If you cannot tolerate the oral form, this drug may be given by injection, though the oral capsules are preferable.

Limit exposure to sunlight and UV light by wearing protective clothing and using a high SPF sunscreen.

Special Populations

Pregnancy/Breast-feeding: These drugs pass into the fetal circulation, and cause miscarriage and reduced fertility in animals. In humans, babies born to mothers taking tacrolimus have had high blood potassium and poor kidney function. There is no reliable experience with sirolimus. When your doctor considers these drugs crucial, their potential benefits must be carefully weighed against their risks. Women who might become pregnant while taking these medicines must begin using reliable contraception before starting tacrolimus and continue at least 12 weeks after treatment has stopped.

These medicines pass into breast milk. Nursing mothers who must take tacrolimus should use infant formula.

Seniors: Seniors may require a reduced dosage of tacrolimus due to loss of kidney function. Seniors may take sirolimus without special precaution.

Generic Name

Tamoxifen Citrate (tuh-MOX-ih-fen SYE-trate) [G]

Brand Name
Soltamox

The information in this profile also applies to the following drug:

Generic Ingredient: Toremifene Citrate
Fareston

Type of Drug
Anti-estrogen.

Prescribed For
Breast cancer. Tamoxifen is also used for painful breasts in women; swollen or painful breasts and breast cancer in men; migraine; and pancreatic, endometrial, and liver-cell cancer.

General Information
Tamoxifen is effective in treating estrogen-positive breast cancer in women. It works by blocking the effects of estrogen in breast tissue. When used together with chemotherapy after mastectomy, tamoxifen can prevent or delay the recurrence of breast cancer. It is used to treat metastatic breast cancer (that which has spread) and to prevent breast cancer in women at high risk. Up to 60% of women whose breast cancer has metastasized may benefit from taking tamoxifen. Toremifene is used only to treat breast cancer, not to prevent it.

Cautions and Warnings
Do not take tamoxifen if you are **allergic** or **sensitive** to any of its ingredients.

Women taking tamoxifen for **ductal carcinoma,** or those at **high risk for breast cancer,** have an increased risk of uterine cancer, stroke, or pulmonary embolism.

Visual difficulties have occurred in people taking tamoxifen for 1 year or more in dosages at least 4 times above the maximum recommended dosage. These include cataracts, loss of color vision, and damage to the retina. A few cases of decreased visual clarity and other vision problems have been reported at normal dosages.

People taking tamoxifen have experienced liver inflammation and, rarely, more serious liver abnormalities. Very high dosages of this drug (15 mg per lb. of body weight) may cause liver cancer.

Women taking tamoxifen have an increased risk of thromboembolic events such as deep vein thrombosis and pulmonary embolism.

Women undergoing **coumarin-type anticoagulant** therapy or those with a history of **heart disease** should not take tamoxifen.

Possible Side Effects

Side effects are generally mild. Lowering drug dosage can sometimes control severe reactions.

▼ Most common: hot flashes, weight changes, fluid retention, vaginal discharge, menstrual changes, headache, and nausea. Increased bone and tumor pain sometimes occur shortly after starting tamoxifen. These may be a sign of a good response to the drug and usually decline rapidly.

▼ Less common: swelling, fatigue, muscle pains, abdominal cramps, vomiting, vaginal bleeding, skin changes, and kidney problems. In men: impotence and lowered sex drive.

▼ Rare: high blood-calcium levels, swelling of the arms or legs, changes in sense of taste, vaginal itching, depression, dizziness, lightheadedness, visual difficulties, and reduced white-blood-cell or platelet count. Ovarian cysts have occurred in premenopausal women with advanced breast cancer who took tamoxifen. Contact your doctor if you experience any side effect not listed above.

Drug Interactions

- The effects of warfarin and other anticoagulant (blood-thinning) drugs may be increased by tamoxifen.
- Tamoxifen may increase blood-calcium levels.

- Bromocriptine may increase tamoxifen blood levels.
- The combination of tamoxifen and cytotoxic agents may increase the risk of blood clots.
- Rifamycins such as rifampin decrease tamoxifen levels.
- Tamoxifen lowers the level of letrozole in the blood.

Food Interactions

Tamoxifen may be taken with food or milk if it upsets your stomach.

Usual Dose

Adult

Tamoxifen: 20–40 a day. Doses higher than 20 mg should be divided and taken morning and evening.

Toremifene: 60 mg once a day.

Child: not recommended.

Overdosage

Symptoms may include breathing difficulties, convulsions, tremors, overactive reflexes, dizziness, and unsteadiness. Take the victim to a hospital emergency room. ALWAYS bring the prescription bottle or container.

Special Information

Take this medication according to your doctor's directions. Inform your doctor if you become very weak or sleepy or if you experience confusion, pain, swelling of the legs, breathing difficulties, blurred vision, bone pain, hot flashes, nausea or vomiting, weight gain, irregular periods, dizziness, headache, or appetite loss. Call your doctor if you vomit shortly after taking a dose of tamoxifen. Your doctor may tell you to take another dose immediately or wait until the next dose.

Women taking tamoxifen should use a condom, diaphragm, or other non-hormonal contraceptive during sexual intercourse until 2 months after treatment is complete.

If you forget a dose, call your doctor. If you cannot reach your doctor, skip the forgotten dose and continue your regular schedule. Do not take a double dose.

Special Populations

Pregnancy/Breast-feeding: Tamoxifen can harm the fetus and cause vaginal bleeding and spontaneous abortion. It should not be taken by any pregnant women. Women of childbearing age taking tamoxifen must use barrier contraception to prevent pregnancy.

Hormonal birth control may not work while taking tamoxifen. Contact your doctor at once if you think you may be pregnant.

It is not known if tamoxifen passes into breast milk. Nursing mothers who must take it should use infant formula.

Seniors: Seniors may take tamoxifen without special restriction.

Generic Name

Tamsulosin (tam-SUE-loe-sin)

Brand Name

Flomax

Type of Drug

Alpha blocker.

Prescribed For

Benign prostatic hyperplasia (BPH).

General Information

Tamsulosin hydrochloride and similar drugs block nerve endings known as alpha$_1$ receptors. In BPH, tamsulosin works by relaxing smooth muscles in the prostate and neck of the bladder. This effect is produced by blocking alpha$_1$ receptors in the affected muscles. Despite the fact that tamsulosin alleviates the urinary symptoms of BPH, the drug's long-term effect on complications of BPH or the need for urinary surgery is not known. Alpha blockers are broken down in the liver.

Cautions and Warnings

Do not take this drug if you are **allergic** or **sensitive** to any of its ingredients or to any alpha blocker.

Tamsulosin may cause dizziness and fainting, especially after the first few doses. This is known as the first-dose effect and may be minimized by limiting the first dose to 1 mg at bedtime. The first-dose effect occurs in about 1% of people and may recur if the drug is stopped for a few days and then restarted.

Rarely, tamsulosin may cause priapism, a persistent, painful erection, which should be treated by a doctor.

Tamsulosin may slightly reduce cholesterol levels and improve the high-density lipoprotein (HDL)/low-density lipoprotein (LDL) ratio, a positive step for people with blood-cholesterol problems.

Red- and white-blood-cell counts may be slightly reduced by other alpha blockers. This effect should be monitored in people taking tamsulosin.

Possible Side Effects

▼ Most common: dizziness, weakness, and headache.

▼ Less common: low blood pressure; rapid heartbeat; abnormal heart rhythms; chest pain; flushing in the face, arms, or legs; fainting; vomiting; dry mouth; diarrhea; constipation; abdominal pain or discomfort; gas; breathing difficulties; stuffy nose; sinus inflammation; cold or flu-like symptoms; cough; bronchitis; worsening of asthma; nosebleed; sore throat; runny nose; shoulder, neck, or back pain; pain in the arms or legs; joint pain; arthritis; muscle pain; blurred vision or other visual disturbances; conjunctivitis (pinkeye); eye pain; nervousness; tingling in the hands or feet; tiredness; anxiety; difficulty sleeping; frequent urination; urinary infection; abnormal ejaculation; itching; rash; sweating; swelling of the face, arms, or legs; and fever.

▼ Rare: depression, reduced sex drive or abnormal sexual function (including priapism), fluid retention, and weight gain. Contact your doctor if you experience any side effect not listed above.

Drug Interactions

- Tamsulosin may interact with beta-blocking drugs to produce a higher rate of dizziness or fainting after taking the first dose of tamsulosin.
- Cimetidine increases blood levels of tamsulosin and should be used with caution.
- The blood-pressure-lowering effect of tamsulosin may be reduced by indomethacin.
- When taken with blood-pressure-lowering drugs, tamsulosin produces severe reduction of blood pressure.
- The blood-pressure-lowering effect of clonidine may be reduced by tamsulosin.
- Drinking alcohol while taking tamsulosin may cause low blood pressure.

Food Interactions

None known.

Usual Dose

Starting dosage—0.4 mg ½ hour after the same meal each day. Dosage may be increased to 0.8 mg a day if there has been no response after 2–4 weeks.

Overdosage

Symptoms may include severe side effects. Take the victim to a hospital emergency room at once. ALWAYS bring the prescription bottle or container.

Special Information

Take tamsulosin exactly as prescribed and do not stop taking it unless directed to do so by your doctor. Avoid over-the-counter drugs that contain stimulants because they may increase your blood pressure.

Tamsulosin may cause dizziness, headache, and drowsiness, especially 2–6 hours after you take your first dose, and these effects may persist after the first few doses. Wait 12–24 hours after taking the first dose before driving or doing any task that requires concentration. You should take it at bedtime to minimize this problem.

Call your doctor if you develop severe dizziness, heart palpitations, priapism, or any bothersome or persistent side effect.

If you forget a dose, take it as soon as you remember. If it is almost time for your next dose, skip the forgotten dose and continue with your regular schedule. If you forget your medication for several days in a row, you will have to begin again at the lower dosage of 0.4 mg a day regardless of the dosage you were taking before.

Special Populations

Pregnancy/Breast-feeding: Tamsulosin is intended only for men. The safety of using tamsulosin during pregnancy and breast-feeding is not known.

Seniors: Seniors may be more sensitive to the action and side effects of tamsulosin.

Generic Name

Tazarotene (tuh-ZAR-oe-tene)

Brand Names

Avage   Tazorac

Type of Drug

Anti-acne.

Prescribed For

Mild to moderate acne and psoriasis. Also prescribed for age- and sun-related skin damage and actinic keratosis, although the advantages of this treatment have not been established.

General Information

Tazarotene is converted to its active form after it is applied to the skin. A retinoid related to vitamin A, tazarotene is in the same family as retinoic acid—the active ingredient in Retin-A anti-acne products.

Cautions and Warnings

Do not use tazarotene if you are **allergic** or **sensitive** to any of its ingredients.

Women who are or might be **pregnant** should not use this drug.

Tazarotene may cause a temporary burning or stinging sensation. It may cause severe burning if applied to eczema. Other skin medications and makeup can make the skin very dry and should be avoided while you are using tazarotene. It may also be advisable to "rest" your skin between using other drugs or makeup and starting tazarotene.

Tazarotene can cause rash, allergy, or a severe toxic reaction, especially if used together with another drug that sensitizes the skin such as a tetracycline antibiotic, a fluoroquinolone, or a phenothiazine sedative.

Possible Side Effects

▼ Most common: peeling skin, a burning or stinging sensation, dry skin, redness, and itching.

▼ Common: irritation, skin pain, cracking, swelling, and skin discoloration.

Drug Interactions

None known.

Usual Dose

Adult: Gently clean your face and apply a thin layer of tazarotene to the affected area every evening.

Child: not recommended.

Overdosage
Accidental ingestion of tazarotene may cause symptoms similar to vitamin A overdose. Call your local poison control center for information about what to do in the case of tazarotene ingestion.

Special Information
Do not get tazarotene gel onto your eyelids or into your eyes or mouth. If eye contact occurs, immediately rinse them thoroughly with water. If skin irritation, redness, itching, or peeling is excessive, stop using tazarotene until your skin is completely healed. Extreme wind or cold may worsen skin irritation.

Applying excessive amounts of tazarotene to your skin can cause redness, peeling skin, or other discomfort.

Special Populations
Pregnancy/Breast-feeding: Tazarotene caused birth defects in lab animals. Women who are or might be pregnant should not use this drug.

It is not known if tazarotene passes into breast milk. Nursing mothers should use infant formula.

Seniors: Seniors may use this drug without special restriction.

Generic Name

Telithromycin (tel-ith-row-MY-sin)

Brand Name
Ketek

Type of Drug
Antibiotic.

Prescribed For
Bacterial infections of the sinus, chronic bronchitis, and pneumonia that develop outside of the hospital and are resistant to other antibiotics. May also be prescribed for infections in other areas of the body.

General Information
Telithromycin is effective against a variety of different common bacteria. When tested against commonly used antibiotics, telithromycin was at least as good as the others and sometimes

better. Telithromycin should only be used to treat infections that are caused by bacteria it can treat.

Telithromycin is related to erythromycin, another antibiotic that has been in use for many years, but is a called a ketolide antibiotic because of its chemical structure. Even though it is related to erythromycin, bacteria that are resistant to erythromycin may still be treated with telithromycin.

Telithromycin is absorbed into the body within an hour after it is taken, but only about half the drug finds its way into the bloodstream. It is broken down in the liver. Patients with liver failure pass more of the drug out of their bodies through their kidneys. People with liver failure can safely use telithromycin with no dosage adjustment. People with severe kidney failure must receive a reduced dose of this drug.

Cautions and Warnings

Do not take telithromycin if you are **allergic** or **sensitive** to any of its ingredients or if you have experienced hepatitis or jaundice with any macrolide antibiotic in the past.

People with **myasthenia gravis** must not use telithromycin because it can worsen this condition, sometimes within a few hours of the first dose of telithromycin. The most common symptom is weakness, and some muscles can be completely wasted by myasthenia gravis over time.

Colitis is possible with nearly any antibacterial agent, including telithromycin, and may range from mild to life threatening.

Telithromycin can affect heart rhythm in some people, leading to an increased risk for severe abnormal rhythms. This drug should be avoided by people with **congenital heart defects** and those with **abnormal heart rhythms**.

Telithromycin can be toxic to the liver, causing jaundice and hepatitis. Liver injury and failure have also occurred. Serious liver injury and 4 deaths due to liver failure have occurred.

Telithromycin has been known to cause visual disturbances or a sudden loss of consciousness. When taking telithromycin, you should not drive or engage in any potentially hazardous activities.

Possible Side Effects

▼ Most common: diarrhea.
▼ Common: nausea and headache.

Possible Side Effects *(continued)*

▼ Less common: visual problems such as difficulty focusing, blurred vision, or double vision; dizziness; vomiting; loose stools; and loss of taste perception.

▼ Rare: allergic reactions, heart palpitations, liver inflammation, myasthenia gravis, and muscle cramps. Other rare side effects can occur in almost any part of the body. Contact your doctor if you experience any side effect not listed above.

Drug Interactions

- Telithromycin can almost double blood levels of cisapride by slowing its breakdown in the liver. This combination can result in dangerously abnormal heart rhythms.
- Telithromycin can increase blood levels of pimozide, an antipsychotic medicine, by preventing its breakdown by the liver. This can expose the patient to serious pimozide side effects. Do not mix these drugs.
- Avoid mixing telithromycin with simvastatin, lovastatin, or atorvastatin. Telithromycin increases the amount of simvastatin absorbed 9 times. This exposes people to a greater chance of simvastatin side effects and muscle damage.
- Telithromycin increases the amount of midazolam absorbed into the blood by several times via slowing its breakdown in the liver. The midazolam dose may have to be reduced to avoid drug side effects. This interaction may also affect other benzodiazepine drugs.
- Telithromycin slows the breakdown of the beta blockers metoprolol and sotalol in the body. Beta-blocker dose adjustments may be needed.
- Telithromycin may increase the effects of warfarin and other blood thinners. Patients taking this combination should have their blood clotting times checked.
- Telithromycin significantly increases the amount of digoxin in the blood, but there are few signs of digoxin toxicity as a result of this interaction. Digoxin levels should be monitored.
- Mixing telithromycin and theophylline produces an increase in theophylline blood levels. This can result in an increase in theophylline side effects such as nausea and vomiting, especially in women. Take these drugs at least one hour apart.

- Telithromycin can increase levels of cyclosporine, ergotamine or dihydroergotamine, tacrolimus, sirolimus, and hexobarbital in the blood, exposing the person taking the combination to drug side effects.
- Itraconazole and ketoconazole substantially increase the amount of telithromycin absorbed into the blood.
- Rifampin, phenytoin, carbamazepine, and phenobarbital reduce the amount of telithromycin in the bloodstream, interfering with its antibacterial action. Avoid these combinations.
- Combining telithromycin with ergot alkaloid derivatives is not recommended.

Food Interactions

This drug may be taken without regard to food or meals.

Usual Dose

Adult: 800 mg (2 tablets) at the same time every day for 5–10 days, depending on the infection. People with severe kidney failure, including dialysis patients, can take 600 mg a day. For patients with both severe kidney and liver disease, the daily dose is 400 mg a day.

Child: not recommended.

Overdosage

Anyone suspected of having taken a telithromycin overdose should be taken to a hospital emergency room for treatment. ALWAYS bring the prescription bottle or container.

Special Information

Use caution when driving, operating machinery, or performing other hazardous activities.

Call your doctor if changes in vision caused by telithromycin affect your daily activities. Avoiding quick changes in viewing between objects in the distance and objects nearby may help to decrease the impact of these visual difficulties.

Telithromycin should only be used to treat bacterial infections. It does not treat viral infections such as the common cold.

It is common to feel better within a day or two of starting telithromycin, but you must continue to take all the medication exactly as it was prescribed in order to get the maximum benefit.

Report any diarrhea to your doctor because of the chance that it can be drug-related.

If you forget to take a dose of telithromycin, take it as soon as you remember, and then continue with your regular dose on the next day. Skipping doses or not completing the full course of therapy can reduce the effectiveness of this antibiotic and increase the chances that bacteria will become resistant to telithromycin. Tell your doctor or pharmacist if you forget more than one dose of telithromycin.

Do not take more than 2 tablets of telithromycin in any 24-hour period.

Be sure to tell your doctor about any other medicines you are taking, including over-the-counter and herbal remedies.

Special Populations

Pregnancy/Breast-feeding: This medication caused birth defects in animal studies. When it is considered crucial by your doctor, its potential benefits must be carefully weighed against its risks. Women who are or might be pregnant should talk with their doctor before taking telithromycin.

Telithromycin passes into breast milk. Nursing mothers who must take it should use infant formula.

Seniors: Seniors can take telithromycin in the same dosage as younger adults.

Generic Name

Temozolomide (tem-oh-ZOHL-oh-mide)

Brand Name
Temodar

Type of Drug
Antineoplastic.

Prescribed For
Brain cancer. Also used for certain kinds of advanced skin cancer.

General Information
Temozolomide is used to treat astrocytoma, a specific type of cancer of the brain, in adults whose tumors have returned after other chemotherapy. Once absorbed, it seems to interfere with the growth of cancer cells, which are then eventually destroyed by the body.

Cautions and Warnings

Do not take this medicine if you are **allergic** or **sensitive** to any of its ingredients or to dacarbazine, another antineoplastic drug.

People taking temozolomide may experience reduced white-blood-cell and platelet counts. These generally occur late in the first treatment cycle and may increase your risk of infection.

People with **impaired liver function** should use temozolomide with caution.

Temozolomide may cause infertility in men.

Possible Side Effects

▼ Most common: headache, fatigue, general weakness, weakness on one side of the body, fever, convulsions, dizziness, diarrhea, nausea, constipation, vomiting, leg or arm swelling, poor muscle coordination, memory loss, sleeplessness, viral infection, and fever.

▼ Common: partial paralysis; anxiety; difficulty swallowing; jerking movements of the face, trunk, arms, or legs; depression; walking unusually; confusion; itching; rash; increased urination; loss of urinary control; urinary infection; appetite loss; abdominal pain; double vision and other visual abnormalities; cough; sore throat; runny nose; respiratory tract infection; muscle aches; breast pain (women); weight gain; and back pain.

▼ Rare: Rare side effects can occur in almost any part of the body. Contact your doctor if you experience any side effect not listed above.

Drug Interactions

- Valproic acid reduces the amount of temozolomide cleared through the kidney. The importance of this interaction is not known.

Food Interactions

Food interferes with the absorption of this drug into the blood. Take it on an empty stomach to reduce nausea and vomiting.

Usual Dose

Adult: 100–200 mg at bedtime. Dosage is adjusted according to body weight and white-blood-cell and platelet counts.

Child: not recommended.

Overdosage

Temozolomide overdose causes drastic reductions in platelets and white blood cells. Overdose victims must be taken to a hospital emergency room at once. ALWAYS bring the prescription bottle or container.

Special Information

Nausea and vomiting usually decline with time and are readily controlled with antinauseant drugs. Antinauseant medication may be taken before or after your temozolomide dose.

Women clear temozolomide from the body more slowly than men and are more likely experience low white-blood-cell and platelet counts in the first cycle of temozolomide treatment.

Exposure to temozolomide powder causes malignant tumors in animals. Be sure that you and others do not inhale the contents of any capsule or get any of the drug on your skin or mucous membranes from a capsule that has been damaged or opened.

Do not open or chew temozolomide capsules. Swallow them whole with a glass of water.

Keep this drug away from children and pets.

If you forget to take a dose of temozolomide, be sure to tell your doctor and continue with your regular schedule on the next day. Do not take a double dose.

Special Populations

Pregnancy/Breast-feeding: Temozolomide will damage a developing fetus. Women who must take it should use an effective contraceptive method and wait 6 months after the treatment is finished before becoming pregnant. Men should not father a child up to 6 months after treatment.

Women who must take temozolomide should use infant formula because temozolomide may pass into breast milk and cause severe reactions in the nursing infant.

Seniors: Seniors are more likely to experience reduced white-blood-cell and platelet counts.

Generic Name

Terbinafine (ter-BIN-uh-feen) Ⓖ

Brand Names

| Desenex Max | Lamisil AT | Lamisil |

Type of Drug

Antifungal.

Prescribed For

Fungal infections of the skin, fingernails, or toenails.

General Information

Terbinafine hydrochloride is a general-purpose antifungal. It can cure common athlete's foot, jock itch, and ringworm faster than other drugs of this type. It is also effective against *Candida* and other fungal infections of the skin. Terbinafine is unique because it accumulates in the skin and continues to kill fungus organisms even after you stop using it. Most other antifungals do not kill the fungus; they only stop it from growing.

Cautions and Warnings

Do not take terbinafine if you are **allergic** or **sensitive** to any of its ingredients.

Kidney or liver disease can increase the amount of terbinafine in your blood by 50%. Rare cases of liver failure have been reported in people without a preexisting liver condition.

Topical terbinafine is only meant to be applied to the skin. Do not put it into your eyes or use it for a vaginal infection. Do not swallow topical terbinafine. Only the capsules are meant for oral use.

Terbinafine should be used only for specific fungal infections and only as prescribed. Rarely, people taking terbinafine have experienced severe eyesight changes or a severe drop in white-blood-cell count, leading to serious infection and fever. Serious skin reactions to terbinafine have been reported; if skin rash occurs, contact your doctor immediately. Call your doctor if anything unusual develops.

Terbinafine use should be discontinued by people with the clinical signs and symptoms of **lupus erythematosus** (fatigue, low-grade fever, aching, weakness, and nausea).

Possible Side Effects

Topical

▼ Most common: itching and irritation of the skin immediately after application.

▼ Less common: burning, irritation, and dryness of the skin.

Possible Side Effects *(continued)*

Oral

▼ Most common: headache.

▼ Common: diarrhea and rash (including psoriasis-type rashes or worsening psoriasis and pinhead-sized pustules).

▼ Less common: upset stomach, abdominal pain, nausea, gas, itching, liver irritation, taste changes, and temporary eyesight changes.

▼ Rare: aching joints and muscles, yellowing of the skin or eyes, loss of appetite, severe reactions of the liver or skin, low white-blood-cell count, and allergic reactions. Contact your doctor if you experience any side effect not listed above.

Drug Interactions

- Cimetidine and terfenadine increase the amount of terbinafine in the blood.
- Do not combine terbinafine and rifampin.
- Terbinafine may reduce the effect of cyclosporine.
- Terbinafine may increase the effect of caffeine.
- Terbinafine may raise blood levels of dextromethorphan, a common ingredient in cough syrups.

Food Interactions

Take terbinafine tablets 1 hour before or 2 hours after eating.

Usual Dose

Cream

   Adult and Child: Apply to affected areas morning and night for 1–4 weeks.

Spray

   Adult and Child: Once or twice a day for 1 week.

Tablets

   Adult: 250 mg a day for 6 or 12 weeks, depending on the condition being treated.

   Child: 125–250 mg a day for 6 weeks, depending on body weight.

Overdosage

Terbinafine overdose may lead to nausea, vomiting, abdominal pain, dizziness, rash, frequent urination, and headache. Overdose victims should be taken to a hospital emergency room. ALWAYS bring the prescription bottle or container.

Special Information

Do not put topical terbinafine in contact with your eyes, nose, mouth, or any other mucous membrane tissues.

Do not stop using terbinafine before your prescription is complete, even if your rash clears up. The full prescription may be necessary to eliminate the fungus.

Do not cover the cream with plastic wrap or anything else that restricts ventilation unless so instructed by your doctor.

Call your doctor if your skin becomes red, burns, itches, blisters, swells, or if oozing develops.

If you forget to administer a dose, do so as soon as you remember. If it is almost time for your next dose, skip the one you forgot and continue with your regular schedule.

Special Populations

Pregnancy/Breast-feeding: The effect of terbinafine during pregnancy is not known. Women who are pregnant should not use terbinafine because the treatment of toenail or fingernail fungal infections can be postponed until after pregnancy.

Terbinafine passes into breast milk. Nursing mothers who must use this drug should use infant formula.

Seniors: Seniors may use terbinafine without special precaution.

Generic Name

Terbutaline (ter-BUE-tuh-leen) Ⓖ

Type of Drug

Bronchodilator.

Prescribed For

Asthma and bronchospasm; also used to treat premature labor.

General Information

Terbutaline sulfate is similar to other bronchodilator drugs, such as metaproterenol and isoetharine, but it has a weaker effect on nerve receptors in the heart and blood vessels. For this reason, it is somewhat safer for people with heart conditions.

Terbutaline tablets begin to work within 30 minutes and continue working for 4–8 hours. Terbutaline injection starts working in 5–15 minutes and lasts for 1½–4 hours.

Cautions and Warnings

Do not take terbutaline if you are **allergic** or **sensitive** to any of its ingredients.

Terbutaline should be used with caution by people with a history of **angina pectoris** (condition characterized by brief attacks of chest pain), **heart disease, high blood pressure, cardiac arrythmia, stroke, seizure, liver or kidney disease, diabetes, thyroid disease, prostate disease,** or **glaucoma**.

Possible Side Effects

▼ Most common: heart palpitations, abnormal heart rhythm, tremors, dizziness and fainting, shakiness, nervousness, tension, drowsiness, headache, nausea and vomiting, and heartburn or upset stomach.

▼ Less common: rapid heartbeat, chest pain and discomfort, angina, weakness, sleeplessness, wheezing, bronchial spasms and difficulty breathing, dry or sore throat, flushing, sweating, and changes in sense of smell and taste.

▼ Rare: hallucinations, rash, seizures, and increased liver enzyme levels. Contact your doctor if you experience any side effect not listed above.

Drug Interactions

- Terbutaline's effects may be increased by monoamine oxidase inhibitor or tricyclic antidepressants, thyroid drugs, other bronchodilator drugs, and some antihistamines.
- The risk of cardiac toxicity may be increased in people taking both terbutaline and theophylline.
- Terbutaline's effectiveness is reduced by beta-blocking drugs such as propranolol.
- Terbutaline may reduce the effects of blood-pressure-lowering drugs, especially reserpine, methyldopa, and guanethidine.
- Use caution when combining terbutaline with potassium-sparing diuretics, especially in higher doses.

Food Interactions

Terbutaline tablets are more effective when taken on an empty stomach—1 hour before or 2 hours after meals—but can be taken with food if they upset your stomach.

Usual Dose

Tablets

Adult and Child (age 15 and over): 2.5–5 mg every 6 hours, 3 times a day. Do not take more than 15 mg within 24 hours.

Child (age 12–14): 2.5 mg 3 times a day. Do not take more than 7.5 mg within 24 hours.

Child (under age 12): not recommended.

Overdosage

Overdose of terbutaline tablets is more likely to trigger changes in heart rate, palpitations, unusual heart rhythms, chest pain, high blood pressure, fever, chills, cold sweats, nausea, vomiting, and dilation of the pupils. Convulsions, sleeplessness, anxiety, and tremors may also develop, and the victim may collapse.

If the overdose was taken within the past 30 minutes, give the victim ipecac syrup—available at any pharmacy—to induce vomiting and to remove any remaining medication from the stomach. Do not give ipecac syrup if the victim is unconscious or convulsing. If symptoms have already begun to develop, the victim should be taken to a hospital emergency room. ALWAYS bring the prescription bottle or container.

Special Information

Do not take more terbutaline than your doctor prescribes. Taking more than you need could actually worsen your symptoms. If your condition worsens rather than improves after taking terbutaline, stop taking it and call your doctor.

Call your doctor immediately if you develop chest pain, palpitations, rapid heartbeat, muscle tremors, dizziness, headache, facial flushing, or urinary difficulty, or if you continue to experience difficulty in breathing after using the medication.

If you forget a dose of terbutaline, take it as soon as you remember. If it is almost time for your next dose, skip the one you forgot and return to your regular schedule. Do not take a double dose.

Special Populations

Pregnancy/Breast-feeding: When used during childbirth, terbutaline can slow or delay labor. Generally, terbutaline should not be taken after the first 3 months of pregnancy; it can cause rapid heartbeat and high blood sugar in the mother, and rapid heartbeat and low blood sugar in the fetus. It is not known if terbutaline causes birth defects in humans, but it has caused defects in pregnant animals. When your doctor considers this drug crucial, its potential benefits must be carefully weighed against its risks.

Terbutaline passes into breast milk. Nursing mothers who must take this drug should use infant formula.

Seniors: Seniors are more sensitive to the effects of terbutaline. Follow your doctor's directions closely and report any side effects at once.

Generic Name

Teriparatide (terr-ih-PAR-a-tide)

Brand Name

Forteo

Type of Drug

Parathyroid hormone.

Prescribed For

Postmenopausal osteoporosis; also used to treat osteopenia (low bone mass) in men.

General Information

Teriparatide is a synthetic form of the human parathyroid hormone, which is involved in maintaining calcium balance in the body. This treatment is the first proven to actually build new bone and improve bone structure in women suffering from osteoporosis. All other osteoporosis drugs change the rate at which calcium is lost from bone, so they slow the rate of bone loss. Studies of teriparatide have shown that people taking it experience significant increases in bone mineral density and suffer fewer bone fractures while they are taking teriparatide as well as after they stop it. Typically, people take teriparatide for 1–2 years to build bone mass and prevent additional fractures.

Cautions and Warnings

Do not take teriparatide if you are **allergic** or **sensitive** to any of its ingredients.

When teriparatide was given to rats, it increased their risk for developing osteosarcoma, a rare but very serious cancer of the bone. This effect has not appeared in humans. People with a **bone disease**, such as **Paget's disease,** a history or risk of **bone cancer,** or **cancer that has spread to the bone** should not take teriparatide.

People known to have an underlying **hypercalcemia disorder** (high blood calcium levels) such as **hyperparathyroidism**, should not use teriparatide.

People who have had **radiation therapy** should not take this drug.

The long-term safety of teriparatide has not been studied past 2 years.

People who have or have had **kidney stones** should use teriparatide with caution because of the risk that it could worsen this condition.

Possible Side Effects

In most cases, studies of teriparatide found that its side effects were similar to people who took an inactive placebo (sugar pill).

▼ Most common: generalized pain and joint pain.

▼ Common: headache, weakness, high blood pressure, nausea, constipation, diarrhea, upset stomach, dizziness, runny nose, coughing, and sore throat.

▼ Less common: neck pain, angina, fainting, vomiting, stomach problems, dental problems, leg cramps, depression, sleeplessness, vertigo, shortness of breath, pneumonia, rash, and sweating.

▼ Rare: difficulty breathing after injection, swelling of the mouth or face, hives, and chest pain. Other rare side effects can occur in almost any part of the body. Contact your doctor if you experience any side effect not listed above.

Drug Interactions

- Teriparatide increases blood levels of calcium and should be used cautiously when combined with digoxin.

- Bisphosphonates reduce the ability of teriparatide to build new bone. Teriparatide alone produces better improvements in bone density than either a bisphosphonate alone or taking the two drugs together.

Food Interactions

You may take this drug without regard to food or meals.

Usual Dose

Adult: 20 mcg a day by subcutaneous injection (under the skin) in the thigh or abdomen (lower stomach area). Teriparatide comes in a "pen" containing 28-days worth of medicine. Teriparatide is a clear and colorless liquid. Do not use if there are particles in it or if the solution is cloudy or colored.

Child: not recommended.

Overdosage

Little is known about the effects of teriparatide overdose. Likely symptoms include high blood calcium, dizziness or fainting, low blood pressure, nausea, vomiting, and headache. Take the victim to a hospital emergency room. ALWAYS bring the prescription bottle or container.

Special Information

Read your pen user manual thoroughly before administering this drug, and re-read it each time you renew your prescription.

Take teriparatide at the same time every day. If you forget to take a dose, take it as soon as you remember. Do not take a double dose and do not take more than one dose a day.

Teriparatide must be injected under the skin. If you cannot inject yourself, you must have someone else do it for you every day.

When you first start taking teriparatide, you should be in a place where you can sit or lie down if you get dizzy. Contact your doctor if dizziness continues.

You must continue taking calcium and/or vitamin D supplements as prescribed by your doctor. Also, regular weight bearing exercise, reducing alcohol consumption, and stopping smoking will help improve your osteoporosis.

Do not use teriparatide after the expiration date printed on the pen and pen packaging. Throw away your teriparatide pen 28 days after you start using it, even if it still contains medicine.

Store this product in the refrigerator. Teriparatide should be injected shortly after you take the pen out of the refrigerator. Replace the cap and put it back into the refrigerator immediately after use.

Special Populations

Pregnancy/Breast-feeding: Teriparatide enters fetal circulation. Pregnant women should not take this drug.

Teriparatide passes into breast milk. Nursing mothers who must take it should use infant formula.

Seniors: Seniors may use this drug without special precaution.

Generic Name

Testosterone (tes-TOS-ter-one) Ⓖ

Brand Names

Androderm	Testim
AndroGel	Testopel
Striant	

The information in this profile also applies to the following drug:

Generic Ingredient: Methyltestosterone Ⓖ

Android	Virilon
Testred	

Type of Drug

Hormone replacement.

Prescribed For

Impotence due to hormone deficiency and testosterone replacement in men who have lost their testicle function or have low blood levels of testosterone. Androgen may be prescribed for boys before they reach puberty to maintain secondary sex characteristics if testosterone is lacking or if puberty is delayed. In women, testosterone may be used to treat metastatic cancer (cancer that has spread from one part of the body to another) and breast enlargement or pain in women who have just given birth. It has also been studied for low sex drive in women.

General Information

Testosterone is the principal androgen (male hormone). In men, testosterone is produced in the testicles. Women make small amounts of testosterone in their ovaries and in the adrenal gland. Testosterone is responsible for the growth and development of male sex organs as well as secondary sex characteristics such as beard, pubic, chest, and underarm hair; vocal cord thickening, which lowers the voice; and muscle and fat distribution. Androgens are also responsible for the adolescent growth spurt.

Weekly testosterone injection of 200 mg, for up to 1 year, has been studied as a reversible male contraceptive.

Cautions and Warnings

Do not take testosterone if you are **allergic** or **sensitive** to any of its ingredients.

The following people should avoid testosterone: **pregnant women, men with breast or prostate cancer,** and people with **heart, liver, or kidney disease,** who may respond to the drug by retaining fluid.

Some **athletes** have taken testosterone in order to improve performance, but this is unsafe and ineffective.

Male hormones may cause very high blood calcium levels in **women with breast cancer** and in **people who are immobilized**; these groups should avoid taking testosterone.

Continuous use of high dosages of male hormones may cause life-threatening liver problems. Liver function should be monitored regularly. Hepatitis and jaundice have occurred with androgen use, but may be reversible when treatment is stopped. Taking male hormones for an extended period of time causes reduced sperm count and semen volume. Men taking testosterone as hormone replacement may develop enlarged breasts.

Testosterone can precipitate an attack of a condition called acute intermittent porphyria (symptoms include abdominal pain, nausea and vomiting, constipation, neurotic or psychotic behavior, and nerve irritation).

Blood cholesterol may rise while you are taking testosterone. People with **heart disease**; those who have had a **stroke** or **transient ischemic attack** (TIA)—"mini-stroke"; and those who have **blood vessel disease**, such as claudication, should be cautious about taking a male hormone.

A man using a scrotal testosterone patch may transfer some hormone to his sexual partner, which may result in unwanted changes in the partner's secondary sex characteristics.

Testosterone may affect glycemic control in people with **diabetes.**

Testosterone must be used with caution in **children.** They should be treated only by specialists who are experienced with testosterone and understand its effects on children's bone development.

Women should inform their doctors of any signs of virilization—a deepening voice, increased hairiness, acne, menstrual problems, and enlarged clitoris—as they may need to stop treatment to prevent irreversible changes.

Possible Side Effects

▼ Most common: women—menstrual irregularities, a deepening voice, hairiness, acne, and enlargement of the clitoris. Men—breast soreness or enlargement, excessive erections, and skin reactions at the site of application.

▼ Common: men and women—swelling of the feet or lower legs, rapid weight gain, water retention, dizziness, headache, tiredness, flushing or redness, bleeding, nausea, vomiting, yellowing of the skin or whites of the eyes, confusion, depression, increased or decreased libido, thirst, increased urination, and constipation. Men—chills, pain in the scrotum or groin, prostate cancer, and difficult urination.

▼ Less common: men and women—mild acne, diarrhea, increased pubic hair, and difficulty sleeping. Men—impotence, irritation or infection of the skin of the scrotum, and decreased testicle size.

▼ Rare: men and women—male pattern baldness, oily skin, jaundice, and changes in liver function tests. Contact your doctor if you experience any side effect not listed above.

Drug Interactions

- Testosterone may increase the effects of anticoagulants (blood thinners) such as warfarin.
- Combining testosterone and imipramine (an antidepressant) may lead to a paranoid reaction.
- Testosterone may interfere with laboratory tests of thyroid function; it does not affect the thyroid gland or normal thyroid function.
- Consult with your doctor if you are taking insulin or other diabetes medications; corticosteroids; or oxyphenbutazone. You may require dosage adjustment or monitoring.

Food Interactions

You may take this drug with food if it upsets your stomach. Food does not interfere with testosterone skin patches or gel.

Usual Dose

Adult (age 18 and over):

Oral Tablets

Men: 10–50 mg a day.

Women: 50–200 mg a day.

Skin Patches: Apply nightly. Testoderm patches should be placed on clean, dry skin of the scrotum. Androderm is applied to clean, dry skin on your back, abdomen, upper arm, or thigh. Androderm dosage starts at one 5 mg or two 2.5 mg patches a night. Dosage may be adjusted to 1–3 patches nightly.

Topical Gel: Apply 5 g (1 tube) to shoulders, upper arms, and/or abdomen once daily to start. May increase to 10 g after 2 weeks. Do not wash site for at least 2 hours after applying.

Striant: Apply to the gums every 12 hours, holding in place for 30 seconds. Do not chew or swallow buccal tabs. Alternate sides of mouth with each application.

Child (under age 18): not recommended.

Overdosage

Symptoms resemble drug side effects. Call your local poison control center or a hospital emergency room for more information. If you seek treatment, ALWAYS bring the prescription package or container.

Special Information

If you develop nausea, vomiting, changes in skin color, or ankle swelling, contact your doctor right away.

Men should report to their doctor frequent or persistent erections, and adolescent males should have their bone development checked every 6 months.

If you are using a testosterone skin patch, apply it as directed by your doctor. The site of Androderm application should be rotated, with an interval of 7 days between application to the same site. The patch should not be applied to oily or irritated skin.

Testosterone gels are flammable and should not be used near an open flame or while smoking.

Take this drug exactly as prescribed. If you forget a dose, take it as soon as possible. If it is almost time for your next dose, skip the dose you forgot and continue with your regular schedule. Do not take a double dose.

Special Populations

Pregnancy/Breast-feeding: Testosterone is not safe for use during pregnancy. Taking this drug during pregnancy, especially during the first 3 months, results in excessive masculinization of the fetus.

It is not known if testosterone passes into breast milk. Nursing mothers who must take it should use infant formula.

Seniors: Seniors who take testosterone may have an increased risk of developing prostate disease, including cancer. A marked increase in sex drive may also develop.

Type of Drug

Tetracycline Antibiotics (teh-tra-SIKE-lene)

Brand Names

Generic Ingredient: Demeclocycline Hydrochloride Ⓖ
Declomycin

Generic Ingredient: Doxycycline Ⓖ

Atridox	Periostat
Doryx	Vibramycin
Monodox	Vibra-Tabs
Oracea	

Generic Ingredient: Minocycline Hydrochloride Ⓖ

Arestin	Minocin
Dynacin	Solodyn

Generic Ingredient: Tetracycline Hydrochloride Ⓖ

Bristacycline	Sumycin

Prescribed For

Infection, including methicillin-resistant Staphylococcus aureus (MRSA); some sexually transmitted diseases; infection of the mouth, gums, and teeth; severe acne; Rocky Mountain spotted fever and other types of fever caused by ticks and lice, including Lyme disease; urinary tract infection; and respiratory infection such as pneumonia or bronchitis. Doxycycline is also prescribed for malaria, rosacea, and to treat and prevent traveler's diarrhea. Tetracycline is also used to treat amebic dysentery. Low-dose tetracycline is the most widely prescribed antibiotic for acne.

General Information

Tetracycline antibiotics are effective against a variety of bacterial infections. They work by interfering with the normal growth cycle of the invading bacteria. This allows the body's normal defenses to fight off the infection. Tetracycline may be substituted for penicillin in people who are allergic to penicillin.

Tetracyclines have been used to treat skin infection but are not considered the first-choice antibiotic. Tetracyclines have been used successfully in the treatment of acne, in low dosages over a long period of time.

Cautions and Warnings

Do not take tetracycline antibiotics if you are **allergic** or **sensitive** to any of their ingredients. If you are allergic to one tetracycline antibiotic, you are probably allergic to them all.

Tetracyclines should not be given to people with **liver or kidney disease** or **certain urinary problems.**

If the antibiotic that your doctor has prescribed does not work, a number of things may have happened. You may not have taken the drug long enough. You may be the victim of a superinfection, in which another organism—usually a fungus—unaffected by the tetracycline antibiotic begins to grow in the same area as the bacteria being treated. If this happens, it may seem like a relapse or new infection. Only your doctor can determine which drug to take for it.

Avoid prolonged exposure to the sun if you are taking high dosages of tetracyclines, especially demeclocycline, because these antibiotics may interfere with your body's normal sun-screening mechanism, making you more prone to severe sunburn.

Tetracyclines should not be used by **children under age 8** because they have been shown to interfere with the development of the long bones and may retard growth. Permanent tooth discoloration may also result.

People taking demeclocycline may experience diabetes insipidus syndrome (symptoms include excessive thirst, urination, and weakness). The severity of this condition depends on the amount of drug taken and is reversible when the drug is withdrawn.

Minocycline may cause lightheadedness, dizziness, or fainting.

Tetracyclines have been associated with pseudotumor cerebri (a condition characterized by increased pressure in the brain—symptoms include headache and blurred vision).

Treatment with antibiotic medications such as tetracycline may cause diarrhea or, more seriously, colitis. Contact your doctor if you develop diarrhea while taking tetracyclines.

People taking doxycycline for **malaria** must understand that that no current antimalarial drug, including doxycycline, guarantees protection against malaria.

Possible Side Effects

▼ Most common: upset stomach, nausea, vomiting, diarrhea, sensitivity of the skin to the sun, and rash.

▼ Less common: hairy tongue and itching and irritation of the anal or vaginal region. If these symptoms appear, call your doctor immediately. Periodic physical examinations and laboratory tests should be given to those who are on long-term tetracycline antibiotic therapy.

▼ Rare: appetite loss, peeling skin, fever, chills, anemia, brown spotting of the skin, reduced kidney function, and liver damage. Contact your doctor if you experience any side effect not listed above.

Drug Interactions

- Tetracyclines may interfere with bactericidal (bacteria-killing) agents such as penicillin. You should not take both kinds of antibiotics for the same infection.
- Do not combine tetracyclines with isotretinoin or methoxyflurane.
- Antacids, mineral supplements, and multivitamins containing bismuth, calcium, zinc, magnesium, or iron may reduce the effectiveness of tetracyclines—with the exception of doxycycline and minocycline. Sodium bicarbonate powder may also be a problem if used as an antacid. Separate doses of an antacid, mineral supplement, vitamin with minerals, or sodium bicarbonate and a tetracycline antibiotic by at least 2 hours.
- Tetracyclines increase the effect of anticoagulant (blood-thinning) drugs such as warfarin. Your anticoagulant dosage may need an adjustment.
- Barbiturates, carbamazepine, and hydantoin antiseizure drugs may reduce doxycycline's effectiveness. More doxycycline or a different antibiotic may be required.

- Cimetidine, ranitidine, and other H_2-antagonists may reduce the effectiveness of tetracyclines.
- Tetracyclines may increase digoxin side effects in a small number of people. This effect may last for months after the tetracycline has been withdrawn. If you are taking this combination, be vigilant for the appearance of digoxin side effects; call your doctor if they develop.
- Tetracyclines may reduce insulin requirements for diabetics. If you are using this combination, be sure to carefully monitor your blood-sugar level.
- Tetracyclines may increase or decrease blood lithium levels.
- These drugs may reduce the effectiveness of contraceptive drugs. Breakthrough bleeding or pregnancy is possible; you should use another method of contraception in addition to a hormonal contraceptive while taking one of these antibiotics.

Food Interactions

Take all tetracycline antibiotics, except for doxycycline and minocycline, on an empty stomach, 1 hour before or 2 hours after meals, and with 8 oz. of water. The antibacterial effect of these antibiotics may be neutralized when they are taken with food, dairy products such as milk or cheese, or antacids. Doxycycline and minocycline may be taken with food or milk. Oracea, a particular brand of doxycycline, should be taken on an empty stomach.

Usual Dose

Demeclocycline
   Adult: 600 mg a day.
   Child (age 9 and over): 3–6 mg per lb. of body weight a day.
   Child (under age 9): not recommended.

Doxycycline
   Adult and Child (age 9 and over; over 100 lbs.): starting dosage—200 mg in 2 doses of 100 mg given 12 hours apart. Maintenance dosage—100 mg a day in 1 or 2 doses. Oracea—40 mg once a day in the morning. For gonorrhea, take 300 mg in 1 dose and then a second 300-mg dose in 1 hour, or 100 mg twice daily for at least 7 days; for syphilis, 100–300 mg for 10 days to 4 weeks. For malaria prevention, take 100 mg a day, beginning 1–2 days before you leave home. Take your medicine every day and continue for

4 weeks after leaving the malaria-infested area. Do not take doxy-cyline for more than 4 consecutive months.

Child (age 9 and over; under 100 lbs.): starting dosage—2 mg per lb. of body weight divided into 2 doses. Maintenance dosage—1 mg per lb. of body weight as a single daily dose. Child's dose for malaria prevention is 1 mg per lb. of body weight as a single daily dose.

Your doctor may double the maintenance dosage for severe in-fection. An increased incidence of side effects is observed with dosages over 200 mg a day.

Minocycline

Adult: starting dosage—200 mg. Maintenance dosage—100 mg every 12 hours. Alternate dosage: starting dosage—100–200 mg. Maintenance dosage—50 mg 4 times a day. Solodyn—45–135 mg a day.

Child (age 9 and over): starting dosage—2 mg per lb. of body weight. Maintenance dosage—1 mg per lb. every 12 hours.

Child (under age 9): not recommended.

Tetracycline

Adult: 250–500 mg 4 times a day.

Child (age 9 and over): 10–20 mg per lb. of body weight a day in 4 equal doses.

Child (under age 9): not recommended.

Tetracycline Ointment and Solution: Apply to affected area morning and night.

Overdosage

Overdose is most likely to affect the stomach and digestive sys-tem. Call your local poison control center or a hospital emergency room for more information. ALWAYS bring the prescription bottle or container.

Special Information

Do not take any antibiotic after the expiration date on the label. De-composed tetracycline may cause serious kidney damage.

Since the action of tetracyclines depends on its concentration within the invading bacteria, it is imperative that you completely follow the doctor's directions and complete the full course of treat-ment prescribed.

Call your doctor if you develop excessive thirst, urination, and weakness; blue-gray discoloration of the skin or mucous membranes (with minocycline); appetite loss; headache; vomiting; changes in vision; abdominal pain with nausea and vomiting; yellowing of the skin or whites of the eyes; or any persistent or intolerable side effect, including dizziness, lightheadedness, or unsteadiness; burning or cramps in the stomach; diarrhea with nausea and vomiting; or itching of the mouth, rectal, or vaginal areas (may indicate the presence of a superinfection). Call your doctor if your child develops tooth discoloration.

Avoid excessive exposure to the sun while taking tetracyclines, especially demeclocycline, because these drugs may cause susceptibility to sunburn.

Tetracyclines may cause dizziness, lightheadedness, or fainting. Be careful when driving or performing any task that requires concentration.

If you are using tetracycline antibiotic topical solution for acne, apply the product generously to your skin until the area to be treated is completely wet. Stinging or burning may occur, but this lasts only a few minutes. Tetracycline antibiotic solution may stain your skin yellow, but the stain usually washes away. Do not apply the solution or cream inside your eyes, nose, or mouth.

If you are taking a tetracycline to prevent malaria, avoid being bitten by mosquitoes by staying in well-screened areas, using mosquito nets, covering the body with clothing, and using an effective insect repellant.

If you miss a dose of an oral tetracycline, take it as soon as possible. If you take the drug once a day and it is almost time for your next dose, space the missed dose and your next dose 10–12 hours apart, then go back to your regular schedule. If you take tetracycline twice a day and it is almost time for your next dose, space the missed dose and your next dose by 5–6 hours, then go back to your regular schedule. If you take the drug 3 or more times a day and it is almost time for your next dose, space the missed dose and your next dose by 2–4 hours, then go back to your regular schedule. Never take a double dose.

Special Populations

Pregnancy/Breast-feeding: Tetracycline should not be taken if you are pregnant, especially during the last 5 months of pregnancy. It interferes with the formation of skull and bone structures in the fetus.

Tetracycline passes into breast milk. It interferes with the development of a child's skull, bones, and teeth. Nursing mothers who must take tetracycline should use infant formula.

Seniors: Seniors, especially those with poor kidney function, are more likely to experience less common side effects.

Generic Name

Thalidomide (thal-IH-doe-mide)

Brand Name
Thalomid

Type of Drug
Immune-system modulator.

Prescribed For
Erythema nodosum leprosum (ENL)—a painful skin condition associated with leprosy. May also be prescribed for multiple myeloma, a blood cancer.

General Information
Thalidomide was approved by the U.S. Food and Drug Administration (FDA) in 1998 for ENL under a very strict distribution system called S.T.E.P.S. (System for Thalidomide Education and Prescribing Safety), as this drug causes serious birth defects. Only doctors who are registered with the S.T.E.P.S. program can prescribe thalidomide. The exact way that thalidomide works is not known, but it appears to suppress excessive amounts of tumor necrosis factor (TNF) and also affects the movement of white blood cells. Thalidomide is also prescribed for leprosy, scleroderma, and other skin conditions, and is being studied for prostate and other cancers.

Cautions and Warnings
Do not use thalidomide if you are **allergic** or **sensitive** to any of its ingredients. A drug sensitivity or allergic reaction to thalidomide (symptoms include rash, fever, rapid heartbeat, and low blood pressure) may be cause to temporarily stop your treatment.

As little as 1 dose of thalidomide can cause birth defects. It should not be taken by **pregnant** women under any circumstances. Women must take a pregnancy test before the drug will be prescribed. Women of childbearing age should use contraceptives 4 weeks prior to, during, and 4 weeks following drug therapy, even if they have a history of infertility. Regular pregnancy tests should be administered throughout treatment. Men taking thalidomide can also transmit the drug through semen. These men should use a condom during intercourse with a pregnant partner or a woman of childbearing age, even if they have had a vasectomy. Using 2 methods of barrier contraception is preferred.

The use of thalidomide in treating multiple myeloma has been associated with an increased risk of developing blood clots, especially if dexamethasone and other drugs are also part of the treatment. Symptoms include shortness of breath, chest pain, or swelling of the arms and legs. Aspirin or another blood-thinning treatment can be used to counter this risk.

Thalidomide should not be used as the sole treatment for ENL by people with **neuritis** (nerve irritation).

Thalidomide frequently causes nerve damage (symptoms include numbness, tingling, or pain in the hands or feet) that may be permanent. It generally occurs after a few months of regular treatment but can also develop after taking thalidomide for a short time.

Thalidomide can cause a rapid drop in white-blood-cell count, increasing the risk of infection.

Thalidomide can increase the level of human immunodeficiency virus (HIV) RNA in people with **AIDS**, but the importance of this finding is unclear.

Thalidomide is generally not recommended for **children under age 18,** though a small number of children have been safely treated with the drug.

Possible Side Effects

▼ Most common: drowsiness, rash, dizziness, impotence, fainting, headache, and stomach pain.

▼ Common: muscle weakness; tingling, burning, numbness, or pain in the hands, arms, feet, or legs; tremors; constipation; diarrhea; nausea; mouth infections; sinus irritation; back pain; fever, alone or with chills and sore throat; infections; and feeling unwell.

▼ Less common: dry mouth, liver inflammation, gas, dry skin, mood change, leg swelling, acne, fungal skin infections,

Possible Side Effects *(continued)*

nail problems, itching, sweating, loss of appetite, tooth pain, anemia, low white-blood-cell count, swollen lymph glands, runny nose, abdominal pain, accidental injuries, and a rigid or painful neck.

▼ Rare: blood in the urine, decreased urination, irregular heartbeat, low blood pressure, and agitation. Other rare side effects can occur in almost any part of the body. Contact your doctor if you experience any side effect not listed above.

Drug Interactions

- Combining thalidomide with alcohol, barbiturates, chlorpromazine, reserpine, sedatives, tricyclic antidepressants, or other nervous system depressants can cause extreme tiredness. Avoid these combinations.
- Combining thalidomide and chloramphenicol, cisplatin, didanosine, ethambutol, ethionamide, hydralazine, isoniazid, lithium, metronidazole, nitrofurantoin, nitrous oxide, phenytoin, stavudine, or vincristine may worsen peripheral neuropathy (symptoms include tingling, burning, numbness, or pain in the hands or feet) or increase your risk of developing it.
- Mixing thalidomide with dexamethasone increases the risk of a life-threatening skin disease involving the separation of the top layer of skin from your body.
- Medications that interfere with contraceptive drugs must be avoided if you are taking thalidomide because they increase the risk of an unwanted pregnancy. These drugs include protease inhibitors—used in the treatment of HIV infection—griseofulvin, rifampin, rifabutin, phenytoin, and carbamazepine.

Food Interactions

For optimal effectiveness, do not take thalidomide with a high-fat meal.

Usual Dose

Adult: 100–400 mg a day at bedtime.
Child: not recommended.

Overdosage

Symptoms are likely to be common side effects. Take the victim to a hospital emergency room. ALWAYS bring the prescription bottle or container.

Special Information

Women of childbearing age who take thalidomide should have weekly pregnancy tests. Women with irregular periods may have to be tested every 2 weeks. Stop taking the drug at once if you are or think you may be pregnant.

Drowsiness is common with thalidomide. Be careful when driving or performing any task that requires concentration.

Thalidomide can make you dizzy or faint if you rise suddenly from a lying position. Sitting up for a few minutes before attempting to stand may help prevent this problem.

Contact your doctor if you experience shortness of breath, chest pain, arm or leg swelling, or numbness, tingling, or burning of the feet or hands.

People taking thalidomide may not donate blood or semen.

Thalidomide can increase your sensitivity to the sun. Use sunscreen and wear protective clothing while taking this drug.

Take this drug exactly as prescribed. Do not stop taking it without your doctor's knowledge. Do not share this medication with anyone else.

If you forget a dose, take it as soon as you remember. If it is almost time for your next dose, skip the one you forgot and continue with your regular schedule. Do not take a double dose.

Special Populations

Pregnancy/Breast-feeding: Women who are or might be pregnant should never take thalidomide, especially during the first 2 months of pregnancy. Women of childbearing age who take thalidomide should use 2 reliable methods of contraception (for example, a contraceptive drug and a condom). Contraception must be used for at least 1 month before treatment is begun, during treatment, and for 1 month after treatment has been completed.

It is not known if thalidomide passes into breast milk, but it could cause serious reactions in a nursing infant. Nursing mothers who must take thalidomide should use infant formula.

Seniors: Seniors may take this drug without special restriction.

Type of Drug

Thiazide Diuretics (THYE-uh-zide dye-ur-RET-iks)

Brand Names

Generic Ingredient: Chlorothiazide Ⓖ
Diuril

Generic Ingredient: Chlorthalidone Ⓖ
Thalitone

Generic Ingredient: Hydrochlorothiazide Ⓖ

Carozide	Loqua
Esidrix	Microzide
Ezide	Oretic
Hydro-Par	

Generic Ingredient: Hydroflumethiazide Ⓖ
Saluron

Generic Ingredient: Indapamide Ⓖ
Lozol

Generic Ingredient: Methyclothiazide Ⓖ
Enduron

Generic Ingredient: Metolazone
Zaroxolyn

Generic Ingredient: Polythiazide
Renese

Prescribed For

Edema associated with congestive heart failure (CHF), cirrhosis of the liver, kidney malfunction, hypertension (high blood pressure), and other conditions where it is necessary to rid the body of excess water.

General Information

Thiazide diuretics increase urine production by affecting the movement of sodium and chloride in the kidney. Thiazide diuretics reduce sodium, magnesium, bicarbonate, chloride, and potassium-ion levels. Calcium elimination is moderated and uric acid is retained as a result of thiazide treatment. Thiazide diuretics may also

raise blood sugar. These drugs are used in the treatment of any disease where it is desirable to eliminate large quantities of water.
Thiazide diuretics are often taken with other drugs to treat high
blood pressure and other conditions. The exact way in which they
reduce blood pressure is not known; sodium elimination is of primary importance. These diuretics begin to work within 2 hours and
produce their effect in 2–6 hours. The differences between thiazide
diuretic drugs lie in duration of effect—6–12 hours for some and
as long as 48–72 hours for others—and quantity of drug absorbed.

Cautions and Warnings

Do not take a thiazide diuretic if you are **allergic** or **sensitive** to
any of its ingredients, to any drugs in this group, or to sulfa drugs.
If you have a history of **allergy** or **bronchial asthma**, you may also
have a sensitivity or allergy to thiazide diuretics. Thiazide diuretics may aggravate **lupus erythematosus** (chronic condition affecting the body's connective tissue).

Thiazides may raise total cholesterol, low-density lipoprotein
(LDL) cholesterol, and total triglyceride levels. They should be used
with caution by people with moderate to high blood-cholesterol or
triglyceride levels. Thiazides should be used with caution if you
have severe **kidney disease** because they may precipitate kidney
failure; only metolazone and indapamide may be safely given in this
group. People with severe **liver disease** should be treated carefully with diuretics because minor changes in electrolyte (body-
fluid) balance may cause hepatic coma.

People with **diabetes** may experience increased blood-sugar
levels and will need dosage adjustments of their antidiabetic
medication.

Switching between brands of metolazone is not recommended.
They are not equivalent.

Possible Side Effects

▼ Most common: Thiazide diuretics cause loss of body potassium. Symptoms of low potassium include dry mouth,
   thirst, weakness, lethargy, drowsiness, restlessness, muscle pain or cramp, muscular tiredness, low blood pressure,
   decreased frequency of urination and decreased urine production, abnormal heart rate, and upset stomach including

Possible Side Effects *(continued)*

nausea and vomiting. Potassium supplements are given to prevent this problem—or you may eat high-potassium foods such as bananas, citrus fruits, melons, and tomatoes.

▼ Less common: appetite loss, abdominal pain, bloating, diarrhea, constipation, dizziness, yellowing of the skin or whites of the eyes, headache, tingling of the toes and fingers, restlessness, changes in blood composition, increased sensitivity to the sun, rash, itching, fever, breathing difficulties, allergic reaction, dizziness when rising quickly from a sitting or lying position, muscle spasm, impotence and reduced sex drive, and blurred vision.

Drug Interactions

- Thiazide diuretics increase the action of other blood-pressure-lowering drugs. Consequently, people with high blood pressure often take more than 1 drug.
- The risk of developing imbalances in electrolytes is increased if you take medicines such as digitalis drugs, amphotericin B, and adrenal corticosteroids while taking a thiazide diuretic.
- If you begin taking a thiazide diuretic, your insulin or antidiabetic dosage may have to be modified.
- Thiazide diuretics may increase the risk of allopurinol side effects.
- Thiazide diuretics may decrease the effects of oral anticoagulant (blood-thinning) drugs.
- Antigout drug dosage may have to be modified since thiazide diuretics raise blood uric-acid levels.
- Thiazide diuretics may prolong the white-blood-cell-reducing effects of chemotherapy drugs.
- Thiazide diuretics may increase the effects of diazoxide, leading to symptoms of diabetes.
- Combining thiazide diuretics and loop diuretics may lead to an extreme diuretic effect and extreme effect on blood-electrolyte levels.
- Thiazide diuretics may increase the action of vitamin D, possibly leading to high blood-calcium levels.
- Propantheline and other anticholinergics may increase the effects of thiazide diuretics.

- Thiazide diuretics increase the risk of lithium side effects.
- Cholestyramine and colestipol block the absorption of thiazide diuretics. Thiazide diuretics should be taken more than 2 hours before cholestyramine or colestipol.
- Methenamine and other urinary agents may reduce the effect of thiazide diuretics.
- Certain nonsteroidal anti-inflammatory drugs (NSAIDs), particularly indomethacin, may reduce the effectiveness of thiazide diuretics. Sulindac, another NSAID, may increase the effect of thiazide diuretics.
- Dosage adjustments of anesthetics may be required while taking thiazide diuretics.

Food Interactions

Thiazide diuretics may be taken with food if they upset your stomach. Your doctor may recommend high-potassium foods like bananas and orange juice to offset the potassium-lowering effect of these drugs.

Usual Dose

Chlorothiazide

Adult: 0.5–1 g 1–2 times a day. Often people respond to intermittent therapy, that is, taking the drug on alternate days or 3–5 days a week. This reduces side effects.

Child (age 6 months and over): 5–10 mg per lb. of body weight a day in 2 equal doses.

Child (under age 6 months): not more than 15 mg per lb. of body weight a day in 2 equal doses.

Chlorthalidone

Adult: 25–100 mg (Thalitone, 30–60 mg) a day, or 100 mg (Thalitone, 60 mg) on alternate days. Some patients may need 150–200 mg (Thalitone, 90–120 mg) at these intervals, or 120 mg Thalitone daily. Hypertension—25 mg (Thalitone, 15 mg) daily, increased if necessary to 50–100 mg (Thalitone, 30–50 mg) once a day.

Child: not recommended.

Hydrochlorothiazide

Adult: 25–200 mg a day depending on the condition being treated. Maintenance dosage—25–100 mg a day. 200 mg a day is sometimes required.

Child (age 6 months and over): 0.5–1 mg per lb. of body weight a day in 2 doses.

Child (under age 6 months): not more than 1.5 mg per lb. of body weight a day in 2 doses.

Hydroflumethiazide
Adult: starting dosage—50–200 mg 1–2 times a day. Maintenance dosage—25–50 mg a day. Daily dosages of more than 100 mg should be divided into separate doses.
Child: not recommended.

Indapamide: 1.25–2.5 mg every morning. Dosage may be increased to 5 mg a day.

Methyclothiazide: 2.5–10 mg a day.

Metolazone: Dosage is individualized. 0.5–20 mg once a day, depending on formulation. Do not switch formulations of metolazone without consulting your doctor.

Polythiazide: 1–4 mg a day.

Overdosage
Symptoms include tingling in the arms or legs, weakness, fatigue, fainting, dizziness, changes in heartbeat, feeling unwell, dry mouth, restlessness, muscle pain or cramp, urinary difficulties, nausea, and vomiting. Take the victim to a hospital emergency room at once. ALWAYS bring the prescription bottle or container.

Special Information
Ordinarily, diuretics are prescribed early in the day to prevent excessive nighttime urination from interfering with sleep.

Thiazide diuretics cause excess urination at first but it subsides after several weeks.

Contact your doctor if you develop muscle pain, sudden joint pain, weakness, cramps, nausea, vomiting, restlessness, excessive thirst, tiredness, drowsiness, increased heart or pulse rate, diarrhea, or dizziness.

Avoid alcohol and other medications while taking a thiazide diuretic, unless directed by your doctor.

Avoid over-the-counter medications for the treatment of coughs, colds, and allergy if you have hypertension or CHF because such medication may contain stimulants.

Thiazide diuretics may cause sensitivity to sunlight. Use sunscreen and wear protective clothing if necessary.

If you forget a dose, take it as soon as you remember. If it is almost time for your next dose, skip the one you forgot and continue with your regular schedule. Do not take a double dose.

Special Populations

Pregnancy/Breast-feeding: Thiazide diuretics enter the fetal circulation and may cause side effects in the newborn such as jaundice, blood problems, and low potassium levels. Diuretics are used to treat specific medical conditions during pregnancy but their routine use during a normal pregnancy is improper. When any of these drugs is considered crucial by your doctor, its potential benefits must be carefully weighed against its risks.

Thiazide diuretics pass into breast milk. Nursing mothers who must take diuretics should use infant formula.

Seniors: Seniors are more likely to have reduced kidney function. Since these drugs leave the body through the kidneys, seniors should use the lowest effective dose and be aware of the possibility of increased side effects, especially dizziness.

Thyroid Hormone Replacements

Brand Names

Generic Ingredient: Levothyroxine Sodium Ⓖ

Levo-T	Synthroid
Levolet*	Thyro-Tabs*
Levothroid	Tirosint*
Levoxyl	Unithroid
Novothyrox*	

*no generic equivalent

Generic Ingredient: Liothyronine Sodium Ⓖ

Cytomel	Triostat

Generic Ingredient: Liotrix Ⓖ
Thyrolar

Generic Ingredient: Thyroid Hormone Ⓖ

Armour Thyroid	Thyrar
S-P-T	Thyroid Strong

Prescribed For

Hypothyroidism (underactive thyroid gland).

General Information

The major differences between these drugs are their sources and hormone content. Thyroid hormone is made from beef and pork thyroid. It is effective but lacks standardization, making it difficult for doctors to control dosage. Synthetic drugs are more desirable because their content is easily standardized, ensuring that you receive the correct amount of hormone.

Basically, there are 2 important thyroid hormones: levothyroxine and liothyronine. Levothyroxine is converted to liothyronine in the body. This process slows the absorption of levothyroxine and lowers the risk of side effects. Liothyronine's potency and its potential for side effects make it less desirable for older adults. Liotrix contains both levothyroxine and liothyronine; since levothyroxine is converted naturally to liothyronine, there is usually no advantage in taking both hormones unless there is a problem with the conversion process. These considerations tend to make levothyroxine the treatment of choice for thyroid hormone replacement.

Cautions and Warnings

Do not use a thyroid hormone replacement if you are **allergic** or **sensitive** to any of its ingredients or to pork.

Thyroid hormone replacements have been prescribed for **weight loss.** Thyroid treatments do not work in people with a normal thyroid status unless large dosages are used—these dosages may produce serious or fatal side effects, especially when taken with appetite-suppressing drugs.

Women, especially post-menopausal women, on long-term thyroid replacement therapy can develop reduced bone density. Using the lowest effective dose helps avoid this effect.

If you have **hyperthyroid disease** (symptoms include headache, nervousness, sweating, rapid heartbeat, chest pain, and other signs of central-nervous-system stimulation) or **high output of thyroid hormone,** you should not use these drugs.

If you have **heart disease** or **hypertension** (high blood pressure), thyroid hormone replacement therapy should not be used unless it is clearly indicated and supervised by your doctor, as it can aggravate the condition. If you develop chest pain or other signs of heart disease while taking this drug, call your doctor immediately.

These drugs should not be used to treat **infertility** unless the person also has hypothyroidism.

Thyroid hormone replacement therapy increases metabolism and may worsen the symptoms of other endocrine system (hormone-related) diseases including **diabetes** and **Addison's disease.** Adjustments in the levels of treatment for these diseases may be needed when you begin using these drugs.

Multiple generic brands of levothyroxine have been approved for use in the U.S. However, unlike other generic products, not all levothyroxine products are equivalent to one another. Three (Levolet, Novothyrox, and Thyro-Tabs) have no acceptable equivalent at all. For this reason, you should not change brands of levothyroxine unless your doctor or pharmacist has verified the equivalency because you may unknowingly switch to a non-equivalent product.

Possible Side Effects

Side effects are rare except during the start of therapy or when dosage is adjusted.

▼ Most common: heart palpitations, rapid heartbeat, abnormal heart rhythms, weight loss, chest pain, hand tremor, headache, diarrhea, nervousness, menstrual irregularity, inability to sleep, sweating, intolerance to heat, and hair loss. These symptoms may be controlled by adjusting dosage.

Drug Interactions

- Antacids, calcium and iron supplements, simethicone, sucralfate, colestipol, and cholestyramine may interfere with the passage of these drugs into the bloodstream. Take your thyroid hormone replacement and these drugs 4–6 hours apart.
- The following drugs may reduce the natural production of thyroid hormone, increasing the need for thyroid replacement: lithium, methimazole, propylthiouracil (PTU), sulfa drugs, and tolbutamide. Amiodarone has been reported to both decrease and increase the production of thyroid hormone.
- Raloxifene interferes with the absorption of levothyroxine. Separate these medicines by 12 hours.
- Avoid taking over-the-counter drugs that contain stimulants— such as many of the products used to treat cough, cold, or

allergy—which affect the heart and may cause symptoms of overdose.

- People with diabetes may need to have their doctors increase their insulin or oral antidiabetic drug dosages when they start taking a thyroid hormone replacement.
- These drugs may reduce the effectiveness of beta blockers. Beta-blocker dosage may need to be increased.
- Dosage reduction of theophylline may be required if you take a thyroid hormone replacement.
- Interferon drugs may reduce thyroid function, increasing or creating the need for thyroid replacement hormone.
- Blood levels of digoxin and similar drugs, and their effectiveness, may be reduced by thyroid hormone replacements.
- Use of carbamazapine, phenytoin, and phenobarbital, may result in a need for increased dosages of levothyroxine.
- Combining tricyclic or SSRI antidepressants with levothyroxine may increase the risk of toxic effects of both drugs.
- These drugs increase the breakdown of vitamin K blood-clotting factors. Anticoagulant dose may have to be reduced.

Food Interactions

Thyroid hormone replacements should be taken as a single dose, preferably at least 30 minutes before breakfast.

Usual Dose

Levothyroxine: starting dosage—as little as 12.5 mcg a day, which is then increased in steps of 12.5–25 mcg once every 2–8 weeks depending upon response. Maintenance dosage—100–300 mcg a day. It is essential to take levothyroxine at the same time each day.

Liothyronine
Adult: 5–100 mcg a day.
Senior and Child: Begin at the low end of the dosage range and increase slowly until the desired effect has been achieved.

Liotrix
Adult: ¼–2 tablets a day, depending on the condition being treated and your response to therapy. Liotrix tablets are rated according to their approximate equivalent to thyroid hormone.
Senior and Child: Begin at the low end of the dosage range and increase slowly until the desired effect has been achieved.

Thyroid Hormone: starting dosage—30 mg a day, which is then increased in 15-mg steps every 2–3 weeks until response is satisfactory. Maintenance dosage—30–120 mg a day.

Overdosage

Symptoms include headache; irritability; nervousness; sweating; rapid heartbeat with unusual stomach rumbling—with or without cramps; chest pain; heart failure; and shock. Take the victim to a hospital emergency room immediately. ALWAYS bring the prescription bottle or container.

Special Information

Thyroid hormone replacement therapy is usually a lifelong treatment, and requires periodic monitoring. Take the drug as prescribed and do not stop taking it unless instructed by your doctor.

Do not switch brands, especially in the case of levothyroxine, without your doctor's or pharmacist's knowledge. Different brands of the same thyroid hormone replacement are not always equivalent.

Many drugs have been reported to affect thyroid hormone levels. Make sure your doctor is aware of every prescription or nonprescription drug and supplement you are taking.

Call your doctor if you develop nervousness, diarrhea, excessive sweating, chest pain, increased pulse rate, heart palpitations, and intolerance to heat—which are signs you may be taking too high a dose—or any bothersome or persistent side effect.

Children beginning thyroid hormone replacement therapy may lose some hair during the first few months, but this is only temporary and the hair generally grows back.

If you forget a dose, take it as soon as you remember. If it is almost time for your next dose, skip the one you forgot and continue with your regular schedule. Do not take a double dose. Call your doctor if you miss 2 or more consecutive doses.

Special Populations

Pregnancy/Breast-feeding: Small amounts of these drugs enter the fetal bloodstream. These medications have not been associated with any problems when used to maintain normal thyroid function in the mother. Pregnant women who have been taking a thyroid hormone replacement should continue their treatment under medical supervision.

Small amounts of these drugs pass into breast milk. Nursing mothers who must take them should consider using infant formula.

Seniors: Seniors, who may be more sensitive to the effects of these drugs, generally require reduced dosage.

Generic Name

Tiagabine (tye-AG-a-bene)

Brand Name

Gabitril

The information in this profile also applies to the following drug:

Generic Ingredient: Gabapentin
Neurontin

Type of Drug

Anticonvulsant and analgesic (pain reliever).

Prescribed For

Partial seizures. Gabapentin may also be used for pain after herpes zoster (shingles) infection, tremors associated with multiple sclerosis, nerve pain, bipolar disorder, hot flashes in women receiving chemotherapy for breast cancer, and for the prevention of migraine headaches.

General Information

The exact way in which tiagabine works is not known but may be related to its ability to improve the activity of GABA, the major inhibitor of nerve transmission in the brain and central nervous system (CNS). This means that tiagabine probably slows GABA-related nerve impulses that lead to a seizure. The medication achieves maximum blood levels in 45 minutes. It is broken down in the liver.

Tiagabine is only prescribed as additional therapy for those already taking other antiepileptic drugs.

Gabapentin is related to GABA, but it does not modify GABA in the body. It may bind directly to receptors in the brain, but has no effect on those receptors commonly affected by other drugs that act on the central nervous system.

Cautions and Warnings

Do not take this drug if you are **allergic** or **sensitive** to any of its ingredients. Several people taking tiagabine have developed a severe rash.

Tiagabine has been associated with seizure development in people without epilepsy. In most cases, those who experienced seizures were also taking other medications including antidepressants, antipsychotics, stimulants, or narcotics. Seizures may also occur with dose increase. If seizures occur in people taking tiagabine who have not had them prior to treatment, the drug should be stopped and patients should be evaluated for an underlying seizure disorder.

People with **liver disease** should take this drug with caution and receive reduced dosages. People with **kidney disease** may require reduced dosages of gabapentin.

Suddenly stopping any antiepileptic drug can increase the chance of a seizures. Dosage should be reduced gradually.

In studies, a small number of people died suddenly while taking gabapentin. It is not known if these deaths were caused by the drug.

A feeling of severe weakness has developed in a small number of people taking tiagabine. The weakness goes away when the medication is reduced or stopped.

Tiagabine may bind to parts of the eye. There is no evidence that this produces long-term effects. Tell your doctor if you experience any changes in vision.

Possible Side Effects

Tiagabine
- ▼ Most common: dizziness, sleepiness, confusion, depression, weakness, nervousness, and nausea.
- ▼ Common: poor concentration, speech or language problems, abdominal or other pain, tremor, sleeplessness, diarrhea, vomiting, sore throat, and rash.
- ▼ Less common: forgetfulness, tingling in the hands or feet, emotional upset, walking unusually, hostility, visual disturbances, agitation, hunger, mouth sores, cough, itching, and flushing.

Gabapentin
- ▼ Most common: tiredness, dizziness, and peripheral edema.
- ▼ Common: fatigue, double vision, blurred vision, and tremors.
- ▼ Less common: weight gain, back pain, upset stomach, dry mouth or throat, constipation, dental problems, muscle aches, runny nose, sore throat, speech problems, memory

---

Possible Side Effects (continued)

loss, depression, abnormal thinking, twitching, itching, abrasions, impotence, and visual disturbances.

▼ Rare: leg swelling, increased appetite, broken bones, poor coordination, low red- and white-blood-cell counts, and flushing. Contact your doctor if you experience any side effect not listed above.

Drug Interactions

- Taking tiagabine with other medications for seizure control, including carbamazepine, phenytoin, phenobarbital, and valproate may affect the amount of each in the blood. Dosage adjustments may be necessary.
- Taking gabapentin with naproxen may increase gabapentin levels in the blood.
- Antacids reduce the absorption of gabapentin; take these drugs at least 2 hours apart.
- Combining gabapentin and hydrocodone may affect each other's blood levels.
- Morphine significantly increases blood levels of gabapentin.

Food Interactions

Take tiagabine with food, but avoid high-fat meals, which slow its absorption. Gabapentin may be taken with or without food.

Usual Dose

Tiagabine

Adult (age 19 and over): starting dosage—4 mg once a day. Dosage may be increased in steps of 4 or 8 mg to 56 mg a day in divided doses.

Child (age 12–18): starting dosage—4 mg once a day. Dosage may be increased in steps of 4 or 8 mg to 32 mg a day in divided doses.

Gabapentin

Adult and Child (age 12 and over): 300–600 mg 3 times a day. Dosage must be reduced in people with kidney disease.

Child (age 3–12): 4.5–7 mg per lb. a day in 3 divided doses to start, increasing gradually over a period of about 3 days to a maximum of 22 mg per lb. a day in divided doses.

Child (under age 3): not recommended.

Overdosage

Tiagabine: Symptoms include tiredness, loss of consciousness, agitation, confusion, difficulty talking, hostility, depression, weakness, and muscle spasm.

Gabapentin: Symptoms include double vision, slurred speech, drowsiness, diarrhea, lethargy, weakness, breathing difficulties, sedation, droopy eyelids, and excitation.

Take the victim to a hospital emergency room. ALWAYS bring the prescription bottle or container.

Special Information

This drug may make you dizzy or tired, or interfere with your concentration. Be extremely careful when driving or performing any task that requires concentration. Avoid alcohol or other nervous system depressants because they increase these effects.

Tell your doctor if you experience changes in vision, rash, or any bothersome or persistent side effect.

If you forget a dose, take it as soon as you remember. If it is almost time for your next dose, take the dose you forgot and space the remaining daily dosage evenly throughout the day. Do not take a double dose.

Special Populations

Pregnancy/Breast-feeding: This medication causes birth defects in laboratory animals. Seizure disorder itself has been associated with an increased risk of birth defects. Discuss with your doctor the need to control seizures and the potential benefits and risks of taking this medication during pregnancy.

Tiagabine may pass into breast milk. It is not known if gabapentin does. Nursing mothers who must take either drug should consider using infant formula.

Seniors: Seniors may take tiagabine without special precaution but may require reduced dosage of gabapentin.

Generic Name

Ticlopidine (tih-KLOE-pih-dene) Ⓖ

Brand Name

Ticlid

Type of Drug

Anticoagulant (blood thinner).

Prescribed For

Reducing risk of stroke; also used to treat intermittent claudication and chronic circulatory occlusion, and to reduce the damage caused by stroke. It is used before open heart surgery to reduce the expected drop in platelet count, during coronary artery bypass surgery or stent placement to improve the chance of success, in some forms of kidney disease to help improve kidney function, and in sickle cell disease to reduce the number and severity of sickle cell attacks.

General Information

Ticlopidine hydrochloride makes blood platelets less "sticky," reducing the risk of blood clotting and the possible consequences of clot formation. It interferes with the functioning of the platelet cell membrane, changing platelet cells irreversibly until they are replaced by new ones. Maximum effect (60–70% reduction in platelet function) is seen 8–11 days after administration of 250 mg of ticlopidine twice a day. In studies, people taking ticlopidine regularly for 2–5 years experienced a 24% reduction in incidence of stroke.

Cautions and Warnings

Do not take ticlopidine if you are **allergic** or **sensitive** to any of its ingredients or have an **active bleeding site such as an ulcer, reduced blood-cell counts,** or severe **liver disease**.

Ticlopidine can cause severe reductions in white-blood-cell counts, greatly increasing the risk of infection. Some cases have been fatal. Your doctor should take white-blood-cell counts 2 weeks after you begin taking ticlopidine and continue testing every 2 weeks for the first 3 months of treatment. Only people showing signs of infection need to be tested after that period. Blood counts usually return to normal 1–3 weeks after you stop taking the drug.

Blood-platelet counts can also be depressed, leading to spontaneous bruising or bleeding. Gastrointestinal (GI) bleeding can also worsen during use of ticlopidine.

Rarely, a potentially fatal syndrome called thrombotic thrombocytopenic purpura (TTP) can occur in people taking ticlopidine. Early signs of TTP are yellow skin or eye color, pinpoint dots (rash) on the skin, fever, weakness on one side of the body, or dark urine. Contact your doctor immediately if you develop any of these symptoms.

Ticlopidine causes an 8–10% increase in blood cholesterol within a month after you start taking the drug.

People being switched from an anticoagulant or thrombolytic to ticlopidine should stop the former drug and allow it to clear the system before starting ticlopidine.

People with severe **kidney disease** may need less ticlopidine.

Possible Side Effects

Side effects occur in more than 50% of all people. About 21% of ticlopidine patients stop taking the drug because of GI side effects.

▼ Most common: diarrhea, nausea, upset stomach, rash, and stomach pain.

▼ Less common: reduced white-blood-cell counts, vomiting, bruising, gas, itching, dizziness, appetite loss, and liver function changes.

Drug Interactions

- Antacids reduce the absorption of ticlopidine. Separate doses by at least 1 hour.
- Taking cimetidine on a regular basis can reduce the clearance of ticlopidine from the body by 50%, increasing the risk of drug toxicity and side effects.
- Combining aspirin and ticlopidine may increase the risk of bleeding. Do not combine these drugs.
- Ticlopidine may slightly reduce blood levels of digoxin. This is not a problem for most people, but dosage adjustment may be needed.
- Ticlopidine reduces the body's clearance of theophylline; your doctor may need to reduce your theophylline dosage.
- Ticlopidine increases the effects of phenytoin and tizanidine. Use caution if taking these drugs simultaneously.

Food Interactions

Ticlopidine should be taken with meals to reduce stomach upset and maximize absorption of the drug. Take it at the same time each day to gain maximum benefit.

Usual Dose

250 mg taken twice a day with food.

Overdosage

Overdose may lead to increased bleeding and liver inflammation. Other possible effects include stomach bleeding, convulsions, breathing difficulties, and low body temperature. Take the victim to a hospital emergency room. ALWAYS bring the prescription bottle or container.

Special Information

Call your doctor if you have fever, chills, sore throat, or other indication of infection; weakness; difficulty speaking; severe or persistent diarrhea; rash; bleeding under the skin; yellowing of the skin or whites of the eyes; dark urine; light-colored stools; or any bothersome or persistent side effect.

Bleeding may be more difficult to stop if you are taking ticlopidine. Be sure your doctor, dentist, and other health care professionals know that you are taking this medication.

If you miss a dose, take it as soon as you can. If it is 4 hours or less until your next dose, skip the missed dose and continue with your regular schedule. Do not take a double dose.

Special Populations

Pregnancy/Breast-feeding: The safety of using ticlopidine during pregnancy is not known. When this drug is considered crucial by your doctor, its potential benefits must be carefully weighed against its risks.

Ticlopidine may pass into breast milk. Nursing mothers who must take it should use infant formula.

Seniors: Seniors may be more sensitive to the effects of ticlopidine.

Generic Name

Timolol (TIM-oe-lol) Ⓖ

Brand Names

Betimol   Istalol
Timoptic

Combination Products

Generic Ingredients: Bendroflumethiazide + Nadolol
Corzide

Generic Ingredients: Dorzolamide + Timolol
Cosopt

The information in this profile also applies to the following drugs:

Generic Ingredient: Nadolol [G]
Corgard

Generic Ingredient: Sotalol [G]
Betapace   Sorine
Betapace AF

Type of Drug

Beta-adrenergic blocking agent.

Prescribed For

High blood pressure, abnormal heart rhythms, prevention of second heart attack or migraine, tremors, stage fright and other anxieties, open-angle glaucoma, and ocular hypertension.

General Information

Timolol is one of many beta-adrenergic blocking drugs, or beta blockers, that interfere with the action of a specific part of the nervous system. Beta receptors are found all over the body and affect many body functions. Each beta blocker has particular characteristics that make it more suitable for certain conditions or people. When applied as eyedrops, timolol reduces ocular pressure (pressure inside the eye) by reducing the production of eye fluids and by slightly increasing the rate at which these fluids flow through and leave the eye.

Cautions and Warnings

Do not take timolol if you are **allergic** or **sensitive** to any of its ingredients or to beta blockers.

You should be cautious about taking timolol if you have **asthma, severe heart failure,** a **very slow heart rate,** or **heart block** (disruption of the electrical impulses that control heart rate) because the drug may aggravate these conditions.

People with **angina** who take timolol for high blood pressure risk aggravating their angina if they suddenly stop taking the drug. These people should have their drug dosage reduced gradually over 1–2 weeks.

Timolol should be used with caution if you have **liver or kidney disease** because your ability to eliminate the drug from your body may be impaired.

People with **asthma** should use timolol with caution, as it may worsen asthma symptoms.

Solatol can increase the risk of ventricular arrhythmias, which are sometimes fatal.

Timolol reduces the amount of blood pumped by the heart with each beat. This reduction in blood flow may aggravate the condition of people with **poor circulation** or **circulatory disease**.

If you are undergoing major surgery, your doctor may want you to stop taking timolol at least 2 days before surgery.

Timolol eyedrops should not be used by people who cannot tolerate oral beta-blocking drugs, such as propranolol.

People with a history of **severe anaphylactic reaction** to allergens may be unresponsive to usual doses of epinephrine while take beta blockers.

Possible Side Effects

Side effects are relatively uncommon and usually mild.

▼ Less common: impotence, unusual tiredness or weakness, slow heartbeat, heart failure, dizziness, breathing difficulties, bronchospasm, depression, confusion, anxiety, nervousness, sleeplessness, disorientation, short-term memory loss, emotional instability, cold hands and feet, constipation, diarrhea, nausea, vomiting, upset stomach, increased sweating, urinary difficulties, cramps, blurred vision, rash, hair loss, stuffy nose, facial swelling, aggravation of lupus erythematosus, itching, chest pain, back or joint pain, colitis, drug allergy (symptoms include fever and sore throat), and liver toxicity.

Drug Interactions

- Timolol may interact with surgical anesthetics to increase the risk of heart problems during surgery. Some anesthesiologists recommend gradually stopping the drug by 2 days before surgery.
- Timolol may interfere with the signs of low blood sugar and with the action of oral antidiabetes drugs.
- Timolol increases the blood-pressure-lowering effects of other blood-pressure-reducing agents, including clonidine, guanabenz, and reserpine; and calcium channel blockers such as nifedipine.
- Aspirin-containing drugs, indomethacin, sulfinpyrazone, and estrogen drugs may interfere with the blood-pressure-lowering effect of timolol.

- Cocaine may reduce the effectiveness of all beta blockers.
- Timolol may worsen the problem of cold hands and feet associated with ergot alkaloids, used to treat migraine. Gangrene is a possibility in people taking both an ergot and timolol.
- Timolol will counteract thyroid hormone replacements.
- Calcium channel blockers, flecainide, hydralazine, contraceptive drugs, propafenone, haloperidol, phenothiazine sedatives (molindone and others), quinolone antibacterials, and quinidine may increase the amount of timolol in the bloodstream and lead to increased timolol effects.
- Timolol should not be taken within 2 weeks of taking a monoamine oxidase inhibitor antidepressant.
- Cimetidine increases the amount of timolol absorbed into the bloodstream from oral tablets.
- Timolol may interfere with the effectiveness of some antiasthma drugs including theophylline and aminophylline, and especially ephedrine and isoproterenol.
- Combining timolol and phenytoin or digitalis drugs may result in excessive slowing of the heart, possibly causing heart block.
- If you stop smoking while taking timolol, your dose may have to be reduced because your liver will break down the drug more slowly afterward.
- Aluminum salts, barbiturates, calcium salts, cholestyramine, colestipol, ampicillin, and rifampin may reduce the effectiveness of timolol.
- Beta blockers may block the effects of epinephrine.

Food Interactions
None known.

Usual Dose
Bendroflumethiazide + Nadolol: starting dosage—2.5–20 mg a day, either in 1 dose or divided into 2 doses. Maintenance dosage—2.5–5 mg a day.

Dorzolamide + Timolol: 1 drop in the affected eye(s) twice a day.

Timolol: 10–60 mg a day divided into 2 doses. For eyedrops, put 1 drop in the affected eye(s) twice a day.

Nadolol: 40–80 mg a day.

Sotalol: 80 mg twice a day.

Overdosage

Symptoms include changes in heartbeat—unusually slow, unusually fast, or irregular—severe dizziness or fainting, breathing difficulties, bluish-colored fingernails or palms, and seizures. The victim should be taken to a hospital emergency room. ALWAYS bring the prescription bottle or container.

Special Information

Timolol is taken continuously. Do not stop taking this drug unless directed to do so by your doctor. Abrupt withdrawal may cause chest pain, breathing difficulties, increased sweating, and unusually fast or irregular heartbeat. When ending timolol treatment, dosage should be reduced gradually over a period of about 2 weeks.

Call your doctor at once if you develop back or joint pain, breathing difficulties, cold hands or feet, depression, rash, or changes in heartbeat. Timolol may produce an undesirable lowering of blood pressure, leading to dizziness or fainting; call your doctor if this happens to you. Call your doctor if you experience persistent or bothersome anxiety, diarrhea, constipation, impotence, headache, itching, nausea or vomiting, nightmares or vivid dreams, upset stomach, trouble sleeping, stuffy nose, frequent urination, unusual tiredness, or weakness.

Timolol can cause drowsiness, dizziness, lightheadedness, or blurred vision. Be careful when driving or performing complex tasks.

It is best to take timolol at the same time each day. If you forget a dose, take it as soon as you remember. If you take timolol twice a day and it is within 4 hours of your next dose, skip the dose you forgot and continue with your regular schedule. Do not take a double dose.

If you forget a dose of timolol eyedrops, administer it as soon as you remember. If it is almost time for your next dose, skip the dose you forgot and continue with your regular schedule. Do not take a double dose.

Special Populations

Pregnancy/Breast-feeding: Infants born to women who took a beta blocker while pregnant had lower birth weights, low blood pressure, and reduced heart rates. Timolol should be avoided by pregnant women.

Timolol passes into breast milk. Nursing mothers who must use it should use infant formula.

Seniors: Seniors may require less of the drug to achieve results. Seniors taking timolol may be more likely to suffer from cold hands and feet, reduced body temperature, chest pain, general feelings of ill health, sudden breathing difficulties, sweating, or changes in heartbeat.

Generic Name

Tipranavir (tih-PRAN-uh-vere)

Brand Name
Aptivus

Type of Drug
Protease inhibitor.

Prescribed For
Advanced human immunodeficiency virus (HIV) infection.

General Information
Tipranavir is prescribed for people with HIV resistant to other drugs. Part of the multidrug "cocktail" responsible for important gains in the fight against acquired immunodeficiency syndrome (AIDS), tipranavir is a member of a group of anti-HIV drugs called protease inhibitors. It is unique because it can enter infected immune cells and work against many strains of HIV that are resistant to other protease inhibitors. Protease inhibitors work at the end of the HIV virus reproduction process, when proteins are "cut" into strands of exactly the correct size to duplicate HIV. An enzyme known as protease cuts the protein. Protease inhibitors prevent the mature HIV virus from being formed by inhibiting this cutting process. Proteins that are cut to the wrong length or those that remain uncut are inactive.

Protease inhibitors revolutionized HIV treatment because, when taken in combination, they reduce the amount of HIV virus in the bloodstream to levels that are often undetectable by current methods—CD_4 (immune system) counts and viral load (amount of virus in the blood) measurements. Multiple-drug therapy has changed the view of HIV from a fatal disease to a manageable chronic illness. However, drug resistance is one of the major challenges that patients and doctors face in the treatment of HIV. Resistance develops when the virus mutates and is no longer suppressed by drugs that were once effective.

Protease inhibitors are always taken with 1 or 2 nucleoside antiviral drugs such as efavirenz, emtricitabine, lamivudine, tenofovir, or zidovudine (AZT). When added to enfurvitide, an HIV fusion inhibitor, the anti-HIV benefit was substantially improved. This drug must also be combined with ritonavir, another protease inhibitor that raises blood levels of tipranavir in the blood by slowing tipranavir's breakdown in the liver.

Cautions and Warnings

Do not take tipranavir if you are **allergic** or **sensitive** to any of its ingredients. Tipranavir is a sulfa drug and people with a **sulfa allergy** may also be allergic to tipranavir.

Tipranavir is broken down in the liver. The combination of tipranavir and ritonavir has been associated with hepatitis B or C and rapid loss of liver function in people with **liver disease,** including some fatalities. Liver function tests must be done when you start treatment and frequently while you are taking the drug. If you develop symptoms of liver problems, such as fatigue, loss of appetite, yellowing of the eyes or skin, or liver tenderness, stop taking this drug and call your doctor.

Mild to moderate rash and unusual sensitivity to the sun occurs in many people taking this drug, especially those also taking an **estrogen** product. Rash accompanied by joint pain or stiffness, throat tightness, or generalized itching should be reported to your doctor.

Tipranavir may raise your blood sugar, worsen your **diabetes,** or bring out latent diabetes. People with diabetes who take tipranavir may need the dosage of their antidiabetes medication adjusted.

People with **hemophilia** may bleed spontaneously after taking a protease inhibitor.

The combination of tipranavir and ritonavir interferes with blood platelets sticking together, slowing the blood-clotting process. This combination should be used with caution in patients who may be at **risk of bleeding from trauma**, **surgery**, or other medical conditions, or who are taking **aspirin**, **blood-thinning drugs**, or high doses of **vitamin E**.

This drug can cause large increases in blood fat levels. Monitoring and treatment is essential.

Redistribution and accumulation of body fat, including obesity, facial thinning, thinning of the arms and legs, "buffalo hump," moon-shaped face, and breast enlargement may occur in people taking HIV therapy. The long-term effects of these changes are unknown.

As your HIV status improves and your immune system becomes more responsive to outside intruders, it may stimulate an unusually severe inflammatory response to an existing infection such as **mycobacterium**, **cytomegalovirus**, **pneumocystis**, **pneumonia**, **tuberculosis**, **herpes zoster**, or **herpes simplex**.

Tipranavir capsules contain alcohol.

The benefits and risks of tipranavir in **children** and in **people who have not previously been treated for HIV** are not known.

HIV virus may become resistant to tipranavir and other HIV therapies. For this reason it is essential that you take tipranavir exactly according to your doctor's directions.

Possible Side Effects

Side effects may become more prominent when tipranavir is combined with antiretroviral drugs.

▼ Most common: diarrhea.

▼ Common: nausea.

▼ Less common: vomiting, abdominal pain, fever, fatigue, weakness, headache, depression, sleeplessness, and rash.

▼ Rare: Rare side effects can occur in almost any part of the body. Contact your doctor if you experience any side effect not listed above.

Drug Interactions

- Do not take amiodarone, astemizole, cisapride, flecainide, pimozide, propafenone, quinidine, or terfenadine with tipranavir because of the possibility of serious and potentially life-threatening effects such as abnormal heart rhythms.
- Rifampin can increase resistance to all protease inhibitors, including tipranavir, reducing their effectiveness.
- Do not take migraine medicines such as dihydroergotamine, ergonovine, ergotamine, or methylergonovine with tipranavir because of the possibility of serious and possible life-threatening reactions due to ergot toxicity.
- Do not take the statin-type drugs simvastatin or lovastatin with tipranavir because of the risk of severe reactions such

as muscle damage and breakdown. Atorvastatin may be taken, but the lowest effective dose should be used.

- Blood levels of tipranavir may be raised by terfenidine, ketoconazole, and itraconazole.
- If you take tipranavir and also take oral antidiabetes drugs, you must carefully monitor blood sugar levels, since dose adjustments may be required.
- Tipranavir cuts levels of ethinyl estradiol, an ingredient in many contraceptive drugs, by ½ and can lead to contraceptive failure. Women taking any contraceptive with an estrogen ingredient should use an alternate means of birth control. Women taking estrogen replacement therapy and tipranavir may find they need to increase their hormone dose to maintain the same benefit.
- Other drugs that may interact with tipranavir and should be carefully monitored by your doctor are calcium channel blockers, desipramine, clindamycin, delavirdine, clarithomycin, and rifabutin.
- If you must take an antacid, take it at least 1 hour before or after you take tipranavir.
- St. John's wort decreases the effectiveness of all protease inhibitors, including tipranavir. Do not combine them.
- Protease inhibitors may drastically increase blood levels of drugs for erectile dysfunction, leading to side effects such as low blood pressure, visual changes, and persistent, painful erection. Dosage reductions are needed.
- Phenobarbital, phenytoin, dexamethasone, carbamazepine, and nevirapine may reduce blood levels of protease inhibitors such as tipranavir.
- Tipranavir can drastically increase the effects of benzodiazepine sedatives such as midazolam and triazolam, leading to prolonged sedation or severe breathing difficulty. Do not take these drugs with tipranavir.
- Blood levels of selective serotonin reuptake inhibitor (SSRI) antidepressants may be increased with tipranavir. SSRI dosage reductions may be needed.
- Immune system suppressants (cyclosporine, sirolimus, and tacrolimus) may be affected by tipranavir. Dosage adjustments may be necessary until blood levels of the immune suppressant have been stabilized.
- Tipranavir reduces the amount of methadone in the blood by ½. Methadone dosage increases may be needed.

- Tipranavir affects meperidine and long-term use of meperidine with tipranavir is not recommended because of the possibility of seizure activity.
- Frequent blood monitoring is suggested if you are taking warfarin, aspirin, or any blood-thinning drug, and begin taking tipranavir.

Food Interactions

Take tipranavir with food to increase the amount of drug absorbed into the blood.

Usual Dose

Adult (age 16 and over): 500 mg taken with 200 mg of ritonavir, twice daily.

Child (under age 16): consult your doctor.

Overdosage

Little is known about the effects of tipranavir overdose. Take the victim to a hospital emergency room. ALWAYS bring the prescription bottle or container.

Special Information

Tipranavir does not cure HIV. It will not prevent you from transmitting the HIV virus to another person; you must still practice safe sex. You may still develop opportunistic infections or other complications associated with advanced HIV disease. The long-term effects of this drug are not known.

It is imperative for you to take this medication exactly according to your doctor's instructions. Missing doses of tipranavir increases the risk that you will become resistant to the drug. If you forget a dose of tipranavir, take it as soon as you remember and continue with your regular schedule. Do not take a double dose.

Special Populations

Pregnancy/Breast-feeding: While animal studies of tipranavir reveal no damage to the fetus, this drug should only be used during pregnancy after carefully weighing its potential benefits against its risks. The manufacturer of this product has established a registry to follow pregnant women who decide to take tipranavir.

It is not known if tipranavir passes into breast milk. Nursing mothers with HIV should always use infant formula, regardless of whether they take this drug, to avoid transmitting the virus to their child.

Seniors: Seniors may take this drug without special precaution.

Generic Name

Tizanidine (tih-ZAN-ih-dene) Ⓖ

Brand Name

Zanaflex

Type of Drug

Skeletal muscle relaxant.

Prescribed For

Spastic muscle movements.

General Information

Tizanidine hydrochloride is prescribed for people who suffer from uncontrolled muscle spasms usually associated with a nervous system condition. It is presumed to work on the central nervous system by affecting nerves that control major muscle systems; it has no direct effect on skeletal muscles. Tizanidine begins working between 1–2 hours after it is taken and lasts for 3–6 hours. Because of its short duration of effect, treatment should be reserved for those times when relief is most important.

Cautions and Warnings

Do not take tizanidine if you are **allergic** or **sensitive** to any of its ingredients.

Tizanidine can cause low blood pressure. This effect usually begins within 1 hour after taking the drug and reaches its height after 2–3 hours. Low blood pressure triggered by tizanidine is associated with slow heart rate, lightheadedness, and dizziness when rising from a sitting or lying position.

About 50% of people taking tizanidine experience some sedation. Sedation usually begins 30 minutes after taking the drug and continues to get worse for about 1 hour. Sedative effects usually start during the first week of treatment or do not occur at all.

Tizanidine may cause liver injury. About 1 in 20 people who take this drug experience some liver inflammation, although most cases resolve once the drug is stopped. Several people have died from liver failure after taking tizanidine; it should be avoided by people with **liver disease**.

Do not switch between tizanidine tablets and capsules. They are not equivalent.

Some people taking tizanidine have experienced hallucinations, delusions, and psychotic symptoms.

Tizanidine should be used with caution by people who have **reduced kidney function**. These people need smaller-than-usual doses.

Possible Side Effects

▼ Most common: dry mouth, sleepiness, tiredness, and weakness.

▼ Common: dizziness.

▼ Less common: uncontrolled muscle movement, nervousness, constipation, sore throat, vomiting, frequent urination, urinary infection, liver inflammation, double vision, flu-like symptoms, runny nose, speech disorders, fever, depression, anxiety, tingling in the hands or feet, rash, sweating, skin sores, diarrhea, abdominal pain, and upset stomach.

▼ Rare: Rare side effects can occur in almost any part of the body. Contact your doctor if you experience any side effect not listed above.

Drug Interactions

- Tizanidine should never be used with fluvoxamine or ciprofloxacin. These combinations can cause serious adverse effects.

- Avoid combining alcohol or any other central-nervous-system depressant and tizanidine because increased sedation may result.

- The addition of Ziluten, fluroquinolones, amiodarone, mexiletine, propafenone, verapamil, cimetidine, famotidine, acyclovir, or ticlopidine may increase the amount of tizanidine in the blood, which can lead to serious adverse effects.

- Women who combine contraceptive drugs and tizanidine should receive reduced dosages of the latter to avoid increased side effects.

- Tizanidine may increase the effects of blood-pressure-lowering drugs.

- Tizanidine may delay the effects of acetaminophen.

Food Interactions

Tizanidine may be taken without regard to food or meals, though it may work faster with food. It should always be taken at the same times of the day and consistently with or without food.

Usual Dose

Adult: 4–8 mg every 6–8 hours as needed, up to 3 doses a day. Do not exceed 24 mg a day.

Child: not recommended.

Overdosage

Little is known about the effects of tizanidine overdose, but it may lead to very slow breathing. Overdose victims should be taken to a hospital emergency room. ALWAYS bring the prescription bottle or container.

Special Information

People taking tizanidine should be careful not to exceed the prescribed dosage since little is known about using higher dosages over an extended period.

Because of the possibility of sedation, be careful when driving or performing any task that requires concentration.

If you take tizanidine on a regular basis and forget a dose, take it as soon as you remember. If it is almost time for your next dose, skip the one you forgot and continue with your regular schedule. Do not take a double dose.

Special Populations

Pregnancy/Breast-feeding: Tizanidine should only be taken during pregnancy if absolutely necessary and after its potential benefits have been carefully weighed against its risks.

Tizanidine may pass into breast milk. Nursing mothers who must take this drug should consider using infant formula.

Seniors: Seniors should use tizanidine with caution.

Generic Name

Tolcapone (TOL-kap-one)

Brand Name

Tasmar

Type of Drug

COMT inhibitor.

Prescribed For

Parkinson's disease.

General Information

Tolcapone is believed to block the effects of an enzyme known as COMT, which is found throughout the body. COMT is an essential part of the process by which natural stimulants or catecholamines are eliminated. This extends levodopa + carbidopa's beneficial effect on Parkinson's disease.

Cautions and Warnings

Do not take tolcapone if you are **allergic** or **sensitive** to any of its ingredients.

Tolcapone can cause liver irritation, injury, and failure, which may be fatal. Liver function should be evaluated every two weeks for the first year of therapy, then every 4–8 weeks. People with **cirrhosis of the liver** should receive about ½ the usual dose. Other forms of liver disease do not affect tolcapone dosage. People with **severe kidney disease** should also use tolcapone with caution.

Tolcapone increases levodopa + carbidopa side effects, including low blood pressure, dizziness or fainting, and uncontrolled muscle movements.

Some people have suffered from hallucinations after initiating therapy with tolcapone.

Diarrhea requiring hospitalization has occurred in people taking tolcapone.

Cases of rhabdomyolysis, a potentially fatal disorder involving destruction of skeletal muscle, have been reported with tolcapone use. It is unclear what role, if any, tolcapone may have had in these cases.

Tolcapone should only be used to treat Parkinson's disease when other therapies are not appropriate or effective. Do not use for more than 3 weeks if no substantial benefit is experienced.

Possible Side Effects

▼ Most common: abnormal muscle movements, sleep disturbances, stiffness, vivid dreams, tiredness, confusion, nausea, appetite loss, diarrhea, vomiting, muscle cramps, dizziness, and fainting.

▼ Common: hallucinations, constipation, dry mouth, abdominal pain, respiratory infections, sweating, falling, and fatigue.

Possible Side Effects (continued)

▼ Less common: loss of balance, changes in muscular activity, tingling in the hands or feet, upset stomach, gas,
arthritis, neck pain, chest pain, low blood pressure, chest
discomfort, breathing difficulties, sinus congestion, flu-like
symptoms, urine discoloration, and difficulty urinating,
▼ Rare: agitation, irritability, hyperactivity, minor skin bleeding, hair loss, a burning sensation, feeling unwell, fever,
cataracts, and eye inflammation. Contact your doctor if
you experience any side effect not listed above.

Drug Interactions

- Do not combine tolcapone and any monoamine oxidase inhibitor antidepressant except selegiline.
- Tolcapone may increase the blood-thinning effects of warfarin; monitoring may be necessary with this combination.
- Tolcapone increases levodopa + carbidopa side effects.

Food Interactions

Take this drug at least 1 hour before or 2 hours after meals.

Usual Dose

Adult: 100–200 mg 3 times a day.
Child: not recommended.

Overdosage

Common symptoms include nausea, vomiting, and dizziness. Take
the victim to a hospital emergency room. ALWAYS bring the prescription bottle or container.

Special Information

Nausea, dizziness or fainting, hallucinations, and other side effects are more likely when you first start taking this drug.

Tolcapone can make you tired and dizzy. Be careful when driving or performing any task that requires concentration.

Your doctor may reduce your dosage of levodopa + carbidopa
when you begin taking tolcapone.

If you forget a dose, take it as soon as you remember. If it is almost time for your next dose, skip the forgotten dose and continue with your regular schedule.

Special Populations

Pregnancy/Breast-feeding: The safety of using tolcapone during pregnancy is not known, though there is a risk that it may be toxic to a pregnant woman. It is always prescribed with levodopa + carbidopa, which is known to cause birth defects. When tolcapone is considered crucial by your doctor, its potential benefits must be carefully weighed against its risks.

Tolcapone may pass into breast milk. Nursing mothers who must take it should consider using infant formula.

Seniors: Seniors may be more sensitive to side effects, especially hallucinations.

Generic Name

Tolterodine (tole-TER-oe-deen)

Brand Names

Detrol   Detrol LA

Type of Drug

Anticholinergic and antimuscarinic.

The information in this profile also applies to the following drugs:

Generic Ingredient: Darifenacin
Enablex

Generic Ingredient: Trospium Chloride
Sanctura   Sanctura XR

Generic Ingredient: Solifenacin
VESIcare

Prescribed For

Overactive bladder.

General Information

These drugs improve bladder control by interfering with nerve receptors that control bladder muscles. By dulling the response of these receptors to nervous system stimulation, tolterodine can prevent bladder muscle contractions and the resulting urgent need to urinate. Tolterodine does not work the same for everyone. Darifenacin, tolterodine, and solifenacin are mostly broken down in the liver. Thus, how you respond to treatment and your dosage depend on your degree of liver function, and some people break down these drugs more slowly than others. Trospium is minimally affected by liver enzymes and is not subject to these limitations.

Cautions and Warnings

Do not take any of these drugs if you are **allergic** or **sensitive** to any of their ingredients.

Caution should be taken with these drugs if you are **retaining urine**, or have a **stomach obstruction**, **severe constipation**, **ulcerative colitis**, **myasthema gravis**, or **narrow-angle glaucoma.**

People with **reduced liver function** should take solifenacin and tolterodine with caution. People with **reduced kidney function** should be cautious about using all of these drugs except darifenacin.

All of these drugs, except darifenacin, may increase heart rate.

Possible Side Effects

Darifenacin

▼ Most common: dry mouth and constipation.
▼ Common: upset stomach and urinary infection.
▼ Less common: dizziness, weakness, dry eyes, abdominal pains, nausea, diarrhea, accidental injuries, and flu infections.
▼ Rare: Other side effects may occur anywhere in the body. Contact your doctor if you experience any side effect not listed above.

Solifenacin

▼ Most common: dry mouth and constipation.
▼ Common: urinary retention.
▼ Less common: nausea, upset stomach, upper abdominal pain, flu infections, sore throat, dizziness, blurred vision, and fatigue.
▼ Rare: vomiting, dry eyes, leg swelling, cough, and high blood pressure. Contact your doctor if you experience any side effect not listed above.

Tolterodine

▼ Most common: dry mouth and headache.
▼ Common: dizziness, fainting, abdominal pain, constipation, diarrhea, upset stomach, nausea, and tiredness.

Possible Side Effects *(continued)*

▼ Less common: sleepiness, visual problems, very dry eyes, bronchitis, coughing, sore throat, runny nose, sinus irritation, respiratory infection, painful urination, frequent urination, urinary retention, joint pain, back pain, chest pain, high blood pressure, fungal infections, flu-like symptoms, and weight gain.

▼ Rare: tingling in the hands or feet, nervousness, itching, rash, dry skin, gas, and vomiting. Contact your doctor if you experience any side effect not listed above.

Trospium

▼ Most common: dry mouth.

▼ Common: constipation.

▼ Less common: upper abdominal pain, aggravated constipation, upset stomach, stomach gas, headache, fatigue, urinary retention, and dry eyes.

▼ Rare: Rare side effects include severe drug reaction, dizziness, rapid heartbeat, palpitations, blurred vision, abdominal swelling, taste changes, dry throat, dry skin, muscle aches due to tissue breakdown, hallucinations, and swelling around the eyes. Contact your doctor if you experience any side effect not listed above.

Drug Interactions

- These drugs increase the effects of one another and other medicines with an anticholinergic effect. Do not take more than one agent for an overactive bladder at one time.
- Fluoxetine may increase tolterodine blood levels and side effects.
- Tolterodine may cause an increase in blood levels of warfarin, escalating anticoagulant effects.
- Clarithromycin, ketoconazole, itraconazole, ritonavir, nelfinavir, clarithromycin, nefazodone, and miconazole can interfere with the breakdown of darifenacin, tolterodine, and solifenacin in the liver. People taking one of these drugs may need only 7.5 mg of darifenacin, 1 mg of tolterodine, or 5 mg of solifenacin each day. Erythromycin, fluconazole, diltiazem, and verapamil may also interact with these drugs, but there is less chance that a dose adjustment will be needed. This

interaction is not likely with trospium, because the liver has only a minimal effect on breaking it down in the body.

- Mixing trospium with digoxin, procainamide, morphine, vancomycin, metformin, or tenofovir may increase blood levels of either or both drugs.
- Darifenacin may increase the amount of tricyclic antidepressant, flecainide, or thioridazine in the blood. These combinations should be avoided.
- Darifenacin may increase blood levels of digoxin, and people taking this combination should be monitored regularly.

Food Interactions

Darifenacin, tolterodine, and solifenacin can be taken with or without food. Trospium should be taken on an empty stomach.

Usual Dose

Darifenacin
Adult: 7.5–15 mg once a day. People with severe liver disease should not take more than 7.5 mg a day.
Child: not recommended.

Solifenacin
Adult: 5–10 mg once a day. People with severe kidney or liver disease should not take more than 5 mg a day.
Child: not recommended.

Tolterodine
Adult: 1–2 mg twice a day. People with liver disease should not take more than 1 mg a day. Extended-release tablets—2–4 mg a day.
Child: not recommended.

Trospium
Adult: 20 mg twice a day at least 1 hour before or 2 hours after meals. Extended-release tablets—one 60-mg tablet a day.
Child: not recommended.

Overdosage

Overdose symptoms usually include severe drug side effects. Take the victim to a hospital emergency room at once. ALWAYS bring the prescription bottle or container.

Special Information

These drugs can blur your vision, or cause dizziness or drowsiness.

Tell your doctor if you have any of the following problems before you start taking one of these drugs: stomach or intestinal problems, constipation, trouble emptying your bladder, a weak urine stream, an eye problem called narrow-angle glaucoma, liver problems, kidney problems, are pregnant or trying to become pregnant, or are breast-feeding.

Heat prostration (fever and heatstroke) is more likely to occur while taking one of these medicines because it reduces your ability to cool your body by sweating.

If you forget a dose, take it as soon as you remember. If it is almost time for your next dose, skip the forgotten dose and continue with your regular schedule. Do not take a double dose.

Special Populations

Pregnancy/Breast-feeding: Large doses of these medicines have caused fetal harm and birth defects in animal studies. If your doctor considers one of these drugs crucial, its potential benefits must be carefully weighed against its risks.

These drugs may pass into breast milk. Nursing mothers who must take them should use infant formula.

Seniors: Seniors may take darifenacin and tolterodine without special precaution. Dosage reduction is required for seniors taking trospium and solifenacin and for people with kidney disease.

Topamax   *see Topiramate, below*

Generic Name

Topiramate   (toe-PI-ruh-mate)

Brand Names

Topamax   Topamax Sprinkle

Type of Drug

Anticonvulsant.

Prescribed For

Partial onset seizures, tonic-clonic seizures, cluster headaches, migraine prevention, infantile spasms, and Lennox-Gastaut syndrome. Topiramate has also been used for alcohol dependence, bipolar disorder, bulimia, and obesity.

General Information

Topiramate has a broad spectrum of antiepileptic activity. It inhibits nerve transmission in the brain and nervous system by blocking sodium channels and the neurotransmitter glutamate, and by increasing the effect of the neurotransmitter gamma-amniobutynic acid (GABA). Topiramate reaches peak blood levels within 2 hours. It passes out of the body through urine.

Cautions and Warnings

Do not take topiramate if you are **allergic** or **sensitive** to any of its ingredients.

People who suddenly stop taking topiramate may worsen their seizures. Anticonvulsant drugs should be reduced gradually.

People taking topiramate may develop reduced bicarbonate levels in their blood (called metabolic acidosis) because it promotes bicarbonate loss through the kidney by inhibiting an enzyme called carbonic anhydrase. **Existing kidney disease, severe respiratory disorders, status epilepticus, diarrhea, surgery**, a **ketogenic diet**, or some other drugs can worsen the degree of acidosis. Common symptoms of metabolic acidosis include rapid breathing, confusion, and lethargy. Other possible symptoms include heart palpitations or chest pain, abnormal heart rhythms, headache, visual changes, difficulty breathing, nausea and vomiting, abdominal pain, diarrhea, appetite changes, weight loss, muscle weakness, bone pain, stupor, and coma.

Some patients receiving topiramate have experienced acute visual disturbances with symptoms of decreased clarity and eye pain. The treatment to reverse this condition is discontinuation of topiramate, according to the treating physician's judgment as to the necessity of the drug.

Topiramate can cause decreased sweating, which may result in body temperature changes that could be dangerous, especially in children.

People with moderate to severe **kidney disease** should receive ½ the usual dose; other dosage adjustments may be needed.

About 1.5% of people taking topiramate develop kidney stones. This effect may be avoided by drinking several glasses of water a day during treatment.

People with **liver disease** may clear topiramate from their bodies more slowly than others do, but the reasons for this are not well understood.

Children taking topiramate are less likely than adults to have slowness in response, difficulty with concentration, speech disorders and language problems. Tiredness and fatigue are the most common side effects of topiramate in children. Children may also experience headache, dizziness, or appetite loss. Stopping topiramate therapy may cause concentration or attention difficulty.

Possible Side Effects

Side effects usually affect the central nervous system and are more likely with increasing drug dose.

▼ Most common: tiredness or fatigue; slow reflexes; slow thought processes; difficulty concentrating; speech or language problems, especially word-finding; dizziness; weakness; poor muscle coordination; tingling in the hands or feet; tremors; nervousness; insomnia; depression; nausea; loss of appetite; respiratory infections; sensitivity to the sun; and visual disturbances, including double vision.

▼ Less common: back or chest pain, leg pain, hot flushes, body odor, swelling, abnormal coordination, agitation, mood changes, aggressive reactions, reduced touch sensation, apathy, emotional instability, depersonalization, itching, rash, hair loss (in children), upset stomach, abdominal pain, constipation, dry mouth, breast pain, menstrual disorders, painful menstruation, sore throat, sinus inflammation, breathing difficulties, eye pain, weight loss, loss of white blood cells, muscle ache, hearing loss, and aggravated convulsions.

▼ Rare: chills, sweating, gum irritation, tongue swelling, blood in the urine, nosebleeds, vision loss, a decrease in sexual desire, severe skin reactions, hepatitis, liver failure, pancreatitis, pemphigus (a chronic autoimmune skin disease), and kidney damage. Other rare side effects can occur in almost any part of the body. Contact your doctor if you experience any side effect not listed above.

Drug Interactions

- Certain other anticonvulsant drugs—phenytoin, carbamaze-pine, and valproic acid—reduce topiramate levels. Using top-iramate with valproic acid may also cause elevated levels of ammonia, resulting in mental symptoms and/or vomiting.
- Topiramate increases the depressive effect of alcohol and other nervous system depressants. Avoid these combinations.
- Combining topiramate with a carbonic-anhydrase inhibitor drug may increase your risk of kidney stones.
- Topiramate may reduce the effect of lithium, risperidone, con-traceptive drugs, and digoxin.
- Combining metformin or pioglitazone with topiramate re-quires careful monitoring of diabetes control.
- Topiramate increases the amount of amitriptyline in the blood. Reductions in amitriptyline dose may be required to avoid drug side effects.
- Hydrochlorothiazide increases the amount of topiramate in the blood.

Food Interactions

None known.

Usual Dose

Adult (age 17 and over): starting dose—25–50 mg a day. Increase gradually to 200 mg twice a day. People with moderate to severe kidney failure should begin with ½ the usual dose. The recom-mended maintenance dose for migraine is 50 mg twice a day.

Child (age 2–16): starting dose—0.5–1.4 mg per lb., up to 25 mg, at night for 1 week. Increase gradually until an optimal response is achieved (2.3–4 mg per lb. per day, divided into 2 doses).

Child (age 2 and under): not recommended.

Overdosage

Overdose is likely to cause convulsions, drowsiness, speech dis-turbance, blurred or double vision, impaired thinking, lethargy, ab-normal coordination, stupor, low blood pressure, abdominal pain, agitation, dizziness, and depression. Overdose victims must be taken to a hospital emergency room immediately. ALWAYS bring the prescription bottle or container.

Special Information

Drink several glasses of water or other fluids every day to avoid developing kidney stones.

Sprinkle capsules may be swallowed whole or may be opened and sprinkled onto a teaspoon of soft food. The mixture should be swallowed at once without chewing.

Call your doctor if you develop heart palpitations or chest pain, headache, visual changes, confusion or other changes in mental status, difficulty breathing, nausea and vomiting, abdominal pain, diarrhea, appetite changes, weight loss, muscle weakness, bone pain, lethargy, stupor, or coma.

Be careful when driving or performing any task that requires concentration.

If you forget a dose, take it as soon as you remember. If it is almost time for your next dose, skip the dose you forgot and continue with your regular schedule. Do not take a double dose.

Special Populations

Pregnancy/Breast-feeding: Animal studies indicate that topiramate may cause birth defects. When this drug is considered crucial by your doctor, its potential benefits must be carefully weighed against its risks.

Animal studies show that topiramate passes into breast milk. Nursing mothers who must take it should consider using infant formula.

Seniors: Lower dosage may be needed because of age-related kidney impairment.

Toprol   see **Metoprolol**, page 713

Generic Name

Tramadol   (TRAM-uh-dol)

Brand Name

Ultram

The information in this profile also applies to the following drug:

Generic Ingredients: Tramadol + Acetaminophen
Ultracet

Type of Drug

Non-narcotic pain reliever.

Prescribed For

Moderate to moderately severe pain.

General Information

Tramadol hydrochloride is a synthetic compound that works in the central nervous system (CNS) to relieve pain. The exact way in which this drug works is unknown, but it binds to opioid receptors and reduces the uptake of 2 important neurohormones, serotonin and norepinephrine, into nerves. Pain relief begins about 1 hour after you take a dose and reaches its maximum effect in 2–3 hours. Like the narcotic pain relievers, tramadol can cause dizziness, tiredness, nausea, constipation, sweating, and itching. Unlike the narcotics, normal doses cause little interference with breathing and do not cause histamine reactions. It has no effect on heart function.

Cautions and Warnings

Do not take tramadol if you are **allergic** or **sensitive** to any of its ingredients or are **intoxicated** with drugs, alcohol, or narcotics. People who must take sedatives or other nervous system depressants should take reduced doses of tramadol.

Large dosages of tramadol may interfere with breathing, especially when combined with alcohol.

Tramadol use should be avoided in people who have had **abdominal conditions** or a **head injury** because the drug may interfere with diagnosing the injury or understanding its severity.

Seizure has occurred in people taking oral doses of 700 mg or intravenous doses of 300 mg. Other factors may increase the risk of seizures, such as **epilepsy,** a history of **seizures, head trauma, metabolic disorder**, and **drug or alcohol withdrawal**.

People who are **dependent on narcotics** and take tramadol may experience withdrawal symptoms.

People with **reduced kidney function** or **liver disease** should receive reduced dosage.

Possible Side Effects

▼ Most common: dizziness or fainting, nausea, constipation, headache, tiredness, vomiting, itching, weakness, sweating, upset stomach, dry mouth, and diarrhea.

▼ Less common: feeling unwell, warmth and flushing, nervousness, anxiety, agitation, euphoria (feeling "high"),

Possible Side Effects *(continued)*

emotional instability, trouble sleeping, abdominal pain, appetite loss, gas, rash, visual disturbances, urinary difficulties, and symptoms of menopause.

▼ Rare: Rare side effects can affect your senses, mental state, heart, stomach and intestines, liver, blood, and urinary tract. Headaches, fainting, and allergies can also occur. Contact your doctor if you experience any side effect not listed above.

Drug Interactions

- Tramadol should be used with caution and in reduced dosages when taking other medications that cause depression of the central nervous system such as opioids, anesthetic agents, narcotics, phenothiazides, or sedatives.
- Rifampin and St. John's wort reduce tramadol's effectiveness.
- Carbamazepine reduces tramadol's effectiveness by ½. This combination should be avoided.
- The combination of tramadol with monoamine oxidase inhibitor antidepressants or selective serotonin reuptake inhibitors (SSRIs) may cause severe reactions and should be used with caution.
- Amitryptiline, erythromycin, fluoxetine, ketoconazole, norfluoxetine, and quinidine may slow the breakdown of tramadol. The full impact of these interactions is not known.
- Tramadol may increase the effects of warfarin and digoxin.

Food Interactions

None known.

Usual Dose

Adult and Child (age 16 and over): 50–100 mg every 4–6 hours; do not exceed 400 mg a day. The lowest effective dose should be used to avoid drug tolerance and dependence. People with cirrhosis should receive 50 mg every 12 hours. People with severe kidney disease should receive no more than 100 mg every 12 hours.

Senior: Do not exceed 300 mg a day.

Child (under age 16): not recommended.

Overdosage

Overdose can be deadly. Symptoms include breathing difficulties and seizure. Take the victim to a hospital emergency room at once. ALWAYS bring the prescription bottle or container.

Special Information

Dizziness or drowsiness may occur. Be careful when driving or performing any task that requires concentration.

Do not drink alcohol while taking tramadol. Hypnotics, opioids, and psychotropic drugs interact adversely with tramadol.

Tramadol can be habit forming. Withdrawal effects are possible if stopped after prolonged treatment.

If you forget a dose, take it as soon as you remember. If it is almost time for your next dose, skip the one you forgot and continue with your regular schedule. Do not take a double dose.

Special Populations

Pregnancy/Breast-feeding: Tramadol is toxic to animal fetuses and passes into the fetal circulation in humans. When this drug is considered crucial by your doctor, its potential benefits must be carefully weighed against its risks.

This drug passes into breast milk. Nursing mothers who must take it should use infant formula.

Seniors: Seniors may be more sensitive to side effects and should not take more than 300 mg a day.

Generic Name

Trandolapril (tran-DOE-luh-pril) Ⓖ

Brand Name

Mavik

Combination Product

Generic Ingredients: Trandolapril + Verapamil
Tarka

Type of Drug

Angiotensin-converting enzyme (ACE) inhibitor.

Prescribed For

High blood pressure, abnormal heart function following a heart attack, and managing post–heart attack patients. Also prescribed for renal failure, kidney hypertension, heart failure, managing people with a high risk of heart disease, diabetic kidney disease, chronic kidney disease, and preventing a second stroke.

General Information

Trandolapril and other ACE inhibitors work by preventing the conversion of a hormone called angiotensin I to another hormone called angiotensin II, a potent blood vessel constrictor. Preventing this conversion relaxes blood vessels, thus reducing blood pressure and relieving symptoms of heart failure. Trandolapril also affects the production of other hormones and enzymes that participate in the regulation of blood-vessel dilation.

Cautions and Warnings

Do not take trandolapril if you are **allergic** or **sensitive** to any of its ingredients. Severe sensitivity reactions can occur in **hemodialysis** patients taking trandolapril and in those undergoing **venom immunization**.

Swelling of the face, extremities, or throat has been known to occur with trandolapril, which can be dangerous (see "Special Information").

Trandolapril may affect kidney function, especially if you have **congestive heart failure.** Your doctor should check your urine for protein content during the first few months of treatment. Dosage adjustment of trandolapril is necessary if you have **reduced kidney function** or **liver cirrhosis**.

Trandolapril may affect white-blood-cell counts, possibly increasing your susceptibility to infection. Your doctor should periodically monitor your blood counts.

Trandolapril may cause serious injury or death to the fetus if taken during **pregnancy**. Pregnant women should not take trandolapril.

People with **impaired liver function** should use trandolapril with caution.

ACE inhibitors may be less effective in some **black patients** with high blood pressure, especially when dietary salt intake is high. Nevertheless, they should still be considered useful blood pressure treatments. Trandolapril, however, may not have reduced efficacy but may require higher doses. Swelling beneath the skin to form welts is more common among black patients.

For additional information about the combination product, see Verapamil, page 1205.

Possible Side Effects

▼ Most common: upset stomach, muscle pain, dizziness, fatigue, headache, nausea, and chronic cough. The cough usually goes away a few days after you stop taking the medication.

▼ Less common: chest tightness or pain, dizziness when rising from a sitting or lying position, fainting, abdominal pain, nausea, vomiting, diarrhea, bronchitis, urinary tract infection, breathing difficulties, weakness, and rash.

▼ Rare: Rare side effects can occur in almost any part of the body. Contact your doctor if you experience any side effect not listed above.

For additional information about the combination product, see Verapamil, page 1205.

Drug Interactions

- The blood-pressure-lowering effect of trandolapril is additive with diuretic drugs and beta blockers. Any other drug that causes a rapid drop in blood pressure should be used with caution if you are taking trandolapril.
- Trandolapril may increase blood potassium levels, especially when taken with dyazide or other potassium-sparing diuretics.
- Trandolapril may increase the effects of lithium; this combination should be used with caution.
- Aspirin and other nonsteroidal anti-inflammatory drugs (NSAIDs) reduce the blood-pressure-lowering effects of trandolapril and other ACE inhibitors. The combination may cause reductions in kidney function.
- Antacids and trandolapril should be taken at least 2 hours apart.
- Capsaicin may trigger or aggravate the cough associated with trandolapril therapy.
- Indomethacin may reduce the blood-pressure-lowering effects of trandolapril.
- Phenothiazine sedatives and antiemetics may increase the effects of trandolapril.
- Severe sensitivity reactions can occur in those taking allopurinol with trandolapril.
- Trandolapril may affect blood levels of digoxin. More digoxin in the blood increases the chance of digoxin-related side

effects, while less digoxin in the blood can compromise its effectiveness.

- Trandolapril may reduce the absorption of tetracycline by about ⅓.
- In rare cases, trandolapril may trigger hypoglycemia in people taking insulin.

For additional information about the combination product, see Verapamil, page 1205.

Food Interactions

You may take trandolapril with food if it upsets your stomach.

Usual Dose

Trandolapril: 1 mg a day; 2 mg a day in black patients. Daily dosage may be adjusted up to 8 mg a day. Daily dosages greater than 4 mg may be taken in 2 doses. A lower starting dose (0.5 mg) may be appropriate when taken with a diuretic, and in patients with kidney or liver problems.

Trandolapril + Verapamil
Adult (age 18 and over): 1 tablet a day.

Overdosage

The principal effect of trandolapril overdose is a rapid drop in blood pressure, as evidenced by dizziness or fainting. Take the overdose victim to a hospital emergency room immediately. ALWAYS bring the prescription bottle or container.

Special Information

Trandolapril may cause a swelling of the face, lips, hands, or feet called angioedema. People with a history of angioedema should not use this drug. This swelling may also affect the larynx (throat) or tongue and interfere with breathing. If this happens, go to a hospital emergency room at once. Call your doctor if you develop sore throat, mouth sores, abnormal heartbeat, chest pain, persistent rash, or loss of taste perception.

Some people who start taking trandolapril after they are already on a diuretic (an agent that increases urination) experience a rapid drop in blood pressure after their first doses or when their dosage is increased. To prevent this from happening, your doctor may tell you to stop taking your diuretic 2 or 3 days before starting trandolapril or to increase your salt intake during that time. The diuretic may then be restarted gradually.

You may get dizzy if you rise too quickly from a sitting or lying position when taking trandolapril. Avoid strenuous exercise or very hot weather, because heavy sweating or dehydration can cause a rapid drop in blood pressure.

While taking trandolapril, avoid over-the-counter diet pills, decongestants, and other stimulants that can raise blood pressure. Also, do not take potassium supplements or salt substitutes containing potassium without consulting your doctor.

If you take trandolapril once a day and forget a dose, take it as soon as you remember. If it is within 8 hours of your next dose, skip the one you forgot and continue with your regular schedule. If you take trandolapril twice a day and miss a dose, take it right away. If it is within 4 hours of your next dose, take 1 dose immediately and another in 5 or 6 hours, then go back to your regular schedule. Never take a double dose.

Special Populations

Pregnancy/Breast-feeding: ACE inhibitors can cause fetal injury or death. Women who are or might be pregnant should not take ACE inhibitors. If you become pregnant, stop taking this drug and call your doctor immediately.

Relatively small amounts of trandolapril pass into breast milk, and the effect on a nursing infant is likely to be minimal. However, nursing mothers who must take this drug should consider using infant formula.

Seniors: Seniors may be more sensitive to the effects of this drug due to age-related losses in kidney or liver function.

Generic Name

Trazodone (TRAY-zoe-done) Ⓖ

Brand Names
Desyrel   Desyrel Dividose

Type of Drug
Antidepressant.

Prescribed For
Depression with or without anxiety. Also used for cocaine withdrawal, alcoholism, panic disorder, agoraphobia (fear of open spaces), insomnia, and aggressive behaviors.

General Information

Trazodone hydrochloride is chemically different from other antidepressants. It is just as effective as other drugs such as tricyclic antidepressants in treating the symptoms of depression. Symptoms can often be relieved as early as 2 weeks after starting trazodone, but 4 or more weeks may be required to achieve maximum benefit.

Cautions and Warnings

Do not use trazodone if you are **allergic** or **sensitive** to any of its ingredients.

Antidepressants have been associated with an increased risk of suicide, especially in **teenagers.** Suicide is always a risk in severely depressed people, who should only be allowed to have minimal quantities of medication in their possession.

Do not use trazodone if you are recovering from a **heart attack.** People with a previous history of **heart disease** should not use trazodone because it may cause abnormal heart rhythms.

Though rare, painful and sustained erections have occurred with trazodone. If this happens, stop taking the drug and call your doctor. One-third of these cases may require surgery or may lead to a permanent inability to achieve erection.

Possible Side Effects

▼ Common: upset stomach, constipation, abdominal pains, a bad taste in the mouth, nausea, vomiting, diarrhea, palpitations, rapid heartbeat, rash, swelling of the arms or legs, blood pressure changes, feeling of paralysis of the body, breathing difficulties, dizziness, anger, hostility, nightmares, vivid dreams, confusion, disorientation, loss of memory or concentration, drowsiness, fatigue, lightheadedness, difficulty sleeping, nervousness, excitement, headache, loss of coordination, tingling in the hands or feet, tremor of the hands or arms, ringing or buzzing in the ears, blurred vision, red, tired, and itchy eyes, stuffy nose or sinuses, loss of sex drive, muscle ache and pain, appetite loss, weight gain or loss, increased sweating, clamminess, and feeling unwell.

▼ Less common: drug allergy, chest pain, heart attack, gas, delusions, hallucinations, agitation, difficulty speaking,

---

Possible Side Effects *(continued)*

restlessness, numbness, weakness, seizures, increased sex drive, reverse ejaculation, impotence, missed or early menstrual periods, increased salivation, anemia, reduced levels of certain white blood cells, muscle twitches, blood in the urine, reduced urine flow, increased urinary frequency, and increased appetite. Trazodone may cause elevations in levels of body enzymes, which are used to measure liver function.

Drug Interactions

- Trazodone may increase digoxin or phenytoin blood levels and the risk of side effects.
- Trazodone may increase the effects of sedatives, alcohol, and other drugs that depress the nervous system.
- Trazodone may cause a small reduction in blood pressure. Your dosage of high blood pressure medication may have to be reduced slightly when you start taking trazodone.
- Clonidine (a drug used to treat high blood pressure) may be inhibited by trazodone. These interactions must be evaluated by your doctor.
- Trazodone may interfere with the effectiveness of warfarin (an anticoagulant).
- Carbamazepine can reduce the amount of trazodone in the blood, decreasing the effectiveness of the drug.
- Little is known about the potential interaction between trazodone and monoamine oxidase inhibitor (MAOI) antidepressants. It is usually recommended that one antidepressant be discontinued 2 weeks before taking another. Caution should be used when combining trazodone and an MAOI.
- Ritonavir, indinavir, delavirdine, ketoconazole, and the phenothiazine sedatives slow the clearance of trazodone, increasing the chance of trazodone side effects such as nausea, low blood pressure, and fainting.
- Mixing venlafaxine with trazodone may result in symptoms of the "serotonin syndrome," including irritability, muscle tightness, shivering, jerking, involuntary movements of the arms and legs, and changes in consciousness.

Food Interactions

Take trazodone with food to increase effectiveness and reduce the risk of upset stomach, dizziness, and lightheadedness.

Usual Dose

Adult: 150 mg a day in divided doses with food, to start. This dose may be increased by 50 mg a day every 3–4 days, to a maximum of 400 mg a day. Severely depressed people may be prescribed as much as 600 mg a day. Trazodone can cause drowsiness, which may require the administration of the major portion of the daily dose near bedtime.

Child: not recommended.

Overdosage

Drowsiness and vomiting are the most frequent symptoms of trazodone overdose. Others include very severe side effects, especially those affecting mood and heart function. Fever may be present at first, but as time passes body temperature will drop below normal. Victims must be taken to a hospital emergency room immediately. ALWAYS bring the prescription bottle or container.

Special Information

Be careful when driving or performing any task that requires concentration. Avoid alcohol or other depressant drugs while taking trazodone.

Call your doctor if you develop any side effect, especially blood in the urine, dizziness, or lightheadedness. Trazodone may cause dry mouth, irregular heartbeat, nausea, vomiting, or breathing difficulties.

If you forget a dose, take it as soon as possible. If it is within 4 hours of your next dose, skip the dose you forgot and go back to your regular schedule. Do not take a double dose.

Special Populations

Pregnancy/Breast-feeding: Trazodone may damage the fetus and generally should not be taken by women who are or might be pregnant. When this drug is considered crucial by your doctor, its potential benefits must be carefully weighed against its risks.

Trazodone passes into breast milk. Nursing mothers who must take it should consider using infant formula.

Seniors: Seniors may be more sensitive to trazodone's effects and should start with lower doses.

Generic Name

Tretinoin (TRET-in-oin) Ⓖ

Brand Names

Atralin	Retin-A
Avita	Retin-A Micro
Renova	Vesanoid

Combination Products

Generic Ingredients: Clindamycin + Tretinoin
Ziana

Generic Ingredients: Fluocinolone Acetonide + Hydroquinone + Tretinoin
Tri-Luma

Generic Ingredients: Mequinol + Tretinoin
Solagé

Type of Drug

Anti-acne; antiwrinkling agent and skin irritant; and antineoplastic.

Prescribed For

Acne and other skin conditions, skin cancer, acute promyelocytic leukemia (APL), wrinkling, and liver spots caused by chronic sun exposure.

General Information

Tretinoin, also known as retinoic acid or vitamin A acid, works against acne by decreasing the cohesiveness of skin cells, causing the skin to peel. Tretinoin is usually not effective in treating severe acne.

Medical research shows that regular application of tretinoin cream to aging skin prevents wrinkling and may even reverse the wrinkling process for some people. Tretinoin causes a temporary "plumping" of the skin when it is applied, peeling the outer layer. This gives the appearance of improved skin and reduced wrinkling. Some tretinoin—about 5%—is absorbed through the skin. When used to treat APL, a blood cancer, tretinoin causes the leukemia cells to mature and reduces the spread of APL cells; the exact way it works is not known.

Cautions and Warnings

Do not use tretinoin if you are **allergic** or **sensitive** to any of its ingredients.

Women who are **pregnant** should not use tretinoin due to the high risk of birth defects.

This drug may increase the skin cancer-causing effects of ultraviolet light. If you apply this drug to your skin, you should allow a "rest period" between uses of tretinoin and other skin irritants or peeling agents. You must also limit sun exposure to treated areas and avoid sunlamps. If you cannot avoid sun exposure, use sunscreen and protective covering.

Do not apply tretinoin close to your eyes, the sides of the nose, or to mucous membrane tissue.

People with APL are at high risk for severe side effects. About 25% of people with APL treated with tretinoin develop a group of symptoms called retinoic acid–APL syndrome. These symptoms include fever, breathing difficulties, weight gain, and fluid in the lungs. Low blood pressure and loss of heart function may also occur.

Forty percent of people who take oral tretinoin develop a rapid increase in white-blood-cell count, which is associated with greater risk of life-threatening complications. Sixty percent of people taking tretinoin develop high blood-cholesterol or triglyceride levels.

Retinoids such as tretinoin have been associated with pseudotumor cerebri (increased pressure in the brain), especially in **children**. Early signs of this problem include swelling in the eyes, headache, nausea, vomiting, and visual difficulties.

There is limited information on children's use of tretinoin, though children ages 1–16 have used this medication.

For more information on the combination product Tri-Luma, see Topical Corticosteroids, page 319.

Possible Side Effects

Skin Products

▼ Most common: burning, stinging, tingling, itching, swelling, peeling, or blistering of the skin; formation of crusts on the skin near the application site; and temporary skin discoloration and greater sun sensitivity. All side effects disappear after the drug has been stopped.

Possible Side Effects *(continued)*

▼ Common: skin irritation.
▼ Less common: dry skin, crusting, and rash.

Capsules

▼ Most common: headache, fever, weakness, and fatigue. These generally go away with time.
▼ Common: skin changes, dry skin and membranes, bone pain and inflammation, itching, sweating, visual disturbances and other eye problems, hair loss, earache or a feeling of fullness in the ears, not feeling well, shivering, bleeding, infection, swelling in the arms or legs, pain, chest discomfort, weight gain, breathing difficulties, pneumonia, wheezing, abdominal pain, diarrhea, constipation, upset stomach, abnormal heart rhythms, blood-pressure changes, vein irritation, dizziness, tingling in the hands or feet, sleeplessness, depression, confusion, and bleeding in the brain.
▼ Less common: muscle aches, pain in the side, skin irritation, facial swelling, loss of color, lymph system problems, asthma, swollen larynx, gas, swollen liver, hepatitis, ulcer, heart failure, heart attack, heart inflammation, kidney problems including kidney failure, painful urination, frequent urination, enlarged prostate, agitation, hallucination, an unusual walk, convulsions, coma, depression, paralysis of the face, and a variety of nervous system problems.
▼ Rare: hearing loss. Contact your doctor if you experience any side effect not listed above.

Drug Interactions

Skin Products

● Other skin irritants will cause excessive sensitivity, irritation, and side effects. Among the substances that cause this interaction are medications that contain sulfur in topical form, resorcinol, benzoyl peroxide, or salicylic acid; abrasive soaps or skin cleansers; cosmetics, creams, or ointments with a severe drying effect; and products with a high alcohol, astringent, spice, or lime content.

- Tretinoin increases the absorption of minoxidil through the skin when they are applied together, leading to lower blood pressure.
- Do not use tretinoin if you are also taking a drug that increases sensitivity to the sun, such as thiazides, tetracyclines, and fluroquinolone antibiotics.

Capsules

- Combining ketoconazole and other drugs that affect systems in the liver with tretinoin causes a substantial increase in tretinoin blood levels.

Food Interactions

Tretinoin capsules are better absorbed when taken with food.

Usual Dose

Skin Products: Wash the affected area thoroughly, then wait 20–30 minutes and apply a small amount of tretinoin at bedtime.

Capsules: Dosage is individualized for each person. Doses are calculated from height and weight.

Overdosage

Ingesting tretinoin is like taking vitamin A and can be extremely dangerous for pregnant women, who should not take more vitamin A than is contained in their prenatal vitamins. Infants who swallow tretinoin should be taken to a hospital emergency room for treatment. ALWAYS bring the prescription bottle or container. Symptoms of accidental ingestion include headache, facial flushing, abdominal pain, dizziness, and weakness. These symptoms have resolved without apparent aftereffects.

Special Information

Your acne may worsen during the first few weeks of treatment because the drug is acting on deeper, hidden lesions. This is beneficial and is not a reason to stop using tretinoin. Results should be seen in 2–3 weeks but may not reach maximum effect for 6 weeks; normal cosmetics can be used during this time.

Keep this drug away from your eyes, nose, mouth, and mucous membranes. Avoid skin exposure to sunlight or sunlamps.

Applying too much tretinoin will cause skin irritation and peeling but will not increase its effectiveness. Use your fingertip, a gauze pad, or a cotton swab when applying tretinoin to acne lesions to reduce the chances of applying too much medication.

You may feel warmth and slight stinging when you apply tretinoin. If you develop a burning sensation, peeling, redness, or are uncomfortable, stop using tretinoin for a short time.

Avoid using depilatories or waxing, or any product which might irritate the skin, while using topical tretinoin.

Extreme weather or wind may cause severe irritation of skin treated with tretinoin.

If you forget a dose of tretinoin, do not apply the forgotten dose. Skip it and continue with your regular schedule. Do not apply a double dose.

Special Populations

Pregnancy/Breast-feeding: At very high doses, tretinoin causes birth defects in animals. A pregnant woman taking tretinoin capsules is likely to deliver a severely deformed infant. When applied to the skin, tretinoin is rapidly broken down. When this drug is considered crucial by your doctor, its potential benefits must be carefully weighed against its risks. Women who need to take tretinoin capsules should be tested for pregnancy before treatment is started. Use 2 reliable forms of contraception while you are taking tretinoin and for 1 month after treatment has ended.

It is not known if tretinoin passes into breast milk. Nursing mothers who must take tretinoin should use infant formula.

Seniors: Seniors may use this product without special restriction.

Generic Name

Triazolam (trye-AY-zuh-lam) Ⓖ

Brand Name

Halcion

The information in this profile also applies to the following drugs:

Generic Ingredient: Quazepam
Doral

Generic Ingredient: Temazepam Ⓖ
Restoril

Type of Drug

Benzodiazepine sedative.

Prescribed For

Insomnia and sleep disturbances.

General Information

Triazolam is a member of the group of drugs known as benzodiazepines. Benzodiazepines work by a direct effect on the brain.
They make it easier to go to sleep and decrease the number of
times you wake up during the night. Triazolam has the shortest
action of drugs in this class. While this virtually eliminates the
"hangover" affect, it may also cause some people to wake up earlier than they would like because the drug has stopped working.
Temazepam is considered to be an intermediate-acting sedative
and generally remains in your body long enough to give you a good
night's sleep with minimal drug hangover.

Cautions and Warnings

Do not take triazolam if you are **allergic** or **sensitive** to any of its
ingredients.

Triazolam has been associated with memory loss, especially
when higher doses are taken. This effect, known as "traveler's amnesia," is most common among people who take this medication
to adjust to **time zone changes** during travel; it may be linked to
the use of alcoholic beverages and to attempts at starting daily
activity too soon after waking up.

If you abruptly stop taking triazolam, you may experience rebound sleeplessness, where sleeplessness is worse during the
first 1–3 nights after you stop the drug than it was before you
started it.

People with **respiratory disease** may experience sleep apnea
(intermittent cessation of breathing during sleep) while taking triazolam. People who have **sleep apnea** should not take triazolam.

People with **kidney or liver disease** should be carefully monitored while taking triazolam. Take the lowest possible dose to help
you sleep.

Clinical **depression** may be increased by triazolam, which can
depress the nervous system. Intentional overdose is more common among depressed people who take sleeping pills than among
those who do not.

All benzodiazepines can be addictive if taken for long periods
of time and can cause drug withdrawal symptoms if suddenly discontinued. Withdrawal symptoms include tremors, muscle cramps,
insomnia, agitation, diarrhea, vomiting, sweating, and convulsions.

Tapering the drug when stopping will help prevent withdrawal symptoms. People with a history of **seizures** should be particularly cautious when stopping use of this drug.

Possible Side Effects

▼ Common: drowsiness, headache, dizziness, talkativeness, nervousness, apprehension, poor muscle coordination, lightheadedness, daytime tiredness, muscle weakness, slowness of movement, drug hangover, and euphoria (feeling "high").

▼ Rare: Rare side effects can affect your heart, stomach and intestines, urinary tract, blood, muscles, and joints. Contact your doctor if you experience any side effect not listed above.

Drug Interactions

- As with all benzodiazepines, the effects of triazolam are enhanced if it is taken with alcohol, antihistamines, sedatives, barbiturates, anticonvulsants, tricyclic antidepressants, monoamine oxidase inhibitor antidepressants, or selective serotonin reuptake inhibitors (SSRIs).
- Contraceptive drugs, cimetidine, disulfiram, itraconazole, ketoconazole, nefazadone, and isoniazid may increase the effect of triazolam by interfering with the drug's breakdown in the liver. Probenecid may also increase triazolam's effect.
- Cigarette smoking, rifampin, and theophylline may reduce the effect of triazolam.
- Triazolam decreases the effectiveness of levodopa + carbidopa.
- Triazolam may increase the amount of zidovudine (an HIV drug—also known as AZT), phenytoin, or digoxin in your blood, increasing the chances of side effects.
- Combining clozapine and benzodiazepines has led to respiratory collapse in a few people. Triazolam should be stopped at least 1 week before starting clozapine treatment.
- The effects of triazolam may be increased by the macrolide antibiotics—azithromycin, erythromycin, and clarithromycin.

Food Interactions

Triazolam may be taken with food if it upsets your stomach. Avoid taking with grapefruit juice or other grapefruit products.

Usual Dose

Quazepam

Adult (age 18 and over): 7.5–15 mg at bedtime. Dosage must be individualized for maximum benefit. Seniors should take the lowest effective dose.

Child (under age 18): not recommended.

Temazepam

Adult: 7.5–30 mg at bedtime. The dose must be individualized for maximum benefit.

Senior: starting dose—7.5 mg at bedtime. Dosage may be increased if needed.

Child (under age 18): not recommended.

Triazolam

Adult (age 18 and over): 0.125–0.5 mg about 30 minutes before sleep.

Senior: starting dose—0.125 mg, then increase in 0.125 mg steps until the desired effect is achieved.

Child (under age 18): not recommended.

Overdosage

The most common symptoms of overdose are confusion, sleepiness, depression, loss of muscle coordination, and slurred speech. Coma may also occur. Overdose victims must be made to vomit with ipecac syrup—available at any pharmacy—to remove any remaining drug from the stomach. Call your doctor or a poison control center before doing this. If 30 minutes have passed since the overdose was taken or if symptoms have begun to develop, the victim must immediately be taken to a hospital emergency room. ALWAYS bring the prescription bottle or container.

Special Information

Never take more triazolam than your doctor has prescribed.

Avoid alcohol and other nervous system depressants while taking triazolam.

Exercise caution while performing tasks that require concentration and coordination. Triazolam may make you tired, dizzy, or lightheaded.

If you take triazolam daily for 3 or more weeks, you may experience some withdrawal symptoms when you stop taking it (see "Cautions and Warnings").

Benzodiazepines, including triazolam, can cause a morning-after "hangover." Do not take triazolam unless circumstances will allow for a full night's sleep and some time before you need to be alert and active.

If you forget to take a dose of triazolam and remember within 1 hour of your regular time, take it as soon as you remember. If you do not remember until later, skip the dose you forgot and continue your regular schedule. Do not take a double dose.

Special Populations

Pregnancy/Breast-feeding: Triazolam should absolutely not be used by pregnant women.

Triazolam passes into breast milk. Nursing mothers who must take it should use infant formula.

Seniors: Seniors are more susceptible to the effects of triazolam.

TriCor   see *Fenofibrate*, page 475

Type of Drug

Tricyclic Antidepressants

Brand Names

Generic Ingredient: Amitriptyline Hydrochloride G

Generic Ingredients: Amitriptyline Hydrochloride + Perphenazine G
Etrafon

Generic Ingredients: Amitriptyline Hydrochloride + Chlordiazepoxide G
Limbitrol   Limbitrol DS

Generic Ingredient: Amoxapine G

Generic Ingredient: Clomipramine Hydrochloride G
Anafranil

Generic Ingredient: Desipramine Hydrochloride G
Norpramin

Generic Ingredient: Doxepin Hydrochloride Ⓖ
Sinequan

Generic Ingredient: Imipramine Ⓖ
Tofranil   Tofranil-PM

Generic Ingredient: Nortriptyline Hydrochloride Ⓖ
Aventyl   Pamelor

Generic Ingredient: Protriptyline Ⓖ
Vivactil

Generic Ingredient: Trimipramine Maleate
Surmontil

Prescribed For

Depression, with or without symptoms of anxiety, agitation, or
sleep disturbance; neurotic or psychotic depressive disorder, depression or anxiety associated with disease or alcoholism (not to
be taken with alcohol); temporary therapy for urine incontinence
in children age 6 and over. Clomipramine is prescribed only for
obsessive compulsive disorder (OCD). These medications may
also be used for chronic pain due to migraine, tension headache,
diabetic neuropathy, tic douloureux, cancer, herpes lesions, and
arthritis; pathologic laughing or weeping caused by brain disease;
bulimia; sleep apnea; peptic ulcer disease; cocaine withdrawal;
panic disorder; eating disorder; premenstrual depression; and skin
problems.

General Information

Tricyclic antidepressants block the passage of stimulant chemicals
—norepinephrine and/or serotonin—in and out of nerve endings,
producing a sedative effect. They also counteract the effects of
the neurohormone acetylcholine. Antidepressants work by causing long-term changes in the way nerve endings function. Tricyclic
antidepressants can elevate mood, increase physical activity and
mental alertness, and improve appetite and sleep patterns after 2–
4 weeks of use.

Tricyclic antidepressants have been used in treating nighttime
bed-wetting but do not produce long-lasting results. The combination of amitriptyline and perphenazine, a sedative, is used to
treat anxiety, agitation, and depression associated with chronic
physical or psychiatric disease. The combination of amitriptyline

and chlordiazepoxide, an antianxiety drug, is used to treat anxiety and depression. Protriptyline may be especially useful for very withdrawn or lethargic depressed people due to its activating properties. Tricyclic antidepressants are broken down in the liver.

Cautions and Warnings

Do not take tricyclic antidepressants if you are **allergic** or **sensitive** to any of their ingredients.

Antidepressants have been associated with an increased risk of suicide, especially in **teenagers** taking them. Suicide is always a risk in severely depressed people, who should only be allowed to have minimal quantities of medication in their possession.

Amoxapine may cause very high fever, muscle rigidity, changes in mental state, irregular pulse or blood pressure, sweating, abnormal heart rhythms, and rapid heartbeat. This group of symptoms is associated with neuroleptic malignant syndrome (NMS), which may be fatal. If these symptoms develop, stop taking your medication at once and call your doctor. Clomipramine may also cause very high fever, especially when used with other drugs; this may also be a sign of NMS.

Amoxapine may increase the risk of potentially irreversible involuntary muscle movements associated with tardive dyskinesia (symptoms include lip smacking or puckering, puffing of the cheeks, rapid or worm-like tongue movements, uncontrolled chewing motions, and uncontrolled arm and leg movements). This condition is more common among the elderly, especially women.

These drugs should not be used if you are recovering from a **heart attack.**

Rapid heartbeat and fainting when rising from a sitting or lying position are problems associated with protryptiline.

These drugs should be taken with caution if you have a history of **epilepsy or other convulsive disorders; seizure** (which may be a special problem with clomipramine); **difficulty urinating; glaucoma; heart disease; liver disease;** or **hyperthyroidism.**

Antidepressants may aggravate the condition of people who are **schizophrenic** or **paranoid** and may cause people with **bipolar (manic-depressive) disorder** to switch phase. These reactions are also possible when changing or stopping antidepressants.

Tricyclic antidepressants should not be combined with monoamine oxidase inhibitor (MAOI) antidepressants except under close medical supervision.

Possible Side Effects

▼ Most common: sedation and anticholinergic effects, including blurred vision; disorientation; confusion; hallucinations; muscle spasm or tremors; seizures or convulsions; dry mouth; constipation, especially in older adults; difficulty urinating; worsening glaucoma; and sensitivity to bright light.

▼ Less common: blood-pressure changes, abnormal heart rate, heart attack, anxiety, restlessness, excitement, numbness and tingling in the extremities, poor coordination, rash, itching, fluid retention, fever, allergy, changes in blood composition, nausea, vomiting, appetite loss, upset stomach, diarrhea, enlargement of the breasts in men and women, changes in sex drive, and blood-sugar changes.

▼ Rare: Rare side effects can occur in almost any part of the body. Contact your doctor if you experience any side effect not listed above.

Drug Interactions

- Combining a tricyclic antidepressant with a monoamine oxidase inhibitor (MAOI) antidepressant may cause high fever, convulsions, and death. Do not take an MAOI until at least 2 weeks after amitriptyline has been discontinued. People who must take both an MAOI and a tricyclic antidepressant require close medical observation.
- Selective serotonin reuptake inhibitors (SSRIs) may increase blood levels of tricyclic antidepressants.
- Tricyclics interact with guanethidine and clonidine (drugs used to treat high blood pressure). Tell your doctor if you are taking any drug for high blood pressure.
- Tricyclics increase the effects of anticholinergic drugs possibly causing severe constipation.
- Barbiturates, charcoal, and rifamycins may decrease the effectiveness of a tricyclic antidepressant.
- Combining a tricyclic antidepressant and a thyroid drug enhances the effects of both, possibly causing abnormal heart rhythms. The combination of reserpine and a tricyclic antidepressant may cause overstimulation.
- Contraceptive drugs and estrogen may increase the effect of a tricyclic antidepressant.

- Smoking may increase the effects of a tricyclic antidepressant.
- Combining a tricyclic antidepressant and cimetidine, methylphenidate, or phenothiazine drugs such as Thorazine and Compazine may cause severe side effects.
- Bupropion, haloperidol, histamine blockers, and valproic acid may increase the effects of tricyclic antidepressants.
- Combining tricyclic antidepressants and carbamazepine may cause decreases in antidepressant blood levels while increasing carbamazepine levels.
- Tricyclic antidepressants may increase the effects of dicumarol, quinolones, grepafloxin, and sparfloxacin, increasing the risk of dangerous heart-related side effects.

Food Interactions

You may take a tricyclic antidepressant with food if it upsets your stomach.

Usual Dose

Amitriptyline

Adult and Child (age 12 and over): 25 mg 3 times a day, increased to 150 mg a day if necessary. Hospitalized patients may take up to 300 mg a day if needed.

Child (under age 12): not recommended.

Senior: Lower dosages are recommended, generally 30–50 mg a day.

Amoxapine

Adult and Child (age 17 and over): 100–400 mg a day. Hospitalized patients may need up to 600 mg a day.

Child (under age 17): not recommended.

Senior: Lower dosages are recommended. People over age 60 usually take 100–300 mg a day.

Clomipramine

Adult: 25–250 mg a day.

Child: 25–200 mg or 1.4 mg per lb. a day, whichever is less.

This drug may be taken at bedtime to minimize daytime sedation.

Desipramine

Adult and Child (age 12 and over): 100–200 mg a day. People taking higher dosages should have regular heart examinations to check for side effects.

Senior and Child (under age 12): Lower dosages are recommended, usually 25–100 mg a day. Doses above 150 mg a day are not recommended for these age groups.

Doxepin

Adult and Child (age 12 and over): Start with 25–75 mg a day, then increase as needed to a maximum daily dose of 150 mg a day for mild to moderate disease and 300 mg a day for more severe anxiety or depression.

Imipramine

Adult: 50–75 mg a day increased to a maximum of 150 mg a day. Hospitalized patients may require dosages up to 300 mg a day.

Child (age 6 and over): 25 mg a day, given 1 hour before bedtime for nighttime bed-wetting. If bed-wetting does not cease within a week, daily dosage is typically increased to 50–75 mg depending on age—more than 75 mg a day increases side effects without increasing effectiveness. Doses are often taken in mid-afternoon and at bedtime. The dosage should be gradually reduced to help prevent bed-wetting from recurring. Doxepin concentrate should be diluted with about 4 oz. of milk, water, or juice just before it is taken. Do not mix with soda or grape juice.

Senior: starting dosage—30–40 mg a day. Maintenance dosage—usually less than 100 mg daily.

Nortriptyline

Adult: 25 mg 3–4 times a day, increased to 150 mg a day if necessary.

Senior and Child (age 13 and over): Lower dosages are recommended, generally 30–50 mg a day.

Child: not recommended.

Protriptyline

Adult: 15–60 mg a day in 3–4 divided doses. Protriptyline must not be taken as a single bedtime dose because of its stimulant effect.

Senior and Child (age 13 and over): Lower dosages are recommended, usually up to 20 mg a day. Seniors taking more than 20 mg a day should have regular heart examinations.

Child (under age 13): not recommended.

Trimipramine

Adult: 75 mg a day in divided doses to start, then increased as necessary to 150–200 mg. The entire daily dosage may be taken at bedtime or divided into several doses a day. Hospitalized adults may receive up to 300 mg a day.

Senior and Child (age 13 and over): starting dosage—50 mg a day. Maintenance dosage—up to 100 mg daily.

Child: not recommended.

Overdosage

Symptoms include confusion, inability to concentrate, hallucinations, drowsiness, lowered body temperature, abnormal heart rate, heart failure, enlarged pupils, convulsions, severely lowered blood pressure, stupor, and coma. Overdose victims should be taken to a hospital emergency room immediately. ALWAYS bring the prescription bottle or container.

Special Information

Avoid alcohol and other depressants while taking any tricyclic antidepressant. Do not stop taking your medication without your doctor's knowledge. Abruptly stopping a tricyclic antidepressant may cause nausea, headache, and feelings of ill health.

Tricyclic antidepressants may cause drowsiness, dizziness, and blurred vision. Be careful when driving or doing any task that requires concentration.

The following symptoms may occur early in treatment or when the drug dosage is adjusted up or down: anxiety, agitation, panic attacks, sleeplessness, irritability, restlessness, hostility, aggressiveness, acting impulsively, a manic reaction, deepening of depression, other unusual changes in behavior, and suicidal thinking. Report anything unusual to your doctor at once.

Call your doctor immediately if you develop seizures, breathing difficulties or rapid breathing, fever and sweating, blood-pressure changes, muscle stiffness, loss of bladder control, or unusual tiredness or weakness.

Dry mouth may lead to an increase in dental cavities and gum bleeding and disease. Maintain good dental hygiene while taking a tricyclic antidepressant.

Discontinue therapy for as long as possible prior to elective surgery.

If your symptoms are unchanged after 6–8 weeks of treatment with an antidepressant, contact your doctor.

These medications may cause sensitivity to the sun. Be sure to wear protective clothing or sunblock if you are exposed to the sun, and avoid prolonged exposure.

When used for nighttime bed-wetting, doxepin and imipramine are often ineffective.

If you forget a dose, skip it and go back to your regular schedule. Do not take a double dose.

Special Populations

Pregnancy/Breast-feeding: Tricyclic antidepressants cross into the fetal circulation. Birth defects including heart, breathing, and urinary problems have been reported when women took a tricyclic antidepressant during the first 3 months of pregnancy. When any of these drugs is considered crucial by your doctor, its potential benefits must be carefully weighed against its risks.

Small amounts of these drugs pass into breast milk. Nursing mothers who must take a tricyclic antidepressant should use infant formula.

Seniors: Seniors are more sensitive to the effects of these drugs, especially abnormal heart rhythms and other cardiac side effects, and often require a reduced dosage.

TriNessa   *see Contraceptives, page 287*

Type of Drug

Triptan-Type Antimigraine Drugs
(TRIP-tan)

Brand Names

Generic Ingredient: Almotriptan
Axert

Generic Ingredient: Eletriptan
Relpax

Generic Ingredient: Frovatriptan
Frova

Generic Ingredient: Naratriptan
Amerge

Generic Ingredient: Rizatriptan
Maxalt   Maxalt-MLT

Generic Ingredient: Sumatriptan
Imitrex

Generic Ingredient: Zolmitriptan
Zomig   Zomig ZMT

Prescribed For

Migraine headache. Sumatriptan injection can be used for cluster headaches.

General Information

Triptan-type drugs are used to alleviate symptoms of migraine, which include severe headaches as well as nausea, vomiting, and increased sensitivity to light and sound. These drugs work by affecting specific serotonin (5-HT) receptors in the brain. This action constricts (narrows) blood vessels in the brain, which are usually dilated (widened) during a migraine attack. Triptan-type drugs mainly interfere with one type of serotonin receptor, known as $5\text{-HT}_{1B/1D}$, and do not affect other serotonin receptors. While these drugs can alleviate symptoms of migraine, they do not prevent attacks.

Triptan-type drugs are only recommended after analgesics (pain relievers)—such as aspirin, acetaminophen, and other nonsteroidal anti-inflammatory drugs (NSAIDs)—have failed to relieve symptoms. If you experience serious, incapacitating migraines more often than twice a month, your doctor may recommend taking other medications on a regular basis to reduce the number and severity of attacks, including beta blockers, calcium channel blockers, tricyclic antidepressants, monoamine oxidase inhibitor (MAOI) antidepressants, methysergide, and cyproheptadine. Triptan-type drugs generally start to relieve migraine symptoms in about 1 hour; rizatriptan works fastest. They are broken down partially in the liver.

Cautions and Warnings

Do not take triptans if you are **allergic** or **sensitive** to any of their ingredients.

These drugs should only be prescribed after you have been diagnosed with migraine (sumatriptan injection may be used for cluster headaches) because they are not effective in treating other types of headache or pain.

Zolmitriptan, eletriptan, and naratriptan should not be used if you have uncontrolled **high blood pressure**.

It is strongly recommended that triptan-type drugs not be taken by people who have or are at risk for **heart disease**, as indicated by high blood pressure, high blood cholesterol, smoking, obesity, diabetes, and a family history of heart disease. If you have any of these risk factors, your doctor must evaluate your heart disease risk before prescribing one of these drugs. People who take triptan-type drugs regularly or who develop risk factors for heart disease should be reevaluated by their doctors. Rarely, serious cardiac problems have occurred after taking one of these drugs. Eletriptan, naratriptan, sumatriptan, and frovatriptan should not be taken by people with **peripheral vascular disease**.

People have experienced chest, neck, or jaw tightness and pain after taking one of these drugs, but these sensations are rarely associated with heart problems.

Do not take these drugs if your headache is different in any way. A change in the characteristics of your headache may signal a much more serious problem. Call your doctor at once.

Strokes and some fatalities have occurred in people taking a triptan-type drug, though they may have happened because a stroke-related headache was treated with a triptan rather than as a symptom of stroke. People with migraine are more likely to have a stroke or bleeding in the brain. Sumatriptan has been associated with seizures.

Rizatriptan must be used with caution by people with severe **kidney problems** or moderate to severe **liver disease**. People with severe kidney or liver disease should not take naratriptan, sumatriptan, or eletriptan.

Frovatriptan accumulates in people with mild to moderate **liver disease,** but blood levels in these people are similar to blood levels in seniors. No dosage adjustment is needed. There is no experience with frovatriptan in people with severe liver disease.

These drugs can collect in the colored part of the eye and cause eye disorders if taken over a long period. Have your eyes checked regularly.

Possible Side Effects

Side effects are usually mild or moderate, do not last long, and are the same in men and women regardless of age. Some

Possible Side Effects *(continued)*

reported side effects (nausea, vomiting, dizziness, fainting, a feeling of ill health, drowsiness, and sedation) are also migraine symptoms. Side effects may increase with dosage, especially tingling in the hands or feet; chest, neck, jaw, or throat tightness or heaviness; dizziness; tiredness; weakness; and nausea. Rare side effects can affect the heart and blood vessels, nervous system, skin, stomach and intestines, urinary and reproductive systems, blood, muscles and bones, eyes, ears, nose, throat, and other parts of the body. Contact your doctor if you experience any side effect not listed below.

Almotriptan
▼ Common: nausea, tiredness, tingling in the hands or feet, dry mouth, and headache.

Eletriptan
▼ Common: weakness, dizziness, sleepiness, and nausea.
▼ Less common: chest, neck, jaw, or throat tightness; dry mouth; upset stomach; flushing; tingling in the hands or feet; abdominal pain or discomfort; and difficulty swallowing.

Frovatriptan
▼ Common: dizziness, tiredness, and headache.
▼ Less common: tingling in the hands or feet, dry mouth, upset stomach, flushing, skeletal pain, and hot or cold sensations.
▼ Rare: heart attack, chest pain, and abnormal heart rhythms. Other rare side effects can occur in almost any part of the body. Contact your doctor if you experience any side effect not listed above.

Naratriptan
▼ Less common: weakness; nausea; tingling in the hands or feet; dizziness; fatigue; drowsiness; pain or pressure in the neck, throat, or jaw; and generalized pain.

Rizatriptan
▼ Common: dizziness, tiredness, fatigue, and nausea.
▼ Less common: tingling in the hands or feet; headache; pain or pressure in the neck, throat, chest, or jaw; generalized pain; and dry mouth.

Possible Side Effects (continued)

Sumatriptan

▼ Common: tingling and nasal discomfort.

▼ Less common: unusual sensations of warmth or cold; flushing; heart palpitations; pain, pressure, or tightness in the jaw, throat, or neck; heaviness, tightness, and pressure in the chest; eye problems; and weakness. At high dosages, agitation, eye irritation, and painful urination may occur.

Zolmitriptan

▼ Most common: dizziness, weakness, sleepiness, tightness in the jaw or neck, tingling, a warm or burning sensation, tiredness, nausea, and fainting.

▼ Less common: diminished sensitivity to stimulation, heart palpitations, chest pain or pressure, sweating, and muscle aches.

Drug Interactions

- Do not take more than 1 triptan-type drug within 24 hours of another.
- Contraceptive drugs increase frovatriptan blood levels and the risk of side effects.
- Ergotamine and dihydroergotamine may add to the effects of triptan-type drugs. Allow at least 24 hours between taking these drugs. Ergotamine reduces the amount of frovatriptan in the blood by about 25%.
- Cimetidine significantly increases blood levels of zolmitriptan.
- Almotriptan and eletriptan should be used with caution with ketoconazole, itraconazole, nefazodone, troleandomycin, clarithromycin, ritonavir, and nelfinavir. Do not use eletriptan within at least 3 days of taking clarithromycin, itraconazole, ketoconazole, nelfinavir, or ritonavir.
- Monoamine oxidase inhibitor (MAOI) antidepressants can increase blood levels of almotriptan, sumatriptan, zolmitriptan, and rizatriptan, and the risk of their side effects. Do not combine these drugs. Stop taking an MAOI at least 2 weeks before starting on almotriptan, sumatriptan, zolmitriptan, or rizatriptan.
- Propranolol may significantly increase frovatriptan, eletriptan, and rizatriptan blood levels.

- Rarely, combining sumatriptan, zolmitriptan, almotriptan, frovatriptan, naratriptan, or rizatriptan with a selective serotonin reuptake inhibitor (SSRI) antidepressant such as fluoxetine, fluvoxamine, or sertraline or a serotonin-norepinephrine reuptake inhibitor (SNRI) such as duloxetine can cause weakness, overly sensitive reflexes, poor coordination, agitation, hallucinations, coma, rapid heartbeat, unstable blood pressure, fever, nausea, vomiting, and diarrhea.
- Naratriptan, rizatriptan, sumatriptan, and zolmitriptan should not be used with sibutramine. A "serotonin syndrome" including tremor, weakness, and altered consciousness may occur.

Food Interactions

These drugs may be taken with or without food.

Usual Dose

Almotriptan

Adult (age 18 and over): 6.25–12.5 mg as soon as migraine symptoms begin or at any time during the attack. If symptoms do not abate, you may take another tablet in 2 hours, but take no more than 12.5 mg a day. The safety of taking more than 4 doses a month has not been established.

Child: not recommended.

Eletripan

Adult (age 18 and over): one 20- or 40-mg tablet when migraine symptoms begin. Repeat again in 2 hours, if needed. Daily dose should not exceed 80 mg.

Child: not recommended.

Frovatriptan

Adult (age 18 and over): one 2.5-mg tablet when migraine symptoms begin. If you experience pain after the first dose has worn off, you may take another 2.5-mg tablet, but be sure you take the second dose at least 2 hours after the first dose. The total daily dose should not exceed three 2.5-mg tablets. The safety of treating more than 4 migraines a month with frovatriptan has not been established.

Naratriptan

Adult (age 18 and over): 1–2.5 mg as soon as migraine symptoms begin or at any time during the attack. If symptoms do not go away, you may take another tablet in 4 hours. Do not take more than 5 mg a day. The safety of treating more than 4 migraines a month with naratriptan has not been established.

Child: not recommended.

Rizatriptan Tablets

Adult (age 18 and over): 5–10 mg as soon as migraine symptoms begin or at any time during the attack. If symptoms do not go away, you may take another tablet in 2 hours. Do not take more than 30 mg a day. People also taking propranolol should take no more than 5 mg of rizatriptan at a time, up to 15 mg a day. The safety of treating more than 4 migraine headaches a month with rizatriptan has been established.

Child: not recommended.

Rizatriptan Tablets (Disintegrating): Dosage is the same as for regular rizatriptan tablets, but these tablets can be taken without fluid. Do not take the tablet out of its protective packaging until just before you swallow it. Make sure your hands are dry and place the tablet on your tongue, where it will dissolve and be swallowed with your saliva. For people with phenylketonuria (PKU disease): orally disintegrating tablets have 1.05 mg of phenylalanine per 5 mg.

Sumatriptan Tablets

Adult (age 18 and over): 25, 50, or 100 mg as soon as migraine symptoms begin or at any time during the attack. If symptoms do not go away, you may take another dose every 2 hours. Do not take more than 200 mg a day. The safety of using sumatriptan for more than 4 headaches a month (on average) has not been established. People with liver disease should take the lowest effective dosage.

Child: not recommended.

Sumatriptan Nasal Spray

Adult (age 18 and over): 1–2 sprays of the 5-mg nasal spray or 1 spray of the 20-mg spray into 1 nostril only (if administering a 10-mg dose, spray 5 mg into each nostril). Higher dosages may increase side effects. The dose may be repeated 2 or more hours later if symptoms return. Do not take more than 40 mg (8 sprays of the 5-mg or 2 sprays of the 20-mg) a day.

Sumatriptan Injection

Adult (age 18 and over): 6 mg as a subcutaneous injection. People not responding to 1 injection are not likely to respond to a second 6-mg injection. Do not take more than 12 mg a day. Single doses larger than 6 mg are not more effective and are not recommended.

Child: not recommended.

Zolmitriptan

Adult (age 18 and over): 1, 1.25, or 2.5 mg as soon as migraine symptoms begin or at any time during the attack. If symptoms do not go away, you may take another tablet in 2 hours; do not take more than 10 mg a day. People with liver disease should take the lowest effective dosage. The safety of treating more than 3 migraine headaches a month with zolmitriptan has not been established. For people with PKU disease: orally disintegrating tablets contain 2.1 mg phenylalanine per 10 mg.

Child: not recommended.

Zolmitriptan Nasal Spray

Adult (age 18 and over): one 5-mg dose into 1 nostril. If headache does not go away, a second dose may be taken. Do not use more than 10 mg in a 24-hour period. The safety of treating more than 4 migraine headaches in a month with zolmitriptan nasal spray has not been established.

Overdosage

Overdose can be expected to cause sedation, convulsions, tremors, swelling, redness in the arms or legs, physical inactivity, slowed breathing, bluish discoloration of the lips or skin under the fingernails, weakness, dilated pupils, paralysis, increased blood pressure, lightheadedness, neck tension, or poor coordination. Take the victim to a hospital emergency room. ALWAYS bring the prescription bottle or container.

Special Information

Tell your doctor if you have had a stroke or high blood pressure, heart disease or a history of heart disease, high cholesterol, circulation problems, diabetes, obesity, or a history of smoking.

Stop taking the drug and contact your doctor at once if you develop shortness of breath; wheezing; heart palpitations; swelling in the eyelids, face, or lips; rash; lumps; hives; severe tightness in the chest or throat; or sudden abdominal pain.

These drugs may make you tired or dizzy. Be careful when driving or performing any task that requires concentration.

These drugs can increase your sensitivity to the sun. Use sunscreen and wear protective clothing.

These drugs are meant only to treat migraine or cluster headaches. They do not work for all types of headache or pain.

Take your medication at the first sign of a migraine—usually pain or aura. You may enhance the effect of the drug if you lie down in a quiet, dark room.

Avoid alcohol because it can worsen your headaches.

Call your doctor if the usual dosage does not relieve 3 consecutive headaches, if your headaches become more frequent or worse, or if you develop chest pain; difficulty swallowing or breathing; high blood pressure; chest pressure, tightness, or heaviness; nausea; vomiting; or any bothersome or persistent side effect.

People taking one of these medicines should have their eyes checked periodically.

Special Populations

Pregnancy/Breast-feeding: Animal studies have shown possible toxic effects on the fetus. When any of these drugs is considered crucial by your doctor, its potential benefits must be carefully weighed against its risks.

Sumatriptan and eletriptan pass into breast milk. Animal studies show that some other triptan-type drugs may pass into breast milk. Nursing mothers who must take any of these drugs should consider using infant formula.

Seniors: Almotriptan, eletriptan, rizatriptan, sumatriptan, and zolmitriptan may be taken without special precaution. Seniors are more likely to develop naratriptan side effects; this drug is not recommended for them. Frovatriptan can raise blood pressure in some seniors, but it generally returns to normal on its own. However, even small increases in blood pressure have been linked to serious risks and should not be ignored.

Tri-Sprintec   *see **Contraceptives**, page 287*

Brand Name

Tussionex Pennkinetic Ⓐ

Generic Ingredients
Hydrocodone + Chlorpheniramine

Type of Drug

Cough suppressant and antihistamine.

Prescribed For

Cough and other symptoms of a cold or other respiratory condition.

General Information

Tussionex Pennkinetic is one of many cough suppressant-antihistamine combinations that may be prescribed to treat a cough or congestion that has not responded to other medication. The narcotic cough-suppressant ingredient in this combination, hydrocodone, is more potent than codeine.

Cautions and Warnings

Do not use Tussionex Pennkinetic if you are **allergic** or **sensitive** to any of its ingredients. Those allergic to codeine may also be allergic to Tussionex Pennkinetic.

Chronic (long-term) use of this drug may lead to drug dependence or addiction.

Tussionex Pennkinetic may cause drowsiness, tiredness, or loss of concentration.

Use with caution if you have a history of **head injury** or **brain tumor, asthma, liver or kidney disease, glaucoma, stomach ulcer, heart disease, hypertension** (high blood pressure)**, thyroid disease, prostatic hypertrophy, urinary problems,** or **diabetes**.

Possible Side Effects

▼ Most common: lightheadedness, dizziness, sleepiness, nausea, vomiting, increased sweating, itching, rash, sensitivity to bright light, chills, and dryness of the mouth, nose, or throat.

▼ Less common: euphoria (feeling "high"), weakness, agitation, uncoordinated muscle movement, disorientation and visual disturbances, minor hallucinations, appetite loss, constipation, facial flushing, rapid heartbeat, palpitations, feeling faint, urinary difficulties, reduced sexual potency, low blood sugar, anemia, yellowing of the skin or whites of the eyes, blurred or double vision, ringing or buzzing in the ears, wheezing, and nasal stuffiness.

Drug Interactions

- Do not use alcohol or other depressant drugs such as anti-histamines, narcotics, antipsychotics, and antianxiety drugs because they increase the depressant effect of Tussionex Pennkinetic.
- This drug should not be combined with monoamine oxidase inhibitor antidepressants.

Food Interactions

Take Tussionex Pennkinetic with food if it upsets your stomach.

Usual Dose

1 tsp. every 12 hours.

Overdosage

Symptoms include depression, slowed breathing, flushing, and upset stomach. Take the victim to a hospital emergency room. ALWAYS bring the prescription bottle or container.

Special Information

This drug causes sedation. Be careful when driving or doing any task that requires concentration.

If you forget a dose, take it as soon as you remember. If it is almost time for your next dose, skip the one you forgot and continue with your regular schedule. Do not take a double dose.

Special Populations

Pregnancy/Breast-feeding: Antihistamines pass into the circulation of the fetus but have not caused birth defects. Taking narcotics during pregnancy may lead to drug dependency in newborns or breathing difficulties if narcotics are used just prior to delivery. When this drug is considered crucial by your doctor, its potential benefits must be carefully weighed against its risks.

The ingredients in this product pass into breast milk and may affect an infant's breathing if abused. Nursing mothers who must take this drug should consider using infant formula.

Seniors: Seniors are more likely to be sensitive to both ingredients in Tussionex Pennkinetic and to experience depressant effects; dizziness, lightheadedness or fainting when rising suddenly from a sitting or lying position; confusion; difficult or painful urination; feeling faint; dry mouth, nose, or throat; nightmares; excitement; nervousness; restlessness; or irritability.

Brand Name

Tussi-Organidin NR 💲

Generic Ingredients

Codeine Phosphate + Guaifenesin 🄶

Other Brand Names

Brontex	Guaituss AC
Cheracol with Codeine	Guaitussin with Codeine
Cheratussin AC	Halotussin AC 💲 🄰
Gani-Tuss NR	Mytussin AC
Glydeine	Robitussin AC 💲
Guaifen AC	

Type of Drug

Cough suppressant and expectorant.

Prescribed For

Cough due to a cold or other upper respiratory infection.

General Information

In Tussi-Organidin NR, codeine is the ingredient that suppresses cough. Guaifenesin, an expectorant, increases the production of mucus and other bronchial secretions, making coughs more productive. Many experts question the effectiveness of guaifenesin, especially for removing the mucus that accumulates during serious respiratory conditions such as bronchitis, bronchial asthma, emphysema, cystic fibrosis, or chronic sinusitis. Drinking plenty of fluid works as well as any expectorant for the average cold or upper-respiratory cough. Expectorants do not suppress your cough.

Cautions and Warnings

Do not take Tussi-Organidin NR if you are **allergic** or **sensitive** to any of its ingredients.

Chronic (long-term) use of codeine may lead to drug dependence or addiction.

Possible Side Effects

▼ Most common: lightheadedness, dizziness, sedation or sleepiness, nausea, vomiting, diarrhea, stomach pain, and sweating.

Possible Side Effects *(continued)*

▼ Less common: euphoria (feeling "high"), weakness, headache, agitation, uncoordinated muscle movements, minor hallucinations, disorientation and visual disturbances, dry mouth, appetite loss, constipation, facial flushing, rapid heartbeat, palpitations, feeling faint, urinary difficulties or hesitancy, reduced sex drive or potency, itching, rash, anemia, lowered blood sugar, and yellowing of the skin or whites of the eyes. Narcotic analgesics (pain relievers) such as codeine may aggravate convulsions in those who have had them.

Drug Interactions

- Codeine has a general depressant effect and may affect breathing. Tussi-Organidin NR should be taken with extreme care in combination with alcohol, sedatives, antihistamines, or other depressant drugs, especially monoamine oxidase inhibitor antidepressants.
- These drugs should not be used with antidepressant medications such as Librium or Prozac.

Food Interactions

Tussi-Organidin NR should be taken with a full glass of water or other fluid.

Usual Dose

2 tsp. every 4 hours as needed for cough relief. Do not take more than 12 tsp. in 24 hours.

Overdosage

Symptoms include breathing difficulties, pinpointed pupils, lack of response to pain stimulation, cold or clammy skin, slow heartbeat, low blood pressure, convulsions, heart attack, or extreme tiredness progressing to stupor and then coma. Take the victim to a hospital emergency room immediately. ALWAYS bring the prescription bottle or container.

Special Information

Codeine is a respiratory depressant and affects the central nervous system (CNS), producing sleepiness, tiredness, or an inability to concentrate. Be careful when driving or doing any task that requires concentration. Report persistent or bothersome side effects to your doctor.

If you take Tussi-Organidin NR 3 or more times a day and forget a dose, take it as soon as you remember. If it is almost time for your next dose, take 1 dose immediately and another in 3 or 4 hours, then go back to your regular schedule. Do not take a double dose.

Special Populations

Pregnancy/Breast-feeding: Taking narcotics during pregnancy may lead to drug dependency in newborns or breathing difficulties in newborns if narcotics are used just prior to delivery. When Tussi-Organidin NR is considered crucial by your doctor, its potential benefits must be carefully weighed against its risks.

Codeine passes into breast milk and may affect an infant's breathing if abused. Nursing mothers who must take Tussi-Organidin NR should consider using infant formula.

Seniors: Seniors are more sensitive to the effects of codeine.

Generic Name

Valacyclovir (val-ay-SYE-kloe-vere) Ⓖ

Brand Name
Valtrex

Type of Drug
Antiviral.

Prescribed For
Herpes zoster (shingles), recurrent genital herpes, and herpes labialis (cold sores).

General Information
Valacyclovir hydrochloride is rapidly converted to the antiviral acyclovir in the liver and intestine after it is absorbed into the blood. Acyclovir, the form valacyclovir takes in order to work, fights the herpes virus by inhibiting and inactivating an enzyme that is key to viral reproduction and by affecting the growing viral DNA chain.

Cautions and Warnings
Do not take valacyclovir if you are **allergic** or **sensitive** to it, acyclovir, or any component of the tablet.

Some people with advanced **HIV disease,** or those who have had a **bone marrow transplant** or an **organ transplant,** developed a potentially fatal condition known as TTP (blood-clotting disorder) while taking valacyclovir. This drug should not be taken by anyone with **HIV** or a **compromised immune system**.

People with **kidney disease** should use caution when taking valacyclovir and may require a reduced dosage.

Possible Side Effects

▼ Most common: headache, diarrhea, dizziness, weakness, constipation, abdominal pain, appetite loss, nausea, and vomiting.

▼ Less common: aching joints, tingling in the hands or feet, stomach gas, fatigue, rash, not feeling well, leg pain, sore throat, a bad taste in the mouth, sleeplessness, and fever.

▼ Rare: Rare side effects can affect behavior and the nervous system, the eyes, gastrointestinal tract, kidney, and skin. Contact your doctor if you experience any side effect not listed above.

Drug Interactions

- Cimetidine and probenecid slow the rate at which valacyclovir is converted to acyclovir, but this does not change valacyclovir's effectiveness. No adjustments in valacyclovir dosage are necessary.
- Cimetidine and probenecid may decrease acyclovir elimination from your body and increase blood drug levels, raising the risk of side effects.
- Combining acyclovir and zidovudine (an HIV drug—also known as AZT) may lead to severe drowsiness or lethargy.

Food Interactions

None known.

Usual Dose

Adult: shingles—1000 mg 3 times a day for 7 days. Genital herpes—1000 mg twice a day for 10 days for initial outbreak, preferably within 48 hours; 500 mg twice a day for 3 days for recurrent outbreaks; and 500 mg a day for prevention of outbreaks. Cold sores—2000 mg twice a day for 1 day. Initiate therapy at earliest onset of symptoms (tingling, itching, or burning). Dosage is reduced in people with kidney disease.

Child (age 12 and under): not recommended.

Overdosage

Little is known about the effects of valacyclovir overdose. It may lead to kidney damage due to deposits of drug crystals in the kidney. Call your local poison control center for more information.

Special Information

Treatment with valacyclovir must be started as soon as possible after shingles is diagnosed. The information on the effectiveness of this drug was gathered from cases in which treatment was begun within 72 hours of diagnosis.

Women with genital herpes have an increased risk of cervical cancer. Check with your doctor about the need for an annual Pap smear.

Herpes may be transmitted even if you do not have symptoms of active disease. Do not have sexual intercourse while visible herpes lesions are present to prevent transmission. A condom should protect against transmission of the herpes virus, but spermicidal products or diaphragms do not. Valacyclovir alone will not prevent herpes transmission.

Call your doctor if valacyclovir does not relieve your symptoms, if side effects become severe, or if you become pregnant or want to begin breast-feeding.

Check with your dentist or doctor about how to take care of your teeth if you notice swelling or tenderness of the gums.

If you forget a dose of valacyclovir, take it as soon as you remember. If it is almost time for your next dose, skip the dose you forgot and continue with your regular schedule. Do not take a double dose.

Special Populations

Pregnancy/Breast-feeding: Acyclovir crosses into the circulation of the fetus. Animal studies have shown that large doses of acyclovir—up to 125 times the human dose—cause damage to both mother and fetus. When this drug is considered crucial by your doctor, its potential benefits must be carefully weighed against its risks.

Acyclovir passes into breast milk. Nursing mothers who must take it should use infant formula.

Seniors: People age 50 and over with shingles tend to have more severe attacks and respond best to valacyclovir treatment if the drug is started within 48–72 hours of the first sign of rash. Seniors with reduced kidney function should receive lower dosages.

Valium   *see Diazepam, page 357*

Generic Name

Valproic Acid (val-PROE-ik) Ⓖ

Brand Names

Depakene	Depakote Sprinkle
Depakote	Stavzor
Depakote ER	

Type of Drug

Anticonvulsant and antimanic.

Prescribed For

Complex partial seizures and simple and complex absence seizures; also used for grand mal, myoclonic, and other seizures; prevention of fever convulsions in children; migraine; anger management; and anxiety or panic attacks.

General Information

Valproic acid is chemically unrelated to other drugs used in the treatment of seizure disorders. It may work by increasing levels of gamma-aminobutyric acid (GABA) and improving its effects in the brain. Valproic acid also has a stabilizing effect on cell membranes within the brain, which may account for some of the drug's other effects. It is broken down in the liver. The information in this profile applies to both forms of the drug: valproic acid (Depakene and Stavzor) and its related compound, divalproex sodium (Depakote). Divalproex sodium is made up of equal quantities of valproic acid and sodium valproate.

Cautions and Warnings

Do not take valproic acid if you are **allergic** or **sensitive** to any of its ingredients. Serious drug reactions involving multiple body systems are rare.

Use this drug with caution if you have a history of **liver problems**. Liver failure, sometimes resulting in death, has occurred in people taking valproic acid. **Children under age 2** are at increased risk for liver failure associated with valproic acid, especially if they are also taking other anticonvulsants or have congenital disorders of metabolism, severe seizure disorders, mental retardation, or organic brain disease. After age 2, the risk of a fatal liver reaction decreases sharply. Ammonia in the bloodstream, another factor that worsens liver disease, may also occur with valproic acid.

If it is going to occur, serious liver disease usually develops during the first 6 months of valproic acid treatment and is often preceded by feeling unwell, weakness, tiredness, facial swelling, appetite loss, yellowing of the skin or whites of the eyes, vomiting, and loss of seizure control. Your doctor should check your liver function before beginning valproic acid treatment and periodically thereafter.

Children and adults taking valproic acid have rarely developed cases of life-threatening pancreatitis (inflammation of the pancreas). Abdominal pain, nausea, vomiting, or appetite loss can be signs of pancreatitis and require immediate medical attention.

Valproic acid can affect platelet function, leading to bruising, bleeding, or changes in blood-clotting function.

Valproic acid should not be taken by those with known **urea cycle disorders.**

Possible Side Effects

Side effects worsen as dosage increases.

▼ Most common: nausea, vomiting, diarrhea, abdominal pain, dizziness, indigestion, sedation or sleepiness, weakness, weight gain, emotional upset, depression, and changes in blood components.

▼ Less common: constipation, increased or decreased appetite, hair loss, change in menstrual periods, headache, loss of eye-muscle control, drooping eyelids, double vision, spots before the eyes, ringing in the ears, loss of muscle control or coordination, and tremors.

Drug Interactions

- Valproic acid may increase the depressive effects of alcohol, sleeping pills, antianxiety drugs, sedatives, phenobarbital, primidone, and other depressant drugs.

- Valproic acid may increase blood levels of zidovudine (an HIV drug also known as AZT).
- Mixing topiramate with valproic acid has led to high blood ammonia levels with or without CNS symptoms, including sudden changes in mental status with tiredness or vomiting. In most cases, symptoms reverse when either drug is stopped.
- Valproic acid may increase the blood concentration and side effects of tricyclic antidepressants, amitriptyline, and nortriptyline.
- Dosages of carbamazepine, clonazepam, diazepam, ethosuximide, lamotrigine, felbamate, and phenytoin may have to be adjusted when you begin taking valproic acid.
- Valproic acid may affect oral anticoagulant (blood-thinning) drugs; your anticoagulant dose may have to be adjusted.
- Aspirin, chlorpromazine, erythromycin, and felbamate may increase the risk of valproic acid side effects by increasing the amount of valproic acid in the blood.
- Rifampin, meropenem, cholestyramine, phenobarbitol, and primidone may reduce the amount of valproic acid in the blood.
- Valproic acid may increase the risk of bleeding or bruising if combined with other drugs that affect platelet "stickiness." These include aspirin, which also increases valproic acid side effects, and other nonsteroidal anti-inflammatory drugs (NSAIDs), dipyridamole, sulfinpyrazone, and ticlopidine.
- Valproic acid may cause false-positive reactions in the urine ketone tests used in diabetes.
- Charcoal tablets interfere with the absorption of valproic acid.

Food Interactions

Food slows the absorption of valproic acid slightly, but you may take it with food if it upsets your stomach. The syrup form can be mixed with food to improve its taste.

Depakote Sprinkle can be taken whole or mixed with 1 tsp. of pudding, applesauce, or other soft food. Swallow the mixture promptly—do not chew.

Usual Dose

Starting dose—125–750 mg, depending on body weight and the condition being treated. Dose may be increased gradually up to 27 mg per lb. per day or until a maximum response is achieved.

Doses of 250 mg or less should be taken at bedtime, and larger doses should be divided throughout the day. Divalproex dosage is expressed in its equivalence to sodium valproate.

Overdosage

Overdose may result in restlessness, hallucinations, flapping tremors of the hands, coma, and death. Call your local poison control center or take the victim to a hospital emergency room immediately. ALWAYS bring the prescription bottle or container.

Special Information

This medication may cause drowsiness. Be careful while driving or performing any task that requires concentration.

Call your doctor at once if you develop nausea, vomiting, abdominal pain, or loss of appetite.

Do not chew or crush the capsules or tablets.

Do not switch brands of valproic acid without your doctor's knowledge. In at least 1 case, seizures resulted when a person was switched to a new product after 3 seizure-free years on another brand of valproic acid.

Valproic acid can cause mouth, gum, and throat irritation or bleeding, and increased risk of mouth infections. Maintain good dental hygiene while taking this drug. Dental work should be delayed if your blood counts are low.

People with a seizure disorder should carry special identification indicating their condition and any drugs being taken.

If you take valproic acid once a day and forget a dose, take it as soon as possible. If you do not remember until the next day, skip the dose you forgot and continue with your regular schedule. If you take valproic acid 2 or more times a day and forget a dose, take it as soon as possible if you remember within 6 hours of your regular time. Take the remaining daily dosage at evenly spaced intervals. Go back to your regular schedule the next day. Never take a double dose.

Special Populations

Pregnancy/Breast-feeding: Taking valproic acid during the first 3 months of pregnancy may increase the risk of birth defects. Pregnant women should take valproic acid only after discussing with their doctors its potential benefits and risks.

Valproic acid passes into breast milk and may affect a nursing infant. Nursing mothers who must take this drug should consider using infant formula.

Seniors: Seniors are more likely to experience side effects due to reduced kidney or liver function and may require lower dosage.

Valtrex   *see **Valacyclovir**, page 1191*

Generic Name

Varenicline   (var-EN-ih-clean)

Brand Name
Chantix

Type of Drug
Nicotinic acid receptor antagonist.

Prescribed For
Smoking cessation.

General Information
Varenicline binds with some of the same receptors that nicotine binds to in the nervous system. This binding satisfies the receptor's need for stimulation at a lower level than nicotine while preventing nicotine from binding to the receptor. The receptor blocked by varenicline is linked to another part of the central nervous system thought to be the basis for the feelings of reward associated with smoking. Preliminary studies indicate varenicline may also be beneficial in alcoholism, which involves the same brain receptors as nicotine addiction. It is eliminated unchanged from the body through the kidney in about 24 hours. Sex, age, race, and length and amount of daily smoking do not alter the effects of varenicline.

Cautions and Warnings
Do not take varenicline if you are **allergic** or **sensitive** to any of its ingredients.

People with **kidney disease** should use this drug with caution and may require a lower dose. It can be removed by dialysis.

People with **diarrhea** should not take varenicline.

Possible Side Effects

Side effects may increase with increased dosage.

▼ Most common: nausea—usually mild or moderate and lasting only a short time, but sometimes lasting for months —headache, sleeplessness, abnormal dreaming, and vomiting.

▼ Common: abdominal pain, gas, upset stomach, constipation, dry mouth, sleep disorders, loss of taste, tiredness or lethargy, not feeling well, weakness, and upper respiratory conditions.

▼ Less common: increased or decreased appetite, vomiting, gastroesophogeal reflux disease, runny nose, breathing difficulty, rash, and itching.

Drug Interactions

- Taking supplemental nicotine (eg, nicotine gum) with varenicline can lead to more nausea, headache, vomiting, dizziness, upset stomach, and fatigue than with nicotine supplements alone.
- Smoking cessation can change the way some drugs are broken down in the body. Insulin, warfarin, and theophylline doses may have to be altered.

Food Interactions

This drug should be taken after meals with a full glass of water.

Usual Dose

Adult (age 18 and over): 0.5 mg a day for the first 3 days of treatment, then 0.5 mg morning and night for 4 days, then 1 mg morning and night for a total of 12 weeks. Stop smoking after 1 week of treatment. People with severe kidney disease may require no more than 0.5 mg twice a day.

Child: not recommended.

Overdosage

There have been only 2 confirmed reports of overdosage with this drug. Symptoms would be expected to be similar to its side effects. Call your local poison control center or a hospital emergency room for more information. ALWAYS bring the prescription bottle or container.

Special Information

Continue to try quitting smoking after the first week of your treatment program, even if you slip up. It may take some time for you to feel comfortable not smoking or for you to stop. An additional 12 weeks of treatment at the full dose is recommended for people who have successfully stopped smoking with varenicline.

If you forget a dose, take it as soon as you remember. If it is almost time for the next dose, skip the one you forgot and continue with your regular schedule. Do not take a double dose.

Special Populations

Pregnancy/Breast-feeding: Animal studies of varenicline have not shown damage to a developing fetus. However, low birth weights and other effects developed in animals given very high doses of the drug. Pregnant women should take this drug only if its potential benefits outweigh the risks.

It is not known if this drug passes into breast milk; however, nursing mothers should either not take varenicline or use infant formula while on this medicine because of the possibility of side effects appearing in the nursing baby.

Seniors: Seniors may require a lower varenicline dosage because of the possibility of age-related reduced kidney function.

Generic Name

Venlafaxine (ven-luh-FAX-ene) Ⓖ

Brand Names

Effexor   Effexor XR

Type of Drug

Antidepressant.

The information in this profile also applies to the following drug:

Generic Ingredient: Duloxetine
Cymbalta

Prescribed For

Venlafaxine is prescribed for major depressive disorder, generalized anxiety disorder, and social anxiety disorder. It is also used to treat premenstrual dyphoric disorder, hot flashes, and post-traumatic stress disorder. Duloxetine is prescribed for major depressive disorder, generalized anxiety disorder, and the management of pain related to diabetes. It is also used to treat fibromyalgia and stress urinary incontinence.

General Information

Chemically different from other antidepressants, these drugs work by inhibiting the ability of nerve endings in the brain to absorb serotonin, norepinephrine and, to a lesser extent, dopamine. They are known as SNRIs (serotonin and norepinephrine reuptake inhibitors). Venlafaxine passes out of the body primarily via the urine. Duloxetine is broken down in the liver. It may take several weeks for these drugs to take effect.

Cautions and Warnings

Do not take venlafaxine or duloxetine if you are **allergic** or **sensitive** to any of their ingredients.

Antidepressants can increase the risk of suicidal thinking and behavior in **children** and **teenagers**. Venlafaxine is not approved for use in children and teenagers. Nevertheless, they are prescribed for and have been studied in this group with some success. Side effects, including the risk of high blood pressure, are similar. The same small weight loss seen in adults was also seen in children but those under age 12 lost more than teens. Children treated with venlafaxine also grew less than those treated with a placebo. In a six-month study, children and teens grew less than would be expected. The difference was greater for those under 12 than for teens.

People taking these drugs should be observed for possible worsening of their condition, suicidal feelings, or unusual behavior changes when treatment is first started and whenever the drug dosage is changed. Symptoms can also occur when people suddenly stop their medicine or quickly lower their daily dose of these medicines.

People with severe **kidney or liver disease** may require reduced dosages of venlafaxine and should not take duloxetine. Heavy drinkers should also not take duloxetine.

People with uncontrolled **narrow-angle glaucoma** should not use duloxetine.

People with a diagnosis of **mania** or **hypomania** (elevated mood, increased activity, decreased need for sleep, grandiosity, racing thoughts) should not take duloxetine.

People with a **seizure disorder** should take duloxetine with caution.

These medicines can raise blood pressure. Venlafaxine can also increase cholesterol levels. If this happens, your dosage of venlafaxine may have to be reduced. Venlafaxine has not been fully studied in people with recent heart attack or unstable heart disease, although a small study revealed no unusual changes in their cardiograms. There was no cardiogram change in a study of people taking duloxetine.

Possible Side Effects

Duloxetine

▼ Most common: nausea, dry mouth, constipation, loss of appetite, headache, dizziness, fatigue, and sleeplessness.

▼ Common: vomiting, diarrhea, loose stools, weakness, tiredness, sweating, anorexia, upset stomach, and viral infection of the nose, throat, sinuses, ears, eustachian tubes, trachea, larynx, or bronchial tubes.

▼ Less common: tremors, hot flushes, fever, blurred vision, anxiety, reduced sex drive, abnormal orgasm, muscle cramps or pain, tremors, weight loss, frequent daytime urination, erectile dysfunction, and delayed or other ejaculation problems including ejaculation failure.

▼ Rare: Rare side effects can affect almost any part of the body. Contact your doctor if you experience any side effect not listed above.

Venlafaxine

Side effects increase with dosage.

▼ Most common: blurred vision, tiredness, dry mouth, headache, sweating, dizziness, sleeplessness, nervousness, tremors, weakness, nausea, constipation, diarrhea, appetite loss, vomiting, impotence, and abnormal ejaculation.

▼ Less common: changes in sense of taste, ringing in the ears, cough, sore throat, dilated pupils, excessive sweating, high blood pressure, rapid heart beat, anxiety, reduced sex drive, agitation, chills, yawning, and inability to experience orgasm.

Possible Side Effects *(continued)*

▼ Rare: Rare side effects can occur in almost any part of the body. Contact your doctor if you experience any side effect not listed above.

Drug Interactions

- Venlafaxine increases blood levels of the beta blocker metoprolol but reduces its blood pressure-lowering effect. Use caution when mixing these drugs.

- Fluvoxamine can increase the amount of duloxetine absorbed by 5 times and elevate the maximum amount in the blood by 2½ times. Cimetidine, ciprofloxacin, fluoxetine, quinidine, quinolone antibiotics, and enoxacin may produce similar effects. Cimetidine can also increase levels of venlafaxine in the blood.

- Duloxetine does not increase the depressant effects of alcohol, but heavy drinkers taking duloxetine are more likely to have damaged their liver and should not take this medicine.

- High levels of stomach acid interfere with duloxetine being absorbed into the blood. Drugs that raise stomach acid will aggravate this effect, but antacids and histamine-2 antagonists like famotidine and ranitidine that lower stomach acidity do not solve the problem. It is not known if proton-pump inhibitors would help.

- Taking an SNRI within 2 weeks of taking a monoamine oxidase inhibitor (MAOI) antidepressant may cause severe and sometimes fatal reactions, including high fever, muscle rigidity or spasm, mental changes, and fluctuations in pulse, temperature, or breathing rate. People stopping venlafaxine should wait at least 1 week before starting an MAOI.

- Clozapine levels may be increased if taken with venlafaxine, with the potential for increased side effects, including seizures.

- Venlafaxine increases blood levels of desipramine and haloperidol significantly.

- Sibutramine, sumatriptan, trazodone, and St. John's wort may cause a "serotonin syndrome," including shivering, spasm, or altered consciousness, if these drugs are taken with duloxetine or venlafaxine.

- Duloxetine and venlafaxine may increase the effects of warfarin.

- Combining venlafaxine and propafenone for severely abnormal heart rhythms may cause psychotic symptoms due to abnormally high levels of venlafaxine in the blood.
- Venlafaxine may decrease levels of indinavir. The significance of this interaction is unknown.

Food Interactions

Take each dose of venlafaxine with food. Duloxetine may be taken without regard to food or meals.

Usual Dose

Duloxetine

Adult: 20–30 mg twice a day. Swallow the tablets whole. Do not chew or crush duloxetine tablets, or sprinkle them on your food.

Child: not recommended.

Venlafaxine

Adult: 75–225 mg a day, divided into 2–3 doses. Some people may benefit from doses up to 375 mg a day. People with severe kidney or liver disease should receive ½ the usual daily dosage. Those with moderate kidney disease may need their daily dosage reduced by only 25%.

Child (under age 18): not recommended.

Overdosage

Symptoms of venlafaxine overdose may include tiredness, mild convulsions, and cardiac effects. There is limited experience with duloxetine overdose. No cases of fatal duloxetine overdose have been reported, but 4 nonfatal cases have occurred in which people took between 300 and 1400 mg. Overdose victims should be taken to a hospital emergency room. ALWAYS bring the prescription bottle or container.

Special Information

Call your doctor if you develop rash, hives, or any other allergic-type reaction.

Venlafaxine may make you tired; be careful when driving or performing any task that requires concentration. Duloxetine may also affect driving and your ability to focus. Alcohol should be avoided when taking these drugs.

If you forget a dose, take it as soon as you remember. If it is almost time for your next dose, skip the dose you forgot and continue with your regular schedule. Do not take a double dose.

Do not suddenly stop taking these drugs. Venlafaxine dosage should be gradually reduced over a 2-week period. People stopping duloxetine may experience dizziness, nausea, headache, tingling in the hands or feet, vomiting, irritability, or nightmares. People taking antidepressants may experience the following side effects when they stop taking them, particularly when they stop suddenly: mood changes, irritability, agitation, dizziness, tingling in the hands or feet, anxiety, confusion, headache, lethargy, emotional instability, insomnia, elevated mood, increased activity, decreased need for sleep, grandiose feelings, racing thoughts, ringing or buzzing in the ears, and seizures. These effects generally clear up on their own, but some have been reported to be severe and may require further attention from your doctor.

Special Populations

Pregnancy/Breast-feeding: Animal studies of venlafaxine and duloxetine suggest they may cause problems for a developing fetus. When your doctor considers these drugs crucial, their potential benefits must be carefully weighed against their risks. Newborn babies exposed to drugs like duloxetine and venlafaxine late in the third trimester of pregnancy have developed complications requiring prolonged hospitalization, respiratory support, and tube feeding.

These drugs pass into breast milk. Nursing mothers who must take them should use infant formula.

Seniors: Seniors may be more sensitive to side effects of venlafaxine. Seniors may take duloxetine without special precautions.

Generic Name

Verapamil (vuh-RAP-uh-mil) [G]

Brand Names

Calan	Verapamil Extended Release
Calan SR	Verelan
Covera-HS	Verelan PM
Isoptin SR	

Combination Product

Generic Ingredients: Trandolapril + Verapamil
Tarka

Type of Drug

Calcium channel blocker.

Prescribed For

Angina pectoris and Prinzmetal's angina, high blood pressure, abnormal heart rhythm, asthma, cardiomyopathy, migraine, nighttime leg cramps, and bipolar (manic-depressive) disorder.

General Information

Verapamil hydrochloride is one of many calcium channel blockers available in the U.S. These drugs block the passage of calcium, an essential factor in muscle contraction, into the heart and smooth muscles. Such blockage of calcium interferes with the contraction of these muscles, which in turn dilates (widens) the veins and vessels that supply blood to them. This dilating effect reduces blood pressure, the amount of oxygen used by the heart muscle, and the risk of blood vessel spasm. Verapamil is therefore useful in treating not only high blood pressure but also angina pectoris (brief attacks of chest pain), a condition related to poor oxygen supply to the heart muscle.

Verapamil affects the movement of calcium only into muscle cells; it has no effect on calcium in the blood.

The sustained-release brands of verapamil should be used only for high blood pressure.

For more information about the combination product Tarka, see Trandolapril, page 1155.

Cautions and Warnings

Do not take verapamil if you are **allergic** or **sensitive** to any of its ingredients.

Verapamil may cause low blood pressure in some people.

People taking a beta-blocking drug who begin taking verapamil may develop heart failure.

Verapamil may cause angina when treatment is first started, when dosage is increased, or if the drug is rapidly withdrawn. This can be avoided by reducing dosage gradually.

People with **heart problems** such as severe congestive heart failure should not take verapamil.

Studies have shown that people taking calcium channel blockers—usually those taken several times a day, not those taken only once daily—have a greater risk of having a heart attack than do people taking beta blockers or other medication for the same purposes. Discuss this with your doctor to be sure you are receiving the best possible treatment.

In small numbers of people, verapamil can lead to an unusual slowing of heart rate.

People with **hypertrophic cardiomyopathy** (progressive weakening and destruction of heart muscle) who are receiving up to 720 mg a day of verapamil are at risk of developing severe cardiac side effects. Most of these effects respond to dosage reduction, and people generally may continue on verapamil at a lower dosage.

People with **kidney disease** or severe **liver disease** should use this drug with caution and may require dosage adjustments.

Verapamil may slow the transmission of nerve impulses to muscle in people with **Duchenne's muscular dystrophy,** possibly causing respiratory muscle failure.

Possible Side Effects

Verapamil generally causes fewer side effects than other calcium channel blockers.

▼ Most common: rash; low blood pressure; slowed heartbeat; heart failure or lung congestion marked by coughing, wheezing, or breathing difficulties; tiredness or weakness; swelling of the ankles, feet, or legs; upper respiratory infection; flu-like symptoms, headache; dizziness; lightheadedness; constipation; and nausea.

▼ Rare: chest pain, rapid or irregular heartbeat, unusual production of breast milk, bleeding or tender gums, fainting, flushing, and feeling warm. Other rare side effects can occur in almost any part of the body. Contact your doctor if you experience any side effect not listed above.

Some people taking verapamil have experienced heart attack and abnormal heart rhythm, but the occurrence of these effects has not been directly linked to verapamil.

Drug Interactions

- If you take verapamil for long periods of time, your dosage of digoxin will have to be lowered by your doctor.
- Disopyramide should not be taken within 48 hours of taking verapamil.
- People taking verapamil together with quinidine may experience very low blood pressure, slow heartbeat, and fluid in the lungs.

- Verapamil's effectiveness and its side effects may be reversed by taking calcium products, including antacids.
- Amiodarone should be used with verapamil with caution.
- Verapamil may increase the effects of benzodiazepines, buspirone, certain statin drugs, imipramine, and prazosin.
- Verapamil should not be taken with dofetilide.
- Verapamil may interact with beta-blocking drugs to cause heart failure, very low blood pressure, or increased angina. Low blood pressure can also result from taking verapamil with fentanyl (a narcotic pain reliever).
- Verapamil may cause unexpected blood pressure reduction in patients also taking other medication to control their high blood pressure.
- Cimetidine and ranitidine increase the amount of verapamil in the blood and may account for a slight increase in its effect.
- The combination of dantrolene and verapamil may lead to high blood-calcium levels and heart muscle depression. If you are taking dantrolene, a calcium channel blocker other than verapamil should be prescribed by your doctor.
- Verapamil may increase the effects of carbamazepine, cyclosporine, tizanidine, and theophylline products, increasing the chance of side effects with those drugs. These combinations should be used with caution.
- Verapamil may decrease the amount of lithium in your body, leading to a possible loss of antimanic control, lithium toxicity, and psychotic symptoms.
- Rifampin, barbiturates, phenytoin and similar antiseizure medicines, vitamin D, and sulfinpyrazone may decrease verapamil's effects.
- Verapamil increases the effects of alcohol.
- Coadministration of verapamil with aspirin may cause increased bleeding.

Food Interactions

Take immediate-release products at least 1 hour before or 2 hours after meals. Take sustained-release products with food if they upset your stomach. Avoid grapefruit juice.

Usual Dose

Verapamil: 120–480 mg a day, according to your condition.

Trandolapril + Verapamil: 1 tablet a day. This sustained-release combination is available in a variety of strengths.

Overdosage

Overdose of verapamil can cause low blood pressure. Symptoms are dizziness, weakness, and slowed heartbeat. If you have taken an overdose of verapamil, call your doctor or go to an emergency room. ALWAYS bring the prescription bottle or container.

Special Information

Call your doctor if you develop abnormal heart rhythm, swelling in the arms or legs, breathing difficulties, increased heart pain, dizziness, lightheadedness, or low blood pressure. Do not stop taking verapamil abruptly.

If you forget to take a dose of verapamil, take it as soon as you remember. If it is almost time for your next dose, skip the one you forgot and continue with your regular schedule. Do not take a double dose.

Special Populations

Pregnancy/Breast-feeding: Verapamil may cause birth defects or interfere with fetal development. When this drug is considered crucial by your doctor, its potential benefits must be carefully weighed against its risks.

Verapamil passes into breast milk. Nursing mothers who must take this drug should use infant formula.

Seniors: Seniors are more sensitive to side effects, especially low blood pressure.

Viagra   see *Erectile Dysfunction Drugs,* page 426

Vigamox   see *Fluoroquinolone Anti-infectives,* page 495

Generic Name

Vorinostat (vah-RIN-oh-stat) Ⓖ

Brand Name

Zolinza

Type of Drug

HDAC inhibitor.

Prescribed For

T-cell lymphoma of the skin.

General Information

Vorinostat is the first HDAC inhibitor to be approved in the U.S. to treat cancer. It is prescribed for people whose lymphoma has persisted, progressed, or recurred on or after 2 systemic treatments for T-cell lymphoma of the skin, which affects fewer than 200,000 Americans. Vorinostat works by inhibiting HDAC enzymes produced in large amounts by certain cancers. In clinical studies of the drug, 25–30% of people taking it responded to treatment. HDAC inhibitors are emerging as a new class of anticancer agents for the treatment of solid and blood cancers.

Cautions and Warnings

Do not take vorinostat if you are **allergic** or **sensitive** to any of its ingredients.

Vorinostat can cause blood clots to form in the lungs or some veins. Anemia and low blood-platelet count may be caused by this drug. Call your doctor if you develop symptoms described in "Special Information," below. Gastrointestinal (GI) bleeding can occur with vorinostat. Nausea, vomiting, and diarrhea that is serious enough to require treatment can also occur.

Vorinostat can cause high blood sugar.

Vorinostat can affect your heart, so your doctor will periodically monitor your heart function.

This drug is broken down in the liver and people with **liver disease** must be treated with caution. It has not been studied in people with **kidney disease**.

Possible Side Effects

About 10% of people taking vorinostat must have their drug dose modified due to a drug side effect.

▼ Most common: diarrhea, fatigue, nausea, low blood-platelet count, appetite loss, weight loss, muscle spasms, hair loss, dry mouth, taste changes, kidney damage, chills, vomiting, constipation, dizziness, anemia, leg swelling, headache, and itching.

Possible Side Effects (continued)

▼ Common: cough, fever, and upper respiratory infections.
▼ Rare: Rare side effects can occur in almost any part of the body. Contact your doctor if you experience any side effect not listed above.

Drug Interactions

- Mixing this drug with warfarin and similar blood-thinning drugs can lead to excessive bleeding.
- Mixing vorinostat with valproic acid can increase the risk of bleeding.

Food Interactions

Take vorinostat with food.

Usual Dose

Adult: 400 mg once a day. Dosage may be reduced to 300 mg once a day for 5 days in a row every week if you have trouble tolerating this drug.

Child (under age 18): Consult your doctor.

Overdosage

Little is known about vorinostat overdose. Overdose victims should be taken to a hospital emergency room. ALWAYS bring the prescription bottle or container.

Special Information

Call your doctor if you develop any of the following symptoms: cough, blood in the sputum, sudden difficulty breathing, rib pain when you take a breath, chest pain, rapid breathing, rapid heart rate, wheezing, clammy skin, bluish skin discoloration, pain in the pelvis area, leg pain, swelling in the legs, a lump (possibly painful) that appears on or near a vein, low blood pressure, dizziness or fainting, sweating, or anxiety. These can be signs that a blood clot formed in a lung or vein.

Drink 2 quarts of liquid every day to avoid becoming dehydrated while taking vorinostat.

If you forget your daily dose of vorinostat, take it as soon as you remember. If it is almost time to take your next dose, skip the forgotten dose and take your next daily dose at the regular time. Do not take a double dose.

Special Populations

Pregnancy/Breast-feeding: Vorinostat can harm a developing fetus. This drug should only be used during pregnancy after carefully weighing its potential benefits against its risks.

It is not known if vorinostat passes into breast milk. Nursing mothers with HIV should always use infant formula, regardless of whether they take this drug, to avoid transmitting the virus to their child.

Seniors: Seniors may be more sensitive to the side effects of vorinostat.

Vytorin   see *Ezetimibe, page 460*

Generic Name

Warfarin   (WOR-far-in) Ⓖ

Brand Names

Coumadin   Jantoven

The information in this profile also applies to the following drug:

Generic Ingredient: Anisindione
Miradon

Type of Drug

Oral anticoagulant (blood thinner).

Prescribed For

Blood clots or coagulation; also prescribed for reducing the risk of small-cell carcinoma of the lung, recurrent heart attack or stroke, and transient ischemic attack (TIA).

General Information

Warfarin prevents the formation of blood clots or coagulation by suppressing the body's production of vitamin-K-dependent factors essential to the coagulation process. If you are taking warfarin, you must take it exactly as prescribed. Notify your doctor at the earliest sign of unusual bleeding or bruising; blood in your urine or stool; or black, tarry stools. Warfarin may be affected by many other drugs, and these interactions may be dangerous (see "Drug Interactions"). One-third of people respond to warfarin in unexpected ways that can be explained by genetic differences. Lab tests are available to help doctors determine the best dose of warfarin for individual patients. Warfarin may also be extremely dangerous if not used properly. Periodic blood-clotting tests are necessary for proper control of warfarin therapy.

Cautions and Warnings

Do not take warfarin if you are **allergic** or **sensitive** to any of its ingredients. Anisindione is usually reserved for people allergic to warfarin.

Warfarin must be taken with care if you have any **blood-clotting disease**. Use of warfarin may be dangerous and should be discussed with your doctor if you have past or planned **eye or nervous system surgery; protein C deficiency**—a hereditary condition; **liver inflammation or disease; kidney disease;** any **infection** being treated with an antibiotic; active **tuberculosis;** severe or prolonged **dietary deficiencies; stomach ulcer or bleeding; bleeding from the genital or urinary areas; high blood pressure;** severe **diabetes; vein irritation; disease of the large bowel,** such as **diverticulitis** or **ulcerative colitis;** and subacute bacterial **endocarditis**.

Anisindione can cause hepatitis and agranulocytosis (a condition characterized by a reduction in the number of white blood cells).

Anticoagulant therapy may increase the release of microplaques into the bloodstream. These microplaques may block very small blood vessels, leading to purple toe syndrome (a condition that occurs when pressure exerted by normal walking leads to bleeding into the skin of your toes). This usually goes away when anticoagulant treatment is stopped, but it may be a sign of a more serious problem present in another part of your body.

Women taking anticoagulants may be at risk of ovarian bleeding when they ovulate.

People taking warfarin must be extremely careful to **avoid cuts, bruises, or other injuries** that may cause internal or external bleeding.

Possible Side Effects

Warfarin

▼ Most common: bleeding, which may occur with usual dosages and even when the results of blood tests used to monitor anticoagulant therapy are normal. If you bleed

Possible Side Effects *(continued)*

abnormally while you are taking anticoagulants, call your
doctor immediately. This includes abnormally heavy menstruation or vaginal bleeding between periods.

▼ Less common: abdominal cramps, nausea, vomiting, diarrhea, fever, anemia, adverse effects on blood components, hepatitis, jaundice (symptoms include yellowing of
the skin or whites of the eyes), itching, rash, hair loss, sore
throat or mouth, red or orange urine, painful or persistent
erection, and purple toe syndrome.

Anisindione
▼ Common: rash.
▼ Less common: headache, sore throat, blurred vision, hepatitis, liver or kidney damage, jaundice (symptoms include
yellowing of the skin or whites of the eyes), red or orange
urine, and changes in blood components.

Drug Interactions

Anticoagulants may have more drug interactions than any other
kind of medication. Your doctor and pharmacist should keep
records of all drugs you take in order to anticipate possible interactions. It is essential that your doctor and pharmacist know about
every medication you are taking, including over-the-counter (OTC)
drugs containing aspirin and herbal medicine.

● Drugs that may increase the effect of warfarin include the following: acetaminophen; aminoglycoside antibiotics; amiodarone; androgen; aspirin and other salicylate drugs; beta
blockers; cephalosporin antibiotics; chloral hydrate; chloramphenicol; chlorpropamide; cimetidine; clofibrate; corticosteroids; cyclophosphamide; dextrothyroxine; diflunisal;
disulfiram; erythromycin; fluconazole; gemfibrozil; glucagon;
hydantoin antiseizure drugs—blood levels of the hydantoins
may also be increased in this interaction; ifosfamide (an influenza virus vaccine); isoniazid; ketoconazole; leflunomide;
loop diuretics; lovastatin; metronidazole; miconazole; mineral
oil; moricizine; nalidixic acid; nonsteroidal anti-inflammatory
drugs (NSAIDs); omeprazole; orlistat; oxandrolone; penicillin;
phenylbutazone; propafenone; propoxyphene; quinidine; qui-

nine; quinolone antibacterials; sulfa drugs; sulfinpyrazone; tamoxifen; tetracycline antibiotics; thioamines; thyroid hormones; and vitamin E.

- Some drugs decrease the effect of warfarin and the interaction may be just as dangerous. Some examples are alcohol, aminoglutethimide, ascorbic acid (vitamin C), barbiturates, carbamazepine, cholestyramine, dicloxacillin, glutethimide, ethchlorvynol, etretinate, meprobamate, griseofulvin, estrogen, contraceptive drugs, chlorthalidone, nafcillin, rifampin, spironolactone, sucralfate, thiazide-type diuretics, trazodone, and vitamin K.

- Warfarin should not be combined with any anticoagulant supplements, including garlic, ginko biloba, chamomile, and ginseng.

Food Interactions

Warfarin is best taken on an empty stomach because food slows the rate at which it is absorbed by the blood. Vitamin K counteracts the effects of warfarin. Avoid eating large quantities of vitamin-K-rich foods, such as spinach and other green, leafy vegetables. Any change in dietary habits or alcohol intake may affect warfarin's action.

Usual Dose

Warfarin: 2–10 mg on the first day, 2–15 mg or more a day thereafter; dosage must be individualized.

Anisindione: 300 mg the first day, 200 mg the second day, 100 mg the third day, and 25–250 mg daily thereafter.

Overdosage

The primary symptom is bleeding. Bleeding may make itself known by the appearance of blood in the urine or stool, an unusual number of black-and-blue marks, oozing of blood from minor cuts, or bleeding from the gums after brushing the teeth. If bleeding does not stop within 10–15 minutes, call your doctor. Your doctor may tell you to skip a dose of warfarin or go to a hospital or doctor's office for blood evaluations, or may give you a prescription for vitamin K, which antagonizes the effect of warfarin. This last approach has some dangers because it may complicate subsequent anticoagulant therapy. If you seek treatment, ALWAYS bring the prescription bottle or container.

Special Information

Do not change warfarin brands without your doctor's knowledge. Different brands may not be equivalent.

Do not stop taking warfarin unless directed to do so by your doctor.

Do not stop or start ANY other medication without your doctor's or pharmacist's knowledge. Avoid alcohol, aspirin and other salicylates, and drastic changes in your diet, since all of these may affect your response.

Call your doctor if you develop unusual bleeding or bruising, red or black tarry stool, or red or dark-brown urine.

Warfarin may turn your urine a red or orange color. This is different from blood in the urine—which causes urine to appear red or brownish in color—and generally happens only if your urine has less acid in it than normal.

If you forget a dose, take it as soon as you remember, then continue with your regular schedule. If you do not remember until the next day, skip the missed dose and continue with your regular schedule. Do not take a double dose. Call your doctor if you miss a dose.

Special Populations

Pregnancy/Breast-feeding: Warfarin is not considered safe for use during pregnancy. It passes into the fetal circulation and causes bleeding, brain and other abnormalities, and stillbirth in 30% of fetuses. In some pregnant women, the benefits of taking warfarin may outweigh its risks, but the drug should not be used during the first 3 months of pregnancy. Pregnant women who need an anticoagulant are often given heparin because it does not cross into the fetal bloodstream.

Warfarin and dicumarol pass into breast milk in an inactive form. Full-term babies are not affected by warfarin but dicumarol may affect a nursing child. The effect on premature babies is not known. Nursing mothers who must take dicumarol should use infant formula.

Seniors: Seniors may be more sensitive to the effects of warfarin and obtain maximum benefit with smaller dosages.

Wellbutrin   *see Bupropion, page 179*

Xalatan *see Prostaglandin Agonists, page 936*

see Prostaglandin Agonists, page 936

Type of Drug

Xanthine Bronchodilators (ZAN-thene)

Brand Names

Generic Ingredient: Aminophylline [G]
Truphylline

Generic Ingredient: Dyphylline [G]
Lufyllin

Generic Ingredient: Oxtriphylline [G]
Choledyl SA

Generic Ingredient: Theophylline [G]

Elixophyllin	Theolair-SR
Quibron-T Dividose	Theo-X
Theo-24	T-Phyl
Theochron	Uniphyl
Theolair	

Prescribed For

Asthma and bronchospasm associated with emphysema, bronchitis, and other diseases; also prescribed for essential tremors and chronic obstructive pulmonary disease (COPD).

General Information

Xanthine bronchodilators are a mainstay of therapy for bronchial asthma and similar diseases. Although the dosage of each of these drugs is different, they all work by relaxing bronchial muscles and helping to reverse spasms. The exact way in which they work is not known.

Some xanthine bronchodilators are sustained-release products that act throughout the day. These minimize potential side effects by avoiding the peaks and valleys associated with immediate-release xanthine drugs. They also allow you to reduce the total number of daily doses.

Initial treatment with a xanthine bronchodilator requires your doctor to take blood samples to assess how much of the drug is in your blood. Dosage adjustments may be required based on these blood tests and on your response to the therapy. Because dyphylline is not eliminated by the liver, it is not subject to many of the drug interactions or limitations placed on the other xanthine bronchodilators.

Cautions and Warnings

Do not use a xanthine bronchodilator if you are **allergic** or **sensitive** to any of their ingredients.

If you have a **stomach ulcer,** congestive **heart failure, heart disease, liver disease, low blood-oxygen levels,** or **high blood pressure,** or are an **alcoholic,** you should use this drug with caution.

People with **seizure disorders** should not take a xanthine bronchodilator unless they are receiving appropriate anticonvulsant medicines.

Theophylline may cause or worsen preexisting **abnormal heart rhythm**. Any change in heart rate or rhythm warrants your doctor's immediate attention.

Status asthmaticus, a medical condition in which the breathing passages are almost completely closed, does not respond to oral bronchodilators. People who experience this condition must be taken to a hospital emergency room at once for treatment.

Serious side effects, including convulsions and serious arrhythmias may be among the initial signs of drug toxicity, and could be fatal. Periodic monitoring of blood levels by your physician is mandatory if you are taking one of these drugs. Do not change your dose without consulting your doctor.

Dosage of dyphylline must be altered in the presence of **kidney failure**.

Xanthine bronchodilators should be used with caution in **children**, who may develop toxic blood levels more easily than adults.

Possible Side Effects

Side effects are directly related to the amount of drug in your blood. As long as you stay in the proper range—below 20 mcg per mL of blood—you should experience few, if any, problems.

▼ Most common: nausea; vomiting; stomach pain; diarrhea; headache; irritability; restlessness; difficulty sleeping; rectal irritation or bleeding, especially with suppositories; and rapid breathing.

Possible Side Effects *(continued)*

▼ Less common: excitability, heartburn, high blood sugar, muscle twitching or spasms, heart palpitations, seizures, brain damage, or death. These effects are more likely when drug levels reach 35 mcg per mL or more.

▼ Rare: vomiting blood, regurgitating stomach contents while lying down, fever, headache, rash, hair loss, and dehydration. Contact your doctor if you experience any side effect not listed above.

Drug Interactions

- Taking 2 xanthine bronchodilators together may increase side effects.

- Xanthine bronchodilators are often given in combination with a stimulant drug such as ephedrine. Such combinations can cause excessive stimulation and should be used only as your doctor specifically directs.

- Reports have indicated that combining erythromycin, clarithromycin, flu vaccine, allopurinol, beta blockers, calcium channel blockers, cimetidine—and, rarely, ranitidine—contraceptive drugs, corticosteroids, disulfiram, ephedrine, interferon, mexiletine, quinolone antibacterials, thiabendazole, or zafirlukast with a xanthine bronchodilator may increase blood levels of the xanthine bronchodilator. Higher blood levels mean the possibility of more side effects. Tetracycline and alcohol may also increase the risk for xanthine bronchodilator side effects.

- The following drugs may decrease theophylline levels: aminoglutethimide, barbiturates, charcoal, ketoconazole, rifampin, sulfinpyrazone, sympathomimetic drugs, and phenytoin and other hydantoin anticonvulsants. The hydantoin level may also be reduced.

- Smoking cigarettes or marijuana makes xanthine bronchodilators less effective by increasing the rate at which your liver breaks them down. This does not apply to dyphylline.

- Drugs that may either increase or decrease xanthine bronchodilator levels include carbamazepine, isoniazid, and furosemide and other loop diuretics. Persons combining a xanthine bronchodilator with one of these drugs must be evaluated individually. Consult your doctor when combining xanthine bronchodilators with any of these drugs.

- People with an overactive thyroid clear xanthine bronchodilators faster and may require a larger dose. People with an underactive thyroid have the opposite reaction. Correcting thyroid function through medical or surgical treatment will normalize your response to a xanthine bronchodilator.
- A xanthine bronchodilator may counteract the sedative effect of diazepam and other benzodiazepines.
- Xanthine bronchodilators may interfere with or interact with a number of different drugs used during anesthesia. Your doctor may temporarily alter your bronchodilator dose or change drugs to avoid this problem.
- Blood lithium levels may be lowered by xanthine bronchodilators.
- Probenecid may increase the effects of dyphylline by interfering with its removal from the body through the kidneys.
- Xanthine bronchodilators may counteract the sedative effects of propofol and zafirlukast.

Food Interactions

To obtain a consistent effect from your medication, take it at the same time each day on an empty stomach, at least 1 hour before or 2 hours after meals.

Theophylline is eliminated from the body faster if your diet is high in protein and low in carbohydrates. Eating charcoal-broiled beef also aids theophylline elimination. Conversely, the rate at which your body eliminates theophylline is reduced by a high-carbohydrate, low-protein diet. You may take some food with a liquid or immediate-release xanthine bronchodilator if it upsets your stomach. Dyphylline is not affected in this way.

Caffeine—a xanthine derivative—may add to the side effects of the xanthine bronchodilators, except dyphylline. Avoid large amounts of caffeine-containing products, such as coffee, tea, cola, cocoa, and chocolate, while taking one of these drugs.

Usual Dose

Aminophylline

Adult (age 16 and over): 100–200 mg every 6 hours. Sustained-release—200–500 mg a day in 1–3 doses.

Child (under age 16): 50–100 mg every 6 hours, or 1–2.5 mg per lb. of body weight every 6 hours.

Dyphylline

Adult: up to 7 mg per lb. of body weight every 6 hours. Dosage is reduced when kidney failure is present.

Child: not recommended.

Oxtriphylline

Adult: about 2 mg per lb. of body weight every 6 hours. Sustained-release—400–600 mg every 12 hours.

Child (age 1–9): 2.8 mg per lb. of body weight every 6 hours.

Theophylline

Adult: up to 6 mg per lb. of body weight a day, in divided doses at 6- or 8-hour intervals, to a maximum daily dose of 900 mg. Sustained-release—same dosage, but taken 1–3 times a day.

Child (age 12–16): up to 8.1 mg per lb. of body weight a day.

Child (age 9–11): up to 9 mg per lb. of body weight a day.

Child (age 1–8): up to 10.8 mg per lb. of body weight a day.

Infant (6–52 weeks): Your doctor will calculate total daily dosage in mg by a formula that factors in age and weight. Under 6 months, give ⅓ the total daily dosage every 8 hours; age 26 weeks–1 year, give ¼ the total daily dosage every 6 hours.

Premature Infant (25 days and over): 0.68 mg per lb. of body weight every 12 hours.

Premature Infant (under 24 days): 0.45 mg per lb. of body weight every 12 hours.

Dosage of xanthine bronchodilators is often calculated on the basis of theophylline equivalents, and must be tailored to your specific condition. The best dose is the lowest that will control your symptoms. Children break down xanthine bronchodilators faster than adults and usually require more drug per lb. of body weight.

Overdosage

The first symptoms of overdose are loss of appetite, nausea, vomiting, nervousness, difficulty sleeping, headache, and restlessness. These symptoms are followed by rapid or abnormal heart rhythm, unusual behavior, extreme thirst, delirium, convulsions, very high temperature, and collapse. These serious toxic symptoms are rarely experienced after overdose by mouth, which generally produces loss of appetite, nausea, vomiting, and stimulation. The overdose victim should be taken to a hospital emergency room immediately. ALWAYS bring the prescription bottle or container.

Special Information

Do not chew or crush coated or sustained-release capsules or tablets. Doing so could result in the immediate release of large amounts of the drug, possibly causing serious side effects.

To ensure consistent effectiveness, take your medication at the same time and in the same way, with or without food, every day.

Call your doctor if you develop nausea, vomiting, heartburn, sleeplessness, jitteriness, restlessness, headache, rash, severe stomach pain, convulsions, or a rapid or irregular heartbeat. Acute drug toxicity may descend abruptly, with little or no warning; serious side effects such as convulsions, life-threatening arrhythmias, and death may result. Periodic monitoring by your physician is mandatory if you are taking a xanthine bronchodilator.

Do not change xanthine bronchodilator brands without notifying your doctor or pharmacist. Different brands of the same bronchodilator may not be identical in their effect on your body.

If you forget to take a dose of your xanthine bronchodilator, take it as soon as you remember. If it is almost time for your next dose, skip the one you forgot and continue with your regular schedule. Do not take a double dose.

Special Populations

Pregnancy/Breast-feeding: Xanthine bronchodilators pass into the fetal circulation. They do not cause birth defects, but they may produce dangerous drug levels in a newborn's bloodstream. Babies born to women who take one of these drugs may be nervous, jittery, and irritable, and may gag or vomit when fed. Pregnant women who must use a xanthine bronchodilator to control asthma or other conditions should talk with their doctors about the risks of this medication.

These drugs pass into breast milk and may cause a nursing infant to be nervous and irritable or to have difficulty sleeping. Nursing mothers who must use one of these drugs should use infant formula.

Seniors: Seniors, especially men age 55 and over, may take longer to clear the xanthine bronchodilators from their bodies. Seniors with heart failure or other cardiac conditions, chronic lung disease, a viral infection with fever, or reduced liver function may require a lower dosage of this medication to account for the clearance effect.

Yasmin see **Contraceptives**, page 287

Generic Name

Zaleplon (zah-LEP-lon)

Brand Name
Sonata

Type of Drug
Hypnotic.

Prescribed For
Insomnia.

General Information
Zaleplon works on the same nerve receptors as the benzodiazepine-type drugs, though it is chemically different from them. Zaleplon usually works within an hour. It is removed from the body relatively quickly and causes little or no "hangover" effect, which may occur with other sleeping pills. Zaleplon is broken down in the liver.

Cautions and Warnings
Do not take zaleplon if you are **allergic** or **sensitive** to any of its ingredients.

People with moderate **liver disease** should take the lowest effective dosage.

Take zaleplon immediately before you go to bed. Taking it during the day causes tiredness and an inability to concentrate and may interfere with normal activities.

People taking zaleplon nightly for an extended period of time may become anxious and have trouble sleeping when they stop the drug.

Difficulty sleeping may be a sign of another physical or psychiatric problem. If zaleplon does not help you, ask your doctor to look for other issues that might be interfering with your sleep and have not yet been discovered. In **depressed** people, taking any hypnotic drug, worsening depression, including suicidal thoughts, is possible.

The effect of zaleplon in people with **respiratory illness** is not known.

Possible Side Effects

In studies, side effects were similar in people taking zaleplon and those taking a placebo (sugar pill).

▼ Most common: headache.

▼ Common: abdominal pain, weakness, muscle aches, memory loss, dizziness, and tiredness.

▼ Less common: fever, difficulty swallowing, tingling in the hands or feet, tremors, eye pain, unusually sensitive hearing, changes in sense of smell, and painful menstrual periods.

▼ Rare: anxiety, feeling unwell, fainting, nosebleeds, visual problems, ear pain, loss of a sense of reality or sense of self, hallucinations, reduced sensitivity to stimulation, increased sensitivity to the sun, appetite loss, and colitis. Other rare side effects can occur in almost any part of the body. Contact your doctor if you experience any side effect not listed above.

Drug Interactions

A number of drug interactions are possible, some of which may not appear below.

- Do not combine zaleplon and diphenhydramine (an over-the-counter antihistamine and sleeping pill).
- Zaleplon increases the depressant effects of alcohol and other nervous system depressants, promethazine, imipramine, and thioridazine.
- Rifampin, phenytoin, carbamazepine, phenobarbital, efavirenz, nevirapine, bartibuates, modafinil, nevirapine, oxcarbazepine, pioglitazone, troglitazone, and St. John's wort may reduce zaleplon's effect by stimulating a liver enzyme that breaks it down.
- Combining zaleplon and cimetidine can almost double zaleplon blood levels. People taking cimetidine regularly for heartburn, ulcers, or stomach acid reduction should begin with the lowest effective dosage of zaleplon.
- Erythromycin, indinavir, nelfinavir, ritonavir, clarithromycin, itraconazole, ketoconazole, nefazodone, saquinavir, telithromycin, aprepitant, fluconazole, verapamil, diltiazem, amiodarone, chloramphenicol, delaviridine, fluvoxamine,

gestodene, imatinib, mibefradil, mifepristone, norfloxacin, norfluoxetine, and voriconazole increase zaleplon's effect by inhibiting an enzyme that breaks it down.

Food Interactions

Take this drug on an empty stomach, at least 2 hours after meals. High-fat meals can reduce its effectiveness. Avoid grapefruit juice and star fruit because they can interfere with the breakdown of zaleplon.

Usual Dose

Adult: 5–10 mg at bedtime.
Senior: Begin with 5 mg nightly and increase if needed.
Child: not recommended.
This medication is usually taken for 7–10 days, and rarely longer than 2–3 weeks.

Overdosage

Symptoms include dizziness, tiredness, and an inability to concentrate or perform complicated tasks and can lead to coma. Take the victim to a hospital emergency room. ALWAYS bring the prescription bottle or container.

Special Information

Sleeping pills sometimes cause memory loss of events that occur during the several hours after a dose. Call your doctor if this happens.

If you see no improvement with this drug in 7–10 days, call your doctor.

Taking zaleplon during the day will make you drowsy and interfere with your concentration and coordination. Use it immediately before bedtime.

If you find that you need a larger dose of zaleplon to help you sleep, you may be developing a tolerance to the drug.

Sometimes, people who stop taking zaleplon after using it for 2 weeks or more have difficulty sleeping or become anxious. These are drug withdrawal symptoms and usually go away after 1 or 2 nights. More severe symptoms are rare.

Special Populations

Pregnancy/Breast-feeding: Taking zaleplon in the weeks just before delivery may cause tiredness or listlessness in newborns. Zaleplon should not be taken during pregnancy.

Small amounts of zaleplon pass into breast milk. Nursing mothers who must take it should use infant formula.

Seniors: Seniors may be more sensitive to side effects.

Generic Name

Zanamivir (zuh-NAM-ih-veer)

Brand Name
Relenza

Type of Drug
Antiviral.

Prescribed For
Influenza A or B viral infection (type A or B flu).

General Information
Zanamivir was the first antiviral agent to be approved for treating flu symptoms. It must be inhaled within 2 days of the beginning of symptoms. It is inhaled directly into the nose and throat, where the influenza virus typically takes hold. Studies of zanamivir in people age 5 and over suggest that people using this product feel better about 1 day sooner. Zanamivir is used to treat and prevent uncomplicated cases of the flu. Treatment is indicated in children age 7 and older, while prevention is indicated in children age 5 and above.

Cautions and Warnings
Do not use zanamivir if you are **allergic** or **sensitive** to any of its ingredients. Stop taking zanamivir if you develop a skin rash or other signs of allergy.

People with **chronic lung problems** like asthma may not benefit from zanamivir inhalations. Also, zanamivir can cause bronchospasm (breathing difficulty) in a small number of people with asthma. Use caution when taking zanamivir if you have any type of **breathing problem**.

People using this drug are still **contagious** and should be careful about spreading the virus to others.

Individual virus particles can become resistant to zanamivir, but it is not yet known if virus infections will become resistant to zanamivir.

The safety of zanamivir in people with **severe liver disease** and in **children under age 5** is not known.

Possible Side Effects

▼ Less common: headache; diarrhea; nausea; vomiting; stuffy nose; nasal irritation; bronchitis; cough; sinus irritation; ear, nose, and throat infections; and dizziness.

▼ Rare: feeling unwell, tiredness, fever, abdominal pain, muscle aches, joint pain, and itching. Contact your doctor if you experience any side effect not listed above.

Drug Interactions
None known.

Food Interactions
None known.

Usual Dose

Adult and Child (age 7 and over): treatment—two 5-mg inhalations twice a day for 5 days. Make sure to take 2 doses on your first day of treatment, even if they are only 2 hours apart. On subsequent days, take zanamivir about 12 hours apart. Prevention (household setting)—one 10-mg inhalation once a day for 10 days.

Child (under age 7): Consult your doctor.

Children under age 12 must be supervised by an adult to be sure that they use the inhaler properly.

Overdosage

Little is known about the effects of zanamivir overdose or accidental ingestion. Call your local poison control center or a hospital emergency room for more information. If you seek treatment, ALWAYS bring the prescription container.

Special Information

Make certain to complete the full 5-day course of zanamivir treatment, even if you start to feel better sooner.

Ask your doctor or pharmacist to instruct you on how to use the Diskhaler device that comes with each 5-day package of zanamivir. The drug comes in a small blister pack that is inserted into the Diskhaler. The blister pack is punctured inside the device and the powdered medication inside is drawn into the throat and nasal passages when you inhale through the Diskhaler.

Make certain that you do not have any food in your mouth when you use this product.

Special Populations
Pregnancy/Breast-feeding
Zanamivir may pass into fetal circulation in extremely small amounts. When this drug is considered crucial by your doctor, its potential benefits must be carefully weighed against its risks.

It is not known if this drug passes into breast milk. Nursing mothers using zanamivir should use infant formula.

Seniors: Seniors may use this product without special restriction. Zanamivir is effective for seniors living at home but did not work in studies of nursing-home residents.

Zetia   *see Ezetimibe, page 460*

see Ezetimibe, page 460

Generic Name

Ziprasidone   (zih-PRAS-uh-done)

Brand Name
Geodon

Type of Drug
Antipsychotic.

Prescribed For
Schizophrenia, acute agitation in schizophrenia, and bipolar disorder.

General Information
Ziprasidone may be prescribed for people who have not been helped by other antipsychotics or for whom other antipsychotics have stopped working. Ziprasidone affects serotonin and dopamine, neurotransmitters in the brain, normalizing their chemical balance and relieving symptoms of schizophrenia.

Cautions and Warnings

Do not take ziprasidone if you are **allergic** or **sensitive** to any of its ingredients.

Ziprasidone should not be used in people with **dementia-related psychosis**. Ziprasidone and other atypical antipsychotic drugs have been associated with deaths. Most are due to heart problems or infection, mostly pneumonia. Ziprasidone can increase blood sugar, worsen **diabetes,** and may push **pre-diabetics** into true clinical diabetes. This effect has been noted with other antipsychotic medicines; coma and death have been reported. People with diabetes and those at risk for diabetes taking ziprasidone must regularly monitor their blood sugars.

Ziprasidone can affect heart function, leading to potentially fatal abnormal heart rhythms called torsade de pointes. Ziprasidone may affect the heart more acutely than other antipsychotic medicines. The chances of developing this abnormal heart rhythm increase if your **blood potassium or magnesium levels** are too low. People with a history of **cardiac arrhythmias** or **serious heart disease** should not take ziprasidone.

Sudden unexplained death has occurred with ziprasidone, as it has with other antipsychotic drugs.

Neuroleptic malignant syndrome (NMS), a potentially fatal group of symptoms associated with ziprasidone and other psychiatric drugs, can occur. NMS consists of very high fever, muscle rigidity, mental changes, irregular pulse or blood pressure, rapid heartbeat, sweating, and abnormal heart rhythm. NMS is potentially fatal and requires immediate medical attention.

Ziprasidone may produce extrapyramidal side effects, including spasm of the neck muscles, rolling back of the eyes, convulsions, difficulty swallowing, and symptoms associated with Parkinson's disease. These side effects usually disappear after the drug has been stopped, although symptoms affecting the face, tongue, or jaw may persist for as long as several years, especially in older adults with a **history of brain damage**. Contact your doctor if you experience any of these side effects.

Antipsychotic drugs, including ziprasidone, may cause involuntary movements of the face and tongue called tardive dyskinesia, which may become permanent. Contact your doctor if you develop any of these side effects.

Ziprasidone should be used with caution in those with **epilepsy** or **a history of seizures**. Antipsychotics can upset the body's temperature-regulating mechanism creating the risk for heat stroke or dehydration.

People with **liver damage or disease** may need to lower dosages of ziprasidone.

Ziprasidone may cause dizziness or fainting when rising from a sitting or standing position, especially when people first start taking the drug.

Possible Side Effects

▼ Most common: sleepiness and nausea.

▼ Common: itching, weakness, headache, rapid heartbeat, dizziness, constipation, nausea, upset stomach, diarrhea, inability to remain in a sitting position, restlessness and a feeling of muscular quivering, extrapyramidal symptoms (see "Cautions and Warnings"), and respiratory conditions.

▼ Less common: accidental injury, rash, fungal infection of the skin, dry mouth, appetite loss, muscle aches, abnormal muscle tone, rigid muscles, runny nose, coughing, and abnormal vision.

▼ Rare: fainting and seizures. Other rare side effects can occur in almost any part of the body. Contact your doctor if you experience any side effect not listed above.

Drug Interactions

- Do not mix ziprasidone with other drugs that can affect the heart. Some drugs to avoid are quinidine, dofetilide, pimozide, sotalol, thioridazine, moxifloxacin, and sparfloxacin.
- Ziprasidone can increase the effects of alcohol, sedatives, and other nervous system depressants.
- Ziprasidone may increase the effect of drugs that lower blood pressure.
- Delavirdine, indinavir, nelfinavir, ritonavir, saquinavir, amiodarone, ciprofloxacin, clarithromycin, diltiazem, erythromycin, fluconazole, fluvoxamine, itraconazole, ketoconazole, mifepristone, nefazodone, norfloxacin, mibefradil, and troleandomycin may increase the amount of ziprasidone in the blood by interfering with its breakdown in the liver.
- Carbamazepine, phenobarbital, phenytoin, and rifampin may reduce ziprasidone blood levels.

- Ziprasidone may antagonize the effects of drugs used to treat Parkinson's disease.

Food Interactions

Avoid grapefruit juice and star fruit as they may interfere with the breakdown of ziprasidone. Take this drug with food.

Usual Dose

Adult: 20–80 mg twice a day. The lowest effective dose is recommended.

Child: not recommended.

Overdosage

In one person who overdosed, the only side effects that developed were minimal sedation, slurring of speech, and a rise in blood pressure that decreased with time. Overdose victims should be taken to a hospital emergency room at once for monitoring and treatment. ALWAYS bring the prescription bottle or container.

Special Information

Avoid alcohol when taking ziprasidone, as with other antipsychotics.

Ziprasidone may take a few weeks to work. Keep taking this drug for as long as your doctor instructs. Do not stop taking ziprasidone if you are feeling better.

Be sure to notify your doctor if you have or had heart disease.

Call your doctor if you become dizzy, faint or have heart palpitations (signs of torsade de pointes), very high fever, muscle rigidity, mental changes, irregular pulse or blood pressure, rapid heartbeat, sweating, or abnormal heart rhythms (signs of NMS).

Rash is common with ziprasidone and may be a sign of a more serious illness. Call your doctor at once if a rash develops.

Some antipsychotics like ziprasidone can interfere with the body's temperature-regulating mechanism. Avoid extreme heat when taking this drug.

Ziprasidone can make you sleepy. Be careful driving and engaging in activities that require coordination and concentration, especially when you first start taking ziprasidone.

If you forget to take a dose of ziprasidone and it is more than 2 hours until your next dose, take the dose you forgot. Otherwise, skip the dose you forgot and continue with your regular schedule. Do not take a double dose.

Special Populations

Pregnancy/Breast-feeding: Ziprasidone may make it more difficult for women to become pregnant. Animal studies suggest that ziprasidone can cause birth defects and fetal death. When this drug is considered crucial by your doctor, its potential benefits must be weighed against its risks.

It is not known if ziprasidone passes into breast milk. Nursing mothers who must take this drug should use infant formula.

Seniors: Older adults may experience more drug side effects.

Zithromax *see Azithromycin, page 131*

Zocor *see Statin Cholesterol-Lowering Agents, page 1052*

Zoloft *see Selective Serotonin Reuptake Inhibitors (SSRIs), page 1020*

Generic Name

Zolpidem (ZOLE-pih-dem) Ⓖ

Brand Names

Ambien   Ambien CR

Type of Drug

Sedative.

Prescribed For

Insomnia.

General Information

Zolpidem is a nonbenzodiazepine sleeping pill that works in the brain in much the same way as do benzodiazepine sleeping pills and sedatives. Unlike the benzodiazepines, however, zolpidem has little muscle-relaxing or antiseizure effects. It is meant for short-term use—7–10 days—and should not be taken regularly for longer than that without your doctor's knowledge. Unlike a benzodi-azepine, zolpidem causes little or no "hangover," and there are no rebound effects after stopping the drug. The CR (controlled-release) formulation was created to address the problem of people not getting a full night's sleep when taking the older, immediate-release product. It does not act as quickly as the older formula-tion because the drug enters the bloodstream much more slowly. Zolpidem is broken down in the liver.

Cautions and Warnings

Do not take zolpidem if you are **allergic** or **sensitive** to any of its ingredients. Rarely, severe allergic reactions have occurred involving swelling of the tongue and throat, nausea, or vomiting. If swelling occurs in the throat, it may be fatal if not treated immediately.

Sleep problems often result from **physical or psychological illnesses**, including worsening of sleep problems, abnormal think-ing, and behavioral changes, including hallucinations, bizarre be-havior, agitation, and depersonalization. Zolpidem does not affect the underlying causes of insomnia. It should be taken only with your doctor's knowledge. If you cannot sleep after 7–10 days of taking zolpidem, contact your doctor.

Studies of zolpidem in **children** ages 6–17 revealed no im-provement in falling asleep and increased risk of side effects, in-cluding an increased risk of hallucinations.

Zolpidem has caused amnesia (memory loss), but this happens mostly at dosages larger than 10 mg a night, and if you do not go to bed immediately after taking the drug.

Sleep driving (driving while not fully awake,

bedtime. Zolpidem may interfere with normal activities the next day, especially if taken with alcohol.

People with **liver disease** require reduced dosage. People with severe **kidney disease** should be monitored for side effects.

Zolpidem should be avoided in the presence of severe **depression,** severe **lung disease, sleep apnea** (condition characterized by intermittent cessation of breathing during sleep), and **drunkenness** or you run the risk of increasing the depressive effects of zolpidem or worsening your overall condition.

Possible Side Effects

Short-Term Use (10 Days or Less)
▼ Most common: headache, drowsiness, dizziness, light-headedness, nausea, and diarrhea.
▼ Less common: chest pain, fatigue, unusual dreams, memory loss, anxiety, nervousness, difficulty sleeping, appetite loss, vomiting, and runny nose.
▼ Rare: Rare side effects can occur in almost any part of the body. Contact your doctor if you experience any side effect not listed above.

Long-Term Use
▼ Most common: headache, dizziness, nausea, drowsiness, and a feeling of being drugged.
▼ Common: allergy symptoms, back pain, flu-like symptoms, lethargy, sensitivity to light, depression, upset stomach, constipation, abdominal pain, muscle and joint pain, upper respiratory infection, sinus irritation, sore throat, rash, urinary infection, heart palpitations, and dry mouth.

Drug Interactions

• A ... turates, ...ing zolpidem with alcohol and other nervous as diazep... sion, tiredn... including sedatives, narcotics, barbi-symptoms. ...es. Taking a benzodiazepine such
• Azole antifunga... selective serotonin ... result in excessive depres-zolpidem's effects an... ...ing difficulties, or similar

...romazine, and ... increase

- Do not combine zolpidem and ritonavir, as this combination may cause severe sedation and respiratory depression.
- Flumazenil may reverse the effects of zolpidem.

Food Interactions

For the most rapid and complete effect, take zolpidem on an empty stomach at least 2 hours after a meal.

Usual Dose

Immediate-Release Zolpidem

Adult (age 18 and over): 10 mg immediately before bedtime. Zolpidem can act very quickly.

Seniors and People With Liver Disease: 5 mg immediately before bedtime.

Child: not recommended.

Controlled-Release (CR) Zolpidem

Adult (age 18 and over): 12.5 mg immediately before bedtime.

Seniors and People With Liver Disease: 6.25 mg immediately before bedtime.

Child: not recommended.

Overdosage

Overdose results in excessive nervous system depression, from unconsciousness to light coma. Combining zolpidem with alcohol or other nervous system depressants may be fatal or affect other body organs. Take the victim to a hospital emergency room at once. ALWAYS bring the prescription bottle or container.

Special Information

Zolpidem may cause tiredness, drowsiness, and an inability to concentrate. Be careful when driving or performing any task that requires concentration on the day following a dose.

People taking zolpidem on a regular basis may develop a drug withdrawal reaction if the medication is stopped suddenly (see "Cautions and Warnings").

If you forget a dose, take it as soon as you remember. If it is almost time for your next dose, skip the forgotten one and continue with your regular schedule. Do not take a double dose.

Special Populations

Pregnancy/Breast-feeding: Animal studies with large do
show that zolpidem may affect the fetus. When this

considered crucial by your doctor, its potential benefits must be carefully weighed against its risks.

Small amounts of zolpidem pass into breast milk. Nursing mothers who must take this drug should use infant formula.

Seniors: Seniors, who are likely to be more sensitive to zolpidem and its side effects, should take the lowest effective dosage.

Generic Name

Zonisamide (zoh-NIS-uh-mide)

Brand Name
Zonegran

Type of Drug
Anticonvulsant.

Prescribed For
Partial seizures.

General Information
Zonisamide was available in Japan for 11 years before it was approved for sale in the U.S. The exact way that this drug works is unknown, but studies suggest it may affect sodium and calcium flow in and out of nerve cells. It does not affect the neurotransmitter GABA, unlike some other anticonvulsant medicines.

Cautions and Warnings
Do not take zonisamide if you are **allergic** or **sensitive** to any of its ingredients or to **sulfa drugs**.

Unexplained skin rash may be a sign of a severe reaction that can be fatal. Contact your doctor immediately if you experience this side effect.

Zonisamide has been associated with serious blood conditions.

Zonisamide has been associated with central nervous system side effects, including depression, psychosis, sleepiness, psychomotor slowing, and difficulty concentrating.

People with severe **kidney disease** may accumulate 1/3 more zonisamide in their blood than others. Lower dosages may be required. Kidney stones are more likely to develop in people taking zonisamide.

People taking zonisamide may be at increased risk of having heat stroke, especially **children**.

People who suddenly stop taking zonisamide may worsen their seizures. Anticonvulsant drugs should be reduced gradually.

Possible Side Effects

▼ Most common: sleepiness, appetite loss, dizziness, headache, nausea, agitation, and irritability.

▼ Common: anxiety, poor muscle coordination, confusion, depression, difficulty concentrating, memory problems, sleeplessness, abdominal pain, and double vision.

▼ Less common: kidney stones, mental slowing, tiredness, unusual eye movements, tingling in the hands or feet, psychotic behavior, constipation, diarrhea, upset stomach, verbal difficulty, taste changes, dry mouth, easy bruising, flu-like symptoms, rash, runny nose, and weight loss.

▼ Rare: Rare side effects can occur in almost any part of the body. Contact your doctor if you experience any side effect not listed above.

Drug Interactions

● Some drugs may reduce the amount of zonisamide in the blood by stimulating enzymes that break it down in the liver. They include carbamazepine, phenobarbital, and phenytoin.

Food Interactions

Zonisamide may be taken with or without food. Avoid drinking grapefruit juice with zonisamide because it can interfere with enzymes that break down the drug.

Usual Dose

100–400 mg a day. Most people taking zonisamide do well with doses in the 100–200 mg range. Higher doses may offer some additional benefit, but they are also associated with an increase in drug side effects.

Overdosage

Overdose symptoms primarily affect the central nervous system, including very low heart rate, coma, low blood pressure, and difficulty breathing. Take the victim to a hospital emergency room. ALWAYS bring the prescription bottle or container.

Special Information

Call your doctor at once if you develop an unexplained skin rash. This may be a sign of a severe reaction.

Sudden back pain, abdominal pain, and blood in the urine may be signs of a kidney stone. Drink plenty of water every day to avoid this problem. Contact your doctor if you experience any of these side effects.

Fever, sore throat, ulcers, and easy bruising can be signs of a blood problem related to zonisamide. Contact your doctor if any of these symptoms develop.

Zonisamide may make you drowsy. Be careful while driving or performing any tasks that require coordination and alertness.

If you forget a dose of zonisamide, take it as soon as you remember. If it is almost time for your next dose, skip the dose you forgot and continue with your regular schedule. Do not take a double dose.

Special Populations

Pregnancy/Breast-feeding: Animal studies of zonisamide have shown it can cause birth defects. Seizure disorder itself has been associated with increased risk of birth defects. Discuss with your doctor the need to control seizure and the potential benefits and risks of taking this medication during pregnancy.

It is not known if zonisamide passes into breast milk. Nursing mothers taking zonisamide should use infant formula or talk to their doctor about switching to a different drug.

Seniors: Seniors may require a lower dose of zonisamide due to normal reductions in kidney or liver function.

Zyprexa   *see **Olanzapine,** page 834*

Zyrtec   *see **Cetirizine,** page 215*

Twenty Questions to Ask Your Doctor and Pharmacist About Your Prescription

Many pharmacies now routinely hand out prescription drug "fact sheets" when a medication is first prescribed. If your pharmacist does not provide you with one, ask him or her for a copy.

1. What is the name of this medication?

2. What results may be expected from taking it?

3. How long should I wait before reporting if this medication does not help me?

4. How does the medication work?

5. What is the exact dosage of the medication?

6. What time of day should I take it?

7. Do alcoholic beverages have an effect on this medication?

8. Do I have to take special precautions with this medication in combination with other prescription medications I am taking?

9. Do I have to take special precautions with this medication in combination with over-the-counter (OTC) or herbal medications?

10. Does food have any effect on this medication?

11. Are there any special instructions I should have about how to use this medication?

12. How long should I continue taking this medication?

13. Is my prescription renewable?

14. For how long a period may my prescription be renewed?

15. Which side effects should I report, and which ones may I disregard?

16. May I save any unused part of this medication for future use?

17. How should I store this medication?

18. How long may I keep this medication without it losing its strength?

19. What should I do if I miss a dose of this medication?

20. Does this medication come in a less expensive, generic form?

Safe Drug Use

- Store your medications in a sealed, light-resistant container to maintain maximum potency, and be sure to follow any special storage instructions listed on your prescription bottle or container, such as "refrigerate," "do not freeze," "protect from light," or "keep in a cool place." Protect all medications from excessive humidity; do not keep them in your bathroom medicine cabinet.
- Make sure each doctor you see knows about all the medications you use regularly, including prescription, over-the-counter (OTC), and herbal medications.
- Keep a record of any bad reaction you have had to a medication.
- Fill each prescription you are given. If you do not fill a prescription, make sure your doctor knows you are not taking the medication.
- Try to fill your prescriptions at the same pharmacy each time. Your pharmacist will keep a record of all your prescription and OTC medications. This listing, called a "Patient Drug Profile," is used to check for potential problems. You may want to keep your own drug profile and take it to your pharmacist for review whenever a new medication is added.
- Do not take extra medication without consulting your doctor or pharmacist.
- Follow the label instructions exactly. If you have any questions, call your doctor or pharmacist.
- Report any unusual symptoms that develop after taking any medication.
- Always read the label before taking your medication. Do not trust your memory.
- Do not share your medication with anyone. Your prescription was written for you and only you. Do not use a prescription medication unless it has been specifically prescribed for you.
- Be sure the label stays on the container until the medication is used or destroyed.
- Keep the label facing up when pouring liquid medication from the bottle so that it is not obscured by spilled medicine.

- For liquid medication, do not forget to shake the bottle, unless directed otherwise.
- If you move to another city, ask your pharmacist to forward your prescription records to your new pharmacy. Carry important medical facts about yourself in your wallet. Such things as drug allergies, chronic diseases (e.g., diabetes), and special requirements may be very useful. Whenever you travel, carry your prescription in its original container.

Safe Use of Eyedrops

To administer eyedrops, lie down or tilt your head back. Hold the dropper above your eye, gently squeeze your lower lid to form a small pouch, and release the drop or drops of medication inside your lower lid while looking up. Release the lower lid, keeping your eye open. Do not blink for 40 seconds. Press gently on the bridge of your nose at the inside corner of your eye for 1 minute to help circulate the drug in your eye. To avoid infection, do not touch the dropper tip to your finger, eyelid, or any other surface. Wait at least 5 minutes before using another eyedrop or eye ointment.

Safety Tips for Self-Injectables

Syringe Storage, Disposal, and Safety

- Store your syringes and needles where others do not have access to them. Some medicines come in prefilled syringes. Store them according to label directions.
- Do not reuse needles or syringes.
- After you have finished using a syringe and needle, cut the needle off and dispose of the needle and syringe in a puncture-resistant, non-see-through container used only for this purpose. Containers specifically designed for needle and syringe disposal can be obtained from a pharmacy.
- Most needles have a device built in so that you may safely cut the needle off. If you do not have one of these devices, you can break the needle off by covering the needle with its protective sheath and working it back and forth until it breaks. Broken needles should be discarded in your disposal device or plastic container.
- Keep containers in areas that are child- and animal-proof.

- When the container is full, seal it securely and throw the entire container away with your regular garbage. Do not throw loose syringes into the garbage.
- Do not put containers filled with used syringes in your recycling bin.
- Do not throw loose needles or lancets into the recycling bin or trash.
- Do not put needles and syringes in soda cans or bottles, glass containers, or milk cartons.
- Do not flush needles or lancets down the toilet.

Choosing an Injection Site

Choose an area for injection where the skin is loose and soft, away from joints, nerves, and bones. Try to avoid the panty or belt line at the waist and the seat portion of your buttocks, as daily activity may irritate these areas.

Good places to use for subcutaneous (under the skin) injection include:

- Arms (outer and upper back portion)
- Abdomen (except around navel and waistline)
- Buttocks (upper outer area)
- Thighs (front and sides except at groin and knee)

Rotating Injection Sites

Change the site where you inject your medicine each time. This helps prevent reactions at the injection site. It also gives the site time to heal from the last injection. Keep a record of where and when you last gave yourself an injection to make sure you do not use the same site too often. If your regular injection areas become tender, talk to your doctor about other possible injection sites.

Self-Injection and Administering Injections to Another Person

- Before you begin, gather your needle and syringe, medicine, alcohol swabs, and cotton balls or gauze pad. Be sure you also have your needle disposal container nearby.
- Do not use an injection solution if it has particles floating in it.
- Certain injection mixtures should not be shaken. Refer to your product patient information for specific instruction.
- Wash your hands.
- Choose an area for injection. Use a different site each day. Do not use any area in which you feel lumps, bumps, firm

knots, or pain. Do not use any area in which the skin is discolored, depressed, scabbed, or has broken open.
- You may use an alcohol swab to clean the skin at the injection site. Let the area air dry. Discard the wipe. Uncap the needle.
- Slowly draw the exact amount of drug prescribed into the syringe, being careful to avoid air bubbles in the solution to be injected.
- Pinch up the skin to prevent injecting the drug into a muscle, and pull back slightly on the plunger to make sure you have not entered a vein.
- Hold the syringe like a pencil or dart and insert the needle at a 45° angle to the skin.
- If blood enters the syringe, remove it and throw it away.
- If no blood enters the syringe, slowly depress the syringe plunger until the contents have been completely injected.
- Hold another alcohol swab on the injection site. Remove the needle from the skin. Gently massage the injection site with a dry cotton ball or gauze pad.
- You may ice the area before and after injection to reduce pain and inflammation.
- If injecting into the leg, extend your leg out to reduce the chance of injecting into a muscle.
- Your doctor, nurse, or pharmacist can help you master this procedure.

Complications of Self-Injection
- You may notice bruising around the injection. This is due to the piercing of tiny blood vessels and is generally not a problem.
- Sometimes harmless but unsightly lumpy areas develop at injection sites. This is due to an increase in fatty tissue at the site of injection, especially when injecting daily insulin. Avoid injecting into these fatty lumps.
- Visible depressions in the skin may develop due to a loss of fat tissue at the injection site.
- To avoid infection at injection sites, always wash your hands before you begin the procedure, do not touch the bare needle before the actual injection, and do not reuse or share needles with another person.
- Call your doctor if an injection site becomes infected. Signs of infection include redness, pain, swelling, and possible oozing. You may apply a non-prescription antibiotic cream or ointment to that area, but your doctor should be aware of this complication.

Medicine and Money

- Make sure you tell the doctor everything about your health problem. More information allows your doctor to provide the most effective treatment.
- Do not hesitate to discuss the cost of medical care with your doctor or pharmacist.
- Generic drugs are usually less expensive than brand-name drugs, whether you pay for them out-of-pocket or have a co-pay with your insurance company. A drug often becomes available generically when its patent has expired, typically 20 years after the patent was granted.
- If you suffer from a chronic condition, you will probably save money by buying in larger quantities.
- Prescription prices vary from pharmacy to pharmacy; it may be worthwhile to comparison shop for the more expensive medications. Internet pharmacies may also have low-cost prescription drugs available, although you must allow additional time for delivery. Many pharmacies will match internet prices, if requested.
- Some insurance companies offer discounted quantities of prescription drugs through a mail-order pharmacy program. Most mail order programs will fill a three-month supply of medication and only charge the co-pay for a two-month supply. Again, extra time must be factored in for delivery.

The Top 200 Prescription Drugs in the United States

RANKED BY NUMBER OF PRESCRIPTIONS DISPENSED FROM JANUARY TO DECEMBER 2006

(Note: Generic drugs by different manufacturers and different formulations of the same drug have been combined.)

1. Hydrocodone + Acetaminophen
2. Levothyroxine
3. Lipitor
4. Metoprolol
5. Lisinopril
6. Amoxicillin
7. Hydrochlorothiazide
8. Atenolol
9. Metformin
10. Azithromycin
11. Alprazolam
12. Furosemide
13. Norvasc
14. Albuterol
15. Potassium Chloride
16. Sertraline
17. Simvastatin
18. Ambien
19. Lexapro
20. Nexium
21. Singulair
22. Zyrtec
23. Ibuprofen
24. Oxycodone + Acetaminophen
25. Warfarin
26. Cephalexin
27. Prednisone
28. Triamterene + Hydrochlorothiazide
29. Clopidogrel
30. Propoxyphene + Acetaminophen
31. Fluoxetine
32. Prevacid
33. Bupropion
34. Lorazepam
35. Paroxetine
36. Amoxicillin + Potassium Clavulanate
37. Advair Diskus
38. Clonazepam
39. Cyclobenzaprine
40. Effexor XR
41. Fosamax
42. Fexofenadine
43. Gabapentin
44. Protonix
45. Tramadol
46. Ciprofloxacin
47. Vytorin
48. Acetaminophen + Codeine
49. Fluticasone
50. Trazodone

51. Diovan
52. Lisinopril + Hydrochlorothiazide
53. Amitriptyline
54. Lovastatin
55. Lotrel
56. Levaquin
57. Glipizide
58. Premarin
59. Enalapril
60. Omeprazole
61. Naproxen
62. Amphetamine + Dextroamphetamine
63. Trimethoprim + Sulfa
64. Valium
65. Zetia
66. Ranitidine
67. Citalopram
68. Fluconazole
69. Diovan HCT
70. Crestor
71. Avandia
72. Actos
73. Digoxin
74. Altace
75. Celebrex
76. Allopurinol
77. Doxycycline
78. Carisoprodol
79. Viagra
80. Clonidine
81. Coreg
82. Yasmin 28
83. Methylprednis Tabs
84. Nasonex
85. Seroquel
86. Tricor
87. Lantus
88. Flomax
89. Isosorbide Mononitrate
90. Actonel
91. Promethazine
92. Verapamil
93. Glyburide
94. Pravastatin
95. Cymbalta
96. Cozaar
97. Oxycodone
98. Omnicef
99. Folic Acid
100. Penicillin
101. Concerta
102. Diltiazem
103. Spironolactone
104. Polyethylene Glycol
105. Risperdal
106. Temazepam
107. Ortho Tri-Cyclen Lo
108. Valtrex
109. Depakote
110. Aciphex
111. Glimepiride
112. Quinapril
113. Moxifloxacin
114. Clindamycin
115. Topamax
116. Meloxicam
117. Hyzaar
118. Xalatan
119. Triamcinolone Acetonide
120. Nitroglycerin
121. Benazepril
122. Metronidazole
123. Metoclopramide
124. Avapro
125. Hydroxyzine
126. Lunesta
127. Estradiol
128. Diclofenac
129. Gemfibrozil
130. Benicar
131. Lyrica
132. Lamictal

133. Doxazosin
134. Combivent
135. Detrol LA
136. Allegra-D
137. Meclizine
138. Glyburide + Metformin
139. Benicar HCT
140. Trinessa
141. Nitrofurantoin
142. Aricept
143. Evista
144. Mirtazapine
145. Nabumetone
146. Spiriva
147. Bisoprolol + Hydrochlorothiazide
148. Tri-Sprintec
149. Propranolol HCl
150. Imitrex
151. Cialis
152. Ortho Evra
153. Acyclovir
154. Minocycline
155. Flovent HFA
156. Butalbital + Acetaminophen + Caffeine
157. Tramadol HCl + Acetaminophen
158. Niaspan
159. Promethazine + Codeine
160. Buspirone
161. Methotrexate
162. Avalide
163. Zyprexa
164. Terazosin
165. Clotrimazole + Betamethasone
166. Quinine
167. Nasacort AQ
168. Strattera
169. Fentanyl
170. NuvaRing
171. Clarinex
172. Skelaxin
173. Sulfamethoxazole + Trimethoprim
174. Patanol
175. Nifedipine
176. Abilify
177. Famotidine
178. Phenytoin
179. Ferrous Sulfate
180. Humalog
181. Phentermine
182. Lithium
183. Atenolol Chlorthalidone
184. Benzonatate
185. Tizanidine
186. Etodolac
187. Aviane
188. Methocarbamol
189. Phenazopyridine
190. Boniva
191. Rhinocort Aqua
192. Nortriptyline
193. Mupirocin
194. Fosinopril
195. Chlorhexidine Glucon
196. Aspirin
197. Tussionex
198. Colchicine
199. Hyoscyamine
200. Felodipine

Index of Generic and Brand-Name Drugs

How to Find Your Medication in *The Pill Book*

- *The Pill Book* lists most medications in alphabetic order by generic name because a medication may have many brand names but has only 1 generic name. Most generic medications produce the same therapeutic effects as their brand-name equivalents but are much less expensive. Drugs that are available generically are indicated by the Ⓖ symbol.

- When a medication has 2 or more active ingredients, it is listed by the most widely known brand name. In a few cases, pill profiles are listed by drug type (e.g., Sulfonylurea Antidiabetes Drugs).

- *The Pill Book* includes the names of the top 100 brand-name drugs (cross-referenced to their generic name) in alphabetic order with the pill profiles.

- Most over-the-counter (OTC) medications are not included in *The Pill Book*. For complete information on OTC medications, refer to *The Pill Book Guide to Over-the-Counter Medications*.

- All brand and generic names are listed in the Index. Brand names are indicated by boldface.

- Sugar-free and alcohol-free brand-name drugs are indicated by the Ⓢ and Ⓐ symbols in the beginning of each pill profile.

A

1%HC, 324
40 Winks, 375
Abacavir, 542, 543
Abilify, 107, plate A

Abilify Discmelt, 107
Acamprosate, 1
Acarbose, 731
Accolate, 626, plate A

AccuHist, 97
AccuNeb, 32
Accupril, 947, plate A
Accuretic, 947
Accutane, 607, plate A
Acebutolol, 3
Aceon, 947
Acephen, 7
Aceta, 7
Acetaminophen, 7, 252, 481, 863, 864, 929, 1152
Acetaminophen Uniserts, 7
Aceta with Codeine, 863
Acetazolamide, 10
Acetohexamide, 1065
Aciphex, 940, plate A
Acitretin, 13
Aclovate, 323
Acrivastine, 95
Acticin, 872
Actifed, 99
Actifed Cold and Allergy, 96
Actiq Lozenge on a Stick, 279
Activella Combipatch, 442
Actonel, 164, plate A
Actonel with Calcium, 164
ACTOplus Met, 528
Actos, 528, plate A
Acular, 828
Acyclovir, 17
Adalat CC, 799, plate A
Adapalene, 20
Adderall, 23, plate A
Adderall XR, 23
Adefovir, 27
Advair Diskus, 304, 1014
Advair HFA, 304, 1014
Advicor, 1052, plate A
Advil, 821
AeroBid, 304
Aerospan HFA, 304
Afeditab CR, 799
Agenerase, 69
Aggrenox, 30, plate A
Agrylin, 74
AK Beta, 151

Akne-mycin, 433
AK-Spore, 785
AK-Spore H.C. Otic, 329
Alacol, 96
Ala-Cort, 324
Alamast, 853
Ala-Scalp, 324
Alavert, 660
Alavert Allergy & Sinus D-12, 98
Alavert Children's, 660
Alaway Eyedrops, 611
Albuterol, 32
Albuterol Sulfate, 597
Alclometasone Dipropionate, 323
Alcortin, 324
Aldactazide, 36, 397, plate A
Aldactone, 36
Aldara, 572
Aldosterone Blockers, 36
Alenaze-D, 96
Alendronate Sodium, 164
Alesse, 287
Aleve, 822
Alferon N, 590
Alfuzosin, 48
Alinia, 808
Aliskiren, 40
Alitretinoin, 43
Allay, 864
Allegra, 215, plate A
Allegra-D, 98, plate B
Allent, 95
AllenVan-S, 98
Aller-Chlor, 97, 224
Allerest PE, 96
Allerfrim, 99
AllerMax, 375
AllerMax Maximum Strength, 375
AllerTan, 97
AlleRx, 97
Alli, 841
Allopurinol, 45
Almotriptan, 1178
Alocril, 334
Alomide Eyedrops, 612

Alora, 441
Alosetron, 88
Alpha Blockers, 48
Alphagan P, 176
Alprazolam, 51
Alprostadil, 55
Alrex, 301
Altabax, 979
Altace, 947, plate B
Altaryl Children's Allergy, 375
Altoprev, 1052
Alupent, 691
Alvesco, 304
Alzide Novo-Spirozine, 397
Amaryl, 1065, plate B
Ambien, 1232, plate B
Ambien CR, 1232
Ambrisentan, 169
Amcinonide, 320, 321
Amerge, 1178
Americet, 481
Amiloride, 397
Aminolevulinic Acid, 57
Aminophylline, 1217
Amiodarone, 59
Amitiza, 668, plate B
Amitriptyline, 1171
Amlexanox, 63
Amlodipine, 65, 81, 663, 1052
Amnesteem, 607
Amoxapine, 1171
Amoxicillin, 857, 940
Amoxil, 857, plate B
Amphetamine Aspartate, 23
Amphetamine Sulfate, 23
Amprenavir, 69
Amrix, 338
Anafranil, 1171
Anagrelide, 74
Anakinra, 76
Analpram-HC, 324
Anaprox, 822
Anaprox DS, 822
Anaspaz, 385
Anastrozole, 78
Anatuss LA, 420

Ancobon, 493, plate B
Andec, 96
Andehist NR Drops, 96
Andehist NR Syrup, 95
Androderm, 1099
AndroGel, 1099
Androgen, 287, 288, 289, 290
Android, 1099
Anexsia, 864
Anexsia 5/500, 864
Anexsia 7.5/650, 864
Anexsia 10/660, 864
Angeliq, 442
Angiotensin II Blockers, 80
Anisindione, 1212
Ansaid, 821, plate B
Antara, 475
Anthelios SX Cream, 87
AntibiOtic, 329
Antiemetics (5HT3 Type), 88
Antihistamine-Decongestant
   Combination Products, 95
Antihistamine Eyedrops, 92
Antispas, 385
Antispasmotic, 385
Antivert, 372, plate B
Antivert 25, 372
Antivert 50, 372
Antrizine, 372
Anusol-HC, 324
Anzemet, 88
Apacet, 7
Apexicon, 320
Apexicon E, 320
Aphthasol, 63
Apidra, 585
Apraclonidine, 101
Aprepitant, 104
Apresoline, 564
Aprodine, 99
Aptivus, 1134
Aquatab D Dosepack, 420
Aranelle, 289
Arava, 620
Arestin, 1103
Arformoterol, 509

Aricept, 237, plates B and C
Aricept ODT, 237
Arimidex, 78
Aripiprazole, 107
Aristocort, 323
Aristocort A, 322
Aristocort Cream and Ointment, 322
Armodafinil, 744
Armour Thyroid, 1118
Aromasin, 455
Arthrotec, 822, plate C
Asacol, 173
Ascomp with Codeine, 868
Asmanex Twisthaler, 304
A-Spas S/L, 385
Aspirin, 30, 110, 484, 487, 868, 869, 929
Aspirin Free Anacin Maximum Strength, 7
Aspirin Free Pain Relief, 7
Astelin, 215
Atacand, 80, plate C
Atacand HCT, 81
Atarax, 567, plate C
Atazanavir, 115
Atenolol, 119
Ativan, 358, plate C
Atomoxetine, 125
Atorvastatin, 65, 1052
Atovaquone, 128
Atralin, 1163
Atretol, 196
Atridox, 1103
Atripla, 543
Atrohist Pediatric, 97
Atropine Sulfate, 385, 751
Atrovent, 597
A/T/S, 433
Augmentin, 857, plate C
Augmentin ES-600, 857
Augmentin XR, 857, plate C
Avage, 1082
Avalide, 81, plate C
Avandamet, 528

Avandaryl, 528
Avandia, 528, plate C
Avapro, 81, plates C and D
Avelox, 495, plate D
Aventyl, 1172
Aviane, 287
Avinza, 279
Avita, 1163
Avobenzone, 87
Avodart, 478
Avonex, 594
Axert, 1178, plate D
Axid, 818, plate D
Axid AR, 818
Axid Pulvules, 818
Aygestin, 679
Azatadine, 95
Azelastine, 92, 215, 838
Azilect, 968
Azithromycin, 131
Azmacort, 304
Azole Antifungals, 134
Azopt, 200
Azulfidine, 1061
Azulfidine EN-Tabs, 1061

B

Baclofen, 140
Bactocill, 857
Bactrim, 1031
Bactrim DS, 1031, plate D
Bactroban, 764
Balsalazide, 173
Bancap HC, 864
Banophen, 375
Banophen Allergy, 375
Baraclude, 417
Barbidonna, 385
Bayer Select Pain Relief Formula, 821
Becaplermin, 143
Beclomethasone Dipropionate, 303, 309
Beconase AQ, 309

Bellatal, 385, 842
Bemote, 361
Benadryl Allergy, 375
Benadryl Children's Allergy, 375
Benadryl Children's Dye Free, 375
Benadryl-D Allergy & Sinus, 98
Benadryl Dye Free Allergy Liquid Gels, 375
Benazepril, 65, 145
Benazepril Hydrochloride, 663
Bendroflumethiazide, 1129
Benicar, 81
Benicar HCT, 81
Bentyl, 361, plate D
Betagan, 151
Betaine, 149
Betamethasone, 313
Betamethasone Dipropionate, 319, 320, 321, 322, 666
Betamethasone Valerate, 321, 322, 323
Betapace, 1130
Betapace AF, 1130
Betaseron, 594
Betatrex, 322
Beta-Val, 322
Betaxolol, 151
Betimol, 1129
Betoptic, 151
Betoptic S, 151
Biaxin, 249, plate D
Biaxin XL, 249, plate D
Bicalutamide, 154
BidHist-D, 95
BiDil, 157
Bimatoprost, 936
Biohist-LA, 97
Bismuth Subcitrate Potassium, 538
Bismuth Subsalicylate, 538
Bisoprolol, 160
Bisphosphonates, 164
Blephamide, 301
Blephamide S.O.P., 301

Bonine, 372
Boniva, 164, plate D
Bosentan, 169
Bowel Anti-Inflammatory Drugs (5-ASA Type), 173
Brevicon, 289
Brimonidine, 176
Brinzolamide, 200
Bristacycline, 1103
Brofed, 95
Bromadrine, 95
Bromadrine PD, 95
Bromanate Elixir, 95
Bromfed, 95
Bromfed-PD, 95
Bromfenac, 828
Bromfenex, 95
Bromfenex PD, 95
Bromhist NR, 95
Bromhist PD, 95
Brompheniramine, 95, 96
Broncholate, 421
Bronkaid, 421
Brontex, 1189
Brovana, 509
Brovex SR, 95
BroveX-D, 96
Budeprion, 179
Budeprion XL, 179
Budesonide, 303, 304, 309, 313, 509
Buffered Aspirin, 110
Bumetanide, 652
Bumex, 652, plate E
Buprenorphine, 774
Bupropion, 179
BuSpar, 183, plate E
Buspirone, 183
Butalbital, 481, 484, 487
Butalgen, 484
Butenafine, 185
Butoconazole Nitrate, 723
Byclomine, 361
Byetta, 457
Bystolic, 119

C

Caduet, 65, 1052, plate E
Caffeine, 481, 484, 487, 868, 929
Calan, 1205, plate E
Calan SR, 1205, plate E
Calcitonin, 187
Calcium Carbonate, 164
Calm-X, 372
Campral, 1
Canasa, 173
Candesartan, 80, 81
Capecitabine, 189
Capex Shampoo, 321
Capital with Codeine, 863
Capoten, 192, plate E
Capozide, 192
Cap-Profen, 821
Captopril, 192
Carafate, 1059
Carbamazepine, 196
Carbatrol, 196
Carbaxefed, 96
Carbaxefed RF, 96
Carbenicillin Indanyl Sodium, 857
Carbic-D, 96
Carbic-DS, 96
Carbidopa, 1042
Carbilev, 1042
Carbinoxamine, 96
Carbiset, 96
Carbiset TR, 96
Carbodec, 96
Carbodec TR, 96
Carbonic-Anhydrase Inhibitors,
　Eyedrops, 200
Carbonyl Iron, 600
Carboxine-PSE, 96
Cardec, 96
Cardec-S, 96
Cardene, 791
Cardene SR, 791
Cardioquin, 950
Cardizem, 369, plate E
Cardizem CD, 369, plate E
Cardizem LA, 369

Cardura, 389, plate F
Cardura XL, 389
Carozide, 1113
Carteolol, 151
Cartia XT, 369, plate F
Carvedilol, 203
Casodex, 154
Cataflam, 821
Catapres, 261, plate F
Catapres-TTS-1, 261
Catapres-TTS-2, 261
Catapres-TTS-3, 261
Caverject, 55
Cedax, 211
Cefaclor, 210
Cefadroxil, 210
Cefdinir, 210
Cefditoren Pivoxil, 211
Cefixime, 211
Cefpodoxime Proxetil, 211
Cefprozil, 211
Ceftibuten, 211
Ceftin, 211
Cefuroxime Axetil, 211
Cefzil, 211, plate F
Celebrex, 206, plate F
Celecoxib, 206
Celestone, 313
Celexa, 1020, plate F
CellCept, 769, plate F
Cenafed, 98
Cena-K, 899
Cenestin, 441
Centany, 764
Cephalexin, 211
Cephalosporin Antibiotics, 210
Cerebyx, 882
Ceron, 96
Cetacort, 324
Ceta-Plus, 864
Cetirizine, 96, 215
Cetrorelix, 671
Cetrotide, 671
Cevimeline, 218
Chantix, 1198, plate F
Cheracol, 1189

Cheratussin AC, 1189
Children's Advil, 821
Children's Benadryl-D Allergy & Sinus, 98
Children's Motrin, 821
Children's Pediacare Nighttime Cough, 375
Chlordiazepoxide, 221
Chlorex A, 97
Chlorex-A12, 97
Chlorothiazide, 1113
Chlorpheniramine, 1186
Chlorpheniramine Maleate, 96, 97, 224
Chlorpheniramine Polistirex, 97
Chlorpheniramine Tannate, 97
Chlorpromazine, 228
Chlorpropamide, 1065
Chlorthalidone, 119, 1113
Chlor-Trimeton, 224
Chlor-Trimeton Allergy 8 Hour, 224
Chlor-Trimeton Allergy 12 Hour, 224
Chlorzoxazone, 232
Cholecalciferol, 164
Choledyl SA, 1217
Cholestyramine, 234
Cholinesterase Inhibitors, 237
Chromagen, 600
Cialis, 426, plate G
Cibalith-S, 648
Ciclesonide, 309
Ciclopirox, 241
Cilostazol, 243
Ciloxan Eyedrops, 495
Cimetidine, 245
Cipro, 495, plate G
Ciprodex, 300
Ciprofloxacin, 300, 495
Cipro XR, 495, plate G
Citalopram Hydrobromide, 1020
Claravis, 607
Clarinex, 660, plate G
Clarinex-D, 98
Clarinex RediTabs, 660

Clarithromycin, 249, 940
Claritin, 660
Claritin 24-Hour Allergy, 660
Claritin Children's Allergy, 660
Claritin-D, 98
Claritin Hives, 660
Claritin Reditabs, 660
Clear-Atadine, 660
Clear-Atadine D, 98
Clemastine, 252
Cleocin, 255
Cleocin T, 255
Climara, 441
Climara Pro, 442
Clinda-Derm, 255
Clindagel, 255
Clindamycin, 255, 1163
Clindesse, 255
Clindets, 255
Clinoril, 822, plate G
Clobetasol Propionate, 320
Clobex, 320
Clocortolone Pivalate, 322
Cloderm, 322
Clomipramine, 1171
Clonazepam, 258
Clonidine, 261
Clopidogrel, 265
Clorazepate, 264
Clorfed, 97
Clorfed II, 97
Clotrimazole, 271, 666
Cloxacillin Sodium, 857
Cloxapen, 857
Clozapine, 274
Clozaril, 274
Codeine, 279
Codeine Phosphate, 487, 863, 868, 924, 925, 1189
Co-Gesic, 864
Cognex, 237
Colazal, 173, plate G
Colchicine, 284
Coldec-D, 96
Coldmist, 420
Coldmist Jr., 420

Coldmist LA, 420
Colesevelam Hydrochloride, 234
Colestid, 234
Colestipol Hydrochloride, 234
Colfed-A, 97
Combivent, 32, 597
Combivir, 543
Combunox, 279, 822
Commit, 794
Compazine, 920, plate G
Compazine Spansule, 920, plate G
Compoz Gel Caps, 375
Compoz Nighttime Sleep Aid, 376
Compro, 920
Comtan, 414, plate G
Concerta, 706, plate G
Condylox, 893
Congess Jr., 420
Congess SR, 421
Congestac, 421
Conjugated Estrogens, 441
Contraceptives, 287
Copaxone, 526
Copegus, 981
Cordarone, 59, plate G
Cordran, 322
Cordran Lotion 0.05%, 323
Cordran Ointment 0.25%, 323
Cordran SP 0.025%, 323
Cordran SP 0.05%, 323
Cordran Tape, 320
Cordron-D, 96
Coreg, 203
Coreg CR, 203, plate G
Corgard, 1130, plate G
Cormax, 320
Cortaid Intensive Therapy, 324
Cortatrigen Ear Drops, 329
Cortef, 314
Cortef Feminine Itch, 324
Corticaine, 324
Corticosteroids, Eye Products, 300
Corticosteroids, Inhalers, 303

Corticosteroids, Nasal, 309
Corticosteroids, Oral, 313
Corticosteroids, Topical, 319
Cortifoam, 324
Cortisone Acetate, 313
Cortisporin Otic, 329
Cortizone-5, 324
Cortizone-10, 324
Cortizone-10 Plus, 324
Cortizone-10 Quickshot, 324
Cortizone for Kids, 324
Corzide, 1129
Cosopt, 200, 331, 1129
Coumadin, 1212, plate H
Covera-HS, 1205, plate H
Cozaar, 81, plate H
CP DEC, 96
Crestor, 1052
Crinone, 680
Crixivan, 574
Crolom, 334
Cromolyn, 334
Cryselle, 288
Cutivate, 321, 322, 323
Cyanocobalamin, 898
Cyclessa, 289
Cyclobenzaprine, 338
Cyclosporine, 341
Cydec, 96
Cymbalta, 1200, plate H
Cyproheptadine Hydrochloride, 224
Cystadane, 149
Cytomel, 1118
Cytospaz, 385
Cytotec, 742

D

Dallergy Drops, 96
Dallergy JR, 96
Dallergy JR Suspension, 97
Dalmane, 503, plate H
Darifenacin, 1144
Darvocet A500, 929
Darvocet-N 50, 929

Darvocet-N 100, 929, plate H
Darvon Compound, 929
Darvon Compound-65, 929
Darvon-N, 929
Darvon Pulvules, 929
Darunavir, 347
Dasatinib, 754
DayHist-1, 252
Daypro, 822, plate H
Daytrana Patch, 706
DDAVP, 355
Declomycin, 1103
Deconamine, 97
Deconamine SR, 97, plate H
Deconomed SR, 97
Deconsal LA, 421
Deconsal II, 421
Deconsal Pediatric, 421
Deferasirox, 352
Delavirdine, 542
Delcort, 324
Delta-Tritex, 321
Delta-Tritex Cream, 322
Demadex, 653
Demeclocycline, 1103
Demerol, 685, plate H
Demulen 1/35, 288
Demulen 1/50E, 288
Denavir, 855
Depade, 773
Depakene, 1194
Depakote, 1194, plate H
Depakote ER, 1194, plate H
Depakote Sprinkle, 1194, plate H
Depo-Provera, 679
Dermabet, 322
Derma-Smoothe/FS Oil, 323
Dermatop E, 322, 323
Desenex Max, 1090
Desipramine, 1171
Desloratadine, 98, 660
Desmopressin, 355
Desogen, 288
Desonate, 322
Desonide, 322, 323
DesOwen, 322, 323

Desoximetasone, 320, 322
Desyrel, 1159, plate H
Desyrel Dividose, 1159, plate I
Detrol, 1144, plate I
Detrol LA, 1144, plate I
Dexamethasone, 300, 313
Dexaphen-SA, 98
Dexbrompheniramine, 98
Dexchlorpheniramine Maleate, 98, 224
Dexedrine, 23
Dexmethylphenidate, 706
Dextroamphetamine Saccharate, 23
Dextroamphetamine Sulfate, 23
Dextromethorphan Hydrobromide, 925
Dextrostat, 23
D-Feda II, 421
DiaBeta, 1066, plate I
Diabinese, 1065, plate I
Diar-Aid, 657
Diastat, 357
Diazepam, 357
Diazepam Intensol, 357
Dibent, 361
Diclofenac, 821, 822, 828
Dicloxacillin Sodium, 857
Dicyclomine, 361
Didanosine, 542
Didronel, 164
Difenoxin Hydrochloride, 751
Differin, 20
Diflorasone Diacetate, 320
Diflucan, 134, plate I
Diflunisal, 821
Digitek, 365
Digoxin, 365
Dihydrocodeine Bitartrate, 868
Dilacor XR, 369, plate I
Dilantin, 882, plate I
Dilantin-125, 882
Dilantin Infatab, 882
Dilantin Kapseals, 882
Dilatrate-SR, 604
Dilomine, 361

Dilt-CD, 369
Diltia XT, 369
Diltiazem, 369
Diltzac, 369
Dimaphen Elixir, 95
Dimenhydrinate, 372
Dimetabs, 372
**Dimetapp Children's ND
　Allergy,** 660
**Dimetapp Cold & Allergy
　Chewable Tablets,** 96
Dimetapp Cold & Allergy Elixir,
　95
Diovan, 81, plate I
Diovan HCT, 81, plate I
Dipentum, 173
Diphen AF, 376
Diphenhist, 376
Diphenhydramine Hydrochloride,
　98, 375
Diphenhydramine Tannate, 98
DiphenMax D, 98
Diprolene, 319, 321
Diprolene AF, 320
Diprosone, 321
Dipyridamole, 30
Disopyramide, 379
Di-Spaz, 361
DisperMox, 857
Ditropan, 850, plate I
Ditropan XL, 850, plate J
Diuril, 1113, plate J
Divigel, 441
Dofetilide, 382
Dolacet, 864
Dolasetron, 88
Dolgic LQ, 481
Dolgic Plus, 481
Donepezil, 237
Donnamar, 385
Donnapine, 385
Donnatal, 385
Donnatal Extencaps, 385
Doral, 1167, plate J
Dormin, 376
Doryx, 1103

Dorzolamide, 200, 331, 1129
Doxazosin, 389
Doxepin, 1172
Doxercalciferol, 392
Doxycycline, 1103
Dramamine, 372
Dricort, 324
Drisdol Liquid, 392
Drixomed, 98
Drixoral Cold & Allergy, 98
Dronabinol, 394
Drosperinone, 442
Drotic, 329
D-Tann, 98
Duetact, 528
Duloxetine, 1200
Duocet, 864
Duonate-12, 98
DuoNeb, 32, 597
Duradyne DHE, 864
Duragesic (Patch), 279
Durasal II, 421
Duratuss AM/PM, 421
Duricef, 210, plate J
Dutasteride, 478
Dutoprol, 713
Dyazide, 397, plate J
Dynacin, 1103
DynaCirc CR, 799
Dynafed, Children's JR, 7
Dynafed EX, 7
Dynafed Extra Strength, 7
Dynex, 421
Dyphylline, 1217
Dytan-D, 98
Dytuss, 376

E

Ear-Eze, 329
E-Base, 433
Ecamsule, 87
EC-Naprosyn, 822
Econazole, 401
Econopred Plus, 301
Ed A-Hist, 96

Ed Chlor-PED, 97
Edecrin, 652
Edex, 55
ED-IN-SOL, 601
ED-SPAZ, 385
E.E.S., 434, plate J
Efalizumab, 402
Efavirenz, 542, 543
Effer-K, 900
Effexor, 1200, plate J
Effexor XR, 1200, plate J
Efidac, 224
Eflornithine, 405
E-Glades, 433
Eldepryl, 1027
Elestat, 92
Elestrin, 441
Eletriptan, 1178
Elidel Cream, 887
Elimite, 872
Elixophyllin, 1217
Elmiron, 861, plate J
Elocon, 321, 322
Emadine, 92
Embeline, 320
Embeline E, 320
Emedastine, 92
Emend, 104
EMLA, 638
**Empirin with Codeine
    No. 3,** 868
**Empirin with Codeine
    No. 4,** 868
Emsam, 1027
Emtricitabine, 542, 543
Emtriva, 542
E-Mycin, 433
Enablex, 1144, plate J
Enalapril, 407, 471, 634
Enbrel, 452
Endafed, 95
Endal, 421
Endal-SR, 421
Endocet, 863
Endocodone, 279
Endometrin Vaginal Insert, 680

Enduron, 1113
Enfuvirtide, 411
Enjuvia, 441
Entacapone, 414, 1042
Entecavir, 417
Entex LA, 421
Entocort EC, 313
Ephedrine Hydrochloride, 421
Epinastine, 92
Epitol, 196
Epivir, 543
Epivir-HBV, 543
Eplerenone, 36
Epoetin, 424
Epogen, 424
Eprosartan, 81
Epzicom, 543, plate K
Equetro, 196
Erectile Dysfunction Drugs, 426
Ergoloid Mesylates, 431
Ertaczo, 271
Eryc, 433
Eryderm, 433
Erygel, 433
EryPed, 434
Ery-Tab, 433, plate K
Erythra-derm, 433
Erythrocin Stearate, 434,
    plate K
Erythromycin, 433
Erythromycin Estolate, 434
Erythromycin Ethylsuccinate, 434
Erythromycin Stearate, 434
Eryzole, 434
Escitalopram Oxylate, 1020
Esgic, 481
Esgic-Plus, 481
Esidrix, 1113
Eskalith, 648, plate K
Eskalith CR, 648
Esomeprazole Magnesium, 939
Estazolam, 438
Esterified Estrogens, 441
Estrace, 441, plate K
Estraderm, 441
Estradiol, 441, 442

Estratest, 441, plate K
Estring, 441
Estrogel, 441
Estrogen, 287, 288, 289, 290, 441
Estropipate, 442
Estrostep 21, 289
Estrostep Fe, 289
Eszopiclone, 449
Etanercept, 452
Ethacrynic Acid, 652
Ethinyl Estradiol, 442
Ethotoin, 882
ETH-Oxydose, 864
Etidronate Disodium, 164
Etodolac, 821
Etonorgestrel, 290
Etrafon, 1171
Etravirine, 543
Evamist Transdermal Spray, 441
Evista, 954, plate K
Evoclin, 255
Evoxac, 218
Exelon, 237, plate K
Exelon Transdermal System, 237
Exemestane, 455
Exenatide, 457
Exforge, 65, 81
Exjade, 352
Extina, 134
Extra Strength CortaGel, 324
Ezetimibe, 460, 1052
Ezide, 1113

F

Factive, 495
Famciclovir, 463
Famotidine, 465
Famvir, 463, plate K
Fansidar, 1061
Farbital, 484
Fareston, 1077

FazaClo Orally Disintegrating Tablets, 274
Felbamate, 468
Felbatol, 468
Feldene, 822, plate K
Felodipine, 471, 634
Femara, 78
Femcet, 481
FemHRT 1/5, 442
Femiron, 600
Femring, 441
Femstat, 723
Femtrace, 441
Fenofibrate, 475
Fenoprofen Calcium, 821
Fentanyl, 279
Fentora Buccal Tablet, 279
Feosol, 600, 601
Feostat, 600
Feratab, 601
Fer-Gen-Sol, 601
Fergon, 601
Fer-In-Sol, 601
Ferretts, 600
Ferrex 150, 601
Ferro-Sequels, 601
Ferrous Fumarate, 600
Ferrous Gluconate, 601
Ferrous Sulfate, 601
Fe-Tinie 150, 601
Feverall, 7
Feverall, Infants, 7
Fexofenadine, 98, 215
Finasteride, 478
Fioricet, 481, plate L
Fioricet with Codeine, 863
Fiorigen, 484
Fiorimor, 484
Fiorinal, 484
Fiorinal with Codeine, 487, 868
Flagyl, 718, plate L
Flagyl ER, 718
Flarex, 301
Flecainide, 490
Flector, 821

Flexeril, 338, plate L
Flomax, 1080, plate L
Flonase, 309
Florone, 320
Florone E, 320
Florvite, 898
Flovent Diskus, 304
Flovent HFA, 304
Floxin, 496, plate L
Floxin Otic, 496
Fluconazole, 134
Flucytosine, 493
Fludrocortisone, 314
Flumadine, 994
Flunisolide, 304, 309
Fluocinolone Acetonide, 321, 322, 323, 1163
Fluocinonide, 320, 321
Fluorometholone, 301
Fluoroquinolone Anti-Infectives, 495
Fluoxetine, 834, 1020
Fluoxymesterone, 501
Fluphenazine Hydrochloride, 228
Flurandrenolide, 320, 322, 323
Flurazepam, 503
Flurbiprofen, 821
Flurbiprofen Sodium, 828
Flurosyn, 323
Flutamide, 507
Flutex, 321, 323
Fluticasone, 1014
Fluticasone Furoate, 309
Fluticasone Propionate, 304, 309, 321, 322, 323
Fluvastatin, 1052
Fluvoxamine Maleate, 1021
Fluxid, 465
FML, 301
FML Forte, 301
Focalin, 706
Focalin XR, 706
Folic Acid, 898
Foradil Aerolizer, 509
Foradil Certihaler, 509

Formoterol, 304, 509
Fortabs, 484
Fortamet, 696
Forteo, 1096
Fortical, 187
Fosamax, 164, plate L
Fosamax Plus D, 164
Fosamprenavir, 69
Fosfomycin, 512
Fosinopril, 514
Fosphenytoin, 882
Fosrenol, 517
Frova, 1178
Frovatriptan, 1178
FS Shampoo, 323
Furadantin, 810
Furosemide, 653
Fuzeon, 411

G

Gabapentin, 1123
Gabitril, 1123
Galantamine, 237
Ganciclovir, 519
Ganirelix Acetate, 671
Gani-Tuss NR, 1189
Gantrisin Pediatric, 1061
Gastrocrom, 334
Gatifloxacin, 495
Gefitinib, 754
Gemfibrozil, 523
Gemifloxacin, 495
Genac, 99
Genahist, 376
Genapap, 7
Genebs, 7
Gengraf, 341
Gentamicin Sulfate, 301
Gen-Xene, 268
Geocillin, 857
Geodon, 1228, plate L
Gerimal, 431
Glatiramer, 526
Gleevec, 754, plate L

Glimepiride, 528, 1065
Glipizide, 1066
Glitazone Antidiabetes Drugs, 528
Glucophage, 696, plate L
Glucophage XR, 696, plate L
Glucotrol, 1066, plate M
Glucotrol XL, 1066, plate M
Glucovance, 1066, plate M
Glumetza, 696
Glyburide, 1066
Glycolax, 895
Glydeine, 1189
Glynase, 1066, plate M
Glyset, 731
Gramicidin, 785
Granisetron, 88
Guaifed, 421
Guaifed-PD, 421
Guaifed-PSE, 421
Guaifed SR, 421
Guaifen AC, 1189
Guaifenesin, 420, 421, 1189
Guaifenex GP, 421
Guaifenex PSE 60, 421
Guaifenex PSE 80, 421
Guaifenex PSE 85, 421
Guaifenex PSE 120, 421
Guaifenex RX, 421
Guaimax-D, 421
Guaipax PSE, 421
Guaitab, 421
Guaituss AC, 1189
Guaituss PE, 421
Guaitussin with Codeine, 1189
Guai-Vent PSE, 421
Guanabenz, 532
Gynazole, 723
Gynecort Female Cream, 324
Gynodiol, 441

H

Habitrol, 794
Halcinonide, 321
Halcion, 1167, plate M

Haldol, 534
Halobetasol Propionate, 320
Halog, 321
Haloperidol, 534
Halotestin, 501, plate M
Halotussin AC, 1189
Hayfebrol, 97
Hectorol Capsules, 392
Helidac, 538
Hemocyte, 601
Hemril, 324
Hepsera, 27
Hexafed, 98
Hi-Cor 1.0, 324
Hi-Cor 2.5, 324
Histade, 97
Histalet, 97
Histamax D, 96
Histatab, 96
Histex, 97
Histex SR, 95
HIV Antivirals, 542
Humalog, 585
Humalog Mix 50/50, 585
Humalog Mix 75/25, 585
Humulin 50/50, 585
Humulin 70/30, 585
Humulin N, 585
Humulin R, 585
Hycet, 864
Hycort, 324
Hydergine, 431
Hydralazine, 564
Hydralazine Hydrochloride, 157
Hydrocet, 864
Hydrochlorothiazide, 36, 40, 81, 145, 160, 192, 397, 407, 514, 645, 702, 713, 748, 932, 947, 1113
Hydrocodone, 1186
Hydrocodone Bitartrate, 822, 864, 868
Hydrocortisone, 314, 324, 329
Hydrocortisone Acetate, 324
Hydrocortisone Butyrate, 323
Hydrocortisone Probutate, 323

Hydrocortisone Valerate, 322, 323
Hydroflumethiazide, 1113
Hydrogenated Ergot Alkaloids, 431
Hydrogesic, 864
Hydro-Par, 1113
Hydroquinone, 1163
Hydro-Ride, 397
HydroSkin, 324
HydroTex, 324
Hydro-Tussin CBX, 96
Hydroxyzine, 567
Hyoscyamine Sulfate, 385
Hyosol, 385
Hyosophen, 385
Hyosyne, 385
Hy-Phen, 864
Hytinic, 601
Hytone, 324
Hytrin, 48, plate M
Hyzaar, 81, plate M

I

Ibandronate Sodium, 164
IB-Stat, 385
Ibuprofen, 821, 822, 868
Ibuprohm, 821
Ibu-Tab, 821
Icar, 600
Iloprost, 569
Imatinib, 754
Imdur, 604, plate M
Imipramine, 1172
Imiquimod, 572
Imitrex, 1179, plate M
Imodium, 657
Imodium A-D, 657
Implanon, 290
Indapamide, 1113
Inderal, 932, plate N
Inderal LA, 932, plate N
Inderide, 932, plate N
Inderide LA, 932
Indinavir, 574

Indochron E-R, 578
Indocin, 578, plate N
Indocin SR, 578
Indomethacin, 578
Infants' Motrin, 821
Infergen, 590
Infliximab, 582
Innofem, 442
Innopran XL, 932
Inspra, 36
Insulin, 585
Insulin Aspart, 585
Insulin Detemir, 585
Insulin Glargine, 585
Insulin Glulisine, 585
Insulin Lispro, 585
Intal, 334
Intelence, 543
Interferon Alpha, 590
Interferon Alpha-2b, 972
Interferon Beta, 594
Intron A, 590
Invega, 996, plate N
Invirase, 1017
Iofed, 95
Iofed PD, 95
Ionsys (Patch), 279
Iosal II, 421
Ipratropium, 32, 597
Iquix Eyedrops, 495
Irbesartan, 81
Ircon, 600
Iressa, 754
Iron Supplements, 600
Isentress, 957
ISMO, 604
Isochron, 604
Isoniazid, 985
Isoptin SR, 1205
Isordil, 604
Isordil Tembids, 604
Isordil Titradose, 604, plate N
Isosorbide Dinitrate, 157, 604
Isosorbide Mononitrate, 604
Isotrate ER, 604

Isotretinoin, 607
Isradipine, 799
Istalol, 1129
Itraconazole, 134
Ivy Soothe, 324

J

Jantoven, 1212
Janumet, 1046
Januvia, 1046, plate N
J-Tan D, 96
J-Tan D PD, 95
Junel Fe 1/20, 287
Junel Fe 1.5/30, 288

K

K+8, 900
K+10, 900
Kadian, 279
Kaletra, 1001, plate N
Kaon, 899
Kaon-Cl-10, 900
Kaon-Cl 20%, 899
Kariva, 288
Kay Ciel, 899, 900
Kaylixir, 899
K+Care, 900
K+Care ET, 900
K-Dur 10, 900
K-Dur 20, 900, plate N
Keflex, 211, plate N
Kemstro, 140
Kenalog, 322, 323
Kenalog Cream, 321
Kenalog-H, 321
Kenonel, 321
Keppra, 631
Kerlone, 151
Ketek, 1084, plate O
Ketoconazole, 134
Ketoprofen, 821
Ketorolac, 828
Ketotifen, 611
Ketozole, 134

K-G Elixir, 899
Kineret, 76
Klonopin, 258, plate O
K-Lor, 900
Klor-Con, 900, plate O
Klor-Con 8, 900
Klor-Con 10, 900
Klor-Con/25, 900
Klor-Con/EF, 900
Klor-Con M10, 900
Klor-Con M15, 900
Klor-Con M20, 900
Klorvess, 899, 900
Klotrix, 900
K-Lyte, 900
K-Lyte/Cl, 900
K-Lyte/Cl 50, 900
K-Lyte DS, 900
Kolyum, 900
K-Pek II, 657
Kronofed-A, 97
Kronofed-A Jr., 97
K-Tab, 900, plate O
K-Tan, 98
K-Tan 4, 98
Kytril, 88, plate O

L

Labetalol, 613
Lamictal, 616, plate O
Lamictal CD, 616
Lamisil, 1090
Lamisil AT, 1090
Lamivudine, 543
Lamotrigine, 616
Lanacort, 324
Lanorinal, 484
Lanoxicaps, 365, plate O
Lanoxin, 365, plates O & P
Lansoprazole, 940
Lanthanum Carbonate, 517
Lantus, 585
Lapitinib, 754
Larotid, 857
Lasix, 653, plate P

Latanoprost, 937
LazerSporin-C, 329
Leflunomide, 620
Lenalidomide, 623
Lescol, 1052, plate P
Lescol XL, 1052
Letairis, 169
Letrozole, 78
Leukotriene Antagonists/
  Inhibitors, 626
Levalbuterol, 33
Levaquin, 495, plate P
Levatol, 714, plate P
Levbid, 386
Levemir, 585
Levetiracetam, 631
Levian, 288
Levitra, 426, plate P
Levlen, 288
Levlite, 287
Levobunolol, 151
Levocabastine, 92, 838
Levocetirizine, 215
Levodopa, 1042
Levofloxacin, 495
Levonorgestrel, 442
Levo-T, 1118
Levolet, 1118
Levothroid, 1118
Levothyroxine Sodium, 1118
Levoxyl, 1118, plate P
Levsin, 386
Levsinex Timecaps, 386
Levulan Kerastick, 57
Lexapro, 1020, plates P & Q
Lexiva, 69
Lexxel, 471, 634, plate Q
Lialda, 173
Librium, 221, plate Q
Lidex, 321
Lidex E, 321
Lidocaine, 638
Lidoderm, 638
Limbitrol, 1171
Limbitrol DS, 1171
Linezolid, 642

Liothyronine Sodium, 1118
Liotrix, 1118
Lipitor, 1052, plate Q
Lipoten, 475
Liquibid D, 421
Liquibid-D 1200, 421
Liquibid-PD, 421
Liquicet, 864
Liquiprin, 7
Lisdexamfetamine Dimesylate,
  23
Lisinopril, 645
Lithane, 648
Lithium Carbonate, 648
Lithium Citrate, 649
Lithobid, 648
Lithonate, 648
Lithotabs, 648
Livostin, 92, 838
LoCHOLEST, 234
LoCHOLEST Light, 234
Locoid, 323
Lodine, 821, plate Q
Lodine XL, 821, plate Q
Lodosyn, 1042
Lodoxamide, 612
Lodrane, 95
Lodrane 12 D, 95
Lodrane 24 D, 95
Lodrane D, 95
Lodrane LD, 95
Loestrin 21 1/20, 287
Loestrin 21 1.5/30, 288
Loestrin 24-FE, 287
Loestrin Fe 1/20, 287
Loestrin Fe 1.5/30, 288
Lofibra, 475
Lo-Hist 12, 96
Lo-Hist LQ, 96
LoHist-PD, 96
Lokara, 322, 323
Lomefloxacin, 495
Loniten, 734
Loop Diuretics, 652
Lo/Ovral, 288
Loperamide, 657

Lopid, 523, plate Q
Lopinavir, 1001
Lopressor, 713, plate Q
Lopressor-HCT, 713
Loprox, 241
Loqua, 1113
Loratadine, 98, 660
Lorazepam, 358
Lorazepam Intensol, 358
Lorcet 10/650, 864
Lorcet-HD, 864
Lorcet Plus, 864, plate Q
Lortab, 864
Lortab 2.5/500, 864
Lortab 5/500, 864
Lortab 7.5/500, 864
Lortab 10/500, 864
Losartan Potassium, 81
Lotemax, 301
Lotensin, 145
Lotensin HCT, 145, plate Q
Loteprednol Etabonate, 301
Lotrel, 65, 663, plate Q
Lotrisone, 666
Lotronex, 88
Lovastatin, 1052
Lozol, 1113, plate R
Lubiprostone, 668
Lufyllin, 1217
Lumigan, 936
Lunesta, 449, plate R
Luteinizing Hormone Inhibitors, 671
Lutera, 287
Luxiq, 323
Luxiq Foam, 321
Lybrel, 287
Lyrica, 914

M

Macrobid, 810, plate R
Macrodantin, 810, plate R
Magnacet, 863
Malathion, 673
Maldec, 96

Mapap, 7
Mapap Children's, 7
Mapap Extra Strength, 7
Mapap Infant Drops, 7
Maprotiline, 738
Maranox, 7
Maraviroc, 676
Margesic, 481, 864
Marinol, 394
Mavik, 1105
Maxair, 33
Maxalt, 1179
Maxalt-MLT, 1179
Maxaquin, 495, plate R
Maxidex, 300
Maxidone, 864
Maxifed, 421
Maxifed G, 421
Maxiflor, 320
Maximum Strength Bactine, 324
Maximum Strength Caldecort, 324
Maximum Strength Cortaid, 324
Maximum Strength Cortaid-Faststick, 324
Maximum Strength KeriCort-10, 324
Maxitrol, 300
Maxivate Lotion, 321
Maxzide, 397
Maxzide-25, 397
Meclizine, 372
Meclofenamate Sodium, 821
Medigesic, 481
Medipren, 821
Medispaz, 386
Medrol, 314
Medroxyprogesterone, 441, 679
Med-RX, 421
Mefenamic Acid, 821
Megace, 679
Megestrol, 679
Meloxicam, 822
Memantine, 683

Menadol, 821
Menest, 441
Meni-D, 372
Menostar, 442
Mentax, 185
Mentax-TC, 185
Meperidine, 685
Meprobamate, 689
Mepron, 128
Mequinol, 1163
Meridia, 1036, plate R
Mesalamine, 173
Metadate, 706
Metadate CD, 706
Metadate ER, 706
Metaglip, 1066, plate R
Metaproterenol, 691
Metaxalone, 694
Metformin, 528, 696, 1046, 1066
Methotrexate, 699
Methyclothiazide, 1113
Methyldopa, 702
Methylin, 706
Methylin ER, 706
Methylphenidate, 706
Methylprednisolone, 314
Methyltestosterone, 441, 1099
Metipranolol, 151
Metoclopramide, 710
Metolazone, 1113
Metoprolol, 713
MetroCream, 718
MetroGel, 718
MetroLotion, 718
Metronidazole, 538, 718
Mevacor, 1052, plate R
Miacalcin, 187
Micardis, 81
Micardis HCT, 81
Miconazole, 723
Micort-HC, 324
Microgestin Fe 1/20, 287
Micro-K Extencaps, 900, plate R
Micro-K 10 Extencaps, 900
Micro-K LS, 900

Micronase, 1066, plate S
Microzide, 1113
Midodrine, 725
Midol Extended Relief, 822
Midol PM, 376
Mifeprex, 728, plate S
Mifepristone, 728
Miglitol, 731
Miles Nervine, 376
Minipress, 911, plate S
Minipress XL, 911
Minirin, 355
Minitran, 813
Minocin, 1103, plate S
Minocycline Hydrochloride, 1103
Minoxidil, 734
Miradon, 1212
Miralax, 895
Mirapex, 903, plate S
Miraphen PSE, 421
Mircette, 288
Mirena, 290
Mirtazapine, 738
Misoprostol, 742, 822
Mobic, 822, plate S
Modafinil, 744
Modicon, 289
Moduretic, 397, plate S
Moexipril, 748
Mometasone Furoate, 304, 321, 322
Mometasone Furoate Monohydrate, 309
Monistat, 723
Monistat-Derm, 723
Monodox, 1103
Monoket, 604
Monopril, 514, plate S
Monopril HCT, 514
Montelukast Sodium, 626
Monurol, 512
Morphine Sulfate, 279
Motofen, 751
Motrin, 821
Motrin IB, 821
Motrin Migraine Pain, 821

Moxifloxacin, 495
M-Oxy, 279, 864
MS Contin, 279
MSIR, 279
Multiple Kinase Inhibitors, 754
Mupirocin, 764
Muromonab-CD3, 766
Muse, 55
Mycelex, 271
Mycophenolate, 769
Mycostatin, 831
Mykacet, 831
Mymethasone, 313
Mytussin AC, 1189

N

Nabumetone, 822
Nadolol, 1129, 1130
Nalex-A, 97
Nalex-A12, 97
Nalfon, 821, plate T
Naloxone, 774, 869
Naltrexone, 773
Namenda, 683, plate T
NapraPAC, 940
Naprelan, 822
Naprosyn, 822
Naproxen/Naproxen Sodium, 822, 940
Naratriptan, 1178
Nardil, 874
Nasabid, 421
Nasabid-SR, 421
Nasacort AQ, 309
Nasarel, 309
Nasatab LA, 421
Nasonex, 309
Nateglinide, 976
ND Clear, 97
Nebivolol, 119
Necon 10/11, 289
Nedocromil, 334
Nefazodone, 778
Nelfinavir, 782
Neocon 0.5/35, 289

Neo-Diaral, 657
Neomycin Sulfate, 300, 301, 329, 785
Neopap, 7
Neoral, 341
Neosol, 386
Neosporin Ophthalmic, 785
Nepafenac, 828
Nephro-Fer, 601
Neupro, 1010
Neurontin, 1123, plate T
Nevanac, 828
Nevirapine, 543
Nexavar, 754
Nexium, 939, plate T
Niacin, 787, 898, 1052
Niacor, 787
Niaspan, 787
Nicardipine, 791
Nicoderm, 794
Nicoderm CQ, 794
Nicorelief, 794
Nicorette, 794
Nicorette DS, 794
Nicotine, 794
Nicotinex, 787
Nicotrol, 794
Nicotrol Inhaler, 794
Nicotrol NS, 794
Nifedical XL, 799
Nifedipine, 799
Niferex, 601
Niferex-150, 601
Nilandron, 154
Nilotinib, 754
Nilstat, 831
Nilutamide, 154
Nimodipine, 805
Nimotop, 805
Niravam, 51
Nisoldipine, 799
Nitazoxanide, 808
Nitrek, 813
Nitrocine, 813
Nitro-Derm, 813
Nitrodisc, 813

Nitro-Dur, 813
Nitrofurantoin, 810
Nitrogard, 813
Nitroglycerin, 813
Nitroglyn, 813
Nitrolingual, 813
Nitromist, 813
Nitrong, 813
NitroQuick, 813
Nitrostat, 813
NitroTab, 813
Nitro-Time, 813
Nizatidine, 818
Nizoral, 134, plate T
NoHist, 96
NoHist A, 97
Nonsteroidal Anti-inflammatory
   Drugs, 821
Nonsteroidal Anti-inflammatory
   Drug Eyedrops, 828
Norco, 864
Norco 5/325, 864
Nordette, 288
Norel LA, 96
Norethindrone, 442, 679
Norfloxacin, 496
Norgestimate, 442
Norinyl 1 + 35, 289
Norinyl 1 + 50, 288
Noritate, 718
Noroxin, 496, plate T
Norpace, 379, plate T
Norpace CR, 379, plate T
Norplant II, 290
Norpramin, 1171, plate T
Nor-Q.D., 290
Nortrel 0.5/35, 289
Nortrel 1/35, 289
Nortriptyline, 1172
Norvasc, 65
Norvir, 1001
Novolin 70/30, 585
Novolin N, 585
Novolin R, 585
Novolog, 585
Novolog Mix 70/30, 585

Novothyrox, 1118
Noxafil, 134
NPH Insulin, 585
NuHist, 97
Nu-Iron, 601
Nu-Iron 150, 601
NuLev, 386
Nutracort, 324
NuvaRing, 290, 442
Nuvigil, 744
Nystatin, 831
Nytol Quick Caps, 376
**Nytol Quick Gels Maximum
   Strength,** 376

O

Octamide, 710
Octicair, 329
Octocrylene, 87
Ocufen, 828
Ocuflox Eyedrops, 496
Ocupress, 151
Ofloxacin, 496
Ogen Cream, 442
Olanzapine, 834
Olmesartan, 81
Olopatadine, 92, 838
Olsalazine, 173
Olux, 320
Olux E, 320
Olux-E Foam, 320
Omeprazole, 940
Omnaris, 309
Omnicef, 210, plate T
Omnipred, 301
Ondansetron, 89
Opana, 279
Opticrom, 334
Optipranolol, 151
Optivar, 92, 838
Oracea, 1103
Oramorph SR, 279
Oraphen-PD, 7
Orapred, 314
Orapred ODT, 314

Oretic, 1113
Orlistat, 841
Ortho-Cept, 288
Orthoclone OKT3 Sterile Solution, 766
Ortho-Cyclen, 288
Ortho-Est, 442
OrthoEvra, 290
Ortho-Micronor, 290
Ortho-Novum 1/35, 289
Ortho-Novum 1/50, 288
Ortho-Novum 10/11, 289
Ortho-Novum 7/7/7, 290
Ortho Tri-Cyclen, 289
Ortho Tri-Cyclen Lo, 289
Or-Tyl, 361
Orvaten, 725
Oseltamivir, 844
Otic-Care, 329
Otocort, 329
Ovcon-35, 289
Ovcon-50, 289
Ovide, 673
Ovral, 289
Oxacillin, 857
Oxaprozin, 822
Oxazepam, 358
Oxcarbazepine, 847
Oxiconazole, 723, 809
Oxistat, 723
Oxtriphylline, 1217
Oxybutynin, 850
Oxycodone Hydrochloride, 279, 822, 863, 864, 868
Oxycodone Terephthalate, 868
OxyContin, 279, 864
Oxydose, 279
OxyFAST, 279, 864
OxyIR, 279, 864
Oxymorphone, 279
Oxytrol, 850

P

Pacerone, 59
Palgic-D, 96

Palgic-DC, 96
Palgic-DS, 96
Paliperidone, 996
Pamelor, 1172, plate U
Panacet 5/500, 864
Panadol, 7
Pandel, 323
Panixine Disperdose, 211
PanMist, 421
PanMist-Jr., 421
PanMist LA, 421
Panretin, 43
Pantoprazole Sodium, 940
Parafon Forte DSC, 232, plate U
Parcopa, 1042
Parnate, 874
Paroxetine Hydrochloride, 1021
Paroxetine Mesylate, 1021
Patanol, 92, 838
Paxil, 1021, plate U
Paxil CR, 1021, plate U
PCE, 433, plate U
PD Hist D, 96
Pediacare Fever, 821
Pediamycin, 434
PediaPhyl D, 97
Pediapred, 314
PediaTan D, 97
Pediatex-D, 96
Pediazole, 434
Pediotic, 329
Pediox S, 224
Pediox Chewable, 97
Peganone, 882
Pegasys, 590
PegIntron, 590
Pemirolast, 853
Penbutolol, 714
Penciclovir, 855
Penicillin Antibiotics, 857
Penicillin V Potassium, 857
Penicillin VK, 857
Penlac, 241
Pentasa, 173
Pentazocine, 864, 869

Pentosan Polysulfate
    Sodium, 861
Pepcid, 465, plate U
Pepcid AC, 465
Pepcid Complete, 465
Pepto Diarrhea Control, 657
Percocet, 863
Percodan, 868
Percodan-Demi, 868
Percolone, 279, 864
Perforomist, 509
Perindopril, 947
Periostat, 1103
Perloxx, 863
Permethrin, 872
Pexeva, 1021
Phenabid, 96
PhenaVent, 421
PhenaVent D, 421
PhenaVent LA, 421
PhenaVent PED, 421
Phenelzine, 874
Phenergan, 924, plate U
Phenergan VC, 98
Phenergan VC Syrup, 925
**Phenergan VC with Codeine
    Syrup,** 925
**Phenergan with Codeine
    Syrup,** 924
**Phenergan with
    Dextromethorphan Syrup,**
    925
Pheniramine, 98
Phenobarbital, 385, 878
Phenylephrine, 96
Phenylephrine Hydrochloride, 96,
    97, 98, 421, 925
Phenylephrine Tannate, 97, 98
Phenyltoloxamine, 97, 98
Phenytek, 882
Phenytoin, 882
Pherazine DM Syrup, 925
**Pherazine VC with Codeine
    Syrup,** 925
**Pherazine with Codeine
    Syrup,** 925

Pimecrolimus, 887
Pindolol, 889
Pioglitazone Hydrochloride, 528
Pirbuterol, 33
Piroxicam, 822
Plan B, 290
Plavix, 265, plate U
Plendil, 471, plate U
Pletal, 243, plate V
Podofilox, 893
Polyethylene Glycol 3350, 895
Polymyxin B Sulfate, 300, 301,
    329, 785
Poly-Pred, 301
Polysaccharide Iron Complex,
    601
Polytabs-F, 898
Polythiazide, 1113
Poly-Vi-Flor, 898
Poly-Vi-Flor with Iron, 898
Ponstel, 821
Posaconazole, 134
Potasalan, 899
Potassium Chloride, 899, 900
Potassium Clavulanate, 857
Potassium Gluconate, 899, 900
Potassium Replacements, 899
Potassium Salt Combination, 900
Pramipexole, 903
Pramlintide, 907
Prandin, 976, plate V
Pravachol, 1052, plate V
Pravastatin, 1052
Prazosin, 911
Precose, 731
Pred Forte, 301
Pred G, 301
Pred Mild, 301
Prednicarbate, 322, 323
Prednisolone, 314
Prednisolone Acetate, 301
Prednisolone Sodium Phosphate,
    301
Prednisone, 314
Prednisone Intensol, 314
Prefest, 442

Pregabalin, 914
Prelone, 314
Premarin, 441, plate V
Premarin Cream, 441
Premphase, 441
Prempro, 441
Prevacid, 940, plate V
Prevalite, 234
Prevpac, 940
Prezista, 347, plate V
Prilocaine, 638
Prilosec, 940, plate V
Prinivil, 645, plate V
Prinzide, 645
ProAir HFA, 32
ProAmatine, 725, plate V
Pro-Banthine, 386
Procainamide, 917
Procardia, 799, plate V
Procardia XL, 799, plates V & W
Prochlorperazine, 920
Procort, 324
Procrit, 424
Proctocream-HC, 324
Proctofoam-HC, 324
Profen, 821
Profen II, 421
Progesterone, 680
Progestin, 287, 288, 289, 290
Prograf, 1071, plate W
Prohist+8, 224
Promethacon, 924
Promethazine, 98, 924, 925
Promethazine VC Plain Syrup, 925
Promethegen, 924
Prometh Plain, 924
Prometh VC Plain, 98
Prometh VC Plain Liquid, 925
Prometh VC with Codeine Liquid, 925
Prometh with Codeine Syrup, 925
Prometh with Dextromethorphan Syrup, 925

Prometrium, 680, plate W
Pronestyl, 917
Propantheline, 386
Propecia, 478
Propoxyphene Hydrochloride, 929
Propoxyphene Napsylate, 929
Propranolol, 932
Proquin XR, 495
Proscar, 478, plate W
Prostaglandin Agonists, 936
ProStep, 794
Protonix, 940, plate W
Proton-Pump Inhibitors, 939
Protopic Ointment, 1071
Protriptyline, 1172
Proventil, 32
Proventil HFA, 32
Provera, 679, plate W
Provigil, 744
Prozac, 1020, plate W
Prozac Weekly, 1020, plate W
PSE CPM, 97
Pseudoephedrine, 95, 96, 97, 98, 252
Pseudoephedrine Hydrochloride, 98, 99, 420
Pseudoephedrine Polistirex, 97
Pseudovent, 421
Pseudovent-PED, 421
Psorcon, 320
Psorcon E, 320
P-Tann D, 97
Pulmicort Flexhaler, 303
Pulmicort Respules, 303
Pylera, 538
Pyrazinamide, 985
Pyridoxine, 898
Pyrilamine, 98
Pyrilamine Tannate, 97, 98
Pyrimethamine, 1061

Q

QDall, 97
QDALL AR, 224

Q-Tapp, 96
Quadra-Hist D Pediatric, 98
Quazepam, 1167
Questran, 234
Questran Light, 234
Quetiapine, 943
Quibron-T Dividose, 1217
Quinaglute Dura-Tabs, 950
Quinapril, 947
Quinaretic, 947
Quinidex Extentabs, 950,
    plate W
Quinidine, 950
Quin-Release, 950
Quixin Eyedrops, 495
QVAR 40, 303
QVAR 80, 303

R

Rabeprazole Sodium, 940
Raloxifene, 954
Raltegravir, 957
Ramelteon, 959
Ramipril, 947
Ranexa, 965
Raniclor, 210
Ranitidine, 962
Ranolazine, 965
Rapamune, 1071
Raptiva, 402
Rasagiline, 968
Razadyne, 237, plate W
Razadyne ER, 237
RE2 + 30, 97
Rebetol, 981
Rebetron, 972
Rebif, 594
Reclomide, 710
Redutemp, 7
Reglan, 710, plate W
Regranex, 143
Relenza, 1226
Relpax, 1178
Remeron, 738, plate W
Remeron SolTab, 738

Remicade, 582
Renagel, 1034
Renese, 1113
Renova, 1163
Renvela, 1034
Repaglinide, 976
Repan, 481
Reprexain, 822, 868
Requip, 1007
Rescon-Ed, 97
Rescon GG, 421
Rescon JR, 96
Rescriptor, 542
Respahist, 96
Respa-1st, 421
Respaire-60 SR, 421
Respaire-120 SR, 421
Restasis Ophthalmic Emulsion,
    341
Restoril, 1167, plate X
Retapamulin, 979
Retin-A, 1163
Retin-A Micro, 1163
Retrovir, 543, plate X
ReVia, 773
Revatio, 426
Revlimid, 623
Reyataz, 115
Rheumatrex, 699
Rhinabid, 96
Rhinabid PD, 96
Rhinacon A, 97
Rhinatate, 97
Rhinatate-NF Pediatric, 97
Rhinatate Pediatric, 97
Rhinocort, 309
Ribasphere, 981
Ribavirin, 972, 981
Riboflavin, 898
Rifadin, 985
Rifamate, 985
Rifampin, 985
Rifater, 985
Rifaximin, 988
Rilutek, 991
Riluzole, 991

Rimactane, 985
Rimantadine, 994
Rimexolone, 301
Riomet, 696
Risedronate Sodium, 164
Risperdal, 996, plate X
**Risperdal M-Tab Orally
    Disintegrating Tablets,** 996
Risperidone, 996
Ritalin, 706
Ritalin LA, 706
Ritalin-SR, 706, plate X
Ritonavir, 1001
Rivastigmine, 237
Rizatriptan, 1179
RMS Suppositories, 279
Robitussin AC, 1189
Robitussin PE, 421
Rogaine, 734
Rondec, 96
Rondec Drops, 96
Rondex, 96
Ropinirole, 1007
Rosiglitazone Maleate, 528
Rosuvastatin, 1052
Rotigotine, 1010
Rowasa, 173
Roxanol, 279
Roxicet, 863
Roxicet 5/500, 863
Roxicodone, 279, 864
Roxilox, 863
Roxiprin, 868
Rozerem, 959, plate X
R-Tanna, 97
R-Tanna 12, 98
Ru-Tuss DE, 421
Ru-Vert-M, 372
Rymed, 421
Ryna-12, 98
Ryna-12 S, 98
Rynatan, 97
Rynatan Pediatric, 97
Rynatan-S Pediatric, 97
RY-T-12, 98

S

Salmeterol, 304, 1013, 1014
Saluron, 1113
Sanctura, 1144, plate X
Sanctura XR, 1144
Sandimmune, 341, plate X
Saquinavir, 1017
Sarafem, 1020
Scopolamine Hydrobromide, 385
Scot-Tussin Allergy, 376
Seasonale, 288
Seasonique, 288
Sectral, 3, plate X
Selective Serotonin Reuptake
    Inhibitors (SSRIs), 1020
Selegiline, 1027
Selzentry, 676
Semprex-D, 95
Septra, 1030
Septra DS, 1031
Serevent, 1013
Serevent Diskus, 1013
Seroquel, 943, plates X & Y
Seroquel XR, 943
Sertaconazole, 271
Sertraline Hydrochloride, 1021
Sevelamer, 1034
Sibutramine, 1036
Siladryl, 376
SilaFed, 99
Silapap, 7
Silapap Children's, 7
Silapap Infants, 7
Sildec, 96
Sildenafil Citrate, 426
Simply Sleep, 376
Simvastatin, 460, 1052
Sinecatechins Ointment, 1039
Sinemet, 1042, plate Y
Sinemet CR, 1042, plate Y
Sinequan, 1172
Singulair, 626, plate Y
Singulair Granules, 626
Sinufed Timecelles, 421

Sinupan, 421
Sinutab, 421
Sinuvent PE, 421
Sirolimus, 1071
Sitagliptin, 1046
Skelaxin, 694, plate Y
Skelid, 164
Sleep-Eze 3, 376
Sleepinol Maximum Strength, 376
Sleepwell 2-Nite, 376
Slo-Niacin, 787
Slow-FE, 601
Snoozefast, 376
Sodium Bicarbonate, 940
Sodium Fluoride, 898
Sodium Oxybate, 1049
Solagé, 1163
Solaraze, 821
Solfoton, 878
Solifenacin, 1144
Solodyn, 1103
Soltamox, 1077
Soluvite, 898
Sominex Original Formula, 376
Sonata, 1223, plate Y
Sonazine, 228
Sorafenib, 754
Soriatane, 13
Sorine, 1130
Sotalol, 1130
Sotret, 607
Sparlon, 744
Spasdel, 386
Spasmolin, 385
Spectazole, 401
Spectracef, 211
Spiriva, 597
Spironazide, 397
Spironolactone, 36, 397
Spirozide, 397
Sporanox, 134
Sprycel, 754, plate Y
S-P-T, 1118
Stagesic, 864

Stalevo, 1042
Stamoist E, 421
Starlix, 976, plate Y
Statin Cholesterol-Lowering Agents, 1052
Stavudine, 543
Stavzor, 1194
Sterapred, 314
Stie-Cort, 324
Stimate, 355
Strattera, 125, plates Y & Z
Striant, 1099
Strifon Forte DSC, 232
Subutex, 774
Suboxone, 774
Sucralfate, 1059
Sudafed PE, 96
Sudafed Sinus & Allergy, 97
Sudafed Sinus Nighttime, 99
Sudal 60/500, 421
Sudal 120/600, 421
Sudal-12, 97
Sudal SR, 421
Sular, 799
Sular CD, 799
Sulfacetamide Sodium, 301
Sulfadiazine, 1061
Sulfadoxine, 1061
Sulfa Drugs, 1061
Sulfamethoprim, 1031
Sulfamethoxazole, 1030
Sulfasalazine, 1061
Sulfatrim Pediatric, 1031
Sulfisoxazole, 434, 1061
Sulfonylurea Antidiabetes Drugs, 1065
Sulindac, 822
Sumatriptan, 1179
Sumycin, 1103, plate Z
Sunitinib, 754
Suprax, 211
Surmontil, 1172, plate Z
Sustiva, 542
Sutent, 754
Sylphen Cough, 376

Symax, 386
Symbicort, 304, 509
Symbyax, 834
Symlin, 907
Synacort, 324
Synalar, 322, 323
Synalar Ointment, 322
Synalar-HP Cream, 322
Synalgos-DC, 868
Syn-RX, 421
Synthroid, 1118, plate Z

T

Tab-Profen, 821
Taclonex, 320
Tacrine, 237
Tacrolimus, 1071
Tadalafil, 426
Tagamet, 245, plate Z
Tagamet HB, 245
Talacen, 864
Talwin Compound, 869
Talwin Nx, 869, plate Z
Tambocor, 490
Tamiflu, 844
Tamoxifen Citrate, 1077
Tamsulosin, 1080
Tanavan, 98
Tapanol, 7
Tarka, 1155, 1205
Tasigna, 754
Tasmar, 1141
Tavist, 252
Tavist-1, 252
Tavist Allergy, 252
Tavist Allergy/Sinus/Headache, 252
Tavist ND, 660
Tazarotene, 1082
Tazorac, 1082
Taztia XT, 369
Tegretol, 196, plate AA
Tegretol-XR, 196, plate AA
Tegrin HC, 324
Tekturna, 40

Tekturna HCT, 40
Teladar, 321
Telbivudine, 417
Telithromycin, 1084
Telmisartan, 81
Temazepam, 1167
Temodar, 1088
Temovate, 320
Temozolomide, 1088
Tempra, 7
Ten-K, 900
Tenofovir, 543
Tenoretic, 119
Tenormin, 119
Terazol, 723
Terazosin, 48
Terbinafine, 1090
Terbutaline, 1093
Terconazole, 723
Teril, 196
Teriparatide, 1096
Testim, 1099
Testopel, 1099
Testosterone, 1099
Testred, 1099
Tetracycline, 538
Tetracycline Antibiotics, 1103
Tetracycline Hydrochloride, 1103
Teveten, 81
Teveten HCT, 81
Texacort, 324
T-Gesic, 864
Thalidomide, 1109
Thalitone, 1113
Thalomid, 1109
Theo-24, 1217
Theochron, 1217
Theolair, 1217
Theolair-SR, 1217
Theophylline, 1217
Theo-X, 1217
TheraFlu Thin Strips Multi Symptom, 376
Thiamine, 898
Thiazide Diuretics, 1113
Thioridazine Hydrochloride, 228

Thorazine, 228
Thrive, 794
Thyrar, 1118
Thyroid Hormone, 1118
Thyroid Hormone Replacements, 1118
Thyroid Strong, 1118
Thyrolar, 1118
Thyro-Tabs, 1118
Tiagabine, 1123
Tiazac, 369, plate AA
Tibamine LA, 97
Ticlid, 1126, plate AA
Ticlopidine, 1126
Tikosyn, 382
Tilade, 334
Tilia Fe, 289
Tiludronate Disodium, 164
Time-Hist, 97
Timolol, 200, 331, 1129
Timoptic, 1129
Tindamax, 718, plate AA
Tinidazole, 718
Tioconazole, 723
Tiotropium Bromide, 597
Tipranavir, 1134
Tirosint, 1118
Tizanidine, 1139
Tobramycin, 300, 301
Tobradex, 300
Tobrasone, 301
Tofranil, 1172
Tofranil-PM, 1172
Tolazamide, 1066
Tolbutamide, 1066
Tolcapone, 1141
Tolectin, 822, plate AA
Tolectin 600, 822
Tolectin DS, 822
Tolinase, 1066, plate AA
Tolmetin Sodium, 822
Tolterodine, 1144
Topamax, 1148, plate AA
Topamax Sprinkle, 1148
Topicort, 320, 321
Topicort LP, 322

Topiramate, 1148
Toprol-XL, 713, plate AA
Toremifene Citrate, 1077
Torsemide, 653
Touro Allergy, 96
Touro LA, 421
T-Phyl, 1217
Tracleer, 169
Tramadol, 1152
Trandate, 613
Trandolapril, 1155, 1205
Tranxene, 268
Tranxene-SD, 268
Tranxene T-Tab, 268, plate AA
Tranylcypromine Sulfate, 874
Travatan Z, 937
Travoprost, 937
Trazodone, 1159
Tretinoin, 1163
Triacet, 321, 323
Triad, 481
Triamcinolone Acetonide, 304, 309, 321, 322, 323, 831
Triaminic Allerchews, 660
Triaminic Thin Strips Cough and Runny Nose, 376
Triamterene, 397
Triazolam, 1167
TriCor, 475, plate BB
Tricyclic Antidepressants, 1171
Triderm, 321, 322
Tridesilon, 322, 323
Trifluoperazine Hydrochloride, 228
Triglide, 475
Tri-K, 900
TriLegest Fe, 289
Trileptal, 847, plate BB
Tri-Levlen, 289
Tri-Luma, 1163
Trimethoprim, 1030
Trimipramine, 1172
Trimox, 857, plate BB
Trinalin Repetabs, 95
TriNessa, 289
Tri-Norinyl, 289
Triostat, 1118

Triotann, 97
Triotann Pediatric, 97
Triotann S, 97
Triotann S Pediatric, 97
Triphasil, 289
Triprolidine Hydrochloride, 99
Triptan-Type Antimigraine Drugs,
    1178–
Triptone, 372
Tri-Sprintec, 289
Tritan, 97
Tri-Tannate Pediatric, 97
Tri-Vi-Flor, 898
Trivora, 289
Trizivir, 543, plate BB
Trospium Chloride, 1144
Truphylline, 1217
Trusopt, 200
Truvada, 543, plate BB
Tussionex Pennkinetic, 1186
Tussi-Organidin NR, 1189
Tuss-LA, 421
Tusstat, 376
Twin-K, 900
Tykerb, 754
Tylenol, 7
Tylenol with Codeine, 863
Tylenol with Codeine No. 2,
    863, plate BB
Tylenol with Codeine No. 3,
    863, plate BB
Tylenol with Codeine No. 4, 863
Tylox, 863, plate BB
Tyzeka, 417

U

UAD, 329
U-Cort, 324
ULTRAbrom, 96
ULTRAbrom PD, 96
Ultracet, 1152, plate BB
Ultram, 1152, plate BB
Ultravate, 320
Uniphyl, 1217

Uniretic, 748
Unisom, 376
Unithroid, 1118
Univasc, 748, plate CC
Uni-Tex 120/10 ER, 96
Uroxatral, 48

V

Vagifem, 442
Vagistat, 723
Valacyclovir, 1191
Valcyte, 519
Valganciclovir, 519
Valium, 357, plate CC
Valnac, 322
Valproic Acid, 1194
Valrelease, 357
Valsartan, 65, 81
Valtrex, 1191, plate CC
Vandazole, 718
Vaniqa, 405
Vanos, 320
Vantin, 211
Vardenafil, 426
Varenicline, 1198
Vaseretic, 407
Vasocidin, 301
Vasotec, 407, plate CC
VaZol-D, 96
V-Dec-M, 421
Veetids, 857, plate CC
Velivet, 289
Venlafaxine, 1200
Ventavis, 569
Ventolin HFA, 32
Veramyst, 309
Verapamil, 1155, 1205
Verapamil Extended Release,
    1205
Verdeso Foam, 322
Veregen, 1039
Verelan, 1205, plate CC
Verelan PM, 1205
Versacaps, 421

Vesanoid, 1163
VESIcare, 1144, plate DD
Vexol, 301
Vfend, 134
Viagra, 426, plate DD
Vibramycin, 1103, plate DD
Vibra-Tabs, 1103, plate DD
Vicodin, 864, plate DD
Vicodin-ES, 864, plate DD
Vicodin-HP, 864
Vicoprofen, 822, 868
Vi-Daylin/F, 898
Videx, 542
Videx EC, 542
Vigamox Eyedrops, 495
Viracept, 782
Viramune, 543
Viravan-T, 98
Viread, 543
Virilon, 1099
Visken, 889
Vistaril, 567
Vitamin A, 898
Vitamin B_1, 898
Vitamin B_2, 898
Vitamin B_3, 898
Vitamin B_6, 898
Vitamin B_{12}, 898
Vitamin C, 898
Vitamin D, 898
Vitamin E, 898
Vitrasert, 519
Vitron-C, 601
Vivactil, 1172
Vivelle, 442
Vivelle-Dot, 442
Voltaren, 821, 828
Voltaren-XR, 821
Vopac, 863
Voriconazole, 134
Vorinostat, 1209
Vospire ER, 32
V-Tann, 98
Vytorin, 460, 1052, plate DD
Vyvanse, 23

W

Warfarin, 1212
WelChol, 234, plate DD
Wellbutrin, 179, plate DD
Wellbutrin SR, 179, plate DD
Wellbutrin XL, 179, plate DD
Westcort, 322, 323
Wygesic, 929

X

Xalatan, 937
Xanax, 51, plate DD
Xanax XR, 51
Xanthine Bronchodilators, 1217
Xeloda, 189
Xenical, 841, plate EE
Xibrom, 828
Xifaxan, 988, plate EE
Xirahist PD, 96
Xodol, 864
Xolegel, 134
Xopenex, 33
Xyrem, 1049
Xyzal, 215

Y

Yasmin, 288
Yaz, 288

Z

Zaditor Eyedrops, 611
Zafirlukast, 626
Zaleplon, 1223
Zanaflex, 1139, plate EE
Zanamivir, 1226
Zantac, 962, plate EE
Zaroxolyn, 1113, plate EE
Zebeta, 160, plate EE
Zegerid, 940
Zelapar, 1027

Zephrex, 421
Zephrex LA, 421
Zerit, 543, plate EE
Zestoretic, 645, plate EE
Zestril, 645, plate FF
Zetia, 460, plate FF
Ziac, 160, plate FF
Ziagen, 542
Ziana, 1163
Zidovudine, 543
Zileuton, 626
Zileuton CR, 626
Ziprasidone, 1228
Zithromax, 131, plate FF
Zmax, 131
Zocor, 1052, plate FF
Zofran, 89
Zofran ODT, 89
Zolinza, 1209
Zolmitriptan, 1179
Zoloft, 1021, plate FF

Zolpidem, 1232
Zomig, 1179, plate FF
Zomig ZMT, 1179
Zonegran, 1236
Zonisamide, 1236
Zovia 1/35E, 288
Zovia 1/50E, 288
Zovirax, 17, plate FF
Zyban, 179, plate FF
Zydone, 864
Zyflo, 626
Zyflo CR, 626
Zylet, 301
Zyloprim, 45
Zymar Eyedrops, 495
Zyprexa, 834, plate FF
Zyprexa Zydis, 834
Zyrtec, 215, plate FF
Zyrtec-D 12-hour, 96,
    plate FF
Zyvox, 642, plate FF

ABOUT THE EDITOR

Educated at Columbia University, Dr. Harold Silverman has been a hospital pharmacist, industry consultant, author, and educator for more than 35 years. Dr. Silverman's professional objective is to help people understand why medicines are prescribed and how to get the most from them.

In addition to *The Pill Book*, Dr. Silverman has also authored *The Women's Drug Store, The Pill Book Guide to Safe Drug Use, The Consumer's Guide to Poison Protection*, and *Travel Healthy*. He is also a co-author of *The Vitamin Book: A No-Nonsense Consumer Guide* and *The Med-File Drug Interactions System*.

Dr. Silverman has contributed more than 70 articles, research papers, and textbook chapters to the professional literature, including *The Merck Manual of Medical Information, Home Edition*. He has taught pharmacology and clinical pharmacy at several universities and has won numerous awards for his work. Dr. Silverman resides in the Washington, D.C. area with his wife Judith Brown and their son Joshua.